Campbell-Walsh-Wein
UROLOGY
TWELFTH EDITION REVIEW

THIRD EDITION

Campbell-Walsh-Wein
UROLOGY
TWELFTH EDITION REVIEW

Alan J. Wein, MD, PhD (Hon), FACS

Founders Professor and Emeritus Chief of Urology
Division of Urology
Director, Residency Program in Urology
Perelman School of Medicine at the University
of Pennsylvania
Penn Medicine
Philadelphia, Pennsylvania

Thomas F. Kolon, MD, FAAP

Howard M. Snyder III MD Chair
in Pediatric Urology
Pediatric Urology Fellowship
Program Director
Children's Hospital of Philadelphia
Professor of Urology in Surgery
Perelman School of Medicine
at the University of Pennsylvania
Philadelphia, Pennsylvania

Editors

**Alan W. Partin,
MD, PhD**

The Jakurski Family Director
Urologist-in-Chief
Chairman, Department
of Urology
Professor, Departments
of Urology, Oncology,
and Pathology
Johns Hopkins Medical
Institutions
Baltimore, Maryland

**Roger R. Dmochowski,
MD, MMHC, FACS**

Professor, Urologic Surgery,
Surgery, and Gynecology
Program Director, Female
Pelvic Medicine and
Reconstructive Surgery
Vice Chair for Faculty Affairs
and Professionalism
Section of Surgical Sciences
Associate Surgeon-in-Chief
Vanderbilt University Medical
Center
Nashville, Tennessee

**Louis R. Kavoussi,
MD, MBA**

Professor and Chair
Department of Urology
Zucker School of Medicine
at Hofstra/Northwell
Hempstead, New York
Chairman of Urology
The Arthur Smith Institute
for Urology
Lake Success, New York

**Craig A. Peters,
MD**

Chief, Pediatric Urology
Children's Health System Texas
Professor of Urology
University of Texas
Southwestern Medical Center
Dallas, Texas

ELSEVIER

Elsevier
1600 John F. Kennedy Blvd.
Ste 1600
Philadelphia, PA 19103-2899

CAMPBELL-WALSH-WEIN UROLOGY TWELFTH EDITION REVIEW,
THIRD EDITION
ISBN: 978-0-323-63969-9

Previous editions copyrighted 2016 and 2012.

Library of Congress Control Number: 2019955903

Senior Content Strategist: Belinda Kuhn
Senior Content Development Specialist: Jennifer Ehlers
Publishing Services Manager: Catherine Jackson
Senior Project Manager: Claire Kramer
Design Direction: Amy Buxton

Printed in Canada

Last digit is the print number: 9   8   7   6   5   4

Working together
to grow libraries in
developing countries

www.elsevier.com • www.bookaid.org

CONTRIBUTORS

Robert Abouassaly, MD
Department of Urology
Glickman Urological and Kidney Institute
Associate Professor of Surgery (Urology)
Cleveland Clinic Lerner College of
  Medicine
Cleveland Clinic
Cleveland, Ohio

Ömer Acar, MD
Department of Urology
College of Medicine
University of Illinois at Chicago
Chicago, Illinois

Mark C. Adams, MD, FAAP
Professor of Urologic Surgery
Division of Pediatric Urology
Department of Urology
Monroe Carell Jr. Children's Hospital at
  Vanderbilt
Vanderbilt University Medical Center
Nashville, Tennessee

**Riyad Tasher Al Mousa, MD, SSCU,
  FEBU, MSHA**
Consultant Urologist/Neuro-urologist
Urology Department
King Fahad Specialist Hospital–Dammam
Dammam, Saudi Arabia

Mohamad E. Allaf, MD
Vice Chairman and Professor of Urology,
  Oncology, and Biomedical Engineering
Director of Minimally Invasive and
  Robotic Surgery
Brady Urological Institute
Department of Urology
Johns Hopkins University School of
  Medicine
Baltimore, Maryland

Christopher L. Amling, MD, FACS
John Barry Professor and Chair
Department of Urology
Oregon Health and Science University
Portland, Oregon

Christopher B. Anderson, MD, MPH
Assistant Professor
Department of Urology
Columbia University Irving Medical Center
New York, New York

Karl-Erik Andersson, MD, PhD
Professor
Aarhus Institute for Advanced Studies
Aarhus University
Aarhus, Jutland, Denmark
Professor
Wake Forest Institute for Regenerative
  Medicine
Wake Forest University School of Medicine
Winston-Salem, North Carolina

Sero Andonian, MD, MSc, FRCS(C), FACS
Associate Professor
Department of Urology
McGill University
Montreal, Québec, Canada

Emmanuel S. Antonarakis, MD
Professor of Oncology and Urology
Johns Hopkins Sidney Kimmel
  Comprehensive Cancer Center
Baltimore, Maryland

Jodi A. Antonelli, MD
Assistant Professor
Department of Urology
University of Texas Southwestern Medical
  Center
Dallas, Texas

Joshua J. Augustine, MD
Associate Professor of Medicine
Cleveland Clinic Lerner College of Medicine
Staff Physician
Glickman Urological and Kidney Institute
Department of Nephrology and
  Hypertension
Cleveland, Ohio

Paul F. Austin, MD
Professor
Department of Urology
Texas Children's Hospital
Baylor College of Medicine
Houston, Texas

Timothy D. Averch, MD, FACS
Clinical Professor and Vice Chair for Quality
Department of Surgery
Palmetto Health USC Medical Group
Columbia, South Carolina

Gina M. Badalato, MD
Assistant Professor of Urology
Columbia University Vagelos College of
  Physicians and Surgeons
Assistant Attending
New York–Presbyterian Hospital
New York, New York

Daniel A. Barocas, MD, MPH, FACS
Associate Professor
Department of Urology
Vanderbilt University Medical Center
Nashville, Tennessee

Julia Spencer Barthold, MD
Principal Research Scientist
Nemours Biomedical Research/Division of
  Urology
Alfred I. duPont Hospital for Children
Wilmington, Delaware
Professor of Urology and Pediatrics
Thomas Jefferson University
Philadelphia, Pennsylvania

Laurence S. Baskin, MD
Frank Hinman Jr., MD, Distinguished
  Professorship in Pediatric Urology
Chief of Pediatric Urology
University of California–San Francisco
  Benioff Children's Hospital
Department of Urology
Mission Hall Pediatric Urology
San Francisco, California

Stuart B. Bauer, MD
Professor of Surgery (Urology)
Department of Urology
Harvard Medical School
Senior Associate in Urology
Department of Urology
Boston Children's Hospital
Boston, Massachusetts

Mitchell C. Benson, MD
Herbert and Florence Irving
  Professor and Chairman Emeritus
Department of Urology
Columbia University
Attending Physician
Department of Urology
New York Presbyterian Hospital–
  Columbia
New York, New York

Sara L. Best, MD
Associate Professor
Department of Urology
University of Wisconsin School of
  Medicine and Public Health
Madison, Wisconsin

Lori A. Birder, PhD
Professor of Medicine and Pharmacology
  and Cell Biology
Renal-Electrolyte Division of Medicine
University of Pittsburgh School of
  Medicine
Pittsburgh, Pennsylvania

Jay T. Bishoff, MD
Director, Intermountain Urological
  Institute
Intermountain Health Care
Salt Lake City, Utah

Trinity J. Bivalacqua, MD, PhD
R. Christian Evenson Professor of Urology
Department of Urology
Johns Hopkins Medicine
Baltimore, Maryland

Marc A. Bjurlin, DO, MSc
Associate Professor
Department of Urology
Lineberger Comprehensive Cancer Center
University of North Carolina at Chapel
  Hill
Chapel Hill, North Carolina

Brian G. Blackburn, MD, FIDSA
Clinical Associate Professor of Internal
    Medicine/Infectious Diseases and
    Geographic Medicine
Stanford University School of Medicine
Stanford, California

Bertil Blok, MD, PhD
Urologist
Department of Urology
Erasmus Medical Center
Rotterdam, the Netherlands

Michael L. Blute, MD
Chief
Department of Urology
Walter S. Kerr Jr., Professor of Urology
Massachusetts General Hospital/Harvard
    Medical School
Boston, Massachusetts

Timothy B. Boone, MD, PhD
Chair, Department of Urology
Houston Methodist Hospital
Professor and Associate Dean
Weill Cornell Medical College and Texas
    A&M College of Medicine
Houston, Texas

Stephen A. Boorjian, MD
Carl Rosen Professor of Urology
Department of Urology
Mayo Clinic
Rochester, Minnesota

Kristy Borawski, MD
Clinical Assistant Professor of Urology
Department of Urology
University of North Carolina at Chapel Hill
Chapel Hill, North Carolina

Michael S. Borofsky, MD
Assistant Professor
Department of Urology
University of Minnesota
Minneapolis, Minnesota

Steven Brandes, MD
Given Foundation Professor of Urology
Department of Urology
Columbia University Medical Center
New York, New York

Michael C. Braun, MD
Chief of Renal Service
Texas Children's Hospital
Professor, Renal Section Chief
Department of Pediatrics
Program Director
Pediatric Nephrology Fellowship Program
Baylor College of Medicine
Houston, Texas

Gregory A. Broderick, MD
Professor of Urology
Mayo Clinic Alix School of Medicine
Department of Urology
Program Director
Urology Residency Program
Mayo Clinic
Jacksonville, Florida

**Elizabeth Timbrook Brown, MD, MPH,
    FACS**
Assistant Professor of Urology
Department of Urology
MedStar Georgetown University
    Hospital
Washington, District of Columbia

Benjamin M. Brucker, MD
Associate Professor
Director of Female Pelvic Medicine and
    Reconstructive Surgery
Departments of Urology and Obstetrics
    and Gynecology
New York University Langone Health
New York, New York

Kathryn L. Burgio, PhD
Professor of Medicine
Division of Gerontology, Geriatrics, and
    Palliative Care
University of Alabama at Birmingham
Associate Director for Research
Birmingham/Atlanta Geriatric Research,
    Education, and Clinical Center
    (GRECC)
Birmingham Veterans Affairs Medical
    Center
Birmingham, Alabama

Arthur L. Burnett II, MD, MBA
Patrick C. Walsh Distinguished Professor
    of Urology
Department of Urology
Johns Hopkins School of Medicine
Baltimore, Maryland

Jeffrey A. Cadeddu, MD
Professor of Urology and Radiology
Department of Urology
University of Texas Southwestern Medical
    Center
Dallas, Texas

Anne P. Cameron, MD, FRCSC, FPMRS
Professor of Urology
University of Michigan
Ann Arbor, Michigan

Steven C. Campbell, MD, PhD
Professor of Surgery
Department of Urology
Cleveland Clinic
Cleveland, Ohio

Douglas A. Canning, MD
Professor of Surgery (Urology)
Perelman School of Medicine
University of Pennsylvania
Chief, Division of Urology
Children's Hospital of Philadelphia
Philadelphia, Pennsylvania

Paolo Capogrosso, MD
IRCCS San Raffaele Hospital
Department of Urology
Vita-Salute San Raffaele University
Milan, Italy

Michael A. Carducci, MD
AEGON Professor in Prostate Cancer
    Research
Sidney Kimmel Comprehensive Cancer
    Center at Johns Hopkins
Johns Hopkins University School of
    Medicine
Baltimore, Maryland

Maude Carmel, MD
Assistant Professor of Urology
University of Texas Southwestern Medical
    Center
Dallas, Texas

Peter R. Carroll, MD, MPH
Professor
Ken and Donna Derr-Chevron
    Distinguished Professor
Taube Family Distinguished Professor
Department of Urology
University of California–San Francisco
San Francisco, California

Clint Cary, MD, MPH
Associate Professor
Department of Urology
Indiana University
Indianapolis, Indiana

Erik P. Castle, MD
Professor of Urology
Department of Urology
Mayo Clinic Arizona
Phoenix, Arizona

Toby C. Chai, MD
Chair of Department of Urology
Boston University School of Medicine
Chief of Urology
Boston Medical Center
Boston, Massachusetts

Charbel Chalouhy, MD
Faculty of Medicine
St. Joseph University
Beirut, Lebanon

Alicia H. Chang, MD, MS
Medical Director
Department of Public Health,
    Tuberculosis Control Program
County of Los Angeles
Los Angeles, California

**Christopher R. Chapple, MD, BSc,
    FRCS (Urol)**
Professor and Consultant Urologist
Department of Urology
The Royal Hallamshire Hospital
Sheffield Teaching Hospitals
Sheffield, United Kingdom

Thomas Chi, MD
Associate Professor
Associate Chair for Clinical Affairs
Department of Urology
University of California–San Francisco
San Francisco, California

John Christodouleas, MD
Professor of Radiation Oncology
Urologic Cancer Program
Penn Medicine
Philadelphia, Pennsylvania

Peter E. Clark, MD
Professor and Chairman
Department of Urology
Atrium Health
Chair, Urologic Oncology
Levine Cancer Institute
Charlotte, North Carolina

Douglass B. Clayton, MD, FAAP
Associate Professor of Urologic Surgery
Division of Pediatric Urology
Department of Urology
Monroe Carell Jr. Children's Hospital at Vanderbilt
Vanderbilt University Medical Center
Nashville, Tennessee

Joshua A. Cohn, MD
Assistant Professor of Urology
Department of Urology
Einstein Healthcare Network
Assistant Professor of Urology
Department of Surgery
Division of Urologic Oncology
Fox Chase Cancer Center
Philadelphia, Pennsylvania

Michael J. Conlin, MD, MCR
Professor
Department of Urology
Portland Veterans Affairs Medical Center
Professor
Department of Urology
Oregon Health and Sciences University
Portland, Oregon

Christopher S. Cooper, MD, FAAP, FACS
Professor
Department of Urology
University of Iowa
Senior Associate Dean of Medical Education
University of Iowa Carver College of Medicine
Iowa City, Iowa

Kimberly L. Cooper, MD
Associate Professor of Urology
Columbia University Vagelos College of Physicians and Surgeons
Associate Attending
New York–Presbyterian Hospital
New York, New York

Lawrence A. Copelovitch, MD
Assistant Professor of Pediatrics
University of Pennsylvania Perelman School of Medicine
Attending Physician
Division of Nephrology
The Children's Hospital of Philadelphia
Philadelphia, Pennsylvania

Hillary L. Copp, MD, MS
Associate Professor, Pediatric Urology
Department of Urology
University of California–San Francisco
San Francisco, California

Nicholas G. Cost, MD
Associate Professor
Department of Surgery
Division of Urology
University of Colorado School of Medicine
Aurora, Colorado

Anthony Costello, MD, AM, FRACS
Professor
Department of Urology
Royal Melbourne Hospital
Parkville, Victoria, Australia

Lindsey Cox, MD
Associate Professor of Urology
Department of Urology
Medical University of South Carolina
Charleston, South Carolina

Paul L. Crispen, MD
Associate Professor
Department of Urology
University of Florida
Gainesville, Florida

Juanita M. Crook, MD, FRCPC
Professor
Department of Radiation Oncology
University of British Columbia
Radiation Oncologist
Center for the Southern Interior
British Columbia Cancer Agency
Kelowna, British Columbia, Canada

Gerald Cunha, PhD
Emeritus Professor, Anatomy and Urology
University of California–San Francisco
San Francisco, California

Douglas M. Dahl, MD, FACS
Associate Professor of Surgery
Harvard Medical School
Chief, Division of Urologic Oncology
Department of Urology
Massachusetts General Hospital
Boston, Massachusetts

Siamak Daneshmand, MD
Associate Professor of Urology
Director of Clinical Research
Keck University of Southern California School of Medicine
Los Angeles, California

Casey A. Dauw, MD
Assistant Professor
Department of Urology
University of Michigan
Ann Arbor, Michigan

Shubha K. De, MD, FRCSC
Alberta Urology Institute
Northern Alberta Urology Centre
Edmonton, Alberta, Canada

Jean J.M.C.H. de la Rosette, MD, PhD
Professor
Department of Urology
Istanbul Medipol University
Istanbul, Turkey

Dirk J.M.K. De Ridder, MD, PhD
Professor
Department of Urology
University Hospitals KU Leuven
Leuven, Belgium

Guarionex Joel DeCastro, MD, MPH
Associate Professor, Urology
Columbia University Medical Center
Department of Urology
New York Presbyterian Hospital/Columbia University
New York, New York

Francisco T. Dénes, MD, PhD
Associate Professor
Chief, Pediatric Urology Unit
Division of Urology
Hospital das Clínicas
Faculdade de Medicina
Universidade de São Paulo
São Paulo, Brazil

Mahesh R. Desai, MS, FRCS, FRCS
Chief Urologist and Managing Trustee
Department of Urology
Muljibhai Patel Urological Hospital
Nadiad, India

David A. Diamond, MD
Urologist-in-Chief
Department of Urology
Boston Children's Hospital
Professor of Surgery (Urology)
Department of Surgery
Harvard Medical School
Boston, Massachusetts

Heather N. Di Carlo, MD
Director, Pediatric Urology Research
Assistant Professor of Urology
The James Buchanan Brady Urological Institute
Johns Hopkins Medical Institutions
Baltimore, Maryland

Colin P.N. Dinney, MD
Chairman and Professor
Department of Urology
University of Texas MD Anderson Cancer Center
Houston, Texas

Roger R. Dmochowski, MD, MMHC, FACS
Professor, Urologic Surgery, Surgery, and
  Gynecology
Program Director, Female Pelvic Medicine
  and Reconstructive Surgery
Vice Chair for Faculty Affairs and
  Professionalism
Section of Surgical Sciences
Associate Surgeon-in-Chief
Vanderbilt University Medical Center
Nashville, Tennessee

Charles G. Drake, MD, PhD
Professor, Medical Oncology and Urology
Department of Medicine
Columbia University
New York, New York

Brian Duty, MD, MBA
Associate Professor
Department of Urology
Oregon Health and Science University
Portland, Oregon

James A. Eastham, MD
Chief, Urology Service
Department of Surgery
Memorial Sloan-Kettering Cancer Center
New York, New York

Scott Eggener, MD
Professor of Surgery and Radiology
University of Chicago
Chicago, Illinois

Mohamed A. Elkoushy, MD, PhD, MSc
Professor, Urology
Faculty of Medicine
Suez Canal University
Ismailia, Egypt

Jonathan Ellison, MD
Assistant Professor of Urology
Medical College of Wisconsin
Children's Wisconsin
Milwaukee, Wisconsin

Sammy E. Elsamra, MD, FACS
Assistant Professor of Surgery (Urology)
Rutgers Robert Wood Johnson Medical
  School
Director of Robotic Surgical Services
Robert Wood Johnson University Hospital
RWJBarnabas Health
New Brunswick, New Jersey

Jonathan I. Epstein, MD
Professor of Pathology, Urology, and
  Oncology
The Reinhard Professor of Urological
  Pathology
Director of Surgical Pathology
The Johns Hopkins Medical Institutions
Baltimore, Maryland

Carlos R. Estrada, MD, MBA
Associate Professor
Department of Surgery
Harvard Medical School
Associate in Urology
Department of Urology
Boston Children's Hospital
Boston, Massachusetts

Jairam Eswara, MD
Attending Surgeon
St. Elizabeth's Medical Center
Clinical Associate Professor
Tufts University School of Medicine
Boston, Massachusetts

Fernando A. Ferrer, MD, FACS, FAAP
Surgeon in Chief
Department of Pediatric Urology
Children's Hospital Omaha
Professor, Surgery (Urology)
University of Nebraska
Omaha, Nebraska

Neil Fleshner, MD, MPH, FRCSC
Professor of Surgery and Martin Barkin
  Chair
Department of Urology
University of Toronto
Surgeon, Uro-Oncology
University Health Network
Toronto, Ontario, Canada

Bryan R. Foster, MD
Associate Professor
Department of Radiology
Oregon Health and Science University
Portland, Oregon

Richard S. Foster, MD
Professor
Department of Urology
Indiana University
Indianapolis, Indiana

Pat F. Fulgham, MD
Surgical Director of Oncology
  Services
Chairman, Department of Urology
Texas Health Presbyterian Dallas
Dallas, Texas

Arvind P. Ganpule, MS, DNB
Vice-Chairman
Department of Urology
Chief, Division of Robotic Surgery
Muljibhai Patel Urological Hospital
Nadiad, India

Kris E. Gaston, MD
Urologic Oncology
Levine Cancer Institute
Charlotte, North Carolina

**John P. Gearhart, MD, FAAP, FACS,
  FRCS**
Chief of Pediatric Urology
Professor of Urology
The James Buchanan Brady Urological
  Institute
Johns Hopkins Medical Institutions
Baltimore, Maryland

Matthew T. Gettman, MD
Professor and Vice-Chair
Department of Urology
Mayo Clinic
Rochester, Minnesota

Reza Ghavamian, MD
Eastern Regional Director of Urology
Department of Urology
Northwell Health
Greenlawn, New York
Professor of Urology
Department of Urology
Zucker School of Medicine at Hofstra/
  Northwell
New Hyde Park, New York

Bruce R. Gilbert, MD, PhD
Professor of Urology
The Smith Institute for Urology
Zucker School of Medicine of Hofstra/
  Northwell
New Hyde Park, New York
Clinical Professor of Urology (Adjunct)
Department of Urology
Weill Cornell Medical College
New York, New York

Timothy D. Gilligan, MD
Associate Professor of Medicine
Solid Tumor Oncology
Cleveland Clinic Lerner College of
  Medicine
Program Director, Hematology/Oncology
  Fellowship
Taussig Cancer Institute
Cleveland Clinic
Cleveland, Ohio

David A. Goldfarb, MD
Professor of Surgery
Cleveland Clinic Lerner College of
  Medicine
Glickman Urological and Kidney
  Institute
Cleveland Clinic
Cleveland, Ohio

Marc Goldstein, MD, DSc (hon), FACS
Matthew P. Hardy Distinguished Professor
  of Urology and Male Reproductive
  Medicine
Department of Urology and Institute for
  Reproductive Medicine
Weill Cornell Medical College of Cornell
  University
Surgeon-In-Chief, Male Reproductive
  Medicine, and Surgery
Department of Urology and Institute for
  Reproductive Medicine
New York Presbyterian Hospital–Weill
  Cornell Medicine
Adjunct Senior Scientist
Population Council
Center for Biomedical Research at
  Rockefeller University
New York, New York

Leonard G. Gomella, MD, FACS
The Bernard W. Godwin Professor of
  Prostate Cancer
Chairman, Department of Urology
Sidney Kimmel Cancer Center
Sidney Kimmel Medical College at
  Thomas Jefferson University
Philadelphia, Pennsylvania

Alex Gomelsky, MD, FACS
B.E. Trichel Professor and Chairman
Department of Urology
Louisiana State University Health
Shreveport, Louisiana

Mark L. Gonzalgo, MD, PhD
Professor and Vice Chairman
Department of Urology
University of Miami Miller School of
    Medicine
Miami, Florida

Michael A. Gorin, MD
Assistant Professor
Department of Urology
Johns Hopkins University School of
    Medicine
Baltimore, Maryland

Tamsin Greenwell, MD, PhD
Consultant Urological Surgeon
University College London Hospitals
London, United Kingdom

Tomas L. Griebling, MD, MPH
John P. Wolf 33-Degree Masonic
    Distinguished Professor of Urology
Department of Urology and The Landon
    Center on Aging
The University of Kansas
Kansas City, Kansas

Khurshid A. Guru, MD
Chair of Urology Department
Director of Robotic Surgery
Robert P. Huben Endowed Professor of
    Urologic Oncology
Roswell Park Comprehensive Cancer Center
Buffalo, New York

Thomas J. Guzzo, MD, MPH
Associate Professor of Urology
The Hospital of the University of
    Pennsylvania
University of Pennsylvania
Philadelphia, Pennsylvania

Jennifer A. Hagerty, DO
Attending Physician
Department of Surgery/Division of Urology
Nemours/AI duPont Hospital for Children
Wilmington, Delaware
Assistant Professor
Department of Urology and Pediatrics
Thomas Jefferson University
Philadelphia, Pennsylvania

Simon J. Hall, MD
Zucker Professor of Urologic Oncology
Smith Institute for Urology
Hofstra/Northwell School of Medicine
Lake Success, New York

Barry Hallner, MD
Associate Program Director, Female Pelvic
    Medicine and Reconstructive Surgery
Assistant Professor
Departments of OB/GYN and Urology
Louisiana State University Health
New Orleans School of Medicine
New Orleans, Louisiana

Ethan J. Halpern, MD
Professor of Radiology and Urology
Sidney Kimmel Cancer Center
Sidney Kimmel Medical College at
    Thomas Jefferson University
Philadelphia, Pennsylvania

Misop Han, MD
David Hall McConnell Professor of
    Urology and Oncology
Department of Urology
Johns Hopkins Medicine
Baltimore, Maryland

Philip Hanno, MD, MPH
Clinical Professor
Department of Urology
Stanford University School of Medicine
Palo Alto, California
Emeritus Professor
Department of Urology
University of Pennsylvania
Philadelphia, Pennsylvania

Siobhan M. Hartigan, MD
Female Pelvic Medicine and Reconstructive
    Surgery Fellow
Department of Urology
Vanderbilt University Medical Center
Nashville, Tennessee

Christopher J. Hartman, MD
Chief of Urology, Forest Hills Hospital
Northwell Health
Associate Program Director, Urology
    Residency Program
Smith Institute for Urology
Assistant Professor of Urology
Zucker School of Medicine at Hofstra/
    Northwell
Hempstead, New York

**Hashim Hashim, MD, MBBS, MRCS
    (Eng), FEBU, FRCS (Urol)**
Consultant Urological Surgeon
Honorary Professor of Urology and
    Director of the Urodynamics Unit
Bristol Urological Institute
Southmead Hospital
Bristol, United Kingdom

Dorota J. Hawksworth, MD
Walter Reed National Military Medical
    Center
Bethesda, Maryland

Sarah Hazell, MD
Resident Physician
Radiation Oncology and Molecular
    Radiation Sciences
Johns Hopkins University School of
    Medicine
Baltimore, Maryland

John P.F.A. Heesakkers, MD, PhD
Urologist
Department of Urology
Radboud University Medical Centre
Nijmegen, The Netherlands

Sevann Helo, MD
Minneapolis Veterans Affairs Medical
    Center
Minneapolis, Minnesota

Amin S. Herati, MD
Assistant Professor of Urology
The James Buchanan Brady Urological
    Institute and Department of Urology
Assistant Professor
Department of Gynecology and Obstetrics
Johns Hopkins University School of
    Medicine
Baltimore, Maryland

C.D. Anthony Herndon, MD, FAAP, FACS
Professor of Surgery
Director of Pediatric Urology
Surgeon in Chief, Children's Hospital of
    Richmond
Division of Urology
Virginia Commonwealth University
Richmond, Virginia

Piet Hoebeke, MD, PhD
Professor of Urology
Dean, Faculty of Medicine and Health
    Sciences
Ghent University
Ghent, Belgium

David M. Hoenig, MD
Professor and Chief
North Shore University Hospital
Smith Institute for Urology
North Shore–Long Island Jewish–Hofstra
    University
Lake Success, New York

Michael Hsieh, MD, PhD
Associate Professor of Urology and
    Pediatrics and Microbiology,
    Immunology, and Tropical Medicine
The George Washington University
Director, Clinic for Adolescent and
    Adult Pediatric OnseT UroLogy
    (CAPITUL)
Children's National Hospital and the
    George Washington University
Washington, District of Columbia

Valerio Iacovelli, MD
Urology Unit
University of Rome Tor Vergata
San Carlo di Nancy General Hospital
GVM Care and Research
Rome, Italy

Stephen V. Jackman, MD
Professor
Department of Urology
University of Pittsburgh
Pittsburgh, Pennsylvania

Joseph M. Jacob, MD, MCR
Assistant Professor
Department of Urology
Upstate Medical University
Syracuse, New York

Micah A. Jacobs, MD, MPH
Associate Professor
Department of Urology
University of Texas Southwestern
Dallas, Texas

Thomas W. Jarrett, MD
Professor and Chairman
Department of Urology
George Washington University
Washington, District of Columbia

Gerald H. Jordan, MD, FACS, FAAP (Hon), FRCS (Hon)
Associate Professor, Urology
Eastern Virginia Medical School
Norfolk, Virginia

Martin Kaefer, MD
Professor of Urology
Indiana University School of Medicine
Indianapolis, Indiana

Kamaljot S. Kaler, MD, FRCSC
Clinical Assistant Professor
University of Calgary
Southern Alberta Institute of Urology
Calgary, Alberta, Canada

Panagiotis Kallidonis, MD, MSc, PhD, FEBU
Assistant Professor Urological Surgeon
Department of Urology
University of Patras
Patras, Greece

Steven Kaplan, MD
Professor and Director, The Men's Health Program
Department of Urology
Icahn School of Medicine at Mount Sinai
New York, New York

Max Kates, MD
Assistant Professor
Department of Urology
Johns Hopkins Medical Institutions
Baltimore, Maryland

Melissa R. Kaufman, MD, PhD, FACS
Associate Professor
Department of Urology
Vanderbilt University
Nashville, Tennessee

Louis R. Kavoussi, MD, MBA
Professor and Chair
Department of Urology
Zucker School of Medicine at Hofstra/Northwell
Hempstead, New York
Chairman of Urology
The Arthur Smith Institute for Urology
Lake Success, New York

Parviz K. Kavoussi, MD, FACS
Reproductive Urologist
Department of Urology
Austin Fertility and Reproductive Medicine
Adjunct Assistant Professor
Department of Psychology
Division of Neuroendocrinology and Motivation
University of Texas at Austin
Austin, Texas
Adjunct Assistant Professor
Department of Urology
University of Texas Health Sciences Center at San Antonio
San Antonio, Texas

Miran Kenk, PhD
Scientific Associate
Department of Surgical Oncology
Princess Margaret Cancer Centre
University Health Network
Toronto, Ontario, Canada

Mohit Khera, MD, MBA, MPH
Professor of Urology
Scott Department of Urology
Baylor College of Medicine
Houston, Texas

Antoine E. Khoury, MD, FRCSC, FAAP
Walter R. Schmid, Professor of Pediatric Urology
Department of Urology
University of California–Irvine
Head of Pediatric Urology
Children's Hospital of Orange County
Orange, California

Eric A. Klein, MD
Andrew C. Novick, Distinguished Professor and Chair
Glickman Urological and Kidney Institute and Cleveland Clinic Lerner College of Medicine
Cleveland Clinic
Cleveland, Ohio

Laurence Klotz, MD, FRCSC, CM
Professor of Surgery
University of Toronto
Urologist, Sunnybrook Health Sciences Centre
Toronto, Ontario, Canada

Bodo E. Knudsen, MD, FRCSC
Associate Professor
Vice Chair Clinical Operations
Department of Urology
Wexner Medical Center
The Ohio State University
Columbus, Ohio

Kathleen C. Kobashi, MD
Chief, Section of Urology
Urology and Renal Transplantation
Virginia Mason Medical Center
Seattle, Washington

Ervin Kocjancic, MD
Lawrence S. Ross Professor of Urology
Vice Chairman
Department of Urology College of Medicine
University of Illinois at Chicago
Chicago, Illinois

Chester J. Koh, MD
Professor of Urology, Pediatrics, and Obstetrics/Gynecology
Baylor College of Medicine
Division of Pediatric Urology
Department of Surgery
Texas Children's Hospital
Houston, Texas

Badrinath Konety, MD, MBA
Chief Executive Officer
University of Minnesota Physicians
Vice Dean for Clinical Affairs
University of Minnesota Medical School
Professor
Department of Urology
University of Minnesota
Minneapolis, Minnesota

Casey Kowalik, MD
Assistant Professor
Department of Urology
University of Kansas Health System
Kansas City, Kansas

Martin A. Koyle, MD, FAAP, FACS, FRCSC, FRCS (Eng)
Division Head, Division of Pediatric Urology
Women's Auxiliary Chair in Urology and Regenerative Medicine
Hospital for Sick Children
Professor of Surgery
University of Toronto
Toronto, Ontario, Canada

Amy E. Krambeck, MD
Michael O. Koch Professor of Urology
Department of Urology
Indiana University
Indianapolis, Indiana

Jessica E. Kreshover, MD
Associate Professor of Urology
The Arthur Smith Institute for Urology
Zucker School of Medicine at Hofstra/Northwell
New Hyde Park, New York

Venkatesh Krishnamurthi, MD
Director, Kidney/Pancreas Transplant Program
Glickman Urological and Kidney Institute Transplant Center
Cleveland Clinic Foundation
Cleveland, Ohio

Ryan M. Krlin, MD, FPMRS
Associate Professor of Urology and
    Gynecology
Department of Urology
Louisiana State University Health New
    Orleans
New Orleans, Louisiana

Alexander Kutikov, MD
Professor and Chief, Urologic Oncology
Fox Chase Cancer Center
Philadelphia, Pennsylvania

Jaime Landman, MD
Professor of Urology and Radiology
Chairman, Department of Urology
University of California, Irvine
Orange, California

Brian R. Lane, MD, PhD
Chief, Urology
Spectrum Health
Associate Professor
Michigan State University College of
    Human Medicine
Grand Rapids, Michigan

David A. Leavitt, MD
Assistant Professor
Department of Urology
Vattikuti Urology Institute
Henry Ford Health System
Detroit, Michigan

Eugene K. Lee, MD
Associate Professor
Department of Urology
University of Kansas Medical Center
Kansas City, Kansas

Gary E. Lemack, MD
Professor of Urology and Neurology
Department of Urology
University of Texas Southwestern Medical
    Center
Dallas, Texas

Thomas Sean Lendvay, MD, FACS
Professor of Urology
University of Washington
Professor of Pediatric Urology
Seattle Children's Hospital
Seattle, Washington

Herbert Lepor, MD
Professor and Martin Spatz Chair
Department of Urology
New York University School of Medicine
Chief, Urology
New York University Langone Health
New York, New York

Evangelos Liatsikos, MD, PhD
Professor and Chairman
Department of Urology
University of Patras
Patras, Greece

Sey Kiat Lim, MBBS, MRCS (Edinburgh), MMed (Surgery), FAMS (Urology)
Senior Consultant and Chief
Department of Urology
Changi General Hospital
Adjunct Associate Professor
Duke–National University of Singapore
    Medical School
Singapore

W. Marston Linehan, MD
Chief, Urologic Oncology Branch
National Cancer Institute
National Institutes of Health
Bethesda, Maryland

Richard Edward Link, MD, PhD
Carlton-Smith Chair in Urologic
    Education
Associate Professor of Urology
Director, Division of Endourology and
    Minimally Invasive Surgery
Scott Department of Urology
Baylor College of Medicine
Houston, Texas

Jen-Jane Liu, MD
Assistant Professor
Director of Urologic Oncology
Department of Urology
Oregon Health and Science University
Portland Oregon

Stacy Loeb, MD
Professor of Urology and Population
    Health
New York University and Manhattan
    Veterans Affairs
New York, New York

Christopher J. Long, MD
Assistant Professor of Urology (Surgery)
Perelman School of Medicine
University of Pennsylvania
Division of Urology
Children's Hospital of Philadelphia
Philadelphia, Pennsylvania

Roberto Iglesias. Lopes, MD, PhD
Assistant Professor
Pediatric Urology Unit
Division of Urology
Hospital das Clínicas
Faculdade de Medicina
Universidade de São Paulo
São Paulo, Brazil

Armando J. Lorenzo, MD, MSc, FRCSC, FAAP, FACS
Staff Paediatric Urologist
Department of Surgery
Division of Urology
Hospital for Sick Children
Associate Professor
Department of Surgery
Division of Urology
University of Toronto
Toronto, Ontario, Canada

Yair Lotan, MD
Professor
Department of Urology
University of Texas Southwestern Medical
    Center
Dallas, Texas

Alvaro Lucioni, MD
Program Director, Female Pelvic Medicine
    Reconstructive Surgery Fellowship
Urology and Renal Transplantation
Virginia Mason Medical Center
Seattle, Washington

Tom F. Lue, MD, ScD (Hon), FACS
Professor of Urology
Department of Urology
University of California–San Francisco
San Francisco, California

Nicolas Lumen, MD, PhD
Professor of Urology
Ghent University Hospital
Ghent, Belgium

Marcos Tobias Machado, MD, PhD
Professor of Urology
Department of Urology
Faculdade de Medicina do ABC
Santo Andre, Brazil

Stephen D. Marshall, MD
Attending Physician
Laconia Clinic Department of Urology
Lakes Region General Hospital
Laconia, New Hampshire

Aaron D. Martin, MD, MPH
Associate Professor
Department of Urology
Louisiana State University Health
    Sciences Center
Department of Pediatric Urology
Children's Hospital New Orleans
New Orleans, Louisiana

Laura M. Martinez, MD
Instructor in Clinical Urology
Department of Urology
Houston Methodist Hospital
Houston, Texas

Timothy A. Masterson, MD
Associate Professor
Department of Urology
Indiana University Medical Center
Indianapolis, Indiana

Surena F. Matin, MD
Professor
Department of Urology
Medical Director
Minimally Invasive New Technology in
    Oncologic Surgery (MINTOS)
University of Texas MD Anderson Cancer
    Center
Houston, Texas

Brian R. Matlaga, MD
Professor
James Buchanan Brady Urological
    Institute
Johns Hopkins Medical Institutions
Baltimore, Maryland

Kurt A. McCammon, MD
Devine Chair in Genitourinary
    Reconstructive Surgery
Chairman and Program Director
Professor
Department of Urology
Eastern Virginia Medical School
Norfolk, Virginia
Devine-Jordan Center for Reconstructive
    Surgery and Pelvic Health
Urology of Virginia PLLC
Virginia Beach, Virginia

James M. McKiernan, MD
Chairman and Professor
Department of Urology
Columbia University Irving Medical Center
New York, New York

Chris G. McMahon, MBBS, FAChSHP
Director
Australian Centre for Sexual Health
Sydney, New South Wales, Australia

Kevin T. McVary, MD
Center for Male Health
Loyola University Medical Center
Maywood, Illinois

Luis G. Medina, MD
Research Fellow
Department of Urology
University of Southern California
Los Angeles, California

Kirstan K. Meldrum, MD
Professor
Department of Surgery
Central Michigan University
Saginaw, Michigan

Matthew J. Mellon, MD, FACS
Associate Professor
Department of Urology
Indiana University
Indianapolis, Indiana

Maxwell V. Meng, MD, FACS
Professor and Chief, Urologic Oncology
Department of Urology
University of California–San Francisco
San Francisco, California

David Mikhail, MD, BSc, FRCSC
Endourology Fellow
Smith Institute for Urology
Northwell Health
New Hyde Park, New York

Nicole L. Miller, MD
Associate Professor
Department of Urology
Vanderbilt University Medical Center
Nashville, Tennessee

Alireza Moinzadeh, MD, MHL
Chair, Department of Urology
Lahey Hospital and Medical Center
Burlington, Massachusetts
Assistant Professor of Urology
Tufts University School of Medicine
Boston, Massachusetts

Robert M. Moldwin, MD
Professor of Urology
The Arthur Smith Institute for Urology
Zucker School of Medicine at Hofstra/
    Northwell
Lake Success, New York

Manoj Monga, MD, FACS
Director, Stevan Streem Center for
    Endourology and Stone Disease
Department of Urology
Cleveland Clinic
Cleveland, Ohio

Francesco Montorsi, MD, FRCS (Hon)
Professor and Chairman
Department of Urology
IRCCS San Raffaele University
Milan, Italy

Daniel M. Moreira, MD, MHS
Assistant Professor
Department of Urology
University of Illinois at Chicago
Chicago, Illinois

Allen F. Morey, MD, FACS
Professor
Department of Urology
University of Texas Southwestern
Dallas, Texas

Todd M. Morgan, MD
Chief of Urologic Oncology
Department of Urology
University of Michigan
Ann Arbor, Michigan

John J. Mulcahy, MD, PhD, FACS
Clinical Professor
Department of Urology
University of Alabama
Birmingham, Alabama

Ravi Munver, MD, FACS
Vice Chairman
Chief of Minimally Invasive and Robotic
    Urologic Surgery
Hackensack University Medical Center
Hackensack, New Jersey
Professor of Urology
Hackensack Meridian School of Medicine
    at Seton Hall University
Nutley, New Jersey

Stephen Y. Nakada, MD, FACS
Professor and Chairman, The David T.
    Uehling Chair of Urology
Department of Urology
University of Wisconsin School of
    Medicine and Public Health
Professor and Chairman
Department of Urology
University of Wisconsin Hospital and Clinics
Madison, Wisconsin

Neema Navai, MD
Associate Professor
Department of Urology
University of Texas MD Anderson Cancer
    Center
Houston, Texas

**Diane K. Newman, DNP, ANP-BC, FAAN,
BCB-PMD**
Adjunct Professor of Urology in Surgery
Division of Urology
Research Investigator Senior
Perelman School of Medicine
University of Pennsylvania
Co-Director, Penn Center for Continence
    and Pelvic Health
Division of Urology
Penn Medicine
Philadelphia, Pennsylvania

Craig S. Niederberger, MD, FACS
Clarence C. Saelhof Professor and Head
Department of Urology
University of Illinois at Chicago College of
    Medicine
Professor
Department of Bioengineering
University of Illinois at Chicago College of
    Engineering
Chicago, Illinois

Victor W. Nitti, MD
Professor of Urology and Obstetrics and
    Gynecology
Shlomo Raz Chair in Urology
Chief, Division of Female Pelvic Medicine
    and Reconstructive Surgery
David Geffen School of Medicine at
    University of California–Los Angeles
Los Angeles, California

Samuel J. Ohlander, MD
Assistant Professor
Department of Urology
University of Illinois at Chicago
Chicago, Illinois

L. Henning Olsen, MD
Professor
Department of Urology
Section of Pediatric Urology
Aarhus University Hospital
Institute of Clinical Medicine
Aarhus University
Aarhus, Denmark

Aria F. Olumi, MD
Professor of Surgery/Urology
Department of Urologic Surgery
Beth Israel Deaconess Medical Center/
    Harvard Medical School
Boston, Massachusetts

**Nadir I. Osman, MBChB (Hons), PhD,
FRCS (Urol)**
Consultant Urologist
Royal Hallamshire Hospital
Sheffield Teaching Hospitals
Sheffield, South Yorkshire

Brandon J. Otto, MD
Assistant Professor of Urology
University of Florida College of Medicine
Gainesville, Florida

Priya Padmanabhan, MD, MPH, FACS
Professor of Urology
Pelvic Reconstruction and Voiding
    Dysfunction
William Beaumont Medical Center
Royal Oak, Michigan

Rodrigo L. Pagani, MD
Assistant Professor
Department of Urology
University of Illinois at Chicago
Chicago, Illinois

Lance C. Pagliaro, MD
Professor of Oncology
Mayo Clinic College of Medicine
Consultant
Division of Medical Oncology
Department of Oncology
Mayo Clinic
Rochester, Minnesota

Ganesh S. Palapattu, MD
The George F. Valassis and Sandy G.
    Valassis Professor and Chair
Department of Urology
University of Michigan
Ann Arbor, Michigan

Drew A. Palmer, MD
Endourology Fellow
Department of Urology
University of North Carolina at Chapel Hill
Chapel Hill, North Carolina

Jeffrey S. Palmer, MD, FACS, FSPU
Director, Genital Reconstruction
Cohen Children's Medical Center of New
    York
Associate Professor of Urology and
    Pediatrics
Zucker School of Medicine at Hofstra/
    Northwell
Long Island, New York

Lane S. Palmer, MD, FACS, FSPU
Chief, Division of Pediatric Urology
Cohen Children's Medical Center of New
    York
Professor of Urology and Pediatrics
Zucker School of Medicine at Hofstra/
    Northwell
Long Island, New York

Meyeon Park, MD, MAS
Associate Professor
Medical Director
UCSF PKD Center of Excellence
Department of Medicine
Division of Nephrology
University of California–San Francisco
San Francisco, California

William P. Parker, MD
Assistant Professor
Department of Urology
University of Kansas Health System
Kansas City, Kansas

Alan W. Partin, MD, PhD
The Jakurski Family Director
Urologist-in-Chief
Chairman, Department of Urology
Professor, Departments of Urology,
    Oncology, and Pathology
Johns Hopkins Medical Institutions
Baltimore, Maryland

Roshan M. Patel, MD
Assistant Clinical Professor
Department of Urology
University of California, Irvine
Orange, California

Margaret S. Pearle, MD, PhD
Professor
Department of Urology and Internal
    Medicine
University of Texas Southwestern Medical
    Center
Dallas, Texas

David F. Penson, MD, MPH
Hamilton and Howd Chair in Urologic
    Oncology
Professor and Chair, Department of Urology
Vanderbilt University Medical Center
Nashville Tennessee

Craig A. Peters, MD
Chief, Pediatric Urology
Children's Health System Texas
Professor of Urology
University of Texas Southwestern
    Medical Center
Dallas, Texas

Curtis A. Pettaway, MD
Professor
Department of Urology
University of Texas MD Anderson Cancer
    Center
Houston, Texas

Janey R. Phelps, MD
Department of Anesthesia
The University of North Carolina at
    Chapel Hill
Chapel Hill, North Carolina

Ryan Phillips, MD, PhD
Resident Physician
Radiation Oncology and Molecular
    Radiation Sciences
Johns Hopkins University School of
    Medicine
Baltimore, Maryland

Phillip M. Pierorazio, MD
Associate Professor of Urology and Oncology
Brady Urological Institute and
    Department of Urology
Johns Hopkins School of Medicine
Baltimore, Maryland

Hans G. Pohl, MD, FAAP
Associate Professor
Department of Pediatrics
Division of Urology
Children's National Medical Center
Washington, District of Columbia

Thomas J. Polascik, MD
Professor of Surgery
Division of Urology
Duke Cancer Institute
Durham, North Carolina

Michel Pontari, MD
Professor and Vice-Chair
Department of Urology
Lewis Katz School of Medicine at Temple
    University
Philadelphia, Pennsylvania

John C. Pope IV, MD
Professor
Departments of Urology and
    Pediatrics
Monroe Carell Jr. Children's Hospital at
    Vanderbilt
Vanderbilt University Medical Center
Nashville, Tennessee

Jay D. Raman, MD, FACS
Professor and Chief
Division of Urology
Penn State Health Milton S. Hershey
    Medical Center
Hershey, Pennsylvania

Ranjith Ramasamy, MD
Director of Reproductive Urology
Department of Urology
University of Miami
Miami, Florida

Ardeshir R. Rastinehad, DO, FACOS
Director, Focal Therapy and Interventional
    Urology
Associate Professor of Radiology and
    Urology
Departments of Urology and Radiology
Icahn School of Medicine at Mount
    Sinai
New York, New York

Yazan F. Rawashdeh, MD
Consultant Pediatric Urologist
Department of Urology
Section of Pediatric Urology
Aarhus University Hospital
Aarhus, Denmark

Pramod P. Reddy, MD
Professor
Division Director, Division of Pediatric
    Urology
Cincinnati Children's Hospital
Cincinnati, Ohio

W. Stuart Reynolds, MD, MPH
Associate Professor
Department of Urology
Vanderbilt University Medical Center
Nashville, Tennessee

Koon Ho Rha, MD, PhD, FACS
Professor
Department of Urology
Urological Science Institute
Yonsei University College of Medicine
Seoul, Republic of Korea

Lee Richstone, MD
Chairman of Urology
Director of Laparoscopic and Robotic
    Surgery
Professor of Urology
Lenox Hill Hospital
New York, New York

Stephen Riggs, MD
Urologic Oncology
Levine Cancer Institute
Charlotte, North Carolina

Richard C. Rink, MD, FAAP, FACS
Emeritus Professor, Pediatric Urology
Riley Hospital for Children Indiana
    University School of Medicine
Faculty, Pediatric Urology
Peyton Manning Children's Hospital at
    Ascension St. Vincent
Indianapolis, Indiana

Michael L. Ritchey, MD
Professor
Department of Urology
Mayo Clinic College of Medicine
Chief Medical Officer
Phoenix Children's Hospital
Phoenix, Arizona

Claus G. Roehrborn, MD
Professor and Chairman
Department of Urology
University of Texas Southwestern Medical
    Center
Dallas, Texas

Ashley E. Ross, MD, PhD
Adjunct Associate Professor
Department of Urology
Johns Hopkins Brady Urological Institute
Baltimore, Maryland

Sherry S. Ross, MD
Department of Urology
The University of North Carolina at
    Chapel Hill
Chapel Hill, North Carolina

Christopher C. Roth, MD
Associate Professor
Department of Urology
Louisiana State University Health Sciences
    Center
Department of Pediatric Urology
Children's Hospital New Orleans
New Orleans, Louisiana

Kyle O. Rove, MD
Assistant Professor
Department of Pediatric Urology
Children's Hospital Colorado
Assistant Professor
Department of Surgery
Division of Urology
University of Colorado
Aurora, Colorado

Eric S. Rovner, MD
Professor
Department of Urology
Medical University of South Carolina
Charleston, South Carolina

Steven P. Rowe, MD, PhD
Assistant Professor of Radiology and
    Radiological Science
Johns Hopkins University School of
    Medicine
Baltimore Maryland

Matthew P. Rutman, MD
Associate Professor of Urology
Columbia University Vagelos College of
    Physicians and Surgeons
Associate Attending
New York–Presbyterian Hospital
New York, New York

Simpa S. Salami, MD, MPH
Assistant Professor
Department of Urology
University of Michigan
Ann Arbor, Michigan

Andrea Salonia, MD, PhD
IRCCS San Raffaele Hospital
Director, Urological Research Institute
Vita-Salute San Raffaele University
Milan, Italy

Edward M. Schaeffer, MD, PhD
Professor and Chair
Department of Urology
Northwestern University Feinberg School
    of Medicine
Chicago, Illinois

Bruce J. Schlomer, MD
Associate Professor
Department of Urology
University of Texas Southwestern
Dallas, Texas

Michael J. Schwartz, MD, FACS
Associate Professor of Urology
The Arthur Smith Institute for Urology
Zucker School of Medicine at Hofstra/
    Northwell
New Hyde Park, New York

Allen D. Seftel, MD
Professor of Urology
Department of Surgery
Cooper Medical School of Rowan
    University
Chief
Division of Urology
Cooper University Health Care
Camden, New Jersey
Adjunct Professor
Department of Surgery
MD Anderson Cancer Center
Houston, Texas

Rachel Selekman, MD, MS
Assistant Professor, Pediatric Urology
Children's National Medical Center
Washington, District of Columbia

Abhishek Seth, MD
Assistant Professor, Urology
Baylor College of Medicine
Houston, Texas

Karen Sandell Sfanos, PhD
Associate Professor
Department of Pathology
Johns Hopkins University School of
    Medicine
Baltimore, Maryland

Paras H. Shah, MD
Assistant Professor of Urology
Albany Medical Center
Albany, New York

Mohammed Shahait, MBBS
Consultant of Urology
Department of Surgery
King Hussein Cancer Center
Amman, Jordan
Leonard Davis Institute of Health
    Economics
University of Pennsylvania
Philadelphia, Pennsylvania

Robert C. Shamberger, MD
Chief, Emeritus
Department of Surgery
Boston Children's Hospital
Robert E. Gross Professor of Surgery
Harvard Medical School
Boston, Massachusetts

Alan W. Shindel, MD, MAS
Associate Professor
Department of Urology
University of California–San Francisco
San Francisco, California

Aseem R. Shukla, MD
Endowed Chair in Minimally Invasive
    Surgery
Division of Pediatric Urology
Children's Hospital of Philadelphia
Associate Professor of Surgery (Urology)
Perelman School of Medicine
University of Pennsylvania
Philadelphia, Pennsylvania

Jay Simhan, MD, FACS
Vice Chairman
Department of Urology
Einstein Healthcare Network
Associate Professor of Urology
Department of Urology
Fox Chase Cancer Center
Philadelphia, Pennsylvania

Brian W. Simons, DVM, PhD
Assistant Professor
Department of Urology
Johns Hopkins University School of Medicine
Baltimore, Maryland

Eila C. Skinner, MD
Professor and Chair
Thomas A. Stamey Research Professor of
    Urology
Department of Urology
Stanford University School of Medicine
Stanford, California

Armine K. Smith, MD
Assistant Professor
Brady Urological Institute
Johns Hopkins University
Assistant Professor
Department of Urology
George Washington University
Washington, District of Columbia

Daniel Y. Song, MD
Professor
Radiation Oncology and Molecular
    Radiation Sciences
Johns Hopkins University School of
    Medicine
Baltimore, Maryland

Rene Sotelo, MD
Professor of Clinical Urology
Department of Urology
University of Southern California
Los Angeles, California

Michael W. Sourial, MD, FRCSC
Assistant Professor
Department of Urology
The Ohio State University
Columbus, Ohio

Anne-Françoise Spinoit, MD, PhD
Pediatric and Reconstructive Urologist
Department of Urology
Ghent University Hospital
Ghent, Belgium

Arun K. Srinivasan, MD
Division of Pediatric Urology
Children's Hospital of Philadelphia
Assistant Professor of Surgery (Urology)
Perelman School of Medicine
University of Pennsylvania
Philadelphia, Pennsylvania

Ramaprasad Srinivasan, MD, PhD
Head, Molecular Cancer Section
Urologic Oncology Branch
Center for Cancer Research
National Cancer Institute
National Institutes of Health
Bethesda, Maryland

Irina Stanasel, MD
Assistant Professor
Department of Urology
University of Texas Southwestern/
    Children's Health
Dallas, Texas

**Andrew J. Stephenson, MD, MBA, FACS,
    FRCS (C)**
Professor
Section Chief and Director, Urologic
    Oncology
Rush Medical College
Chicago, Illinois

Julie N. Stewart, MD
Assistant Professor
Department of Urology
Houston Methodist Hospital
Houston, Texas

John Stites, MD
Minimally Invasive and Robotic Urologic
    Surgery
Hackensack University Medical Center
Hackensack, New Jersey

Douglas W. Storm, MD
Assistant Professor
Department of Urology
University of Iowa Hospitals and Clinics
Iowa City, Iowa

Douglas W. Strand, PhD
Assistant Professor
Department of Urology
University of Texas Southwestern Medical
    Center
Dallas, Texas

Li-Ming Su, MD
David A. Cofrin Professor of Urologic
    Oncology
Chairman, Department of Urology
University of Florida College of
    Medicine
Gainesville, Florida

**Chandru P. Sundaram, MD, FACS, FRCS
    Eng**
Dr. Norbert and Louise Welch Professor of
    Urology
Vice Chair (QI)
Director, Minimally Invasive Surgery and
    Residency Program
Department of Urology
Indiana University School of Medicine
Indianapolis, Indiana

Samir S. Taneja, MD
The James M. Neissa and Janet Riha Neissa
    Professor of Urologic Oncology
Professor of Urology and Radiology
Director, Division of Urologic
    Oncology
Department of Urology
New York University Langone Health
New York, New York

Nikki Tang, MD
Assistant Professor
Department of Dermatology
Johns Hopkins University
Baltimore, Maryland

Gregory E. Tasian, MD
Assistant Professor of Urology and
    Epidemiology
University of Pennsylvania Perelman
    School of Medicine
Attending Physician
Division of Urology
The Children's Hospital of Philadelphia
Philadelphia, Pennsylvania

**Kae Jack Tay, MBBS, MRCS (Ed), MMed
    (Surgery), MCI, FAMS (Urology)**
Consultant
Department of Urology
Singapore General Hospital
SingHealth Duke–National University of
    Singapore Academic Medical Center
Singapore

John C. Thomas, MD, FAAP, FACS
Professor of Urologic Surgery
Division of Pediatric Urology
Department of Urology
Monroe Carell Jr. Children's Hospital at
    Vanderbilt
Vanderbilt University Medical Center
Nashville, Tennessee

J. Brantley Thrasher, MD, FACS
Professor Emeritus of Urology
University of Kansas Medical Center
Kansas City, Kansas
Executive Director
American Board of Urology
Charlottesville, Virginia

Edouard J. Trabulsi, MD, FACS
Professor and Vice Chair
Department of Urology
Sidney Kimmel Cancer Center
Sidney Kimmel Medical College at
    Thomas Jefferson University
Philadelphia, Pennsylvania

Chad R. Tracy, MD
Professor of Urology and Radiology
Department of Urology
University of Iowa
Iowa City, Iowa

Paul J. Turek, MD
Director
The Turek Clinic
San Francisco, California

Mark D. Tyson, MD, MPH
Urologic Oncologist
Department of Urology
Mayo Clinic Arizona
Phoenix, Arizona

Robert G. Uzzo, MD, MBA, FACS
Professor and Chairman
Department of Surgery
G. Willing "Wing" Pepper Chair in Cancer
    Research
Adjunct Professor of Bioengineering
Temple University College of Engineering
Fox Chase Cancer Center–Temple
    University Health System
Lewis Katz School of Medicine
Temple University
Philadelphia, Pennsylvania

Brian A. VanderBrink, MD
Associate Professor
Division of Urology
Cincinnati Children's Hospital
Cincinnati, Ohio

Alex J. Vanni, MD
Associate Professor
Department of Urology
Lahey Hospital and Medical Center
Burlington, Massachusetts

David J. Vaughn, MD
Professor of Medicine
Division of Hematology/Oncology
Department of Medicine
Abramsom Cancer Center at the
    University of Pennsylvania
Philadelphia, Pennsylvania

Vijaya M. Vemulakonda, MD, JD
Associate Professor and Director of Research
Division of Urology
Department of Surgery
University of Colorado School of
    Medicine
Attending Pediatric Urologist
Children's Hospital Colorado
Aurora, Colorado

Manish A. Vira, MD
System Chief of Urologic Oncology
Northwell Health Cancer Institute
Smith Institute for Urology
Lake Success, New York
Associate Professor of Urology
Zucker School of Medicine at Hofstra/
    Northwell
Hempstead, New York

Ramón Virasoro, MD
Associate Professor
Department of Urology
Eastern Virginia Medical School
Norfolk, Virginia
Fellowship Co-Director
Department of Urology
Universidad Autonoma de Santo Domingo
Santo Domingo, Dominican Republic

Alvin C. Wee, MD
Assistant Professor of Surgery
Cleveland Clinic Lerner College of
    Medicine
Director, Kidney Transplant Program
Glickman Urological and Kidney Institute
Cleveland Clinic
Cleveland, Ohio

Elias Wehbi, MD, MSc, FRCSC
Assistant Professor
Department of Urology
University of California–Irvine
Children's Hospital of Orange County
Orange, California

Alan J. Wein, MD, PhD (Hon), FACS
Founders Professor and Emeritus Chief of
    Urology
Division of Urology
Director, Residency Program in Urology
Perelman School of Medicine at the
    University of Pennsylvania
Penn Medicine
Philadelphia, Pennsylvania

Dana A. Weiss, MD
Assistant Professor of Urology
    in Surgery
University of Pennsylvania
Attending Physician
Children's Hospital of Philadelphia
Philadelphia, Pennsylvania

Jeffrey P. Weiss, MD
Professor and Chair
Department of Urology
State University of New York Downstate
    Health Sciences University
Attending Surgeon
Veterans Affairs New York Harbor
    Healthcare System
Brooklyn, New York

Robert M. Weiss, MD
Donald Guthrie Professor of Surgery/
    Urology
Department of Urology
Yale University School of Medicine
New Haven, Connecticut

R. Charles Welliver, Jr., MD
Department of Urology
Albany Medical Center
Albany, New York

Hunter Wessells, MD, FACS
Professor and Nelson Chair
Department of Urology
Affiliate Member
Harborview Injury Prevention and
    Research Center
University of Washington School of
    Medicine
Seattle, Washington

Duncan T. Wilcox, MD, MBBS
Surgeon in Chief, Ponzio Family Chair of
    Pediatric Urology
Department of Pediatric Urology
Children's Hospital Colorado
Aurora, Colorado

J. Christian Winters, MD, FACS
H. Eustis Reily Professor and Chairman
Department of Urology
Louisiana State University Health New
    Orleans
New Orleans, Louisiana

Anton Wintner, MD
Instructor of Surgery
Harvard Medical School
Associate Residency Program Director
Department of Urology
Massachusetts General Hospital
Boston, Massachusetts

J. Stuart Wolf, Jr., MD
Professor and Associate Chair for Clinical
    Integration and Operations
Surgery and Perioperative Care
Dell Medical School of the University of
    Texas at Austin
Austin, Texas

Christopher E. Wolter, MD
Assistant Professor
Department of Urology
Mayo Clinic Arizona
Phoenix, Arizona

Dan Wood, PhD, MB BS, FRCS (Urol)
Consultant in Adolescent and
    Reconstructive Urology
University College London Hospitals
London, United Kingdom

Michael E. Woods, MD
Professor of Urology
Department of Urology
Loyola University Medical Center
Maywood, Illinois

Hailiu Yang, MD
Resident Physician
Department of Urology
Cooper University Hospital
Camden, New Jersey

Richard Nithiphaisal Yu, MD, PhD
Department of Urology
Assistant Professor of Surgery (Urology)
Boston Children's Hospital and Harvard
    Medical School
Boston, Massachusetts

Joseph Zabell, MD
Assistant Professor
Department of Urology
University of Minnesota
Minneapolis, Minnesota

Mark R. Zaontz, MD
Professor of Urology (Surgery)
Perelman School of Medicine
University of Pennsylvania
Division of Urology
Children's Hospital of Philadelphia
Philadelphia, Pennsylvania

Rebecca S. Zee, MD, PhD
Assistant Professor
Division of Urology
Children's Hospital of Richmond
Virginia Commonwealth University
Richmond, Virginia

HOW TO USE THIS STUDY GUIDE

This study guide is designed to provide the reader with a comprehensive review of urology based on the text *Campbell-Walsh-Wein Urology*, twelfth edition. Each chapter includes a series of questions and possible answers, explanations for each answer, and a collection of chapter review points. Within the answer explanations, text of particular importance has been indicated in blue. If the reader knows the blue text and the chapter review points, he or she will know the majority of important points for that particular chapter. Moreover, if the questions are understood and the emphasized points are remembered, then the reader will have a thorough understanding of the important aspects of each chapter.

It is important to note that some of the questions are not of the format used in standardized tests such as the Qualifying Examination of the American Board of Urology. The proper format for examination questions is a question that asks for the one best possible answer out of five. While many questions in this review guide are in this format, some additional formats are used for teaching purposes. For example, "all of the following are true except" allows the author to provide the reader with four true statements regarding the question, and "more than one answer may be correct" also allows the author to make several points. Both formats serve to broaden the reader's knowledge.

We hope that this study guide will be helpful to both the resident or fellow in training and the practicing clinician in refreshing knowledge as well as in preparing for a urology examination.

Alan J. Wein, MD, PhD (Hon), FACS
Founders Professor and Emeritus Chief of Urology
Division of Urology
Director, Residency Program in Urology
Perelman School of Medicine at the University of Pennsylvania
Penn Medicine
Philadelphia, Pennsylvania

Thomas F. Kolon, MD, FAAP
Howard M. Snyder III MD Chair in Pediatric Urology
Pediatric Urology Fellowship Program Director
Children's Hospital of Philadelphia
Professor of Urology in Surgery
Perelman School of Medicine at the University of Pennsylvania
Philadelphia, Pennsylvania

CONTENTS

1   Evaluation of the Urologic Patient: History and Physical Examination

Sammy E. Elsamra

QUESTIONS

1. Pain associated with a stone in the ureter is the result of:
   a. obstruction of urine flow with distention of the renal capsule.
   b. irritation of the ureteral mucosa by the stone.
   c. excessive ureteral peristalsis in response to the obstructing stone.
   d. irritation of the intramural ureter.
   e. urinary extravasation from a ruptured calyceal fornix.

2. The most common cause of gross hematuria in a patient older than 50 years is:
   a. renal calculi.
   b. infection.
   c. bladder cancer.
   d. benign prostatic hyperplasia.
   e. trauma.

3. The most common cause of pain associated with gross hematuria is:
   a. simultaneous passage of a kidney stone.
   b. ureteral obstruction due to blood clots.
   c. urinary tract malignancy.
   d. prostatic inflammation.
   e. prostatic enlargement.

4. All of the following are typical lower urinary tract symptoms associated with benign prostatic hyperplasia EXCEPT:
   a. urgency.
   b. frequency.
   c. nocturia.
   d. dysuria.
   e. weak urinary stream.

5. The most likely cause of continuous incontinence (loss of urine at all times and in all positions) is:
   a. enterovesical fistula.
   b. noncompliant bladder.
   c. detrusor hyperreflexia.
   d. vesicovaginal fistula.
   e. sphincteric incompetence.

6. All of the following are potential causes of anejaculation EXCEPT:
   a. sympathetic denervation.
   b. pharmacologic agents.
   c. bladder neck and prostatic surgery.
   d. androgen deficiency.
   e. cerebrovascular accidents.

7. What percentage of patients with multiple sclerosis will present with urinary symptoms as the first manifestation of the disease?
   a. 1%
   b. 5%
   c. 10%
   d. 15%
   e. 20%

8. What important information is gained from pelvic bimanual examination that cannot be obtained from radiologic evaluation?
   a. Presence of bladder mass
   b. Invasion of bladder cancer into perivesical fat
   c. Presence of bladder calculi
   d. Presence of associated pathologic lesion in female adnexal structures
   e. Mobility/fixation of pelvic organs

9. With which of the following diseases is priapism most commonly associated?
   a. Peyronie disease
   b. Sickle cell anemia
   c. Parkinson disease
   d. Organic depression
   e. Leukemia

10. What is the most common cause of cloudy urine?
    a. Bacterial cystitis
    b. Urine overgrowth with yeast
    c. Phosphaturia
    d. Alkaline urine
    e. Significant proteinuria

11. Conditions that decrease urine specific gravity include all of the following EXCEPT:
    a. increased fluid intake.
    b. use of diuretics.
    c. decreased renal concentrating ability.
    d. dehydration.
    e. diabetes insipidus.

12. Urine osmolality usually varies between:
    a. 10 and 200 mOsm/L.
    b. 50 and 500 mOsm/L.
    c. 50 and 1200 mOsm/L.
    d. 100 and 1000 mOsm/L.
    e. 100 and 1500 mOsm/L.

13. Elevated ascorbic acid levels in the urine may lead to false-negative results on a urine dipstick test for:
    a. glucose.
    b. hemoglobin.
    c. myoglobin.
    d. red blood cells.
    e. leukocytes.

14. Hematuria is distinguished from hemoglobinuria or myoglobinuria by:
    a. dipstick testing.
    b. the simultaneous presence of significant leukocytes.
    c. microscopic presence of erythrocytes.
    d. examination of serum.
    e. evaluation of hematocrit.

15. The presence of one positive dipstick reading for hematuria is associated with significant urologic pathologic findings on subsequent testing in what percentage of patients?
    a. 2%
    b. 10%
    c. 25%
    d. 50%
    e. 75%

16. The most common cause of glomerular hematuria is:
    a. transitional cell carcinoma.
    b. nephritic syndrome.
    c. Berger disease (immunoglobulin A nephropathy).
    d. poststreptococcal glomerulonephritis.
    e. Goodpasture syndrome.

17. The most common cause of proteinuria is:
    a. Fanconi syndrome.
    b. excessive glomerular permeability due to primary glomerular disease.
    c. failure of adequate tubular reabsorption.
    d. overflow proteinuria due to increased plasma concentration of immunoglobulins.
    e. diabetes.

18. Transient proteinuria may be due to all of the following EXCEPT:
    a. exercise.
    b. fever.
    c. emotional stress.
    d. congestive heart failure (CHF).
    e. ureteroscopy.

19. Glucose will be detected in the urine when the serum level is above:
    a. 75 mg/dL.
    b. 100 mg/dL.
    c. 150 mg/dL.
    d. 180 mg/dL.
    e. 225 mg/dL.

20. The specificity of dipstick nitrite testing for bacteriuria is:
    a. 20%.
    b. 40%.
    c. 60%.
    d. 80%.
    e. >90%.

21. All of the following are microscopic features of squamous epithelial cells EXCEPT:
    a. large size.
    b. small central nucleus.
    c. irregular cytoplasm.
    d. presence in clumps.
    e. fine granularity in the cytoplasm.

22. The number of bacteria per high-power microscopic field that corresponds to colony counts of 100,000/mL is:
    a. 1.
    b. 3.
    c. 5.
    d. 10.
    e. 20.

23. Pain in the flaccid penis is usually due to:
    a. Peyronie disease.
    b. bladder or urethral inflammation.
    c. priapism.
    d. calculi impacted in the distal ureter.
    e. hydrocele.

24. Chronic scrotal pain is most often due to:
    a. testicular torsion.
    b. trauma.
    c. cryptorchidism.
    d. hydrocele.
    e. orchitis.

25. Terminal hematuria (at the end of the urinary stream) is usually due to:
    a. bladder neck or prostatic inflammation.
    b. bladder cancer.
    c. kidney stones.
    d. bladder calculi.
    e. urethral stricture disease.

26. Enuresis is present in what percentage of children at age 5 years?
    a. 5%
    b. 15%
    c. 25%
    d. 50%
    e. 75%

27. All of the following in the medical history suggest that erectile dysfunction is more likely due to organic rather than psychogenic causes EXCEPT:
    a. sudden onset.
    b. peripheral vascular disease.
    c. absence of nocturnal erections.
    d. diabetes mellitus.
    e. inability to achieve adequate erections in a variety of circumstances.

28. All of the following should be routinely performed in men with hematospermia EXCEPT:
    a. cystoscopy.
    b. digital rectal examination.
    c. serum prostate-specific antigen (PSA) level.
    d. genital examination.
    e. urinalysis.

29. Pneumaturia may be due to all of the following EXCEPT:
    a. diverticulitis.
    b. colon cancer.
    c. recent urinary tract instrumentation.
    d. inflammatory bowel disease.
    e. ectopic ureter.

30. Which of the following disorders may commonly lead to irritative voiding symptoms?
    a. Parkinson disease
    b. Renal cell carcinoma
    c. Bladder diverticula
    d. Prostate cancer
    e. Testicular torsion

ANSWERS

1. **a. Obstruction of urine flow with distention of the renal capsule.** Pain is usually caused by acute distention of the renal capsule, usually from inflammation or obstruction.
2. **c. Bladder cancer.** The most common cause of gross hematuria in a patient older than age 50 is bladder cancer.
3. **b. Ureteral obstruction due to blood clots.** Pain in association with hematuria usually results from upper urinary tract hematuria with obstruction of the ureters with clots.
4. **d. Dysuria.** Dysuria is painful urination that is usually caused by inflammation.
5. **d. Vesicovaginal fistula.** Continuous incontinence is most commonly due to a urinary tract fistula that bypasses the urethral sphincter or an ectopic ureter.
6. **e. Cerebrovascular accidents.** Anejaculation may result from several causes: (1) androgen deficiency, (2) sympathetic denervation, (3) pharmacologic agents, and (4) bladder neck and prostatic surgery.
7. **b. 5%.** In fact, 5% of patients with previously undiagnosed multiple sclerosis present with urinary symptoms as the first manifestation of the disease.
8. **e. Mobility/fixation of pelvic organs.** In addition to defining areas of induration, the bimanual examination allows the examiner to assess the mobility of the bladder; such information cannot be obtained by radiologic techniques such as computed tomography (CT) and magnetic resonance imaging (MRI), which convey static images.
9. **b. Sickle cell anemia.** Priapism occurs most commonly in patients with sickle cell disease but can also occur in those with advanced malignancy, coagulation disorders, and pulmonary disease, as well as in many patients without an obvious cause.
10. **c. Phosphaturia.** Cloudy urine is most commonly caused by phosphates in the urine.
11. **d. Dehydration.** Conditions that decrease specific gravity include (1) increased fluid intake, (2) diuretics, (3) decreased renal concentrating ability, and (4) diabetes insipidus.
12. **c. 50 and 1200 mOsm/L.** Osmolality is a measure of the amount of solutes dissolved in the urine and usually varies between 50 and 1200 mOsm/L.
13. a. **Glucose.** False-negative results for glucose and bilirubin may be seen in the presence of elevated ascorbic acid concentrations in the urine.
14. **c. Microscopic presence of erythrocytes.** Hematuria can be distinguished from hemoglobinuria and myoglobinuria by microscopic examination of the centrifuged urine; the presence of a large number of erythrocytes establishes the diagnosis of hematuria.

15. **c. 25%.** Investigators at the University of Wisconsin found that 26% of adults who had at least one positive dipstick reading for hematuria were subsequently found to have significant urologic pathologic findings.
16. **c. Berger disease (immunoglobulin A nephropathy).** IgA nephropathy, or Berger disease, is the most common cause of glomerular hematuria, accounting for about 30% of cases.
17. b. **Excessive glomerular permeability due to primary glomerular disease.** Glomerular proteinuria is the most common type of proteinuria and results from increased glomerular capillary permeability to protein, especially albumin. Glomerular proteinuria occurs in any of the primary glomerular diseases such as IgA nephropathy or in glomerulopathy associated with systemic illness such as diabetes mellitus.
18. **e. Ureteroscopy.** Transient proteinuria occurs commonly, especially in the pediatric population, and usually resolves spontaneously within a few days. It may result from fever, exercise, or emotional stress. In older patients, transient proteinuria may be due to CHF.
19. **d. 180 mg/dL.** This so-called renal threshold corresponds to a serum glucose level of about 180 mg/dL; above this level, glucose will be detected in the urine.
20. **e. >90%.** The specificity of the nitrite dipstick test for detecting bacteriuria is greater than 90%.
21. **d. Presence in clumps.** Squamous epithelial cells are large, have a central small nucleus about the size of an erythrocyte, and have an irregular cytoplasm with fine granularity.
22. **c. 5.** Therefore five bacteria per high-power field in a spun specimen reflect colony counts of about 100,000/mL.
23. **b. Bladder or urethral inflammation.** Pain in the flaccid penis is usually secondary to inflammation in the bladder or urethra, with referred pain that is experienced maximally at the urethral meatus.
24. **d. Hydrocele.** Chronic scrotal pain is usually related to noninflammatory conditions such as a hydrocele or varicocele, and the pain is usually characterized as a dull, heavy sensation that does not radiate.
25. **a. Bladder neck or prostatic inflammation.** Terminal hematuria occurs at the end of micturition and is usually secondary to inflammation in the area of the bladder neck or prostatic urethra.
26. **b. 15%.** Enuresis refers to urinary incontinence that occurs during sleep. It occurs normally in children as old as 3 years but persists in about 15% of children at age 5 and about 1% of children at age 15.
27. **a. Sudden onset.** A careful history will often determine whether the problem is primarily psychogenic or organic. In men with psychogenic impotence, the condition frequently develops rather quickly, secondary to a precipitating event such as marital stress or change or loss of a sexual partner.
28. **a. Cystoscopy.** A genital and rectal examination should be done to exclude the presence of tuberculosis, a PSA assessment and digital rectal examination should be done to exclude prostatic carcinoma, and a urinary cytologic assessment should be done to exclude the possibility of transitional cell carcinoma of the prostate.
29. **e. Ectopic ureter.** Pneumaturia is the passage of gas in the urine. In patients who have not recently had urinary tract instrumentation or a urethral catheter placed, this is almost always due to a fistula between the intestine and bladder. Common causes include diverticulitis, carcinoma of the sigmoid colon, and regional enteritis (Crohn disease).
30. **a. Parkinson disease.** The second important example of nonspecific lower urinary tract symptoms that may occur secondary to a variety of neurologic conditions is irritative symptoms resulting from neurologic disease such as cerebrovascular accident, diabetes mellitus, or Parkinson disease.

CHAPTER REVIEW

1. IPSS score: 0 to 7 mild symptoms, 8 to 19 moderate symptoms, 20 to 35 severe symptoms.
2. Renal pain radiates from the flank anteriorly to the respective lower quadrant and may be referred to the testis, labium, or medial aspect of the thigh. The pain is colicky (fluctuates). It may be associated with gastrointestinal symptoms due to reflex stimulation of the celiac ganglion.
3. Patients with slowly progressive urinary obstruction with bladder distention often have no pain, despite residual volumes in excess of a liter.
4. Pain of prostatic origin is poorly localized.
5. Scrotal pain may be primary or referred. Pain referred to the testicle originates in the retroperitoneum, ureter, or kidney.
6. Hematuria, particularly in adults, should be regarded as a symptom of malignancy until proven otherwise.
7. Adults normally arise no more than twice a night to void. Urine production increases at night (recumbent position) in older patients and those with cardiac disease, particularly CHF.
8. Postvoid dribbling: Urine escapes into the bulbar urethra and then leaks at the end of micturition. This may be alleviated by perineal pressure following voiding.
9. Those who present with microscopic hematuria and irritative voiding symptoms should be suspected of having carcinoma in situ of the bladder until proven otherwise.
10. Continuous incontinence is most commonly due to ectopic ureter, urinary tract fistula, or totally incompetent sphincter.
11. Hematospermia almost always resolves spontaneously and is rarely associated with any significant urologic pathology.
12. When urinary obstruction is associated with fever and chills, it should be regarded as a urologic emergency.
13. It is always worthwhile to obtain the previous operative report in patients who are to be operated on.
14. If the patient is uncircumcised, the foreskin must be retracted for inspection of the glans.
15. The testes are normally 6 cm in length and 4 cm in width.
16. If one obtains a stool guaiac test (hemoccult) as a screen for colon cancer, two subsequent stool specimens must be obtained for an adequate test. If the hemoccult is positive, the patient should be on a red meat–free diet for 3 days before collection of three specimens.
17. A male urologist should always perform a female pelvic examination with a female nurse in attendance.
18. The bulbocavernosus reflex tests the integrity of this spinal cord reflex involving S2 to S4.
19. A positive dipstick for blood in the urine indicates hematuria, hemoglobinuria, or myoglobinuria. Hematuria is distinguished from hemoglobinuria and myoglobinuria by microscopic examination of the centrifuged urine and identification of red blood cells (more than three red blood cells per high-power field is abnormal).
20. Hematuria of nephrologic origin is frequently associated with proteinuria and dysmorphic erythrocytes.
21. Anticoagulation at normal therapeutic levels does not predispose patients to hematuria.
22. The most accurate method to diagnose urinary tract infection is by microscopic examination of the urine and identifying pyuria and bacteria. This is confirmed by urine culture.
23. The chief complaint is the focus of the visit and is the reason the patient seeks consultation. It should be the lead sentence in the history and physical (H&P).
24. A family history should always include questions about renal and prostate cancer, renal cysts, and stone disease.
25. Priapism occurs most commonly in patients with sickle cell disease but can also occur in those with advanced malignancy, coagulation disorders, or pulmonary disease, as well as in many patients without an obvious cause.
26. On urine dipstick, false-negative results for glucose and bilirubin may be seen in the presence of elevated ascorbic acid concentrations in the urine.
27. Glomerular proteinuria is the most common type of proteinuria and results from increased glomerular capillary permeability to protein, especially albumin. Glomerular proteinuria occurs in any of the primary glomerular diseases such as IgA nephropathy or in glomerulopathy associated with systemic illness such as diabetes mellitus.
28. Five bacteria per high-power field in a spun specimen reflect colony counts of about 100,000/mL.
29. An important example of nonspecific lower urinary tract symptoms that may occur secondary to a variety of neurologic conditions is irritative symptoms resulting from neurologic disease such as cerebrovascular accident, diabetes mellitus, and Parkinson disease.
30. The renal threshold for glucose corresponds to a serum glucose level of about 180 mg/dL; above this level, glucose will be detected in the urine.

2 Evaluation of the Urologic Patient: Testing and Imaging

Erik P. Castle, Christopher E. Wolter, and Michael Woods

QUESTIONS

1. What is the most common cause of cloudy urine?
   a. Bacterial cystitis
   b. Urine overgrowth with yeast
   c. Phosphaturia
   d. Alkaline urine
   e. Significant proteinuria

2. Conditions that decrease urine specific gravity include all of the following EXCEPT:
   a. increased fluid intake.
   b. use of diuretics.
   c. decreased renal concentrating ability.
   d. dehydration.
   e. diabetes insipidus.

3. Urine osmolality usually varies between:
   a. 10 and 200 mOsm/L.
   b. 50 and 500 mOsm/L.
   c. 50 and 1200 mOsm/L.
   d. 100 and 1000 mOsm/L.
   e. 100 and 1500 mOsm/L.

4. Elevated ascorbic acid levels in the urine may lead to false-negative results on a urine dipstick test for:
   a. glucose.
   b. hemoglobin.
   c. myoglobin.
   d. red blood cells.
   e. leukocytes.

5. Hematuria is distinguished from hemoglobinuria or myoglobinuria by:
   a. dipstick testing.
   b. the simultaneous presence of significant leukocytes.
   c. microscopic presence of erythrocytes.
   d. examination of serum.
   e. evaluation of hematocrit.

6. The presence of one positive dipstick reading for hematuria is associated with significant urologic pathologic findings on subsequent testing in what percentage of patients?
   a. 2%
   b. 10%
   c. 25%
   d. 50%
   e. 75%

7. The most common cause of glomerular hematuria is:
   a. transitional cell carcinoma.
   b. nephritic syndrome.

   c. Berger disease (immunoglobulin A nephropathy).
   d. poststreptococcal glomerulonephritis.
   e. Goodpasture syndrome.

8. The most common cause of proteinuria is:
   a. Fanconi syndrome.
   b. excessive glomerular permeability due to primary glomerular disease.
   c. failure of adequate tubular reabsorption.
   d. overflow proteinuria due to increased plasma concentration of immunoglobulins.
   e. diabetes.

9. Transient proteinuria may be due to all of the following EXCEPT:
   a. exercise.
   b. fever.
   c. emotional stress.
   d. congestive heart failure.
   e. ureteroscopy.

10. Glucose will be detected in the urine when the serum level is above:
    a. 75 mg/dL.
    b. 100 mg/dL.
    c. 150 mg/dL.
    d. 180 mg/dL.
    e. 225 mg/dL.

11. The specificity of dipstick nitrite testing for bacteriuria is:
    a. 20%.
    b. 40%.
    c. 60%.
    d. 80%.
    e. >90%.

12. All of the following are microscopic features of squamous epithelial cells EXCEPT:
    a. large size.
    b. small central nucleus.
    c. irregular cytoplasm.
    d. presence in clumps.
    e. fine granularity in the cytoplasm.

13. The number of bacteria per high-power microscopic field that corresponds to colony counts of 100,000/mL is:
    a. 1.
    b. 3.
    c. 5.
    d. 10.
    e. 20.

14. All of following is true of uroflowmetry EXCEPT:
    a. Qmax >20 mL/s is not consistent with obstruction.
    b. Qmax, mean flow rate, and voided volume are parameters obtained from this study.
    c. 80 mL voided volume is adequate for uroflowmetry.
    d. the study can be performed in sitting and standing positions.
    e. uroflowmetry cannot diagnose the location of obstruction.

15. The following should be given to uncomplicated patients undergoing simple flexible diagnostic cystourethroscopy:
    a. single-dose oral antibiotic following procedure
    b. 3 days of oral antibiotics following procedure
    c. 3 days of oral antibiotics starting the day prior to procedure
    d. nothing
    e. single intramuscular injection of ceftriaxone following procedure

16. What is the most appropriate initial workup for asymptomatic microscopic hematuria (AMH)?
    a. Flexible cystoscopy, urinary cytology, CT urogram, and UroVysion FISH
    b. Flexible cystoscopy and CT urogram
    c. CT urogram and NMP22
    d. Flexible cystoscopy, urinary cytology, and CT urogram
    e. Flexible cystoscopy, renal ultrasound, and urinary cytology

ANSWERS

1. **c. Phosphaturia.** Cloudy urine is most commonly caused by phosphates in the urine.
2. **d. Dehydration.** Conditions that decrease specific gravity include (1) increased fluid intake, (2) diuretics, (3) decreased renal concentrating ability, and (4) diabetes insipidus.
3. **c. 50 and 1200 mOsm/L.** Osmolality is a measure of the amount of solutes dissolved in the urine and usually varies between 50 and 1200 mOsm/L.
4. **a. Glucose.** False-negative results for glucose and bilirubin may be seen in the presence of elevated ascorbic acid concentrations in the urine.
5. **c. Microscopic presence of erythrocytes.** Hematuria can be distinguished from hemoglobinuria and myoglobinuria by microscopic examination of the centrifuged urine; the presence of a large number of erythrocytes establishes the diagnosis of hematuria.
6. **c. 25%.** Investigators at the University of Wisconsin found that 26% of adults who had at least one positive dipstick reading for hematuria were subsequently found to have significant urologic pathologic findings.
7. **c. Berger disease (immunoglobulin A nephropathy).** IgA nephropathy, or Berger disease, is the most common cause of glomerular hematuria, accounting for about 30% of cases.
8. **b. Excessive glomerular permeability due to primary glomerular disease.** Glomerular proteinuria is the most common type of proteinuria and results from increased glomerular capillary permeability to protein, especially albumin. Glomerular proteinuria occurs in any of the primary glomerular diseases such as IgA nephropathy or in glomerulopathy associated with systemic illness such as diabetes mellitus.
9. **e. Ureteroscopy.** Transient proteinuria occurs commonly, especially in the pediatric population, and usually resolves spontaneously within a few days. It may result from fever, exercise, or emotional stress. In older patients, transient proteinuria may be due to congestive heart failure.
10. **d. 180 mg/dL.** This so-called renal threshold corresponds to a serum glucose level of about 180 mg/dL; above this level, glucose will be detected in the urine.
11. **e. >90%.** The specificity of the nitrite dipstick test for detecting bacteriuria is greater than 90%.
12. **d. Presence in clumps.** Squamous epithelial cells are large, have a central small nucleus about the size of an erythrocyte, and have an irregular cytoplasm with fine granularity.
13. **c. 5.** Therefore 5 bacteria per high-power field in a spun specimen reflect colony counts of about 100,000/mL.
14. **c. 80 mL voided volume is adequate for uroflowmetry.** The minimum voided volume that is accepted as a requirement for considering an adequate assessment is at least 100 mL.
15. **d. Nothing.** For patients undergoing simple diagnostic flexible cystoscopy no antibiotic prophylaxis is recommended unless there are extenuating risk factors for infection or recent orthopedic implantation of artificial joints. Refer to American Urological Association (AUA) recommendations on antibiotic prophylaxis for urological procedures.
16. **b. Flexible cystoscopy and CT urogram.** For the initial workup of AMH, routine urine cytology is not necessary. Cytology is generally utilized in patients with a history of bladder cancer undergoing surveillance or the index of suspicion of a high-grade lesion is present.

CHAPTER REVIEW

1. A catheterized urine specimen should be obtained in the female patient with a history of recurrent urinary tract infections or suspected contaminated specimen.
2. Hematuria should be stratified into glomerular, nonglomerular, medical, and surgical causes.
3. A dipstick alone is inadequate for the diagnosis of microscopic hematuria.
4. Asymptomatic microscopic hematuria is defined as three or greater RBC/HPF on a properly collected urinary specimen in the absence of an obvious benign cause.
5. Urine dipstick positive for only leukocyte esterase or nitrites but not both should be confirmed with microscopic analysis and urine culture.
6. Serum creatinine and glomerular filtration rate should be ordered when renal obstruction of nephrologic disease is suspected.
7. Prostate-specific antigen is a very sensitive test for prostate conditions such as BPH and prostatitis and correlates most often with prostate volume.
8. Urine cytology is not recommended during the initial evaluation and screening for asymptomatic microscopic hematuria.
9. Urine cytology is very specific for high-grade urothelial carcinoma.
10. Uroflowmetry and assessment of postvoid residual should be ordered when lower urinary tract obstruction is suspected.
11. Urodynamic studies provide information on disorders of storage and voiding.
12. Routine use of antimicrobial prophylaxis is not recommended for office cystourethroscopy, urodynamics, or cystography in the patient without risk factors.
13. Renal ultrasonography can provide basic screening information on the presence of hydronephrosis and medical renal disease but is not an adequate stand-alone study for the workup of hematuria.
14. CT without contrast of the abdomen and pelvis is the gold standard for detecting urinary stones.
15. A KUB is a useful and easy test for the follow-up of existing non-emergent radio opaque urinary stones.

3

Urinary Tract Imaging: Basic Principles of CT, MRI, and Plain Film Imaging

Jay T. Bishoff and Ardeshir R. Rastinehad

QUESTIONS

1. The measure of the potential adverse health effects of ionizing radiation in sieverts (Sv) is known as:
   a. radiation exposure.
   b. absorbed dose.
   c. equivalent dose.
   d. effective dose.
   e. relative radiation levels.

2. The relative radiation level associated with abdominal computed tomography (CT) without and with contrast is:
   a. none.
   b. minimal, less than 0.1 mSv.
   c. low, 0.1 to 1.0 mSv.
   d. moderate, 1 to 10 mSv.
   e. high, 10 to 100 mSv.

3. Bladder filling may precipitate autonomic dysreflexia in patients with a spinal cord injury above:
   a. S2.
   b. L4.
   c. T10.
   d. T12.
   e. T6.

4. Radiation exposure diminishes as the square of the distance from the radiation source. An exposure of 9 mSv at 1 foot from the source would be how much at 3 feet from the source?
   a. 0.09 mSv
   b. 1 mSv
   c. 3 mSv
   d. 9 mSv
   e. 27 mSv

5. Type 2 diabetics on oral metformin biguanide hyperglycemic therapy are at risk for biguanide lactic acidosis after exposure to intravascular radiologic contrast media if they:
   a. discontinue metformin 48 hours before the study.
   b. have severe renal insufficiency and take metformin the day of the study.
   c. are given a saline injection while taking metformin.
   d. have normal kidney function and fail to stop metformin 48 hours before the study.
   e. decrease metformin dose and increase other antihyperglycemic agents on the day of the study.

6. All of the following are true EXCEPT:
   a. Patients with a history of asthma are at greater risk of having an adverse reaction to contrast media.
   b. Severe allergic reactions are not dose dependent.
   c. Hyperosmolar contrast media are more likely to cause contrast reactions than are iso-osmolar agents.
   d. The mechanism of action associated with severe idiosyncratic anaphylactoid (IA) reactions is an immunoglobulin E (IgE) antibody reaction to the contrast media.
   e. Severe cardiac disease is a risk factor for an adverse reaction to contrast media.

7. After rapidly assessing airway, breathing, and circulation, the medical treatment of choice for a severe, life-threatening adverse drug reaction following exposure to contrast media is:
   a. subcutaneous injection of epinephrine 0.5 mg of 1:10,000 epinephrine.
   b. intravenous injection of 100 mg of methylprednisone.
   c. 0.01 mg/kg of epinephrine (1:10,000 concentration), given intramuscularly in the lateral thigh.
   d. intravenous diphenhydramine, 50 mg.
   e. 0.01 mg/kg of epinephrine (1:1000 concentration), given intramuscularly in the lateral thigh.

8. Which of the following is NOT a risk factor for developing contrast-induced nephropathy (CIN)?
   a. Type 2 diabetes mellitus
   b. Dehydration
   c. Hypertension
   d. Ventricular ejection fraction less than 50%
   e. Chronic kidney disease (CKD) (glomerular filtration rate [GFR] < 60 mL/min)

9. Nephrogenic systemic fibrosis (NSF) is:
   a. a rare genetic condition exacerbated by the use of gadolinium-based contrast medium (GBCM).
   b. immediately evident after exposure to gadolinium in 10% of exposed patients.
   c. fibrosis of the skin, subcutaneous tissue, and skeletal muscle seen in patients with chronic hypertension exposed to gadolinium contrast medium.
   d. not seen in patients with GFR greater than 60 mL/min/1.73 m^2.
   e. mainly seen in dialysis patients exposed to gadolinium contrast medium.

10. During a diuretic renal scintigraphy:
   a. the diuretic is administered approximately 2 minutes after peak activity is seen in the collecting system.
   b. a $T_{1/2}$ of greater than 14 minutes is consistent with obstruction.
   c. ^{99m}Tc-DMSA is the most sensitive for obstruction and determination of GFR.

   d. intestinal or gallbladder activity should never be seen with ^{99m}Tc-MAG3.

   e. a $T_{1/2}$ of less than 10 minutes is consistent with a nonobstructed system.

11. Positron emission tomography (PET):

   a. has a higher diagnostic accuracy than CT for seminoma and nonseminoma testis cancer following chemotherapy.

   b. is sensitive and specific for detection of postchemotherapy teratoma.

   c. can be used with high positive predictive value within 2 weeks of completion of chemotherapy for bulky lymph adenopathy.

   d. has greater predictive value of primary disease in metastatic urothelial carcinoma than magnetic resonance imaging (MRI).

   e. is able to detect local or systemic recurrence of prostate cancer in 74% of patients with prostate-specific antigen recurrence.

12. What is the minimum estimated GFR for use of gadolinium-based contrast agents?

   a. Less than 30 mL/min/1.73 m^2

   b. Greater than 50 mL/min/1.73 m^2

   c. Greater than 35 mL/min/1.73 m^2

   d. Greater than 30 mL/min/1.73 m^2

   e. There are no restrictions for patients with renal insufficiency.

13. In magnetic resonance (MR) images using T2-weighted sequences, fluid appears as:

   a. dark.

   b. bright.

   c. low signal.

   d. signal void.

   e. indeterminate.

14. What lesions may have a high signal (bright) on T2-weighted MRI of the adrenal gland?

   a. Pheochromocytoma

   b. Metastasis

   c. Adrenal cortical carcinoma (ACC)

   d. None of the above

   e. All of the above

15. MR chemical shift imaging (CSI) for adrenal adenoma takes advantage of which of the following phenomena to aid in the diagnosis?

   a. Water and fat within the same voxel signals are canceled out in opposed-phase imaging.

   b. Opposed-phase imaging will exhibit a high signal (bright).

   c. Intracellular lipid content within an adenoma is low.

   d. Intravenous contrast is required.

   e. All of the above.

16. Oncocytoma typically has been characterized by a central scar. Which other renal lesion may also exhibit a central scar on T2-weighted images?

   a. Clear cell carcinoma

   b. Angiomyolipoma

   c. Chromophobe carcinoma

   d. Transitional cell carcinoma

   e. No other renal masses exhibit a central scar.

17. Which renal mass exhibits signal drop on opposed phase imaging?

   a. Papillary renal cell

   b. Chromophobe carcinoma

   c. Angiomyolipoma

   d. Clear cell carcinoma

   e. Transitional cell carcinoma

18. What signal characteristics do kidney stones exhibit on MR urography?

   a. High signal on T2-weighted images

   b. Low signal on T2-weighted images

   c. Signal void

   d. High signal on T1-weighted images

   e. Low signal on T1-weighted images

19. Multiparametric imaging of the prostate consists of anatomic and functional sequences. Match the correct pair.

   a. Anatomic: Diffusion-weighted imaging

   b. Functional: T1- and T2-weighted images

   c. Anatomic: Dynamic contrast enhanced sequences

   d. Functional: Apparent diffusion coefficient maps

   e. All of the above

ANSWERS

1. **d. Effective dose.** The distribution of energy absorption in the human body will be different based on the body part being imaged and a variety of other factors. The most important risk of radiation exposure from diagnostic imaging is the development of cancer. The effective dose is a quantity used to denote the radiation risk (expressed in sieverts) to a population of patients from an imaging study.

2. **e. High, 10 to 100 mSv.** The average person living in the United States is exposed to 6.2 mSv of radiation per year from ambient sources, such as radon, cosmic rays, and medical procedures, which account for 36% of the annual radiation exposure (NCRP, 2012). The recommended occupational exposure limit to medical personnel is 50 mSv per year (NCRP, 2012). The effective dose from a three-phase CT of the abdomen and pelvis without and with contrast may be as high as 25 to 40 mSv.

3. **e. T6.** Autonomic dysreflexia, also known as hyperreflexia, means an overactivity of the autonomic nervous system that can result in an abrupt onset of excessively high blood pressure. Persons at risk for this problem generally have spinal cord injury level above T6. Autonomic dysreflexia can develop suddenly, is potentially life threatening, and is considered a medical emergency. If not treated promptly and correctly, it may lead to seizures, stroke, and even death.

4. **b. 1 mSv.** Maintaining the maximum practical distance from an active radiation source significantly decreases exposure to medical personnel.

5. **b. Have severe renal insufficiency and take metformin the day of the study.** Patients with type 2 diabetes mellitus on metformin may have an accumulation of the drug after administering intravascular radiologic contrast medium (IRCM), resulting in biguanide lactic acidosis presenting with vomiting, diarrhea, and somnolence. This condition is fatal in approximately 50% of cases (Wiholm, 1993).[a]

---

[a] Sources referenced can be found in *Campbell-Walsh-Wein Urology, 12th Edition*, on the Expert Consult website.

Biguanide lactic acidosis is rare in patients with normal renal function. Consequently in patients with normal renal function and no known comorbidities, there is no need to discontinue metformin before IRCM use, nor is there a need to check creatinine following the imaging study.

6. **d. The mechanism of action associated with severe idiosyncratic anaphylactoid (IA) reactions is an immunoglobulin E (IgE) antibody reaction to the contrast media.** The IA reactions are most concerning because they are potentially fatal and can occur without any predictable or predisposing factors. Approximately 85% of IA reactions occur during or immediately after injection of IRCM and are more common in patients with a prior adverse drug reaction to contrast media; patients with asthma, diabetes, impaired renal function, or diminished cardiac function; and patients on beta-adrenergic blockers (Spring et al., 1997).

7. **e. 0.01 mg/kg of epinephrine (1:1000 concentration), given intramuscularly in the lateral thigh.** Rapid administration of epinephrine is the treatment of choice for severe contrast reactions. Epinephrine can be administered intravenously (IV) 0.01 mg/kg body weight of 1: 10,000 dilution or 0.1 mL/kg slowly into a running IV infusion of saline and can be repeated every 5 to 15 minutes as needed. If no IV access is available, the recommended intramuscular dose of epinephrine is 0.01 mg/kg of 1:1000 dilution (or 0.01 mL/kg to a maximum of 0.15 mg of 1:1000 if body weight is <30 kg; 0.3 mg if weight is >30 kg) injected intramuscularly in the lateral thigh.

8. **d. Ventricular ejection fraction less than 50%.** The most common patient-related risk factors for CIN are CKD (creatinine clearance <60 mL/min), diabetes mellitus, dehydration, diuretic use, advanced age, congestive heart failure, age, hypertension, low hematocrit, and ventricular ejection fraction less than 40%. The patients at highest risk for developing CIN are those with both diabetes and preexisting renal insufficiency.

9. **d. Not seen in patients with GFR greater than 60 mL/min/1.73 m².** Patients with CKD but GRF greater than 30 mL/min/1.73 m² are considered to be at extremely low or no risk for developing NSF if a dose of GBCM of 0.1 mmol/kg or less is used. Patients with GFR greater than 60 mL/min/1.73 m² do not appear to be at increased risk of developing NSF, and the current consensus is that all GBCM can be administered safely to these patients.

10. **e. a $T_{1/2}$ of less than 10 minutes is consistent with a nonobstructed system.** Transit time throughout the collecting system in less than 10 minutes is consistent with a normal, nonobstructed collecting system. A $T_{1/2}$ of 10 to 20 minutes shows mild to moderate delay and may be a mechanical obstruction. The patient's perception of pain after diuretic administration can be helpful for the treating urologist to consider when planning surgery in the patient with middle to moderate obstruction. A $T_{1/2}$ of greater than 20 minutes is consistent with a high-grade obstruction.

11. **a. Has a higher diagnostic accuracy than CT for seminoma and nonseminoma testis cancer following chemotherapy.** There are data on the use of PET/CT in testis cancer, where PET/CT was found to have a higher diagnostic accuracy than CT for staging and restaging in the assessment of a CT-visualized residual mass following chemotherapy for seminoma and nonseminomatous germ cell tumors (Hain et al., 2000; Albers et al., 1999).

12. **d. Greater than 30 mL/min/1.73 m².** NSF occurs in patients with acute or chronic renal insufficiency with a GFR less than 30 mL/min/1.73 m².

13. **b. Bright.** High signal on T2-weighted images. Fluid exhibits a low signal on T1-weighted images.

14. **e. All of the above.** Traditional teaching reported the lightbulb sign to be consistent with pheochromocytoma. However, metastasis and ACC also have a high signal on T2-weighted images. Furthermore, Varghese and colleagues reported that 35% of pheochromocytomas demonstrated low T2 signal, contrary to conventional teaching. Therefore the conventional teaching of the "lightbulb sign" is incorrect.

15. **a. Water and fat within the same voxel signals are canceled out in opposed-phase imaging.** MR CSI is performed on T1-weighted images. Opposed-phase imaging will demonstrate a low signal (dark) if fat and water occupy the same voxel. Adrenal adenomas have high intracytoplasmic fat. CSI is performed without the use of intravenous contrast.

16. **c. Chromophobe carcinoma.** Chromophobe carcinoma exhibits a high signal on T2-weighted images.

17. **d. Clear cell carcinoma.** Microscopic intracytoplasmic lipids have been found in 59% of clear cell carcinomas, which allows it to be differentiated from other renal cell carcinoma cell types.

18. **c. Signal void.** Nephrolithiasis/calcification on MR imaging has no signal characteristics; therefore it appears as a void on imaging.

19. **d. Functional: Apparent diffusion coefficient maps.** Multiparametric MRI refers to the use of anatomic sequences (T1-weighted images, T2 triplanar [axial, sagittal, and coronal] images) and functional sequences (diffusion-weighted imaging/apparent diffusion coefficient maps, dynamic contrast-enhanced MRI, spectroscopy). The combined approach has reported negative and positive predictive values to be greater than 90% in detecting prostate cancer.

CHAPTER REVIEW

1. Absorbed dose for therapy is measured in units called gray (Gy); 1 rad = 0.01 Gy, or 1 centigray (cGy) = 1 rad.
2. The amount of energy absorbed by a tissue for diagnostic purposes is referred to as the equivalent dose and is measured in sieverts (Sv). Exposure of the eyes and gonads to radiation has a more significant biologic impact than exposure of other parts of the body. The occupational safety limit is 50 mSv. Exposure time during fluoroscopy should be minimized by the use of short bursts of fluoroscopy; positioning the image intensifier as close to the patient as feasible substantially reduces scatter radiation.
3. There are four basic types of iodinated contrast media: (1) ionic monomer, (2) nonionic monomer, (3) ionic dimer, (4) nonionic dimer.
4. IA reactions are potentially fatal, are not dose dependent, and are more common in patients with a history of adverse reactions to contrast media, those with asthma or diabetes, those with impaired renal and cardiac function, and those on β-adrenergic blockers.
5. It is common to have nausea, flushing, pruritus, urticaria, headache, and occasionally emesis after administration of contrast media.
6. Patients at high risk for adverse allergic reactions should be medicated with steroids, given 12 to 24 hours before the injection of contrast media, as well as antihistamines.
7. For retrograde pyelography, it is useful to dilute contrast media by half with sterile saline, which facilitates identifying filling defects in the collecting system. There is a low

CHAPTER REVIEW—cont'd

risk of contrast reactions in patients in whom a retrograde or loopogram is performed.

8. Metformin does not need to be held before contrast administration in a patient with normal renal function and no comorbidities.

9. The risk of developing contrast-induced nephropathy is increased in patients with decreased renal function (GFR < 60 mL/min), diabetes mellitus, dehydration, advanced age, congestive heart failure, liver disease, and cardiac ejection fraction less than 40%.

10. TcDTPA is primarily filtered by the glomerulus. It is a good agent to assess renal function.

11. Because TcDMSA is both filtered by the glomerulus and secreted by the proximal tubule, it localizes in the renal cortex and is a good agent for assessing cortical scarring and ectopic renal tissue.

12. TcMAG3 is cleared mainly by tubular secretion; it has a limited ability to access renal function.

13. A $T_{1/2}$ less than 10 minutes suggests an unobstructed system. A $T_{1/2}$ greater than 20 minutes is consistent with renal obstruction.

14. A positive bone scan is not specific for cancer. Moreover, the volume of cancer cannot be quantitated on bone scan. Patients with widely metastatic disease may have diffuse uptake (hyper scan) and no discrete lesions.

15. Glucose, choline, and amino acids have been used as imaging agents for PET scans.

16. ^{18}F-fluorodeoxyglucose (FDG) is used as an imaging agent in PET scanning and takes advantage of the fact that tumors have increased glycolysis and decreased dephosphorylation. This scan is useful in testicular germ cell tumors, particularly seminomas, in determining residual viable tumor following chemotherapy.

17. The Hounsfield units scale assigns a value of −1000 Hounsfield units for air. Dense bone is assigned a value of +1000 Hounsfield units, and water is assigned 0 Hounsfield units.

18. With the exception of some indinavir stones, all renal and ureteral calculi may be detected by helical CT.

19. The advantage of MRI is high-contrast resolution of soft tissue on T1-weighted images. Fluid has a low signal and appears dark on T1-weighted images; on T2-weighted images, fluid has a high signal and appears bright. Gadolinium increases the brightness of T1-weighted images. Hemorrhage within a cyst results in a high signal on T1-weighted images. MRI is the imaging modality of choice for patients with iodine contrast allergies.

20. The risk of developing NSF after gadolinium administration is increased in patients with GFRs less than 30 mL/min.

21. Adrenal adenomas have high lipid content and may be differentiated from adrenal cancers or metastatic disease by specialized CT or MRI scans.

22. Thirty-five percent of pheochromocytomas do not enhance on T2-weighted images.

23. MRI and CT are excellent imaging studies to determine the presence and extent of renal vein and vena cava tumor thrombus. Uptake of gadolinium by the thrombus on MRI differentiates tumor from bland (blood clot) thrombus.

24. Prostate MRI coupled with an assessment of dynamic contrast uptake and washout increases the diagnostic accuracy for detecting cancer.

25. MR spectroscopy for prostate cancer is based on decreased citrate levels and increased creatine and choline levels.

26. Bladder filling in patients with spinal cord injuries higher than T6 may precipitate autonomic dysreflexia.

27. Radiation exposure diminishes as the square of the distance from the radiation source.

4   Urinary Tract Imaging: Basic Principles of Urologic Ultrasonography

Bruce R. Gilbert and Pat F. Fulgham

QUESTIONS

1. The maximum excursion of a wave above and below the baseline is known as its:
   a. wavelength.
   b. frequency.
   c. period.
   d. cycle.
   e. amplitude.

2. The artifact that occurs when an ultrasound wave strikes an interface at a critical angle and is refracted with limited reflection is:
   a. reverberation artifact.
   b. increased through-transmission artifact.
   c. edging artifact.
   d. comet-tail artifact.
   e. aliasing artifact.

3. Which ultrasound mode allows for detection and characterization of the velocity and direction of motion?
   a. Harmonic scanning
   b. Color Doppler
   c. Power Doppler
   d. Spatial compounding
   e. Gray-scale ultrasonography

4. If the kidney is less echogenic than the liver, the kidney is described as:
   a. hyperechoic.
   b. hypoechoic.
   c. isoechoic.
   d. anechoic.
   e. echogenic.

5. The sonographic hallmark of testicular torsion is:
   a. the "blue dot" sign.
   b. epididymal edema.
   c. paratesticular fluid.
   d. increased epididymal blood flow.
   e. absence of intratesticular blood flow.

6. Ultrasound waves are examples of:
   a. radio waves.
   b. mechanical waves.
   c. electromagnetic waves.
   d. ionizing radiation.
   e. light waves.

7. The most important determinant of axial resolution is:
   a. impedance.
   b. speed of propagation.
   c. acoustic power.
   d. frequency.
   e. number of foci.

8. Increasing frequency results in a loss of:
   a. absorption.
   b. axial resolution.
   c. lateral resolution.
   d. depth of penetration.
   e. mechanical index.

9. When sound waves encounter the interface between two tissues with large differences in impedance, the waves are:
   a. increased in frequency.
   b. decreased in frequency.
   c. reflected.
   d. refracted.
   e. reverberated.

10. When a tissue appears darker than the surrounding tissue on ultrasound it is said to be relatively:
    a. hypoechoic.
    b. hyperechoic.
    c. hypodense.
    d. isoechoic.
    e. anechoic.

11. The focal zone represents the area of best:
    a. lateral resolution.
    b. axial resolution.
    c. echogenicity.
    d. blood flow.
    e. tissue penetration.

12. Increasing the gain has the effect of:
    a. increasing amplitude of the sound waves.
    b. increasing acoustic power.
    c. increasing thermal index.
    d. increasing mechanical index.
    e. increasing transducer sensitivity.

13. One way to improve the visualization of deep structures is to:
    a. increase the frequency.
    b. decrease the frequency.
    c. increase the wave velocity.
    d. decrease the gain.
    e. employ Doppler flow.

14. The best frequency for performing external renal ultrasound in most adults is:
    a. 3.5 to 5 MHz.
    b. 6 to 7 MHz.

c. 7.5 to 8.4 MHz.

d. 8.5 to 9.9 MHz.

e. None of the above.

15. A simple cyst of the kidney would not display which of the following characteristics?

a. Bright back wall

b. Increased through transmission

c. Anechoic interior

d. Edging artifact

e. Hyperechoic internal nodule

16. Which of the following is correct?

a. Measuring bladder volume requires three-dimensional scanning.

b. A nearly empty bladder is desirable for bladder scanning.

c. A curved array transducer is preferred for bladder ultrasound in most patients.

d. Ureteroceles are usually poorly visualized because the membrane is thin.

e. Bladder ultrasound is a sensitive screening exam for suspected bladder tumors.

17. Which of the following are evaluable by transabdominal bladder ultrasound?

a. Urine volume

b. Bladder wall characteristics

c. Stones or diverticulum

d. Dilated ureters

e. All of the above

18. Scrotal ultrasound for the evaluation of possible testicular torsion may include all of the following but must include:

a. B-mode ultrasound.

b. multiple scrotal views.

c. Doppler flow studies.

d. simultaneous bilateral views.

e. harmonic scanning.

19. The most important limitation of ultrasound in attempting to characterize complex renal cysts as benign or malignant is:

a. refraction.

b. inability to evaluate enhancement.

c. lack of axial resolution.

d. increased through-transmission with artifact.

e. reverberation artifact.

20. A complete transrectal ultrasound of the prostate should include an evaluation of:

a. rectal wall.

b. seminal vesicles and ejaculatory ducts.

c. bladder.

d. prostate.

e. all of the above.

21. Which of the following would not typically be visible in a sagittal midline prostate ultrasound?

a. Middle lobe of the prostate

b. Central zone

c. Ejaculatory duct

d. Tip of right seminal vesicle

e. Apex of the prostate

22. Characteristics of prostate cancer as demonstrated on transrectal ultrasound of the prostate may include:

a. hypoechogenicity.

b. hyperechogenicity.

c. prostate asymmetry.

d. increased vascularity.

e. all of the above.

23. The single most important determinant of patient safety in ultrasound utilization is:

a. multifrequency probes.

b. good documentation.

c. an informed operator.

d. periodic equipment inspection.

e. Doppler capability.

24. The disinfection level protocol required for transrectal ultrasound probes following needle biopsy is:

a. low.

b. moderate.

c. high.

d. critical.

e. none of the above.

25. For patient safety it is preferable to maximize and limit:

a. acoustic power, exam duration.

b. acoustic power, gain.

c. gain, acoustic power.

d. gain, use of cine function.

e. images, description.

ANSWERS

1. **e. Amplitude.** In ultrasound physics it is crucial to understand the concept of amplitude. The amplitude of an ultrasound wave represents its relative energy state, and it is the amplitude of the returning sound wave that determines the pixel brightness to be displayed on a monitor during real-time gray-scale imaging.

2. **c. Edging artifact.** Echo reflection is the primary mechanism whereby sound waves are returned to a transducer. It is important to understand how the angle of insonation affects the reflection and refraction of sound waves. There is a critical angle at which waves will travel along an interface rather than being returned to the probe. When this angle is encountered, it provides a dark or hypoechoic "shadow" called an "edging artifact." A reverberation artifact is one caused by multiple transits of a sound wave between the transducer and the reflecting object. Increased through-transmission artifact is caused by decreased attenuation of sound waves as they travel through a fluid-filled structure. Comet-tail artifact is seen as the result of the interaction between sound waves and fluid and gas filled structures such as the bowel. Aliasing artifact is seen with Doppler ultrasonography.

3. **b. Color Doppler.** Doppler ultrasonography is important for evaluating motion and flow. The critical difference between color Doppler and power Doppler is that color Doppler is able to evaluate both flow velocity and direction. Power Doppler evaluates integrated amplitude of the returning sound waves. Although gray-scale ultrasonography does permit the evaluation of motion, it does not permit the characterization of velocity or direction. Harmonic scanning and spatial compounding are modes that allow the selective evaluation or combination of reflected frequencies in ways that improve image quality.

4. **b. Hypoechoic.** In describing ultrasound images, it is important to use correct terminology. Descriptive terms involving echogenicity are relative terms. A hyperechoic or hypoechoic structure is being described in relation to the echogenicity of a reference standard. In most cases the reference standard is the liver. In the adult the normal kidney is hypoechoic relative to the normal liver in approximately 75% of patients.

5. **e. Absence of intratesticular blood flow.** The absence of intratesticular blood flow is the classic sonographic finding in testicular torsion. However, there are many documented cases of some preserved intratesticular blood flow even in cases with significant torsion. Therefore testicular torsion remains a clinical diagnosis. Epididymal edema, paratesticular fluid, and increased epididymal blood flow may be seen with testicular torsion but may also be seen with other clinical conditions. The blue dot sign is a classic physical finding in torsion of the appendix testis.

6. **b. Mechanical waves:** Mechanical waves are represented graphically as a sine wave alternating between a positive and negative direction from the baseline. Sound waves as they propagate through human tissue produce areas of returning compression and rarefaction.

·7. **d. Frequency:** Axial resolution is directly dependent on the frequency of sound waves. The higher the sound wave's frequency is, the better the axial resolution.

8. **d. Depth of penetration:** The optimal ultrasound image requires tradeoffs between resolution and depth of penetration. High-frequency transducers of 6 to 10 MHz may be used to image structures near the surface of the body (e.g., testis, pediatric kidney) with excellent resolution. However, deeper structures (e.g., right kidney, bladder) require lower frequencies of 3.5 to 5 MHz to penetrate. Such images will have poorer axial resolution.

9. **c. Reflected:** The shape and size of the object and the angle at which the advancing wave strikes the object are critical determinants of the amount of energy reflected. The amount of energy reflected from an interface is also influenced by the **impedance** of the two tissues at the interface. Impedance is a property that is influenced by tissue stiffness and density. It is the difference in impedance that allows an appreciation of interfaces between different types of tissue.

10. **a. Hypoechoic:** The liver is usually used as a benchmark for echogenicity. A hypoechoic area is described as "darker" on B-mode ultrasound.

11. **a. Lateral resolution:** Lateral resolution refers to the ability to identify separately objects that are equidistant from the transducer. Lateral resolution is a function of the focused width of the ultrasound beam and is a characteristic of the transducer. The location of the narrowest beam width can be adjusted by the user. The more focused the beam is, the better the lateral resolution at that location. Thus image quality can be enhanced by locating the narrowest beam width (focus or focal zone) at the depth of the object or tissue of interest

12. **e. Increasing transducer sensitivity:** The gain control on the console of the ultrasound machine permits the user to increase or decrease the sensitivity of the transducer to reflected sound waves.

13. **b. Decrease the frequency:** The optimal ultrasound image requires trade-offs between resolution and depth of penetration. High-frequency transducers of 6 to 10 MHz may be used to image structures near the surface of the body (e.g., testis, pediatric kidney), with excellent resolution. However, deeper structures (e.g., right kidney, bladder) require lower frequencies of 3.5 to 5 MHz to penetrate. Such images will have poorer axial resolution.

14. **a. 3.5 to 5 MHz:** Deeper structures (e.g., right kidney, bladder) require lower frequencies of 3.5 to 5 MHz to penetrate.

15. **e. Hyperechoic internal nodule:** A simple cyst is an example of a structure that is well circumscribed, with an anechoic interior and through transmission.

16. **c. A curved array transducer is preferred for bladder ultrasound in most patients:** A curved array transducer is of lower frequency (3.5–6 MHz) and provides greater depth of penetration but with less axial resolution. It is most often the transducer of choice for imaging the kidney and urinary bladder.

17. **e. All of the above:** Urine volume, bladder wall characteristics, the presence of calculi or diverticulum, and the presence of dilated ureters just outside the bladder are all evaluable by transabdominal bladder ultrasound.

18. **c. Doppler flow studies:** Caution should be used when interpreting Doppler flow studies in the evaluation of suspected testicular torsion. The hallmark of testicular torsion is the absence of **intratesticular** blood flow. Paratesticular flow in epididymal collaterals may appear within hours of torsion. Comparison with the contralateral testis should be performed to ensure that the technical attributes of the study are adequate to demonstrate intratesticular blood flow.

19. **b. Inability to evaluate enhancement:** Unlike computed tomography (CT), currently ultrasound cannot evaluate enhancement. Once it is approved by the US Food and Drug Administration (FDA) for this purpose, contrast-enhanced ultrasound will allow the detection of enhancement of renal masses by ultrasound.

20. **e. All of the above:** When evaluating the prostate, surrounding structures need to be assessed. Rectal lesions (including cancer), dilated seminal vesicles, and/or ejaculatory ducts as well as bladder pathology should all be evaluated for a complete examination.

21. **d. Tip of right seminal vesicle:** In a midline sagittal view the tips of the seminal vesicles are not normally visualized on ultrasound. An axial projection needs to be obtained to be able to measure the length of each seminal vesicle.

22. **e. All of the above:** Although excellent resolution and tissue characteristics is possible with transrectal ultrasound a diagnosis of prostate cancer is not often able to be made with ultrasound alone.

23. **c. An informed operator:** The ALARA (as low as reasonably achievable) principle is intended to limit the total energy imparted to the patient during an examination. This can be accomplished by (1) keeping power outputs low, (2) using appropriate scanning modes, (3) limiting examination times, (4) adjusting focus and frequency, and (5) using the cine function during documentation. All of these are dependent upon an informed sonographer.

24. **d. Critical:** Any time body fluids or tissues come in contact with an ultrasound transducer, critical or high-level disinfection protocols must be strictly adhered to.

25. **c. Gain, acoustic power:** Unlike gain, which refers to amplification of the acoustic signal returning to the transducer, acoustic power is the amount of acoustic energy applied to the tissue. The biologic effects of ultrasound in terms of power are in the milliwatt range. High levels generate heat and cavitation, which might result in tissue damage.

CHAPTER REVIEW

1. One cycle per second is known as 1 hertz (Hz). High-frequency ultrasonic transducers of 6 to 10 MHz are used to image structures near the surface. Deeper structures require lower frequencies of 3.5 to 5 MHz. Axial resolution improves with increasing frequency, and depth of penetration decreases with increasing frequency.

2. Resistive index is the peak velocity minus the end-diastolic velocity over the peek systolic velocity. This is measured using the color flow Doppler with spectral display and is used to characterize renal artery stenosis, ureteral obstruction, and penile arterial insufficiency.

3. By convention, the liver is used as a benchmark for echogenicity. By convention, the cephalad aspect of the structure is to the left of the image.

4. Ultrasonography may produce injury due to mechanical effects caused by cavitation or by heat generation.

5. With the exception of some indinavir stones, all renal and ureteral calculi may be detected by helical CT.

6. The advantage of magnetic resonance imaging (MRI) is high-contrast resolution of soft tissue on T1-weighted images. Fluid has a low signal and appears dark on T1-weighted images; on T2-weighted images, fluid has a high signal and appears bright. Gadolinium increases the brightness of T1-weighted images. Hemorrhage within a cyst results in a high signal on T1-weighted images.

5 Urinary Tract Imaging: Basic Principles of Nuclear Medicine

Michael A. Gorin and Steven P. Rowe

QUESTIONS

1. ^{99m}Tc-diethylenetriaminepentaacetic acid (^{99m}Tc-DTPA) undergoes renal clearance by which mechanism?
   a. Glomerular filtration
   b. Active tubular secretion
   c. Anion exchange
   d. Both A and B
   e. All of the above

2. ^{99m}Tc-mercaptoacetyltriglycine (^{99m}Tc-MAG3) undergoes renal clearance by which mechanism?
   a. Glomerular filtration
   b. Active tubular secretion
   c. Anion exchange
   d. Both A and B
   e. All of the above

3. ^{99m}Tc–dimercaptosuccinic acid (^{99m}Tc-DMSA) undergoes renal clearance and is endocytosed by cells of which part of the nephron?
   a. Glomerulus
   b. Proximal tubule
   c. Distal tubule
   d. Ascending loop of Henle
   e. Collecting duct

4. When performing ^{99m}Tc-MAG3 renography, the relative function of each kidney is determined by measuring the area under the time activity curve between what two time points post injection?
   a. 1 to 3 minutes
   b. 3 to 5 minutes
   c. 5 to 10 minutes
   d. 10 to 15 minutes
   e. 15 to 20 minutes

5. Which radiotracer is ideally suited for imaging renal scaring?
   a. ^{99m}Tc-DTPA
   b. ^{99m}Tc-MAG3
   c. ^{99m}Tc-DMSA
   d. ^{67}Ga-citrate
   e. ^{99m}Tc–sulfur colloid

6. 2-Deoxy-2-[^{18}F]fluoro-D-glucose (^{18}F-FDG) is phosphorylated by which glycolytic enzyme, trapping it inside metabolically active cells?
   a. Hexokinase
   b. Glucokinase
   c. Phosphofructokinase
   d. Pyruvate kinase
   e. Phosphoglucose isomerase

7. Which urologic malignancy is poorly imaged with ^{18}F-FDG positron emission tomography (PET)?
   a. Bladder cancer
   b. Penile cancer
   c. Prostate cancer
   d. Renal cell carcinoma
   e. Seminomatous germ cell tumor

8. What is the half-life of the radionuclide ^{18}F?
   a. 20.3 minutes
   b. 109.8 minutes
   c. 68.0 minutes
   d. 4.17 days
   e. 78.4 hours

9. Which of the following PET radiotracers for prostate cancer imaging is an amino acid analog?
   a. ^{18}F-DCFPyL
   b. ^{68}Ga-PSMA-11
   c. ^{11}C-choline
   d. ^{68}Ga-RM2
   e. ^{18}F-FACBC

10. Which protein is highly expressed by clear cell renal cell carcinoma (RCC) but not other renal tumor types and serves as a target for molecular imaging of this malignancy?
    a. GLUT1
    b. PSMA
    c. GRPR
    d. CAIX
    e. ASCT2

11. Which radiotracer has the highest specificity for imaging prostate cancer?
    a. ^{18}F-DCFPyL
    b. ^{67}Ga-citrate
    c. ^{11}C-choline
    d. ^{18}F-FDG
    e. ^{18}F-FACBC

12. ^{18}F-FDG PET is recommended for which application in men with testicular cancer?
    a. Initial cancer staging of patients with elevated postorchiectomy tumor markers
    b. Initial cancer staging of patients with negative postorchiectomy tumor markers
    c. Postchemotherapy imaging of a residual retroperitoneal mass in men with a seminomatous germ cell tumor
    d. Postchemotherapy imaging of a residual retroperitoneal mass in men with a nonseminomatous germ cell tumors
    e. Post-treatment surveillance in patients with negative markers

ANSWERS

1. **a. Goluerular filtration.** ^{99m}Tc-DPTA is a single-photon radiotracer that is excreted in the urine and can be used to determine renal split function and to assess for functional obstruction. ^{99m}Tc-DTPA is extracted by the kidneys through glomerular filtration. The drug then quickly moves through the renal tubules and is excreted in the urine without being reabsorbed.

2. **b. Active tubular secretion.** ^{99m}Tc-MAG3 is a single-photon radiotracer that is excreted in the urine and can be used to determine renal split function and to assess for functional obstruction. ^{99m}Tc-MAG3 is protein bound in circulation and undergoes clearance exclusively through tubular secretion. ^{99m}Tc-MAG3 imaging is therefore not impacted by impaired glomerular filtration.

3. **b. Proximal tubule.** ^{99m}Tc-DMSA is cleared from the plasma primarily by glomerular filtration. Once within the lumina of the renal tubules, ^{99m}Tc-DMSA undergoes receptor-mediated endocytosis by the proximal tubular cells. The receptors responsible for the endocytosis of ^{99m}Tc-DMSA are megalin and cubilin.

4. **a. 1 to 3 minutes.** Dynamic renal imaging is performed in two phases. In the first phase, known as the perfusion phase, renal plasma flow to each individual renal unit is measured and compared with flow within the aorta. Activity should be detected in the regions of interest overlying the kidneys within several seconds of detection in the aorta. The relative function of each kidney is determined by measuring the area under the time activity curves between 1 and 3 minutes post injection of the radiotracer.

5. **c. ^{99m}Tc-DMSA.** Because this radiotracer undergoes endocytosis by the proximal tubular cells, it is ideally suited for imaging cortical processes such as acute pyelonephritis and renal scaring.

6. **a. Hexokinase.** ^{18}F-FDG is a glucose analog that is taken up by metabolically active cells via GLUT transporters. Once within the cell, ^{18}F-FDG is phosphorylated by the glycolytic enzyme hexokinase, preventing diffusion back across the cell membrane. The trapped ^{18}F-FDG molecules, which are missing a 2-hydroxyl group, cannot undergo further glycolytic metabolism and remain intact allowing for their detection with PET imaging.

7. **c. Prostate cancer.** ^{18}F- FDG is taken up by malignant cells, which commonly shunt energy production toward anaerobic metabolism, a phenomenon referred to as the Warburg effect. A number of genitourinary malignancies, including urothelial carcinoma, renal cell carcinoma, squamous cell carcinoma of the penis, and testicular germ cell tumors, can be successfully imaged with ^{18}F-FDG PET. Prostate cancer is unique in that it does not show increased levels of glycolysis and therefore is poorly visualized with ^{18}F-FDG PET.

8. **b. 109.8 minutes.** The half-lives of other commonly used radionuclides for PET imaging can be found in Table 5.2.

9. **a. 18F-FACBC.** This radiotracer functions as a substrate for the amino acid transporters LAT1 and ASCT2, which are overexpressed by multiple malignancies including prostate cancer.

10. **d. CAIX.** This cell surface protein is near universally expressed by clear cell RCC but not other renal tumor histologies. CAIX is upregulated following loss of the von Hippel-Lindau *(VHL)* gene, which is a defining event in the pathogenesis of clear cell RCC.

11. **a. 18F-DCFPyL.** PET radiotracers targeting prostate-specific membrane antigen (PSMA) have the highest specificity for prostate cancer imaging. Of the radiotracers listed, 18F-DCF-PyL is the only PSMA-targeted radiotracer. A summary of other radiotracer used for prostate cancer imaging can be found in Table 5.3.

12. **c. Postchemotherapy imaging of a residual retroperitoneal mass in men with a seminomatous germ cell tumor.** Guidelines from the European Association of Urology endorse the use of ^{18}F-FDG PET for men with a residual mass following treatment of a seminoma with chemotherapy. Using ^{18}F-FDG PET in this manner helps to differentiate fibrosis from residual active tumor. For patients with non-seminomatous germ cell tumors, ^{18}F-FDG PET imaging is not indicated because there appears to be no clinical benefit for PET in the detection of viable tumor over the combination of computed tomography (CT) and serum markers.

CHAPTER REVIEW

1. The most commonly used radiopharmaceutical agents for nuclear imaging of the kidneys are technetium ^{99m}Tc-diethylenetriaminepentaacetic acid (^{99m}Tc-DTPA), ^{99m}Tc- mercaptoacetyltriglycine (MAG3), and ^{99m}Tc–dimercaptosuccinic acid (DMSA).
2. ^{99m}Tc-DTPA and ^{99m}Tc-MAG3 are used to measure renal blood flow, determine differential renal function, and to evaluate for the presence and degree of renal obstruction.
3. ^{99m}Tc-DTPA is cleared by glomerular filtration, whereas ^{99m}Tc-MAG3 is cleared by tubular secretion.
4. ^{99m}Tc-MAG3 is the preferred at most centers over ^{99m}Tc-DTPA because it has a higher extraction efficiency and is less impacted by changes in renal function.
5. ^{99m}Tc-DMSA is retained by cells of the proximal renal tubules and is used to evaluate for infection and the presence renal scarring.
6. ^{99m}Tc-DTPA and ^{99m}Tc-MAG3 can also be used to evaluate renovascular hypertension, transplant graft function, and vesicoureteral reflux.
7. Molecular imaging of cancer is most commonly performed using the positron emission tomography (PET) radiotracer 2-deoxy-2-(^{18}F)fluoro-D-glucose (^{18}F-FDG)
8. A number of genitourinary malignancies can be successfully imaged with ^{18}F-FDG PET, albeit with varying degrees of clinical utility beyond conventional anatomical imaging techniques.
9. Because ^{18}F-FDG is excreted in the urine, imaging with this radiotracer is typically performed to detect distant sites of disease.
10. ^{18}F-FDG has little role in imaging prostate cancer and a number of other radiotracers have been developed for this purpose.
11. Radiotracers targeting PSMA are the most promising class of agents for prostate cancer imaging and in many parts of the world have become the new standard of care for imaging this malignancy.
12. One of the most well-established indications for ^{18}F-FDG PET imaging is in the detection of residual seminomatous germ cell tumors following chemotherapy.

6 Assessment of Urologic and Surgical Outcomes

David F. Penson and Mark D. Tyson

QUESTIONS

1. When assessing disease-specific mortality, researchers need to be aware that this outcome is subject to:
   a. detection bias.
   b. attribution bias.
   c. problems with loss to follow-up.
   d. all of the above.
   e. b and c.

2. Which of the following is NOT one of the four requirements for a valid surrogate endpoint as described by Prentice?
   a. Treatment is associated with the true endpoint.
   b. The surrogate endpoint is associated with the true endpoint.
   c. The full effect of treatment on the true endpoint is explained by the surrogate endpoint.
   d. The surrogate endpoint can reliably be measured using highly objective methods.
   e. Treatment is also associated with the surrogate endpoint.

3. With regard to patient-centered outcomes:
   a. clinicians can reliably assess these outcomes from the doctor–patient interaction.
   b. there are very few validated and reliable questionnaires available for use in urology.
   c. health-related quality of life is an important outcome to measure, but only function need be assessed to get a full portrait of this outcome.
   d. patient-centered questionnaires are developed using the principles of psychometric test theory.
   e. none of the above.

4. Which of the following methods has not been suggested as a technique to assess patient experience of pain?
   a. Collect verbal or written descriptions of the pain
   b. Query patient's caregiver regarding patient's pain level.
   c. Have subject rate pain via its effect on observable behavior.
   d. Use analogue techniques in which the patient compares his/her pain with an experimentally induced stimulus of a known intensity in a laboratory setting.
   e. All of the above can be used to assess pain levels.

5. When a scale has a coefficient α of 0.90, one can be assured that the scale has high degree of:
   a. alternate form reliability.
   b. test-retest reliability.
   c. internal consistency reliability.
   d. intraobserver reliability.
   e. interobserver reliability.

6. If a urologist were designing an instrument to measure cancer-specific quality of life following prostatectomy, how would she design an experiment to assess test-retest reliability?
   a. She could administer the questionnaire before and after the operation.
   b. She could administer the questionnaire to her patients and a group of age-matched healthy controls.
   c. She could use a differently worded questionnaire to obtain the same information.
   d. She could administer the questionnaire to the same patient twice in the same week and compare the results.
   e. She could administer the questionnaire to the same patient twice at an interval of one year and compare the results.

7. Of the following types of validity, which one often takes many years of instrument use by numerous investigators to adequately assess?
   a. Face validity
   b. Content validity
   c. Concurrent validity
   d. Predictive validity
   e. Construct validity

8. The use of uroflow results in validating a new survey instrument that measures disease-specific HRQOL in benign prostatic hyperplasia (BPH) patients is an example of:
   a. concurrent validity.
   b. content validity.
   c. construct validity.
   d. predictive validity.
   e. face validity.

9. A patient undergoes a radical cystectomy. On post-operative day #2, he aspirates and requires emergent intubation and transfer to the ICU. He is started on intravenous antibiotics and is extubated on post-operative day #4. The remainder of his hospital course in unremarkable and he is discharged on post-operative day #8. The complication he experienced is a Clavien-Dindo grade:
   a. II.
   b. IIIa.
   c. IIIb.
   d. IVa.
   e. IVb.

10. A patient with kidney cancer has a single target lesion, a 5-cm bony metastases. She is treated with a tyrosine kinase inhibitor (TKI). The lesion is reduced in size and is now 4 cm on imaging. According to the RECIST criteria, this is considered a:
    a. complete response.
    b. partial response.
    c. stable disease.
    d. non-CR/non-PD.
    e. progressive disease.

ANSWERS

1. **e. b and c.** When assessing disease-specific mortality, researchers need to be aware that this outcome is subject to attribution bias and problems with loss to follow-up.
2. **d. The surrogate endpoint can reliably be measured using highly objective methods.** It is not a requirement for a valid surrogate endpoint that it can reliably be measured using highly objective methods.
3. **d. Patient-centered questionnaires are developed using the principles of psychometric test theory.** For patient-centered outcomes, patient-centered questionnaires are developed using the principles of psychometric test theory.
4. **e. All of the above can be used to assess pain levels.** Collecting verbal or written descriptions of the pain, querying the patient's caregiver regarding the patient's pain level; having the subject rate pain via its effect on observable behavior; and using analogue techniques in which the patient compares his/her pain with an experimentally induced stimulus of a known intensity in a laboratory setting are all methods to assess patient pain.
5. **c. Internal consistency reliability.** When a scale has a coefficient alpha of 0.90, the scale has a high degree of internal consistency reliability.
6. **d. She could administer the questionnaire to the same patient twice in the same week and compare the results.** A urologist wishing to measure cancer-specific quality of life following prostatectomy could design an experiment to assess test-retest reliability by administering the questionnaire to the same patient twice in the same week and comparing the results.
7. **e. Construct validity.** Construct validity often takes many years of instrument use by numerous investigators to adequately assess.
8. **a. Concurrent validity.** The use of uroflow results in validating a new survey instrument that measures disease-specific HRQOL in BPH patients is an example of concurrent validity.
9. **d. IVa.** The patient's complication is Clavien-Dindo grade IVa.
10. **c. Stable disease.** This is considered stable disease per RECIST criteria.

CHAPTER REVIEW

1. The effectiveness of health services delivery and treatment can be measured across three distinct dimensions: structure, process, and outcomes. Structure and process measures are easier to assess but outcomes tend to be most meaningful to clinicians and patients.
2. Mortality is the "hardest" endpoint one can assess in urology. That being said, it can be subject to bias. Specifically, studies using overall mortality can still be subject to lead- and length-time bias, and studies using disease-specific mortality may be subject to attribution bias.
3. While there are many proxy endpoints in urology, few meet all four requirements for being a valid surrogate endpoint. Despite this, urologists routinely use proxy endpoints in research and clinical practice.
4. There are a number of published and widely accepted criteria for defining disease progression and surgical complications in urology. While these urologists should use these reporting systems whenever possible, they should also remember that the use of these systems does not completely eliminate the potential for bias in research due to study design and other factors.
5. Frailty, functional status, and comorbidity are important potential confounders that should be considered in urologic research. There are numerous standardized tools available to capture these variables.
6. There are numerous patient-reported outcome tools available to assess symptoms and quality of life in patients with urologic diseases. Physicians and researchers should always use validated and reliable patient-centered tools when possible.

7 Ethics and Informed Consent

Vijaya M. Vemulakonda

QUESTIONS

1. The Hippocratic Oath does not include the ethical principle of:
   a. beneficence.
   b. non-maleficence.
   c. patient privacy.
   d. patient autonomy.
   e. accountability to the profession.

2. Important events leading to the modern framework of medical ethics include:
   a. The Nuremburg Trials.
   b. The Tuskegee Syphilis Studies.
   c. The Milgram Experiments.
   d. all of the above.
   e. none of the above.

3. The most important of the four basic principles of modern medical ethics is:
   a. justice.
   b. autonomy.
   c. beneficence.
   d. non-maleficence.
   e. none of the above.

4. The term bioethics was first coined by:
   a. Veatch.
   b. Potter.
   c. Beauchamp and Childress.
   d. Jonsen, Siegler, and Winslade.
   e. none of the above.

5. The Four Box Method does not:
   a. provide a systematic approach to apply ethical principles to specific clinical situations.
   b. include consideration of medical indications, patient preferences, quality of life, and other contextual features.
   c. create a venue for discussion of relative risks and benefits of potential treatment options.
   d. provide definitive answers to ethically challenging situations.
   e. none of the above

6. Clinical informed consent originated in:
   a. The Hippocratic Oath.
   b. 19th-century negligence laws.
   c. The Nuremburg Code.
   d. 20th-century battery laws.

7. Under current informed consent requirements, physicians are obligated to provide:
   a. information about the most common risks of a procedure.
   b. information that a "reasonable physician" would provide.
   c. information that a "reasonable person" would want to know.
   d. a written document detailing risks and benefits of the procedure.

8. The element of informed consent that is most often lacking is:
   a. description of the clinical problem, proposed treatment, and alternatives.
   b. discussion of the risks and benefits of the proposed treatment.
   c. assessment of the patient's understanding of the information provided by the medical provider.
   d. solicitation of the patient's preferences for treatment.

9. Exceptions to the informed consent requirement do not include:
   a. an unconscious 25-year-old patient who sustained multiple gunshot wounds.
   b. a 75-year-old patient with Alzheimer dementia who is being evaluated for benign prostatic hyperplasia (BPH) and has a previously identified surrogate decision maker.
   c. a 3-year-old patient who is accompanied by his parents for circumcision evaluation.
   d. a conscious 25-year-old patient who sustained multiple gunshot wounds.
   e. none of the above.

10. Issues thought to be associated with lack of patient understanding of consent include all EXCEPT:
    a. language of the surgical consent form is above the average patient reading level.
    b. patients may misunderstand the risks posed by surgery.
    c. patients idealize surgeons and defer to surgeon recommendations.
    d. patients may not recall the information contained within a surgical consent form.
    e. none of the above.

11. Use of decision aids have been associated with all of the following EXCEPT:
    a. improved knowledge of the procedure.
    b. improved assessment of risk.
    c. increased patient participation in the decision-making process.
    d. increased decisional conflict.
    e. none of the above.

ANSWERS

1. **d. Patient autonomy.** Although the Hippocratic Oath includes the concepts of benefiting and avoiding harm to patients as well as protecting patient privacy, it does not include the concept of patient autonomy, which emerged in the 20th century.

2. **d. All of the above.** The Nuremburg trials revealed the involuntary experiments of Dr. Josef Mengele and other Nazi doctors

on concentration camp detainees, resulting in pain, debilitation, and death of subjects. The trials led to the development of the Nuremburg code, which reinforced the need for voluntary consent, need to minimize harm, absence of other methods to obtain data, and need to terminate studies early if evidence of potential harm in a clinical research study. The Tuskegee studies were performed from 1932 to 1972 in Tuskegee, Alabama, to study the natural history of syphilis, with investigators withholding antibiotic treatment even after the discovery of the efficacy of penicillin to treat the disease. The study raised issues of adequate knowledge for consent, need to avoid coercion for participation, and need to terminate studies early if the investigator has knowledge of preventable harm. The Milgram experiments, which were conducted in 1963 at Yale by psychologist Stanley Milgram, encouraged subjects to administer fake electrical shocks to unseen participants. Recorded responses to the shocks were played, including screaming and silence suggestive of possible unconsciousness. Subjects were encouraged to continue to escalate shocks despite these responses, with the majority of subjects administering maximal shocks, leading to psychological trauma in many participants. The study raised concerns about use of deception in research and lack of adequate safeguards against harm. All of these events led to heightened scrutiny and development of heightened standards for medical research.

3. **e. None of the above.** According to Beauchamp and Childress, the four basic principles of autonomy, beneficence, non-maleficence, and justice should be considered equal in weight.

4. **b. Potter.** Van Rensselaer Potter first coined the term *bioethics* in 1970, described as the "study of the moral relationship between humans and their social and physical world."

5. **d. Provide definitive answers to ethically challenging situations.** Although the Four Box Method allows for systematic consideration of ethically complex clinical situations and creates a vehicle for discussions regarding treatment, it may also oversimplify ethical problems and does not always provide clear "right" and "wrong" answers to address ethical concerns.

6. **d. 20th-century battery laws.** Although now considered within the scope of negligence, informed consent was first described by state courts in early 20th-century battery cases and was considered to be grounded in the right to bodily integrity. The Nuremburg code recommended expansion of the right to informed consent to medical research.

7. **c. Information that a "reasonable person" would want to know.** Although battery law required disclosure of risks and early negligence law required disclosure of what a "reasonable and prudent" physician would do, the current standard is what a reasonable person would want to know (Canterbury vs. Spence, 1972). The informed consent process requires both information from the physician and demonstrated understanding by the patient but does not require written documentation.

8. **c. Assessment of the patient's understanding of the information provided by the medical provider.** Although all four elements are needed for a comprehensive informed consent, the majority of informed consents are incomplete with the element of assessing patient understanding of the information provided being the most commonly missed.

9. **d. A conscious 25-year-old patient who sustained multiple gunshot wounds.** In emergency settings where there is a significant threat to patient life or well-being, consent is presumed. However, this waiver of consent does not extend to the conscious patient even if refusal of treatment is life-threatening (In re Quackenbush 1978).

10. **e. None of the above.** All of the options have been posed as limitations to patient understanding of consent. The information provided in consent forms often is above the 12th-grade level, although the majority of patients have reading levels below the 8th-grade level. Additionally, patients who report reading consent forms may not recall the information contained in the document. Additionally, patients often underestimate their risks compared to other people or may use heuristics to make decisions that lead to a misunderstanding of the risks involved. Finally, patients often accept surgical recommendations without meaningful participation in the decision-making process due to idealization of the surgeon and his or her judgment.

11. **d. Increased decisional conflict.** Decision aids have been associated with improved knowledge about procedures, reduced decisional conflict, improved patient participation in the decision, and improved assessment of risk.

CHAPTER REVIEW

1. Although the scope of medical ethics continues to evolve, the basic ethical principles of autonomy, beneficence, non-maleficence, and justice remain the foundation of ethical medical practice.

2. Informed consent is essential to the practice of surgery with limited exceptions.

3. Despite the goal of ensuring adequate understanding of the nature, risks, benefits, and alternatives of surgery to facilitate a meaningful decision, the informed consent process is often incomplete. It is therefore the responsibility of the surgeon to make every effort to facilitate patient understanding and participation in the decision-making process.

8   Principles of Urologic Surgery: Perioperative Care

Simpa S. Salami

QUESTIONS

1. A 64-year-old man is found to have an 8-cm left renal mass and presents to the office for evaluation regarding laparoscopic radical nephrectomy. He has a history of hypertension, non–insulin-dependent diabetes, and 30-pack-year history of tobacco use, which he quit 10 years ago. He has a strong family history of heart disease (father died at the age of 55 years from a myocardial infarction). Further questioning reveals that he does not regularly exercise but is able to walk up three flights of stairs without shortness of breath. Before surgery, to minimize the risk of complications, the patient should:

   a. undergo routine preoperative testing with complete blood count, basic metabolic panel, electrocardiogram, and chest radiograph.

   b. be referred to cardiology consultation to determine if further testing is necessary.

   c. undergo noninvasive cardiac stress testing.

   d. undergo pulmonary function testing to determine the need for preoperative bronchodilators.

   e. be started on a perioperative β blocker to reduce the risk of perioperative myocardial ischemia.

2. With regard to unique patient populations, which of the following statements is TRUE?

   a. Although elderly patients have an increased perioperative risk, recent larger trials have not found age to be an independent risk factor for perioperative morbidity and mortality.

   b. Morbidly obese patients should undergo open rather than laparoscopic surgery because of increased risk of pulmonary complications.

   c. In a pregnant patient presenting with urolithiasis, operative intervention should be delayed, if possible, until the second trimester.

   d. A patient who presents with a 30-pound weight loss over the previous 3 months should be started on parenteral feedings immediately postoperatively after elective surgery.

   e. In patients with liver disease, the primary determinant of postoperative risk is degree of liver function enzyme abnormality.

3. A 74-year-old man with muscle-invasive bladder cancer is scheduled for radical cystectomy and ileal conduit urinary diversion. Preoperative urine culture shows no growth at 72 hours. The most important factor in the prevention of surgical site infection in this patient is:

   a. preoperative bowel preparation with oral antibiotics (Nichols prep) and sodium phosphate solution (Fleet).

   b. administration of 2 g cefoxitin 1 hour before incision.

   c. continuation of perioperative antibiotics for 48 hours following surgery.

   d. preoperative hair removal with mechanical clippers and proper sterile preparation of the operative field.

   e. optimization of comorbid illness and nutritional status.

4. According to current guidelines in the prevention of thromboembolic complications, a 78-year-old male with a recent history of colon cancer, medical history of hypertension, coronary artery disease (postoperative angioplasty with two coronary stents), and chronic renal insufficiency (creatinine, 2.9 mg/dL) undergoing laparoscopic transabdominal surgery should have pneumatic compression stockings and:

   a. early ambulation.

   b. aspirin and early ambulation.

   c. low-molecular-weight heparin.

   d. low-molecular-weight heparin and aspirin.

   e. unfractionated heparin and aspirin.

5. A 72-year-old woman with a history of asthma, mild congestive heart failure, and breast cancer is to undergo cystoscopy and placement of a midurethral sling. Of the following agents, the best choice for anesthesia induction would be:

   a. inhaled halothane.

   b. intravenous thiopental.

   c. inhaled desflurane.

   d. inhaled sevoflurane.

   e. intravenous succinylcholine.

6. A 56-year-old man with autoimmune disease is scheduled to undergo robotic-assisted laparoscopic radical prostatectomy. Which of the following represents the best choice for managing his chronic exogenous steroid therapy?

   a. Discontinue prior to surgery

   b. Discontinue prior to surgery and resume post-operatively

   c. Discontinue prior to surgery, administer stress dose steroid before the induction of anesthesia, and continue post-operatively until home medication is resumed

   d. Continue patient's oral medication at the current dosage through surgery

   e. Increase the dose of patient's oral medication prior to surgery and reduce back to baseline dose after surgery.

ANSWERS

1. **e. Be started on preoperative β blocker to reduce the risk of perioperative myocardial ischemia.** This choice is best given the patient's multiple risk factors. Although cardiac stress testing may be considered, the patient's ability to climb three flights of stairs indicates a capacity of greater than 4 metabolic equivalents (METs) and therefore a low risk of significant coronary artery disease. Although routine preoperative testing is performed widely, there is no evidence that routine testing reduces the risk of perioperative complications.

2. **c. In a pregnant patient presenting with urolithiasis, operative intervention should be delayed, if possible, until the second trimester.** The second trimester represents the least anesthetic risk to the mother and fetus with regard to

spontaneous abortion and teratogenicity. Although controversy exists as to the exact etiology, several recent trials have found age to be an independent predictor of morbidity on multivariate analyses. Laparoscopic surgery is the preferred approach in morbidly obese patients secondary to the reduced risk of pulmonary and wound complications. Literature suggests that severely malnourished patients (>20 pounds weight loss in 3 months) significantly benefit from 7 to 10 days of enteral (not parenteral) feedings *before* elective surgery. The primary determinants of the degree of severity in patients with cirrhosis are hepatic function and severity of clinical manifestations.

3. **b. Administration of 2 g cefoxitin 1 hour before incision.** Administration of appropriate antibiotics within 60 minutes of incision has been shown to significantly decrease the incidence of surgical site infections. Recent meta-analyses from the colorectal literature indicate that mechanical bowel preparation does not decrease the risk of postoperative infections. Unless in the presence of active infection, perioperative antibiotics should be stopped 24 hours after incision to decrease the risk of *Clostridium difficile* colitis. Although preoperative hair removal and optimization of nutritional status and comorbid illness improve surgical outcomes, there is no specific evidence that this reduces surgical site infections.

4. **e. Unfractionated heparin and aspirin.** The clinical scenario describes a patient with high to highest risk of venous throm-

boembolism. Such a patient would require both mechanical and pharmacologic prophylaxis. In a patient with renal insufficiency, unfractionated heparin is a better choice than low-molecular-weight heparin. There is no evidence that aspirin is effective in the prevention of venous thromboembolism, but in a patient with coronary stents, aspirin is important in the prevention of stent thrombosis in the perioperative period.

5. **d. Inhaled sevoflurane.** This is an excellent choice for rapid induction in this patient secondary to its odorless and bronchodilation properties. Halothane can adversely affect left ventricular function and should be used with caution in patients with congestive heart failure. Desflurane has a pungent odor and is more suitable for maintenance of anesthesia during prolonged procedures. Intravenous thiopental can increase airway reactivity and is not appropriate in patients with asthma. Succinylcholine is appropriate for neuromuscular blockade and not commonly used for induction.

6. **c. Discontinue prior to surgery, administer stress dose steroid before the induction of anesthesia, and continue post-operatively until home medication is resumed.** Patients who have a depressed hypothalamic pituitary adrenal axis due to exogenous steroids should receive 50 to 100 mg of intravenous hydrocortisone before the induction of anesthesia and 25 to 50 mg every 8 hours thereafter until the patient's medication is resumed. Simply discontinuing the patient's steroid medication can result in adrenal crisis due to adrenal insufficiency post-operatively.

CHAPTER REVIEW

1. One must always determine whether a woman in the childbearing years is pregnant before a surgical procedure. A urine pregnancy test is a simple method to do this.
2. The American Society of Anesthesiologists' classification is a significant predictor of operative mortality.
3. Preoperative cardiac evaluation is meant to identify serious coronary artery disease, heart failure, symptomatic arrhythmias, and the presence of a pacemaker or defibrillator. Major clinical predictors of cardiovascular risk are a recent myocardial infarction (within 1 month), unstable angina, evidence of an ischemic burden, decompensated heart failure, significant arrhythmias, and severe valvular disease.
4. A patient's ability to climb two flights of stairs is a good assessment of adequate functional capacity.
5. Patients with an FEV_1 of less than 30% predicted are at high risk for complications.
6. Smoking must be discontinued at least 8 weeks before surgery to be effective in reducing risk.
7. Perioperative β blockade is associated with a reduced risk of death among high-risk patients undergoing major noncardiac surgical procedures. However, more recent data bring this into question.
8. Patients who have a depressed hypothalamic pituitary adrenal axis due to exogenous steroids should receive 50 to 100 mg of intravenous hydrocortisone before the induction of anesthesia and 25 to 50 mg every 8 hours thereafter until the patient's medication is resumed.
9. In the elderly, delirium can be the first clinical sign of hypoxia or of metabolic or infectious complications.
10. In the pregnant patient, postoperative pain is best managed with narcotic analgesics.
11. A preoperative electrocardiogram should be obtained in all patients older than 40 years and in those with a significant cardiac history.
12. It is important to remember that for prophylaxis of venous thromboembolic disease and the use of antibiotic and mechanical bowel preps before intestinal surgery, the studies are often based on data obtained from nonurologic patients. The urologist must consider this when the procedure being performed is significantly different from the standard general surgical operation on which the data

are based. This is particularly true for bowel preparation, as urologic reconstructive procedures often require opening the isolated intestinal segment to be used in the procedure, exposing the entire contents to the operative field.
13. Parenteral antibiotics should be given within 60 minutes before intestinal surgery.
14. Nitrous oxide inhalation anesthesia results in bowel distention.
15. The half-life of warfarin is 36 to 42 hours, and it is recommended that warfarin be stopped 5 days before the surgical event.
16. Aspirin and clopidogrel are irreversible inhibitors of platelet function and should be discontinued 7 to 10 days before surgery if bleeding risk is to be minimized.
17. For moderate- to high-risk groups on anticoagulation therapy, a therapeutic bridge is performed using unfractionated or low-molecular-weight heparin. These may be stopped 4 or 12 hours, respectively, before the procedure and instituted shortly after its completion.
18. The indications for fresh frozen plasma are immediate reversal of warfarin and replacement of specific clotting factors.
19. The most common cause of transfusion-related fatality is transfusion-related acute lung injury (TRALI).
20. Hypothermia results in increased blood loss and an increased incidence of wound infection.
21. If hair is to be removed, it should preferably be removed immediately before the surgical event with mechanical clippers.
22. The need for postoperative parenteral nutrition should be anticipated in patients undergoing major urologic procedures involving the use of bowel. If it is likely the patient will not be able to take an adequate caloric intake orally by 7 to 10 days, postoperative parenteral nutrition should be instituted.
23. The second trimester represents the least anesthetic risk to the mother and fetus with regard to spontaneous abortion and teratogenicity.
24. Severely malnourished patients (>20 pounds weight loss in 3 months) significantly benefit from 7 to 10 days of enteral (not parenteral) feedings *before* elective surgery.
25. In a patient with renal insufficiency, unfractionated heparin is a better choice than low-molecular-weight heparin.

9 Principles of Urologic Surgery: Incisions and Access

David Mikhail and Simon J. Hall

QUESTIONS

1. Which of the following is not considered an indication for an open abdominal approach (as opposed to minimally invasive)?
   a. Multiple prior abdominal surgeries
   b. Complex renal mass with caval thrombus
   c. Previous abdominal hernia repair with mesh
   d. Patient with multiple comorbidities
   e. Surgeon's preference and experience

2. Following a motor vehicle crash (MVC), a 35-year-old male is found to have a significant right-sided renal hilar injury on imaging. He becomes hemodynamically unstable, despite intravenous fluid resuscitation and massive transfusion protocol. The decision is made to take him to the OR. What incision should you use?
   a. Flank incision
   b. Complete midline incision
   c. Chevron incision
   d. Subcostal incision
   e. Thoracoabdominal incision

3. Which approach of abdominal wall fascial closure has been shown to have a higher rate of abdominal wall hernias?
   a. Rapidly absorbable suture, running continuous closure
   b. Rapidly absorbable suture, interrupted closure
   c. Slowly absorbable suture, running continuous closure
   d. Slowly absorbable suture, interrupted closure

4. A 25-year-old patient has been cleared to donate her left kidney to her cousin who recently was started on dialysis for end-stage renal disease. She is seeing you for pre-surgical consultation. You inform her you will be performing the nephrectomy laparoscopically and will be extracting the kidney through _____ because this has been shown to have _____.
   a. extension of the inferior port site; lower morbidity and incisional hernia rates
   b. extension of the midline port site; decreased pain scores and complications
   c. pfannenstiel incision; lower morbidity and incisional hernia rates
   d. pfannenstiel incision; decreased pain scores and complications
   e. extension of the superior most port site; decreased pain scores and complications

5. A 45-year-old female had deceased donor renal transplant placed 5 years ago. She has been noncompliant with immunosuppressive medications and the allograft has failed. She has developed peri-allograft abscess, and the allograft must be removed. Which incision is best for renal allograft nephrectomy?
   a. Lower midline
   b. Inguinal incision
   c. Subcostal incision
   d. Gibson incision
   e. Flank incision

6. Which incision is rarely used due to high risk of nerve injuries and ventral hernias?
   a. Midline incision
   b. Paramedian incision
   c. Thoraco-abdominal incision
   d. Pfannenstiel incision
   e. Gibson incision

7. Which of the following is NOT an advantage of the thoracoabdominal incision as an approach to large renal tumors?
   a. Exposure of adjacent thorax
   b. Exposure of retroperitoneum
   c. Early vascular control
   d. Large incision
   e. Access to inferior vena cava (IVC) for advanced disease/caval thrombus

8. Which is the second muscle layer incised in a typical flank incision?
   a. External oblique
   b. Internal oblique
   c. Serratus anterior
   d. Latissimus dorsi
   e. Transversalis

9. Which of the following is not considered a true flank incision approach?
   a. 12th rib supracostal
   b. 11th rib transcostal
   c. Subcostal
   d. 9th rib supracostal

10. Which nerve must be carefully handled to avoid injury during surgery in the inguinal canal?
    a. Femoral nerve
    b. Sciatic nerve
    c. Genitofemoral nerve
    d. Ilioinguinal nerve
    e. Lateral femoral cutaneous nerve

11. Which incision was used for the first-ever planned nephrectomy?
    a. Thoracoabdominal incision
    b. Flank incision
    c. Posterior lumbodorsal incision
    d. Subcostal incision
    e. Gibson incision

12. Which are NOT considered benefits of the dorsal lumbotomy approach compared to flank incisions?
    a. Rib and muscle sparing
    b. Less postoperative pain
    c. Decreased hospitalization
    d. Better surgical exposure for vascular control
    e. Decreased intra-peritoneal complications

13. Which of the following is NOT a border of the lumbodorsal region?
    a. 12th rib–superiorly
    b. Quadratus lumborum–inferiorly
    c. Spinal processes–medially
    d. Iliac crest–inferiorly
    e. Line between anterior superior iliac spine (ASIS) and costal margin–laterally

14. Which superficial muscles are NOT encountered during a dorsal lumbotomy approach?
    a. Internal oblique
    b. External oblique
    c. Latissimus dorsi
    d. Sacrospinalis
    e. Quadratus lumborom

ANSWERS

1. **d. Patient with multiple comorbidities.** With an aging and more complex population, having multiple comorbidities on its own is not an indication for open surgery compared to minimally invasive surgery. Answers a, b, c, and e are all considered relative indications for open surgery. Patients with multiple previous abdominal procedures are more likely to have adhesions and difficulties establishing a pneumoperitoneum. Complicated renal tumors with caval thrombi, although possible to do laparoscopically, should be considered for open surgery. A large abdominal wall mesh could significantly complicate a minimally invasive approach, and surgeon skill and preference is another important consideration for an open approach.

2. **b. Complete midline incision.** Trauma nephrectomies should always be approached with a laparotomy or complete midline incision. The other approaches would not be appropriate in this clinical setting.

3. **a. Rapidly absorbable suture, running continuous closure.** In a 2002 meta-analysis of closure techniques for midline abdominal incisions, Riet et al. found that continuous rapidly absorbable sutures had significantly more incisional hernias than slowly absorbable or non-absorbable sutures. No difference in hernia rates between slowly absorbable and non-absorbable sutures. (Reference: van 't Riet M, Steyerberg EW, Nellensteyn J, Bonjer HJ, Jeekel J: Meta-analysis of techniques for closure of midline abdominal incisions. *Br J Surg* 89:1350–1356, 2002.)

4. **c. Pfannenstiel incision; lower morbidity and incisional hernia rates.** A prospective study comparing Pfannenstiel incision versus port site expansion for nephrectomies showed that morbidity and length of stay were shorter in the pfannensteil group, while a meta-analysis for extractions in laparoscopic bowel surgery showed lower hernia rates with pfannensteil. (References: Binsaleh S, Madbouly K, Matsumoto ED, Kapoor A: a prospective randomized study of pfannenstiel versus expanded port site incision for intact specimen extraction in laparoscopic radical nephrectomy. *J Endourol* 29[8]:913–918, 2015; Lee L, Abou-Khalil M, Liberman S, Boutros M, Fried GM, Feldman LS: Incidence of incisional hernia in the specimen extraction site for laparoscopic colorectal surgery: systematic review and meta-analysis. *Surg Endosc* 31[12]:5083–5093, 2017)

5. **d. Gibson incision.** Renal transplants and renal allograft nephrectomies are performed through a traditional Gibson incision, which gives extraperitoneal access to the iliac vessels and bladder.

6. **b. Paramedian incision.** Paramedian incisions have been described as an extra-peritoneal approach to nephroureterectomies and pediatric bladder augmentations. They are lateral to the rectus and are rarely used due to risks of nerve injury and ventral hernias.

7. **d. Large incision.** The thoracoabdominal incision, although considered to be a large invasive incision, provides the added benefit of significantly improved exposure, ability to achieve early vascular control, and access to major vessels (including the IVC) and organs for advanced renal tumors.

8. **b. Internal oblique.** The muscle and fascial layers encountered in a traditional flank incision, from skin to abdomen, are the external oblique, internal oblique, and transversalis muscles.

9. **d. 9th rib supracostal.** True flank incisions include the 12th rib supracostal, 11th rib transcostal, and subcostal approaches. Going above this level is often in the context of a thoraco-abdominal incision rather than a true flank incision.

10. **d. Ilioinguinal nerve.** The ilioinguinal nerve runs in the inguinal canal alongside the spermatic cord and should be identified upon opening and closure of an inguinal incision above the inguinal ligament. The genital branch of the genitofemoral nerve is present with the cord structures but is not exposed in the inguinal canal. The other nerves listed do not run through the inguinal canal.

11. **c. Posterior lumbodorsal incision.** The first-ever planned nephrectomy was performed in 1870 through a posterior lumbodorsal incision by Simon. This incision had multiple benefits over other open approaches. These include lack of muscle or rib distortion, faster convalescence, and decreased intra-peritoneal complications.

12. **d. Better surgical exposure for vascular control.** The dorsal lumbotomy approach, although not as common now, did boast multiple advantages over subcostal or anterior abdominal approaches. These include faster convalescence, less pain, less musculoskeletal complications (flank bulge), decreased hospitalization, and less intra-peritoneal complications. The major disadvantage was limited surgical exposure to the renal hilum and vessels for vascular control.

13. **b. Quadratus lumborum–inferiorly.** The borders of the lumbodorsal region are the 12th rib superiorly, iliac crest inferiorly, spinous processes of vertebral columns medially, and a line between the ASIS (anterior superior iliac spine) and costal margin laterally. The incision is generally made directly over the quadratus lumborum, but it is not a border of this region.

14. **a. Internal oblique.** The superficial muscles encountered are the sacrospinalis (medially), latissimus dorsi (posteriorly), and external oblique (anteriorly). The incision is deepened through the lumbodorsal fascia where the sacrospinalis muscle is encountered and a "Y" should be made around it (Fig. 9.1). The incision is made directly over the quadratus lumborum muscle over the lateral part of the sacrospinalis muscle slightly obliquely toward the iliac crest or sacroiliac joint. The internal oblique muscle is not encountered during this incision.

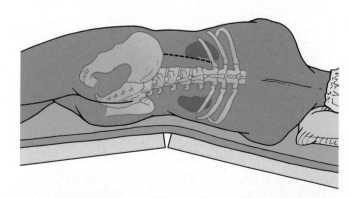

Fig. 9.1 Lumbodorsal incision. Once the iliac crest, the 12th rib, and the spinal processes have been located, the sacrospinalis muscle can be identified easily, and the surgeon can then locate the quadratus lumborum. This muscle goes from the medial part of the 12th rib to the middle third of the iliac crest; its upper third is under the sacrospinalis muscle. The skin incision is made over the quadratus lumborum muscle and begins at the costovertebral angle, over the lateral part of the sacrospinalis muscle, and with a slightly oblique course extends down to the iliac crest, 3 to 5 cm in front of the anterior margin of the sacrospinalis muscle. Modified from Pansadora V: Surgical atlas: the posterior lumbotomy, surgery illustrated. *BJU Int* 95:1121–1131, 2005.

CHAPTER REVIEW

1. There remain several indications for open surgical approaches in urology. Decisions regarding open versus minimally invasive approaches depend on complexity/size of pathology, patient preferences, and surgeon's skill set.

2. Knowledge of the abdominal wall musculature and anatomy are important to avoid key vessels and nerves when making incisions. These can usually be avoided by staying in the midline.

3. Anterior abdominal incisions can be used to access pelvic, intraperitoneal, retroperitoneal, and extraperitoneal structures. Urologists most commonly use a lower midline incision for access to the bladder and prostate.

4. There are many open approaches to the kidney, each with their own advantages and disadvantages. Usually the kidney is approached via anterior or flank incisions, however dorsal incisions were a traditional approach which are being explored again by some groups.

5. Dorsal lumbotomy incisions traditionally have some advantages over anterior abdominal incisions, but with current minimally invasive options, this incision is used far less commonly. The lumbodorsal region is bordered between the 12th rib superiorly, iliac crest inferiorly, spinous processes medially, and an imaginary line between the ASIS and costal margin laterally.

6. Inguinal incisions can be above or below the inguinal ligament depending on the indication. They give access to contents of the spermatic cord, testicle, and ilio-inguinal lymph nodes.

7. Adult circumcisions are commonly performed through a two-incision technique on either side of the prepuce.

8. Meticulous hemostasis is necessary for scrotal and penile incisions as one can have significant bruising and bleeding complications.

9. Perineal incisions might become more common for various pelvic procedures with the development of new robotic technology.

10. A complete midline incision (laparotomy incision) is used for trauma nephrectomies. Gibson incisions are used for transplants and transplant nephrectomies.

11. When closing abdominal fascia, one should not use rapidly absorbable sutures as these have been linked to higher hernia rates.

12. Pfannenstiel incisions are better for specimen extractions than extension of a port site during minimally invasive procedures.

13. Thoracoabdominal incisions are usually made above the 9th to 10th rib bed, although they can be modified through the 8th rib bed and combined with a subcostal incision along with the standard longitudinal abdominal incision. A chest tube is not always required unless a parietal pleural injury is suspected.

14. Penile fractures can be approached through a degloving technique or by directly incising onto the suspected injury if the region is confirmed with imaging.

15. With advancements in minimally invasive surgery and surgical technique, many incisions are being revisited for modern indications. These include lumbodorsal approach for partial nephrectomies and the perineal incision for robotic prostatectomies or cystectomies. Although the operative modality might have changed, all the incisions in this chapter should be known by urologists to have a plethora of options for any pathology.

Principles of Urologic Surgery: Intraoperative Technical Decisions

Manish A. Vira and Christopher J. Hartman

QUESTIONS

1. The most appropriate indication for blood product transfusion is:
   a. packed red blood cells for an 82-year-old male with coronary artery disease and hematocrit of 31%.
   b. fresh frozen plasma for a 69-year-old patient with an international normalized ratio (INR) of 1.6 scheduled to undergo laparotomy for a small bowel obstruction.
   c. platelet transfusion for a 78-year-old male with chronic renal insufficiency who was scheduled to undergo partial nephrectomy and found to have a platelet count of 55,000 on preoperative testing.
   d. packed red blood cells for a healthy 22-year-old male with a stable large retroperitoneal hematoma after motor vehicle accident and hematocrit of 21%.
   e. Fresh frozen plasma for a 64-year-old female during resection of a large renal mass with inferior vena cava thrombus who experiences significant blood loss requiring 4 U of packed red blood cell transfusion.

2. To reduce the risk of iatrogenic injury to a patient in the operating room, the patient should:
   a. be maintained with core body temperature between 36°C and 38°C throughout the perioperative period.
   b. be instructed to bathe with an antiseptic solution the night before surgery.
   c. be secured to the operating room table with fixed shoulder braces for procedures in steep Trendelenburg.
   d. be positioned in the lithotomy position one leg at a time to ensure safe flexion of the hips.
   e. be positioned and draped by the operating room staff before arrival of the surgeon.

3. In a patient undergoing an exploratory laparotomy for pelvic abscess following radical cystectomy, the best method of abdominal fascial closure is with:
   a. polyglycolic acid (Dexon) suture with continuous closure.
   b. silk suture with continuous closure.
   c. polypropylene (Prolene) suture with interrupted closure.
   d. polyglactin (Vicryl) suture with interrupted closure.
   e. polydioxanone suture (PDS) with continuous closure.

4. A patient undergoing an open radical cystectomy with ileal conduit urinary diversion has a platelet count of 78,000/mm^3 prior to the procedure. During the surgery, diffuse oozing of blood is noted in the pelvis after the bladder is removed. The least appropriate hemostatic agent to use would be:
   a. An oxidized regenerated cellulose agent (Fibrillar, Surgicel, Nu-Knit).
   b. Microfibrillar collagen (Avitene).
   c. A topical thrombin agent (Thrombin-JMI, Evithrom, Recothrom).
   d. A fibrin sealant (Tisseel, Evicel, Evarrest).
   e. A tissue adhesive (BioGlue).

5. A patient undergoing an open radical nephrectomy is noted to have a temperature of 35°C 3 hours into the procedure. Studies have demonstrated that this patient is at an increased risk of all of the following in the perioperative period except:
   a. increased bleeding.
   b. transfusion requirements.
   c. surgical site infection.
   d. prolonged hospital stay.
   e. renal insufficiency.

6. To avoid peripheral neuropathy during a robotic radical cystectomy in Trendelenburg position, the surgeon should make sure to:
   a. flex the patient's hips in lithotomy at no more than 70 degrees.
   b. abduct the patient's hips to between 45 and 55 degrees.
   c. pad the lateral knee to avoid excessive compression against the stirrups.
   d. tightly wrap the patient's arms at his or her side to prevent inadvertent crushing injuries from robotic arms.
   e. loosely secure the patient's shoulders to the table to avoid brachial plexus injury.

ANSWERS

1. **c. Platelet transfusion for a 78-year-old male with chronic renal insufficiency who was scheduled to undergo partial nephrectomy and found to have a platelet count of 55,000 on preoperative testing.** This patient has moderate thrombocytopenia with likely platelet dysfunction secondary to uremia undergoing a high-bleeding-risk procedure; therefore platelet transfusion is indicated. Current indications for packed red blood cell transfusion are maintenance of hematocrit of greater than 30% in patients with high risk of myocardial ischemia or in patients with hematocrit 21% to 30% with signs of inadequate oxygen-carrying capacity. Fresh frozen plasma transfusion is indicated only in the presence of active bleeding rather than isolated INR elevation or large-volume transfusion.

2. **a. Be maintained with core body temperature between 36°C and 38°C throughout the perioperative period.** Hypothermia by as little as 1°C has been shown to increase surgical site infection and postoperative complications. There is no evidence that showering with an antiseptic solution the night before surgery decreases the incidence of wound infection. Fixed shoulder braces have been associated with an increased risk of brachial plexus injury and should not be used in the operating room. Both legs should be positioned simultaneously when placing patients in the dorsal lithotomy position. Everyone in the operating room is responsible for patient safety, and therefore the surgeon should always be present for patient positioning.

3. **e. Polydioxanone suture (PDS) with continuous closure.** Continuous closure with PDS (slowly absorbable) suture has been shown to have the lowest wound failure rates. In the presence of infection, braided sutures (silk and Vicryl) should be avoided to prevent secondary wound infection and failure. Although nonabsorbable sutures may be used, these have been associated with increased postoperative patient discomfort. Fast-absorbing sutures (such as Dexon) should not be used in continuous fascial closure because of increased wound failure risks.
4. **b. Microfibrillar collagen (Avitene).** Microfibrillar collagen acts by enhancing platelet aggregation. Its efficacy is reduced in patients with thrombocytopenia and therefore may not stop bleeding in patients with thrombocytopenia as well as other hemostatic agents. Each of the other choices would be an acceptable hemostatic agent to use to in this case.
5. **e. Renal insufficiency.** Numerous studies have demonstrated that hypothermia may lead to complications and adverse effects in the perioperative period. Bleeding was found in one study to lead to an increased estimated blood loss of 16% and a 22% increase in transfusion requirements. In addition, hypothermia was associated with a threefold increased risk of wound infection and a 2.6-day increase in hospitalization. Renal insufficiency and other end-organ impairment have not been demonstrated in patients with minor degrees of hypothermia in the perioperative period.
6. **c. Pad the lateral knee to avoid excessive compression against the stirrups.** Numerous injuries leading to neuropathy can occur during prolonged surgery in the Trendelenburg position. Of particular concern is injury to the brachial plexus from improper shoulder positioning, radial nerve injury from prolonged pressure on the radial nerve, and lower extremity nerve injuries from improper positioning in lithotomy stirrups. In general, the hips should be flexed at 80 to 100 degrees with 30- to 45-degree abduction. Tightly wrapping the patient's arms at his or her side imposes the risk of injury to the radial nerve. Only loosely securing the patient's shoulders to the table may prevent brachial plexus injuries, but it also puts the patient at risk of a fall off the table during the course of the procedure.

CHAPTER REVIEW

1. The two primary reasons for hypothermia in the operating room are peripheral vasodilation that occurs with anesthetic agents and radiation of heat as the body interacts with the environment.
2. Normothermia is defined as a core temperature between 36°C and 38°C, and either hypothermia or hyperthermia may have adverse perioperative outcomes, including increased blood loss and increased incidence of surgical site infection.
3. Strategies to maintain normothermia include patient warming blankets, warmed intravenous and irrigation fluids, warmed CO_2 insufflation during laparoscopy, and an increase in ambient operating room temperature.
4. Commonly used skin antiseptic solutions for sterile skin preparation include alcohol, povidone-iodine, and chlorhexidine-based solutions, none of which has proven to be superior to the others in reducing SSI.
5. If hair is to be removed, it should preferably be removed immediately before the surgical procedure with clippers.
6. Three commonly occurring and preventable injuries in the operating room are retractor-associated injuries, thermal injuries, and patient position–related injuries.
7. Peripheral neuropathy may result from improper patient positioning and is often secondary to excessive stretch, prolonged compression, or ischemia of a nerve.
8. When positioning in lithotomy, care should be taken to manipulate both lower extremities simultaneously with flexion of the hips at 80 to 100 degrees with 30- to 45-degree abduction.
9. Current indications for packed red blood cell transfusion include hematocrit lower than 21%, maintenance of hematocrit of greater than 30% in patients with high risk of myocardial ischemia, or in patients with hematocrit 21% to 30% with signs of inadequate oxygen-carrying capacity.
10. Platelet transfusion may be beneficial in patients with severe thrombocytopenia ($<50,000/mm^3$) who are undergoing a planned surgical procedure, or in patients with moderate thrombocytopenia ($50,000/mm^3$ to $100,000/mm^3$) who are undergoing a high-risk procedure or have evidence of platelet dysfunction.
11. The indications for fresh frozen plasma are immediate reversal of warfarin, replacement of specific clotting factors, and evidence of bleeding in the setting of an INR greater than 1.5.
12. Adjunct hemostatic agents may be broadly classified as dry matrix agents or biologically active agents.
13. Oxidized regenerated cellulose agents (Fibrillar, Surgicel, Nu-Knit) aid in surgical hemostasis by activating the body's natural clotting cascade.
14. Topical thrombin agents (Thrombin-JMI, Evithrom, Recothrom) and the combination of thrombin sealants with a gelatin matrix (Floseal and Surgiflo) are not inhibited by urine and additionally resist stone formation within the urinary tract, making them advantageous hemostatic agents for use in urologic surgery.
15. Numerous studies have shown that surgical drains may not be of benefit in the perioperative period and may cause pain and lead to an increased risk of SSI; therefore the routine use of surgical drains is not recommended outside of specific indications to do so.
16. The surgical scar regains 3% of strength at 1 week, 20% at 3 weeks, and 80% at 3 months.
17. Nonabsorbable sutures should be avoided when contact with urine is anticipated, such as during urinary tract anastomosis, because this increases the risk of stone development.
18. The risk of incisional hernia formation is not increased between slowly absorbable and nonabsorbable suture material in continuous versus interrupted fascial closures, although closure with nonabsorbable suture material was associated with increased wound pain.
19. Rapidly absorbable sutures used for continuous fascia closure are associated with an increased incidence of incisional hernias.
20. Fascia dehiscence generally occurs 7 to 10 days postoperatively but may occur up to 30 days after surgery.
21. In the presence of infection, braided sutures (Vicryl, Mersilene) should be avoided for wound closure.
22. Using staples for skin closure as opposed to sutures has been shown to decrease incision closure time, reduce the risk of wound infection, and has resulted in nonsignificant differences in cosmetic outcomes and patient satisfaction with wound appearance.

11 Lower Urinary Tract Catheterization

Joseph M. Jacob and Chandru P. Sundaram

QUESTIONS

1. The male urethra is ___ cm long.
   a. 15
   b. 13
   c. 24
   d. 20

2. The anterior male urethra is surrounded by ____
   a. the bulbospongiosus muscle.
   b. corpus spongiosum.
   c. both a and b.
   d. none of the above.

3. The female urethra is approximately ____ cm long
   a. 4
   b. 6
   c. 8
   d. 10

4. A 16-Fr catheter is approximately ____ cm in outer diameter.
   a. 16
   b. 10.4
   c. 8.7
   d. 5.3

5. _____ is the most rigid catheter material.
   a. Latex
   b. Silicone
   c. Polyvinylchloride (PVC)
   d. None of the above

6. Suprapubic catheter placement with a guide wire is the _____ technique.
   a. cystotomy
   b. Seldinger
   c. Lowsley
   d. trocar

7. The most common cause of inability to catheterize an Indiana pouch is ____.
   a. perforation
   b. catheter malfunction
   c. overdistension
   d. none of the above

8. A urostomy should never be catheterized.
   a. T
   b. F

9. Patients after bladder neck reconstruction should never be catheterized per urethra.
   a. T
   b. F

10. Catheter-associated urinary tract infection is the most common type of health care–associated infection
    a. T
    b. F

11. The incidence of bladder cancer in spinal cord patients with chronic catheters is _____.
    a. 1%
    b. 2%
    c. 3%
    d. 4%
    e. 6%

ANSWERS

1. **d. 20.** The male urethra is 18 to 20 cm. The anterior urethra is 16 cm.
2. **c. Both a and b.** The anterior male urethra is surrounded by both corpus spongiosum and bulbospongiosus muscle at the bulbar urethra.
3. **a. 4.** The female urethra is approximately 4 cm long
4. **d. 5.3.** To calculate French size approximately, divide by 3.
5. **a. Latex.** Rigidity from least to greatest: latex, silicone, PVC. This is important to understand, and different catheter materials may be more appropriate for different clinical situations.
6. **b. Seldinger.** The Seldinger technique involves gaining access into the bladder with a 21-gauge needle. I wire is placed once urine return is identified. Various catheters or kits can be used to place a catheter over the wire. The Lowsley retractor is a modified male urethral sound that can be used to place a suprapubic catheter. There are trocars that can be placed under vision with a cystoscope that can accommodate a catheter once the inner section is removed and the sheath left in place.
7. **c. Overdistension.** Overdistension is the most common reason for catheterization difficulty. If the catheter is forced, a perforation in the channel will be likely. A 21-gauge needle can be placed into the reservoir. After drainage, a catheter will usually pass without difficulty.
8. **b. F.** Catheterizing a urostomy gently can be performed without risk. Occasionally, catheterizing the stoma may be therapeutic in cases such as stomal stenosis or parastomal hernia.
9. **a. T.** A history of bladder neck reconstruction is one of the few contraindications to urethral catheterization.
10. **a. T.** Unfortunately, this is true based on a Centers for Disease Control and Prevention report. Decreasing catheter use should decrease the hospital-acquired infection rates.
11. **a. 1%.** There are retrospective studies that do show what appears to be an increased risk of bladder cancer. Some recommend surveillance after 8 years of chronic catheterization.

CHAPTER REVIEW

1. There are many indications for urethral catheterization and many sizes and types of catheters that can be used.
2. As the French size increases, the diameter of the catheter lumen increases.
3. Catheter rigidity will vary by material.
4. Three-way hematuria catheters should be used if clot retention is suspect.
5. The urologist should be prepared to attain lower urinary drainage in almost all situations.
6. The clinician should closely review the patient's history and prior operative reports prior to instrumenting the lower urinary tract.
7. If benign prostatic hyperplasia (BPH) is expected, the practitioner should use an 18-Fr Coudé catheter for lower urinary tract drainage.
8. A history of bladder neck repair or closure are a contraindication to urethral catheterization.
9. Catheter placement should be avoided in patients with an artificial urinary sphincter (AUS). A 12-Fr catheter should be used after deactivation of the sphincter if necessary.
10. Catheter-associated urinary tract infections are the most common hospital-acquired infection.
11. Catheters may lead to trauma, stricture, and erosion.
12. Chronic catheterization can lead to bladder inflammation and increase the risk of bladder cancer.

12 Fundamentals of Upper Urinary Tract Drainage

Casey A. Dauw and J. Stuart Wolf, Jr.

QUESTIONS

1. Percutaneous nephrostomy is not indicated for:
   a. instillation of intracavitary topical therapy for urothelial carcinoma.
   b. Whitaker test.
   c. management of fungal bezoars.
   d. urinary retention.
   e. ureteral injury.

2. Relative to retrograde ureteral stent placement, percutaneous nephrostomy:
   a. has a lower success rate.
   b. requires less anesthesia.
   c. is preferred in cases of ureteral obstruction owing to malignancy.
   d. is less commonly complicated by bacteriuria after indwelling for 1 week.
   e. is associated with worse health-related quality-of-life scores.

3. Which of the following is correct regarding the orientation of the kidney?
   a. The right kidney is slightly cephalad to the left kidney.
   b. The longitudinal axis is 45 degrees from vertical, with the lower pole lateral to the upper pole.
   c. The longitudinal axis is 45 degrees from vertical, with the lower pole anterior to the upper pole.
   d. The apposition of the colon to the kidney is greatest on the left side at the upper pole.
   e. Immediately posterior to the kidneys are the quadratus lumborum muscle, the psoas muscle, and the diaphragm.

4. Which of the following is correct regarding the intrarenal collecting system?
   a. Paired anterior and posterior calyces enter the infundibula approximately 90 degrees from each other.
   b. Compound calyces are most common in the lower pole
   c. Most kidneys have three distinct infundibula: the upper, middle, and lower.
   d. There are 8 to 16 minor calyces.
   e. There is a consistent relationship between anterior and posterior calyces and their medial-lateral position on anterior-posterior radiography.

5. The correct order of the division of the intrarenal branches of the renal artery is:
   a. segmental, arcuate, interlobar (infundibular), interlobular.
   b. segmental, arcuate, interlobular, interlobar (infundibular).
   c. segmental, interlobar (infundibular), arcuate, interlobular.
   d. interlobular, segmental, interlobar (infundibular), arcuate.
   e. segmental, interlobular, interlobar (infundibular), arcuate.

6. To reduce the risk of infectious complications from percutaneous renal surgery:
   a. all patients should receive prophylactic antimicrobials.
   b. urine cultures should be obtained on all patients.
   c. urine must be sterile before the procedure.
   d. gentamicin is an acceptable single agent for antimicrobial prophylaxis.
   e. ampicillin/sulbactam is not an acceptable single agent for antimicrobial prophylaxis.

7. To reduce the risk of hemorrhagic complications associated with percutaneous renal access, the minimum recommended preoperative cessation period for:
   a. herbal medications is 2 weeks.
   b. clopidogrel is 10 days.
   c. aspirin is 5 days.
   d. warfarin is 5 days.
   e. nonsteroidal inflammatory agents is 1 day.

8. Which of the following have NOT been demonstrated in randomized controlled clinical trials to reduce pain associated with percutaneous renal access?
   a. Tract infiltration with local anesthetic
   b. Intercostal nerve block
   c. Thoracic paravertebral block
   d. Balloon dilation compared with semirigid plastic dilation of the access tract
   e. Smaller, compared with larger, caliber postprocedure nephrostomy tubes

9. An advantage of the supine versus prone position for percutaneous renal surgery is:
   a. improved pulmonary mechanics.
   b. a large horizontal working surface.
   c. easier entry into upper pole calyces.
   d. easier entry into posterior calyces.
   e. reduced pressure in the collecting system.

10. Access into which site provides the optimal versatility and safety for percutaneous renal surgery in the prone position?
    a. Upper pole posterior calyx
    b. Upper pole infundibulum
    c. Renal pelvis
    d. Middle calyx
    e. Lower pole anterior calyx

11. Techniques for retrograde assistance for percutaneous renal access include all but which of the following?
    a. Straight ureteral catheter to inject air
    b. Ureteral access sheath to facilitate drainage

c. Ureteroscopy to retrieve guidewire

d. Retrograde approach to percutaneous access

e. Retrograde placement of externalized (single pigtail) ureteral stent for drainage

12. Compared with an 18-gauge needle, the 21-gauge needle for percutaneous renal access:

a. should not be used by inexperienced operators.

b. requires a 0.025-inch guidewire.

c. cannot be directed as easily.

d. entails less risk of loss of access.

e. is more traumatic.

13. Compared with ultrasonography, fluoroscopy for percutaneous renal access:

a. is less suited in the morbidly obese.

b. provides more rapid evaluation of the entire kidney.

c. cannot be used to monitor tract dilation.

d. visualizes the access needle better.

e. is preferred in transplant kidneys.

14. The "triangulation" technique for fluoroscopic percutaneous renal access:

a. increases radiation exposure to the operator's hands compared with the "eye-of-the-needle" technique.

b. cannot be performed in malrotated kidneys.

c. is not as dependent on retrograde assistance as the "eye-of-the-needle" technique.

d. is less suitable than the "eye-of-the-needle" technique in morbidly obese patients.

e. continuously monitors depth of needle penetration.

15. Dilation of the tract for percutaneous renal surgery is:

a. not effective with a balloon dilator in hypermobile kidneys.

b. most effective with semirigid dilator.

c. least expensive with metal dilators.

d. most rapid with metal dilators.

e. easiest with a one-shot semirigid dilator.

16. When considering percutaneous renal surgery in horseshoe kidneys:

a. upper pole access is dangerous.

b. lower pole access is preferred in most cases.

c. computed tomography can be misleading.

d. the puncture site is more lateral than in normal kidneys.

e. lower hemorrhage rates than in normal kidneys can be expected.

17. When considering percutaneous renal surgery in transplant kidneys:

a. retrograde assistance is difficult.

b. fluoroscopy is more useful than ultrasonography for initial access.

c. the typical hypermobility renders tract dilation difficult.

d. semirigid plastic dilators should not be used.

e. secondary procedures are usually required.

18. Foley catheters for postprocedure nephrostomy drainage:

a. do not need to be secured at the skin.

b. can have a ureteral catheter passed through the end.

c. should have the balloon filled with dilute contrast material.

d. stay more securely in the kidney than Malecot catheters.

e. are less likely to become infected than Malecot catheters.

19. The Cope retention mechanism:

a. is used in nephroureteral stents.

b. is used in internal ureteral stents.

c. is more secure than a balloon catheter.

d. requires cutting the tube to disengage.

e. should not be used in more than one access site.

20. Alternatives to a nephrostomy tube after percutaneous renal surgery include all EXCEPT:

a. maintenance of the working sheath.

b. an internal ureteral stent that is removed cystoscopically.

c. an internal ureteral stent with an attached string that exits out the flank.

d. a ureteral stent externalized out the urethra.

e. no drainage tube at all.

21. A postoperative nephrostomy tube:

a. offers greater assurance of upper urinary tract drainage than an internal ureteral stent.

b. should be placed in the dilated access site.

c. does not maintain the percutaneous access tract unless >18 Fr.

d. reduces postoperative bleeding.

e. is associated with pain unrelated to tube diameter.

22. A small-caliber (8 to 18 Fr) compared with a large-caliber (20 to 24 Fr) nephrostomy tube after percutaneous renal surgery is associated with:

a. equivalent pain.

b. more urinary leakage.

c. less postprocedure blood loss.

d. less need for removal in the radiology suite.

e. earlier hospital discharge.

23. Adjuncts intended to enhance hemostasis of the percutaneous tract include all EXCEPT:

a. direct cauterization of the tract.

b. microwave treatment of the tract.

c. cryotreatment of the tract.

d. insertion of oxidized cellulose.

e. instillation of fibrin glue.

24. Compared with internal ureteral stents after percutaneous renal surgery, nephrostomy tubes are associated with:

a. reduced need for a second procedure for removal.

b. greater technical success rate.

c. greater narcotic use.

d. fewer complications.

e. less urinary leakage from skin entry site.

25. Following an unremarkable percutaneous nephrolithotomy, there is nonpulsatile bleeding from the tract when the sheath is removed around a 12-Fr nephrostomy tube. The next step is:

a. replace the nephrostomy tube with an 18-Fr Malecot catheter.

b. replace the nephrostomy tube with a ureteral stent and suture the skin.

c. irrigate the nephrostomy tube.

d. occlude the nephrostomy tube and apply pressure to the incision.

e. replace the nephrostomy tube with a Kaye nephrostomy tamponade balloon.

26. During a percutaneous resection of a 2-cm upper pole urothelial neoplasm, there is sudden hemorrhage from the resection site. The next step is:
    a. continue with the procedure if vision is adequate.
    b. insert a percutaneous nephroureteral stent.
    c. instill gelatin granules plus thrombin into the collecting system.
    d. place an 18-Fr Councill catheter with the balloon inflated at the injury site.
    e. prepare the patient for selective angioembolization.

27. A 65-year-old man calls the office 1 week after percutaneous nephrolithotomy complaining of bright red blood in the urine on his last two urinations. He is otherwise feeling well. He should next:
    a. check the percutaneous access site and come to the hospital if there is external bleeding.
    b. force fluids and call back if bleeding persists.
    c. take aminocaproic acid (Amicar).
    d. apply pressure to the percutaneous access site.
    e. come to the hospital.

28. Which of the following has NOT been reported to cause renal pelvic perforation in association with percutaneous renal surgery?
    a. Wire passage
    b. Tract dilation
    c. Massive hemorrhage
    d. Use of resectoscope
    e. Ultrasonic lithotripsy

29. Two days after percutaneous endopyelotomy in a 65-year-old woman, nephrostography reveals contrast entering the colon. The next step is to:
    a. perform exploratory laparotomy.
    b. maintain the nephrostomy tube in place and insert a ureteral stent.
    c. maintain the nephrostomy tube in place and insert a colostomy tube.
    d. back out the nephrostomy tube into the colon and insert a new nephrostomy tube.
    e. start parenteral feeding, after appropriate tube insertions.

30. Injury to which organ during percutaneous renal surgery can often be managed with little additional interventions?
    a. Liver
    b. Spleen
    c. Duodenum
    d. Jejunum
    e. Gallbladder

31. Regarding pleural injuries in association with percutaneous renal surgery:
    a. access below the 12th rib results in hydropneumothorax in 1% to 2% of cases.
    b. supra-12th rib punctures (the 11th intercostal space) result in hydropneumothorax in 20% to 40% of cases.
    c. supra-11th rib punctures (the 10th intercostal space) result in hydropneumothorax in 50% to 75% of cases.
    d. combined with distal ureteral obstruction, a nephropleural fistula can occur.
    e. thoracostomy to water seal drainage and suction is recommended.

32. Irrigation fluid during percutaneous renal surgery:
    a. is not absorbed systemically unless there is significant venous injury.
    b. should be normal saline except during percutaneous nephrolithotomy.
    c. can have fatal consequences.
    d. should not be glycine.
    e. will not create a defined extrarenal collection.

33. A 55-year-old woman has an oral temperature of 38.5°C on the first night after an uncomplicated percutaneous nephrolithotomy for a partial staghorn renal calculus. A nephrostomy tube is in place. She is hemodynamically stable. The preoperative urine culture had grown a pansensitive *Proteus* sp., and she had received oral trimethoprim sulfamethoxazole for 2 weeks preoperatively. One gram of cefazolin had been administered on call to the operating room. The next step is:
    a. observation.
    b. culture aspirate from nephrostomy tube and irrigate nephrostomy tube.
    c. Doppler ultrasonography of lower extremities and/or pulmonary embolus-protocol computed tomography scan.
    d. administer broad-spectrum antibiotics.
    e. culture urine and blood, obtain chest radiograph, and administer broad-spectrum antibiotics.

34. Following percutaneous renal surgery, loss of renal function is:
    a. approximately 5% of ipsilateral function per access site.
    b. minimal in the absence of vascular injury.
    c. greater than after shock wave lithotripsy.
    d. less in pelvic compared with orthotopic kidneys.
    e. greater in solitary compared with nonsolitary kidneys.

35. With regard to ureteral stents, which factors have been associated with improved patient tolerance?
    a. Ureteral stent length
    b. Ureteral stent diameter
    c. Stent material
    d. Distal stent tip architecture (pigtail vs. Polaris)
    e. None of the above

ANSWERS

1. **d. Urinary retention.** Obstruction of the lower urinary tract is best treated by drainage of the bladder rather than the kidney, unless secondary obstruction of the upper tract has developed that is refractory to vesical drainage. The other indications are appropriate ones for percutaneous nephrostomy.
2. **b. Requires less anesthesia.** Percutaneous nephrostomy can be done under local anesthesia, as opposed to retrograde ureteral stent placement, which usually requires at least intravenous sedation, and commonly general or regional anesthesia. Percutaneous nephrostomy has a greater initial success rate than retrograde ureteral stent placement, at least when the collecting system is dilated. Percutaneous nephrostomy is commonly associated with bacteriuria and has health-related quality-of-life scores that are equivalent to those associated with retrograde ureteral stent placement. Ureteral stents provide satisfactory drainage in most cases of ureteral obstruction owing to malignancy.
3. **e. Immediately posterior to the kidneys are the quadratus lumborum muscle, the psoas muscle, and the diaphragm.** The upper poles are anterior to attachments of the diaphragm. It is the left kidney that is slightly cephalad to the right one.

The second two statements are correct, except that the angulation is 30 degrees rather than 45 degrees. The apposition of the colon to the kidney varies with location; it is greatest on the left side but at the lower rather than upper pole.

4. **a. Paired anterior and posterior calyces enter the infundibula approximately 90 degrees from each other.** The paired anterior and posterior calyces enter approximately 90 degrees from each other. Although compound calyces are common in the lower pole, they are almost always present in the upper pole. In approximately two-thirds of kidneys, there are only two major calyceal systems (upper and lower). There are 5 to 14 minor calyces in each kidney. Because variation is considerable, the lateral-medial orientation of the calyces on anteroposterior radiography cannot be used to reliably determine which calyces are posterior.

5. **c. Segmental, interlobar (infundibular), arcuate, interlobular.**

6. **a. All patients should receive prophylactic antimicrobials.** The American Urological Association recommends periprocedural antimicrobial prophylaxis for all cases of percutaneous renal surgery. Urine cultures are considered standard only in patients where bacteriuria is likely; in other cases a screening urinalysis likely is adequate, with urine culture when the urinalysis is suspicious. The urine cannot be sterilized in some patients, especially in the presence of an externalized urinary catheter or an infected calculus, and the goal in these situations is only to suppress the bacterial count before intervention. Aminoglycosides (e.g., gentamicin) are acceptable for antimicrobial prophylaxis when combined with another agent. Ampicillin/sulbactam, first- and second-generation cephalosporins, and fluoroquinolones are acceptable single agents for antimicrobial prophylaxis.

7. **d. Warfarin is 5 days.** The recommended preoperative cessation periods are as follows: herbal medicines, 1 week; clopidogrel, 5 days; aspirin, 1 week; warfarin, 5 days; nonsteroidal inflammatory agents, 3 to 7 days.

8. **d. Balloon dilation compared with semirigid plastic dilation of the access tract.** There is no evidence that balloon dilation is associated with less pain compared with semirigid plastic dilation of the access tract. All of the other maneuvers have been demonstrated in randomized controlled clinical trials to reduce pain associated with percutaneous renal access.

9. **e. Reduced pressure in the collecting system.** The angle of the sheath is more horizontal in the supine compared with the prone position for percutaneous renal surgery, which reduces pressure in the collecting system (the volume also is reduced, which is a disadvantage). When padding is appropriate, pulmonary mechanics are better in the prone position. The prone position also provides a large horizontal working surface and easier entry into posterior and upper pole calyces compared to the supine position.

10. **a. Upper pole posterior calyx.** This offers the most versatile access to the intrarenal collecting system, and as long as the entry is below the 11th rib, the advantages generally outweigh the risks. Percutaneous access into an infundibulum or the renal pelvis poses a greater risk of vascular injury than calyceal entry. Middle calyceal access provides good access to the ureter but usually does not provide good access to the upper and lower calyces. In the prone position an anterior calyx offers little access to the rest of the kidney.

11. **e. Retrograde placement of externalized (single pigtail) ureteral stent for drainage.** This can be performed at the conclusion of the procedure for drainage as an alternative to a nephrostomy tube, but it is not useful before access because the pigtail might interfere with the procedure and it would not have any advantage over a straight ureteral catheter or an occlusion balloon catheter. The other choices are all well-described techniques of retrograde assistance for percutaneous renal access.

12. **e. Is more traumatic.** A 21-gauge needle is not as easy to direct as an 18-gauge needle because it is more flexible. A 21-gauge needle requires a 0.018-inch guidewire, and because of this extra step (exchanging the 0.018-inch guidewire for a 0.035-inch guidewire) there is a greater risk of loss of access. Compared with an 18-gauge needle, the 21-gauge needle is less traumatic; this is its primary advantage, and it is for this reason that the 21-gauge needle should be used when the operator is less experienced or if minimizing trauma is paramount.

13. **d. Visualizes the access needle better.** It is easier to see a needle and monitor tract dilation with fluoroscopy than with ultrasonography. Percutaneous access is always more difficult in the morbidly obese, and ultrasonography is no better than fluoroscopy in this situation. Ultrasonography is more portable, can more rapidly evaluate different views of the kidney, and is preferred in settings in which retrograde access cannot be attained or is difficult to attain (kidneys above urinary diversions, transplanted kidneys, kidneys above a completely obstructed ureter, etc.).

14. **e. Continuously monitors depth of needle penetration.** The "triangulation" technique monitors depth of needle placement in all fluoroscopic views, whereas the "eye-of-the-needle" technique assesses depth only at the final step. If the fluoroscopy field is collimated down and the needle is held with a hemostat, sponge forceps, or purpose-built needle holder, then radiation exposure to the operator's hands can be avoided with both techniques. Retrograde assistance is useful with any fluoroscopic percutaneous renal access, and both techniques are more difficult in morbidly obese patients.

15. **c. Least expensive with metal dilators.** Metal dilators are least expensive on a per-case basis because they are reusable. The metal dilators are also the most effective dilators. It is uncertain which are the safest dilators, at least in terms of association with hemorrhage. The balloon dilators are more effective in hypermobile kidneys than other techniques and also more rapid than sequential passage of metal or semirigid dilators. The one-shot semirigid dilator technique requires considerable manual force to create the tract.

16. **e. Lower hemorrhage rates than in normal kidneys can be expected.** The rate of major hemorrhagic complications during percutaneous renal surgery in horseshoe kidneys (4.3%) is less than in normal kidneys (6% to 20%). Upper pole access is useful, and direct lower pole access is usually not possible. Cross-sectional imaging is useful in assessing the anatomy of horseshoe kidneys. The initial entry into a horseshoe kidney usually is more medial than in normal kidneys.

17. **a. Retrograde assistance is difficult.** Because of the site of ureteral implantation in the bladder, retrograde assistance for percutaneous renal surgery in transplant kidneys is difficult. Given this, ultrasonography is more useful than fluoroscopy for guiding initial access. Semirigid plastic and metal dilators are often more useful than balloon dilators because of the perinephric scarring, which makes the transplant kidney quite fixed in place rather than hypermobile. Despite the challenges, percutaneous renal surgery in transplant kidneys has a high success rate, and secondary procedures are usually not required.

18. **d. Stay more securely in the kidney than Malecot catheters.** Malecot tubes are the easiest to pull out, and circle nephrostomy tubes are the hardest. All tubes should be secured at the skin to reduce the risk of at least one mechanism of tube removal. A ureteral catheter can be passed through the end hole of a Councill catheter; a Foley catheter does not have this end hole. Saline or water should be used to inflate the balloon, because the more viscous contrast material might hinder emptying of the balloon when removal is attempted. All nephrostomy tubes, even ones with robust internal retention devices, should be fixed to the skin externally with a suture or other mechanism. There is no evidence that Foley and Malecot catheters differ in propensity for infection.

19. **a. Is used in nephroureteral stents.** The Cope retention mechanism is used in the renal pelvic portion of nephroureteral stents. According to one study, the Cope retention mechanism

is more secure than Malecot wings but does not retain as well as a balloon. It is more secure than a passive pigtail retention mechanism owing to the string that holds the coil in place. There is no evidence that more than one Cope-type nephrostomy tube should not be used.

20. **a. Maintenance of the working sheath.** The stiff working access sheath would be a poor choice for postprocedure collecting system drainage. All of the other options have been described.

21. **a. Offers greater assurance of upper urinary tract drainage than an internal ureteral stent.** Drainage of upper urinary tract after percutaneous renal surgery is adequate with an internal ureteral stent in most cases (or with no tube at all in selected cases), but when hemorrhage occurs, the larger caliber of a nephrostomy tube provides better drainage of the upper urinary tract collecting system than an internal ureteral stent. The nephrostomy tube does not have to be placed in the dilated access site (i.e., it can be placed at a new site), although that is common practice. Although redilation may be required, any external nephrostomy tube maintains the percutaneous access tract. There is actually less hemorrhage when a postoperative nephrostomy tube is omitted. Most studies suggest that the pain associated with nephrostomy tubes is related to tube diameter, with smaller-caliber tubes causing less pain.

22. **d. Less need for removal in the radiology suite.** The removal of larger tubes occasionally can be followed by immediate hemorrhage; this is rare with smaller tubes. Therefore large-caliber nephrostomy tubes should be removed in a radiology suite where there is the opportunity for immediate replacement of the tube. Small-caliber tubes can be removed safely at the bedside after a period of clamping to assess clinically for distal ureteral obstruction. A number of studies have compared the impact of nephrostomy tube diameter after percutaneous renal surgery. Only one study found no benefit to the smaller tube. Otherwise, consistent advantages of the small-caliber tubes were less pain, less urinary leakage, and no change in postprocedure blood loss. There is no consistent evidence that small-caliber tubes are associated with shorter duration of hospitalization compared with large-caliber tubes.

23. **b. Microwave treatment of the tract.** Microwave treatment of the tract would be difficult with current instruments. The other options have all been described. Other hemostatic agents that have been inserted/instilled into the tract include gelatin sponge and gelatin granules plus thrombin.

24. **c. Greater narcotic use.** Most randomized controlled trials comparing internal ureteral stents to large-caliber nephrostomy tubes after percutaneous renal surgery have shown reduced narcotic use in the stented patients. The difference is less significant when a small-caliber nephrostomy tube is used. Depending on physician preference, both internal ureteral stents (if attached to a string that exits via the flank) and small-caliber nephrostomy tubes can be removed at the bedside. Randomized controlled trials comparing internal ureteral stents to nephrostomy tubes have not revealed any difference in technical success rates, complication rates, or incidence of urinary leakage from the skin entry site.

25. **d. Occlude the nephrostomy tube and apply pressure to the incision.** The first step in this situation is to occlude the nephrostomy tube and apply pressure to the incision. Let the collecting system clot off, and do not irrigate until the following morning. This management is successful in the majority of cases. If bleeding persists, then insert a Kaye nephrostomy tamponade balloon. An 18-Fr Malecot catheter will be no more effective than the 12-Fr Cope nephrostomy tube. Irrigation is not useful, and removing the nephrostomy tube altogether is ill advised.

26. **a. Continue with the procedure if vision is adequate.** If the procedure can be continued with acceptable vision, then the blood loss cannot be great. However, if vision is lost, then the procedure must be aborted. If so, then inserting and occluding

a nephrostomy tube, as well as applying pressure to the incision so that the collecting system clots off, will suffice in most cases. If this is not successful, then place a Councill catheter and attempt to inflate the balloon at the injury site. Instillation of gelatin granules plus thrombin into the collecting system can create a clot that is difficult to manage. Selective angioembolization is required only when an arterial injury does not respond to less intensive management, or if the injury is obviously a significant one that will not respond to these maneuvers.

27. **e. Come to the hospital.** Any report of bright red blood in the urine after percutaneous renal surgery should prompt hospital admission. This man likely has an arteriovenous fistula or arterial pseudoaneurysm. The conservative measures are not likely to be helpful, and aminocaproic acid (Amicar) is contraindicated in the setting of upper tract hemorrhage.

28. **c. Massive hemorrhage.** The renal pelvis will clot off before the pressure from hemorrhage would rupture it. Any manipulation during percutaneous renal surgery can cause renal pelvic perforation.

29. **d. Back out the nephrostomy tube into the colon and insert a new nephrostomy tube.** The main principle of care of a colon injury associated with percutaneous renal surgery is prompt and separate drainage of the colon and urinary collecting system. If detected postoperatively, the simplest management is to back the nephrostomy tube out of the kidney and into the colon to serve as a colostomy, and then obtain separate access to the upper urinary tract, with either a new percutaneous access that does not traverse the colon or a retrograde-placed ureteral stent. Parenteral feeding is usually not required, and for the typical extraperitoneal injury, open surgical repair usually is needed only if the patient develops peritonitis or sepsis.

30. **a. Liver.** Although splenic injuries have been managed conservatively, the need for surgical intervention is more likely than with liver injuries. Injuries to small bowel or the biliary system require prompt treatment.

31. **d. Combined with distal ureteral obstruction, a nephropleural fistula can occur.** Nephropleural fistula (urinothorax) is a direct and persistent communication between the intrarenal collecting system and the intrathoracic cavity, which can follow percutaneous renal access of the upper urinary tract in the setting of pleural transgression. Some degree of distal ureteral obstruction usually contributes to the problem. The rates of pleural injures for infra-12th rib, supra-12th rib, and supra-11th rib punctures are approximately less than 0.5%, 5%, and 25%, respectively. Thoracostomy is not necessary for all patients with hydrothorax. If one is needed, then a small-caliber tube with a Heimlich valve is all that is required in the absence of lung injury.

32. **c. Can have fatal consequences.** Intravascular hemolysis from the extravasated water irrigant can be fatal. The irrigant for percutaneous renal surgery should be saline, with the exception of glycine or similar nonelectrolytic isotonic fluids when monopolar electrocautery is used. Intravascular or extravascular extravasation of fluid from continued irrigation in the setting of a large venous injury or collecting system perforation can lead to clinically significant sequelae including volume overload and extrarenal fluid collections that require drainage.

33. **a. Observation.** Preoperative and perioperative management of this patient has been appropriate. In this setting, most patients with fever after percutaneous nephrolithotomy do not have infection. If the fever is an isolated postoperative one, then standard postoperative care (early ambulation, use of incentive spirometry, etc.) is all that is needed. If the fever does not resolve promptly, then appropriate diagnostic evaluation and initiation of antimicrobial therapy and other supportive care are indicated.

34. **b. Minimal in the absence of vascular injury.** The kidney suffers little permanent damage after uncomplicated percutaneous renal surgery. If there is significant loss of function, it is usually owing to disastrous vascular injury or the

angioembolization used to treat hemorrhage. Loss of renal function associated with percutaneous renal surgery is less than or equal to the loss associated with shock wave lithotripsy. There is no evidence that damage to the kidney is any more or less in pelvic, orthotopic, solitary, or nonsolitary kidneys.

35. **e. None of the above.** Randomized controlled trials have failed to show association between stent length, diameter, material, or architecture and impact on patient tolerability.

CHAPTER REVIEW

1. Percutaneous nephrostomy and retrograde ureteral stents are generally equivalent in their capacity to resolve fever in patients with upper urinary tract obstruction. However, obstruction complicated by infection is an emergency, and in the unstable patient, percutaneous drainage may be more efficacious.
2. The colon can be lateral or posterior to the right and left kidney.
3. A guidewire that enters the kidney percutaneously and exits the urethra via the meatus (through and through access) may be the only guidewire used when operating on the upper urinary tract. However, in all other situations, two guidewires—a safety and a working guidewire—are required. No matter what the access, it is always prudent to have a safety guidewire in addition to the working guidewire.
4. It is imperative that the dilators do not pass too far into the collecting system because this results in renal pelvic injury.
5. Percutaneous nephrostomy is generally the preferred approach for endoscopy of the obstructed collecting system in the transplanted kidney.
6. Approximately 1% of percutaneous procedures are complicated by delayed hemorrhage. Delayed hemorrhage is usually due to arteriovenous fistulas or arterial pseudoaneurysms. The preferred management is selective angioembolization.
7. Renal arteries are end arteries and result in loss of the segment of renal parenchyma they supply when occluded. Renal veins communicate with each other.
8. Complications of percutaneous nephrostomy include hemorrhage, collecting system injury, colon injury, pleural injury, neuromuscular injuries, air embolism, and infundibular stenosis.
9. Although compound calyces are common in the lower pole, they are almost always present in the upper pole.
10. The recommended preoperative cessation periods are as follows: herbal medicines, 1 week; clopidogrel, 5 days; aspirin, 1 week; warfarin, 5 days; nonsteroidal inflammatory agents, 3 to 7 days.
11. The main principle of care of a colon injury associated with percutaneous renal surgery is prompt and separate drainage of the colon and urinary collecting system. The simplest management is to back the nephrostomy tube out of the kidney and into the colon to serve as a colostomy, and then obtain separate access to the upper urinary tract, either with a new percutaneous access that does not traverse the colon or with a retrograde-placed ureteral stent.
12. Intravascular hemolysis from the extravasated water irrigant can be fatal. The irrigant for percutaneous renal surgery should be saline, with the exception of glycine or similar nonelectrolytic isotonic fluids when monopolar electrocautery is used.

13 Principles of Urologic Endoscopy

Brian Duty and Michael J. Conlin

QUESTIONS

1. Patients undergoing diagnostic cystoscopy should receive prophylactic antibiotics if they have any of the following risk factors except:
   a. poor nutritional status.
   b. anatomic anomalies.
   c. hypertension.
   d. corticosteroid use.
   e. smoking history.

2. Compared with reusable flexible ureteroscopes, single-use flexible ureteroscopes have been shown to have:
   a. decreased active deflection.
   B. comparable visibility.
   c. well-established cost savings.
   d. decreased durability.
   e. longer procedure time.

3. Techniques that have been shown to improve flexible cystourethroscopy tolerance in men include all of the following except:
   a. allowing the patient to observe the procedure.
   b. having the patient empty his bladder before the procedure.
   c. playing classical music during the procedure.
   d. using lidocaine lubricating gel.
   e. increasing the hydrostatic pressure of the irrigant during scope passage.

4. Indications for ureteroscopy include all of the following except:
   a. obstructing ureteral calculus.
   b. filling defect of the renal pelvis.
   c. 1.2-cm renal calculus in the lower pole.
   d. ureteropelvic junction obstruction with a large crossing vessel present.
   e. 1.5-cm midureteral stricture.

5. Which of the following statements about ureteroscopy are true?
   a. Ureteral access sheaths decrease intrarenal pressure during ureteroscopy.
   b. Flexible ureteroscopes accept working instruments 3.6 Fr in diameter.
   c. Normal saline should be used for irrigation during ureteroscopy.
   d. A preoperative antibiotic is needed only in high-risk patients.
   e. a and c.

6. Compared with white-light endoscopy, narrow-band imaging has been shown to:

   a. predict favorable response to bacillus Calmette Guérin (BCG) intravesical therapy.
   b. accurately differentiate between low- and high-grade lesions.
   c. obviate the need for re-resection in patients with high-grade tumors involving the lamina propria.
   d. significantly improve detection accuracy of muscle-invasive lesions.
   e. improve detection of noninvasive lesions, including carcinoma in situ.

7. Which of the following statements are true?
   a. The holmium laser is absorbed in 3 cm of water.
   b. Water is the preferred irrigant for ureteroscopy because of improved visibility.
   c. Baskets made of nitinol are more "kink resistant" compared with stainless steel.
   d. Balloon dilation of the intramural ureter is usually necessary before flexible ureteroscopy.
   e. Compared with fiberoptic flexible ureteroscopes, digital flexible ureteroscopes less frequently require the use ureteral access sheaths.

8. Techniques to minimize staff radiation exposure include all of the following except:
   a. using "last image hold" setting.
   b. using fixed fluoroscopy units.
   c. surgeon control of the foot pedal.
   d. using image collimation.
   e. using pulse fluoroscopy mode.

ANSWERS

1. **c. Hypertension.** The American Urological Association's Best Practice Policy Statement on Antimicrobial Prophylaxis did not recommend routine antibiotic administration for diagnostic cystourethroscopy. This recommendation was based on the recognition that some randomized studies have shown antibiotic prophylaxis reduces bacteriuria and symptomatic infection rates, whereas others have not. However, antibiotic administration was advocated by the panel for patients with host factors increasing their risk of infection. These include advanced age, anatomic anomalies, poor nutritional status, smoking, chronic corticosteroid use, immunodeficiency, chronic indwelling hardware infected with endogenous or exogenous material, distant coinfection, and prolonged hospitalization.

2. **b. Comparable visibility.** One of the early studies evaluating disposable ureteroscopes was a cadaveric study comparing the LithoVue to nondisposable fiberoptic and digital ureteroscopes. The researchers found the LithoVue to be comparable in visibility and scope maneuverability.

3. **b. Having the patient empty his bladder before the procedure.** A variety of prospective studies have been performed with the aim of improving patient tolerance during office-based diagnostic flexible cystourethroscopy. A meta-analysis of four randomized trials involving 411 patients found that patients receiving lidocaine gel were 1.7 times less likely to experience moderate to severe pain during the procedure. Results of a randomized trial involving 151 men indicated that increasing the hydrostatic pressure of the irrigation solution during passage of the scope through the membranous urethra was associated with significantly less discomfort on an analog pain scale. In another study, men who were allowed to watch the procedure had significantly less pain on a 100-mm visual analog scale. Last, 70 men were randomly assigned to hear either no music or classical music during cystourethroscopy. Patients listening to classical music had significantly less pain, greater satisfaction, lower postprocedure pulse rates, and lower systolic blood pressures.

4. **d. Ureteropelvic junction obstruction with a large crossing vessel present.** All of the options are common indications for ureteroscopy except ureteropelvic junction obstruction due to a large crossing vessel. Although ureteropelvic junction obstruction can be managed with ureteroscopic endopyelotomy, patients with a large crossing vessel are better treated by laparoscopic pyeloplasty.

5. **e. a and c.** Auge and colleagues measured the pressure within the renal pelvis and proximal, mid, and distal ureter before and after ureteral access sheath placement in five patients who had previously undergone nephrostomy tube placement. The pressure within the collecting system was found to be significantly lower at each location following access sheath placement.

6. **e. Improve detection of noninvasive lesions, including carcinoma in situ.** Narrow-band imaging uses only blue (415 nm) and green (540 nm) wavelengths to image the urothelium compared with white-light endoscopy, which uses the entire visible light spectrum. Blue and green wavelengths are strongly absorbed by hemoglobin, improving visibility of urothelial capillaries, small papillary lesions, and carcinoma in situ. A meta-analysis of eight studies including 1022 patients found that narrow-band imaging improves detection accuracy of noninvasive lesions, including carcinoma in situ.

7. **c. Baskets made of nitinol are more "kink resistant" compared with stainless steel.** Nitinol has a variety of advantageous properties compared with stainless steel. Nitinol is more biocompatible, has greater torquability and improved "memory," and is more resistant to kinking. These properties make it ideal for stone basket construction. Holmium laser energy is absorbed by 3 mm of water. Saline is the preferred irrigation solution because of the decreased risk of "transurethral resection syndrome" compared with hypotonic solutions. The need for ureteral dilation has decreased over time with the advent of smaller-diameter ureteroscopes. However, digital models have larger tip and shaft diameters, making them more likely to need ureteral dilation or access sheath placement compared with their fiberoptic counterparts.

8. **b. Using fixed fluoroscopy units.** All endourologic procedures using fluoroscopy should operate on the ALARA principle (as low as reasonably achievable). Techniques that have been shown to minimize radiation exposure include surgeon control of the foot pedal, using "last image hold," image collimation, and pulsed fluoroscopy mode. Compared with fixed units, mobile C-arm fluoroscopy machines are able to position the image intensifier closer to the patient, thereby reducing exposure while improving image quality.

CHAPTER REVIEW

1. Rigid cystourethroscopes are manufactured in sets consisting of an optical lens, bridge, sheath, and obturator.
2. Flexible cystourethroscopes are available in fiberoptic, standard-definition and high-definition digital models.
3. Cystourethroscope sizes are expressed using the French gauge system, with 1 Fr equaling a third of a millimeter in circumference.
4. The smallest-diameter cystourethroscope that can be used to perform the procedure should be selected to decrease the risk of genitourinary tract trauma.
5. Antimicrobial prophylaxis is not recommended for diagnostic cystourethroscopy unless patient-related risk factors are present.
6. Increasing the hydrostatic pressure during scope passage and allowing men to observe the procedure have been prospectively shown to improve patient comfort during flexible cystourethroscopy.
7. Semirigid ureteroscopy is used below the iliac vessels and flexible ureteroscopy above.
8. Semirigid ureteroscopes with two working channels permit better irrigation and the added safety of being able to pass a lithotripsy device through one channel when needing to fragment a stone engaged in a basket in the other channel.
9. Flexible ureteroscopes must be straight when passing a laser fiber or the working channel will be damaged.
10. The golden rule of safe laser lithotripsy: "Do not step on the pedal if you cannot see the tip of the fiber in contact with the stone."
11. Stone baskets made of nitinol maintain their shape, resist kinking, and allow disengagement of stones more reliably that stainless steel baskets.
12. Ureteral access sheaths facilitate repeated passage of flexible ureteroscopes and decrease the intrapelvic pressure during ureteroscopy.
13. Mobile C-arm fluoroscopy is preferred because of greater mobility, improved image quality, and less scatter radiation exposure to the surgeon compared with urology tables with fixed fluoroscopy units.
14. A routine preoperative antibiotic should be given to all patients undergoing ureteroscopy.
15. Normal saline should be used as irrigation during ureteroscopy to prevent absorption of a hypotonic solution.

Roshan M. Patel, Kamaljot S. Kaler, and Jaime Landman

QUESTIONS

1. Absolute contraindications to laparoscopic surgery include all of the following EXCEPT:
   a. uncorrectable coagulopathy.
   b. hemodynamic instability.
   c. significant abdominal wall infection.
   d. suspected malignant ascites.
   e. extensive prior abdominal or pelvic surgery.

2. Of the following, which is considered a relative contraindication to laparoscopic surgery?
   a. Generalized peritonitis
   b. Massive hemoperitoneum
   c. Intestinal obstruction with intention to treat
   d. Extensive prior abdominal or pelvic surgery
   e. Abdominal wall infection

3. The most effective preoperative preparation for patients undergoing routine laparoscopic renal surgery is:
   a. a 3-day mechanical bowel preparation if an extraperitoneal or retroperitoneoscopic approach is anticipated.
   b. a mechanical bowel preparation and antibiotic preparation with neomycin and metronidazole.
   c. for most uncomplicated patients, a clear liquid diet and a light mechanical bowel preparation the day before surgery.
   d. both an antibiotic and 3-day mechanical bowel preparation in patients who have had previous abdominal surgery if one anticipates encountering dense intra-abdominal adhesions.
   e. intravenous antibiotics 1 hour before surgery.

4. Which of the following statements regarding enhanced recovery after surgery (ERAS) protocol is TRUE?
   a. They reduce hospital stay by 30% but have no effect on complication rates.
   b. They reduce hospital stay by 30% and decrease complication rates by 50%.
   c. They decrease admission rates and have no effect on hospital stay.
   d. They increased healthcare costs.
   e. They have no effect on complication rates and decrease healthcare costs.

5. Which of the following is TRUE regarding operating table padding?
   a. The unaugmented operating room table mattress is best for reducing pressure.
   b. Shoulder support and braces should always be used.
   c. Gel padding is better than egg crate padding.
   d. Kidney rest should always be used for more than 30 minutes.
   e. Egg crate padding is equivalent to gel padding and both are better than the unaugmented bed.

6. Which of the following statements regarding pneumoperitoneum insufflation is TRUE?
   a. CO_2 as an insufflant can be dangerous because it can support combustion.
   b. CO_2 is most commonly used because it is insoluble in the blood.
   c. In patients with chronic respiratory disease, CO_2 is advantageous because it does not accumulate in the bloodstream.
   d. Argon gas would be an ideal insufflant because of its low cost and poor solubility in blood.
   e. Nitrous oxide has previously been used for insufflation; however, it is no longer routinely used because of the potential for intra-abdominal explosion.

7. When a patient undergoing renal laparoscopy with a potential for extensive adhesions due to multiple prior abdominal surgeries, which of the following access techniques is recommended for obtaining a pneumoperitoneum and access to the abdomen for laparoscopy?
   a. Closed technique with Veress needle
   b. Closed technique with blind trocar insertion
   c. Open-access technique
   d. Hand-port access
   e. EndoTip entry

8. Of the following access locations, which port site most often requires formal closure with a fascial and peritoneal suture?
   a. 5-mm nonbladed ports
   b. 5-mm bladed ports
   c. 10- to 12-mm bladed ports placed on the midclavicular line
   d. 10- to 12-mm nonbladed ports placed on the midclavicular line
   e. 10- to 12-mm nonbladed ports placed on the anterior axillary line

9. Which of the following pneumoperitoneum pressures is associated with the least perturbation in cardiac parameters (i.e., change in stroke volume)?
   a. 12 mm Hg
   b. 15 mm Hg
   c. 18 mm Hg
   d. 21 mm Hg
   e. 24 mm Hg

10. Which of the following is a common physiologic effect that has been observed after the establishment of pneumoperitoneum?
    a. Increase in diaphragmatic motion
    b. Increase in disturbances of gastrointestinal motility
    c. Alkalosis
    d. Decrease in urinary output
    e. Increase in mesenteric vessel blood flow

11. Which of the following intra-abdominal structures is most commonly the site of injury in laparoscopic surgery?
    a. Bowel injury
    b. Vascular injury
    c. Liver injury
    d. Splenic laceration
    e. Bladder injury

12. What is a characteristic of a blunt trocar, compared with a bladed trocar?
    a. The blunt trocar requires formal closure of the port site regardless of its size.
    b. The blunt trocar takes less force to insert than the bladed trocar.
    c. The blunt trocar decreases the chance of injury to the epigastric vessels.
    d. The blunt trocar should only be placed in the midline.
    e. The blunt trocar eliminates possible trocar injury to the bowel.

13. All of the following are treatment options for a gas embolism during laparoscopy are true EXCEPT:
    a. Hyperventilate the patient with 100% oxygen.
    b. Immediately cease insufflation.
    c. Place the patient in a head-down position.
    d. Advance a central venous line into the right side of the heart.
    e. Place the patient in a right lateral decubitus position with the left side up.

14. Pneumomediastinum, pneumothorax, and pneumopericardium associated with laparoscopy are a result of:
    a. gas leaking along major blood vessels through congenital defects in the diaphragm.
    b. gas passing through secondary enlargement of openings in the diaphragm.
    c. diffusion of gas across the peritoneum and diaphragm.
    d. a and b.
    e. a and c.

15. If the Veress needle has been unintentionally placed in the iliac artery during creation of the pneumoperitoneum for insufflation of the abdomen, which of the following is the best course of action to minimize further patient injury?
    a. Remove the Veress needle, and proceed to open the abdomen.
    b. Remove the Veress needle, and then proceed with insufflating at a different location.
    c. Leave the Veress needle in place, and open the abdomen.
    d. Leave the Veress needle in place, and proceed with insufflation of the abdomen at a different location.
    e. Call for a vascular surgery consult.

16. What is the most effective management option if trocar injury to the iliac artery should occur during the placement of the first trocar?
    a. Remove the trocar, and open the abdomen immediately.
    b. Remove the trocar immediately, and proceed with reinsufflation of the abdomen and placement of the trocar at an alternate site.
    c. Leave the trocar in place, consult a vascular surgeon, and convert to open laparotomy.
    d. Leave the trocar in place, and proceed with insufflation of the abdomen and placement of another port at an alternate site.
    e. Remove the obturator, and immediately flush the port with fibrin glue.

17. Laparoscopic surgery can potentially cause thermal bowel injury during as a direct result from all of the following EXCEPT:
    a. capacitive coupling.
    b. insulation failure.
    c. inappropriate direct activation.
    d. electrode resistance.
    e. coupling to another instrument.

18. When a postoperative bladder injury is diagnosed following laparoscopy, what is the most effective method of treatment?
    a. Transurethral indwelling Foley catheter if it is an intraperitoneal injury of the bladder
    b. Open repair if it is an extraperitoneal injury of the bladder
    c. Laparoscopic or open repair if it is an intraperitoneal injury to the bladder
    d. Laparoscopic repair if it is an extraperitoneal injury to the bladder
    e. Transurethral injection of fibrin glue into the bladder injury site if it is an extraperitoneal injury to the bladder

19. Hypercarbia during laparoscopy may be related to all of the following EXCEPT:
    a. severe chronic respiratory disease.
    b. subcutaneous emphysema.
    c. increased insufflation pressures.
    d. prolonged operative time.
    e. radical nephrectomy.

20. Possible advantages of retroperitoneal laparoscopy include all of the following EXCEPT:
    a. less need for lysis of adhesions.
    b. decreased risk of paralytic ileus.
    c. decreased risk of port-site hernias.
    d. direct rapid access to the renal hilum.
    e. technically easier to learn.

21. In comparison with transperitoneal pelvic node dissection, which of the following incidence rates are higher after extraperitoneal pelvic lymph node dissection?
    a. Urinoma
    b. Lymphocele
    c. Bowel injury
    d. Laparoscopic repair if it is an extraperitoneal injury to the bladder
    e. Shoulder/hip pain

22. All of the following instruments might be part of a hemorrhage control tray EXCEPT:
    a. laparoscopic needle drivers.
    b. laparoscopic Satinsky clamp and accompanying trocar.
    c. Lapra-Ty clip applier and 6-inch length of 3-0 absorbable suture.
    d. hemostatic agents (fibrin glue, gelatin matrix thrombin, etc.) plus laparoscopic applicators.
    e. laparoscopic renal biopsy forceps.

23. Which of the following hemostatic agents requires a 20-minute setup time before use?
    a. Tisseel
    b. FloSeal
    c. CrossSeal

d. BioGlue

e. CoSeal

24. Which of the following relationships is true for port placement for laparoscopic suturing?

    a. The angle produced by the horizontal plane and the instruments should be greater than 55 degrees, and the angle between the needle drivers should be less than 25 degrees.

    b. The angle produced by the horizontal plane and the instruments should be less than 55 degrees, and the angle between the needle drivers should be between 25 and 45 degrees.

    c. The angle produced by the horizontal plane and the instruments should be greater than 55 degrees, and the angle between the needle drivers should be greater than 45 degrees.

    d. The angle produced by the horizontal plane and the instruments should be less than 55 degrees, and the angle between the needle drivers should be less than 25 degrees.

    e. The angle produced by the horizontal plane and the instruments should be greater than 55 degrees, and the angle between the needle drivers should be between 25 and 45 degrees.

25. During a procedure using the da Vinci Robotic System, the robot malfunctions and one of the grasping forceps is closed on a vital structure. The system is completely unresponsive. The appropriate action to safely disengage the instrument from the vital structure is to:

    a. use the surgeon's console to override the system and robotically disengage the grasper.

    b. remove the robotic instrument from the robotic arm.

    c. use the sterile Allen wrench provided by the company to manually disengage the instrument and then remove it from the robotic arm.

    d. use a handheld laparoscopic instrument to pry open the jaws of the robotic instrument.

    e. unplug the surgeon's console and robotic tower, plug them back in, and restart the system.

26. Insufflation should never commence after placement of the Veress needle unless all of the following signs for proper peritoneal entry are confirmed EXCEPT?

    a. negative aspiration.

    b. easy irrigation of saline.

    c. negative pressure test.

    d. positive drop test.

    e. normal advancement test.

27. Insufflation of the abdomen is most commonly conducted using carbon dioxide because it is:

    a. noncombustible.

    b. rapidly absorbed.

    c. inexpensive.

    d. colorless.

    e. all of the above.

28. Helium is a useful insufflant in patients with:

    a. coronary artery disease.

    b. peripheral vascular disease.

    c. pulmonary disease.

    d. inflammatory bowel disease.

    e. chronic kidney disease.

29. Which of the following are signs of bowel insufflation with the Veress needle?

    a. Asymmetric abdominal distention

    b. Flatus

    c. High pressures reached after a large amount of CO_2 is insufflated

    d. a and c

    e. a and b

30. The diagnosis of air embolism is usually made by the anesthesiologist based on an initial abrupt:

    a. increase in end-tidal CO_2.

    b. decrease in end-tidal CO_2.

    c. increase in oxygen saturation.

    d. increase in mean arterial pressure.

    e. decrease in airway pressures.

31. Laparoscopic virtual reality (VR) trainers have been shown to:

    a. increase the operating time and improve the operative performance of surgical trainees with limited laparoscopic experience when compared with no training or with box-trainer training.

    b. decrease the operating time and improve the operative performance of surgical trainees with limited laparoscopic experience when compared with no training or with box-trainer training.

    c. decrease the operating time and improve the operative performance of surgical trainees with extensive laparoscopic experience when compared with no training or with box-trainer training.

    d. a and b.

    e. a and c.

32. When the patient is positioned in the modified flank position, the risk of developing rhabdomyolysis from flank pressure is increased by all of the following EXCEPT:

    a. body mass index (BMI) greater than 25.

    b. elevation of the kidney rest.

    c. age less than 45 years.

    d. male gender.

    e. full table flexion.

33. When using a laparoscopic stapling device, the 2.0-mm or 2.5-mm staple cartridges are preferred for:

    a. bowel.

    b. bladder.

    c. ureter.

    d. vascular (renal artery or vein).

    e. a and d.

34. All of the following represent options for port site fascial closure EXCEPT:

    a. retractors and direct vision.

    b. Endo Stitch.

    c. Carter-Thomason needlepoint suture passer.

    d. disposable Endo Close suture carrier.

    e. angiocatheter technique.

35. The basic principles of Hem-o-Lok clip placement include all of the following EXCEPT:

    a. incomplete circumferential dissection of the vessel.

    b. visualization of the curved tip of the clip around and beyond the vessel.

c. confirmation of the tactile snap when the clip engages.

d. during transaction of vessels, only a partial division is performed initially to confirm hemostasis before complete transaction.

e. no cross clipping.

36. Balloon trocars are advantageous because they can help reduce the risk of:

a. air embolism.

b. alkalosis.

c. subcutaneous emphysema.

d. hypothermia.

e. all of the above.

37. To avoid local or distant transmitted thermal injury during monopolar electrosurgery, certain precautions must be followed, including:

a. checking the insulation of the electrosurgical instrument carefully for damage.

b. not activating the electrosurgical probe unless the metal part is in complete view.

c. not activating the probe unless it is in direct contact with the tissue to be incised.

d. never using a metal trocar in conjunction with an outer plastic retaining ring.

e. all of the above.

ANSWERS

1. **e. Extensive prior abdominal or pelvic surgery.** Absolute contraindications for laparoscopic surgery include uncorrectable coagulopathy, intestinal obstruction, abdominal wall infection, massive hemoperitoneum or hemoretroperitoneum, generalized peritonitis or retroperitoneal abscess, and suspected malignant ascites.

2. **d. Extensive prior abdominal or pelvic surgery.** When extensive intra-abdominal or pelvic adhesions are suspected, close attention must be given to access into the abdomen, whether this is by Veress needle (Ethicon Endo-Surgery, Blue Ash, OH) or some open-access technique. The Palmer point (subcostal midclavicular line) on the left side is preferred. Alternatively, in these patients, a retroperitoneal approach may be preferable to a transperitoneal approach, but this is only a relative contraindication to performing laparoscopic surgery. All of the other options listed are absolute contraindications to laparoscopic surgery.

3. **e. Intravenous antibiotics 1 hour before surgery.** For extraperitoneoscopy and retroperitoneoscopy, no bowel preparation is necessary. Similarly, for transperitoneal laparoscopic/robotic procedures not involving the use of bowel segments for urinary tract reconstruction, a mechanical bowel preparation is not necessary. A recent large-scale propensity score-matched analysis demonstrated no benefit for mechanical bowel preparation in operative time, postoperative stay, or overall complications for patients undergoing laparoscopic nephrectomy.

4. **b. They reduce hospital stay by 30% and decrease complication rates by 50%.** These protocols have resulted in shorter hospital stay by 30%, a reduction in complications by 50%, decrease in readmission rates, and thus reducing healthcare costs.

5. **a. The unaugmented operating room table mattress is best for reducing pressure.** Use of the kidney rest was believed to be the most detrimental, and its use beyond 20 to 30 minutes was discouraged. Male patients with a BMI of 25 or higher undergoing laparoscopic surgery in the lateral position with the kidney rest elevated and the table completely flexed are at highest risk of developing rhabdomyolysis from flank pressure. In this study the unaugmented operating table mattress was superior to egg crate or gel padding as an augmenting surface material; of note, egg crate padding was equal or superior to the more expensive gel padding. Support or braces should never be used in Trendelenburg position, due to risk of brachial plexus injury.

6. **e. Nitrous oxide has previously been used for insufflation however, it is no longer routinely used because of the potential for intra-abdominal; explosion.** Most commonly, CO_2 is used as the insufflant because it does not support combustion and is very soluble in blood. However, in patients with chronic respiratory disease, CO_2 may accumulate in the bloodstream to dangerous levels. In these patients, helium may be used for insufflation once the initial pneumoperitoneum has been established with CO_2. The drawback of helium is that, like air, it is much less soluble in the blood than is CO_2. However, its use averts problems with hypercarbia. Other gases that were once used for insufflation, including room air, oxygen, and nitrous oxide, are no longer routinely used because of their potential side effects, such as air embolus or intra-abdominal explosion and potential to support combustion.

7. **c. Open-access technique.** Pneumoperitoneum can be more easily and, in one's early experience, more safely established using an open technique, especially in patients with multiple prior surgeries, who are at high risk for intra-abdominal adhesions. However, its use involves making a larger incision and increases the chances of port-site gas leakage during the procedure. Studies in general surgery have shown the open technique to be as efficient as a closed approach. Insertion should be performed in an unscarred quadrant of the abdomen. If there is no scar-free area, then an open technique should be used.

8. **c. 10- to 12-mm bladed ports placed on the midclavicular line.** All bladed port sites that are greater than 5 mm should be formally closed, independent of location.

9. **a. 12 mm Hg.** Recent studies support a pneumoperitoneum pressure of 12 mm Hg, because this results in no perturbation in cardiac parameters (i.e., no change in stroke volume) versus a pressure of 15 mm Hg. Working at lower pneumoperitoneum pressures has also been found to reduce postoperative pain. In addition, a marked reduction in oliguria has been associated with working at 10 mm Hg pressure.

10. **d. Decrease in urinary output.** Because of increased intra-abdominal pressure from the pneumoperitoneum, diaphragmatic motion is limited. Laparoscopic surgery causes less significant disturbances of the gastrointestinal motility pattern compared with open surgery. Insufflation with CO_2 results in variable amounts of gas absorption, thereby raising the PCO_2 in the blood and creating an acidosis. Increased intra-abdominal pressure was found to be associated with a significant decrease in urinary output secondary to decreased blood flow to the renal cortex with an associated decrease in renal vein blood flow of up to 90% at 15 mm Hg.

11. **b. Vascular injury.** The most common site of injury during laparoscopic surgery, in reports in the literature, is vascular in origin, occurring in 2.8% of patients, followed by bowel injury at 1.1%. The most often injured intra-abdominal organ was the bowel, at an incidence of 1.2%.

12. **c. The blunt trocar decreases the chance of injury to the epigastric vessels.** The use of only blunt trocars decreases the chance of injury to the epigastric vessels by fivefold. Indeed, studies have shown the risk of inferior epigastric injury or port site herniation is fivefold less with blunt versus sharp trocars. In addition, a recent meta-analysis demonstrated a lower relative risk of trocar site bleeding (3% vs. 9%) and overall complications (3% vs. 10%) with blunt compared with bladed trocars.

13. **e. Place the patient in a right lateral decubitus position with the left side up.** The treatment for a suspected gas embolism

is immediate cessation of insufflation and prompt desufflation of the peritoneal cavity. The patient is turned into a **left lateral decubitus** head-down position (i.e., right side up) to minimize right ventricular outflow problems. The patient is hyperventilated with 100% oxygen. Advancement of a central venous line into the right side of the heart with subsequent attempts to aspirate the gas may rarely be helpful. Use of hyperbaric oxygen and cardiopulmonary bypass have also been reported.

14. **d. a and b.** Gas leaking along major blood vessels through congenital defects or secondary enlargement of openings in the diaphragm may lead to pneumomediastinum, pneumopericardium, and pneumothorax.

15. **d. Leave the Veress needle in place, and proceed with insufflation of the abdomen at a different location.** If vascular injury should occur with the Veress needle, the needle should be left in place to identify the area of injury, and insufflation of the abdomen can be reperformed at an alternate site and then the laparoscope inserted to identify the area of injury and to observe this as the Veress needle is removed to control any hemorrhage that may occur from the site. Note this is different than a trocar vessel injury.

16. **c. Leave the trocar in place, consult a vascular surgeon, and convert to open laparotomy.** A trocar injury to a major arterial vessel is a potentially life-threatening complication. The trocar should remain in place to tamponade the bleeding and also identify the area of injury once the abdomen is opened. The patient's blood should be typed and crossmatched, and immediate laparotomy should be performed and the site of vascular injury identified. A vascular surgery consult may be needed.

17. **d. Electrode resistance.** Electrosurgically induced thermal injury may occur through of one of four mechanisms: inappropriate direct activation; coupling to another instrument; capacitive coupling; and insulation failure.

18. **c. Laparoscopic or open repair if it is an intraperitoneal injury to the bladder.** When bladder injury is diagnosed postoperatively, the surgeon must determine whether the perforation is extraperitoneal or intraperitoneal. Extraperitoneal injury, without any complicating additional problems, may be treated by simple placement of a transurethral indwelling Foley catheter. Intraperitoneal injury is an indication for subsequent laparoscopic or open repair.

19. **e. Radical nephrectomy.** The potential for developing hypercarbia exists during both transperitoneal and preperitoneal laparoscopic procedures. Conceivably, this assumes greater importance in patients with preexisting airway and cardiovascular compliance. Vigilant perioperative anesthetic management is essential to prevent the development of potential complications related to CO_2 buildup. A rise in end-tidal CO_2 should prompt the anesthesiologist to adjust the respiratory rate and tidal volume to enhance CO_2 elimination. Simultaneously, the insufflation pressure of CO_2 should be decreased by the surgeon or, if need be, the operation should be halted and the abdomen desufflated until the end-tidal CO_2 returns to an acceptable level.

20. **e. Technically easier to learn.** Retroperitoneoscopy is associated with unique anatomic orientation and a relatively restricted initial working area compared with transperitoneal laparoscopy. This results in a steeper learning curve.

21. **b. Lymphocele.** Absence of the peritoneal absorptive surface after extraperitoneoscopic lymphadenectomy may increase the risk of development of postoperative lymphocele

22. **e. Laparoscopic renal biopsy forceps.** The contents of a hemorrhage tray for laparoscopic surgery include the following:
    - Laparoscopic Satinsky clamp (Medline Industries Inc., Mundelein, IL)
    - 10-mm suction/irrigation tip
    - Endo Stitch device with a 4-0 absorbable suture
    - Lapra-Ty clip (Ethicon US, LLC, CA) applier and a packet of Lapra-Ty clips

- 6-inch length of 4-0 vascular suture on an SH needle with a Lapra-Ty clip preplaced on the end
- Two laparoscopic needle drivers
- Topical hemostatic agent of choice

23. **a. Tisseel.** Tisseel (Baxter, Glendale, CA) is a form of fibrin glue containing fibrinogen, calcium chloride, aprotinin, and thrombin. It is useful as a topical hemostatic agent as well as a tissue glue, but it has a 20-minute setup time and thus must be prepared well in advance of potential use.

24. **b. The angle produced by the horizontal plane and the instruments should be less than 55 degrees, and the angle between the needle drivers should be between 25 and 45 degrees.** Frede and colleagues performed an in vitro experiment performing laparoscopic suturing while varying trocar relationship to the horizontal plane and the distance between the two instrument trocars. They found that suturing was easiest when the angle between the horizontal plane and the instruments was less than 55 degrees and the angle between the two instruments was between 25 and 45 degrees.

25. **c. Use the sterile Allen wrench provided by the company to manually disengage the instrument and then remove it from the robotic arm.** In the event of a system failure of the da Vinci Robotic System (Intuitive Surgical, Sunnyvale, CA) during which the robotic arms are rendered nonfunctional, instrument jaws can be manually opened using a sterile Allen wrench provided by the company for this purpose.

26. **c. Negative pressure test.** Several tests can be performed in an attempt to confirm proper placement of the Veress needle within the peritoneal cavity before insufflation, to reduce the risk of insufflation-related complications. These tests include: the aspiration/irrigation/aspiration test, the advancement test, and the drop test. Insufflation should never be initiated unless all of the signs for proper peritoneal entry (negative aspiration, easy irrigation of saline, negative aspiration of saline, positive drop test, and normal advancement test) have been confirmed.

27. **e. All of the above.** CO_2 is the most commonly used insufflant for laparoscopic surgery and is favored by most laparoscopists thanks to its properties (colorless, noncombustible, very soluble in blood, and inexpensive).

28. **c. Pulmonary disease.** Helium is an inert and noncombustible insufflant. Initial studies performed in various animal models showed favorable effects on arterial partial pressure of CO_2 and pH with no evidence of hypercarbia. These results were corroborated by clinical studies. Therefore helium is particularly useful for the patient with pulmonary disease in whom hypercarbia would be poorly tolerated.

29. **e. a and b.** If entry into the bowel is not recognized at the time of irrigation and aspiration through the Veress needle, then the surgeon may insufflate the small or large bowel. The first sign of this problem is asymmetric abdominal distention followed by flatus and insufflation of only a small amount of CO_2 (< 2 L) before high pressures are reached.

30. **a. Increase in end-tidal CO_2.** The diagnosis of CO_2 gas embolism is usually made by the anesthesiologist based on an abrupt increase of end-tidal CO_2 accompanied by a sudden decline in oxygen saturation and then a marked decrease in end-tidal CO_2. Sometimes, a "millwheel" precordial murmur can be auscultated. In addition, the anesthesiologist may notice foaming of a blood sample, if drawn, owing to the presence of insufflated CO_2.

31. **b. Decrease the operating time and improve the operative performance of surgical trainees with limited laparoscopic experience when compared with no training or with box-trainer training.** VR trainers are computer-based simulators that offer the opportunity to practice laparoscopic and robotic skills through specific tasks, as well as whole procedures. VR trainers have been shown to improve the skills of trainees helping to prepare them for better performance during live

surgery. A recent systematic review demonstrated that VR training appears to decrease the operating time and improve the operative performance of surgical trainees with limited laparoscopic experience when compared with no training or with box-trainer training.

32. **c. Age less than 45 years.** Male patients with a BMI greater than 25 undergoing laparoscopic surgery in the lateral position with the kidney rest elevated and the table completely flexed are at highest risk of developing rhabdomyolysis due to flank pressure.

33. **d. Vascular (renal artery or vein).** Various stapling devices are available for tissue occlusion and division. Each staple load cartridge is color-coded depending on the size of the staples: 2.0-mm staples (gray) or 2.5-mm staples (white) are preferred for vascular (renal vein or renal artery) stapling, whereas 3.8-mm (blue) and 4.8-mm (green) are used in thicker tissues (ureter, bowel, bladder).

34. **b. Endo Stitch.** The Endo Stitch (Covidien, Mansfield, MA) device is an innovative, disposable 10-mm instrument that facilitates laparoscopic suture placement and knot tying, not port site closure.

35. **a. Incomplete circumferential dissection of the vessel.** The basic principles of Hem-o-Lok (Teleflex, Morrisville, NC) placement include the following:
   - Complete circumferential dissection of the vessel
   - Visualization of the curved tip of the clip around and beyond the vessel, often with curved end of the clip placed between artery and vein
   - Confirmation of the tactile snap when the clip engages
   - No cross clipping
   - Not squeezing clip handles too hard (compared with the application of metal clips)
   - Careful removal of the applier after application given; the tips are sharp and can cause a laceration of nearby vessels (e.g., renal vein)

   - During transection of vessels, only a partial division is performed initially to confirm hemostasis before complete transection
   - Minimum of two clips placed on the patient side of the renal hilar vessel

36. **c. Subcutaneous emphysema.** Once the balloon cannula is positioned in the abdominal cavity, the balloon is inflated; the cannula is pulled upward until the balloon is snug on the underside of the abdominal wall. Next, the soft foam or rubber collar on the outside surface of the cannula is slid down until it is snug on the skin and locked in place. This process creates an excellent seal, precluding gas leakage and subcutaneous emphysema.

37. **e. All of the above.** Several actions can be taken by the surgeon to lessen the risks of a thermal complication. First, electrosurgical instruments must be carefully inspected before use for any "breaks" in the insulation; if these are found, the instrument must be sent for recoating. Second, electrosurgical instruments should never be left untended within the abdomen; when not in use, they must be removed from the abdomen. Third, only the primary surgeon should control electrode activation. Fourth, isolation of the area to be cauterized from the surrounding tissues, as well as use of bipolar electrocautery, reduces the risk of thermal spread and injury to other tissues. Fifth, the electrosurgical device should never be activated unless the entire extent of the metal portion of the instrument is in view. Sixth, problems of capacitive coupling can be precluded by not creating a situation in which a mixture of conducting and nonconducting elements are used by the surgeon (e.g., metal trocars combined with plastic retainers). Last, an active electrode monitoring system (Encision, Boulder, CO) is extremely helpful, as any sudden break in the insulation of the electrosurgical instrument results in immediate shutdown of the electrosurgical current, thereby precluding an electrosurgical injury.

CHAPTER REVIEW

1. Careful patient selection and identification of contraindications for laparoscopic and robotic procedures are vital for successful outcomes. A meticulous past history, focusing on prior surgeries, and physical examination, detailing the location and extent of all abdominal scars, are the initial steps in patient evaluation for minimally invasive surgery.

2. Contraindications to laparoscopic or robotic surgery include uncorrectable coagulopathy, intestinal obstruction unless treatment is intended, significant abdominal wall infection, massive hemoperitoneum or hemoretroperitoneum, generalized peritonitis, and suspected malignant ascites.

3. A checklist ensuring that all essential equipment is present and operational should be completed just before initiating the pneumoperitoneum. Additional items to check when using the da Vinci Robotic System include ensuring that all plugs for the console, vision cart, and patient-side cart are plugged into different circuits and that all cables connecting these carts are connected properly.

4. After placement of the Veress needle, insufflation should never be initiated unless all of the signs for proper peritoneal entry (negative aspiration, easy irrigation of saline, negative aspiration of saline, positive drop test result, and normal advancement test) have been confirmed.

5. The open technique is recommended specifically when extensive adhesions are anticipated.

6. Noncutting dilating trocars have superseded bladed trocars because they are safer. These trocars enter the abdomen by spreading the abdominal wall musculature, rather than cutting it, and therefore there is less chance of injuring an abdominal wall vessel and the resulting entry site is less prone to subsequent herniation.

7. Carbon dioxide is the most commonly used insufflant because it is noncombustible and rapidly absorbed in the blood.

8. Helium is potentially useful for the patient with pulmonary disease in whom hypercarbia would be poorly tolerated.

9. Intra-abdominal pressures during laparoscopy should not be allowed to exceed 20 mm Hg over extended periods, and a working pressure of 10 to 12 mm Hg is recommended.

10. Early in one's experience with laparoscopic and robotic surgery, it is wise to apply the minimally invasive approach to low-risk surgical candidates of normal body habitus.

11. The first sign of gas embolism is an abrupt increase of end-tidal CO_2 accompanied by a sudden decline in oxygen saturation and then a marked decrease in end-tidal CO_2.

12. Electrosurgically induced thermal bowel injury may occur through one of four mechanisms: inappropriate direct activation; coupling to another instrument; capacitive coupling; and insulation failure.

13. Careful planning of trocar placement is essential to avoid crossing swords, striking handles, rollover, and robotic arm collisions.

14. Laparoscopic VR trainers have been shown to improve the skills of trainees, helping to prepare them for better performance during live surgery.

15. VR robotic trainers have been shown to have face, content, and construct validity.

15   Basic Energy Modalities in Urologic Surgery

Michael W. Sourial, Shubha K. De, Manoj Monga, and Bodo E. Knudsen

QUESTIONS

1. What is the mechanism electrosurgery uses to affect tissues?
   a. Current is delivered to the tip of the instrument, causing it to heat and affect the tissue.
   b. Current is delivered to the tissue directly, causing it to heat.
   c. Current is conducted through a fluid medium to affect the tissue.
   d. Electrons are excited, creating increased light energy, which directly affects the tissue.

2. What is the mechanism electrocautery uses to affect tissues?
   a. Current is delivered to the tip of the instrument, causing it to heat and affect the tissue.
   b. Current is delivered to the tissue directly, causing it to heat.
   c. Current is conducted through a fluid medium to affect the tissue.
   d. Electrons are excited, creating increased light energy, which directly affects the tissue.

3. When cautery is set to "pure cut," the current is:
   a. interrupted but mainly on.
   b. interrupted but mainly off.
   c. continuous.
   d. continuous but oscillates between high and low voltage.
   e. variable in both intermittency and voltage.

4. An argon beam coagulator:
   a. works by igniting a column of argon gas.
   b. uses an argon laser to diffusely coagulate tissues.
   c. should be used in direct contact with the tissue's surface.
   d. should be used in a dry environment.
   e. uses a column of argon gas that passes over an electrode.

5. Bipolar and monopolar cautery differ in that:
   a. monopolar does not require a dispersive electrode.
   b. monopolar can be used at much higher voltages.
   c. bipolar does not require a dispersive electrode.
   d. bipolar can be used at much higher voltages.
   e. there are no differences.

6. The LigaSure and Gyrus PK both show benefits over the Thunderbeat and Ultrashears in that they:
   a. are able to produce less smoke and keep a clear visual field.
   b. seal vessels faster and with higher burst pressures.
   c. function more reliably in wet environments.
   d. are cheaper and reusable.
   e. show no benefits and are inferior products.

7. The wavelength for the holmium:YAG (Ho:YAG) laser is:
   a. 488 nm—blue; 514 nm—green.
   b. 1064 nm.
   c. 1318 nm.
   d. 2140 nm.
   e. 2640 nm.

8. Stone fragmentation via Ho:YAG lasers occurs by:
   a. cavitation bubble collapse and resulting shock waves.
   b. fluid jets created by rapid heating of the surrounding fluid.
   c. pneumatic activity of the laser tip against the stone.
   d. direct energy absorption.
   e. ultrasonic thermal ablation of the stone surface.

9. The major downside of pneumatic lithotripsy in the ureter is:
   a. cost.
   b. ureteral injury.
   c. poor visualization.
   d. stone retropulsion.
   e. all of the above.

10. Which instruments can be used through flexible ureteroscopy?
    a. Electrohydraulic lithotripsy (EHL), pneumatic, ultrasonic
    b. Laser, ultrasonic, combination (pneumatic and ultrasonic)
    c. Ultrasonic, laser, EHL
    d. Combination (pneumatic and ultrasound), laser, EHL
    e. All modalities

ANSWERS

1. **b. Current is delivered to the tissue directly, causing it to heat.** Electrosurgery uses radiofrequency current in the range of 400,000 to 600,000 Hz to pass through tissue and create the desired effects. The generators deliver more than 100 W of power to the tissue at voltages ranging from 100 to 5000 V. While the current is delivered to the tissue, the tissue is heated and the effect occurs. This is in contrast to electrocautery, in which the instrument itself is heated and then applied to the tissue.

2. **a. Current is delivered to the tip of the instrument, causing it to heat and affect the tissue.** In contrast to electrosurgery, where radiofrequency current in the range of 400,000 to 600,000 Hz passes through tissue and create the desired effects, with electrocautery the tip of the instrument is heated and then applied to the tissue to create the desired effect.

3. **c. Continuous.** Pure cut uses continuous delivery, whereas coagulation uses interrupted delivery. Generators will also usually provide "blended" modes that modify the degree of interruption to gain the desired effect.

4. **e. Uses a column of argon gas that passes over an electrode.** The argon beam coagulator works by adding a column of argon gas that passes over the electrode; electrosurgical energy ionizes the argon gas and helps to displace the blood in the surgical field. Because argon is a noble gas, the current from the electrode is effectively transmitted to the underlying tissue.

5. **c. Bipolar does not require a dispersive electrode.** Unlike monopolar systems in which a circuit is created by delivering

the energy via an electrode and then removed from the patient using a dispersive electrode (grounding pad), bipolar delivery does not require a dispersive electrode. Rather, the active and return electrodes are integrated in the delivery handpiece. The tissue contained between the electrodes is the target tissue.

6. **b. Seal vessels faster, and with higher burst pressures.** A comparison study comparing the vessel sealing times and thermal spread of two bipolar vessel sealing systems (LigaSure and Gyrus PK), as well as an ultrasonic devise (Ethicon Harmonic Scalpel), was performed. This demonstrated that the two bipolar systems had faster vessel sealing times with higher burst pressures compared with the ultrasonic device. However, the ultrasonic device had less thermal spread and smoke production (Lamberton et al., 2008).[a]

7. **d. 2140 nm.** Ho:YAG laser is a 2140-nm pulsed laser that is used for both soft tissue and lithotripsy applications in urology. The 2140-nm wavelength is strongly absorbed in water, traveling only approximately 0.5 mm in the fluid medium, making it ideal for the urologic environment. Both the argon (488 nm—blue; 514 nm—green) and Nd:YAG (1064 nm, 1318 nm) lasers use two different wavelengths.

8. **d. Direct energy absorption.** Previous laser technologies (Ruby, Nd:YAG) used photoacoustic or photomechanical processes, where light energy created shock waves that fragmented stones. In contrast, the Ho:YAG laser uses photothermal lithotripsy, which involves direct light energy absorption ("photo") by stone surfaces, causing rapid temperature ("thermal") increases, before significant heat diffusion can occur. A "Moses effect" occurs by the rapid vaporization of fluid creating a vapor channel between the fiber tip and stone's surface, allowing for more direct energy transfer. Interstitial water may also become vaporized, leading to fragment ejection; however, these forces are not great enough to directly lead to stone fracture.

9. **d. Stone retropulsion.** Pneumatic lithotripsy uses ballistic forces to transfer kinetic energy from a handheld probe to the stone surface. Repetitive strikes (12 Hz LithoClast, 15 to 30 Hz Electrokinetic lithotripter) from the probe tip act as a jackhammer, fragmenting stones at the point of contact. Stone migration is a significant disadvantage when treating ureteric stones because the probe's ballistic effect can propel stones in capacious ureters into the kidney. Retropulsion has been reported in as much as 10% of distal and 40% of proximal stones treated with pneumatic lithotripsy. In a four-way comparison of intracorporeal lithotripters on iatrogenic urothelial trauma, pneumatic probes were found to be the least traumatic (compared with laser, ultrasonic, and EHL). Pneumatic lithotripters are currently one of the most cost effective because of their durability and use of reusable probes.

10. **c. Ultrasonic, laser, EHL.** Because of their mechanisms of action, EHL probes and laser fibers can fragment stones while being flexed; 200-μm laser fibers can be readily flexed 270 degrees in flexible ureteroscopes, whereas thin EHL probes (1.9 Fr) are flexible enough to reach the lower pole while conducting electrical pulses for spark discharge. Thin ultrasonic probes can be moderately deflected using flexible scopes; however, these wirelike probes lack a lumen for suction and suffer from significant dampening and reduced efficiency with flexion. Any amount of torque applied to pneumatic lithotrites significantly reduces the jackhammer-like movements and reduces fragmentation potential. Similarly, combination lithotrites cannot be flexed, nor are they available in sizes compatible with ureteroscopy.

---

[a] Sources referenced can be found in *Campbell-Walsh-Wein Urology, 12th Edition*, on the Expert Consult website.

CHAPTER REVIEW

1. When alternating current is used, the term for resistance is impedance; impedance increases when charring occurs.
2. Lasers with shorter wavelengths have a much greater amount of scatter than those with longer wavelengths.
3. The depth of tissue penetration for Nd:YAG is 10 mm, KTP 1 to 2 mm, Ho:YAG 0.4 mm, and CO_2 no significant penetration.
4. The electrohydraulic probe produces a spark that creates a shock wave; one should place the probe 1 mm away from the stone.
5. Stone composition and surface characteristics affect the efficiency of EHL, with uric acid stones taking the most time to fragment.
6. The pneumatic device is the only modality that does not cut through wire, such as a safety guidewire or stone basket.
7. The ultrasonic probe results in vibration at the end of the probe that is transferred to the stone, causing it to fracture.
8. Ho:YAG laser stone fragmentation is primarily due to a photothermal effect.
9. Laser lithotripsy produces the smallest fragments and is useful for all stone compositions.
10. The argon beam coagulator works by adding a column of argon gas that passes over the electrode, and then electrosurgical energy ionizes the argon gas and helps to displace the blood in the surgical field. Because argon is a noble gas, the current from the electrode is effectively transmitted to the underlying tissue.
11. Bipolar delivery does not require a dispersive electrode (grounding pad). The active and return electrodes are integrated in the delivery handpiece.
12. The bipolar systems for sealing tissue have faster vessel sealing times with higher burst pressures compared with the ultrasonic device. However, the ultrasonic device has less thermal spread and smoke production.
13. Pneumatic probes are the least traumatic to ureteral tissue compared with laser, ultrasonic, and EHL.

16 Evaluation and Management of Hematuria

Stephen A. Boorjian, Jay D. Raman, and Daniel A. Barocas

QUESTIONS

1. According to AUA guidelines, microhematuria sufficient to trigger a diagnostic evaluation is defined as:
   a. a positive chemical test (urine dipstick) showing small, moderate, or large blood on one properly collected specimen.
   b. a positive chemical test (urine dipstick) showing small, moderate, or large blood on at least two of three properly collected specimens.
   c. a positive chemical test (urine dipstick) showing large blood on one properly collected specimen.
   d. urine microscopy showing three or more red blood cells per high-powered field on one properly collected urine specimen.
   e. urine microscopy showing three or more RBC/HPF on at least two of three properly collected urine specimens.

2. The likelihood of finding a malignancy in a patient with microhematuria is influenced by all of the following EXCEPT:
   a. age.
   b. gender.
   c. use of anticoagulants.
   d. tobacco use.
   e. degree of hematuria.

3. According to AUA guidelines, the proper initial assessment of a 50-year-old patient with asymptomatic microhematuria includes:
   a. blood pressure measurement, serum creatinine level, cystoscopy, and computed tomography (CT) urogram.
   b. urine cytology, cystoscopy, and CT urogram.
   c. urine cytology, blue-light cystoscopy, and any upper tract imaging.
   d. urine cytology and renal/bladder ultrasound.
   e. no evaluation is necessary unless microhematuria is persistent/recurrent or hematuria is visible.

4. In the evaluation of patients with microhematuria, cystoscopy may be safely avoided if:
   a. there are no associated symptoms in a patient of any age.
   b. the patient is under 35 years of age and without symptoms or risk factors for malignancy.
   c. the patient is taking aspirin or warfarin.
   d. the cytology is negative.
   e. the patient has a history of urinary tract infection and hematuria is still present after treatment.

5. Patients presenting with gross hematuria in the absence of recent trauma or concurrent infection who are on anticoagulation medications should be evaluated with:
   a. urinalysis, urine cytology, and cystoscopy only.
   b. CT urogram, with cystoscopy only if symptomatic.
   c. no evaluation necessary.
   d. assessment of anticoagulation status, and evaluation only if supra-therapeutic.
   e. urine cytology, cystoscopy, CT urogram.

6. The metabolite of oxazaphosphorine chemotherapeutic agents which is responsible for hemorrhagic cystitis is:
   a. Mesna.
   b. Acrolein.
   c. Formalin.
   d. Gemcitabine.
   e. Methotrexate.

7. Use of intravesical alum for hemorrhagic cystitis should be avoided in patients with:
   a. a history of malignancy.
   b. a history of detrusor instability.
   c. active gross hematuria.
   d. renal insufficiency.
   e. vesicoureteral reflux.

8. The molecular pathophysiology linking BPH and hematuria is exemplified by the identification of which of the following in the prostate tissue from men with BPH:
   a. decreased microvessel density
   b. androgen-independent angiogenesis
   c. elevated VEGF expression
   d. reduced cell proliferation
   e. diminished blood flow

9. A 65-year-old man with a history of BPH has recurrent gross hematuria. The patient is clinically stable, with no transfusion requirement, no clots in urine, and no difficulty with bladder emptying. A hematuria evaluation with CT urogram, cystoscopy, and urine cytology is otherwise unremarkable. The best next step in management is:
   a. five-alpha reductase inhibitor.
   b. alpha-blocker therapy.
   c. prostatic artery embolization (PAE).
   d. channel TURP.
   e. trial of antibiotic therapy.

10. A 35-year-old man presents with complaint of penile pain and immediate detumescence during intercourse. Physical examination notes blood at the urethral meatus. The next step should be:
    a. immediate operative exploration.
    b. CT scan of pelvis.
    c. retrograde urethrography.
    d. obtain serum coagulation parameters.
    e. conservative management with serial examinations.

11. A 55-year-old woman presents with intermittent gross hematuria 2 weeks after undergoing a right partial nephrectomy for a 4-cm solid enhancing renal mass. She is afebrile with stable

vital signs. She is able to void to completion and her urine is red without clots. Her creatinine is 1.1 mg/dL. The next step should be:

a. surgical exploration.

b. renal angiography.

c. continuous bladder irrigation.

d. observation.

e. noncontrast CT scan of the abdomen/pelvis.

ANSWERS

1. **d. Urine microscopy showing three or more red blood cells per high-powered field on one properly collected urine specimen.** The presence of three of more RBCs/HPF on a single urine microscopy is associated with malignancy in 2.3-5.5% of patients. Chemical tests for hematuria detect the peroxidase activity of erythrocytes using benzidine, and can render false results in the presence of dehydration, myoglobinuria, high doses of vitamin C, improper technique, and other factors. While higher levels of microhematuria (>25 RBCs/HPF) are known to be associated with higher rates of malignancy on evaluation, setting the threshold higher than three RBCs/HPF or requiring more than one positive urinalysis would lead to an unknown number of missed opportunities for diagnosis.

2. **c. Use of anticoagulants.** Increasing age, male gender, and tobacco use are risk factors for urologic cancers and specifically for urothelial carcinoma. In addition, while there is little data to distinguish among thresholds of two, three, four, or five RBCs/HPF, it is clear that a high level of microhematuria (>25 RBCs/HPF) is associated with a greater likelihood of malignancy. By contrast, patients using anticoagulant medications or anti-platelet medications have a similar risk of malignancy compared to those who do not use these medications. Therefore such patients should be evaluated comparably to those who do not use anticoagulants or anti-platelet agents.

3. **a. Blood pressure measurement, serum creatinine level, cystoscopy, and computed tomography (CT) urogram.** The AUA suggests that adult patients presenting with asymptomatic microhematuria should undergo evaluation to determine the cause. Blood pressure measurement and serum creatinine level may help identify patients who require concurrent nephrologic workup, and creatinine level also helps determine patient eligibility for contrast imaging. The evaluation of asymptomatic hematuria includes imaging (preferably with CT urogram), and cystoscopy in patients 35 and older and those under 35 with risk factors for malignancy.

4. **b. The patient is under 35 years of age and without symptoms or risk factors for malignancy.** The AUA guidelines (Fig. 16.1) call for use of cystoscopy for evaluation of hematuria in all patients 35 years of age and older (Recommendation). The risk of malignancy is very low in persons under 35 years of age, such that the potential benefits of cystoscopy may be outweighed by the very small risks associated with the procedure. Therefore it is an option to omit cystoscopy in patients under the age of 35, provided that the patient does not have risk factors for a urologic malignancy.

5. **e. Urine cytology, cystoscopy, CT urogram.** Given the increased frequency with which clinically significant findings are associated with gross hematuria, the recommended evaluation

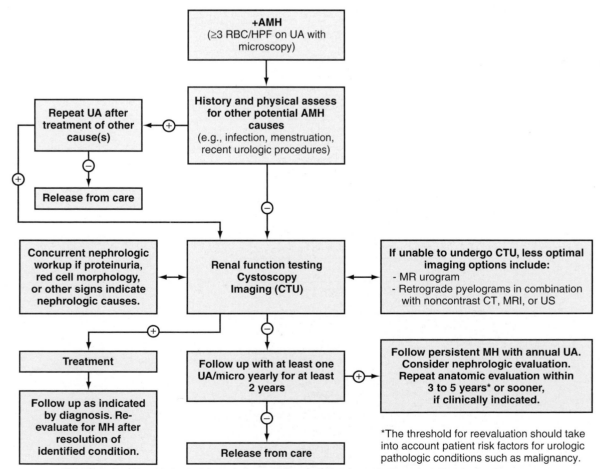

Fig. 16.1 American Urological Association guideline algorithm for evaluation of adult patients with asymptomatic microhematuria. *AMH,* Asymptomatic microhematuria; *CT,* computed tomography; *CTU,* computed tomography urogram; *HPF,* high-power field; *MH,* microhematuria; *MR,* magnetic resonance; *MRI,* magnetic resonance imaging; *RBC,* red blood cell; *UA,* urinalysis; *US,* ultrasound.

in this setting is relatively uniform. That is, patients presenting with gross hematuria in the absence of antecedent trauma or culture-documented urinary tract infection should be evaluated with a urine cytology, cystoscopy, and upper tract imaging, preferably CT urogram. Importantly, patients who develop hematuria who are on anticoagulation medications should undergo a complete evaluation in the same manner as patients not taking such medications, as the prevalence of hematuria, as well as the likelihood of finding genitourinary cancers, among patients with hematuria on anticoagulation has been reported to be no different from patients not taking such medications.

6. **b. Acrolein.** Bladder toxicity from oxazaphosphorine chemotherapeutic agents results from renal excretion of the metabolite acrolein, which is produced by the liver and which stimulates bladder mucosal sloughing and subsequent tissue edema/fibrosis. Mesna (2-mercaptoethane sulfonate), which binds to acrolein and renders it inert, has been suggested for prophylaxis against cyclophosphamide-induced hemorrhagic cystitis.

7. **d. Renal insufficiency.** Alum may be considered for first-line intravesical therapy among patients with hemorrhagic cystitis (**Fig. 16.2**) failing initial supportive measures. However, while cell penetration and therefore overall toxicity of this agent are low, systemic absorption may nevertheless occur and may result in aluminum toxicity, with consequent mental status changes, particularly among patients with renal insufficiency. Meanwhile, prior to intravesical administration of silver nitrate or of formalin, a cystogram should be obtained to evaluate for the presence of vesicoureteral reflux.

8. **c. Elevated VEGF expression.** The etiology for BPH-related hematuria has been thought to be increased prostatic vascularity due to higher microvessel density in hyperplastic prostate tissue. This noted increase in microvessel density has in turn been linked to higher levels of VEGF. Moreover, as the pathophysiology of BPH-related bleeding has been postulated as increased cell proliferation stimulating increased vascularity, efforts to suppress prostate growth via androgen ablation have been explored. Indeed, both estrogens and antiandrogens have, in small case re-

ports, been associated with decreased prostate bleeding, presumably through the repression of androgen-stimulated angiogenesis and the induction of programmed cell death within the prostate.

9. **a. Five-alpha reductase inhibitor.** Treatment with five-alpha reductase inhibitors has been associated with decreased VEGF expression, prostate microvessel density, and prostatic blood flow. Clinically, multiple series have demonstrated efficacy of finasteride for BPH-related hematuria, with symptom improvement or resolution consistently noted in approximately 90% of patients. As such, in otherwise stable patients, finasteride represents a reasonable first-line therapy for BPH-related gross hematuria after the completion of an initial diagnostic evaluation. Channel TURP has typically been utilized in the setting of prostate cancer, while a "standard" TURP or an alternative form of such endoscopic prostate tissue removal/destruction may be used for patients with persistent bleeding from BPH despite conservative therapies and/or endoscopic fulguration, particularly when additional indications for BPH surgery coexist. In cases with persistent bleeding despite TURP or in the significantly comorbid patient, prostatic artery embolization can be considered.

10. **c. Retrograde urethrography.** The clinical scenario is consistent with an acute penile fracture. Blood at the meatus raises suspicion for concomitant urethral injury that requires investigation by retrograde urethrography prior to planned operative repair. Conservative management poses the risk of untreated urethral and corporal injury that can result in urethral stricture disease and erectile dysfunction.

11. **b. Renal angiography.** The clinical scenario is consistent with a renal arteriovenous malformation (AVM). Renal angiography may be both diagnostic and therapeutic in this scenario with ability to coil or embolize this abnormal vascular communication. Observation and bladder irrigation do not address the underlying causative factor while non-contrast CT imaging fails to delineate the vascular anatomy. Surgical exploration has a high likelihood of renal loss and is reserved for cases refractory to angiographic modalities.

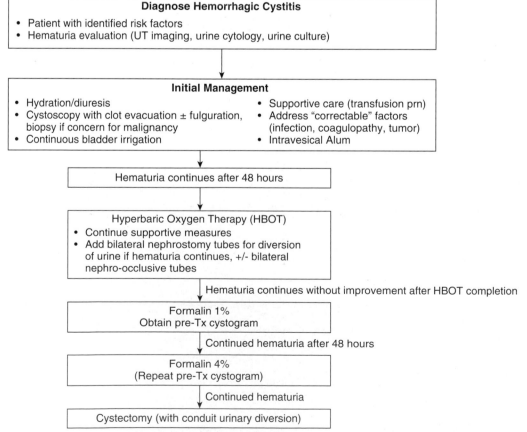

Fig. 16.2 Management algorithm for patients with hemorrhagic cystitis. *HBOT*, Hyperbaric oxygen therapy; *Tx*, treatment; *UT*, upper tract.

CHAPTER REVIEW

1. Microscopic hematuria (MH) is defined by the AUA guidelines as three or more RBCs/HPF, identified on one or more occasions on urine microscopy. Urine dipstick testing is insufficient for the diagnosis of MH.
2. MH is quite common, with a prevalence of approximately 6.5% of adults, varying according to the characteristics of the population.
3. Malignancy has been detected in approximately 3.5% of patients evaluated for asymptomatic MH. The risk of malignancy diagnosis is greater in patients with higher degrees of hematuria, male gender, and/or risk factors for malignancy, and lower in absence of these risk factors.
4. Evaluation of adults with microscopic hematuria includes a history and physical examination, renal function testing, and upper tract imaging for all patients.
5. White light cystoscopy is recommended in the evaluation of asymptomatic MH for patients 35 years of age or older and/or those with risk factors for malignancy.
6. CT urogram is the preferred imaging modality for the evaluation of hematuria.
7. Urine cytologic examination and biomarkers are not indicated in the initial evaluation of asymptomatic MH.
8. Patients with a negative complete evaluation can be released from care if subsequent urinalyses confirm resolution of MH. Reevaluation should be considered in patients with persistent/recurrent MH and those with an incomplete initial evaluation.
9. Oxazaphosphorine chemotherapeutic agents have been linked to the development of hemorrhagic cystitis through exposure of the metabolite acrolein to the urothelium.
10. Alum may be used as a first-line intravesical therapy for hemorrhagic cystitis in patients without renal dysfunction.
11. Formalin is a highly effective form of intravesical therapy for hemorrhagic cystitis. A cystogram should be obtained before therapy to ensure no vesicoureteral reflux.
12. HBOT has been associated with response rates of 80% to 100% for patients with hemorrhagic cystitis.
13. BPH represents the most common cause of GH in men older than 60 years.
14. 5α-Reductase inhibitors may be used for BPH-related GH, with potential improvement having been noted within weeks after instituting therapy.
15. Androgen deprivation may be effective for patients with locally advanced prostate cancer with GH.
16. Angioembolization and/or urinary diversion represent salvage options for management for patients with refractory hematuria, pending clinical status.
17. Urethral bleeding should be suspected with blood at the meatus and/or initial hematuria.
18. A concern for traumatic urethral injury should prompt retrograde urethrogram.
19. Urinary findings suggestive of a glomerular or tubulointerstitial medical renal disease include the presence of RBC casts in the urinary sediment, dysmorphic RBCs, and proteinuria.
20. In patients with GH after a recent renal procedure, expeditious angiography should be considered to allow for the diagnosis and management of renal AVM.

17 Complications of Urologic Surgery

Reza Ghavamian and Charbel Chalouhy

QUESTIONS

1. During posterior dissection in a robotic salvage radical prostatectomy, an inadvertent rectal injury is encountered. Gross fecal spillage is seen in the surgical field. What does a good management strategy include?

    a. Closure of rectal mucosa and serosa with non-absorbable sutures

    b. Open conversion, colostomy, and delayed repair

    c. Broad-spectrum antibiotics are advised for up to 1 month postoperatively

    d. Primary closure and omental flap

    e. Open approach to radical prostatectomy is preferable in this case given the lower incidence of injuries

2. Which of the following has the greatest effect on pseudoaneurysm development following partial nephrectomy?

    a. The open approach versus minimally invasive (1% vs. 5%)

    b. Patients with higher nephrometry score are at increased risk

    c. Early unclamping even in the presence of arterial bleed

    d. Tumor depth has no impact on incidence of pseudoaneurysm

    e. Deep suture repair through the renal parenchyma is the best preventative measure

3. When obtaining pneumoperitoneum with the VERESS needle:

    a. the angle of entry for the needle should be near 90 degrees for people with normal body mass index (BMI).

    b. the angle of entry for the needle should be near 45 degrees for people with high BMI.

    c. the most commonly injured vessel is the right iliac vein.

    d. the most commonly injured vessel is the left common iliac vein.

    e. this access modality has been increasingly abandoned and replaced by optical trocars.

4. What is true about urine leaks after partial nephrectomy?

    a. They are more likely to cause ileus during open surgery

    b. 90% of patients will require readmission.

    c. The mean postoperative day for presentation is 18 days.

    d. Longer warm ischemia times are directly related to the development of urine leaks.

    e. This complication is more common in minimally invasive surgery.

5. Once all attempts for conservative management have failed for ureteral complications, it is agreed that:

    a. waiting 6 weeks for surgical repair allowing inflammation to subside is reasonable.

    b. early surgical repair can be achieved when discovered early within 3 weeks.

    c. urinomas do not have to be drained to prevent reaccumulation.

    d. there is no increased risk for stricture.

    e. robotic approach for Boari flap and psoas hitch should be avoided.

6. During Psoas hitch procedure, the most commonly injured structure is:

    a. obturator nerve.

    b. ilio-inguinal nerve.

    c. pudendal nerve.

    d. sympathetic nerves.

    e. genito-femoral nerve.

7. Brachial plexus injuries can be prevented by:

    a. adequate padding of the arms.

    b. arm positioning in external rotation and posterior shoulder displacement.

    c. avoiding excess arm abduction of greater than 90 degrees.

    d. preferring modified lateral to lateral positions.

    e. limiting axillary rolls.

ANSWERS

1. **b. Open conversion, colostomy, and delayed repair.** A good management strategy in this case includes open conversion, colostomy, and delayed repair.

2. **b. Patients with higher nephrometry score are at increased risk.** Patients with higher nephrometry score are at increased risk for pseudoaneurysm development following partial nephrectomy.

3. **d. The most commonly injured vessel is the left common iliac vein.** When obtaining pneumoperitoneum with the Veress needle, the most commonly injured vessel is the left common iliac vein.

4. **d. Longer warm ischemia times are directly related to the development of urine leaks.** Longer warm ischemia times are directly related to the development of urine leaks after partial nephrectomy.

5. **a. Waiting 6 weeks for surgical repair allowing inflammation to subside is reasonable.** Once all attempts for conservative management have failed for ureteral complications, it is agreed that waiting 6 weeks for surgical repair allowing inflammation to subside is reasonable.

6. **e. Genito-femoral nerve.** The most commonly injured structure during Psoas hitch procedure is the genito-femoral nerve.

7. **c. Avoiding excess arm abduction of greater than 90 degrees.** Avoiding excess arm abduction of greater than 90 degrees can prevent brachial plexus injuries.

CHAPTER REVIEW

1. A wide array of physiologic, urinary, vascular, bowel, and visceral complications can occur with all forms of urologic operations.
2. With the wide adoption of laparoscopic and robotic surgery in urology, unique sets of complications are encountered.
3. As more complex operations are performed in a minimally invasive fashion, the rate of complications can increase.
4. Some complications after laparoscopic and robotic procedures can present in an atypical and delayed fashion.
5. A high index of suspicion is necessary for prompt and timely intraoperative and postoperative diagnosis and management.
6. The most important aspect of complication management is complication prevention with adequate planning, attention to detail, and meticulous surgical technique.

Urologic Considerations in Pregnancy

Melissa R. Kaufman

QUESTIONS

1. Decreased cardiac output in pregnant patients undergoing urologic surgery may be ameliorated by the following maneuver:
   a. Aggressive intraoperative fluid resuscitation
   b. Administration of alpha receptor agonists
   c. Use of only regional anesthesia
   d. Right-side elevation allowing displacement of the uterus off the vena cava
   e. High lithotomy position to increase venous return from lower extremities

2. Changes in renal tubular function during pregnancy result in alterations of urine chemistries EXCEPT for:
   a. glycosuria.
   b. proteinuria.
   c. pyuria.
   d. albuminuria.
   e. calcinuria.

3. Symptomatic physiologic hydronephrosis of pregnancy should be primarily managed by:
   a. percutaneous nephrostomy.
   b. conservative measures.
   c. antibiotic prophylaxis.
   d. ureteral stent.
   e. Alpha-blocker therapy.

4. Which of the following statements is FALSE regarding imaging in pregnant patients?
   a. Ultrasound and magnetic resonance imaging are the techniques of choice.
   b. Routine imaging with magnetic resonance imaging (MRI) should employ use of gadolinium contrast.
   c. Radiation from computed tomography (CT) scan is usually at a dose lower than that associated with fetal harm.
   d. Safety of nuclear medicine studies is dependent on the isotope utilized.
   e. None of the above.

5. Current practice recommendations for pregnant women undergoing nonobstetric surgery include:
   a. Anesthetic agents should be avoided due to teratogenic effects.
   b. Elective surgery is best accomplished in the first trimester.
   c. Use of fetal heart rate monitoring during the first trimester to influence delivery decisions.
   d. Surgery should be performed at an institution with neonatal and pediatric services.
   e. None of the above.

6. Which of the following statements regarding stone disease in pregnancy is TRUE?
   a. Approximately 30% of pregnant women with symptomatic calculi pass the stone spontaneously.

   b. Stone events in pregnancy carry an increased risk of maternal and fetal morbidity.
   c. Complication rates of ureteroscopy in pregnant women is 27%.
   d. Ureteroscopy and stent placement should always be performed without fluoroscopic guidance.
   e. None of the above.

7. Counseling of female patients with myelomeningocele (MMC) desiring pregnancy includes:
   a. Women with MMC in general are considered to have normal fertility.
   b. There is no risk of genetic transmission of neural tube defects to the offspring.
   c. Patients with preexisting renal insufficiency do not have increased risk during pregnancy of worsening renal function.
   d. Women with MMC do not require folic acid supplementation during conception.
   e. None of the above.

8. All of the following regarding placenta percreta are correct EXCEPT:
   a. Prior cesarean section is the predominant risk factor for abnormal placentation.
   b. Biopsy prior to surgical intervention is indicated for placenta percreta.
   c. A multidisciplinary team is mandated to deliver specialized care.
   d. Preoperative counseling should include discussion of ureteral catheters, stents, urinary tract injury, or possible extirpative surgery with urinary diversion.
   e. None of the above.

ANSWERS

1. **d. Right-side elevation allowing displacement of the uterus off the vena cava.** CO in pregnancy is dependent on maternal position and standard techniques for urology may pose unintended consequences. In the supine position, CO in the pregnant woman decreases by up to 30% at term as compared to a lateral recumbent position. Prevention of potential acute drops in venous return and CO may require avoidance of supine and lithotomy positions when feasible with right-side elevation to displace the uterus to the left. Placement of a wedge may be logistically challenging but achieving a 15- to 20-degree left tilt should reduce uterine compression of the inferior vena cava.

2. **c. Pyuria.** Marked change in renal tubular function during pregnancy results in a variety of alterations of urine chemistries that may be encountered by the urologist although elevation of ketones is not typical. Indeed, glycosuria during pregnancy is exceedingly common, with 10- to 100-fold increase in urinary glucose excretion described. Proteinuria and albuminuria additionally manifest during pregnancy and may increase as the gestation advances. Calcinuria doubles during pregnancy. Although women may display pyuria due to contamination or superimposed infection, it is not a consistent finding during gestation.

3. **b. Conservative measures.** In general, ureteral stent insertion in symptomatic gestational hydronephrosis does not generally add benefit over conservative treatment and should be reserved for complicated cases or additional pathologic obstructions. Conservative measures include analgesia, position, and intravenous fluids and failure included signs of evolving infection or deteriorating renal function. Parameters that may increase the likelihood of surgical treatment with ureteral stenting for symptomatic hydronephrosis include maximal anterior-posterior renal pelvis diameter, parity, C-reactive protein level, white blood cell count, and pain on a visual analog scale. Rarely is percutaneous nephrostomy required, and there is not a role for antibiotics outside of acute infection. Alpha blockers are likewise not indicated for relief of colic from physiologic hydronephrosis.

4. **b. Routine imaging with magnetic resonance imaging (MRI) should employ use of gadolinium contrast.** This statement is false. The American College of Obstetricians and Gynecologists (ACOG) have outlined clinical guidelines to drive management decisions and determine the diagnostic imaging modality which provides the optimal risk/benefit ratio in many situations. The use of gadolinium contrast with MRI should be limited; it may be used as a contrast agent in the pregnant woman only if it significantly improves diagnostic performance and is expected to improve fetal or maternal outcomes.

5. **d. Surgery should be performed at an institution with neonatal and pediatric services.** Recommendations from the ACOG provide the urologist guidance regarding considerations for nonobstetric surgery during pregnancy. Overall, consultation with an obstetrician should be obtained to ensure pertinent aspects of maternal physiology are considered along with potential need for fetal monitoring. If possible, nonurgent surgery should be performed in the second trimester when preterm contractions and spontaneous abortion are least likely.

6. **b. Stone events in pregnancy carry an increased risk of maternal and fetal morbidity.** Of pregnant patients with symptomatic calculi, 50% to 80% will pass their stones spontaneously when treated conservatively with hydration and analgesia. However, a stone event in pregnancy does carry with it an increased risk of maternal and fetal morbidity, so patients should be followed closely for recurrent or persistent symptoms. Ureteroscopy in pregnancy carries an overall complication rate of 8.3%, with no significant difference in rates of urinary tract complications compared to the non-pregnant population. Although methods to reduce fetal radiation exposure should be employed, rarely would endoscopic procedures need to be performed without the aid of fluoroscopy.

7. **a. Women with MMC in general are considered to have normal fertility.** Females with MMC are considered to have normal fertility with up to 70% of those who conceive having successful pregnancies. With regard to transmission, the threat is identical if the affected parent is male or female; however, the incidence in female offspring is 1 in 13 and diminishes to 1 in 50 for male children. However, if both parents are affected, the neural tube defect transmission rate increases dramatically to 15%. Foremost is recognition that the greatest risk factor for worsening renal function in pregnant women with or without urinary reconstruction is preexisting renal insufficiency. Notably, compared to routine supplementation of women without MMC of 0.4 mg folic acid per day, **doses of 4 to 5 mg/ day have been advocated for the MMC patient desirous of fertility.**

8. **b. Biopsy prior to surgical intervention is indicated for placenta percreta.** With knowledge of the potential risk factors for abnormal placentation, the clinician may choose to proceed with cystoscopic evaluation of such patients to evaluate the posterior bladder wall and significant invasion. Biopsy of the hypervascular tissue visualized in the bladder is discouraged. Assembly of a multidisciplinary team is currently recommended standard of care to reduce maternal and fetal morbidity and mortality. Suggested involvement includes an appropriate anesthesiologist, obstetrician, experienced pelvic surgeon such as a gynecologic oncologist, intensivist, maternal-fetal medicine specialist, interventional radiologist, and as required additional surgical subspecialties such as urology and general surgery. Preoperative planning by the urologist should include appropriate counseling of the patient with regard to placement of ureteral catheters or stents as well as potential manifestations of substantial injury or need for extirpative surgery for urologic organs and urinary diversion. Prior cesarean delivery appears to be the predominant risk factor due to abnormal implantation in the myometrial scar with compromised vascularity. Advanced maternal age is additionally contributory with women over 35 years of age accounting for 57% of placental adhesive disorders.

CHAPTER REVIEW

1. Management of symptomatic physiologic hydronephrosis in the absence of other pathologies such as calculi remains a dilemma for the consulting urologist. Ureteral stent insertion in symptomatic gestational hydronephrosis does not generally add benefit over conservative treatment and should be reserved for complicated cases or additional pathologic obstructions.

2. Ultrasonography and MRI are the imaging techniques of choice for the pregnant patient, but they should be used prudently and only when use is expected to answer a relevant clinical question or otherwise provide medical benefit to the patient. With few exceptions, radiation exposure through radiography, CT scan, or nuclear medicine imaging techniques is at a dose much lower than the exposure associated with fetal harm. If these techniques are necessary in addition to ultrasonography or MRI or are more readily available for the diagnosis in question, they should not be withheld from a pregnant patient.

3. A pregnant woman should never be denied indicated surgery, regardless of trimester. If possible, nonurgent surgery should be performed in the second trimester when preterm contractions and spontaneous abortion are least likely.

4. Due to the tendency for the gravid uterus to compress the IVC, optimizing venous return often requires placing the pregnant surgical patient in a left lateral decubitus position when feasible. This left lateral position should be modified and considered during open, laparoscopic, and endoscopic procedures.

5. Of pregnant patients with symptomatic calculi, the majority will pass their stones spontaneously when treated conservatively with hydration and analgesia. However, for patients requiring intervention, ureteroscopy may be performed with no significant difference in rates of urinary tract complications compared to the non-pregnant population.

6. Most patients with congenital conditions affecting the lower urinary tract have normal fertility and should have prenatal counseling. Complexities of pregnancy in the population with prior urinary diversion require an individualized approach. Mode of delivery is dependent on prior urinary reconstructions and patient preference, although in most cases cesarean section is preferred for the bladder exstrophy patient.

7. Since pregnant women with asymptomatic bacteriuria (ASB) remain at higher risk for development of symptomatic lower or upper urinary tract infections that may precipitate adverse fetal outcomes such as decreased birth weight and premature labor, consensus opinions indicate that pregnant women should be screened for ASB and positive cultures should be treated.

8. Women diagnosed antenatally with placenta percreta should be referred to a tertiary care center and managed by a multidisciplinary team that includes urologists, general surgeons, obstetric anesthesiologists, interventional radiologists, and intensivists. Urologists should carefully counsel patients regarding complexities of management and outcomes for urinary tract injury including possible urinary diversion.

19 Intraoperative Consultation

Michael J. Schwartz and Jessica E. Kreshover

QUESTIONS

1. A colorectal surgeon calls you for intraoperative consultation. She believes that the right ureter "looks denuded" and wants your opinion on management. There is no prior history of radiation therapy to the abdomen or pelvis. You scrub into the surgery, inspect the field, and find a partial-thickness injury to approximately ⅓ of the circumference of the distal right ureter. No free fluid is present. The surgeon states that cautery may have been used in the area during dissection but is not sure. Retrograde pyelogram shows no extravasation. The best option for management is:

   a. perform cystoscopy and insertion of right ureteral stent.

   b. perform primary suture imbrication of the injured area and cover with omentum.

   c. debride and reimplant the right ureter with or without a Boari flap or psoas hitch.

   d. remove the segment of injured ureter and perform uretero-ureterostomy.

   e. replacement of the right distal ureter with ileum.

2. A bladder injury has been identified by an obstetrician immediately after tertiary cesarean delivery and you are called to evaluate and repair the injury intraoperatively. You arrive 20 minutes later, and when you arrive, the obstetrician shows you the 2-cm cystotomy that he closed while waiting for you. He reports that a catheter tip (14 F) had been visible through a small cystotomy at the anterior bladder dome. Your next step is:

   a. dictate an intraoperative consultation stating that the bladder had been injured and repaired by the obstetrician and no further urologic evaluation was required.

   b. leave a pelvic drain and larger catheter in place.

   c. cystoscopy to inspect the closure.

   d. scrub in to explore the bladder and visually inspect the closure.

   e. reopen the cystotomy and enlarge it as needed to inspect the ureteral orifices before closing and irrigating the bladder.

3. Your former co-resident calls by phone after causing an avulsion injury of the proximal left ureter during ureteroscopy for a ureteropelvic junction (UPJ) stone. The patient is stable. Your colleague is proposing a laparoscopic nephrectomy while the patient is under anesthesia, as he is concerned that repairing the ureter would require open surgery and possibly fail. He is very uncomfortable with performance of a primary repair himself and concerned about possible stricture development. He is on call and his partner, whom he would typically ask to help, is out of town until tomorrow. He asks if you agree with nephrectomy. You:

   a. disagree. He should perform primary ureteroureterostomy over a stent.

   b. disagree. He should discuss options with the family including primary repair, ureteral replacement (ileal ureter), autotransplant, and nephrectomy. The family should make the decision and he should proceed with their choice.

   c. disagree. He should speak with the family, temporize the patient with a nephrostomy, awaken the patient, and wait for available colleague comfortable with ureteroureterostomy to assist.

   d. agree. Nephrectomy holds no risk of stricture or other reparative procedures. It is the best and lowest-risk option.

   e. agree, but counsel him to present this to the patient's family as the best option before proceeding.

4. Gross hematuria is noted in the catheter drainage bag by the anesthesiologist just after a colorectal surgeon has completed a proctocolectomy for Crohn's disease and creation of a J-pouch. The 43-year-old male patient's abdomen is closed. You arrive to find the surgical drapes taken down, the patient in lithotomy still under anesthesia, and a catheter in place draining red urine. After prepping and draping the patient, you perform a cystoscopy and find two bleeding areas that appear to be at sites of perforations along the posterior bladder wall. After cauterizing the bleeding to improve your vision, you inspect the bladder and find no other injury. Your next step is to:

   a. perform bilateral retrograde studies and a cystogram.

   b. inject biologic glue via the cystoscope at the two sites and leave a large catheter for drainage.

   c. reopen the abdomen and repair the bladder perforations.

   d. leave large catheter and start continuous bladder irrigation.

   e. reopen the abdomen, repair the bladder, and dissect out the ureters bilaterally for visual inspection.

5. During a laparoscopic hysterectomy for a large benign fibroid uterus, the distal right ureter is cauterized with a bipolar cautery instrument and appears segmentally devascularized. There is no free fluid in the field. The patient is stable. After performing cystoscopy and left retrograde pyelogram to assess for bladder and contralateral ureteral injury, you find no other abnormality and recommend right ureteral reimplant. However, the gynecologist is strongly opposed to reimplant and insists on stent insertion, as the continuity of the ureter has not been disrupted. What is your next step?

   a. Defer to the primary surgeon, as she has a preexisting relationship with the patient and retains ultimate decision-making authority, even if you disagree.

   b. Offer the option of ureteroureterostomy over a stent, which would eliminate the need for the reimplant the gynecologist wants to avoid.

   c. Do nothing immediately, but defer and awaken the patient to allow her to participate in the decision for stent or reimplant.

   d. Perform the ureteral reimplant, involving the hospital medical director if necessary. The reimplant is in the patient's best interest, and deferring the decision is likely in this case only to cause harm.

   e. Agree to the stent, but insist that it remain in place for 6 to 8 weeks, as you are concerned about stricture or fistula formation otherwise.

ANSWERS

1. **c. Debride and reimplant the right ureter with or without a Boari flap or psoas hitch.** Although there is no extravasation, with a potential thermal injury, the extent of the injury may not be immediately apparent. As injury is within the distal $1/3$ of the ureter, reimplantation should be undertaken to minimize the much greater potential morbidity associated with delayed recognition.

2. **e. Reopen the cystotomy and enlarge it as needed to inspect the ureteral orifices before closing and irrigating the bladder.** Need to ensure appropriate closure as well as inspect for concomitant injuries. Relying upon the other surgeon to complete the assessment is not meeting the expected role of the consultant.

3. **c. Disagree. He should speak with the family, temporize the patient with a nephrostomy, awaken the patient, and wait for available colleague comfortable with ureteroureterostomy to assist.** It is important for surgeons to balance recognition of their own limitations with prioritizing the best interests of the patient. In this case, there is an available temporizing measure that will allow the surgeon to act in the best interest of the

patient and avoid unnecessary risk to the patient by performing a surgery outside of his own skillset. Performing a nephrectomy would not be the standard of care in a patient with presumably normal renal function being treated for a ureteral stone.

4. **a. Perform bilateral retrograde studies and a cystogram.** As there is potential need for reopening the patient and repairing the bladder in this case, performance of imaging to assess the ureters and bladder is a critical step that will direct the extent of exploration required. If the retrograde studies are normal, this will remove the need for ureteral exploration and minimize the time for any additional repair needed. The cystogram would also help determine if the bladder injury is extraperitoneal or intraperitoneal, influencing the decision for reopening and repairing the bladder.

5. **d. Perform the ureteral reimplant, involving the hospital medical director if necessary. The reimplant is in the patient's best interest, and deferring the decision is likely in this case only to cause harm.** The decision maker for an intraoperative consultation is the consultant. In this instance, knowing the potential harm that may occur with a delayed injury, it is in the patient's best interest to perform ureteral reimplant.

CHAPTER REVIEW

1. The intraoperative consultation enters the physician into a new patient-physician relationship, and full disclosure regarding the reason for consultation is critical.
2. When possible, all relevant stakeholders should be included when difficult intraoperative decisions are to be made.
3. When considering whether to temporize or attempt definitive action at intraoperative consultation, current patient condition, procedure morbidity, long-term consequences, and reversibility should all be thoroughly considered.
4. Complex reconstructions, with selected exceptions, are best deferred with temporizing measures until such time that the patient is able to participate in shared decision making.
5. Documentation of intraoperative consultations should be fact-based and include the consultant's primary observations and assessment.
6. When bladder injury is found, it is important to ensure there is no concomitant injury to the ureters or ureteral orifices.
7. When a bladder injury is suspected but not visualized, a cystotomy may be performed to facilitate identification of the area of injury.
8. Early recognition of ureteral injury is important, as failure to do so carries significant morbidity.
9. If ureteral injury is suspected but not visualized, imaging and/or endoscopic assessments should be performed to confirm presence or absence of injury.
10. Consultation for ureteral catheter placement should be reserved for the preoperative setting and for appropriately selected cases.

SECTION A Development and Prenatal Urology

20 Embryology of the Human Genitourinary Tract

Laurence S. Baskin and Gerald Cunha

QUESTIONS

1. The fetal kidneys develop from which of the following embryonic structures?
   a. Paraxial (somite) mesoderm
   b. Intermediate mesoderm
   c. Neural tube
   d. Lateral mesoderm

2. At what gestational time point does the metanephros development begin?
   a. 2 weeks
   b. 3 weeks
   c. 4 weeks
   d. 5 weeks

3. Which of the following statements is TRUE of the metanephric development?
   a. It requires the reciprocal inductive interaction between Müllerian duct and metanephric mesenchyme.
   b. The calyces, pelvis, and ureter derive from the differentiation of the metanephric mesenchyme.
   c. Older, more differentiated nephrons are located at the periphery of the developing kidney, whereas newer, less differentiated nephrons are found near the juxtamedullary region.
   d. In humans, although renal maturation continues postnatally, nephrogenesis is completed by birth.

4. The fused lower pole of the horseshoe kidney is trapped by which of the following structures during the ascent?
   a. Inferior mesenteric artery
   b. Superior mesenteric artery
   c. Celiac artery
   d. Common iliac artery

5. The homozygous gene disruption (gene knockout) in which of the following molecules does NOT lead to a significant renal maldevelopment in mice?
   a. WT-1
   b. Pax-2
   c. GDNF
   d. p53

6. Which of the following statements is NOT TRUE of GDNF?
   a. It is a ligand for the RET receptor tyrosine kinase.
   b. GDNF gene knockout mice demonstrate an abnormal renal development.
   c. It is expressed in the metanephric mesenchyme but not in the ureteric bud.
   d. GDNF arrests the ureteric bud growth in vitro.

7. The bladder trigone develops from which of the following structures?
   a. Mesonephric ducts
   b. Müllerian ducts
   c. Urogenital sinus
   d. Metanephric mesenchyme

8. The urachus involutes to become:
   a. verumontanum.
   b. the median umbilical ligament.
   c. appendix testicle.
   d. epoophoron.

9. Which of the following statements is NOT TRUE of bladder development?
   a. The bladder body and trigone is derived from the urogenital sinus and not the terminal portion of the mesonephric ducts.
   b. Bladder compliance seems to be low during early gestation, and it gradually increases thereafter.
   c. Epithelial-mesenchymal inductive interactions appear to be necessary for proper bladder development.
   d. Histologic evidence of smooth muscle differentiation begins near the bladder neck and proceeds toward the bladder dome.

10. The primordial germ cell migration and the formation of the genital ridges begin at which time point during gestation?
    a. Third week
    b. Fifth week
    c. Seventh week
    d. Ninth week

11. Which of the following statements is NOT TRUE of the paramesonephric (müllerian) ducts?
    a. Both male and female embryos form paramesonephric (müllerian) ducts.
    b. In male embryos, the paramesonephric ducts degenerate under the influence of the MIS (müllerian-inhibiting substance) produced by the Leydig cells.
    c. In male embryos, the paramesonephric ducts become the appendix testis and the prostatic utricle.
    d. In female embryos, the paramesonephric ducts form the female reproductive tract, including fallopian tubes, uterus, and upper vagina.

12. Which of the following structures in the male reproductive tract develops from the urogenital sinus?
    a. Vas deferens
    b. Testis
    c. Prostate
    d. Appendix epididymis

13. Which of the following statements is NOT TRUE of normal prostate development?

    a. It requires the conversion of testosterone into dihydrotestosterone by 5α-reductase.

    b. It is dependent on epithelial-mesenchymal interactions under the influence of androgens.

    c. It is first seen at the 10th to 12th week of gestation.

    d. It requires the effects of MIS.

14. In female embryos, the remnants of the mesonephric ducts persist as the following structures EXCEPT:

    a. epoophoron.

    b. paroophoron.

    c. hymen.

    d. Gartner duct cysts.

15. Which of the following statements is NOT TRUE of the external genitalia development?

    a. The appearance of the external genitalia is similar in male and female embryos until the 8th week.

    b. The external genital appearance of males who are deficient in 5α-reductase is similar to that of females.

    c. In males, the formation of distal glandular urethra may occur by the fusion of urethral folds proximally and the ingrowth of ectodermal cells distally.

    d. In females, the urethral folds become the labia majora, and the labioscrotal folds become the labia minora.

16. The testicles descend to the level of internal inguinal ring by which time point during gestation?

    a. Sixth week

    b. Third month

    c. Sixth month

    d. Ninth month

17. Which of the following statements is NOT TRUE of the sex-determining region of the Y chromosome (SRY)?

    a. Its expression triggers the primitive sex cord cells to differentiate into the Sertoli cells.

    b. Approximately 25% of sex reversal conditions in humans are attributable to SRY mutations.

    c. It is located on the short arm of the Y chromosome.

    d. It causes the regression of mesonephric ducts.

ANSWERS

1. **b. Intermediate mesoderm.** Mammals develop three kidneys in the course of intrauterine life. The embryonic kidneys are, in order of their appearance, the pronephros, the mesonephros, and the metanephros. The first two kidneys regress in utero, and the third becomes the permanent kidney. In terms of embryology, all three kidneys develop from the intermediate mesoderm.

2. **c. 4 weeks.** The definitive kidney, metanephros, forms in the sacral region as a pair of new structures, called the ureteric buds, sprouts from the distal portion of the nephric duct and comes in contact with the blastema of metanephric mesenchyme at about 4 weeks.

3. **d. In humans, although renal maturation continues postnatally, nephrogenesis is completed by birth.** It requires the inductive interaction between the ureteric bud and metanephric mesenchyme. The calyces, pelvis, and ureter derive from the ureteric bud. Older, more differentiated nephrons are located in the inner part of the kidney near the juxtamedullary region. In humans, although renal maturation continues to take place postnatally, nephrogenesis is completed before birth.

4. **a. Inferior mesenteric artery.** The inferior poles of the kidneys may fuse, forming a horseshoe kidney that crosses over the ventral side of the aorta. During ascent, the fused lower pole becomes trapped under the inferior mesenteric artery and thus does not reach its normal site.

5. **d. p53.** Mutant WT-1 mice do not form ureteric buds, and in Pax-2 gene knockout mice, no nephric ducts, müllerian ducts, ureteric buds, or metanephric mesenchyme form, and the animals die within 1 day of birth because of renal failure. Ureteric bud formation is impaired in glial cell line–derived neurotrophic factor (GDNF) knockout mice, but p53 gene knockout mice do not demonstrate significant renal developmental anomaly.

6. **d. GDNF arrests the ureteric bud growth in vitro.** GDNF promotes ureteric bud growth in vitro. Although the importance of RET in kidney development was clearly demonstrated, it is only recently that its ligand, GDNF, has been identified. GDNF is a secreted glycoprotein that possesses a cystine-knot motif. GDNF is expressed within the metanephric mesenchyme prior to ureteric bud invasion, and ureteric bud formation is impaired in GDNF knockout mice.

7. **c. Urogenital sinus.** With use of the cell lineage studies the trigone was found to form mostly from bladder smooth muscle cells with only a minor contribution from the ureters. This is in contrast to the classic hypothesis where the trigone is formed from an extension of the ureteral development into the bladder.

8. **b. The median umbilical ligament.** By the 12th week, the urachus involutes to become a fibrous cord, which becomes the median umbilical ligament.

9. **d. Histologic evidence of smooth muscle differentiation begins near the bladder neck and proceeds toward the bladder dome.** Between the 7th and 12th weeks, the surrounding connective tissues condense and smooth muscle fibers begin to appear, first at the region of the bladder dome and later proceeding toward the bladder neck.

10. **b. Fifth week.** During the fifth week, primordial germ cells migrate from the yolk sac along the dorsal mesentery to populate the mesenchyme of the posterior body wall near the 10th thoracic level. In both sexes, the arrival of primordial germ cells in the area of future gonads serves as the signal for the existing cells of the mesonephros and the adjacent coelomic epithelium to proliferate and form a pair of genital ridges just medial to the developing mesonephros.

11. **b. In male embryos, the paramesonephric ducts degenerate under the influence of the MIS (müllerian-inhibiting substance) produced by the Leydig cells.** A new pair of ducts, called the paramesonephric (müllerian) ducts, begins to form just lateral to the mesonephric ducts in both male and female embryos. These ducts arise by the craniocaudal invagination of thickened coelomic epithelium, extending all the way from the third thoracic segment to the posterior wall of the developing urogenital sinus. The caudal tips of the paramesonephric ducts adhere to each other as they connect with the urogenital sinus between the openings of the right and left mesonephric ducts. The cranial ends of the paramesonephric ducts form funnel-shaped openings into the coelomic cavity (the future peritoneum). As developing Sertoli cells begin their differentiation in response to the SRY (sex-determining region of the Y chromosome), they begin to secrete MIS, which causes the paramesonephric (müllerian) ducts to regress rapidly between the 8th and 10th weeks. Small müllerian duct remnants can be detected in the developed male as a small tissue protrusion at the superior pole of the testicle, called the appendix testis, and as a posterior expansion of the prostatic urethra, called the prostatic utricle. In female embryos, MIS is absent, so the müllerian ducts do not regress and instead give rise to fallopian tubes, uterus, and vagina.

12. **c. Prostate.** Vas deferens and appendix epididymis all develop from the mesonephric ducts. Testis from the gonadal ridge. The prostate and bulbourethral glands develop from the urogenital sinus.

13. **d. It requires the hormonal effects of MIS.** The prostate gland begins to develop during the 10th to 12th week as a cluster of

endodermal evaginations budding from the pelvic urethra (derived from the urogenital sinus). These presumptive prostatic outgrowths are induced by the surrounding mesenchyme, and this process depends on the conversion of testosterone into dihydrotestosterone by 5α-reductase. Similar to renal and bladder development, prostatic development depends on mesenchymal-epithelial interactions but under the influence of androgens. There is no evidence that MIS plays a direct role in prostate development.

14. **c. Hymen.** In the absence of MIS and androgens, the mesonephric (wolffian) ducts degenerate and the paramesonephric (müllerian) ducts give rise to the fallopian tubes, uterus, and upper two-thirds of the vagina. The remnants of mesonephric ducts are found in the mesentery of the ovary as the epoophoron and paroophoron, and near the vaginal introitus and anterolateral vaginal wall as Gartner duct cysts. The hymen develops from the endodermal membrane located at the junction between the vaginal plate and the definitive urogenital sinus, which is the future vestibule of the vagina.

15. **d. In females, the urethral folds become the labia majora, and the labioscrotal folds become the labia minora.** The early development of the external genital organ is similar in both sexes until 8 weeks gestation. Early in the fifth week, a pair of swellings called cloacal folds develops on either side of the cloacal membrane. These folds meet just anterior to the cloacal membrane to form a midline swelling called the genital tubercle. During the cloacal division into the anterior urogenital sinus and the posterior anorectal canal, the portion of the cloacal folds flanking the opening of the urogenital sinus becomes the urogenital folds, and the portion flanking the opening of the anorectal canal becomes the anal folds. A new pair of swellings, called the labioscrotal folds, then appears on either side of the urogenital folds. In the absence of dihydrotestosterone, the primitive perineum does not lengthen, and the labioscrotal and urethral folds do not fuse across the midline in the female embryo. The phallus bends inferiorly, becoming the clitoris, and the definitive urogenital sinus becomes the vestibule of the vagina. The urethral folds become the labia minora, and the labioscrotal folds become the labia majora. The external genital organ develops in a similar manner in genetic males who are deficient in 5α-reductase and therefore lack dihydrotestosterone.

16. **b. Third month.** The testicle reaches the level of internal inguinal ring by the third month and passes through the inguinal canal to reach the scrotum between the seventh and ninth months.

17. **d. It causes the regression of mesonephric ducts.** When the Y-linked master regulatory gene, called SRY, is expressed in the male, the epithelial cells of the primitive sex cords differentiate into Sertoli cells, and this critical morphogenetic event triggers subsequent testicular development. Analysis of DNA narrowed the location of the SRY to a relatively small region within the short arm of the chromosome. It is now clear that only about 25% of sex reversals in humans can be attributed to disabling mutations of the SRY.

CHAPTER REVIEW

1. The glomerulus, proximal tubule, loop of Henle, and distal tubule are derived from the metanephric mesenchyme.
2. The remainder of the collecting system is formed from the ureteric bud.
3. The Weigert-Meyer rule states that the most lateral and cephalad ureteric orifice arises from the lower pole and may demonstrate reflux whereas the most medial and caudad orifice drains the upper pole and may be associated with a ureterocele.
4. Sertoli cells produce müllerian-inhibiting substance, which causes regression of the müllerian ducts.
5. Testosterone is secreted by the Leydig cells and stimulates the wolffian ducts to form the vas deferens and seminal vesicles.
6. The prostate and bulbourethral glands develop from the urogenital sinus.
7. Circulating androgens play a critical role in the development of the prostate.
8. When 5α-reductase is deficient, prostatic growth and development is severely compromised.
9. In the absence of müllerian-inhibiting substance and androgens, the wolffian ducts degenerate and the müllerian ducts give rise to the fallopian tubes, uterus, and upper two-thirds of the vagina.
10. Boys with spina bifida have a 23% incidence of cryptorchidism.
11. If the *SRY* gene complex is translocated to an X chromosome, an XX female will have male characteristics.
12. The renin-angiotensin system is important for the normal development and growth of the kidney.
13. Circulating androgens and the conversion of testosterone to dihydrotestosterone (DHT) are critical to the normal development of the prostate and male external genitalia.
14. A defect in the WT1 gene may result in hypospadias, cryptorchidism, and ambiguous genitalia (disorders of sex development).
15. Defects in the androgen receptor result in abnormal masculinization of the external genitalia.
16. Abdominal pressure appears to be important for the transit of the testis through the inguinal canal and into the scrotum.
17. The embryonic kidneys are, in order of their appearance, the pronephros, the mesonephros, and the metanephros. The first two kidneys regress in utero, and the third becomes the permanent kidney.
18. Older, more differentiated nephrons are located in the inner part of the kidney near the juxtamedullary region.
19. Primordial germ cells migrate from the yolk sac along the dorsal mesentery to populate the mesenchyme of the posterior body wall near the 10th thoracic level.
20. Sertoli cells begin their differentiation in response to the SRY (sex-determining region of the Y chromosome); they begin to secrete MIS, which causes the paramesonephric (müllerian) ducts to regress.
21. Müllerian duct remnants in the male include the prostatic utricle and the appendix testis.

21 Urologic Aspects of Pediatric Nephrology

Michael C. Braun and Chester J. Koh

QUESTIONS

1. The mature nephron segments arise from which embryonic precursors?
   a. Pronephros
   b. Mesonephros
   c. Mesonephric duct
   d. Metanephros
   e. A combination of the mesonephros and metanephros

2. In term infants, which of the following are fully mature?
   a. Glomerular filtration rate (GFR)
   b. Tubular maturation
   c. Nephrogenesis
   d. Renal growth
   e. Renal sodium regulation

3. A 10-year-old healthy boy is found on routine physical examination to have asymptomatic microscopic hematuria. Urinalysis reveals yellow urine with a specific gravity of 1.020, pH 6, no protein, and moderate amount of blood. The microscopic examination shows 5 to 6 red blood cells (RBCs) per high-powered field and no white blood cells, bacteria, or crystals. The most appropriate next step would be:
   a. renal ultrasonography.
   b. spot urine calcium and creatinine determinations.
   c. urine culture.
   d. measurement of serum creatinine.
   e. repeat urinalysis in 2 weeks.

4. Urine protein excretion can be assessed qualitatively and quantitatively; which of the following represents abnormal urine protein excretion?
   a. A term infant with a urine protein to creatinine ratio (UPC) of 0.6 mg/mg
   b. A 13-year-old girl with a UPC of 1.0 mg/mg
   c. A first morning urine sample with a UPC of 0.1 mg/mg
   d. A 24-hour urine collection in a 15-year-old male with 150 mg of total protein
   e. A 12-hour urine collection with 3.1 mg/m^2/h of protein

5. A 6-year-old boy presents with generalized swelling and weight gain. His blood pressure is normal and his urinalysis notes clear yellow urine, a specific gravity of 1.030, pH 5.5, 3+ protein, and trace blood. Laboratory testing shows a creatinine of 0.2 mg/dL, an albumin of 1.8 gm/dL, a cholesterol of 350 mg/dL, and a spot UPC of 10 mg/mg. The most likely cause of his nephrotic syndrome is:
   a. congenital nephrotic syndrome.
   b. focal segmental glomerulosclerosis.
   c. membranous nephropathy.
   d. mesangial proliferation.
   e. minimal change disease.

6. An 8-year-old boy is seen in the emergency room with new-onset headaches and gross hematuria. He has no history of fever, dysuria, joint pains, rash, or abdominal pain. He had a sore throat 2 weeks before, which resolved with antibiotics. His blood pressure is 125/90 mm Hg, and his physical examination is remarkable for 1+ lower extremity edema. The urinalysis notes tea-colored urine with a specific gravity = 1.025, pH = 6.5, large blood, and 2+ protein. His diagnostic evaluation should include all of the following EXCEPT:
   a. computed tomography (CT) of the abdomen and pelvis.
   b. comprehensive metabolic panel.
   c. C3 determination.
   d. antistreptolysin O (ASO)/DNase B titer.
   e. microscopic examination of the urine.

7. The causes of hypocomplementemic nephritis in children include all of the following EXCEPT:
   a. poststreptococcal glomerulonephritis.
   b. membranoproliferative glomerulonephritis.
   c. lupus nephritis.
   d. antineutrophil cytoplasmic antibody (ANCA)–associated glomerulonephritis.
   e. C3 glomerulopathy.

8. A 6-year-old girl is seen in the emergency room with complaints of abdominal and joint pains with gross hematuria. Her blood pressure is normal. Her physical examination is remarkable for a raised red rash on her lower legs and buttocks, mild abdominal pain on palpation, and bilateral ankle pain with minimal swelling. Her urinalysis noted tea-colored urine with a specific gravity of 1.020, pH 6.5, 3+ blood, and 2+ protein; urine microscopy showed numerous RBC cast. Her most likely diagnosis is:
   a. Henoch-Schönlein purpura (HSP).
   b. Postinfectious glomerulonephritis.
   c. Hemolytic uremic syndrome (HUS).
   d. Alport syndrome.
   e. ANCA-associated glomerulonephritis.

9. A 3-year-old boy presents to clinic with failure to thrive. His blood pressure is normal. His initial evaluation is remarkable for a serum sodium of 144 meq/L, potassium of 2.5 meq/L, a chloride of 105 meq/L, a HCO$_3$ of 9 meq/L, and a phosphorus of 4.5 mg/dL. A urinalysis notes a specific gravity = 1.005, pH = 7.0, and no blood or protein. A renal ultrasound shows normal renal size and shape with findings consistent with nephrocalcinosis. His most likely diagnosis is:
   a. Fanconi syndrome.
   b. proximal renal tubular acidosis (RTA).
   c. Bartter syndrome.
   d. Dent disease.
   e. distal RTA.

10. A 4-year-old girl is referred to clinic because her mother was recently diagnosed with cystic renal disease and a polycystin-1 mutation. Likely findings on ultrasound in this child could include all of the following EXCEPT:

    a. normal renal ultrasound.

    b. a unilateral renal cyst.

    c. hepatic fibrosis.

    d. multiple unilateral cysts.

    e. multiple bilateral renal cysts.

11. A 10-year-old boy is seen in the emergency department with the new onset of left-sided flank pain, gross hematuria, and vomiting. His blood pressure is 100/65 mm Hg, and the physical examination reveals right costovertebral angle tenderness. The urinalysis shows brown urine with a specific gravity = 1.030, pH = 7, large amount of blood, and 2+ protein. The next step in diagnostic evaluation of choice should be:

    a. high-resolution CT of abdomen/pelvis without contrast.

    b. microscopic examination of the urine.

    c. cystoscopy.

    d. abdominal ultrasound.

    e. serum electrolyte determination.

12. Common causes of hyperoxaluria include all of the following EXCEPT:

    a. vitamin C excess.

    b. short gut syndrome.

    c. oxylate-rich diets.

    d. alanine:glyoxylate aminotransferase deficiency.

    e. adenine phosphoribosyltransferase (APRT) deficiency.

13. A 15-year-old boy has a blood pressure of 120/80 mm Hg during routine examination. The child is calm, and a properly sized blood pressure cuff was used for blood pressure measurement. The family history is strongly positive for essential hypertension and diabetes mellitus. His physical examination is unremarkable except for a body mass index (BMI) of 29 kg/m². The best next step in management is to:

    a. repeat blood pressure measurement in 1 to 2 weeks.

    b. obtain a fasting lipid profile.

    c. perform Doppler renal ultrasonography.

    d. obtain peripheral vein renin levels.

    e. obtain 24-hour ambulatory blood pressure monitoring (ABPM).

14. A 12-year-old boy is sent to the emergency department for evaluation of vomiting and decreased urination. He has a blood urea nitrogen (BUN) level = 40 mg/dL and a creatinine = 1.8 mg/dL. His urinary sodium level = 20 meq/L, fractional excretion of sodium (FE_{Na}) = 0.8%, and urinary osmolality = 600 mOsm/kg. The most likely cause of his elevated creatinine is:

    a. posterior urethral valves.

    b. dehydration.

    c. interstitial nephritis.

    d. Hemolytic uremic syndrome.

    e. acute urinary tract infection (UTI).

15. Common complications of advanced chronic kidney disease in children include all of the following EXCEPT:

    a. growth hormone deficiency.

    b. protein malnutrition.

    c. erythropoietin deficiency.

    d. metabolic acidosis.

    e. 1,25 vitamin D insufficiency.

16. A 5-year-old-boy with posterior urethral valves since birth has renal function that has slowly declined, with a current creatinine = 1.7 mg/dL. His growth is impaired, with height and weight less than the third percentile. The most appropriate management strategy is:

    a. referral for initiation of transplant evaluation.

    b. urologic evaluation for urethral obstruction.

    c. repeat urodynamics in expectation of preemptive transplantation.

    d. optimization of nutritional intake and recombinant growth hormone therapy.

    e. G-tube placement.

17. The most common cause of pediatric renal allograft loss is:

    a. primary anastomotic failure.

    b. recurrent obstructive uropathy.

    c. antibody mediated rejection.

    d. acute cellular rejection.

    e. chronic allograft nephropathy.

ANSWERS

1. **d. Metanephros.** The metanephros forms the mature nephron segments. The pronephros undergoes complete involution, while residual segments of the mesonephros, the mesonephric duct, forms portions of the urinary tract.

2. **c. Nephrogenesis.** Nephrogenesis is complete by 34 to 36 weeks post conception, whether in utero or ex utero. Tubular maturation, including urinary sodium regulation, continues for weeks to months post partum. GFR reaches adult levels by 2 years of age, whereas renal growth continues until the post-pubertal period.

3. **e. Repeat urinalysis in 2 weeks.** In a healthy asymptomatic child, isolated microscopic hematuria can occur in up to 1% of school-age children. With repeat measure, less than 25% will have persistent hematuria. Should the microscopic hematuria be persistent, then screening studies of renal function, renal structure, urinary calcium excretion, and possible infection are indicated.

4. **b. A 13-year-old girl with a UPC of 1.0 mg/mg.** A UPC of greater than 1.0 mg/mg is abnormal. Normal urine protein excretion as measured by UPC is less than 0.7 mg/m in a newborn and less than 0.2 mg/mg in older children. A 24-hour protein collections in adolescents and adults should be less than 200 mg/24 h or in younger children less than 4 mg/m²/h. A UPC of greater than 2.0 mg/mg defines nephrotic range proteinuria.

5. **e. Minimal change disease.** The most common cause of nephrotic syndrome in childhood is minimal change disease. Congenital nephrotic syndrome by definition is seen in children younger than 3 months of age. Membranous nephropathy and mesangial proliferation are seen less frequently in childhood, whereas focal segmental glomerulosclerosis (FSGS) become increasing common during adolescence and late childhood.

6. **a. Computed tomography (CT) of the abdomen and pelvis.** A child presenting with symptomatic hypertension and gross hematuria is strongly suggestive of acute glomerulonephritis. The prior history of pharyngitis is consistent with poststreptococcal-associated disease. Examination of the urine sediment for signs of glomerulonephritis (cellular casts) and documentation of renal function and electrolytes, as well as elevated antistreptolysin O titer and decreased C3, are recommend to confirm the diagnosis. Abdominal CT scans play no role in the initial evaluation of suspected acute glomerulonephritis.

7. **d. Antineutrophil cytoplasmic antibody (ANCA)–associated glomerulonephritis.** Serum complement levels are very useful in narrowing the differential diagnosis in acute glomerulonephritis. Low C3 and C4 levels are seen in lupus nephritis and membranoproliferative glomerulonephritis (MPGN), whereas low C3 and normal C4 levels are seen in postinfectious glomerulonephritis (PIGN) and C3 glomerulonephritis (C3GN). Complement levels are normal in patients with ANCA-associated glomerulonephritis.

8. **a. Henoch-Schönlein purpura (HSP).** HSP is a systemic vasculitis that is characterized by purpuric rash, commonly on legs and buttocks, abdominal pain, arthritis, and nephritis. HUS is commonly seen in association with bloody diarrhea. Alport syndrome is not commonly seen with systemic complaints, whereas PIGN is usually preceded by either pharyngitis or impetigo. ANCA-associated glomerulonephritis, although rare is childhood, can be seen in older children or adolescents, and systemic complaints including fever are common.

9. **e. Distal RTA.** Failure to thrive in an infant in association with hyperchloremic acidosis (nonanion gap) is strongly suggestive of RTA. Nephrocalcinosis is a common finding in distal RTA, as is the very low HCO_3 level. With proximal RTA or Fanconi, HCO_3 levels are typically in the 12 to 14 meq/L range, and hypophosphatemia, low-grade proteinuria, and glycosuria are commonly seen. Dent disease does not present with RTA, and Bartter syndrome is defined by metabolic alkalosis.

10. **c. Hepatic fibrosis.** Hepatic fibrosis is a feature commonly seen in autosomal recessive polycystic kidney disease (AR-PKD). Mutations in polycystin-1 are associated with autosomal dominant polycystic kidney disease (ADPKD). Renal ultrasound findings in childhood can be highly variable and range from "normal" to severe bilateral cystic disease.

11. **d. Abdominal ultrasound.** This clinical scenario is most consistent with acute presentation of a renal or ureteral stone. Ultrasound imaging to rule out hydronephrosis and to identify presence of a stone is the best first step. Intervention for drainage is not indicated until appropriate analgesics have been initiated. CT imaging is unlikely to add further information and exposes the child to radiation.

12. **e. Adenine phosphoribosyltransferase (APRT) deficiency.** Hyperoxaluria can be primary, in the case of alanine:glyoxylate aminotransferase deficiency, or secondary due to excessive oxalate intake, vitamin C (a precursor of oxalate), or hyperabsorption in the case of short gut syndrome. APRT deficiency is an autosomal recessive disorder of adenine metabolism linked with recurrent dihydroxyadenine stones.

13. **a. Repeat blood pressure measure in 1 to 2 weeks.** Repeat the measurement next week in the office. This child's blood pressure is elevated, and measurement should be repeated and possible hypertension confirmed. ABPM could be considered and is recommended; however, availability is a challenge and is more practically performed after repeated office measurements. Therefore the blood pressure should be remeasured in the office. If hypertension is confirmed, the workup will include a complete metabolic panel, lipid profile, echocardiogram, and renal ultrasonography. Angiography and selective renin levels can be considered in case of severe or recalcitrant hypertension.

14. **b. Dehydration.** The initial evaluation of patients with suspected acute kidney injury (AKI) should include urinary indices including urine sodium, osmolality, and creatinine. A low urine sodium (<25 meq/L) or a FeNa of less than 1% is consistent with "prerenal" AKI, or renal hypoperfusion as seen with dehydration of vomiting and/or diarrhea. An elevated BUN and creatinine due to posterior urethral valves, interstitial nephritis, or UTIs are due to "intrinsic" renal disease, and urinary sodium and FeNa (>1%) are typically elevated.

15. **a. Growth hormone deficiency.** Patients with chronic kidney disease (CKD) have growth failure due to abnormalities in growth hormone activity rather than true growth hormone deficiency. Protein malnutrition, anemia from erythropoietin deficiency, chronic metabolic acidosis, and an inability to convert 25 vitamin D to active 1,25 vitamin D are all common feature of advanced CKD in children.

16. **d. Optimization of nutritional intake and recombinant growth hormone therapy.** Impairment of growth is a common feature of CKD even at an early stage, regardless of etiology. Aggressive management of nutritional needs is often insufficient, and therapy with recombinant growth hormone is indicated in the majority of patients.

17. **e. Chronic allograft nephropathy.** The most common cause of renal transplantation loss in children is chronic allograft nephropathy. Primary anastomotic failure is very rare, and recurrent obstructive uropathy in most patients can be managed with medical or surgical interventions. Acute cellular rejection, although common, is typically responsive to immunomodulation. Antibody-mediated rejection is increasing being recognized as a cause of graft failure.

CHAPTER REVIEW

1. Congenital anomalies of the kidney and urinary tract (CAKUT) are the most common causes of end-stage renal disease (ESRD) in children.
2. Prenatal and neonatal GFR is significantly lower than adult GFR levels.
3. The maintenance of the balance of sodium is an important function of the neonatal kidney.
4. The newborn kidney has a limited capacity to excrete potassium and tends to have higher serum potassium values than older children.
5. Isolated microscopic hematuria is reported to occur in approximately 1% of school-age children.
6. Most children with microscopic hematuria will have spontaneous resolution within 1 year of presentation.
7. Gross hematuria and a urinalysis with no RBCs but a positive heme dipstick is strongly suggestive of hemoglobinuria or myoglobinuria.
8. It is important to recognize that urine contains protein under physiologic conditions and especially with fever and exercise.
9. Transient proteinuria accounts for more than 75% of patients with isolated proteinuria.
10. If a patient with proteinuria has evidence of systemic disease or glomerular nephritis, testing should include C3, C4, and antinuclear antibody (ANA) screening.
11. Corticosteroids will induce a remission in the vast majority of children with nephrotic syndrome.
12. Focal segmental glomerulosclerosis is seen in the majority of children with steroid-resistant nephrotic syndrome.
13. Minimal change nephrotic syndrome is the most common cause of nephrotic syndrome in childhood.
14. Immunoglobulin A (IgA) nephropathy is the most common primary cause of glomerulonephritis throughout the world.
15. HUS is a common cause of severe AKI in a previously healthy young child.
16. The hallmark of **RTA** is hyperchloremic metabolic acidosis (normal anion gap acidosis).
17. Children with distal RTA classically have hyperchloremic metabolic acidosis, hypokalemia, hypercalciuria, and nephrocalcinosis.
18. Hypokalemic metabolic alkalosis is the defining feature of Bartter syndrome.
19. RTA associated with hyperkalemia is also known as type 4 RTA.
20. Urologic anomalies are seen in up to 25% of patients with multicystic dysplastic kidney (MCDK), including renal hypoplasia/dysplasia, vesicoureteral reflux (VUR), and ureteropelvic junction (UPJ) obstruction.

CHAPTER REVIEW—cont'd

21. ARPKD is caused by a mutation in the PKHD1 gene.
22. ADPKD is due to mutations in the polycystin-1 (PKD-1) or polycystin-2 (PKD2) genes.
23. Urolithiasis remains underdiagnosed because many children are asymptomatic at the time of diagnosis.
24. Calcium stones are currently the most prevalent stones in children.
25. Cystinuria results in decreased tubular reabsorption of cystine, ornithine, arginine, and lysine.
26. The increase in the prevalence in pediatric hypertension in recent years is closely linked to increasing obesity rates in children.
27. Up to a quarter of patients have normal blood pressures outside of the office setting ("white coat" hypertension).
28. Therapeutic lifestyle changes are the initial intervention of choice for patients with primary hypertension without end-organ damage.
29. Hospitalized pediatric patients with AKI have a nearly 15-fold increased mortality risk compared with patients without AKI.
30. Prerenal AKI requires prompt and vigorous fluid resuscitation with isotonic fluids.
31. Continuous renal replacement therapy (CRRT) has become the standard of care because it delivers slow continuous correction of fluid overload and electrolyte imbalances.
32. Causes of CKD in children are very different from those that cause CKD in adults and vary by age group within the pediatric population.
33. The most common cause of anemia with CKD is a deficiency of erythropoietin.
34. With CKD, kidney function declines in a nonlinear fashion, as the later stages are associated with a more rapid progression.
35. Peritoneal dialysis is the most common initial modality for dialysis in children younger than 9 years of age and less than 20 kg.
36. The unique benefits of renal transplantation include improved growth, neurocognitive development, and quality of life.
37. The risk for acute cellular rejection in the first year after pediatric renal transplantation is less than 10% in living donor transplants.
38. The risk for acute cellular rejection in the first year post transplant is approximately 15% in deceased donor transplants.

Perinatal Urology

C.D. Anthony Herndon and Rebecca S. Zee

QUESTIONS

1. A newborn girl has prenatally detected left A1 urinary tract dilation (UTD) with 8-mm anteroposterior diameter APD on third-trimester US. A renal ultrasound (US) is obtained on day of life (DOL) 3, which demonstrates left P1 UTD. What is the most likely cause of this condition?
   a. Vesicoureteral reflux (VUR)
   b. Transient dilation
   c. Ureteropelvic junction (UPJ) obstruction
   d. Ureterovesical junction (UVJ) obstruction
   e. Ectopic ureteral insertion

2. A circumcised newborn boy with prenatally detected A2-3 UTD receives a renal ultrasound on DOL 3 that is normal. What is the best next step?
   a. Discharge from urologic care
   b. Voiding cystourethrogram (VCUG)
   c. Repeat US in 3 to 6 months
   d. Start prophylactic antibiotics
   e. Renal scintigraphy

3. Which of the following is accurate with regard to prenatal intervention for lower urinary tract obstruction (LUTO)?
   a. Improved survival; unchanged long-term renal function
   b. Decreased survival; improved long-term renal function
   c. Unchanged survival; improved long-term renal function
   d. Improved survival; decreased long-term renal function
   e. Decreased survival; unchanged long-term renal function

4. A fetus is diagnosed with lumbosacral myelomeningocele. After having an informed discussion of risks and benefits, the pregnant mother would like you to discuss the urologic benefits of prenatal intervention with her. Which of the following is the best answer?
   a. Prenatal intervention improves urodynamic parameters, need for clean intermittent catheterization (CIC), and reconstruction in most patients who undergo prenatal myelomeningocele closure.
   b. Prenatal intervention has not shown a benefit to urodynamic parameters, nor does it decrease the need for CIC and for urinary reconstruction.
   c. The risks outweigh the benefits, and prenatal intervention should never be performed.
   d. Prenatal intervention for myelomeningocele can be done at any center that has a pediatric neurosurgeon and pediatric urologist.
   e. Postnatal intervention is associated with a lower incidence of preterm labor.

5. A 6-week-old circumcised boy is referred to your office for A1 prenatal UTD. His postnatal US at DOL 2 demonstrated central calyceal dilation with an APD of 11 mm (P1). The ureter and bladder appeared normal. An US repeated today is unchanged (P1). He is otherwise healthy. What is his most likely outcome?

   a. He has a UPJ obstruction and requires surgery.
   b. He should have a VCUG and a technetium-mercaptoacetyl-triglycine (Tc-MAG3) Lasix renal scan before further discussion
   c. His UTD is most likely to resolve within the next 2.5 years.
   d. His UTD will resolve, but the timing is unknown.
   e. He should start prophylactic antibiotics to prevent an infection.

6. Which of the following is correct with regard to VUR and UTD?
   a. All patients who present with P2 UTD should undergo VCUG.
   b. UTD correlates in a linear fashion with VUR.
   c. All patients with VUR will demonstrate UTD to some degree on postnatal US.
   d. VUR will occur more commonly in females.
   e. VCUG is recommended in patients with increased risk of UTI.

7. Which of the following is TRUE regarding the link between UTD and UTI?
   a. There is no correlation between degree of dilation and risk of UTI.
   b. Gender does not impact risk of UTI.
   c. Recent data fail to demonstrate the efficacy of prophylactic antibiotics to prevent UTI in patients with UTD.
   d. All patients with UTD should be started on prophylactic antibiotics at birth.
   e. The event rate of UTI in patients with UTD is high.

8. A newborn with P3 UTD undergoes a MAG3 Lasix renal scan at 3 months of age. Which of the following is TRUE?
   a. Indications for surgery include decreased differential function (<40%), delayed $t_{1/2}$ (>20 minutes), and significant retention on delayed upright imaging.
   b. MAG3 Lasix renal scan provides sufficient anatomic detail to identify the insertion point of an ectopic ureter.
   c. A MAG3 Lasix renal scan is an accurate measure of glomerular filtration rate (GFR).
   d. Dehydration does not impact the results of the study.
   e. Furosemide (Lasix) should be given at the exact same time interval after radionuclide administration for every patient.

9. An uncircumcised newborn boy with UTD A2-A3 presents to your clinic at 4 weeks of age. He is on amoxicillin and has not experienced any UTIs. He has been otherwise healthy. A repeat US today demonstrates peripheral calyceal dilation, APD 20 mm, 10-mm dilation of distal right ureter, and a normal bladder. VCUG is negative for reflux. What is the next best step?
   a. Transition to trimethoprim/sulfamethoxazole prophylaxis
   b. Perform MAG3 scan
   c. Repeat US in 3 months
   d. Recommend newborn circumcision
   e. Stop prophylaxis

10. Pediatric urology is urgently consulted for evaluation of an abnormal scrotum in a 2-day-old neonate. The primary team reports that the newborn examination was normal at birth and has changed in the past 2 hours. On exam, the right testis is tender, firm, and overlying skin is discolored. The left testis is normal. The neonate is fussy. What is the next step?

    a. Elective contralateral septopexy

    b. Scrotal US with Doppler

    c. Initiate antibiotics

    d. Serial scrotal examination

    e. Emergent surgical exploration

ANSWERS

1. **b. Transient dilation.** A majority of UTD is transient (41%–88%). Normal values for UTD are less than 7 mm at greater than 28 weeks. This prenatal US with 8-mm anteroposterior diameter of renal pelvic diameter (APRPD) in the third trimester would represent low risk, or A1 disease. UPJ obstruction is the second most common cause of UTD. VUR accounts for 10% to 20% UTD and other causes account for less than 10% of UTD. A postnatal US after 48 hours of age is recommended.

2. **c. Repeat US in 3 to 6 months.** If the first postnatal US demonstrates no dilation after 48 hours of age, a US should be repeated in 3 to 6 months to confirm that UTD has resolved. Up to 28% of UTD may be detected after initial negative US. An informed discussion should be performed with the family to discuss therapeutic options. VCUG should not be performed as the risk of UTI from reflux is currently low in the absence of dilation in a circumcised boy. Similarly, prophylactic antibiotics and renal scintigraphy are not warranted given the low risk of infection.

3. **a. Improved survival; unchanged long-term renal function.** Several publications have shown that prenatal intervention for LUTO improves survival without a significant effect on renal function. Prenatal intervention for LUTO is most beneficial for those patients who present with oligohydramnios early in the second trimester to facilitate pulmonary development after 27 weeks' gestation.

4. **b. Prenatal intervention has not shown a benefit to urodynamic parameters, nor does it decrease the need for CIC and for urinary reconstruction.** A multicenter trial was published in 2011 that randomized patients to prenatal closure versus postnatal closure of myelomeningocele. The study reported that prenatal closure decreased the need for ventriculoperitoneal shunting, as well as motor and cognitive functioning. However, prenatal closure did not affect urodynamic parameters or the need for CIC or urinary reconstruction compared to postnatal closure.

5. **c. His UTD is most likely to resolve within the next 2.5 years.** Most patients with P1 UTD will resolve within 30 months of birth. This patient has P1 UTD and should be observed with serial ultrasound alone. Guidelines suggest that VCUG should be performed at the discretion of the clinician but should not universally be applied. UPJ obstruction is unlikely with low-risk upper tract dilation. Prophylactic antibiotics and additional imaging studies such as VCUG and MAG3 scans should be reserved for those patients who are at the highest risk of infection, which includes females, uncircumcised males, high-grade dilation (SFU [Society of Fetal Urology] grades 3–4), and ureteral dilation.

6. **e. VCUG is recommended in patients with increased risk of UTI.** VCUG is recommended for any patient with P3 UTD or high risk. P2 and P3 risk categories both include an APRPD greater than or equal to 15 mm, peripheral calyceal dilation, or ureteral abnormality. P2 patients may undergo VCUG at discretion of the clinician. P3 or high risk is distinguished by any abnormality of renal parenchymal thickness, renal parenchymal appearance, or abnormality of the bladder. Therefore a patient with P3 UTD or high risk should undergo a follow-up US at 1 month and a VCUG and should be started on prophylactic antibiotics. Renal scintigraphy can be performed at the clinician's discretion. VCUG can be performed on an outpatient basis. VUR will be present in up to 31% of patients screened with UTD, will occur more commonly in males, and will be high grade and bilateral. Upper tract dilation correlates poorly with presence of VUR. One-quarter of patients with VUR on postnatal VCUG will have no dilation on a postnatal US.

7. **c. Recent data fail to demonstrate the efficacy of prophylactic antibiotics to prevent UTI in patients with UTD.** A recent meta-analysis of 11 studies failed to show a benefit of continuous prophylactic antibiotics (CAP) on preventing UTI in patients with prenatal UTD. The degree of UTD is predictive of risk of UTI. Risk factors for UTI include female gender, uncircumcised status, and higher grades of UTD. PA are recommended only for those at higher risk (P2 and P3). The incidence of UTI is low (8%–19%), which makes it difficult to study UTI rates in the UTD population.

8. **a. Indications for surgery include decreased differential function (<40%), delayed t½ (>20 minutes), and significant retention on delayed upright imaging.** Sussman et al. reported that indications for surgery in an otherwise asymptomatic patient include decreased split differential function, delayed drainage, or significant retention on delayed upright imaging. A limitation of a MAG3 renal scan is that it does not provide high-resolution imaging of the genitourinary (GU) system. The best imaging modality to assess the insertion point of an ectopic ureter would be magnetic resonance (MR) urogram. MAG3 is not filtered through the glomerulus. Rather, it is handled by the proximal tubule and therefore is not an accurate measure of GFR. Dehydration of the patient may affect the results of a MAG3 scan. Administration of Lasix should be individualized for each patient at the height of tracer uptake within the collecting system.

9. **d. Recommend newborn circumcision.** Uncircumcised status and ureteral dilation are risk factors for UTI in this male patient with P2 intermediate risk UTD. An informed discussion should be held with the family to discuss risk of UTI, risk of circumcision, and continued prophylaxis. The patient is too young to be transitioned to Bactrim, which should not be administered prior to 2 to 3 months of age. Similarly, prophylactic antibiotics should not be discontinued in this patient. Renal scintigraphy may be performed at the clinician's discretion, but recommendation for circumcision should not be delayed to assess renal drainage and function.

10. **e. Emergent surgical exploration.** An acute postnatal change in scrotal examination suggests a postnatal torsion. Up to 44% of postnatal torsion can be salvaged with emergent exploration and septopexy. In prenatal torsion, the postnatal exam will not change from birth. The testis will be a solid, nontender mass and demonstrate absence of flow on Doppler US. The affected testis is not salvageable in prenatal torsion. Most pediatric urologists would perform contralateral septopexy on an urgent basis in patients with a diagnosis of prenatal torsion to prevent asynchronous contralateral torsion. Scrotal US with Doppler may have a role if the diagnosis is unclear, but surgical exploration should not be delayed if the clinician has made a diagnosis of postnatal torsion. Serial scrotal examinations are not warranted, because postnatal torsion can be diagnosed clinically and should be addressed as a surgical emergency. Likewise, there is no role for antibiotics, because this clinical picture is not consistent with an infectious process.

66 PART III Pediatric Urology

CHAPTER REVIEW

1. The initial screening maternal ultrasound is performed at approximately 20 weeks' gestation. Low-risk pregnancies average two scans and high-risk four scans throughout pregnancy.
2. Urinary tract dilation represents the second most common condition detected prenatally and occurs in 1% to 3% of pregnancies.
3. Ultrasound cannot reliably predict the severity of disease for all urologic conditions. It tends to correlate best with obstructive lesions such as UPJ obstruction or posterior urethral valves (PUV) and less with vesicoureteral reflux.
4. Prenatal detection of urologic disease affords the opportunity for the family to meet with a specialist prior to delivery to become informed of the anticipated course and natural history of the suspected diagnosis.
5. An inverse relationship exists between the severity of UTD and incidence of urologic disease.
6. APD demonstrates a linear relationship for obstructive lesions such as UPJ obstruction and PUV.
7. An APD of 15 in the third trimester demonstrates reasonable positive predictive value for the need for surgery for UPJ obstruction.
8. The SFU hydronephrosis grading system consists of a five-point grading system that is based on calyceal dilation and integrity of the parenchyma.
9. The UTD grading system consists of a combination of APD and SFU systems with the additional inclusion of the lower urinary tract and uses a standardized reporting system and risk stratification.
10. Prenatal intervention for LUTO appears to improve perinatal survival but does not reliably impact long-term renal function.
11. Parental consultation for fetal myelomeningocele closure should take place at a center with expertise in fetal surgery that offers a multidiscipline approach.
12. Fetal surgery for myelomeningocele appears to improve motor/cognitive skills and decrease the need for VP shunting but does not offer definitive benefit to bladder function.
13. Clinical predictors of poor outcome are oligohydramnios less than 27 weeks EGA, renal cortical cysts, and increased echogenicity.
14. Prenatal intervention for LUTO appears to improve perinatal survival but does not reliably impact long-term renal function.
15. Fetal cystoscopy affords the opportunity to establish the diagnosis and provide treatment for LUTO.
16. Fetal cystoscopy may offer a short-term advantage for overall renal function when compared with vesicoamniotic shunting, but long-term renal data do not exist.
17. The initial postnatal US should be obtained at 48 hours to account for intravascular depletion that occurs in the initial postnatal period secondary to third spacing, which later becomes mobilized to the intravascular space.
18. UTD classification assigns three levels of risk: P1 UTD (SFU 2) (low risk) APD 10 < 15 mm, P2 UTD (SFU 3) (intermediate risk) APD greater than 15 mm and peripheral calyceal dilation, P3 (SFU 4) (high risk) APD greater than 15 mm and/or positive values for other data points.
19. The degree of APD dilation correlates poorly with the presence and degree of VUR in patients with prenatal UTD.
20. Recommendations for VCUG for prenatal UTD should be based on risk of UTI in the absence of concerns for LUTO.
21. Complete resolution of P1 UTD should occur in most patients by 4 years of age.
22. For P1 UTD (SFU 2), PA and VCUG are not recommended.
23. For P2 UTD (SFU 3), the use of PA and VCUG is left to the discretion of the physician.
24. For P3 UTD (SFU 4), PA and VCUG are recommended, as well as a MAG3 renal scan.
25. The degree of dilation is predictive of risk of UTI in patients with prenatal UTD.
26. Risk factors for UTI for prenatal UTD include female, intact foreskin, high-grade kidney dilation, ureteral dilation, and VUR.
27. Prophylactic antibiotics are recommended for those at risk of UTI, including P2 UTD (SFU 3) and P3 UT (SFU 4).
28. Most patients with prenatal UTD will have transient dilation with reported resolution rates between 41% and 88%.
29. Prenatal APD dilation of 15 mm in third semester is predictive of the need for surgery.
30. VUR is reported in up to 31% of patients with prenatal UTD and will occur most commonly in males that have bilateral high-grade disease.
31. Multicystic dysplastic kidney (MCDK) does not pose an increased risk to Wilms tumor and can be safely observed in most patients.
32. Duplication anomalies may be associated with VUR to the lower pole moiety, which may influence decisions for intervention to the obstructed upper pole moiety.
33. Megaureter will resolve spontaneously in a majority of patients. However, surgical intervention is indicated for recurrent UTI, decreased function, or increasing UTD. Temporizing diverting procedures are recommended for younger than 1 year of age.
34. Fetal closure of myelomeningocele appears to increase motor/cognitive skills and decrease the need for a VP shunt, but it does not improve urologic symptoms and urodynamic parameters or decrease the need for urinary reconstruction.
35. A urologic source for abdominal distention in the newborn includes urinary ascites, urinary obstruction (upper and lower tract), renal mass (cystic and solid), and, rarely, a retroperitoneal mass (adrenal).
36. Urinary retention may occur with LUTO and may occur in males with PUV or females with urogenital (UG) sinus or cloacal anomaly.
37. Renal tumors are uncommon in the newborn period, and the most common is congenital mesoblastic nephroma.
38. The newborn with ambiguous genitalia (including any newborn "male" with bilateral nonpalpable testes) should prompt an evaluation for electrolyte disturbance due to classical salt wasting congenital adrenal hyperplasia.
39. Gross hematuria in the neonate is not common and should be evaluated with a urinalysis and Doppler abdominal ultrasound.
40. The acuity of neonatal testicular torsion will dictate the need for emergent exploration.

23   Urologic Evaluation of the Child

Rachel Selekman and Hillary L. Copp

QUESTIONS

1. Which one of the following patients does NOT need to be seen emergently?
   a. A newborn with hydronephrosis in a solitary kidney
   b. A 4-year-old boy with acute right scrotal pain
   c. A 12-year-old girl with microscopic hematuria found during a routine examination
   d. An 8-year-old boy with sickle cell anemia and a 5-hour history of priapism
   e. A male newborn with a distended bladder, bilateral hydronephrosis, and respiratory insufficiency

2. Which of the following is a potential complication of neonatal circumcision?
   a. Wound infection
   b. Meatal stenosis
   c. Cicatrix
   d. Death
   e. All of the above

3. The pediatric kidney is particularly susceptible to trauma due to:
   a. relatively increased renal size.
   b. limited visceral adipose tissue.
   c. limited chest wall protection.
   d. increased mobility.
   e. all of the above.

4. What is the optimal timing of spinal ultrasonography during screening for occult spinal dysraphism?
   a. Before 6 months of age
   b. 6 months to 2 years of age
   c. At any age before puberty
   d. At any age
   e. Never. Ultrasound (US) is not useful to screen for spinal dysraphism.

5. What is the most commonly detected etiology for asymptomatic microscopic hematuria in children?
   a. Fibroepithelial polyp
   b. Hypercalciuria
   c. Poststreptococcal glomerulonephritis
   d. Uncomplicated urinary tract infection
   e. Hyperuricosuria

6. Findings associated with the Beckwith-Wiedemann syndrome include:
   a. macroglossia.
   b. hepatosplenomegaly.
   c. nephromegaly.
   d. macrosomia.
   e. all of the above.

7. A voiding cystourethrogram (VCUG) is essential in the diagnosis of which clinical condition?
   a. Ureteropelvic junction obstruction
   b. Primary obstructive megaureter
   c. Posterior urethral valves
   d. Nephrolithiasis
   e. Renal mass

8. When should a child with suspected congenital adrenal hyperplasia be tested?
   a. Before discharge from the nursery
   b. At the first well-baby visit
   c. At 6 months of age
   d. At puberty
   e. Only if undergoing general anesthesia

9. All of the following statements about the pediatric abdominal examination are true EXCEPT:
   a. renal pathology is the source of as many as two-thirds of neonatal abdominal masses.
   b. abdominal distention at birth or shortly afterward suggests either obstruction or perforation of the gastrointestinal tract.
   c. the abdominal wall is normally strong, especially in infants with hydronephrosis.
   d. a solid flank mass may be due to renal venous thrombosis.
   e. in cloacal exstrophy, an omphalocele is superior to the cecal plate and lateral bladder halves with prolapsed ileum in the midline.

10. Which of the following statements is FALSE about cutaneous markers of occult spinal dysraphism?
    a. Forty percent of patients with atypical presacral dimples have associated occult spinal dysraphism.
    b. A combination of two or more congenital midline skin lesions is the strongest marker of occult spinal dysraphism.
    c. A presacral dimple less than 2.5 cm from the anal verge at birth may indicate spina bifida or cord tethering.
    d. Sacral hypertrichosis may be associated with spinal dysraphism.
    e. All of the above are true.

11. Sexual abuse can be associated with which of the following physical examination findings?
    a. Bruised vaginal mucosa in a prepubertal child
    b. Penile discharge
    c. A normal genital and perineal examination
    d. a and c
    e. a, b, and c

12. Urethral meatal stenosis in the infant occurs most commonly:
    a. as a result of birth trauma.
    b. after urinary tract infection.
    c. after a VCUG.
    d. after healing of the inflamed, denuded glans after circumcision.
    e. from penile adhesions.

13. In newborns with ambiguous genitalia, palpation of a gonad rules out which difference of sexual development (DSD/intersex)?
    a. Ovotesticular disorder
    b. Mixed gonadal dysgenesis
    c. Partial androgen insensitivity
    d. Pure gonadal dysgenesis
    e. Persistent müllerian duct syndrome

14. Secondary urinary incontinence is defined as:
    a. diurnal and nocturnal enuresis.
    b. incontinence associated with urinary tract infection.
    c. urinary incontinence associated with constipation.
    d. urinary incontinence after a dry interval greater than 6 months.
    e. urinary incontinence associated with a neurologic condition.

15. A newborn should have a scrotal hydrocele surgically corrected in the neonatal period if:
    a. it is large.
    b. it is changing in volume.
    c. it accompanies a symptomatic hernia.
    d. a, b, and c.
    e. b and c.

ANSWERS

1. **c. A 12-year-old girl with microscopic hematuria found during a routine examination.** In the absence of other symptoms, microscopic hematuria in children is not an emergency. Bilateral hydronephrosis or hydronephrosis in a solitary kidney represents neonatal emergencies and should be evaluated as soon as possible. Acute scrotal pain should always be considered testicular torsion until proven otherwise. Boys with sickle cell anemia are at increased risk for priapism and should always be treated immediately to decrease the long-term sequelae associated with priapism.
2. **e. All of the above.** Wound infections, meatal stenosis, removal of too much/too little prepuce, cicatrix, and even death are all potential complications of neonatal circumcision.
3. **e. All of the above.** The pediatric kidney is particularly susceptible to trauma due to limited visceral adipose tissue, limited chest wall protection, relatively increased renal size, and increased mobility of the kidney.
4. **a. Before 6 months of age.** Ossification of the posterior elements after 6 months of age prevents an acoustic US window. After 6 months, spinal magnetic resonance imaging (MRI) is recommended when an occult spinal dysraphism is suspected.
5. **b. Hypercalciuria.** Most microscopic hematuria in children is transient and the source is not identified. The most commonly identified etiology of asymptomatic microhematuria in children is hypercalciuria.
6. **e. All of the above.** Beckwith-Wiedemann syndrome is caused by a mutation on chromosome 11p15.5. Clinical features include macroglossia, nephromegaly, organomegaly (hepatosplenomegaly), macrosomia (gigantism), and hemihypertrophy. Many of the affected infants have hypoglycemia in the first few days of life. Patients are at increased risk for specific tumors (e.g., adrenal carcinoma, Wilms tumor, hepatoblastoma, and rhabdomyosarcoma).
7. **c. Posterior urethral valves.** The diagnosis of posterior urethral valves requires visualization of the urethra during voiding. Bladder diverticula, a pronounced bladder neck, dilated posterior urethra, vesicoureteral reflux, and valve leaflets can all be associated with posterior urethral valves and are visible on VCUG. Ureteropelvic junction obstruction and primary obstructive megaureter are both obstructions above the level of the urethra and are usually evaluated with ultrasonography and a mercaptoacetyltriglycine (MAG3) renal scan or magnetic resonance urogram. Nephrolithiasis is typically evaluated using ultrasonography and computed tomography (CT) scan when necessary. Renal mass is initially evaluated by US, then MRI.
8. **a. Before discharge from the nursery.** Congenital adrenal hyperplasia may result in salt wasting, a medical emergency. Therefore neonates with ambiguous genitalia must be quickly evaluated and stabilized, prior to discharge home.
9. **c. The abdominal wall is normally strong, especially in infants with hydronephrosis.** Renal pathology accounts for approximately two-thirds of abdominal masses found in the neonate. Solid masses include neuroblastoma, congenital mesoblastic nephroma, teratoma, and renal enlargement due to renal venous thrombosis. The abdominal wall is normally weak in premature infants and on occasion in those with hydronephrosis.
10. **c. A presacral dimple less than 2.5 cm from the anal verge at birth may indicate spina bifida or cord tethering.** The lower back should be examined for any evidence of cutaneous markers of occult spinal dysraphisms that may account for abnormal bladder function. In a series of 207 neonates with sacral and presacral cutaneous stigmata, 40% of patients with atypical dimples were found to have occult spinal dysraphism. An "atypical" presacral dimple is defined as a dimple that is off center, more than 2.5 cm from the anal verge at birth, or deeper than 0.5 cm. Sacral hair tuft (hypertrichosis) may also be associated with spinal dysraphism.
11. **e. a, b, and c.** Although penile discharge and bruised vaginal mucosa can reflect sexual abuse, the possibility of sexual abuse should not be dismissed in the absence of physical examination findings. Only 11% of girls evaluated in a sexual abuse clinic demonstrated suggestive physical examination findings.
12. **d. After healing of the inflamed, denuded glans after circumcision.** Meatal stenosis is not unusual after circumcision. It may result from contraction of the meatus after healing of the inflamed, denuded glans tissue that occurs after retraction of the foreskin or from damage to the frenular artery at the time of circumcision.
13. **d. Pure gonadal dysgenesis.** Particular attention to the symmetry of the examination is important if intersex/difference of sex development is thought to exist. A symmetric gonadal examination (gonads palpable on each side or impalpable on both sides) suggests a global disorder, such as congenital adrenal hyperplasia or androgen insensitivity. When a gonad is palpable, female congenital adrenal hyperplasia (ovaries are not palpable) and pure gonadal dysgenesis (bilateral streak gonads are not palpable) are ruled out.
14. **d. Urinary incontinence after a dry interval greater than 6 months.** Although urinary incontinence can be associated with infection, constipation, and neurologic disease, secondary urinary incontinence is defined as occurring after a dry interval greater than 6 months.
15. **e. b and c.** A hydrocele that changes in volume suggests a patent processus vaginalis. These infants are at risk for an inguinal hernia. The processus vaginalis is less likely to close after birth. If a hernia has been symptomatic, it should be corrected in the newborn period. A large scrotal hydrocele may still resorb and get smaller with time—distinction must be made from an abdominoscrotal hydrocele.

CHAPTER REVIEW

1. The most common malignant abdominal tumor in infants is a neuroblastoma, followed by Wilms tumor.
2. Undescended testes are present in 30% of preterm neonates and 3% of full-term neonates; the testis will likely not descend after 6 months of age.
3. The most common prepubertal testicular/paratesticular tumor is teratoma, followed by rhabdomyosarcoma, epidermoid cyst, yolk sac tumor, and germ cell tumor, in that order.
4. Very few children hold urine and not stool. Conversely, children who retain stool nearly always retain urine.
5. Gross hematuria in the newborn is an emergency because it may indicate renal venous thrombosis or renal artery thrombosis.
6. In general, blunt renal trauma is treated nonoperatively, except when there is a major vascular avulsion or extensive urinary extravasation.
7. In the newborn, the foreskin is adherent to the glans, and adhesions should not be separated unless a circumcision is performed.
8. A positive dipstick for blood requires a microscopic examination. Absence of red blood cells in the microscopic examination indicates hemoglobinuria or myoglobinuria.
9. Continuous leakage of urine in a girl should suggest ectopic ureter.
10. Infants younger than 6 months of age and uncircumcised male infants are at increased risk for urinary tract infections.
11. A patients with a myelomeningocele is at increased risk for latex allergy.
12. Most microscopic hematuria in children is transient, and the source is not identified. The most commonly identified etiology of asymptomatic microhematuria in children is hypercalciuria.
13. Beckwith-Wiedemann syndrome is caused by a mutation on chromosome 11p15.5. Clinical features include macroglossia, nephromegaly, organomegaly (hepatosplenomegaly), macrosomia (gigantism), and hemihypertrophy. Many of the affected infants have hypoglycemia in the first few days of life. These individuals are at increased risk for adrenal carcinoma, Wilms tumor, hepatoblastoma, and rhabdomyosarcoma.
14. Renal pathology accounts for approximately two-thirds of abdominal masses found in the neonate.
15. If a difference of sex development (intersex) is thought to exist, a symmetric gonadal examination (gonads palpable on each side or impalpable on both sides) suggests a global disorder, such as congenital adrenal hyperplasia or androgen insensitivity. If the gonads are nonpalpable, congenital adrenal hyperplasia is likely.
16. A hydrocele that changes in volume suggests a patent processus vaginalis.

24 Pediatric Urogenital Imaging

Hans G. Pohl

QUESTIONS

1. All of the following statements regarding prenatal sonography are true EXCEPT:
   a. amniotic fluid contains fetal urine before 10 weeks of age.
   b. amniotic fluid contains fetal urine by 10 to 12 weeks of age.
   c. urine fills the fetal bladder by 20 weeks of age.
   d. the fetal bladder never completely empties despite normal bladder cycling.
   e. in the fetal kidney, prominent corticomedullary differentiation can be confused for hydronephrosis.

2. All of the following statements about postnatal ultrasound findings of hydronephrosis are true EXCEPT:
   a. hydronephrosis may be obstructive or nonobstructive
   b. hydronephrosis is always an indication of obstruction.
   c. hydronephrosis can be more fully evaluated by functional imaging to identify obstruction.
   d. hydronephrotic pelvicalyceal system can be differentiated from renal cysts based on whether the fluid spaces do not or do communicate.
   e. autosomal recessive polycystic kidneys are characterized by homogeneously bright kidneys that are enlarged.

3. Identify the false statement about imaging for urinary tract infection.
   a. Sonography is very sensitive for the detection of vesicoureteral reflux.
   b. Sonography is not very sensitive for the detection of acute pyelonephritis.
   c. Sonography should be considered during acute infection when the patient fails to respond to antibiotic treatment.
   d. Contrast-enhanced sonography may soon supplant voiding cystourethrogram (VCUG) as a means to diagnose vesicoureteral reflux.
   e. Dimercaptosuccinic acid (DMSA) renal scan is highly accurate for the detection of acute pyelonephritis and renal scarring.

4. Identify the false statement about imaging the acute scrotum.
   a. Surgical exploration for torsion should not be delayed to obtain scrotal imaging if the history and physical examination suggests that diagnosis.
   b. Salvageability of the testicle based on sonographic appearance is difficult to predict.
   c. Epididymo-orchitis and spontaneous detorsion can *both* demonstrate hyperemia on sonography.

   d. Torsion of the appendix testis can be seen as an enlarged and avascular lower pole testicular nodule with surrounding hyperemia.
   e. Most prepubertal testicular masses are benign.

5. The four "key elements" to a successful diuresis renogram for the evaluation of hydronephrosis are:
   a. hydration, selection of the appropriate region of interest, bladder drainage as appropriate, timing of diuretic administration.
   b. sedation, selection of the appropriate region of interest, bladder drainage as appropriate, timing of diuretic administration.
   c. hydration, selection of the appropriate region of interest, bladder drainage as appropriate, timing of diuretic administration to occur exactly when furosemide is administered.
   d. hydration, selection of the appropriate region of interest, catheterization of the bladder on completion of the test, timing of diuretic administration.
   e. hydration, selection of the region of interest tightly around the renal cortex, bladder drainage as appropriate, timing of diuretic administration.

ANSWERS

1. **a. Amniotic fluid contains fetal urine before 10 weeks of age.** Amniotic fluid does not contain fetal urine before 10 weeks of age.

2. **b. Hydronephrosis is always an indication of obstruction.** Hydronephrosis is not always an indication of obstruction.

3. **a. Sonography is very sensitive for the detection of vesicoureteral reflux.** Sonography is not sensitive for the detection of vesicoureteral reflux.

4. **d. Torsion of the appendix testis can be seen as an enlarged and avascular lower pole testicular nodule with surrounding hyperemia.** Torsion of the appendix testis is not seen as an enlarged and avascular lower pole testicular nodule with surrounding hyperemia.

5. **a. Hydration, selection of the appropriate region of interest, bladder drainage as appropriate, timing of diuretic administration.** The four key elements to a successful diuresis renogram are hydration, selection of the appropriate region of interest, bladder drainage as appropriate, and timing of diuretic administration.

CHAPTER REVIEW

1. Sonography is the initial examination to perform for suspect obstruction, as well as being helpful for longitudinal follow-up.
2. Based upon the sonographic findings, ancillary imaging (such as voiding cystourethrography and/or diuresis renography) might be considered.
3. A normal infant renal sonogram can be confused with mature hydronephrosis because of hypoechoic renal pyramids with a distinct corticomedullary junction.
4. Diagnosis of obstruction in children with diuresis renography requires review of all parameters of the test because variations in technique can skew results considerably.
5. Sonographically, multicystic dysplastic kidney (MCDK) is characterized by echolucent spaces (cysts) of varying sizes that are randomly distributed throughout the kidney with a paucity of renal parenchyma that is hyperechoic.
6. Autosomal recessive polycystic kidney disease (ARPKD) typically affects both kidneys and is characterized by enlarged and echogenic parenchyma.
7. Autosomal dominant polycystic kidney disease (ADPKD) typically affects both kidneys and is characterized by replacement of the renal parenchyma by cysts.
8. Although patient age and hallmark sonographic features suggest the diagnosis of renal masses, contrast-enhanced computed tomography (CT) scan of the abdomen should follow.
9. Numerous guidelines have been published on the radiographic evaluation following pediatric urinary tract infection, and sonography is used as an initial screening modality despite its low yield.
10. A normal sonogram is insufficient to risk-stratify a child with a febrile urinary tract infection (UTI) and is not a good predictor for vesicoureteral reflux (VUR).
11. The "bottom-up" approach relies on VCUG—following US—to identify all cases of VUR that may result in overtreatment of low-grade VUR.
12. The "top-down" approach replaces screening US with a DMSA renal scan to identify acute pyelonephritis and/or renal scarring. Proponents of this algorithm recommend VCUG only in response to abnormal DMSA scans as an indicator of high-risk patients.
13. Abdominal sonography is useful as part of the acute trauma evaluation and compares favorably to contrast-enhanced CT scans. Sonography should be considered for the longitudinal evaluation of known renal injuries, particularly to assess resolution of perinephric hematomas or urinomas.
14. Ionizing radiation is used to evaluate genitourinary trauma, frequently with the addition of intravenous or intraluminal iodinated contrast.
15. Radiographic evaluation is incomplete unless delayed views of the renal parenchyma and collecting system are obtained on CT scan, or lateral projections of the bladder, bladder neck, and urethra.
16. In addition to careful history and physical examination, scrotal sonography provides much of the information needed to discriminate between inflammation, neoplasm, trauma, and testicular torsion.
17. Nuclear scintigraphy may be used to evaluate testicular torsion but provides little additional information over what can be gleaned from sonography.
18. Sonography for the undescended testis is unreliable and should not be used, perhaps with the exception of seeking the inguinal undescended testis in an overweight boy.

25 Infection and Inflammation of the Pediatric Genitourinary Tract

Christopher S. Cooper and Douglas W. Storm

QUESTIONS

1. The primary symptom in a 3-month-old that leads to the diagnosis of a pediatric urinary tract infection (UTI) is:
   a. diarrhea.
   b. frequency.
   c. fever.
   d. jaundice.
   e. foul-smelling urine.

2. Which of the following factors would not increase the probability of a UTI in a febrile girl?
   a. Age less than 12 months
   b. Temperature 39°C or higher
   c. African American race
   d. Absence of other source of infection
   e. Recent previous UTI

3. A false-negative urinary nitrite test for UTI may be caused by all of the following EXCEPT:
   a. gram-positive bacterial UTI.
   b. urinary retention.
   c. dilute urine.
   d. yeast infection.
   e. frequent urination.

4. Which of the following tests has the highest sensitivity for UTI?
   a. Leukocyte esterase
   b. Urinary nitrite
   c. Urinary nitrate
   d. Serum procalcitonin
   e. Urine protein

5. Which of the following statements is FALSE regarding dimercaptosuccinic acid (DMSA) renal scan?
   a. The maximum sensitivity for detection of acute pyelonephritis is within 1 week from the onset of symptoms.
   b. Demonstration of irreversible renal damage and scar may require a renal scan at least 1 year after pyelonephritis.
   c. The risk of an abnormal scan increases with increased grades of vesicoureteral reflux (VUR).
   d. The estimated radiation dose is approximately 1 mSv.
   e. DMSA is bound to the glomerular basement membrane, providing excellent cortical imaging but slow excretion.

6. Which of the following statements regarding imaging is most likely to be broadly accepted?
   a. All children with febrile UTI require a voiding cystourethrogram (VCUG).
   b. All children with a febrile UTI require a renal ultrasound.
   c. All children with fever persisting longer than 48 hours after appropriate antibiotics require a renal and bladder ultrasound.
   d. All children with a febrile UTI require a DMSA.
   e. All children with fever persisting longer than 18 hours after appropriate antibiotics require a computed tomography (CT) scan.

7. The most common pediatric uropathogen is:
   a. *Escherichia coli.*
   b. *Klebsiella.*
   c. *Proteus.*
   d. *Enterobacter.*
   e. *Citrobacter.*

8. Ampicillin should be strongly considered for use with neonates because of the increased incidence of which uropathogen?
   a. *E. coli*
   b. *Klebsiella*
   c. *Pseudomonas*
   d. *Enterococcus*
   e. *Staphylococcus aureus*

9. Which of the following antibiotics would NOT be a good choice for a child with suspected pyelonephritis?
   a. Fluoroquinolones
   b. Trimethoprim
   c. Cephalosporin
   d. Nitrofurantoin
   e. Gentamicin

10. Which of the following antibiotics is contraindicated in children younger than 6 weeks?
    a. Trimethoprim-sulfamethoxazole
    b. Amoxicillin-clavulanate
    c. Cephalexin
    d. Piperacillin
    e. Tobramycin

11. Which of the following have been identified as risk factors for UTI?
    a. Constipation
    b. Bladder dysfunction
    c. High-grade VUR
    d. Female gender, older than 1 year
    e. All of the above

12. Which of the following is NOT true regarding renal scars?
    a. Increased incidence occurs with delayed treatment of a UTI
    b. May be indistinguishable on renal scan from renal dysplasia
    c. Most frequently seen in midportion of the kidney parenchyma
    d. Involve a loss of renal parenchymal tissue
    e. Have been associated with an increased risk of hypertension

13. Children with significant bilateral renal scars require:
    a. prophylactic antibiotics.
    b. renin-angiotensin antagonists.
    c. dietary modification.
    d. long-term assessment of proteinuria.
    e. none of the above.

14. Which of the following statements regarding recurrent UTIs is FALSE?
    a. The risk of a recurrent UTI is higher in a boy with an initial UTI who is younger than 1 year than in one who is older than 1 year.
    b. Ten percent to 30% of children will develop at least one recurrent UTI.
    c. The recurrence rate is highest within the first 3 to 6 months following a UTI.
    d. The more frequent and more recurrent a child's UTIs, the more likely the child is to have subsequent UTIs.
    e. The risk of renal scars increases with recurrent UTIs.

15. In children aged 0 to 24 months who present with a fever, which of the following signs/symptoms are not useful in suspecting that they may have a UTI as the cause of their fever?
    a. Fever greater than 40°C
    b. Vomiting
    c. History of a previous UTI
    d. Suprapubic tenderness
    e. Uncircumcised penis

16. Which of the following statements is FALSE?
    a. Virulent bacteria that cause UTIs are otherwise known as uropathogenic bacteria.
    b. Virulent bacteria possess different adaptations and fitness factors that allow them to subvert or hijack host defenses and reside in an environment in which they would not normally preside.
    c. Virulent bacteria have mechanisms that allow the bacteria to initially attach to urogenital mucosal surfaces and then interact with these tissues by setting off cascades of signaling and other immunologic response events and subsequently invade the bladder.
    d. Commensal bacteria cannot cause UTIs.
    e. Commensal bacteria are defined as lacking the virulent traits that would allow bacteria to subvert a host's immune defenses.

17. Which of the following is NOT considered a bacterial virulence trait?
    a. Properties that improve bacterial adherence
    b. Properties that allow bacterial nourishment in otherwise adverse environments
    c. Flagellar attachments that allow bacteria to move more quickly
    d. Properties that protect bacteria from the host's immune response
    e. Toxins that allow bacteria to invade host cells

18. Which of the following statements is FALSE?
    a. In children younger than 1 year, UTIs are more common in boys than girls.
    b. After 1 year, UTIs are more prevalent in females than males, except in elderly individuals.
    c. It has been estimated that 7% of girls and 2% of boys suffer a UTI by the age of 6 years.
    d. Three percent to 5% of febrile children have a UTI.
    e. In sexually active teenagers, there is a female predominance of UTIs.

19. Which of the following is a TRUE statement?
    a. Circumcision reduces the rate of UTI development in the first 12 months of life by almost 20-fold.
    b. Circumcision reduces the rate of UTI development in the first 6 months of life by almost 5-fold.
    c. Circumcision reduces the rate of UTI development in the first 6 months of life by almost 10-fold.
    d. Circumcision reduces the rate of UTI development in the first 18 months of life by almost 5-fold.
    e. Circumcision does not reduce the rate of UTI.

20. Which of the following statements is FALSE regarding the role that VUR plays in pediatric UTI development?
    a. VUR has been identified in 1% to 2% of all newborns.
    b. VUR is found in 25% to 40% of children after their first episode of UTI.
    c. In children who are found to have a DMSA-proven episode of pyelonephritis, 66% will be found to have VUR.
    d. Kidneys associated with higher-grade VUR (grades III and IV) are twice as likely to have pyelonephritic changes on DMSA scan.
    e. Obtaining a VCUG in only those children with an abnormal DMSA scan may miss 15%–30% of children with dilating VUR.

21. A 9-year-old female referred for treatment of multiple afebrile UTIs suffers from urinary urgency and is known to prolong using the toilet. She suffers from day and nighttime urinary incontinence. She also has a bowel movement only every few days that is typically hard and painful. She underwent a renal ultrasound that showed normal upper tracts and a thick-walled bladder. A VCUG was performed that showed grade II left VUR and a spinning top urethra. Which of the following statements regarding treatment of this child is TRUE?
    a. The use of anticholinergics in this child would not help to resolve her VUR.
    b. Biofeedback would be of no use in this patient because it has not been shown to improve VUR resolution and further UTI development.
    c. Treatment of her constipation may improve her day and nighttime urinary incontinence and help to reduce the incidence of recurrent UTIs.
    d. The implementation of a timed voiding schedule would not be appropriate because this child requires urgent surgical therapy for treatment of her VUR to prevent further UTI development.
    e. Treatment of her dysfunctional elimination should not be considered because she has VUR.

22. Multiple studies demonstrate that _____ of individuals who intermittently catheterize develop chronic bacteria and/or pyuria and most are asymptomatic.
    a. 40% to 80%
    b. 50% to 90%
    c. 30% to 60%
    d. 10% to 25%
    e. 45% to 85%

23. Which of the following statements is FALSE?
    a. Catheter-associated UTI is the second most common nosocomial infection, accounting for more than 1 million cases each year in U.S. hospitals and nursing homes.
    b. The risk of UTI increases with the length of time that the catheter is in place.
    c. Nosocomial UTIs typically necessitate one extra hospital day per patient and nearly 1 million extra hospital days annually.

d. The best way to avoid a catheter-related UTI and its related cost is the judicious use of urinary catheters and to remove urethral catheters in hospitalized patients as soon as they are no longer medically necessary.

e. In children, nosocomial UTIs account for 6% to 18% of nosocomial infections on pediatric hospital services.

24. A 9-year-old female presents with fevers, nausea, vomiting, and flank pain and is shown to have a culture-proven UTI. If she underwent a DMSA scan, how likely is it that the scan would show changes associated with pyelonephritis?

    a. 95% to 100%

    b. 50% to 66%

    c. 60% to 75%

    d. 70% to 85%

    e. 10% to 25%

25. Which of the following statements is FALSE regarding why bacteria within a biofilm may be difficult to eradicate with antibiotics?

    a. Antibiotics often fail to penetrate the full depth of a biofilm.

    b. Organisms within a biofilm often grow quickly, resulting in resistance to the antibiotics.

    c. Antimicrobial binding proteins are poorly expressed in these biofilm bacteria.

    d. Bacteria within a biofilm activate many genes that alter the cell envelope, the molecular targets, and the susceptibility to antimicrobial agents.

    e. Bacteria in a biofilm can survive in the presence of antimicrobial agents at a concentration 1000 to 1500 times higher than the concentration normally necessary to kill non–biofilm-associated bacteria in the same species.

26. A girl who presents for a preschool physical is found to have more than 105 colony-forming units (CFU)/mL E. coli on a urine culture. She has never previously suffered a UTI and is asymptomatic. How should she be treated?

    a. Three-day course of antibiotics

    b. Urodynamics and kidney-ureter-bladder (KUB) radiography for evaluation of occult voiding dysfunction and constipation

    c. Renal ultrasound and VCUG

    d. No treatment or further evaluation is necessary.

    e. A catheterized urine specimen should be obtained to verify that this is truly a UTI.

27. Which of the following statements is FALSE?

    a. Recurrent UTIs can be subdivided into unresolved bacteriuria, bacterial persistence, and reinfection.

    b. Unresolved bacteriuria is most commonly caused by inadequate bacterial therapy.

    c. Bacterial persistence and reinfection occur after sterile urine has been documented after previous UTI therapy.

    d. In cases of bacterial reinfection, typically a nidus causing the infection has not been eradicated.

    e. Asymptomatic bacteriuria (ASB) is defined as the presence of two consecutive urine specimens yielding positive cultures (more than 105 CFU/mL) of the same uropathogen in a patient who is free of any infectious symptoms.

28. Which of the following is TRUE regarding a renal abscess?

    a. Individuals presenting with a renal abscess commonly are more ill than patients with just pyelonephritis.

    b. In as many as 30% of renal abscess cases, the urine culture may be negative.

    c. CT appears to be the most sensitive and specific imaging modality in making the diagnosis of a renal abscess.

    d. Associated early CT findings include a poorly defined area of low attenuation or decreased enhancement or a striated, wedge-shaped zone of increased or decreased enhancement.

    e. Ultrasound can detect an abscess as small as 2 cm and usually appears as a sonolucent area containing low-amplitude echoes.

29. Which of the following defines a UTI?

    a. If a suprapubic aspiration was performed, then recovery of any organisms defines a UTI.

    b. For catheterized specimens, recovery of at least 10,000 CFU/mL is required to define a UTI.

    c. If the specimen was collected via a clean catch method, 50,000 CFU/mL are required.

    d. If a suprapubic aspiration was performed, then recovery of at least 10,000 CFU/mL organisms defines a UTI.

    e. No matter how the culture is collected, the presence of 10,000 CFU/mL defines a UTI.

ANSWERS

1. **c. Fever.** Although all of the choices may be symptoms of a UTI in infants and young patients and UTI should be considered as a possible diagnosis, after the neonatal period fever is usually the primary symptom that leads to the diagnosis of a pediatric UTI.

2. **c. African American race.** The probability of a UTI in girls has been shown to be at least 1%, and 2% if they had two or more, or three or more, of the following risk factors, respectively: white race, age younger than 12 months, temperature at or above 39°C, fever lasting 2 days or more, or absence of another source of infection (Gorelick and Shaw, 2000).[a] In addition, children with a previous UTI are at increased risk for UTI. Children younger than 6 years with a documented UTI have been noted to have a 12% risk of recurrence per year in a community-based study (Conway et al., 2007).

3. **b. Urinary retention.** Urinary nitrite is reduced from dietary nitrates in the urine by gram-negative enteric bacteria. This conversion requires several hours to occur; thus a first morning urine sample gives the best sensitivity with this test. Frequent urination, as is often the case in infants and small children, may not permit enough time for the urine in the bladder to undergo significant conversion of nitrates to nitrites and therefore result in a false-negative nitrite test more frequently than in older children (Mori et al., 2010). A dilute urine may also generate a false-negative test. Other reasons for a false-negative test include infection with gram-positive organisms that do not reduce nitrates.

4. **a. Leukocyte esterase.** Leukocyte esterase has a relatively high sensitivity but low specificity. Urinary nitrite has a very high specificity. Urinary nitrite is formed by bacterial enzymatic reduction of urinary nitrate. Procalcitonin may be useful in identifying children with acute pyelonephritis.

5. **e. DMSA is bound to the glomerular basement membrane and providing excellent cortical imaging but slow excretion.** All other statements are true. DMSA is injected intravenously and taken up by the kidney, bound to the proximal renal tubular cells, and excreted very slowly in the urine, providing good and stable imaging of the renal cortex.

6. **c. All children with fever persisting longer than 48 hours after appropriate antibiotics require a renal and bladder ultrasound.** There is a lack of consensus among various guidelines around the world on what routine imaging, if any, is required with a febrile UTI. However, significant clinical improvement including defervescence routinely takes at least 24 hours after beginning antibiotics (Hoberman et al., 1999). Ninety percent of children

---

[a]Sources referenced can be found in *Campbell-Walsh-Wein Urology, 12th Edition,* on the Expert Consult website.

will have a normal body temperature within 48 hours of the start of therapy, but if the child is not improving after 48 hours, a renal and bladder ultrasound should be strongly considered.

7. **a. *Escherichia coli.*** *E. coli* remains the most common pediatric uropathogen (>80% of UTIs).

8. **d. *Enterococcus.*** Neonates and young infants should be covered for *Enterococcus* species when choosing empiric antibiotics, because the incidence of infections with this uropathogen is higher in early infancy than at a later age (Beetz and Westenfelder, 2011). *Enterococcus* is frequently sensitive to ampicillin and first-generation cephalosporins.

9. **d. Nitrofurantoin.** Nitrofurantoin has poor tissue penetration and should not be used for febrile UTI/pyelonephritis.

10. **a. Trimethoprim-sulfamethoxazole.** Trimethoprim-sulfamethoxazole (TMP-SMX) is contraindicated in premature infants and newborns younger than 6 weeks. Sulfonamides may compete for bilirubin binding sites on albumin and cause neonatal hyperbilirubinemia and kernicterus, so TMP-SMX is avoided in the first 6 weeks of life.

11. **e. All of the above.** All of the listed options have been identified as risk factors. Boys in the first year of life have a higher incidence of UTIs than girls.

12. **c. Most frequently seen in midportion of the kidney parenchyma.** Pyelonephritic scarring occurs most commonly in the poles of the kidney and is associated with compound papillae (Hannerz et al., 1987).

13. **d. Long-term assessment of proteinuria.** Although certain children with significant bilateral renal scars may benefit from a, b, or c, on a routine basis, children with significant bilateral renal scars or reduction of renal function warrant long-term follow-up for assessment of hypertension, renal function, and proteinuria. Recent studies suggest that proteinuria not only may be a clinical feature of chronic kidney disease but may hasten its progression. The use of renin-angiotensin antagonists may slow the progression of chronic kidney disease in some of these patients (Wong et al., 2009).

14. **a. The risk of a recurrent UTI is higher in a boy with an initial UTI who is younger than 1 year than in one who is older than 1 year.** For boys younger than 1 year, 18% will develop a recurrent infection, usually within the next year. If the initial infection is in a boy older than 1 year, his risk of a reinfection increases to 32%. A similar trend is noted in girls younger than and older than 1 year of age, who have a recurrence risk of 26% and 40%, respectively (Winberg et al., 1974).

15. **b. Vomiting.** Vomiting has been shown to be nonspecific in predicting the presence of a UTI in patients aged 0 to 24 months of age. The remainder of the symptoms/signs are more specific for predicting the presence of a UTI.

16. **d. Commensal bacteria cannot cause UTIs.** Although virulent bacteria do account for the majority of UTIs, commensal bacteria may also cause a small percentage of UTIs.

17. **c. Flagellar attachments that allow bacteria to move more quickly.** Flagellae are considered a normal component of some bacteria and not necessarily a virulence trait. The remainder of the statements are true regarding virulence factors.

18. **b. After 1 year, UTIs are more prevalent in females than males, except in elderly individuals.** UTIs are more common in boys compared with girls younger than 1 year of age. After 1 year, UTIs are more common in females and remain so, even in elderly individuals.

19. **c. Circumcision reduces the rate of UTI development in the first 6 months of life by almost 10-fold.** Although controversial, several studies have demonstrated that the risk of UTI appears to correlate with a period during the first 6 months of life when there is an increased amount of uropathogenic bacteria colonizing the prepuce, which appears to decrease and resolve by 5 years.

20. **c. In children who are found to have a DMSA-proven episode of pyelonephritis, 66% will be found to have VUR.** Although we continually question whether VUR may be present in a child who has suffered a pyelonephritic infection, it is important to remember that the majority of children who have suffered from pyelonephritis do not have VUR. Rushton et al. (1992) found that in children suffering DMSA-proven pyelonephritis, only 37% are found to have VUR.

21. **c. Treatment of her constipation may improve her day and nighttime urinary incontinence and help to reduce the incidence of recurrent UTIs.** This child suffers from dysfunctional bowel and bladder issues that are known to contribute to UTI development and VUR. Treatment of her bladder issues with antimuscarinics, biofeedback, and timed voiding would be appropriate, along with therapies to treat her constipation, before considering surgical therapy. In fact, these conservative therapies often will eliminate the need for any surgery for VUR treatment.

22. **a. 40% to 80%.** Of individuals who intermittently catheterize, 40% to 80% develop chronic bacteriuria and/or pyuria. Most of these individuals are asymptomatic and do not require antibiotic prophylaxis or treatment.

23. **a. Catheter-associated UTI is the second most common nosocomial infection, accounting for more than 1 million cases each year in U.S. hospitals and nursing homes.** Catheter-associated UTIs are the most common nosocomial infections affecting children. The risk increases with the duration that the catheter is in place. The best way to avoid these infections is to use urinary catheters judiciously and to remove them from hospitalized patients as soon as they are no longer medically necessary.

24. **b. 50% to 66%.** We use signs and symptoms such as fever, flank pain, nausea, and vomiting to clinically define a pyelonephritic UTI. However, it is important to remember that acute changes on a DMSA renal scan at the time of a UTI is currently the "gold standard" for indicating that a child truly has pyelonephritis. When a patient presents with these pyelonephritic symptoms, a DMSA scan is positive only 50% to 66% of the time.

25. **b. Organisms within a biofilm often grow quickly, resulting in resistance to the antibiotics.** Bacteria within a biofilm have been found to grow at a slower than normal rate, making them more resistant to antibiotic therapy.

26. **d. No treatment or further evaluation is necessary.** ASB occurs in 0.8% of preschool girls and even fewer preschool boys. Children in this age group who are without VUR and/or other genitourinary abnormalities do not require antibiotics to clear their bacteria because they do not appear to be at any risk for recurrent symptomatic infections, renal damage, or impaired renal growth.

27. **d. In cases of bacterial reinfection, typically a nidus causing the infection has not been eradicated.** Typically, a nidus causing a UTI has not been eradicated in cases of bacterial persistence, not bacterial reinfection.

28. **c. CT appears to be the most sensitive and specific imaging modality in making the diagnosis of a renal abscess.** Individuals presenting with a renal abscess often have symptoms similar to those of patients with pyelonephritis. In as many as 20% of renal abscess cases, the urine culture may be negative. Ultrasound can detect an abscess as small as 1 cm, which usually appears as a sonolucent area containing low-amplitude echoes. CT appears to be the most sensitive and specific imaging modality in making the diagnosis of a renal abscess.

29. **a. If a suprapubic aspiration was performed, then recovery of any organisms defines a UTI.** For catheterized specimens, recovery of at least 50,000 CFU/mL is required to define a UTI, and 100,000 CFU/mL are required if the specimen was collected via a clean catch method.

CHAPTER REVIEW

1. UTIs cause abnormally elevated renal pelvic pressures.
2. Clinical symptoms correlate poorly with bacterial localization in the urinary tract.
3. Microbial lipopolysaccharides trigger urothelial receptors (Toll-like receptors) to activate the innate local immune system, activating cytokines, chemokines, and neutrophils.
4. For children, when performing intermittent catheterization, neither sterile or single-use lubricated catheters nor antimicrobial prophylaxis is recommended.
5. In teenage females, sexually transmitted infections may progress to pelvic inflammatory disease, infertility, and chronic pelvic pain.
6. Suprapubic bladder aspiration is the most reliable method of determining whether a UTI is present.
7. Elevated C-reactive protein and procalcitonin have been associated with acute pyelonephritis.
8. Children with glucose-6-phosphate dehydrogenase deficiency should not be given nitrofurantoin.
9. Children with gross polynephritic nephropathy (reflux nephropathy) have a 10% to 20% risk of hypertension.
10. Significant proteinuria is a routine finding in patients with VUR who have progressive deterioration of renal function.
11. Adenovirus is the most common cause of acute viral hemorrhagic cystitis in children.
12. Any catheter that has been left in place for more than 4 days will result in infected urine.
13. Mechanisms possessed by bacteria to promote their ability to cause a UTI include bacterial adhesion facilitated by pili, access to iron, production of hemolysin, capsular polysaccharides that interfere with the host's ability to detect antigen, and biofilms.
14. Age of first UTI, a mother with a history of UTI, and the presence of certain blood group antigens are risk factors for women for recurrent UTIs.
15. Bladder and bowel dysfunction (dysfunctional elimination syndrome) contribute to UTI. Correcting the dysfunction reduces the recurrence of UTI and improves VUR resolution.
16. Urethritis can be caused by *Neisseria gonorrhoeae*, *Chlamydia trachomatis*, and *Ureaplasma urealyticum*.
17. More than 5 to 10 white blood cells per high-power field is required for the diagnosis of UTI; a positive culture confirms the diagnosis.
18. A febrile UTI in a newborn or young infant requires hospitalization and parenteral antibiotics.
19. For a febrile UTI, antibiotics should be given for 7 to 14 days; for afebrile cystitis, a 2- to 4-day course is sufficient.
20. Renal dysplasia occurs with VUR and on DMSA scan dysplasia may be mistaken for a renal scar.
21. Urinary nitrite is reduced from dietary nitrates in the urine by gram-negative enteric bacteria. This conversion requires several hours to occur; thus a first morning urine gives the best sensitivity with the nitrite dipstick test. Frequent voiding may cause a false-negative test.
22. Neonates and young infants should be covered for *Enterococcus* species when choosing empiric antibiotics.
23. In the first year of life, boys have a higher incidence of UTIs than girls.
24. Pyelonephritic scarring occurs most commonly in the poles of the kidney and is associated with compound papillae.
25. Of individuals who intermittently catheterize, 40% to 80% develop chronic bacteriuria and/or pyuria. Most of these individuals are asymptomatic and do not require antibiotic prophylaxis or treatment.
26. For catheterized specimens, recovery of at least 50,000 CFU/mL is required to define a UTI and 100,000 CFU/mL is required if the specimen was collected via a clean catch method.

26 Core Principles of Perioperative Management in Children

Sherry S. Ross and Janey R. Phelps

QUESTIONS

1. Current U.S. Food and Drug Administration (FDA) guidelines for the administration of anesthesia agents to children are as follows:

   a. Repeated or lengthy use of general anesthetic and sedation drugs during surgeries or procedures in children younger than 3 years or in pregnant women during their third trimester may affect the development of children's brains.

   b. Repeated or lengthy use of general anesthetic and sedation drugs during surgeries or procedures in children younger than 2 years or in pregnant women during their third trimester may affect the development of children's brains.

   c. Repeated or lengthy use of general anesthetic and sedation drugs during surgeries or procedures in children younger than 3 years or in pregnant women during their second trimester may affect the development of children's brains.

   d. Repeated or lengthy use of general anesthetic and sedation drugs during surgeries or procedures in children younger than 3 years may affect the development of children's brains.

   e. Repeated or lengthy use of general anesthetic and sedation drugs during surgeries or procedures in children younger than 2 years or in pregnant women during their second trimester may affect the development of children's brains.

2. Which is true regarding pain in children?

   a. Discussion of pain expectations with children and parents influences pain associated with procedures.

   b. Child life specialists are experts in the education and procedure preparation of children and families through various techniques that help overcome anxiety and should be used in the perioperative setting to help decrease child and parental anxiety.

   c. Preoperative anxiety in children is predictive of postoperative pain levels and behaviors.

   d. a and c

   e. a, b, and c

3. Which of the following concerning pain assessment in children is FALSE?

   a. Self-assessment of pain is considered the "gold standard" for pain assessment.

   b. Self-assessment measurements to rate pain are not present in children less than 2 years old.

   c. Self-assessment in children include: validated in children include Pieces of Hurt (3–6 years), Faces scale (4–12 years), Oucher scale (4–12 years), visual analog scale (8–16 years).

   d. Objective pain scales are available for premature infants (e.g., Premature Infant Pain Profile [PIPP]), neonates, and nonverbal and cognitively impaired children.

   e. Pain should be described in terms of intensity, location, duration, modifiable interventions, and quality.

4. NPO (nothing by mouth [nil per os]) status recommendations in children include:

   a. There should be an 8-hour period between the intake of full meals prior induction of general anesthesia, regional anesthesia, or sedation/analgesia.

   b. Children may consume formula, nonhuman milk, or a light meal up to 6 hours prior to needed anesthesia.

   c. There should be a 4-hour period of time between the consumptions of breast milk and administration of general anesthesia, regional anesthesia, or sedation/analgesia.

   d. Children may have clear liquids up to 2 hours before elective procedures requiring anesthesia administration since risk of aspiration is low.

   e. All of the above.

5. Children may have dietary requirements outside the normal parameters. Which of the following is a false statement?

   a. Children on a ketogenic diet should receive carbohydrate-free fluids.

   b. Enteral feeds are considered a fatty meal and should be stopped 8 hours prior to anesthesia induction.

   c. Children with diabetes may be affected by volume depletion during preoperative fasting coupled with the discontinuation of outpatient diabetes medications. This may result in preoperative hypoglycemia.

   d. Metformin should be discontinued 24 hours prior to surgery because it has a long half-life, which increases the risk of lactic acidosis in the presence of dehydration, hypoxemia, or poor tissue perfusion.

   e. Medications that should be taken on the morning of surgery include antiseizure, gastrointestinal reflux, and asthma medications.

6. Which of the following is true concerning perioperative laboratory evaluation?

   a. Urologic procedures where the urinary tract is opened electively are considered clean contaminated and increase the risk of postoperative infection.

   b. Routine laboratory evaluation has little use and is not cost effective.

   c. For female patients of childbearing age, a preoperative urine pregnancy test is recommended.

   d. The American Academy of Pediatrics recommended preoperative chest x-ray as part of routine preoperative assessment.

   e. a, b, and c.

7. Perioperative considerations in premature infants include:

   a. Respiratory function in the premature infant is challenging due to inadequate surfactant levels, especially in children born less than 36 weeks, resulting in high oxygen consumptions and low pulmonary functional residual capacity, as well as tracheomalacia.

   b. Premature infants have a high risk of apnea, which can result in death.

   c. Premature infants have an increased risk of retinopathy and blindness in the presence of supplemental oxygen so the overall goal is oxygen saturation percentage ranging in the low 90s.

d. Neonates have a higher potential for large fluid losses due to higher rates of evaporation from skin and surgical wound sights, as well as decreased ability to concentrate urine.

e. b, c, and d.

8. Regarding children with renal insufficiency, which of the following is true?

a. Infants and children under the age of 6 years typically have kidney insufficiency due to acquired abnormalities such as immunoglobulin A (IgA) nephropathy.

b. Children with chronic kidney disease (CKD) have an increased potential for anemia due to decreases in the renal production of erythropoietin and increases in ureas, which decreases red blood cell production.

c. Elevations in urea platelet dysfunction, which increases the risk of thrombus.

d. Cardiac function is typically normal in patients with CKD.

e. Electrolyte abnormalities in children with CKD are often abnormal. Abnormalities such as hypernatremia can increase the risk of cardiac arrhythmias.

9. Which of the follow is a true statement?

a. Patients with CKD 2 have mild impairment of renal function but are able to excrete drugs and metabolites, so they do not require medication adjustments. However, they should be monitored closely for effects of NSAIDs on renal function and for worsening renal deterioration.

b. The most important factor in the perioperative management of children with sickle cell disease is dehydration, especially during the preoperative NPO status.

c. In the presence of high-inspired oxygen levels during anesthesia, patients treated with the chemotherapeutic agent bleomycin can develop pulmonary toxicity, which can be fatal.

d. b and c only.

e. All of the above.

10. Which of the following statements are true concerning children under anesthesia for surgical procedures?

a. Spina bifida patients with lesions at T5 to T8 are at an increased risk of autonomic dysreflexia with noxious stimuli. This can lead to uncontrolled hypertension, bradycardia, stroke, and potentially death.

b. Spina bifida patients have an increased risk of latex allergies.

c. Symptoms of severe latex allergy include bronchoconstriction, vasodilation and subsequent hypotension, increased capillary permeability, coronary vasoconstriction, and myocardial depression.

d. Children with congenital adrenal hyperplasia can have epinephrine and cortisol deficiency, which may result in hypoglycemia.

e. All of the above.

11. Which of the following is a false statement?

a. For postoperative pain management in the septic child, peripheral nerve blocks may be effective and avoid the systemic effects of opioid in a hemodynamically unstable patient.

b. Pediatric trauma victims should always be considered to have a full stomach, and rapid sequence induction should be the gold standard.

c. Infection-induced inflammation of the upper respiratory mucosa will result in airway hyperreactivity, which increases secretions and airway irritability during anesthesia and can persist for 2 to 8 weeks following infection.

d. The American Urological Association guidelines state that if urologic surgery is planned in the presence of an existing infection, antibiotics should be administered with the goal of a sterilized operative field.

e. All of the above.

12. Which of the following are true?

a. The most common cause of perioperative fever in children involves an infectious etiology, which is most commonly a viral upper respiratory tract infection.

b. Preoperative urine cultures should be obtained preoperatively if a sterilized field is required and can be obtained.

c. Blood transfusion can result in a nonspecific fever up to 1 week after transfusion.

d. Preoperative UTI, especially if recurrent, is recognized as a high-risk factor for postoperative infection.

e. All of the above.

13. Which of the following statements are true?

a. The ERAS (Early Recovery After Surgery) pathway uses several components, which include avoiding prolonged fasting, early enteral nutrition, preoperative oral carbohydrate loading, early mobilization, and enhanced efforts in patient education. These are yet to be established in pediatric patients.

b. In the preoperative setting, administration of antibiotics should allow time for adequate serum and tissue concentrations prior to incision.

c. Neuromuscular blocking agents and β-lactam antibiotics are the main triggers of perioperative anaphylactic reactions.

d. Treatment of perioperative anaphylaxis includes stopping the suspected drug immediately, 100% oxygen administration, Trendelenburg position, fluid therapy, and epinephrine.

e. All of the above.

14. Which of the following is true concerning malignant hyperthermia?

a. Malignant hyperthermia is a common disorder

b. Malignant hyperthermia is a potentially fatal hypermetabolic disorder that is triggered by acetylcholine and inhaled anesthetics.

c. Signs of malignant hyperthermia include hypocarbia, sinus bradycardia, masseter muscle spasm, and hyperthermia.

d. If malignant hyperthermia is suspected, the triggering agent should be stopped, anesthesia backup should be requested, anesthesia machine should be exchanged, and an arterial line should be placed, as well as a Foley catheter.

e. Late signs include severe metabolic alkylosis, hypokalemia, generalized muscle rigidity, and rhabdomyolysis.

15. Which of the following is true concerning the postoperative period?

a. Respiratory events only include hypoxia and airway obstruction.

b. Most postoperative cardiac events in children are preventable.

c. Emergency delirium occurs only in children between the ages of 2 to 8.

d. Patients with high preoperative anxiety are at increased risk of postoperative emergence delirium.

e. b and d.

ANSWERS

1. **a. Repeated or lengthy use of general anesthetic and sedation drugs during surgeries or procedures in children younger than 3 years or in pregnant women during their third trimester may affect the development of children's brains.**

2. **e. a, b, and c.** Discussion of pain expectations with children and parents influences pain associated with procedures. Child life specialists are experts in the education and procedure preparation of children and families through various techniques that help to overcome anxiety and should be used in the perioperative setting to help decrease child and parental anxiety. Preoperative anxiety in children is predictive of postoperative pain levels and behaviors.

3. **b. Self-assessment measurements to rate pain are not present in children less than 2 years old.** "Self-assessment measurements to rate pain are not present in children less than 2 years old" is a false statement.

4. **e. All of the above.** NPO status recommendations in children include all of the listed options.

5. **c. Children with diabetes may be affected by volume depletion during preoperative fasting coupled with the discontinuation of outpatient diabetes medications. This may result in preoperative hypoglycemia.** "Children with diabetes may be affected by volume depletion during preoperative fasting coupled with the discontinuation of outpatient diabetes medications. This may result in preoperative hypoglycemia" is a false statement.

6. **e. a, b, and c.** All of the listed options are true.

7. **e. b, c, and d.** Premature infants have a high risk of apnea, which can result in death. Premature infants have an increased risk of retinopathy and blindness in the presence of supplemental oxygen, so the overall goal is oxygen saturation percentage ranging in the low 90s. Neonates have a higher potential for large fluid losses due to higher rates of evaporation from skin and surgical wound sites, as well as decreased ability to concentrate urine.

8. **b. Children with chronic kidney disease (CKD) have an increased potential for anemia due to decreases in the renal production of erythropoietin and increases in urea, which decreases red blood cell production.**

9. **e. All of the above.** All of the listed options are true.

10. **e. All of the above.** All of the listed options are true.

11. **e. All of the above.** All of the listed options are true.

12. **e. All of the above.** All of the listed options are true.

13. **e. All of the above.** All of the listed options are true.

14. **d. If malignant hyperthermia is suspected, the triggering agent should be stopped, anesthesia backup should be requested, anesthesia machine should be exchanged, and an arterial line should be placed, as well as a Foley catheter.**

15. **e. b, and d.** Most postoperative cardiac events in children are preventable. Patients with high preoperative anxiety are at increased risk of postoperative emergence delirium.

CHAPTER REVIEW

1. Families should be informed of current FDA recommendations including what is known and what studies are currently underway to allow thoroughly informed consent.

2. Anesthesia risks include nausea, vomiting, bronchospasm, laryngospasm, stridor, emergence delirium, and postanesthesia maladaptive behaviors.

3. NPO violation significantly increases risk of gastric aspiration and pneumonitis.

4. Premature infants have a significantly increased risk of perioperative complications.

5. Spina bifida patients have the potential for multiple comorbidities that should be considered perioperatively.

6. Autonomic dysreflexia is life threatening, and the pediatric urologist should know signs and symptoms of onset.

7. Antibiotics are the mainstay of sepsis treatment and should be administered as soon as possible. Cultures should be obtained if possible.

8. Urine cultures should be obtained preoperatively when indicated and positive cultures treated with antibiotics based on sensitivities.

9. Antibiotics are the mainstay to prevent surgical site infections. Selection of antimicrobial should consider the site and potential source of infection.

10. Pain management is important to discuss with anesthesia for intraoperative and postoperative management.

11. Perioperative complications most often occur in the immediate postoperative period.

12. Postoperative pain control is important for optimal surgical outcomes. A multimodal drug approach is recommended.

13. Proper administration and disposal of unused narcotics are necessary to prevent overdoses with these medications.

27 Principles of Laparoscopic and Robotic Surgery in Children

Thomas Sean Lendvay and Jonathan Ellison

QUESTIONS

1. Which of the following is *true* regarding cosmetic benefits of minimally invasive surgery in children?
   a. Incisional scars will contract over time as the children grow longitudinally.
   b. Parents have no preference toward clinical outcomes (success and complications) over cosmetic appears of incisions when weighing open versus minimally invasive approach.
   c. Size of the incisions are not as important as location of the incision as it relates to cosmetic outcomes.
   d. Cosmetic benefits of single-port laparoendoscopic surgery are durable over several years.
   e. No validated questionnaires exist to assess bother as related to incisional scarring following surgical interventions.

2. Which of the following procedures has not been shown to have a length of stay benefit for minimally invasive approaches as compared with the open surgical counterpart?
   a. Pyeloplasty
   b. Ureteral reimplant
   c. Hernia/hydrocele
   d. Appendicovesicostomy
   e. Augmentation enterocystoplasty

3. Which of the following is false regarding cardiovascular implications of pneumoperitoneum?
   a. Bradycardia may be seen upon insufflation.
   b. Tachyarrhythmia may be seen secondary to a sympathetic response of pneumoperitoneum.
   c. Cardiac index is decreased at insufflation pressures as low as 10 mm Hg.
   d. Left ventricular ejection fraction does not appear to be impacted by pneumoperitoneal changes, although myocardial workload may increase.
   e. Mortality is no different in laparoscopic approaches for children with congenital cardiac defects as compared with healthy children, despite the cardiovascular implications of pneumoperitoneum.

4. With pneumoperitoneum, which of the following physiological changes is incorrectly described?
   a. Increase in end-tidal CO_2
   b. Increase in dynamic pulmonary compliance
   c. Increase in systemic vascular resistance
   d. Increase in intracranial pressure
   e. Decrease in urine output

5. Which of the following statements appropriately reflects the impact of the pneumoperitoneum on the immune response?
   a. Polymorphonuclear cells and macrophages, as well as levels of interleukin-6 (IL-6), are increased locally due to the effect of pneumoperitoneum across the entire abdominal wall, as compared with open surgery.
   b. Pediatric patients have a greater degree of benefit toward a blunted immune response following laparoscopy as compared with adult patients.

   c. Peritoneal signs following laparoscopy are heightened as compared with open surgery, likely owing to the local acidotic environment following CO_2 insufflation.
   d. Systemic C-reactive protein (CRP) and IL-6 levels are decreased following laparoscopy as compared with open surgery.
   e. Insufflation with room air results in a lessened inflammatory response as compared with CO_2 gas.

6. Which of the following is/are an absolute contraindication to minimally invasive surgery?
   a. Size less than 4 kg
   b. Inability to tolerate pneumoperitoneum
   c. Age less than 3 months
   d. Prior abdominal surgery
   e. a and c

7. Which of the following is true regarding peritoneal access via the umbilicus?
   a. A fascial hernia is rarely identified.
   b. Due to the fascial support at the umbilicus, a port site in this location does not usually require closure.
   c. The umbilicus is a reliable indicator of the location of the aortic bifurcation, which will lie superior to the umbilicus.
   d. Trendelenburg positioning does not alter the relation between the umbilicus and the aortic bifurcation.
   e. None of the above.

8. A comparison of open and Veress access techniques has revealed:
   a. an increased risk of visceral injury with open access.
   b. an increased risk of vascular injury with Veress access.
   c. an increased risk of failed access with Veress access.
   d. an increased risk of failed access with open access.
   e. an increased risk of port site hernia with open access.

9. Port site hernias in children:
   a. have not been reported in trocar sites smaller than 5 mm.
   b. may present with lethargy and a bulge in the absence of peritoneal signs.
   c. are at an increased risk at the umbilical site.
   d. are a lower risk complication after robotic-assisted procedures.
   e. b and c.

10. The blood vessel most likely injured by Veress needle access at the umbilicus, as shown in Fig. 27.1, is:
    a. left common iliac vein.
    b. right common iliac vein.
    c. right common iliac artery.
    d. vena cava.
    e. aorta.

11. Pulmonary air embolus:
    a. may be prevented by using CO_2 insufflation.
    b. is a common complication with rare catastrophic outcome.

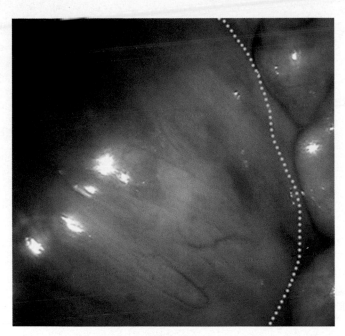

Fig. 27.1

   c. may present with increased or decreased end-tidal CO_2.

   d. likely results from direct absorption of insufflation gas via the peritoneum.

   e. can be managed best by repositioning the patient prone.

12. All of the following factors are aid in training of minimally invasive surgeons EXCEPT:

   a. training standardization across centers.

   b. standardized assessments of robotic and laparoscopic surgical skills.

   c. certified curriculum for surgical training.

   d. well-validated low- and high-fidelity simulation.

   e. use of surgical "warm-up."

ANSWERS

1. **c. Size of the incisions are not as important as location of the incision as it relates to cosmetic outcomes.** Validated instruments to assess scar both do exist and have been used to show that families show preference over location of scar (i.e., prefer more inconspicuous positions), as well as that the benefits cosmetically from a single-site incisional approach are not significantly better than standard laparoscopic approaches after 18 months of follow-up. Families would prefer optimal clinical outcomes to cosmetic appearance, although if equal, families would choose a minimally invasive approach for their child.

2. **c. Hernia/hydrocele.** Although a combination of prospective observational trials, randomized controlled trials, and retrospective cohort analyses have shown length of stay benefits for minimally invasive pyeloplasty, ureteral reimplantation, appendicovesicostomy, and augmentation enterocystoplasty, no such data exist showing benefit for hernia/hydrocele repairs. In fact, pain scores may be higher following laparoscopic hernia/hydrocele repairs as compared with open inguinal incisions, potentially due to the stress of pneumoperitoneum. Thus the benefit of convalescence and postoperative pain from a minimally invasive approach is likely proportional to the burden of the alternative open approach.

3. **e. Mortality is no different in laparoscopic approaches for children with congenital cardiac defects as compared with healthy children, despite the cardiovascular implications of pneumoperitoneum.** Vagal nerve stimulation can result in initial bradycardia, which may be managed with atropine

or glycopyrrolate but is typically self-limited. Cardiac index decreases with pneumoperitoneum greater than 10 mm Hg, likely due in part to increased intraabdominal and intrathoracic pressure on the venous return. This may result in an increased work of the myocardium as a compensatory response, which is why the left ventricular ejection fraction remains stable in spite of the cardiovascular changes. However, mortality is increased for children with congenital cardiac defects undergoing laparoscopic procedures as compared with healthy children, indicating a need for close hemodynamic monitoring and consideration of a specialized cardiac anesthesia team for these procedures.

4. **b. Increase in dynamic pulmonary compliance.** End-tidal CO_2 will increase from both an increased absorption of insufflated CO_2 gas and a decrease in minute ventilation from upward pressure on the diaphragm. Systemic vascular resistance increases, which drives a sympathetic response. Both of these changes likely contribute to a decrease in glomerular filtration rate and thus a decrease in urine output. Intracranial pressure also increases, although in most cases not to a clinically relevant degree. Dynamic pulmonary compliance will decrease, likely secondary to upward mobilization of the diaphragm and a decrease in the overall tidal volumes; often these changes necessitate ventilator manipulations to maintain appropriate ventilation.

5. **d. Systemic C-reactive protein (CRP) and IL-6 levels are decreased following laparoscopy as compared with open surgery.** Systemic and local inflammatory responses are blunted with insufflation, a result that appears to be in part due to the use of CO_2 gas, which elicits a lessened immune response as compared with insufflation with room air or open surgery. This blunted immune response results in lower pain and fatigue levels postoperatively but also may blunt peritoneal signs in the event of a visceral injury. Thus the surgeon must have a high index of suspicion for visceral injury in the absence of an acute abdomen, if the child otherwise appears ill.

6. **b. Inability to tolerate pneumoperitoneum.** Inability to tolerate pneumoperitoneum and inability of the surgeon to perform the procedure in a minimally invasive fashion are the only two absolute contraindications to a minimally invasive approach in children. Children less than a week of age have safely undergone robotic and laparoscopic-assisted procedures in experienced hands. Although prior abdominal operations may increase the risk for conversion to open surgery, these patients may also experience a differential benefit to a minimally invasive approach if performed successfully.

7. **e. None of the above.** Fascial openings are commonly observed in children and even found in up to 25% of adults at the umbilicus. However, the variance of the fascial support necessitates closure of the umbilical port sites in children. The umbilicus is a poor indicator of the location of the aortic bifurcation, which may fall inferior to the umbilicus in up to 40% of patients, a proportion that may even increase should the patient be placed in Trendelenburg position. The implication of this fact is that the surgeon should take care in blind trocar placement at the umbilicus as major vascular structures including the aorta and vena cava are at risk of injury in that approach.

8. **c. An increased risk of failed access with Veress access.** Major complications with access are rare regardless of technique chosen. Thus no difference is observed in major vascular or visceral injury with either open or Veress access technique. However, Veress access does appear to be associated with a higher risk for access failure as compared with the open technique. Port site hernia risk has not been formally assessed in most studies.

9. **b. May present with lethargy and a bulge in the absence of peritoneal signs.** Port site herniation of omentum has been reported in a 3-mm port site, indicating the importance of closure of all laparoscopic and robotic ports in children. Unlike adults, there does not appear to be a protective location for port site hernia comparing midline, umbilical, and lateral port site location. The blunted inflammatory response post-pneumoperitoneum can mute peritoneal signs even when a port site herniation poses risk of compromise to incarcerated intestine.

10. **a. Left common iliac vein.** This photo represents a retroperitoneal hematoma from venous injury, the dotted line representing the extent of the hematoma bulge. Although the umbilicus is a poor marker of the aortic bifurcation, most commonly the left common iliac vein is found as the most superior blood vessel in this location, crossing over the iliac artery. Recognition of a vascular injury at the time of Veress access is imperative as dilation with a trocar in this situation could result in life-threatening hemorrhage.

11. **c. May present with increased or decreased end-tidal (CO_2)** Although traditionally described as presenting with an increase in end-tidal CO_2, vascular collapse with either increased or decreased end-tidal CO_2 at the onset of insufflation should prompt concern for a pulmonary air embolus. This rare but life-threatening event may be managed by placing the patient in the left lateral decubitus position, thereby encour

aging migration of the air embolus out of the right pulmonary vein back into the right atrium. Up to 10% of insufflated gas initially may be nitrogen or oxygen, even when using CO_2 insufflation, emanating from the insufflation tubing. Thus flushing the tubing is recommended, especially in infants where the volume of ventilator dead space might be quite low.

12. **a. Training standardization across centers.** Although a certified training curriculum (Fundamentals in Laparoscopic Surgery) exists and is commonly applied across general surgery training sites, there is not a standardized laparoscopic or robotic curriculum for urologic surgeons. However, standardized assessments, a combination of low- and high-fidelity surgical simulators, and surgical warm-ups are all tools that can aid in training the newest generation of minimally invasive urologic surgeons, as well as maintaining expertise and skill in those already practicing.

CHAPTER REVIEW

1. A diminished postoperative inflammatory response may result in postoperative complications such as visceral injury presenting without peritoneal signs.

2. Because of the risk of herniation, closure of all port sites in the pediatric population following minimally invasive surgery is recommended.

3. Infants pose anatomic and physiologic challenges such as limited working space, a pliable abdominal wall, and cardiopulmonary changes with insufflation.

4. Benefits of smaller laparoscopic instrumentation must be weighed against potential limited versatility of the smallest instruments currently on the market.

5. Novel instrumentation, robotic technology, and augmented intelligence will continue to further the efficiency and safety of minimally invasive surgery.

6. Surgeon simulation, standardized evaluation and feedback, and warm-up preparation before surgery may all play a role in enhancing a surgeon's preparedness for minimally invasive surgery.

28

Clinical and Urodynamic Evaluation of Lower Urinary Tract Dysfunction in Children

Duncan T. Wilcox and Kyle O. Rove

QUESTIONS

1. Under what conditions is a uroflow reading valid and interpretable?
   a. Postvoid residual (PVR) < 100 mL
   b. Voided volume > 150 mL
   c. Voided volume > 50 mL
   d. Electromyography (EMG) lag time < 6 seconds
   e. Any voided volume if there is no PVR

2. What are the five reference uroflow curve types?
   a. Stuttering, bell shaped, peaked, plateau, intermittent
   b. Staccato, intermittent, bell shaped, plateau, tower
   c. Tower, peaked, stuttering, normal, flat
   d. Plateau, intermittent, high, normal, staccato
   e. Continuous staccato, bell shaped, normal, inverted

3. EMG lag time less than 2 seconds corresponds to what potential patient presentation?
   a. Normal voiding and bell-shaped uroflow curve
   b. Overactive bladder and tower uroflow curve
   c. Primary bladder neck dysfunction and plateau uroflow curve
   d. Underactive bladder and staccato uroflow curve
   e. Incontinence without PVR

4. What is a normal EMG lag time?
   a. <2 seconds
   b. 2 to 6 seconds
   c. >6 seconds
   d. 10 seconds
   e. >12 seconds

5. EMG lag time greater than 6 seconds typically corresponds to what potential patient presentation?
   a. Normal voider and bell-shaped uroflow curve
   b. Overactive bladder and tower uroflow curve
   c. Primary bladder neck dysfunction and plateau uroflow curve
   d. Underactive bladder and staccato uroflow curve
   e. Controlled (external sphincter) incontinence

6. Which are valid methods to define functional bladder capacity?
   a. Voided volume on uroflow + PVR
   b. (Age + 2) × 30 mL
   c. Smallest voided volume on voiding diary
   d. Largest voided volume on voiding diary
   e. a + d

7. What is the significance of debris visualized within the bladder or collecting system on ultrasound?
   a. This is a normal finding
   b. Concern for ureterocele
   c. Increased risk of symptomatic urinary tract infection
   d. Increased risk of positive urine culture regardless of symptoms
   e. Urothelial tumor

8. What test is recommended for all patients who present with lower urinary tract symptoms and no prior urologic diagnosis?
   a. Urinalysis
   b. Urodynamics
   c. Serum creatinine
   d. Uroflow
   e. Renal bladder ultrasound

9. Which cutaneous finding over the sacral spine on exam is at highest risk for diagnosis of occult spinal dysraphism (tethered cord)?
   a. Cutaneous dimple less than 2.5 cm from anus
   b. Hemangioma
   c. Dermal sinus tract
   d. Symmetric bifid gluteal cleft
   e. hypertrichosis

10. What imaging modality is the gold standard for diagnosing spinal dysraphism?
    a. Computed tomography (CT) scan
    b. Ultrasound
    c. Positron emission tomography (PET) scan
    d. Magnetic resonance imaging (MRI)
    e. Videourodynamics

11. Under which conditions would it be appropriate to consider ultrasound of the spine to rule out spinal dysraphism?
    a. Newborn with open myelomeningocele
    b. 6-month-old with deviated gluteal cleft
    c. 3-year-old with gait problems and secondary enuresis
    d. Healthy 12-month-old with normal exam and cutaneous dimple 2 cm from the anal verge
    e. Family history of a tethered cord

12. What test/treatment is recommended in patients with lower urinary tract dysfunction who fail first-line, conservative therapies (e.g., behavioral modification, timed voiding, avoidance of bladder irritants)?

a. 7-day bowel and bladder diary or 48-hour frequency-volume chart

b. Formal videourodynamics

c. Treatment with antimuscarinics

d. Treatment with α-blocker

e. Intradetrusor injection of botulinum toxin

13. Lower urinary tract dysfunction is associated with which of the following?

a. Constipation

b. Neuropsychiatric issues

c. Urinary tract infections

d. Vesicoureteral reflux

e. All of the above

14. What is an appropriate fill rate on cystometrogram for a pediatric patient?

a. 5 mL/min

b. 10 mL/min

c. 15 mL/min

d. 20% of expected bladder capacity per minute

e. 5% to 10% of expected bladder capacity per minute

15. What finding(s) may be reduced on urodynamics when performed under sedation?

a. Detrusor overactivity

b. Compliance

c. Detrusor leak point pressure

d. Bladder capacity

e. Internal sphincter control

ANSWERS

1. **c. Voided volume > 50 mL.** Uroflowmetry is affected by multiple parameters. However, the validity of a test is generally affected by voided volumes. For many studies of pediatric uroflowmetry, 50 mL is the cutoff for validity. In adults, a higher value is used (>150 mL). Ideally, a voided volume greater than 50 mL and less than 115% of expected bladder capacity generates the best results. Volumes greater than 115% of expected capacity may also produce uroflow results that are spurious or misleading.

2. **b. Staccato, intermittent, bell shaped, plateau, tower.** The Standardization Committee of the International Children's Continence Society published a list of terminology standardization in the Journal of Urology in 2014. This important document lists common terms used to describe voiding dysfunction and the requisite testing performed on these patients.

3. **b. Overactive bladder and tower uroflow curve.** EMG lag times of 2 to 6 seconds are considered normal. Times less than 2 seconds are prevalent in patients with overactive bladder. Times greater than 6 seconds indicate primary bladder neck dysfunction.

4. **b. 2 to 6 seconds.** EMG lag times of 2 to 6 seconds are considered normal and associated with a bell-shaped voiding curve. Times less than 2 seconds are prevalent in patients with overactive bladder. Times greater than 6 seconds indicate primary bladder neck dysfunction.

5. **c. Primary bladder neck dysfunction and plateau uroflow curve.** EMG lag times of 2 to 6 seconds are considered normal. Times less than 2 seconds are seen with bladder hyperactivity. Times greater than 6 seconds indicate primary bladder neck dysfunction associated with a uroflow curve that plateaus or flattens after an initial rise.

6. **e. a + d.** Functional bladder capacity is a measure of day-to-day capacity of a patient's bladder. This number should reflect how much a particular patient's bladder holds when full. This is reflected by both (a) voided volume on uroflow + PVR and (d) smallest voided volume on voiding diary. (b) corresponds to the patient's estimated bladder capacity (if older than 1 year). (d) does not reflect any clinically useful measure of the bladder.

7. **d. Increased risk of positive urine culture regardless of symptoms.** Studies looking at the association of debris on ultrasound have shown increased association with positive culture. These findings should be interpreted with caution in asymptomatic patients.

8. **a. Urinalysis.** American Urological Association (AUA) guidelines for work-up of lower urinary tract symptoms recommend a urinalysis to rule out the presence of a urinary tract infection. None of the other options are recommended for initial testing in new patients seen for lower urinary tract symptoms.

9. **b. Hemangioma.** The risk of occult spinal dysraphism is different for each of the listed lesions. From lowest risk to highest, they are: simple cutaneous dimple, symmetric bifid gluteal, hypertrichosis (hair tuft), dermal sinus tract, and hemangioma.

10. **d. Magnetic resonance imaging (MRI).** MRI is the most sensitive and specific test to rule out any form of spinal dysraphism. Spinal ultrasound can be used for neonates up to age 6 months in whom there is suspicion for dysraphic conditions, but this imaging modality has lower sensitivity. There is no role for CT or PET scans or videourodynamics for the diagnosis of possible dysraphism.

11. **b. 6-month-old with deviated gluteal cleft.** There is debate between use of ultrasound and MRI to rule out spinal dysraphism. MRI is more sensitive but more expensive than ultrasound. For skin findings associated with spina bifida, lesions with low likelihood of diagnosis of spina bifida (like deviated gluteal cleft) may be more appropriate to use ultrasound if testing is being considered. Inconclusive or positive ultrasounds can then be followed up with an MRI to confirm the diagnosis.

12. **a. 7-day bowel and bladder diary or 48-hour frequency-volume chart.** Elimination diaries can pinpoint a number of issues that may not be elicited during a clinical encounter, including low functional capacity, infrequent voiding, nocturia, and polydipsia. This should be used prior to more invasive evaluation or treatment.

13. **e. All of the above.** Constipation, neuropsychiatric issues, urinary tract infections, and vesicoureteral reflux are commonly associated with lower urinary tract dysfunction.

14. **e. 5% to 10% of expected bladder capacity per minute.** Pediatric patients have varied bladder capacities, so fill rates relative to expected bladder capacity should be considered. As such, absolute fill rates (e.g., 20 mL/min) might be too fast for a neonate with a bladder capacity of 80 mL. The recommended fill rate is 5% to 10% of expected capacity per minute.

15. **a. Destrusor overactivity.** Studies have demonstrated that the only parameter reliably affected by sedation or anesthesia is detrusor overactivity. That is, if it were present normally, it would not be present on a sedated urodynamics study. Compliance, detrusor leak point pressure (dLPP), and bladder capacity are not generally affected.

CHAPTER REVIEW

1. History and physical should be performed to ascertain whether the patient has primarily a storage or emptying disorder. Further workup and treatment are then tailored as needed.

2. The important components of a complete history should include symptomatology, voiding frequency, bowel function, prior urinary tract infections, relevant family history, maternal prenatal history including screening ultrasonography, birth history, developmental milestones including toilet training, neuropsychiatric conditions, past medical and surgical history, social history, diet, and review of systems.

3. Seven-day bowel and bladder diaries and 48-hour frequency volume charts are invaluable in diagnosing simple and complex lower urinary tract voiding dysfunction.

4. Validated questionnaires can be used to assess symptoms (dysfunctional voiding score system [DVSS], dysfunctional voiding and incontinence score system [DVISS], and incontinence symptom index-pediatric [ISI-P]), quality of life (Pediatric Incontinence Questionnaire [PinQ]), and behavioral changes in response to underlying urinary dysfunction (Child Behavior Checklist [CBCL] and short screening instrument for psychological problems in enuresis [SSIPPE]).

5. Particular attention should be paid to the lower back on physical examination with both visual inspection (examine for dimples, deviations of the gluteal cleft, hair tufts, dermal sinuses and vascular malformations) and palpation (presence of sacrum, rule out mass).

6. Children presenting with lower urinary tract symptoms should have urinalysis testing, with important test details including the specific gravity, protein or glucose, and the presence of white, red blood cells, or bacteria.

7. Isolated malodorous urine in the general population lacks sensitivity and specificity to detect positive urine culture in an otherwise asymptomatic patient.

8. Blood testing is not recommended unless there are specific concerns for concomitant upper tract disease.

9. Noninvasive urodynamics includes modalities like uroflowmetry, patch electromyography, and pelvic ultrasound.

10. Uroflowmetry provides useful information regarding flow characteristics during urination, including shape or pattern. Qmax is the most relevant quantitative variable when assessing bladder outflow.

11. Ultrasonography is another useful adjunct, noninvasive exam that can provide a number of different clinically important variables, including prevoid and postvoid bladder volumes to calculated a PVR, bladder wall thickness, rectal diameter, and presence of debris.

12. EMG provides for assessing coordination between the bladder and external sphincter to determine whether voiding is synergistic or dyssynergic and can also be used in conjunction with uroflowmetry to determine the lag time.

13. Urodynamics is the "gold standard" for evaluation and diagnosis of lower urinary tract dysfunction.

14. Universal strategies of antibiotic prophylaxis or urine cultures prior to urodynamics do not appear to be effective at preventing postprocedure urinary tract infection, which occurs 1.4% of the time.

15. Special considerations in pediatric urodynamics include use of sedation for catheter placement and/or the procedure itself and bladder fill rate, accounting for the varied expected bladder capacities across a wide range of patient ages and sizes.

29 Management Strategies for Vesicoureteral Reflux

Antoine E. Khoury and Elias Wehbi

QUESTIONS

1. The estimated prevalence of vesicoureteral reflux (VUR) in children with a urinary tract infection (UTI) is:
   a. 1%.
   b. 3%.
   c. 5%.
   d. 10%.
   e. 30%.

2. Which of the following statements regarding reflux is FALSE?
   a. Antenatally detected reflux is associated with a male preponderance.
   b. Antenatally detected reflux is usually low grade in boys as compared with that in girls.
   c. Antenatally detected reflux is usually bilateral in boys as compared with that in girls.
   d. When reflux is detected antenatally, renal impairment is frequently present at birth and is likely due to congenital dysplasia.
   e. The majority of reflux detected later in life occurs in females.

3. Which of the following statements regarding VUR in regard to the patient's race is TRUE?
   a. The incidence of VUR is equal in children of all races.
   b. The disparity in the incidence of VUR with respect to race becomes clearer in adulthood.
   c. The frequency of detected VUR is lower in female children of African descent.
   d. African and white infants have a similar incidence of reflux diagnosed on the basis of antenatal hydronephrosis.
   e. There is a clear understanding regarding the predisposition to reflux because many of the studies have included patients from different countries around the world.

4. Which of the following statements is FALSE in regard to the diagnosis and treatment of sibling VUR?
   a. On the basis of clinical judgment and the presence or absence of urinary tract infection (UTI), the patient's age should be taken into account in regard to the decision to proceed with intervention to diagnose sibling reflux.
   b. It is reasonable to prescribe antibiotic prophylaxis while the decision to diagnose sibling reflux is being made.
   c. Once sibling reflux has been diagnosed, the indications for correction differ from those for treating reflux in the general pediatric population diagnosed after UTI.
   d. Siblings who are younger than 5 years with normal imaging studies of the kidneys can be managed on the basis of clinical judgment, and it is not absolutely necessary to obtain a voiding cystogram.
   e. Siblings younger than 5 years who present with cortical renal defects have the most to lose by febrile UTIs in the presence of VUR.

5. Primary reflux is a congenital anomaly of the ureterovesical junction with a deficiency of the
   a. longitudinal muscle of the extravesical ureter, which results in an inadequate valvular mechanism.
   b. longitudinal muscle of the intravesical ureter, which results in an inadequate valvular mechanism.
   c. circumferential muscle of the extravesical ureter, which results in an inadequate valvular mechanism.
   d. circumferential muscle of the intravesical ureter, which results in an inadequate valvular mechanism.
   e. longitudinal and circumferential muscles of the intravesical ureter, which results in an inadequate valvular mechanism.

6. What is the accepted ratio of tunnel length to ureteral diameter found in most normal children without reflux?
   a. 5:1
   b. 4:1
   c. 3:1
   d. 2:1
   e. 1:1

7. Which of the following statements is TRUE regarding children with nonneurogenic neurogenic bladders?
   a. Constriction of the urinary sphincter occurs during voiding in a voluntary form of detrusor-sphincter dyssynergia.
   b. Gradual bladder decompensation and myogenic failure result from incomplete emptying.
   c. Gradual bladder decompensation and myogenic failure result from increasing amounts of residual urine.
   d. All of the above.
   e. None of the above.

8. Which of the following statements is TRUE in regard to secondary VUR?
   a. The most common cause of anatomic bladder obstruction in the pediatric population is posterior urethral valves, and VUR is present in a great majority of these children.
   b. Anatomic obstruction of the bladder is a common cause of secondary VUR in female patients.
   c. Patients with neurofunctional etiology for secondary VUR benefit from immediate surgical intervention to try to correct VUR.
   d. A sacral dimple or hairy patch on the lower back is not a significant finding in regard to the evaluation and treatment of VUR.
   e. The most common structural obstruction in male and female patients is the presence of a ureterocele at the bladder neck.

9. The complex anatomic relationships required of the ureterovesical junction may gradually be damaged by
   a. a decrease in bladder wall compliance.
   b. detrusor decompensation.
   c. incomplete emptying.
   d. subureteric injection of a bulking agent.
   e. a, b, and c.

10. What does the initial management of functional causes of reflux involve?
    a. Transurethral cystoscopic treatment
    b. Medical treatment
    c. Observation only
    d. Laparoscopic repair
    e. Videourodynamics

11. Signs or symptoms of bladder dysfunction include
    a. dribbling.
    b. urgency.
    c. incontinence.
    d. "curtsying" behavior in girls.
    e. all of the above.

12. Treatment of bladder dysfunction and detrusor overactivity regardless of its severity or cause is directed at:
    a. dampening overactive detrusor contractions.
    b. dilating the urethral sphincter.
    c. lowering intravesical pressures.
    d. a and c.
    e. all of the above.

13. There is a strong association between the presence of reflux in patients with neuropathic bladders and intravesical pressures of greater than:
    a. 10 cm H_2O.
    b. 20 cm H_2O.
    c. 40 cm H_2O.
    d. 60 cm H_2O.
    e. 80 cm H_2O.

14. Bladder infections and their accompanying inflammation can also cause reflux by:
    a. lessening compliance.
    b. elevating intravesical pressures.
    c. distorting and weakening the ureterovesical junction.
    d. all of the above.
    e. none of the above.

15. Which system provides the current standard for grading reflux on the basis of the appearance of contrast in the ureter and upper collecting system during voiding cystourethrography?
    a. The Heikel and Parkkulainen system
    b. The International Classification system
    c. The Dwoskin and Perlmutter system
    d. The National Classification System
    e. The Dwoskin and Parkkulainen system

16. Which of the following is TRUE regarding accurately grading reflux with coexistent obstruction of the ipsilateral ureteropelvic junction (UPJ)?
    a. It is not possible.
    b. It is facilitated by obtaining a mercaptoacetyltriglycine (MAG3) lasix renal scan.
    c. It is facilitated by obtaining a renal bladder ultrasound.
    d. It is facilitated by obtaining a magnetic resonance urogram.
    e. It is facilitated by obtaining a radionuclide cystogram.

17. Which of the following is TRUE regarding the presence of fever?
    a. It represents eventual renal scarring.
    b. It correlates with greater than 100,000 bacterial colony-forming units.

    c. It may not always be a reliable sign of upper urinary tract involvement.
    d. It increases the likelihood of discovering VUR.
    e. c and d.

18. Complete evaluation including a voiding cystourethrogram (VCUG) and ultrasound are required for which of the following patients?
    a. An uncircumcised male infant with a febrile illness and a positive urine culture obtained through a bagged specimen
    b. A 3-year-old girl admitted to the hospital with pneumonia and found to have *Escherichia coli* on a urine culture without pyuria detected by microscopic analysis
    c. A female patient with recurrent culture and urinalysis proven to have afebrile UTIs and later found to have scarring on a dimercaptosuccinic acid (DMSA) scan
    d. Any child older than 5 years with documented UTIs
    e. None of the above

19. Which of the following is required for screening of older girls who present with asymptomatic bacteriuria?
    a. Renal bladder ultrasound
    b. VCUG
    c. VUDS
    d. DMSA renal scan
    e. No screening studies are required

20. Which of the following is TRUE regarding cystography?
    a. Cystography performed with a Foley catheter or while the patient is under anesthesia produces static studies that inaccurately screen for reflux or sometimes exaggerate its degree because of bladder overfilling.
    b. Cystography performed in the presence of excessive hydration may mask low grades of reflux because diuresis can blunt the retrograde flow of urine.
    c. Cystography may show reflux only during active infection when cystitis weakens the ureterovesical junction with edema or by increasing intravesical pressures.
    d. Cystography obtained during active infection will underestimate the grade of reflux because the endotoxins produced by some gram-negative organisms can paralyze ureteral smooth muscle.
    e. a, b, and c.

21. Radionuclide cystography:
    a. provides similar anatomic detail to that obtained with fluoroscopic cystography.
    b. is an accurate method for detecting and following reflux.
    c. is associated with more radiation exposure than is fluoroscopic cystography.
    d. is a less sensitive test than fluoroscopic cystography.
    e. provides more anatomic detail than fluoroscopic cystography.

22. Ultrasonography of the kidneys and bladder:
    a. is the diagnostic study of choice to initially evaluate the upper urinary tracts of patients with suspected or proven VUR.
    b. can effectively rule out reflux.
    c. should be performed every 2 to 3 years in patients with reflux who are medically managed.
    d. is the study of choice for assessing renal function.
    e. showing intermittent dilatation of the renal pelvis or ureter confirms the presence of reflux.

23. What is the best study for the detection of pyelonephritis and cortical renal scarring?
    a. Diethylenetriaminepentaacetic acid (DTPA) renal scan
    b. DMSA renal scan
    c. MAG3 renal scan
    d. computed tomography (CT) urogram
    e. Renal ultrasound

24. Which of the following is TRUE regarding urodynamic studies?
    a. They may be indicated in any child suspected of having a secondary cause for reflux (valves, neurogenic bladder, non-neurogenic neurogenic bladder, voiding dysfunction).
    b. They should be performed without the use of prophylactic antibiotics in children with secondary reflux.
    c. They help to direct therapy in patients with secondary reflux.
    d. They are more accurate when performed under sedation.
    e. a and c.

25. Which of the following is TRUE in regard to the evaluation of VUR?
    a. Routine cystoscopy is indicated in the workup of patients with VUR.
    b. The radiation doses with modern digital techniques have improved the anatomic detail, but the radiation dose with VCUG remains significantly higher than that of a radionuclide cystogram.
    c. Grading of reflux by VCUG and radionuclide cystography is similar and comparable between the two imaging modalities.
    d. Ultrasonography provides an alternative means of evaluating the presence or absence of VUR.
    e. Uroflowmetry is a valuable tool in the workup of a patient with VUR.

26. During ureteral development, a ureteral bud that:
    a. is medially (caudally) positioned from a normal takeoff at the trigone offers an embryologic explanation for primary reflux.
    b. is laterally (cranially) positioned from a normal takeoff at the trigone offers an embryologic explanation for primary reflux.
    c. fails to meet with the renal blastema offers an embryologic explanation for primary reflux.
    d. is laterally (cranially) positioned is often obstructed.
    e. fails to meet with the renal blastema is often obstructed.

27. In regard to the diagnosis of renal scars based on renal scintigraphy, which of the following is TRUE?
    a. An area of photopenia detected during an acute episode of pyelonephritis always represents renal scar.
    b. Photopenic areas may result from postinfection renal scarring and some renal dysplasia.
    c. Ultrasound is a sensitive and accurate diagnostic modality for renal scarring.
    d. Areas for photopenia detected during an acute episode of pyelonephritis that later resolve on a subsequent renal scan represent resolution of renal scarring.
    e. All of the above.

28. Which of the following is TRUE regarding hypertension?
    a. In children and young adults, it is most commonly caused by reflux nephropathy.
    b. It is not related to the grade of reflux or severity of scarring.
    c. It is not associated with abnormalities of Na⁺,K⁺-ATPase activity.

    d. All of the above.
    e. None of the above.

29. Which of the following factors might contribute to the effects of reflux on renal growth?
    a. The congenital dysmorphism often associated with but not caused by reflux
    b. The number and type of urinary infections and their resultant nephropathy
    c. The quality of the contralateral kidney and its implications for compensatory hypertrophy
    d. The grade of reflux in the affected kidney
    e. All of the above

30. Which of the following statements is FALSE in regard to bladder and bowel dysfunction (BBD) and VUR?
    a. BBD lowers VUR resolution rates.
    b. BBD is associated with higher recurrence rates of VUR after successful endoscopic correction.
    c. BBD reduces the success rate of endoscopic implantation of dextranomer/hyaluronic copolymer (Dx/HA) and open surgical correction of VUR.
    d. BBD is associated with higher breakthrough infection rates.
    e. BBD is associated with an increased incidence of UTI after surgery.

31. The anatomy of patients with ureteral duplication typically follows the Weigert-Meyer rule, in which the upper pole ureter enters the bladder:
    a. distally and medially, and the lower pole ureter enters the bladder proximally and laterally.
    b. proximally and medially, and the lower pole ureter enters the bladder distally and laterally.
    c. distally and laterally, and the lower pole ureter enters the bladder proximally and medially.
    d. proximally and laterally, and the lower pole ureter enters the bladder distally and medially.
    e. superior to the lower pole ureter.

32. Which of the following is not found to be associated with higher success rate of endoscopic correction of VUR?
    a. Volume of bulking agent used
    b. Surgeon experience
    c. Volcano-shaped mound with no hydrodistention
    d. Negative intraoperative cystography
    e. Utilization of the double hydrodistention-implantation technique

33. Which of the following accurately describes the state of the bladder during pregnancy?
    a. Urine volume decreases in the upper collecting system while the physiologic dilatation of pregnancy evolves.
    b. Bladder tone increases because of edema and hyperemia.
    c. Bladder changes predispose the patient to bacteriuria.
    d. All of the above.
    e. None of the above.

34. During pregnancy, the presence of VUR in a system already prone to bacteriuria may lead to increased morbidity. What is an additional risk factor?
    a. Renal scarring
    b. Tendency toward urinary infections
    c. Hypertension
    d. Renal insufficiency
    e. All of the above

35. Which of the following statements is considered to be FALSE regarding reflux management?

    a. Spontaneous resolution of VUR is common.

    b. High-grade VUR has a higher resolution rate when diagnosed in the newborn as compared with diagnosis in childhood.

    c. Reflux of sterile urine is a benign process that does not lead to significant renal damage.

    d. The 2014 *New England Journal of Medicine* Randomized Intervention for Children with Vesicoureteral Reflux (RIVUR) study reported a 0.5% incidence of adverse reaction to prophylactic antibiotics and a 2% incidence of adverse reaction to the placebo.

    e. Reflux cannot be accurately graded in patients with posterior urethral valves.

36. Common to each type of open surgical repair for reflux is the creation of:

    a. a valvular mechanism that enables ureteral compression with bladder filling and contraction.

    b. a mucosal tunnel for reimplantation having adequate muscular backing.

    c. a tunnel length of three times the ureteral diameter.

    d. a ureteral orifice aimed toward the trigone/bladder neck.

    e. all of the above.

37. Complete ureteral duplications with reflux can be best managed surgically by:

    a. separating the ureters and reimplanting them separately.

    b. a common sheath repair in which both ureters are mobilized with one mucosal cuff.

    c. performing an upper to lower ureteroureterostomy and reimplanting the lower ureter.

    d. performing a lower to upper ureteroureterostomy and reimplanting the upper ureter.

    e. none of the above.

38. Early postoperative obstruction can occur after a ureteral reimplant due to:

    a. edema.

    b. subtrigonal bleeding.

    c. a twist or angulation of the ureter.

    d. blood clots.

    e. all of the above.

39. If early postoperative obstruction occurs after a ureteral reimplant, the next step is:

    a. immediate nephrostomy tube placement.

    b. immediate placement of a ureteral stent.

    c. initial observation and diversion for unabating symptoms.

    d. placement of both a nephrostomy tube and a ureteral stent.

    e. reoperation.

40. Which of the following is TRUE regarding persistent reflux after ureteral reimplantation?

    a. It may be due to unrecognized secondary causes of reflux such as neuropathic bladder and severe voiding dysfunction.

    b. It seldom results from a failure to provide adequate muscular backing for the ureter within its tunnel.

    c. It may be repaired surgically by using minor submucosal advancements.

    d. It should be repaired immediately with a subureteric bulking agent.

    e. None of the above.

41. Which of the following is TRUE regarding the treatment of VUR?

    a. Since the widespread acceptance of endoscopic treatment, the indications for surgical correction differ between the open endoscopic and laparoscopic approaches.

    b. Long-term follow-up data support the durability of endoscopic injection therapy.

    c. All injection materials provide a similar success rate and are just as easily injected under similar circumstances.

    d. The accuracy of the needle entry point during endoscopic injection as well as the needle placement are important components for the success of the surgical procedure.

    e. The learning curve for endoscopic injection is similar to the learning curve for open surgical reimplantation.

42. Which of the following is TRUE regarding the laparoscopic approach for ureteral reimplantation?

    a. The advantages of this approach versus open surgery include smaller incisions, less discomfort, and quicker convalescence.

    b. As with other laparoscopic procedures, experience is essential to the success of this approach.

    c. Costs may be increased because of lengthier surgery and the expense of disposable equipment.

    d. It is associated with a success rate higher than that of open surgery.

    e. a, b, and c.

43. After discontinuation of continuous antibiotic prophylaxis (CAP) in toilet-trained children, who is likely to develop recurrent UTI?

    a. Patients with higher grades of VUR

    b. Uncircumcised male children

    c. Children with BBD

    d. All of the above

    e. a and c only

44. Which patients were more likely to have febrile or symptomatic recurrences in the RIVUR trial?

    a. Children with grade III or IV reflux at baseline

    b. Patients presenting with febrile index infection

    c. The presence of BBD at baseline

    d. All of the above

    e. a and c only

45. The 2011 American Academy of Pediatrics guidelines for management of the initial UTI in febrile infants and children 2 to 24 months of age recommend obtaining:

    a. a renal and bladder ultrasound and a VCUG during the febrile episode.

    b. a renal and bladder ultrasound and a VCUG 3 weeks after the febrile episode has resolved.

    c. a DMSA renal scan and, if positive, a VCUG.

    d. a renal and bladder ultrasound after confirmation of UTI by a properly collected urine specimen for culture and analysis.

    e. waiting for the second infection before performing any radiological testing.

ANSWERS

1. **e. 30%.** A meta-analysis of studies of children undergoing cystography for various indications has indicated that the prevalence of VUR is estimated to be 30% for children with UTIs and approximately 17% in children without infection.

2. **b. Antenatally detected reflux is usually low grade in boys as compared with that in girls.** Reflux detected due to workup of antennal hydronephrosis is usually high grade and bilateral in boys as compared with that in girls.

3. **c. The frequency of detected VUR is lower in female children of African descent.** One of the clear differences that has been established with several studies is the relative 10-fold lower frequency of vesicoureteral reflux in female children of African descent.

4. **c. Once sibling reflux has been diagnosed, the indications for correction differ from those for treating reflux in the general pediatric population diagnosed after UTI.** If undertaken, imaging of the kidneys first, as well as the patient's age and history of UTI, can offer counsel with regard to the approach to sibling reflux screening. However, in any sibling in whom reflux is diagnosed, the indications for treatment remain the same as for general reflux in the pediatric population.

5. **b. Longitudinal muscle of the intravesical ureter, which results in an inadequate valvular mechanism.** Primary reflux is a congenital anomaly of the ureterovesical junction in which a deficiency of the longitudinal muscle of the intravesical ureter results in an inadequate valvular mechanism.

6. **a. 5:1.** In Paquin's novel study, a 5:1 tunnel length–ureteral diameter ratio was found in normal children without reflux.

7. **d. All of the above.** On the far end of this spectrum are children with nonneurogenic neurogenic bladders. Here, constriction of the urinary sphincter occurs during voiding in a voluntary form of detrusor-sphincter dyssynergia. Gradual bladder decompensation and myogenic failure result from incomplete emptying and increasing amounts of residual urine.

8. **a. The most common cause of anatomic bladder obstruction in the pediatric population is posterior urethral valves, and VUR is present in the great majority of these children.** This diagnosis is obviously limited to male patients; consequently female patients have a lower incidence of anatomic bladder obstruction. The most common structural obstruction in female patients is the presence of a ureterocele that prolapses and obstructs the bladder neck. Between 48% and 70% of patients with posterior urethral valves have vesicoureteral reflux, and relief of obstruction appears to be responsible for resolution of the reflux in a good number of those patients. The presence of a neurologic disorder should prompt the clinician to treat on the basis of the primary etiology as opposed to proceeding with immediate surgical correction. One important aspect of the physical examination in children who present with VUR is detection of potential occult spinal dysraphism, which includes a thorough physical examination looking for sacral dimples, hairy patches, or gluteal cleft abnormalities.

9. **e. a, b, and c.** A decrease in bladder wall compliance, detrusor decompensation, and incomplete emptying gradually damages the complex anatomic relationships required of the ureterovesical junction. Subureteric injection of various bulking materials has not been shown to compromise UVJ function.

10. **b. Medical treatment.** The initial management of functional causes of reflux is medical. It is imperative that clinicians inquire about and determine the voiding patterns of children with reflux.

11. **e. All of the above.** In addition to a careful physical examination, signs or symptoms of bladder dysfunction include dribbling, urgency, and incontinence. Girls often exhibit curtsying behavior and boys will squeeze the penis in an attempt to suppress bladder contractions.

12. **d. a and c only.** Treatment of bladder dysfunction and detrusor overactivity, regardless of its severity or cause, is directed at decreasing overactive detrusor contractions and lowering intravesical pressures. Urethral dilation does not have a role in the routine treatment of bladder dysfunction.

13. **c. 40 cm H_2O.** There is a strong association between intravesical pressures of greater than 40 cm H_2O and the presence of reflux in patients with myelodysplasia and neuropathic bladders, although upper tract damage can also be seen in lower bladder pressures.

14. **d. All of the above.** Bladder infections (UTIs) and their accompanying inflammation can also cause reflux by lessening compliance, elevating intravesical pressures, and distorting and weakening the ureterovesical junction.

15. **b. The International Classification System.** The Heikel and Parkkulainen system gained popularity in Europe a few years before the Dwoskin and Perlmutter system became widely accepted in the United States. The International Classification System, devised in 1981 by the International Reflux Study, represents a melding of the two. It provides the current standard for grading reflux on the basis of the appearance of contrast in the ureter and upper collecting system during voiding cystourethrography.

16. **a. It is not possible.** Accurate grading of reflux is impossible with coexistent ipsilateral obstruction.

17. **e. c and d.** The presence of fever may be an indicator of upper urinary tract involvement but is not always a reliable sign. However, if fever (and presumably pyelonephritis) is present, the likelihood of discovering VUR is significantly increased. Fever can be associated with less than 100,000 bacterial colonies. Fever and pyelonephritis does not always lead to renal scarring.

18. **c. A female patient with recurrent culture and urinalysis proven to have afebrile UTIs and later found to have scarring on a dimercaptosuccinic acid (DMSA) scan.** The presence of culture-proven UTIs in the setting of an abnormal renal scan should raise the question of VUR; it is reasonable to proceed with a VCUG and ultrasound in those patients. The other clinical scenarios include a patient without pyuria and a clear alternative source for her fever as well as an infant diagnosed with UTI with a specimen obtained through a bagged collection. In those children the diagnosis of UTI should be questioned before proceeding with evaluation through cystogram and renal ultrasonography. Patients older than 5 years should not undergo immediate VCUG just on the basis of the presence of a UTI.

19. **e. No screening studies are required.** Although a renal bladder ultrasound may be helpful in some cases, it is not required in all older children who present with asymptomatic bacteriuria or UTIs that manifest solely with lower tract symptoms (afebrile simple cystitis). Cystography is reserved for those with abnormal upper tracts or recalcitrant infections. The initial focus should be more on voiding and bowel habits and fluid intake.

20. **e. a, b, and c.** Excessive hydration may mask low grades of reflux because diuresis can blunt the retrograde flow of urine. Some reflux is demonstrated only during active infections when cystitis weakens the ureterovesical junction with edema or by increasing intravesical pressures. In addition, cystograms obtained during active infections can overestimate the grade of reflux because the endotoxins produced by some gram-negative organisms can paralyze ureteral smooth muscle and exaggerate ureteral dilatation.

21. **b. Is an accurate method for detecting and following reflux.** Nuclear cystography is the scintigraphic equivalent of conventional cystography. Although the technique does not provide the anatomic detail of fluoroscopic studies, it is an accurate method for detecting and following reflux.

22. **a. Is the diagnostic study of choice to initially evaluate the upper urinary tracts of patients with suspected or proven vesicoureteral reflux.** Ultrasonography is the diagnostic study of choice to initially evaluate the upper urinary tracts of

patients with suspected or proven VUR. However, the appearance of the kidneys on ultrasound does not correlate with the absence or presence of reflux or with its grade.

23. **b. DMSA renal scan.** Renal scintigraphy with technetium-99m–labeled DMSA is the best study for detection of pyelonephritis and the cortical renal scarring that sometimes results.

24. **e. a and c.** Urodynamic studies may be indicated in any child suspected of having a secondary cause for reflux (e.g., valves, neurogenic bladder, nonneurogenic neurogenic bladder, voiding dysfunction), and they help to direct therapy. Sedation or anesthesia may change bladder function.

25. **e. Uroflowmetry is a valuable tool in the workup of a patient with VUR.** Evaluation of the lower urinary tract cannot solely rely on imaging studies because reflux is considered to be a dynamic phenomenon. Uroflowmetry provides valuable information in the clinical assessment of these patients. Modern management of reflux does not include routine evaluation through cystoscopy. The radionuclide cystogram has historically been described as a technique that requires a significantly lower dose of radiation than a regular VCUG, but the advances with modern digital techniques have significantly narrowed the difference between these two imaging modalities. Unfortunately, ultrasound cannot reliably detect the presence or absence of VUR.

26. **b. Is laterally (cranially) positioned from a normal takeoff at the trigone offers an embryologic explanation for primary reflux.** As Mackie and Stevens have suggested, a ureteral bud that is laterally (cranially) positioned from a normal takeoff at the trigone offers an embryologic explanation for primary reflux, whereas those inferiorly (caudally) positioned are often obstructed.

27. **b. Photopenic areas may result from postinfection renal scarring and some renal dysplasia.** Vesicoureteral reflux, particularly reflux of higher grades, may result in renal dysplasia, which often appears scintigraphically identical to postinfection pyelonephritic scars. During an episode of active pyelonephritis, the renal scan may show an area of photopenia that later, if it persists, represents renal scarring secondary to the infection. Neither renal scan nor ultrasonography can accurately differentiate between renal dysplasia and renal scarring.

28. **a. In children and young adults it is most commonly caused by reflux nephropathy.** Reflux nephropathy is the most common cause of severe hypertension in children and young adults, although the actual incidence is unknown.

29. **e. All of the above.** Factors that might contribute to the effects of reflux on renal growth include the congenital dysmorphism often associated with reflux (30% of cases) but not caused by it; the number and type of urinary infections and their resultant nephropathy; the quality of the contralateral kidney and its implications for compensatory hypertrophy; and the grade of reflux in the affected kidney.

30. **c. BBD reduces the success rate of endoscopic implantation of dextranomer/hyaluronic copolymer (Dx/HA) and open surgical correction of VUR.** However, BBD is associated with an increased incidence of UTI after surgery.

31. **a. Distally and medially, and the lower pole ureter enters the bladder proximally and laterally.** The anatomy of patients with ureteral duplication typically follows the Weigert-Meyer rule, wherein the upper pole ureter enters the bladder distally and medially and the lower pole ureter enters the bladder proximally and laterally.

32. **d. Negative intraoperative cystography.** Studies have not consistently shown increased outcome success with the volume of the bulking agent, surgeon experience, or techniques of volcano-shaped mound with no hydrodistention or the double hydrodistention-implantation technique.

33. **c. Bladder changes predispose the patient to bacteriuria.** Bladder tone decreases because of edema and hyperemia, which are changes that predispose the patient to bacteriuria.

In addition, urine volume increases in the upper collecting system as the physiologic dilation of pregnancy evolves.

34. **e. All of the above.** It seems logical to assume that during pregnancy, the presence of VUR in a system already prone to bacteriuria would lead to increased morbidity. Maternal history also becomes a factor if past reflux, renal scarring, and a tendency to develop urinary infections are included. Women with hypertension and an element of renal failure are particularly at risk.

35. **d. The 2014 *New England Journal of Medicine* Randomized Intervention for Children with Vesicoureteral Reflux (RIVUR) study reported a 0.5% incidence of adverse reaction to prophylactic antibiotics and a 2% incidence of adverse reaction to the placebo.** Adverse reactions to antibiotics were reported in 2% of *both* the antibiotic prophylaxis and placebo groups.

36. **a. A valvular mechanism that enables ureteral compression with bladder filling and contraction.** Common to each technique is the creation of a valvular mechanism that enables ureteral compression with bladder filling and contraction, thus reenacting normal anatomy and function. A successful ureteroneocystostomy provides a submucosal tunnel for reimplantation having sufficient length and adequate muscular backing. A tunnel length of five times the ureteral diameter is cited as necessary for eliminating reflux.

37. **b. A common sheath repair in which both ureters are mobilized with one mucosal cuff.** Approximately 10% of children undergoing antireflux surgery have an element of ureteral duplication. The most common configuration is a complete duplication that results in two separate orifices. This is best managed by preserving a cuff of bladder mucosa that encompasses both orifices. Because the pair typically share blood supply along their adjoining wall, mobilization as one unit with a "common sheath" preserves vascularity and minimizes trauma.

38. **e. All of the above.** Early after surgery, various degrees of obstruction can be expected of the reimplanted ureter. Edema, subtrigonal bleeding, and bladder spasms all possibly contribute. Mucus plugs and blood clots are other causes. Most postoperative obstructions are mild and asymptomatic and resolve spontaneously. More significant obstructions are usually symptomatic. Affected children typically present 1 to 2 weeks after surgery with acute abdominal pain, nausea, and vomiting.

39. **c. Initial observation and diversion for unabating symptoms.** The large majority of perioperative obstructions subside spontaneously, but placement of a nephrostomy tube or ureteral stent sometimes becomes necessary for unabating symptoms.

40. **a. It may be due to unrecognized secondary causes of reflux such as neuropathic bladder and severe voiding dysfunction.** Other than technical errors, failure to identify and treat secondary causes of reflux is a common cause of the reappearance of reflux. Foremost among these secondary causes are unrecognized neuropathic bladder and severe voiding dysfunction.

41. **d. The accuracy of the needle entry point during endoscopic injection as well as the needle placement are important components for the success of the surgical procedure.** The learning curve for endoscopic injection is believed to be different from that of open surgical reimplantation, but studies have not been carried out comparing these two surgical approaches for correction of VUR. Treatment is currently based on the same indications, and these indications do not differ between the different types of intervention.

42. **e. a, b, and c.** The advantages of this approach versus open surgery include smaller incisions, less discomfort, brief hospitalizations (although many centers now perform open reimplants on an outpatient basis), and quicker convalescence. As with other laparoscopic procedures, a learning curve must be climbed and experience is essential to the success of this approach. Laparoscopic reimplantation requires a team

with at least two surgeons; the repair is converted from an extraperitoneal to an intraperitoneal approach; operative time is longer than with open techniques (although with experience it is now becoming gradually shorter); and cost is increased because of lengthier surgery and the expense of disposable equipment.

43. **e. a and c only.** Uncircumcised male children older than 1 year do not appear to be at higher risk for development of recurrent UTI after discontinuation of CAP.

44. **d. All of the above.** Children with grade III or IV reflux at baseline and patients presenting with febrile index infection and the presence of BBD at baseline were considered event modifiers in the RIVUR trial and appeared to benefit from CAP.

45. **d. A renal and bladder ultrasound after confirmation of UTI by a properly collected urine specimen for culture and analysis.** A VCUG is recommended only if the renal and bladder ultrasound is abnormal or if the child develops a second infection.

CHAPTER REVIEW

1. Approximately one-third of the siblings of patients with reflux will have reflux.
2. Reflux that is inherited is thought to be due to an autosomal dominant pattern.
3. There is a frequent association of constipation and encopresis with reflux and UTIs.
4. If both the ureteropelvic junction (UPJ) and ureterovesical junction (UVJ) require operative repair, the UPJ should be repaired first.
5. There is an association of renal maldevelopment with high grades of reflux.
6. The cardinal renal anomalies associated with reflux are multicystic dysplastic kidney and renal agenesis.
7. Women with UTIs and reflux who have undergone reimplantation will still be at significant risk for UTIs during pregnancy and should be monitored.
8. Almost 80% of low-grade and half of grade III reflux will resolve spontaneously.
9. Sterile reflux is benign.
10. Cohen's cross-trigonal technique of ureteral reimplantation is particularly well suited for small bladders and thick-walled bladders.
11. There is a 10% to 15% incidence of contralateral reflux after unilateral reflux is repaired.
12. Prophylactic bilateral reimplantation for unilateral reflux is not indicated.
13. Reflux is unlikely to be of any clinical significance in the absence of infection in a patient with normal bladder function.
14. The greatest risk for postinfection renal scarring is in the first year of life.
15. Reflux associated with a paraureteral diverticulum resolves at a similar rate to primary reflux.
16. There is a 10-fold lower frequency of vesicoureteral reflux in female children of African descent.
17. The endoscopic repair of reflux is less invasive and less durable than the open surgical repair.
18. A 5:1 tunnel length–ureteral diameter ratio should be achieved in antireflux surgery for best results.
19. Bladder infections (UTIs) and their accompanying inflammation can also cause reflux by lessening compliance, elevating intravesical pressures, and distorting and weakening the ureterovesical junction.
20. Modern management of reflux does not include routine evaluation through cystoscopy.
21. Vesicoureteral reflux, particularly reflux of higher grades, may be associated with renal dysplasia, which often appears scintigraphically identical to postinfection pyelonephritic scars.
22. Reflux nephropathy is the most common cause of severe hypertension in children and young adults.
23. In a duplex system where one ureter refluxes and surgical reconstruction is indicated, both ureters should have a common sheath reimplantation because the paired ureters typically share blood supply along their adjoining wall, and mobilization as one unit with a "common sheath" preserves vascularity and minimizes trauma.
24. Failure to identify and treat secondary causes of reflux is a common cause of the reappearance of reflux following correction. Foremost among these secondary causes are unrecognized neuropathic bladder and severe voiding dysfunction.

30 Bladder Anomalies in Children

Aaron D. Martin and Christopher C. Roth

QUESTIONS

1. All are true regarding the embryologic development of the urinary system **EXCEPT** which?
   a. Between the fourth and sixth weeks of gestation, the uro-rectal septum divides the endodermal cloaca into a ventral urogenital sinus and a dorsal rectum.
   b. Around the fourth to fifth month of gestation, the allantoic duct and ventral cloaca involute as the bladder descends into the pelvis.
   c. The obliterated urachus becomes the median umbilical ligament and connects the apex of the bladder with the umbilicus.
   d. Definitive nephrons within the embryologic kidneys will begin urine production around the 12th week of gestation, and the first signs of lower urinary tract anomalies may become evident.
   e. Unlike the case in males, the entire female urethra is derived from the pelvic part of the urogenital sinus.

2. Which of the following statements best describes visualization of the fetal bladder?
   a. Transabdominal imaging is more sensitive than transvaginal imaging for early detection of the fetal bladder.
   b. The fetal bladder typically empties every 15 to 20 minutes, and nonvisualization of the bladder necessitates prolonged inspection to make sure that a full bladder was not missed.
   c. At 10 weeks of gestation the bladder will be visualized in 25% of fetuses.
   d. At 13 weeks of gestation the bladder will be visualized in 50% of fetuses.
   e. During the first trimester the normal bladder diameter is 12 mm or less.

3. In prenatally detected bladder anomalies,
   a. the incidence of bladder agenesis is approximately 1 per 600,000 gestations.
   b. bladder agenesis is most common in males.
   c. bladder exstrophy is most often associated with nonvisualization of the bladder and oligohydramnios.
   d. most cases of bladder exstrophy are diagnosed prenatally.
   e. visualization of the bladder is expected to be normal in cases of bilateral renal dysplasia.

4. Regarding megacystis,
   a. the bladder is dilated secondary to high-grade reflux.
   b. this finding indicates that lower urinary tract obstruction (LUTO) is present.
   c. during the first trimester a normal bladder should be 6 mm or less.
   d. beyond the first trimester a bladder that fails to empty after 15 minutes is abnormal.
   e. this finding is always associated with a dilated posterior urethra.

5. Genetic evaluation of a fetus with megacystis is likely to demonstrate:
   a. a definitive genetic diagnosis in most cases.
   b. a decreased rate of expected genetic anomalies based on maternal age.
   c. a decreased rate of expected genetic anomalies based on nuchal translucency.
   d. trisomy 13 or 18.
   e. none of the above.

6. Improved outcomes for megacystis have been noted when all are present **EXCEPT** which?
   a. Aneuploidy
   b. Initial bladder dilation of 12 mm or less
   c. Resolution of megacystis by 23 weeks of gestational age
   d. Normal amniotic fluid levels
   e. Isolated bladder findings without associated congenital anomalies

7. Megacystis microcolon intestinal hypoperistalsis (MMIH) syndrome:
   a. is best described as the most common cause of megacystis on routine surveillance.
   b. is most often detected prenatally by the gastrointestinal findings.
   c. has more morbidity for urologic than enteric sequelae.
   d. has no known survivors beyond the neonatal period.
   e. is suspected of being secondary to dysfunction of actin smooth muscle.

8. Bladder duplication will usually be associated with:
   a. duplex ureters and collecting systems.
   b. duplication of the urethra.
   c. less than 25% incidence of gastrointestinal (GI) anomalies.
   d. diurnal continence.
   e. genital anomalies.

9. Which statement is most accurate regarding congenital bladder diverticula?
   a. A majority are diagnosed prenatally.
   b. Most occur through a hiatus in the bladder wall and consist of mucosal lining only.
   c. The reported incidence is 20% of the population.
   d. A cystogram offers little information over ultrasound imaging.
   e. Most diverticula will require surgical resection.

10. Diverticula secondary to connective tissue disorders:
    a. usually present as a single diverticulum.
    b. have walls composed of smooth muscle as well as mucosa.
    c. are best managed surgically before symptoms.

d. have an unlikely chance of recurrence after resection.

e. are often associated with increased incidence of urothelial tumors.

11. Regarding urachal anomalies,

a. urachal squamous cell carcinoma has been reported in some children.

b. most cases of a patent urachus are associated with bladder outlet obstruction.

c. resection of a urachal cyst is not recommended after treatment of a prior infection.

d. a patent omphalomesenteric duct can mimic a patent urachus.

e. surgical management is best performed with minimally invasive surgery.

12. Which statement best describes noninflammatory bladder conditions?

a. Bladder hemangiomas are often multiple.

b. Bladder hemangiomas often require radical resection.

c. Bladder hemangiomas are associated with Klippel-Trenaunay or Sturge-Weber syndrome.

d. Fibroepithelial polyps are the most common cause of bladder masses in children.

e. Fibroepithelial polyps are difficult to treat endocscopically.

13. Nephrogenic adenoma:

a. is more common in children than in adults.

b. often demonstrates malignant transformation.

c. rarely recurs after local treatment.

d. is best treated by a partial cystectomy.

e. can be seen as a reaction to infection or urolithiasis.

14. When the diagnoses of cystitis cystica and eosinophilic cystitis is being considered, it is important to note that:

a. cystitis cystica more commonly occurs in males.

b. eosinophilic cystitis can be treated with steroids, antihistamines, and antibiotics.

c. eosinophilic cystitis more commonly occurs in females.

d. eosinophilic cystitis in young children will almost always progress.

e. cystitis cystica treatment typically includes steroids.

ANSWERS

1. **d. Definitive nephrons within the embryologic kidneys will begin urine production around the 12th week of gestation, and the first signs of lower urinary tract anomalies may become evident.** Definitive nephrons within the embryologic kidneys will actually begin to produce urine prior to the 12th week of gestation. It is around the 10th week of gestation that the first signs of lower urinary tract anomalies may become evident.

2. **b. The fetal bladder typically empties every 15 to 20 minutes and nonvisualization of the bladder necessitates prolonged inspection to make sure that a full bladder was not missed.** The timing of ultrasound findings is important and due to the frequent cycling of the normal fetal bladder. Careful observation is needed prior to determining that a bladder is not visualized.

3. **a. The incidence of bladder agenesis is approximately 1 per 600,000 gestations.** Bladder agenesis incidence is approximately 1 per 600,000 and is more common in females. Bladder exstrophy is typically associated with normal amniotic fluid levels, and most cases are diagnosed postnatally.

4. **c. During the first trimester a normal bladder should be 6 mm or less.** Megacystis commonly refers to a finding on imaging and has a varied differential beyond dilation secondary to reflux. It may or may not be associated with bladder outlet obstruction. During the first trimester, the definition of megacystis is based on size, with the normal bladder being 6 mm or less in size. Beyond the first trimester, megacystis is defined as a bladder that does not empty during 45 minutes of observation.

5. **d. Trisomy 13 or 18.** Genetic testing in patients with the finding of megacystis is not universal, and most cases will not have a genetic diagnosis. When genetic testing is performed, the most common anomalies are trisomy 13 and 18. Genetic anomalies in patients with megacystis exceed the expected rates when maternal age and nuchal translucency are controlled for.

6. **a. Aneuploidy.** When genetic testing is performed, positive findings are associated with poor outcomes. All other factors listed are predictors of improved outcomes.

7. **e. Is suspected of being secondary to dysfunction of actin smooth muscle.** MMIH is a rare cause of megacystis and is most often detected by the bladder findings. The urologic sequelae are significant, although morbidity is most often due to enteric complications. Although MMIH was once thought to be incompatible with life, survival beyond the neonatal period is now well documented.

8. **e. Genital anomalies.** Most cases of bladder duplication will be associated with genital anomalies and the urethra may or may not be duplicated. Over 25% will have GI anomalies, and continence is difficult to predict based on the anatomy alone.

9. **b. Most occur through a hiatus in the bladder wall and consist of mucosal lining only.** A cystogram is the definitive test for diagnosing bladder diverticula; most instances are diagnosed only following symptomatic presentation. The reported incidence is 1.7%, and most cases will not require surgical resection.

10. **b. Have walls composed of smooth muscle as well as mucosa.** Diverticula associated with connective tissue disorders will often present with multiple diverticula, and the typical histology will show smooth muscle and mucosa in the wall of the diverticulum. Surgical management can be chosen when symptomatic, and recurrence is to be expected.

11. **d. A patent omphalomesenteric duct can mimic a patent urachus.** Adenocarcinoma of urachal anomalies has been reported in adults and is rare in children, but this is not true of squamous cell carcinoma. Most cases of a patent urachus are not associated with bladder outlet obstruction. Resection of a urachal cyst is recommended after treatment of a prior infection. Surgical management of urachal anomalies can be effectively performed with either open or minimally invasive surgery.

12. **c. Bladder hemangiomas are associated with Klippel-Trenaunay or Sturge-Weber syndrome.** Hemangiomas are often singular and can be associated with known syndromes. Fortunately, simple resection can be curative. Fibroepithelial polyps are rare causes of bladder masses and can usually be managed simply with endoscopic resection.

13. **e. Can be seen as a reaction to infection or urolithiasis.** This mostly benign lesion is usually described as a reaction to infection, lithiasis, or injury. Nephrogenic adenomas are more common in adults than in children. Recurrence after resection (usually cystoscopic rather than open) reaches 80%, with a latency of 4 years.

14. **b. Eosinophilic cystitis can be treated with steroids, antihistamines, and antibiotics.** Eosinophilic cystitis occurs more commonly in boys. When it occurs in young children, it will often be self-limited. Inflammatory cells with numerous eosinophils are seen throughout all layers of the biopsy and can be treated with a combination of steroids, antihistamines, and antibiotics. Cystitis cystica occurs more commonly in females and antibiotics are a component of treatment.

CHAPTER REVIEW

1. Persistent megacystis in the background of oligohydramnios is concerning for LUTO; megacystis that resolves prior to delivery may not have any postnatal sequelae.
2. MMIH syndrome may present with megacystis noted only prenatally.
3. Nondilated anomalies are the most severe forms of congenital urologic malformations, such as bladder exstrophy. Normal amniotic fluid levels are usually found.
4. Bladder agenesis is compatible with life only if the ureters drain ectopically.
5. Children with connective tissue disorders can have multiple bladder diverticula that may have to be treated owing to stasis-related infections or stones.
6. Urachal anomalies are usually detected postnatally because of umbilical drainage.
7. Infected urachal remnants are treated with antibiotics, followed by surgical excision.
8. Urachal remnants can be confused for a persistent omphalomesenteric duct on preoperative workup.
9. Asymptomatic incidentally found urachal remnant excision should be discussed with family because of the potential for malignant transformation in adulthood.
10. Acquired bladder diverticula can become large enough to cause urinary obstruction or create stasis leading to recurrent urinary tract infections.
11. After resection of nephrogenic adenomas, routine cystoscopy is necessary because of an 80% recurrence rate in children.
12. Cystitis cystica can mimic a bladder tumor but is benign and is best treated with long-term antibiotic prophylaxis.
13. Eosinophilic cystitis has no "typical" appearance and requires biopsy for diagnosis.
14. Cyclophosphamide therapy can lead to hemorrhagic cystitis. For prevention, mesna is given simultaneously, and oral sodium pentosan polysulfate shows promise.

31 Exstrophy-Epispadias Complex

John P. Gearhart and Heather N. Di Carlo

QUESTIONS

1. What is the live birth incidence of classic bladder exstrophy?
   a. 1 in 1000
   b. 1 in 10,000
   c. 1 in 50,000
   d. 1 in 70,000
   e. 1 in 100,000

2. What is the live birth risk of bladder exstrophy in the offspring of individuals with bladder exstrophy and epispadias?
   a. 1 in 70
   b. 1 in 300
   c. 1 in 500
   d. 1 in 700
   e. 1 in 1000

3. The main theory of embryologic maldevelopment in exstrophy is that of:
   a. underdevelopment of the cloacal membrane, preventing medial migration of the mesoderm tissue and proper lower abdominal wall development.
   b. overdevelopment of the cloacal membrane, preventing medial migration of the mesodermal tissue and proper lower abdominal wall development.
   c. infiltration of ectoderm into the cloacal membrane.
   d. infiltration of mesoderm into the cloacal membrane.
   e. invasion of endoderm into the cloacal membrane.

4. In evaluating the skeletal defects of bladder exstrophy, Sponseller and colleagues (1995)[a] found that with classic bladder exstrophy, there are changes in the orientation of the pelvic bones. These include:
   a. external rotation of the posterior aspect of the pelvis of 12 degrees on each side.
   b. retroversion of the acetabulum.
   c. an 18-degree rotation of the anterior pelvis.
   d. a 30% shortening of the pubic rami in addition to a significant pubic symphyseal diastasis.
   e. all of the above.

5. Which of the following statements is TRUE regarding hernias in children with exstrophy?
   a. Identification at the time of initial closure is not possible.
   b. They are usually unilateral.
   c. They are noted in 80% of boys and 10% of girls.
   d. The orientation of the pelvic bones makes them infrequent.
   e. A patent processus vaginalis is rarely noted.

6. Which of the following statements is TRUE regarding the male genital defect in exstrophy?
   a. The posterior length of the corporeal bodies was 30% shorter than that in healthy controls.
   b. The diameter of the posterior corporeal segments was less than that in healthy controls.
   c. The shortening of the penis was due entirely to the pubic diastasis.
   d. The anterior corporeal segments are 50% shorter than those of healthy control participants.
   e. The angle between the corpora cavernosa is markedly reduced in boys with exstrophy.

7. Which of the following statements best describes findings regarding the prostate in exstrophy?
   a. Volume weight and the cross-sectional area appeared healthy compared with published results from control subjects.
   b. The prostate extended circumferentially around the urethra in all patients with exstrophy.
   c. Free prostate-specific antigen (PSA) values were greater than in healthy controls, indicating recurrent injury from infection.
   d. The vas deferens and seminal vesicles were abnormal due to the effect of the exstrophic bladder.
   e. Total PSA values were not measurable in men with exstrophy.

8. Which of the following accurately describes the vagina in the female patient with bladder exstrophy?
   a. It is shorter than normal and of smaller caliber.
   b. The vaginal orifice is displaced posteriorly because of the anterior exstrophic bladder.
   c. It is shorter than normal but of normal caliber.
   d. It is longer than normal and of wider caliber.
   e. The cervix enters the posterior vaginal wall.

9. Findings regarding the structure and innervation of the exstrophic bladder included the following:
   a. The density and binding affinity of the muscarinic receptors were similar to norms.
   b. There was a decreased ratio of collagen to muscle in the exstrophic bladder.
   c. There were more myelinated nerve profiles, indicating a later developmental stage.
   d. A threefold increase in the amount of type I collagen was noted.
   e. Study of vasoactive intestinal polypeptide, protein gene product 9.5, and calcitonin gene–related peptide indicated the presence of dysinnervation.

[a]Sources referenced can be found in *Campbell-Walsh-Wein Urology, 12th Edition*, on the Expert Consult website.

10. Which of the following statements best describes bladder function in patients with bladder exstrophy?

    a. After reconstruction, normal cystometrograms are noted in 10% to 25% of patients who are continent.

    b. Before bladder neck reconstruction, 80% of patients had compliant and stable bladders.

    c. Involuntary contractions were rarely noted after bladder neck reconstruction.

    d. After bladder neck reconstruction, 90% of patients maintained normal bladder compliance.

    e. After successful closure, ultrastructure remains abnormal in the majority.

11. The characteristic prenatal appearance of bladder exstrophy includes which of the following?

    a. Absence of bladder filling

    b. Low-set umbilicus

    c. Widening of the pubic ramus

    d. Diminutive genitalia

    e. All of the above

12. Newborn patient selection for immediate reconstruction is based on:

    a. examination of the bladder in the nursery without anesthesia.

    b. complete lack of any surface defects on examination.

    c. indentation of the bladder under anesthesia or outward bulging when the child cries.

    d. size of the phallus at birth.

    e. extent of the pubic diastasis.

13. Fundamental steps in the modern staged reconstruction of bladder exstrophy include all of the following EXCEPT

    a. Early closure of the bladder, posterior urethra, and abdominal wall

    b. Early epispadias repair at around age 1 year

    c. Conversion of the bladder exstrophy to complete epispadias

    d. Bladder neck reconstruction before the epispadias repair to provide early continence

    e. Ureteral reimplantation at the time of bladder neck reconstruction

14. What is the best treatment option at the time of birth in a child whose bladder template is judged to be too small to undergo closure?

    a. Excision of the bladder with a nonrefluxing colon conduit

    b. Immediate closure with epispadias repair to provide resistance and allow the bladder to grow

    c. Delaying closure by 4 to 6 months with reassessment to see if the bladder will grow

    d. Bladder closure, augmentation, ureteral reimplantation, and a continence procedure

    e. An osteotomy to improve the potential for successful closure

15. Combined osteotomy was developed for all of the following reasons EXCEPT

    a. This approach allows placement of an external fixator device.

    b. Superior cosmesis is provided by this approach.

    c. There is no need to turn the patient to perform an osteotomy.

    d. Pubic approximation is easier.

    e. There is less risk of malunion of the iliac wing and also less blood loss.

16. Complications associated with osteotomy and immobilization techniques include all of the following EXCEPT

    a. Skin ulceration is associated with use of mummy wrapping.

    b. Failure of the bladder and abdominal wall closure is associated with the use of spica casting.

    c. High rates of failure of reconstruction are associated with the use of osteotomy and external fixation.

    d. Transient femoral nerve palsy is associated with the use of osteotomy.

    e. Delayed union of the iliac wings may occur after the use of posterior osteotomy.

17. Which of the following statements is TRUE regarding the various described approaches to bladder exstrophy reconstruction?

    a. The Warsaw approach includes bladder neck reconstruction at the time of initial bladder closure.

    b. The Erlangen approach includes all of the features of reconstruction of the exstrophy in a single procedure.

    c. The Seattle approach (Complete Primary Repair of Exstrophy [CPRE]) includes bladder neck reconstruction as part of the complete reconstruction of exstrophy.

    d. Combined bladder closure and epispadias repair is performed in cases of primary exstrophy repair at birth.

    e. The Warsaw approach uses the Young repair as the preferred method for epispadias reconstruction.

18. After initial primary bladder closure in the newborn, what should be done if there are recurrent urinary tract infections?

    a. Voiding cystourethrogram

    b. Computed tomography (CT) scan of the bladder

    c. Ureteral reimplantation

    d. Prophylaxis modified

    e. Cystoscopy

19. After successful bladder closure, management should include all the following EXCEPT

    a. Calibration of the urethral outlet 4 weeks after closure to ensure free drainage

    b. Ultrasound evaluation of the kidneys and bladder

    c. Intermittent antibiotics for urinary tract infections

    d. Complete bladder drainage by suprapubic tube clamping

    e. Yearly cystoscopic evaluation

20. In a patient with bladder exstrophy who undergoes more than one closure of the bladder and urethral defect, what is the chance of having adequate bladder capacity for later bladder neck reconstruction?

    a. 10%

    b. 20%

    c. 30%

    d. 60%

    e. 75%

21. The key concepts in the reconstruction of epispadias include all of the following EXCEPT

    a. Correction of ventral chordee

    b. Urethral reconstruction

    c. Glans reconstruction

    d. Penile skin coverage

    e. Penile lengthening

22. Information gleaned from most major series of bladder neck reconstruction indicates that the most important factor to predict success and eventual continence after bladder neck reconstruction is:
    a. the age of the child.
    b. the number of prior bladder infections.
    c. the number of attempts at bladder closure.
    d. bladder capacity.
    e. vesicoureteral reflux.

23. After bladder neck reconstruction, within what time period do the majority of patients achieve daytime continence?
    a. 2 months
    b. 6 months
    c. 1 year
    d. 2 years
    e. 4 years

24. After a failed attempted bladder closure in the newborn period, what time period should elapse before a secondary repair is attempted?
    a. 2 months
    b. 6 months
    c. 12 months
    d. 18 months
    e. 2 years

25. All of the following statements are TRUE regarding the results of modern staged reconstruction of exstrophy EXCEPT
    a. The onset of eventual continence and continence rates were unchanged in those who had initial successful closure.
    b. The modified Cantwell-Ransley repair has replaced the Young technique because there is less urethral tortuosity and fistula rates are lower.
    c. The incidence of fistula formation was 12% at 3 months after epispadias repair.
    d. Continence is more likely in those patients undergoing initial closure before 72 hours of age or those who have closure after 72 hours of age with osteotomy.
    e. Continence rates are higher in those who have a capacity of 85 mL or more at the time of bladder neck reconstruction.

26. Which of the following statements is TRUE regarding exstrophy failures?
    a. After successful secondary closure, 90% of patients develop dryness and voided continence.
    b. Dehiscence after complete primary repair may be associated with corporal, urethral, and other major soft tissue loss.
    c. Bladder prolapse can be managed with minimal outlet procedures because this is considered a mild failure.
    d. Because the results of reclosure are poor, immediate resection of the bladder plate followed by neobladder construction is the preferred management.
    e. Posterior urethral stricture is usually a late complication occurring 4 to 6 years after initial closure.

27. Bladder neck reconstruction is designated as a failure if a 3-hour dry interval is not achieved within 2 years after surgery. Management of such failure is with the use of:
    a. collagen injection, which can lead to dryness.
    b. artificial urinary sphincter with small bladder capacity.
    c. bladder neck transection, augmentation cystoplasty, and continent diversion.

d. repeat bladder neck reconstruction in relatively tight bladder necks.
    e. repeat bladder neck reconstruction in bladder instability.

28. The risks of ureterosigmoidostomy in the exstrophy population include:
    a. pyelonephritis and hyperchloremic acidosis.
    b. pyelonephritis, hyponatremia, and rectal incontinence.
    c. low incidence for eventual development of cancer.
    d. poor outcomes with upper tract deterioration.
    e. prolapse of the abdominal stoma.

29. What is the live birth incidence of cloacal exstrophy?
    a. 1 in 20,000
    b. 1 in 100,000
    c. 1 in 400,000
    d. 1 in 600,000
    e. 1 in 1,000,000

30. All of the following statements regarding neurospinal abnormalities in cloacal exstrophy are true EXCEPT
    a. Thoracic defects may be noted in 10% of patients.
    b. The embryologic basis for the neurospinal defect has been identified as failure of neural tube closure.
    c. Autonomic bladder innervation is derived from a more medial location.
    d. Innervation of the duplicated corporal bodies arises from the sacral plexus and courses medial to the hemibladders.
    e. Functional defects can include minimal lower extremity function.

31. Which of the following is TRUE regarding cloacal exstrophy?
    a. The bones in a child with cloacal exstrophy are markedly different microscopically from those of healthy controls.
    b. In the presence of a normal bowel length, there is low probability for the development of short-gut syndrome.
    c. The most common Müllerian anomaly noted is partial uterine duplication.
    d. Cardiovascular and pulmonary anomalies are frequently noted.
    e. The most common upper urinary tract anomaly noted is multicystic dysplastic kidney.

32. What is the incidence of omphalocele associated with cloacal exstrophy?
    a. 20%
    b. 40%
    c. 60%
    d. 75%
    e. 95%

33. In the patient with cloacal exstrophy, hindgut remnants should be preserved in order to:
    a. enlarge the bladder.
    b. permit vaginal reconstruction.
    c. allow either bladder augmentation or vaginal reconstruction.
    d. provide additional length of bowel for fluid absorption.
    e. allow later anal pull-through surgery.

34. Current research regarding gender in cloacal exstrophy indicates that:
    a. psychosexual evaluation indicates that patients have a marked female shift in development.

b. patients have feminine childhood behavior but develop masculine gender identity.

c. histology of the testis at birth is abnormal; therefore removal has been recommended.

d. gender is based on quality of functional reconstruction rather than on karyotype.

e. a functional and cosmetically acceptable phallus can now be constructed.

35. What is the live birth incidence of male epispadias?

a. 1 in 72,000

b. 1 in 117,000

c. 1 in 150,000

d. 1 in 250,000

e. 1 in 400,000

36. What is the incidence of reflux in patients with complete epispadias?

a. 10% to 20%

b. 30% to 40%

c. 50%

d. 70%

e. 90%

37. In the complete epispadias group, what is the predominant indicator of eventual continence?

a. Length of the urethral groove

b. Lack of spinal abnormalities

c. Bladder capacity at the time of bladder neck reconstruction

d. Age at bladder neck reconstruction

e. Age at epispadias repair and degree of resistance provided

38. All of the following are true regarding exstrophy-epispadias variants EXCEPT

a. The presence of musculoskeletal defects characteristic of the complex, with a normal urinary tract, is termed *pseudoexstrophy*.

b. The bladder is completely exstrophied in the superior vesical fissure variant.

c. With "covered" exstrophy, an isolated ectopic bowel segment has frequently been noted.

d. An isolated segment of bladder is left on the abdominal wall, with a complete urinary tract within the bladder in duplicate exstrophy.

e. A common embryologic origin has been postulated for developments of all of the variants.

39. Sexual function and libido in male and female exstrophy patients are:

a. normal in males, abnormal in females.

b. normal only in males.

c. normal in both males and females.

d. normal only in females.

e. abnormal in both males and females.

40. What is the most common complication after pregnancy in female exstrophy patients?

a. Premature labor

b. Rectal prolapse

c. Preeclampsia

d. Cervical and uterine prolapse

e. Oligohydramnios

41. Psychologic studies of male and female children with bladder exstrophy find that:

a. all have clinical psychopathology.

b. they do not have clinical psychopathology.

c. most have significant depression because of the condition.

d. many children have gender dysphoria.

e. half of males and half of females have clinical psychopathology.

42. Single-stage reconstruction by using the complete primary exstrophy repair technique offers several advantages versus staged reconstruction EXCEPT

a. The possibility of correcting the penile, bladder, and bladder neck abnormalities of bladder exstrophy with one operation.

b. The ability to achieve urinary continence without bladder neck reconstruction.

c. Correction of vesicoureteral reflux at the time of surgery.

d. Lower complication rates than previous attempts at single-stage reconstruction.

e. Initiation of bladder cycling early in life.

43. Single-stage reconstruction by using the complete primary exstrophy repair technique relies on which of the following to achieve continence?

a. Reestablishment of normal anatomic relationships

b. Bladder neck reconstruction at the time of primary surgery

c. Osteotomy at the time of single-stage reconstruction

d. Simultaneous epispadias repair

e. None of the above

44. The following postoperative factors have been shown to increase the success of reconstruction for bladder exstrophy EXCEPT

a. Immobilization with external fixators, Buck traction, a spica cast, or a mummy wrap

b. Antibiotic therapy

c. Prolonged status of nothing by mouth (NPO) to avoid abdominal distention

d. Urinary diversion through ureteral stenting and suprapubic urinary drainage

e. Adequate nutritional support

45. Single-stage reconstruction by using the complete primary exstrophy repair technique can be safely performed because:

a. the neurovascular bundles of the corpus cavernosal bodies lie laterally rather than dorsally on the bodies.

b. the cavernosal bodies and urethral wedge are not actually separated from each other in this technique.

c. the blood supply to the cavernosal bodies and that to the urethral wedge are independent of each other.

d. the blood supply is quickly reestablished once the components are "reassembled."

e. the distal vascular communications between the corpora and urethral wedge are preserved.

46. The proximal limit(s) of dissection by using the complete primary exstrophy repair technique is/are:

a. the intersymphyseal band.

b. the muscles of the pelvic floor.

c. the rectum.

d. the corpora spongiosa.

e. the endopelvic fascia.

47. Factors that mitigate against use of a single-stage reconstruction technique for cloacal exstrophy include the presence of:

    a. a large omphalocele.

    b. a wide pubic diastasis.

    c. a concomitant myelomeningocele.

    d. a small bladder plate.

    e. all of the above.

48. Complications of the complete primary exstrophy repair technique include:

    a. myogenic bladder failure.

    b. testicular atrophy.

    c. urethrocutaneous fistula.

    d. hip dislocation.

    e. epispadias.

ANSWERS

1. **c. 1 in 50,000.** The incidence of bladder exstrophy has been estimated as between 1 in 10,000 and 1 in 50,000 live births.
2. **a. 1 in 70.** Shapiro determined that the risk of bladder exstrophy in the offspring of individuals with bladder exstrophy and epispadias is 1 in 70 live births, a 500-fold greater incidence than in the general population.
3. **b. Overdevelopment of the cloacal membrane, preventing medial migration of the mesodermal tissue and proper lower abdominal wall development.** The theory of embryonic maldevelopment in exstrophy held by Marshall and Muecke is that the basic defect is an abnormal overdevelopment of the cloacal membrane. This theory of embryonic maldevelopment was held by Marshall and Muecke to explain the basic defect in exstrophy patients.
4. **e. All of the above.** Sponseller and colleagues found that patients with classic bladder exstrophy have a mean external rotation of the posterior aspect of the pelvis of 12 degrees on each side, retroversion of the acetabulum, and a mean 18-degree external rotation of the anterior pelvis along with 30% shortening of the pubic rami.
5. **c. They are noted in 80% of boys and 10% of girls.** Connelly and colleagues, in a review of 181 children with bladder exstrophy, reported inguinal hernias in 81.8% of boys and 10.5% of girls.
6. **d. The anterior corporeal segments are 50% shorter than those of healthy control participants.** With the use of magnetic resonance imaging (MRI) to examine adult men with bladder exstrophy and comparison of these results with those from age- and race-matched control participants, it was found that the anterior corporeal length in male patients with bladder exstrophy is almost 50% shorter than that in healthy control participants.
7. **a. Volume weight and the cross-sectional area appeared healthy compared with published results from control participants.** The volume, weight, and maximal cross-sectional area of the prostate appeared normal compared with published results from control subjects.
8. **a. It is shorter than normal and of smaller caliber.** The vagina is shorter than normal, hardly greater than 6 cm in depth, but of normal caliber.
9. **a. The density and binding affinity of the muscarinic receptors were similar to norms.** Muscarinic cholinergic receptor density and binding affinity were measured in control participants and in patients with classic bladder exstrophy. The density of the muscarinic cholinergic receptors in both the control and exstrophy groups was similar, as was the binding affinity of the muscarinic receptor. Therefore it was thought by the authors that the neurophysiologic composition of the exstrophied bladder is not grossly altered during its anomalous development.

10. **b. Before bladder neck reconstruction, 80% of patients had compliant and stable bladders.** Diamond and colleagues (1999), looking at 30 patients with bladder exstrophy at various stages of reconstruction, found that 80% of patients had compliant and stable bladders before bladder neck reconstruction.
11. **e. All of the above.** In a review of 25 prenatal ultrasonographic examinations with the resulting birth of a newborn with classic bladder exstrophy, several observations were made: (1) absence of bladder filling; (2) a low-set umbilicus; (3) a widened pubis ramus; (4) diminutive genitalia; and (5) a lower abdominal mass that increases in size while the pregnancy progresses and as the intra-abdominal viscera increase in size.
12. **c. Indentation of the bladder under anesthesia or outward bulging when the child cries.** In minor grades of exstrophy that approach the condition of complete epispadias with incontinence, the bladder may be small yet may demonstrate acceptable capacity, either by bulging when the baby cries or by indenting easily when touched by a sterile gloved finger in the operating room with the child under anesthesia.
13. **d. Bladder neck reconstruction before the epispadias repair to provide early continence.** The most significant changes in the management of bladder exstrophy have been (1) early bladder, posterior urethral, and abdominal wall closure, usually with osteotomy; (2) early epispadias repair; (3) reconstruction of a continent bladder neck and reimplantation of the ureters; and (4) definition of strict criteria for the selection of patients suitable for this approach. Bladder neck repair usually occurs when the child is 4 to 5 years of age, has an adequate bladder capacity, and, most important, is ready to participate in a postoperative voiding program.
14. **c. Delaying closure by age 4 to 6 months with reassessment to see if the bladder will grow.** Ideally, waiting for the bladder template to grow for 4 to 6 months in the child with a small bladder is not as risky as submitting a small bladder template to closure in an inappropriate setting, resulting in dehiscence and allowing the fate of the bladder to be sealed at that point.
15. **c. There is no need to turn the patient to perform an osteotomy.** Combined osteotomy was developed for three reasons: (1) osteotomy is performed with the patient in the supine position, as is the urologic repair, thereby avoiding the need to turn the patient; (2) the anterior approach to this osteotomy allows placement of an external fixator device and intrafragmentary pins under direct vision; and (3) the cosmetic appearance of this osteotomy is superior to that of the posterior iliac approach.
16. **c. High rates of failure of reconstruction associated with the use of osteotomy and external fixation.** Successful closure was noted in 97% of those immobilized with an external fixator and modified Buck traction.
17. **b. The Erlangen approach includes all of the features of reconstruction of the exstrophy in a single procedure.** This method is truly a "complete repair" because it accomplishes all of the facets of exstrophy reconstruction in a single procedure. Surgical repair is, however, performed at 8 to 10 weeks of age, when the infant is larger and has had the opportunity to be medically stabilized.
18. **e. Cystoscopy.** An important caveat is that if there are recurrent urinary tract infections or if the bladder is distended on an ultrasonographic study, cystoscopy should be performed and the posterior urethra should be carefully examined anteriorly for erosion of the intrapubic stitch, which may be the cause of the recurrent infections.
19. **c. Intermittent antibiotics for urinary tract infections.** Before removal of the suprapubic tube 4 weeks after surgery, the bladder outlet is calibrated by a urethral catheter or a urethral sound to ensure free drainage. A complete ultrasound examination is obtained to ascertain the status of the renal pelves and ureters, and appropriate urinary antibiotics are administered because all patients will have reflux postclosure. Residual urine is estimated by clamping the suprapubic tube, and

specimens for culture are obtained before the patient leaves the hospital and at subsequent intervals to detect infection and ensure that the bladder is empty.

20. **d. 60%.** In one study, if a patient underwent two closures, the chance of having an adequate bladder capacity for bladder neck reconstruction was 60%.

21. **a. Correction of ventral chordee.** Regardless of the surgical technique chosen for reconstruction of the penis in bladder exstrophy, four key concerns must be addressed to ensure a functional and cosmetically pleasing penis: (1) correction of dorsal chordee, (2) urethral reconstruction, (3) glanular reconstruction, and (4) penile skin closure.

22. **d. Bladder capacity.** The most important long-term factor gleaned from a review of all these series is the fact that bladder capacity at the time of bladder neck reconstruction is an important determinant of eventual success.

23. **c. 1 year.** The vast majority of patients achieve daytime continence in the first year after bladder neck reconstruction.

24. **b. 6 months.** Dehiscence—which may be precipitated by incomplete mobilization of the pelvic diaphragm and inadequate pelvic immobilization postoperatively, wound infection, abdominal distention, or urinary tube malfunction—necessitates a 6-month recovery period before a second attempt at closure.

25. **a. The onset of eventual continence and continence rates were unchanged in those who had initial successful closure.** The importance of a successful initial closure is emphasized by Oesterling and Jeffs (1987) and by Husmann and colleagues (1989), who found that the onset of eventual continence was quicker and the continence rate higher in those who underwent a successful initial closure with or without osteotomy.

26. **b. Dehiscence after complete primary repair may be associated with corporeal, urethral, and other major soft tissue loss.** Dehiscence and prolapse have also been reported after the "complete repair" and may be associated with glandular, corporeal, urethral plate, and other major soft tissue loss.

27. **c. Bladder neck transection, augmentation cystoplasty, and continent diversion.** A majority of bladder neck failures require eventual augmentation or continent diversion. The artificial urinary sphincter has been used with some success in patients who have a good bladder capacity. However, in most of these failures the bladder capacity is small and augmentation will be required. At the time of reoperative surgery, the bladder neck is transected proximal to the prostate with a Mitrofanoff substitution, a continence procedure such as an artificial sphincter or collagen injection is performed, or both are performed. In our extensive experience with failed bladder neck reconstruction, most of the patients have had several surgeries and must be dry. In such cases the most suitable alternative is bladder neck transection, augmentation, and a continent urinary stoma (Gearhart et al., 1995b; Hensle et al., 1995).

28. **a. Pyelonephritis and hyperchloremic acidosis.** However, this form of diversion should not be offered until one is certain that anal continence is normal and after the family has been made aware of the potentially serious complications including pyelonephritis, hyperchloremic acidosis, rectal incontinence, ureteral obstruction, and delayed development of malignancy.

29. **c. 1 in 400,000.** Fortunately cloacal exstrophy is exceedingly rare, occurring in 1 in 200,000 to 400,000 live births.

30. **b. The embryologic basis for the neurospinal defect has been identified as failure of neural tube closure.** The embryologic basis for the neurospinal defects associated with cloacal exstrophy has been postulated to be secondary to problems with the disruption of the tissue of the dorsal mesenchyme rather than failure of neural tube closure (McLaughlin et al., 1995). Alternatively, it has been suggested that the defects that lead to the formation of cloacal exstrophy may lead to the developing spinal cord and vertebrae being pulled apart (Cohen, 1991).

31. **c. The most common Müllerian anomaly noted was partial uterine duplication.** This anomaly is reported to be as high as 95% (Diamond, 1990). The vast majority of these patients had partial uterine duplication, predominantly a bicornate uterus.

32. **e. 95%.** In Diamond's series, the incidence of omphalocele was 88%, with a majority of all series reporting 95% or greater.

33. **d. Provide additional length of bowel for fluid absorption.** With the recognition of the metabolic changes in patients with ileostomy, an attempt is always made to use the hindgut remnant to provide additional length of bowel for fluid absorption.

34. **e. A functional and cosmetically acceptable phallus can now be constructed.** Most authors recommend assigning gender consistent with the karyotypic makeup of the individual if at all possible. This policy can be supported by a report indicating that the histology of the testis at birth is normal (Mathews et al., 1999a). Furthermore, with the evolution of techniques for phallic reconstruction, a functional and cosmetically acceptable phallus can now be constructed (Husmann et al., 1989).

35. **b. 1 in 117,000.** Male epispadias is a rare anomaly, with a reported incidence of 1 in 117,000 males.

36. **b. 30% to 40%.** The ureterovesical junction is inherently deficient in complete epispadias, and reflux has been reported between 30% and 40% in a number of series.

37. **c. Bladder capacity at the time of bladder neck reconstruction.** In the epispadias group, much as in the exstrophy group, bladder capacity is the predominant indicator of eventual continence.

38. **b. The bladder is completely exstrophied in the superior vesical fissure variant.** In the superior vesical fissure variant of the exstrophy complex, the musculature and skeletal defects are exactly the same as those in classic exstrophy; however, the persistent cloacal membrane ruptures only at the uppermost portion, and a superior vesical fistula that actually resembles a vesicostomy results. Bladder extrusion is minimal and is present only over the normal umbilicus.

39. **c. Normal in both males and females.** Sexual function and libido in exstrophy patients are normal.

40. **d. Cervical and uterine prolapse.** The main complication after pregnancy was cervical and uterine prolapse, which occurred frequently.

41. **b. They do not have clinical psychopathology.** The conclusion of this long-term study was that children with exstrophy do not have clinical psychopathology.

42. **c. Correction of vesicoureteral reflux at the time of surgery.** In most applications of the primary exstrophy repair technique, correction of vesicoureteral reflux is not performed, although some have reported performing ureteral reimplantation. All of the other elements are considered advantages of the primary repair.

43. **a. Reestablishment of normal anatomic relationships.** The fundamental basis of the primary repair technique is to reposition the bladder neck and urethral complex into the normal pelvic position more posteriorly than at birth. This permits more normal function of the pelvic floor in maintenance of continence. The other factors do not contribute as significantly to continence.

44. **c. Prolonged status of nothing by mouth (NPO) to avoid abdominal distention.** It is not necessary to maintain an NPO status after primary repair because this will compromise nutrition. If an ileus develops, appropriate decompression and management are necessary because abdominal distention strains the repair. All other factors contribute to a successful outcome.

45. **c. The blood supply to the corpus cavernosal bodies and that to the urethral wedge are independent of each other.** Because the three elements of the penis, the two corpora, and the urethral wedge are fully separated in the penile disassembly, their vasculature must be proximal, which it is; that accounts for the success of this method. Nevertheless, preservation of these proximal vascular supplies is essential.

46. **b. The muscles of the pelvic floor.** The limit of dissection along the penile structures is the pelvic floor, which is then split to permit repositioning of the bladder neck complex posteriorly.
47. **e. All of the above.** All of these factors would indicate that an attempt to perform a primary repair would be at high risk for failure, predominantly by dehiscence. Several of these factors may be present at one time.
48. **c. Urethrocutaneous fistula.** The most common complication after primary repair is development of a urethrocutaneous fistula on the ventrum of the penis. Other complications can include corporeal devascularization, hydronephrosis, and hypospadias.

CHAPTER REVIEW

1. The male-to-female ratio for exstrophy is 2.3:1.
2. The risk of bladder exstrophy in family members is increased.
3. Rectal prolapse frequently occurs in untreated exstrophy patients who have widely separated symphyses. It disappears after exstrophy closure.
4. If rectal prolapse occurs after closure, bladder outlet obstruction should be suspected.
5. The autonomic nerves are displaced laterally in patients with exstrophy.
6. Reflux occurs in 100% of patients with exstrophy; inguinal hernias are common.
7. An ectopic isolated bowel segment may be present in the lower abdominal wall.
8. Osteotomy is rarely performed in newborns unless the diastasis is greater than 4 cm.
9. The most reliable predictors of urinary continence are the size of the bladder template at birth and successful primary closure.
10. Approximately 75% of patients with exstrophy are continent after repair. Continence is defined as 3 hours of dryness.
11. Cloacal exstrophy consists of exstrophy of the bladder; complete phallic separation; wide diastasis of the pubis; exstrophy of the terminal ileum, which lies between the two halves of the bladder; rudimentary hindgut; imperforate anus; omphalocele; and, not infrequently, associated spinal defects. Spinal defects are not common in patients who have only exstrophy.
12. In adolescents and adults with exstrophy, concerns in the male are length, appearance, and deviation of the penis. In the female, concerns are the appearance of the external genitalia, adequacy of the vaginal opening, and uterine prolapse.
13. Women with exstrophy have delivered children; however, a frequent complication after pregnancy is cervical and uterine prolapse.
14. Closure of exstrophy: (1) reshapes the pelvis, (2) redistributes the levator group, and (3) smooths the contour of the pelvic floor.
15. At birth the exstrophy patient should have the umbilical cord secured with silk rather than an umbilical clamp to prevent trauma to the exposed bladder, and the bladder should be covered with a nonadherent film to minimize trauma and prevent desiccation of the bladder mucosa.
16. Bladder spasms must be controlled in the postoperative period following closure of the exstrophy.
17. Patients with epispadias may have associated vesicoureteral reflux and inguinal hernias, although the incidence is not as high as it is in bladder exstrophy.
18. The factor most likely to cause long-term disability in the reconstructed cloacal exstrophy patient is the associated neurologic deficit.
19. The basic defect in exstrophy is an abnormal overdevelopment of the cloacal membrane, preventing medial migration of the mesenchymal tissue and proper lower abdominal wall development.
20. Anterior corporal length in male patients with bladder exstrophy is almost 50% shorter than that of healthy control participants.
21. Bladder neck repair usually occurs when the child is 4 to 5 years old; has an adequate bladder capacity; and, most important, is ready to participate in a postoperative voiding program.
22. In a closed exstrophy patient, recurrent urinary tract infections should prompt evaluation for erosion of the anterior pubic stitch into the bladder or urethra.
23. A majority of bladder neck failures require eventual augmentation or continent diversion.
24. At birth, most recommend assigning gender that is consistent with karyotypic makeup of the individual if at all possible.

32 Prune-Belly Syndrome

Francisco T. Dénes and Roberto Iglesias Lopes

QUESTIONS

1. The common antenatal ultrasonographic findings of a fetus with prune-belly syndrome are all of the following EXCEPT:
   a. oligohydramnios.
   b. empty scrotal sac.
   c. hydroureteronephrosis.
   d. distended bladder.
   e. ambiguous genitalia.

2. Which of the following is the most appropriate indication for antenatal intervention in a fetus with prune-belly syndrome?
   a. Distended bladder
   b. Bilateral hydroureteronephrosis
   c. Pulmonary hypoplasia
   d. Progressive oligohydramnios
   e. Urinary ascites

3. Common findings in the urinary tract of patients with prune-belly syndrome include all of the following EXCEPT:
   a. renal dysplasia.
   b. ureteropyelocaliectasis.
   c. vesicoureteral reflux.
   d. elevated bladder neck.
   e. urachal diverticulum.

4. Common nonurinary findings in patients with prune-belly syndrome include all of the following EXCEPT:
   a. flaccid abdomen due to nonhomogeneous deficiency of the abdominal musculature.
   b. intestinal obstruction.
   c. impalpable testes.
   d. pectus carinatum.
   e. pulmonary deficiency.

5. Which of the following organ systems are MOST likely to impact the early life of the patient with prune-belly syndrome?
   a. Cardiac
   b. Urinary
   c. Pulmonary
   d. Endocrine
   e. Orthopedic

6. Considering the prognosis of untreated patients with prune-belly syndrome, which statement is FALSE?
   a. Most patients present some degree of urinary tract dilatation.
   b. Recurrent urinary tract infection increases the risk of renal damage.
   c. The intra-abdominal testes may descend spontaneously before puberty.

   d. Abdominal wall laxity may be associated with ineffective cough and respiratory illnesses.
   e. Bladder emptying may improve spontaneously with time.

7. Considering the dilatation of the upper urinary tract of patients with prune-belly syndrome, which of the following statements is TRUE?
   a. The degree of dilation is not proportional to the abdominal wall laxity.
   b. Pyelocaliceal dilatation is never associated with ureteropelvic junction obstruction.
   c. Histologically, the thickened ureteral wall has an increased number of muscular cells.
   d. Ureteral dilation is proportional to the degree of vesicoureteral reflux.
   e. All statements above are correct.

8. Considering the lower urinary tract of patients with prune-belly syndrome, which of the following statements is TRUE?
   a. The thickened and enlarged bladder has poor compliance and uninhibited bladder contractions.
   b. Elevated bladder pressures occur due to detrusor-sphincter dyssynergia.
   c. Large postvoid residuals occur due to poorly contractile detrusor and diminished bladder sensation.
   d. Reduction cystoplasty reduces permanently the postvoid residual.
   e. All statements above are correct.

9. Considering the characteristics of the urethra of prune-belly syndrome patients, which of the following statements is TRUE?
   a. The posterior urethra is dilated due to distal obstruction.
   b. The lack of bladder neck hypertrophy is typical of the posterior urethral dilatation.
   c. Megalourethra is a frequent finding and is due to distal obstruction.
   d. Hypospadias is commonly associated.
   e. Prostatic hyperplasia is associated with upper tract dilatation.

10. Regarding abdominal undescended testes in prune-belly syndrome, which of the following statements is CORRECT?
    a. The testes must be brought down to the scrotum at the age of 2 years if spontaneous descent hasn't occurred before then.
    b. Due to the position of the testes, the Fowler-Stephens technique is always necessary.
    c. In cases of successful orchidopexy, the testes maintain endocrine function but are incapable of preserving spermatogenesis.
    d. Most patients require hormonal supplementation in adulthood.
    e. None of the statements are correct.

11. Considering the management of patients with prune-belly syndrome, which of the statements is CORRECT?

    a. The spontaneous improvement of the urinary tract dilatation with time is the basis for the clinical management, particularly in grade III prune belly syndrome (PBS) patients.

    b. In newborns with significant dilatation and vesicoureteral reflux, early ureterostomy is always indicated.

    c. Continuous antibiotic prophylaxis and antimuscarinic drugs are necessary in all patients, to preserve the upper urinary tract.

    d. Only patients with persistently elevated postvoid residuals must undergo internal urethrotomy.

    e. All statements are correct.

12. Considering the surgical management of PBS patients, which of the statements is CORRECT?

    a. Abdominoplasty must be planned and performed after urinary tract reconstruction is completed.

    b. The surgical and anesthesiologic risks are elevated when orchidopexy and abdominoplasty are performed simultaneously with the urinary tract reconstruction before puberty.

    c. Vesicoureteral reflux can be corrected with the Gregoir-Lich procedure in most cases.

    d. Even when reduction cystoplasty is performed, significant postvoid results may remain or recur.

    e. All statements are false.

ANSWERS

1. **e. Ambiguous genitalia.** Although not present in all cases, the common findings in the antenatal ultrasound in prune-belly syndrome are urinary tract dilatation with a large, full bladder, and abnormal abdominal circumference. The penis is normal to fetal age, but the scrotum is empty due to abdominal cryptorchidism. There are no reports of association of PBS with ambiguous genitalia.

2. **d. Progressive oligohydramnios.** Bilateral hydronephrosis with a distended bladder is usually well tolerated and does not represent a definitely obstructed urinary tract. Therefore, no antenatal intervention is necessary. The presence of isolated urinary ascites or pulmonary hypoplasia also does not warrant drainage of the fetal bladder. Nevertheless, the association of those findings with a progressively decreased amniotic fluid most probably represents an obstructed bladder due to an atretic urethra associated with functioning kidneys, which can be treated by bladder decompression.

3. **d. Elevated bladder neck.** In prune-belly syndrome, the kidneys may present variable degrees of renal dysplasia, with substitution of the normal parenchyma by cystic structures. This may affect one or both kidneys, in a pattern that is not proportional to the patient's abdominal flaccidity, the degree of dilatation of the urinary tract, or the presence of vesicoureteral reflux. When bilateral dysplasia occurs, survival is compromised. Hydroureteronephrosis is also variable, but in general does not impact in the initial renal function. Vesicoureteral reflux occurs in two-thirds of the patients, eventually associated with more dilated lower ureteral segments. Urachal diverticulum is present frequently, usually with thick musculofibrotic walls. In more rare cases, associated with an atretic urethra, the urachus can be completely patent to the umbilicus, in this case functioning as an efficient bladder drainage that helps preserve the upper urinary tract function. The posterior urethra is dilated, but contrary to patients with posterior urethral valves, the bladder neck is wide open, making it difficult to characterize the transition between the posterior urethra and the base of the bladder.

4. **b. Intestinal obstruction.** The abdominal flaccidity is the hallmark of the syndrome. It affects unevenly the medial and inferior segments of the abdomen, but in some patients the lateral aspects are more compromised. The musculo-aponeurotic layer of the abdominal wall is very deficient, with a very thin layer of muscle cells interwoven with aponeurotic tissue that hardly exert any contraction and support to respiration, therefore impairing pulmonary function. The lack of adequate abdominal muscular anchoring and support is responsible for the cases that present with pectus carinatum or scavatum. The lack of intra-abdominal pressure due to the weakness of the abdominal wall musculature is one of the causes of abdominal cryptorchidism. Despite eventually described intestinal abnormalities, obstruction doesn't occur primarily, being reported as a complication of intraperitoneal surgical procedures.

5. **c. Pulmonary.** Significant cardiac, orthopedic, and endocrine abnormalities that impact early patient survival are infrequent. Urinary tract abnormalities may be significant, particularly if kidney function is impaired due to bilateral dysplasia. Hydroureteronephrosis, vesicoureteral reflux, and difficult bladder emptying are also important factors, but are rarely fatal in early infancy. More frequently, it is the pulmonary hypoplasia due to oligohydramnios, often aggravated by the lack of abdominal muscle support, that impacts survival, thereby requiring prolonged respiratory support.

6. **c. The intra-abdominal testes may descend spontaneously before puberty.** The abdominal testes are situated high in the intra-abdominal cavity, usually laying upon the dilated distal ureteral folds. The inguinal region and the scrotum are empty. There is no description of spontaneous descent of the testes to the inguinal or scrotal position in a patient with the full spectrum of prune-belly syndrome, and the lack of abdominal pressure is one of the factors that preclude this descent.

7. **a. The degree of dilation is not proportional to the abdominal wall laxity.** The dilation of the upper urinary tract can be significant in one or both sides but has no correlation with the intensity of abdominal wall flaccidity. There are cases where the transition from the renal pelvis to the upper ureter may be considerably narrow, due to thickened renal pelvic or ureteral walls secondary to increased collagen, suggesting stenosis. Sometimes the ureteral folds at this segment may also cause significant difficulty to the drainage of the renal pelvis. The lower ureteral dilatation is usually more intense than that of the upper ureter, independent of the presence of vesicoureteral reflux.

8. **c. Large postvoid residuals occur due to poorly contractile detrusor and diminished bladder sensation.** The bladder usually has thick walls due to increase in collagen and a decrease in smooth muscle cells. Functionally, it has a large capacity with increased compliance but decreased sensitivity and poor contraction. Voiding pressures are usually low, and adequate bladder emptying is achieved only with the help of increased abdominal pressure. Significant postvoid residuals can be seen in many patients. In the case of a very large bladder, a reduction cystoplasty can decrease the postvoid residual, but the long-term effects of this procedure are not consistent.

9. **b. The lack of bladder neck hypertrophy is typical of the posterior urethral dilatation.** The characteristic dilatation of the posterior urethra is mostly due to the lack of support by prostatic tissue, dilatation being present even in the presence of a normal distal urethra. The lack of bladder neck hypertrophy distinguishes prune-belly syndrome from posterior urethral valves, where increased bladder pressures are observed. The presence of megalourethra in the penile urethral segment is not associated with distal stenosis, but is due to the segmental lack of support by the spongiosum.

10. **e. None of the statements is correct.** As in nonsyndromic cryptorchidism, the adequate time for orchidopexy is between 6 and 18 months of age. There is no formal indication to

anticipate or postpone the procedure in patients with prune-belly syndrome, except when another major procedure, such as abdominoplasty or urinary tract reconstruction, is being planned for an earlier or later period. As in all children with abdominal undescended testes, the orchidopexy can be successfully carried out without the Fowler-Stephens technique before the second year of age. In adult patients who underwent early successful orchidopexy, the hormonal function is normally preserved, with no need of hormonal supplementation. The presence of sperm in the ejaculate or postmasturbation urine in adult patients has been well documented, and shows potential fertility with assisted reproduction techniques.

11. **a. The spontaneous improvement of the urinary tract dilatation with time is the basis for the clinical management, particularly in grade III prune belly syndrome (PBS) patients.** As in cases of primary megaureter and vesicoureteral reflux, a considerable functional and anatomic improvement of the upper urinary tract is expected. Continuous antibiotic prophylaxis must be employed in the more vulnerable patients to prevent pyelonephritic injuries to the kidneys. As there is no increased detrusor activity or hypertrophic bladder neck in these patients, there is no indication for the use of antimuscarinic drugs or alpha-blockers. Upper urinary tract diversion in cases of evident upper urinary tract obstruction is rarely indicated, as urinary tract reconstruction is indicated in these cases. Persistent and elevated postvoid residual must be treated by timed voiding and/or clean intermittent catheterization.

12. **d. Even when reduction cystoplasty is performed, significant postvoid results may remain or recur.** Whenever necessary, urinary tract reconstruction can be performed simultaneously with abdominoplasty, orchidopexy, and circumcision. It has been documented that the procedure has acceptable rates of surgical and anesthetic complications even in infants. The urinary tract reconstruction aims to decrease the ureteral redundancy by removing the distal, more dilated ureteral segments and reimplanting them in the bladder. At the same time, removal of the urachal diverticulum and part of the noncontractile bladder dome is usually performed, but it doesn't prevent the persistence or recurrence of significant postvoid residual.

CHAPTER REVIEW

1. Hydroureteronephrosis is often to a severe degree; however, the calyceal morphology may be well preserved.
2. The proximal portion of the ureters has more normal muscle than the distal portions.
3. The bladder is large with a pseudodiverticulum at the urachus and a wide bladder neck opening into a dilated prostatic urethra.
4. Megalourethra is more commonly seen in PBS than any other syndrome. With the scaphoid variety, the ventral urethra dilates with voiding, whereas with the fusiform variety, the entire phallus dilates with voiding.
5. Infertility is thought to be due to a combination of testicular histologic abnormalities, structural defects of the ducts and prostatic abnormalities, and retrograde ejaculation.
6. Pulmonary hypoplasia can result from severe oligohydramnios related to renal dysplasia, or severe bladder outlet obstruction, and may result in newborn demise.
7. Despite being one of the hallmarks of the syndrome, the abdominal flaccidity has no direct relationship with the intensity of the urologic abnormalities and doesn't impair the short- and long-term survival of the patient. Together with the orthopedic abnormalities, if significant and left untreated, it may cause a decrease in the quality of life in the adolescent and adult patients.
8. A team consisting of neonatology, nephrology, urology, and other specialties such as cardiology is necessary.
9. A voiding cystourethrogram (VCUG) is indicated in the neonatal period if there is renal insufficiency or evidence of bladder outlet obstruction and only after antibiotic prophylaxis.
10. A chest x-ray to evaluate for pneumothorax, pneumomediastinum, and pulmonary hypoplasia is necessary.
11. Baseline assessment of renal function should include renal and bladder ultrasonography, blood urea nitrogen (BUN), creatinine, and electrolytes.
12. Circumcision is advisable in the absence of a structural penile abnormality.
13. Early intervention is indicated for evidence of bladder outlet obstruction and preferably with a percutaneous suprapubic tube.
14. Upper urinary tract reconstruction is controversial but clearly indicated for evidence of declining renal function in the presence of recurrent upper tract infections or progression of the hydroureteronephrosis.
15. Orchidopexy is best performed early in life because this affords the most likely prospect of a successful single-stage procedure, as well as the perspective of preservation of germ cells.
16. Abdominal wall reconstruction has demonstrated improved bladder emptying, a more effective cough, and improved defecation, though long-term utility for appearance is still debatable.

33 Posterior Urethral Valves

Aseem R. Shukla and Arun K. Srinivasan

QUESTIONS

1. A newborn infant with a history of antenatal hydronephrosis and oligohydramnios is evaluated with a renal/bladder ultrasound and voiding cystourethrogram. All of the following are characteristic findings of posterior urethral valves EXCEPT:
   a. hypertrophy and apparent elevation of the bladder neck.
   b. multiple bladder diverticula
   c. bladder perforation with small amount of urinary extravasation causing ascites.
   d. rupture of an upper pole calyceal fornix causing distortion of the renal capsule.
   e. all of the above.

2. All of the following are true regarding antenatal diagnosis and management of posterior urethral valves EXCEPT:
   a. Thickened dilated bladder with bilateral upper tract dilation are pathognomonic findings.
   b. Significant renal cortical dysplasia is a contraindication to antenatal intervention.
   c. Vesicoamniotic shunting has been shown to improve renal failure rates.
   d. Early reports suggest that fetal cystoscopy and valve ablation might offer better outcomes than vesicoamniotic shunting.
   e. Antenatal interventions should only be offered in select cases as outcomes are not universally predictable.

3. A 6-month-old child with a history of posterior urethral valves has a serum creatinine of 1.4 mg/dL. He has a dilated, thick-walled bladder and hydroureteronephrosis on sonography and evidence of dilating vesicoureteral reflux with no remnant valves on voiding cystourethrography. Which of the following BEST explains the renal impairment noted in this child?
   a. Increased intravesical storage pressures transmitted to the ureter, renal pelvis, and glomerular units causing architectural and functional changes
   b. High-grade vesicoureteral reflux
   c. Repeated afebrile urinary tract infections
   d. Family history
   e. Likely misdiagnosis of hydronephrosis for concurrent autosomal dominant polycystic kidney disease

4. A newborn diagnosed with posterior urethral valves is noted on VCUG to have unilateral high-grade vesicoureteral reflux into the right kidney that has no measurable renal function on nuclear renography. The left kidney displays normal uptake and excretion of nuclear tracer. Which of the following best characterizes this boy's renal status?
   a. Better long-term renal function due to protective effect of reflux into dysplastic right kidney
   b. No better or worse long-term renal function, still requiring close observation
   c. High risk of febrile urinary tract infections will require early nephroureterectomy of nonfunctioning renal unit
   d. Plan early right ureteral reimplantation to reduce risk of pyelonephritis
   e. None of the above

5. All of the following findings on antenatal imaging should raise suspicion of posterior urethral valves EXCEPT:
   a. thickened bladder wall.
   b. bilateral pelvicaliectasis with ureterectasis.
   c. oligohydramnios.
   d. ambiguous genitalia.
   e. dilated posterior urethra (keyhole sign).

6. The most common cause of early neonatal mortality in a baby affected by posterior urethral valves is:
   a. urinary sepsis.
   b. end-stage renal disease not amenable to dialysis.
   c. pulmonary hypoplasia.
   d. urinary ascites due to calyx forniceal rupture.
   e. necrotizing enterocolitis.

7. A 3-year-old circumcised boy presents with urinary incontinence, stranguria, and occasional afebrile urinary tract infections. A renal ultrasound reveals moderate bilateral hydroureteronephrosis. The next most appropriate urological evaluation for this child would be:
   a. ordering a repeat renal ultrasound in 6 months.
   b. treatment of dysfunctional elimination syndrome with timed voiding and laxative.
   c. beginning an alpha receptor blocker.
   d. Botox injection to the external urethral sphincter.
   e. voiding cystourethrogram.

8. Fetal intervention for obstructive uropathy secondary to posterior urethral valves has been shown to:
   a. diminish the incidence of end-stage renal disease.
   b. be associated with a high rate of fetal demise.
   c. lead to improved pulmonary function in the neonate.
   d. be most effective when accomplished by open fetal surgery.
   e. be associated with neonatal respiratory failure.

9. A premature neonate with a weight of 2500 g with impaired renal function and bilateral hydroureteronephrosis (right greater than left) is diagnosed with posterior urethral valves. After 1 week of bladder catheterization, a plan is made to proceed to the operating room for valve ablation. Cystoscopy is precluded by the small genitalia. Which of the following is the preferred initial surgical option?
   a. Creation of a vesicostomy
   b. Bilateral proximal loop ureterostomy
   c. Cystotomy with antegrade valve ablation
   d. Suprapubic tube placement until child is old enough for valve ablation
   e. Bilateral percutaneous nephroureteral stent placement

10. A 4-year-old boy with a history of ablation of posterior urethral valves in infancy is volitionally voiding with no incontinence, stable renal function, and no urinary tract infections. He has high-grade vesicoureteric reflux on the left side with stable hydroureteronephrosis that has not changed since infancy. What is the best management for this child?

    a. Cross-trigonal ureteral reimplantation

    b. Vesicostomy

    c. Conservative management with timed voiding and anticholinergic therapy

    d. Cystoscopy with subureteral injection of Deflux

    e. Both a and d are correct

11. In cases of posterior urethral valves, the bladder transitions through three contractility patterns in childhood. Choose the correct order for the changes in bladder contractility.

    a. Detrusor hyperreflexia with high intravesical pressure; improved compliance with reduced intravesical pressures; high-capacity bladder and hypocontractility

    b. High-capacity bladder and hypocontractility; detrusor hyperreflexia with high intravesical pressure; improved compliance with reduced intravesical pressures

    c. Improved compliance with reduced intravesical pressures; high-capacity bladder and hypocontractility; detrusor hyperreflexia with high intravesical pressure

    d. High-capacity bladder and hypocontractility; improved compliance with reduced intravesical pressures; detrusor hyperreflexia with high intravesical pressure

    e. Detrusor hyperreflexia with high intravesical pressure; high-capacity bladder and hypocontractility; improved compliance with reduced intravesical pressures

12. All of the following are associated with the development of the valve bladder syndrome EXCEPT:

    a. High voiding pressures

    b. Incomplete bladder emptying with high post-void residuals

    c. Renal tubular and glomerular impairment

    d. Previous history of vesicostomy

    e. Bilateral hydroureteronephrosis

13. A child with a history of posterior urethral valves ablation suffers renal impairment and, ultimately, progresses to end-stage renal disease. All of the factors below likely characterized his clinical course EXCEPT:

    a. nadir creatinine at 1 year of life.

    b. renal dysplasia with or without vesicoureteral reflux.

    c. recurrent urinary tract infections.

    d. valve bladder syndrome.

    e. all of the above.

14. A 13-year-old boy with a history of posterior urethral valves progresses to end-stage renal disease and is a candidate for renal transplant. Of the complications listed below, which one may be most likely to occur in a child with a history of posterior urethral valves?

    a. Acute graft rejection

    b. Vesicoureteral reflux

    c. Chronic graft rejection

    d. Ureteral obstruction at site of ureteroneocystostomy

    e. All of the above

15. In a child with urethral duplication, all of the following are true EXCEPT:

    a. In a case of duplicated urethra, the ventral urethra is morphologically more normal in terms of caliber and function.

    b. Not all urethral duplications require surgical correction.

    c. Most children with urethral duplication present with incontinence.

    d. Children with urethral duplication are not at high risk for urinary tract infection.

    e. Can occur in both genders.

16. An 8-year-old boy presents with a few drops of blood at the urethral meatus at the end of voiding intermittently, over the past 3 months. Which of the following is true regarding the diagnosis of urethrorrhagia?

    a. Presents classically as painful hematuria

    b. Associated with an increased risk of urinary tract infection

    c. Cystoscopy is essential to locate a bladder or urethral source of bleeding and rule out the presence of a neoplasm.

    d. May be associated with dysfunctional elimination syndrome

    e. Renal and bladder ultrasonography is diagnostic

ANSWERS

1. **c. Bladder perforation with small amount of urinary extravasation causing ascites.** Fetal and neonatal lower urinary tract obstruction due to posterior urethral valves may transmit enough pressure to the upper urinary tract to cause a rupture of a calyceal fornix causing urine to be trapped within the renal capsule or cause ascites, in rare cases. However, bladder perforation is not a characteristic of posterior urethral valves, since the process actually leads to significant bladder wall hypertrophy.

2. **c. Vesicoamniotic shunting has been shown to improve renal failure rates.** Thickened dilated bladder and bilateral upper tract dilation imply posterior urethral valves with high sensitivity. Criteria for intervention include favorable urinary chemistry, a singleton pregnancy, normal karyotype, and absence of significant dysplasia. Antenatal intervention includes vesicoamniotic shunting and fetal cystoscopic ablation. Vesicoamniotic shunting is associated with an increased incidence of live births in the severely affected fetus, but is not correlated with decreasing the risk of renal failure. Early reports suggest fetal cystoscopy and ablation are more accurate in diagnosing valve patients and thus have better outcomes. Experience in antenatal intervention is early and varied and hence should only be offered in highly selected cases.

3. **a. Increased intravesical storage pressures transmitted to the ureter, renal pelvis, and glomerular units causing architectural and functional changes.** Sustained increases in intravesical storage pressure over prolonged time intervals transmit these pressures to the ureter, renal pelvis, and, ultimately, glomerular units. Of the options provided, this is the most likely etiology of renal insufficiency in this child.

4. **b. No better or worse long-term renal function, still requiring close observation.** Contrary to previous assumptions, the so-called vesicoureteric reflux and dysplasia (VURD) syndrome is not a renal protective phenomenon. These children often have evidence of renal dysplasia detectable in the solitary functioning kidney, increasing the likelihood of significant long-term renal impairment.

5. **d. Ambiguous genitalia.** All of the aforementioned findings are characteristic findings of posterior urethral valves on antenatal imaging, except ambiguous genitalia. Posterior urethral valves are not associated with external genital anomalies.

6. **c. Pulmonary hypoplasia.** While the focus in posterior urethral valves is too often on the lower urinary tract and kidneys, the most profound complication and cause of perinatal mortality in infants affected by severe lower urinary tract obstruction remains pulmonary hypoplasia.

7. **e. Voiding cystourethrogram.** Despite the ubiquity of antenatal imaging today, delayed presentation of posterior urethral valves after 6 months of age is not uncommon. A high index of

suspicion for posterior urethral valves must be assumed when a boy presents with lower urinary tract symptoms, especially recurrent urinary tract infections, but also overflow incontinence, gross hematuria, renal dysfunction, and, less commonly, ejaculatory dysfunction.

8. **c. Lead to improved pulmonary function in the neonate.** Fetal intervention for posterior urethral valves has not been shown to lower the incidence of end-stage renal disease, but, in properly selected cases, it can offer the benefit of improved neonatal pulmonary function. Neonates with severe obstructive uropathy die of respiratory failure due to a noncompliant and hypoplastic lung.

9. **a. Creation of a vesicostomy.** In the low-birth-weight infant with renal impairment and whose urethra will not accommodate an infant cystoscope, a vesicostomy is the ideal first option. The vesicostomy allows decompression of the obstructed system, allows continued bladder cycling, and is easily managed with diapers. Upper tract diversion is a reasonable option, but does require bilateral incisions and also a complex follow-up surgery that can risk injury to the developing ureters.

10. **c. Conservative management with timed voiding and anticholinergic therapy.** Vesicoureteral reflux in children with posterior urethral valves is a common finding and should be understood to be a consequence of neonatal obstruction and the secondarily elevated bladder pressures. Management of this child should be centered on the lower urinary tract with attention to timed voiding, double voiding, and anticholinergics as necessary. Ureteral reimplantation is an option in atypical cases where urinary tract infections continue despite maximal bladder therapy.

11. **a. Detrusor hyperreflexia with high intravesical pressure; improved compliance with reduced intravesical pressures; high-capacity bladder and hypocontractility.** The bladder evolves through three distinct contractility patterns through childhood: (1) detrusor hyperreflexia in infancy and early childhood; (2) decreasing intravesical pressures and improved compliance bladder in childhood; (3) increased capacity bladder with hypocontractility and atony in adolescence.

12. **d. Previous history of vesicostomy.** The theory of the valve bladder syndrome holds that while the bladder initially compensates for outlet obstruction by generating high voiding pressures, it begins to experience higher volumes of urine due to increasing urine production as the child grows. The polyuria

due to nephrogenic diabetes insipidus secondary to evolving renal impairment augments the urine volumes entering a bladder that is increasingly unable to empty completely. As the post-void residuals increase, the bladder no longer enjoys periods of complete relaxation, and the detrusor fibers are continuously in a state of partial or complete stretch, beginning a cascade of gene expression and phenotypic changes that further impair contractility of the bladder. Creation of a vesicostomy does not impair bladder contractility.

13. **e. All of the above.** Risk factors known to affect the prognosis of an infant diagnosed with posterior urethral valves include age at diagnosis, renal dysplasia with or without vesicoureteral reflux, nadir creatinine during first year of life, recurrent urinary tract infections, and bladder dysfunction.

14. **d. Ureteral obstruction at site of ureteroneocystostomy.** The thickened bladder wall of posterior urethral valve patients may contribute to the significantly increased incidence of ureteral obstruction on univariate and multivariate analysis compared to a non–posterior urethral valve transplant cohort, but recent studies saw no risk of increased graft loss or patient death despite ureteral obstruction, stenting, or dilation.

15. **c. Most children with urethral duplication present with incontinence.** Most children with urethral duplication are continent since most duplications occur distal to the urethral sphincter. Although more common in boys, rare reports of female urethral duplications are seen in the literature. Urinary tract infection is not commonly seen in urethral duplication. Blind ending duplications or duplications where both urethra end in or near the orthotopic location do not need surgical correction. Clinical presentation with significant functional abnormalities require surgical reconstruction.

16. **d. May be associated with dysfunctional elimination syndrome.** Urethrorrhagia presents classically as bleeding at the end of urination, or with a blood stain in the underwear with no association of pain. It is not associated with urinary tract infection. Diagnosis is clinically rendered, based on history and examination and exclusion of other potential causes of gross hematuria. Cystoscopy is not essential for diagnosis, and there are no diagnostic radiological imaging exams. There is a significant association with voiding dysfunction, and improving voiding parameters have been shown to improve symptoms and resolve urethrorrhagia.

CHAPTER REVIEW

1. Type 1 valves are the most common variant of posterior urethral valves, and appear as leaflets that arise from the verumontanum and fuse anteriorly just proximal to the external urethral sphincter.
2. Type 3 valves present as a congenitally obstructing membrane that is likely perforated at the time of the initial postnatal catheterization.
3. The incidence of posterior urethral valves is between 1.6 and 2.1 per 10,000 births.
4. There is an emerging understanding of the genetic basis for posterior urethral valves, particularly associated with chromosome 11 and copy number variants.
5. The renal dysfunction, vesicoureteral reflux, and voiding dysfunction seen in children with posterior urethral valves is mediated by a dysfunctional bladder.
6. Renal impairment in posterior urethral valve patients is due to renal dysplasia and obstructive uropathy.
7. The vesicoureteral reflux and dysplasia (VURD) syndrome confers no protective benefit on long-term renal prognosis. Antenatal diagnosis is primarily by fetal ultrasound sometimes aided by fetal MRI. Combination of thickened dilated bladder with upper tract dilation along with oligohydramnios has a high sensitivity for posterior urethral valves.
8. Postnatal diagnosis is with ultrasound and finding confirmed by fluoroscopic voiding cystourethrogram. More recently, contrast-enhanced voiding ultrasonogram is emerging as a good alternative.
9. Biochemical evaluation centers on electrolyte and creatinine values. Nadir creatinine value is an effective prognostic indicator for long-term kidney function.
10. Up to 50% of infants with posterior urethral valves are diagnosed in the antenatal period.
11. Severity of obstruction can be objectively assessed by the volume of amniotic fluid, degree of renal dysplasia, and fetal urinary markers.
12. Vesicoamniotic shunting may have a survival benefit for the infant in select cases, but there is no clear benefit in the risk for renal failure.
13. Antenatal finding of a thickened bladder and bilateral ureterectasis should be evaluated with early postnatal ultrasound and voiding cystourethrogram.
14. VCUG in valve patient will show bladder wall irregularity, hypertrophied, elevated bladder neck, and dilated and elongated posterior urethra.
15. The most common cause of early mortality in infants with posterior urethral valves is pulmonary hypoplasia.
16. Cystoscopy with valve ablation is the preferred initial treatment for posterior urethral valves.
17. Vesicostomy does not inhibit bladder cycling, as the bladder continues to contract, but is reserved for select cases where valve ablation is not possible.
18. High urinary diversion offers no renal protective benefit and requires a complex secondary procedure to reverse the diversion.
19. Circumcision should be encouraged as a prophylactic measure for any boy with posterior urethral valves, and especially any boy with a history of urinary tract infection.
20. The focus of management for vesicoureteral reflux in a child with valves should be centered on the bladder, and ureteral reimplantation is rarely offered.
21. The bladder evolves through three patterns in boys with valves: (1) detrusor hyperreflexia in infancy and early childhood; (2) decreasing intravesical pressures and improved compliance bladder in childhood; (3) increased capacity bladder with hypocontractility and atony in adolescence.
22. Videourodynamics is completed in boys with valves especially when there is a clinical change, such as increasing upper tract dilation or recurrent urinary tract infections.
23. Overnight bladder drainage is considered in the scenario of increasing post-void residuals, urinary tract infections, or worsening hydronephrosis and renal function.
24. An antenatal vesicoamniotic shunt can be considered in select patients with bladder wall thickening, hydroureteronephrosis, and oligohydramnios. While it may reduce the severity of pulmonary hypoplasia, the procedure confers no protection from renal impairment.
25. A nadir serum creatinine at 1 year of less than 0.8 mg/dL confers a significantly decreased risk of developing end-stage renal disease.
26. Transplantation into a valve-affected bladder may carry a higher risk of ureteral obstruction, but there is no increased risk of graft loss compared to controls.
27. Anterior urethral valves and urethral atresia are less common causes of lower urinary tract obstruction (LUTO), and long-term outcomes can be similar to those of posterior urethral valves if the neonate survives.
28. Dysfunctional voiding causing a turbulent urinary flow may lead to urethrorrhagia.
29. Treatment for urethrorrhagia should focus on improving voiding habits and conservative management, reserving cystoscopy for refractory cases, and when there is significant straining during voiding.
30. An infant diagnosed with anorectal malformation should undergo a renal ultrasound as well as VCUG due to the high risk of associated genitourinary anomalies.

34

Neuromuscular Dysfunction of the Lower Urinary Tract in Children

Carlos R. Estrada and Stuart B. Bauer

QUESTIONS

1. Which of the following is an acquired form of neuromuscular dysfunction of the lower urinary tract?
   a. Myelomeningocele
   b. Cerebral palsy
   c. Lipomeningocele
   d. Sacral agenesis
   e. Anorectal malformation

2. What is the primary goal in management of neuromuscular dysfunction of the lower urinary tract?
   a. Achievement of urinary continence
   b. Achievement of fecal continence
   c. Preservation of renal function
   d. Facilitation of sexual function
   e. Avoidance of urinary tract infection

3. The International Children's Continence Society (ICCS) recommends more frequent evaluation of children during periods of high rates of somatic growth when spinal cord tethering is more likely. These two development periods are:
   a. newborn to toddler AND toddler to adolescent.
   b. newborn to toddler AND adolescent to adult.
   c. newborn to toddler AND adulthood.
   d. toddler to adolescent AND adolescent to adult.
   e. toddler to adolescent AND adulthood.

4. The ICCS's indications for repeat investigations prior the routinely scheduled follow-up for neuromuscular dysfunction of the lower urinary tract do NOT include:
   a. urinary tract infections.
   b. development or worsening of hydronephrosis.
   c. worsening continence.
   d. change in lower extremity function.
   e. improved continence.

5. Which of the following may compromise bladder emptying in neuromuscular dysfunction of the lower urinary tract?
   a. Low capacity
   b. Low compliance
   c. Detrusor overactivity
   d. Detrusor sphincter dyssynergia
   e. Low outlet resistance

6. Initial minimally invasive treatment options to address inadequate bladder storage in neuromuscular dysfunction in children usually involves:
   a. overnight indwelling catheter drainage.
   b. antimuscarinics and clean intermittent catheterization (CIC).

   c. percutaneous cystostomy tube.
   d. endoscopic injection of botulinum toxin.
   e. robotic-assisted augmentation cystoplasty.

7. The use of antimuscarinics for the treatment of detrusor over-activity in children does NOT result in the following:
   a. Increased bladder capacity
   b. Decreased number of bladder contractions
   c. Decreased number of incontinence episodes
   d. Decreased number of catheterizations
   e. Decreased volume to first bladder contraction

8. A possible predictor of poor clinical response to intravesical injection of botulinum toxin injection is preexisting:
   a. low maximum cystometric capacity.
   b. detrusor overactivity.
   c. more than five episodes of incontinence per day.
   d. poor detrusor compliance.
   e. previous botulinum toxin injections.

9. Which of the following increases the risk of developing lower urinary tract stones in children with bladder augmentation?
   a. Use of the ileal segment
   b. Routine bladder irrigation with water or saline
   c. Use of an antimuscarinic
   d. Catheterization of the urethra, rather than an abdominal stoma
   e. A mobile patient

10. The presentation of bladder malignancy in those with a history of bladder augmentation does NOT include:
    a. presenting with advanced disease.
    b. presenting at an older age than is typical for bladder malignancies.
    c. presenting with atypical symptoms such as vague abdominal pain, urosepsis or increased frequency of urinary tract infection (UTI), difficult catheterization, and renal failure.
    d. presenting with a time lag of a minimum of 10 years after a bladder augmentation.
    e. presenting with atypical signs such as new hydronephrosis and bladder wall thickening.

11. Which of the following is the preferred approach to increase bladder capacity in children with neuromuscular dysfunction of the lower urinary tract?
    a. Autoaugmentation
    b. Enteric augmentation with a gastric segment
    c. Tissue engineered bladder substitute
    d. Enteric augmentation with an ileal segment
    e. Enteric augmentation with an ileal-cecal segment

12. Worsening of bladder function after isolated bladder neck procedures including implantation of an artificial urinary sphincter or bladder neck fascial sling is more common in those with:
    a. preexisting detrusor overactivity and poor compliance.
    b. preexisting low maximum cystometric capacity.
    c. surgery in the post-pubertal period.
    d. detrusor sphincter dyssynergia.
    e. history of prior bladder neck outlet procedures.

13. Which of the following is NOT an acceptable method of managing high-grade vesicoureteral reflux in children with neuromuscular dysfunction of the lower urinary tract?
    a. CIC
    b. Antimuscarinics
    c. Antibiotic prophylaxis
    d. Ureteral re-implantation
    e. Bladder emptying by the Credé maneuver

14. Prenatal surgery for children with myelomeningocele compared to standard post-natal closure has been noted to result in:
    a. an increased risk of fetal death and need for cerebrospinal fluid shunting.
    b. worsening of mental development and motor function at 30 months.
    c. fewer pregnancy complications.
    d. a lower risk of preterm labor.
    e. no improvement in bladder function.

15. Indications for the initiation of CIC in the newborn with myelomeningocele do NOT include:
    a. post-void residual urine measurement of 3 mL after the Credé maneuver.
    b. post-void residual urine measurement of 10 mL after spontaneous voiding.
    c. the presence of detrusor sphincter dyssynergia on urodynamic studies.
    d. the presence of hydronephrosis and high-grade vesicoureteral reflux with poor bladder emptying.
    e. poor bladder compliance with bladder filling pressures greater than 40 cm of water.

16. The highest risk for the development of urinary tract deterioration in children with myelodysplasia is in those with initial urodynamic findings of:
    a. detrusor sphincter synergy.
    b. detrusor sphincter dyssynergy.
    c. complete denervation.
    d. low maximum cystometric capacity.
    e. detrusor overactivity.

17. The gold standard for measuring renal function in children with spina bifida is:
    a. serum creatinine.
    b. glomerular filtration rate as estimated by the Schwarz formula.
    c. glomerular filtration rate as estimated by the Schwartz formula.
    d. serum cystatin C.
    e. nuclear renography.

18. Sexual function and satisfaction in men with myelomeningocele is better with the following condition:
    a. Living with their parents
    b. Severe incontinence

    c. A sacral level lesion of the neural tube defect
    d. A thoracic level lesion of the neural tube defect
    e. The presence of hydrocephalus

19. The most common finding associated with an occult neural tube defect is:
    a. a cutaneous abnormality overlying the lower spine.
    b. high-arched feet.
    c. claw or hammer toes.
    d. abnormal gait.
    e. absent perineal sensation.

20. In a 1-year-old child, definitive diagnosis of an occult neural tube defect can be made by:
    a. spinal ultrasound.
    b. urodynamic studies demonstrating findings consistent with neurogenic bladder dysfunction.
    c. magnetic resonance imaging of the spine.
    d. documentation of resolution of abnormal urodynamic findings after a detethering procedure.
    e. abnormal electromyography of the external urinary sphincter.

21. Which of the following is UNLIKELY to be noted in a child with neuromuscular dysfunction of the lower urinary tract secondary to sacral agenesis?
    a. Urinary incontinence
    b. A maternal history of diabetes mellitus or gestational diabetes
    c. Flattened buttocks and a short, low gluteal cleft
    d. Absent perineal sensation
    e. Vesicoureteral reflux and recurrent urinary tract infections

22. Urodynamic studies of children with an anorectal malformation should be performed in all of the following circumstances EXCEPT:
    a. a bony malformation of the spine or a spinal cord defect.
    b. hydronephrosis.
    c. vesicoureteral reflux.
    d. urinary or fecal incontinence.
    e. a low insertion of the fistulous site.

23. The following statement concerning bladder function in children with cerebral palsy is TRUE:
    a. They achieve nighttime urinary continence first.
    b. They achieve urinary continence at the same age as their age-adjusted peers.
    c. Lower urinary tract symptoms are more common in younger children.
    d. The most common urinary tract symptom is monosymptomatic nocturnal enuresis.
    e. Clinical symptoms of recurrent UTI and detrusor sphincter dyssynergia (retention, interrupted stream, and hesitancy) are associated with upper urinary tract deterioration.

24. The most common presenting urinary symptom in children with transverse myelitis is:
    a. urinary incontinence.
    b. urinary tract infection.
    c. urinary retention.
    d. urinary frequency.
    e. urinary urgency.

ANSWERS

1. **b. Cerebral palsy.** Cerebral palsy is the only acquired disease process on the list. The remainder are congenital.
2. **c. Preservation of renal function.** Although the other listed goals have important clinical and social implications, preservation of renal function is the primary goal of treatment. Achievement of urinary/fecal continence, sexual function, and avoidance of urinary tract infection are secondary goals of treatment.
3. **b. Newborn to toddler AND adolescent to adult.** The correct combination of growth periods in which the rate of somatic growth is highest is in the newborn to toddler and adolescent to adult age group. This recommendation is due to the fact that the highest rate of spinal cord tethering, and thus a change in bladder/bowel function, is during periods of highest somatic growth.
4. **e. Improved continence.** Urinary tract infections, hydronephrosis, worsening continence, and a change in lower extremity function are more likely to indicate a significant change in bladder function than improved continence.
5. **d. Detrusor sphincter dyssynergia.** Detrusor sphincter dyssynergia is the only entity listed that may compromise bladder emptying. All other listed options would facilitate or encourage early bladder emptying.
6. **b. Antimuscarinics and clean intermittent catheterization (CIC).** The beneficial effects of early initiation of antimuscarinics and CIC are well established. The other listed options would be considered to be more invasive or less established methods of intervention.
7. **e. Decreased volume to first bladder contraction.** Antimuscarinics in children result in increased bladder capacity, fewer bladder contractions, less incontinence, and catheterizations. The question is worded negatively; (e) is correct as antimuscarinics would be expected to increase the volume to first bladder contraction, rather than to decrease it.
8. **d. Poor detrusor compliance.** Kask et al. (2013) demonstrated that preexisting poor detrusor compliance predicts a poor clinical response to intravesical injection of botulinum toxin. One could postulate that the histologic changes that are present after the development of poor detrusor compliance are not amenable to the effects of botulinum toxin.
9. **a. Use of the ileal segment.** The use of an ileal segment has been shown to increase the risk of lower urinary tract stones. Catheterization through the urethra, rather than via an abdominal stoma, is associated with fewer lower urinary tract stones, presumably because of better drainage. A mobile patient and routine bladder irrigation decrease the risk of stones. The use of an antimuscarinic should not affect stone formation.
10. **b. Presenting at an older age than is typical for bladder malignancies.** Those with bladder augmentation present at a younger age, with atypical symptoms and advanced disease, usually with a minimum 10-year lag time between augmentation and presentation of bladder malignancy.
11. **d. Enteric augmentation with an ileal segment.** Lack of improvement in urodynamic and clinical symptoms, along with a high failure rate, makes autoaugmentation an undesirable option. Gastric segments are associated with more symptomatic side effects (such as hematuria dysuria syndrome) and metabolic complications than ileal segments. It is recommended to avoid the ileal-cecal segment in children with neural tube defects because it may aggravate bowel dysfunction. Phase II studies of tissue-engineered bladder revealed no improvement in urodynamic parameters and serious adverse events. Thus, the ileal segment is the most desirable for enteric augmentation.
12. **a. Preexisting detrusor overactivity and poor compliance.** Isolated bladder neck procedures such as artificial urinary sphincter and bladder neck repairs have been noted to lead to worsening of bladder function in up to 30% of patients, especially those with preexisting detrusor overactivity and poor compliance. The remaining answers have not been associated with worsening of bladder function after isolated bladder neck procedures.
13. **e. Bladder emptying by the Credé maneuver.** Children with a reactive external urinary sphincter will have a reflex response of increased external urethral tone in response to the Credé maneuver that can aggravate reflux and thus is contraindicated in this group. The other listed options are all reasonable methods of managing vesicoureteral reflux in those with neuromuscular dysfunction of the lower urinary tract.
14. **e. No improvement in bladder function.** Prenatal surgery for children with myelomeningocele compared to standard post-natal closure has been noted to decrease the need for cerebrospinal fluid shunting, improve neuromotor function, and increase pregnancy complications and the risk for preterm labor. The correct answer is there is no improvement in lower urinary tract function with prenatal versus postnatal closure.
15. **a. Post-void residual urine measurement of 3 mL after the Credé maneuver.** A post-void residual urine measurement on 3 mL after the Credé maneuver is within normal limits and does not require the initiation of CIC. All other possible answers are indications for the initiation of CIC.
16. **b. Detrusor sphincter dyssynergy.** Within the first 3 years of life, over 70% of children with detrusor sphincter dyssynergy will have urinary tract deterioration, whereas less than one-quarter of those with synergy or complete denervation will have deterioration. Low maximum cystometric capacity and detrusor overactivity have not been associated with upper tract deterioration.
17. **e. Nuclear renography.** Although all possible answers are means of measuring renal function in children with myelodysplasia, nuclear renography is considered to be the gold standard.
18. **c. A sacral level lesion of the neural tube defect.** Lesions above the sacral spinal cord, hydrocephalus, incontinence, and living with your parents are associated with less sexual function and satisfaction compared to men with a sacral level lesion.
19. **a. A cutaneous abnormality overlying the lower spine.** A cutaneous abnormality overlying the spine such as a skin dimple, tuft of hair, skin tag, lipoma, vascular malformation, or asymmetric gluteal cleft is noted in 90% of those with occult neural tube defect. The other listed answers are also noted as part of this entity but their occurrence is much less frequent.
20. **c. Magnetic resonance imaging of the spine.** Spinal ultrasound may be utilized prior to ossification of vertebral bones (3 months of age). After this time point, magnetic resonance imaging of the spine is required for definitive diagnosis of an occult neural tube defect.
21. **d. Absent perineal sensation.** Most children with sacral agenesis have preserved perineal sensation, thus they are UNLIKELY to have absent perineal sensation. The other listed answers are all potential presenting features of a child with sacral agenesis.
22. **e. A low insertion of the fistulous site.** Urodynamic evaluation in those with anorectal malformation is indicated if there is suggestion of possible spinal cord tethering (bony malformation of the spine or spinal cord defect) or signs and/or symptoms that might indicate a neurogenic defect such as hydronephrosis, vesicoureteral reflux, or urinary/fecal incontinence. Although spinal cord defects may be present in up to a third of those with a low insertion of the fistula site, a low insertion site itself is not an indication for urodynamic study.
23. **e. Clinical symptoms of recurrent UTI and detrusor sphincter dyssynergia (retention, interrupted stream, and hesitancy) are associated with upper urinary tract deterioration.** Children with cerebral palsy usually achieve daytime dryness first, at an age later than their age-adjusted peers. Lower urinary tract symptoms become more prevalent in children with cerebral palsy as they age. The most common symptom in these children is incontinence. Clinical symptoms of recurrent UTI and detrusor sphincter dyssynergia are associated with upper urinary tract deterioration and may warrant investigation with renal/bladder ultrasound and urodynamic studies.
24. **c.** The most common presenting urinary symptom of transverse myelitis is urinary retention. Ninety-five percent of children in the acute phase of the disease will have urinary retention.

CHAPTER REVIEW

1. Renal ultrasonography and measurement of residual urine are performed as early as possible after birth. Initial evaluation can be compared with findings on subsequent assessments, so that early signs of deterioration of urinary tract function and drainage, or of progressive neurologic denervation, can be detected.

2. Infants at risk for urinary tract deterioration as a result of a poorly compliant or overactive detrusor or outflow obstruction from detrusor-sphincter dyssynergia need to be identified. This determines the need to initiate prophylactic measures before any deterioration in upper urinary tract architecture and function take place.

3. Three categories of lower urinary tract (LUT) dynamics may be detected: synergic (26%), dyssynergic with and without poor detrusor compliance (37%), and complete denervation (36%).

4. Early intervention with CIC and antimuscarinics improves urodynamic parameters and decreases the rate of UTI, vesicoureteral reflux (VUR), upper urinary tract deterioration, and the incidence of end-stage renal disease.

5. Cystatin C is superior to serum creatinine in monitoring renal function in children with neural tube defects. Renography is the gold standard for estimating glomerular filtration rate (GFR).

6. Determinants of risk of renal dysfunction in spina bifida include: detrusor sphincter dyssynergia, high detrusor pressures, detrusor overactivity, febrile UTIs, and vesicoureteral reflux. These entities should be actively managed to minimize risk of renal functional decline.

7. The primary goal of management is preservation of renal function. Secondary goals of management include urinary/fecal continence, avoidance of urinary tract infection, and facilitation of sexual function and fertility.

8. Preservation of renal function is achieved by maintaining low bladder filling pressures and active management of vesicoureteral reflux and avoidance of urinary tract infection.

9. The International Children's Continence Society recommendations for follow-up are based on developmental stages and the relative risk for secondary spinal cord tethering.

10. The CDC-endorsed multicenter collaborative has published a protocol for the management of patients with neurogenic bladder ages from birth to 5 years.

11. Minimally invasive approaches should precede the use of more invasive therapies to address bladder failure to store urine efficiently or empty effectively. Antimuscarinic therapy and CIC are the mainstay of therapy.

12. Bladder filling pressures should be maintained below 30 cm H_2O as much as possible to prevent upper urinary tract deterioration.

13. Intravesical injection of botulinum toxin is well tolerated and avoids the need for more invasive treatment options in a high proportion of children with minimal side effects.

14. Enterocystoplasty is an effective option to prevent upper urinary tract deterioration but comes with a high risk of complications.

15. Patients undergoing isolated bladder neck procedures (artificial urinary sphincter and bladder neck sling) may develop detrusor overactivity and poor compliance that leads to upper urinary tract deterioration, mandating close follow-up.

16. Low-grade reflux in those who are emptying well without outlet resistance can be managed with antibiotic prophylaxis alone. High-grade reflux or those who do not empty well also require CIC.

17. Those with poor compliance with or without hydronephrosis should be started on antimuscarinics.

18. The Credé maneuver is contraindicated in patients with reflux who have a reactive external urethral sphincter.

19. Indications for antireflux surgery are similar to those for children without neurogenic bladder. Success rates are similar if effective bladder emptying is addressed.

20. Children with an occult neural tube defect often present after age 3 or 4 years with incontinence or constipation. They may present with new urologic symptoms after a growth spurt related to tethering of the spinal cord. Most have a cutaneous abnormality overlying the spine.

21. Radiologic examination of the spine, MRI, and renal US are indicated in the initial evaluation. A spinal US may be used as a screening investigation prior to MRI in those less than 3 months of age.

22. Urodynamic studies should be done before and after spinal cord detethering.

23. Intervention with spinal cord detethering early in life is associated with better outcomes than when done at a later age.

24. Spinal cord abnormalities including a tethered spinal cord, thickened or fatty filum terminale, and a lipoma occur in 18% to 50% of patients with an anorectal malformation.

25. The incidence of LUTS in children with cerebral palsy is 16% to 94%, and the most common symptom is urinary incontinence.

26. In patients with spinal cord injury, there is an acute phase of spinal shock wherein the bladder is often acontractile and the urethral sphincter nonreactive; with resolution of spinal shock, an overactive detrusor and bladder-sphincter dyssynergy most commonly develop.

27. Patients with a cervical or thoracic spine lesion above T6 are likely to exhibit autonomic dysreflexia during bladder filling and detrusor contractions.

35

Functional Disorders of the Lower Urinary Tract in Children

Paul F. Austin and Abhishek Seth

QUESTIONS

1. A 9-year old girl presents to the office with a chief complaint of daytime urinary incontinence. She denies dysuria, hematuria, or enuresis. She has never had a urinary tract infection (UTI) and there is no history of hydronephrosis. Her mother states that toilet training occurred at 2 years of age and was "easy." A clean-catch urinalysis has been obtained by her pediatrician and is completely normal. When characterizing the incontinence, she states that she completely soaks her clothes, necessitating a change in wardrobe. She denies urgency or frequency and otherwise voids every 2 to 3 hours during the day. She states that the episodes are often associated with laughing at a funny joke or movie. She denies any issues with constipation. Assuming physical examination and voiding diary are normal, which of the following would be a reasonable first-line treatment strategy?

   a. Acupuncture

   b. Biofeedback

   c. Hypnosis

   d. Imipramine

   e. Oxybutynin

2. A 4-year-old girl presents to the office with a chief complaint of labial adhesions, dysuria, daytime urinary incontinence, and recurrent UTIs. Her mother states that toilet training was completed at 20 months and that there were no issues with this. Based on history and completed voiding diary, her elimination pattern is normal. Her mother states that during the past 3 months, however, she has noted that her underpants are damp and that this is often noted within a few minutes of the child having voided. They deny any urgency or frequency. She recently has been complaining of severe dysuria with two urinalyses (UAs) in the past 4 weeks demonstrating 5 to 10 white blood cells per high-power field (WBCs/hpf). Urine cultures have all been negative, and antibiotics have not helped with symptomatology. Physical examination reveals superficial labial adhesions with moderately erythematous external genitalia. Noninvasive urodynamics with pelvic ultrasound and uroflowmetry reveal a bell-shaped curve and an empty bladder with normal wall thickness. There is a small amount of fluid noted in the vagina. While the child climbs down off of the examining room table, there is involuntary leakage of urine. Repeat pelvic ultrasound reveals that the vaginal vault is empty. What is the most likely diagnosis?

   a. Bladder-bowel dysfunction

   b. Dysfunctional voiding

   c. Urge urinary incontinence

   d. Vaginal reflux

   e. Vesicoureteral reflux (VUR)

3. An 8-year-old boy is brought in by his grandmother, who recently obtained guardianship due to parental divorce and the biological mother's recent untimely death. She states that his teachers have been complaining that for the last 4 months he spends most of his time in the restroom, asking to use the bathroom approximately every 15 minutes. He has had some occasional dysuria, but no hematuria or fevers. They deny any UTIs or daytime urinary incontinence. He has occasional constipation, but this is readily corrected with fruit juice and he generally has one soft, smooth bowel movement daily. He is generally able to sleep through the night without having to wake to void, and they deny enuresis. The element in the history that will most often be able to distinguish pollakiuria from overactive bladder (OAB) is:

   a. a recent life event.

   b. male versus female gender.

   c. no history of UTIs.

   d. no urinary incontinence.

   e. the child does not wake to void.

4. Lower urinary tract (LUT) dysfunction is associated with which of the following?

   a. Constipation

   b. Neuropsychiatric issues

   c. UTIs

   d. VUR

   e. All of the above

5. The purported mechanism of action for botulinum toxin in the treatment of children and adolescents with dysfunctional voiding is:

   a. reducing the frequency and intensity of uninhibited detrusor contractions during the filling phase of the bladder.

   b. smooth muscle relaxation at the bladder neck.

   c. paralysis of striated muscle of the external sphincter.

   d. stabilization of the motor end plate, inhibiting spinal cord feedback loops.

   e. none of the above.

6. A 7-year-old girl presents to your office with a 6-month history of recurrent UTIs, daytime urinary incontinence, urgency, dysuria, and enuresis. Mother states that her daughter will have wet underwear and clothes 3 to 4 times per week. She is also wet 5 out of 7 nights per week. Mother states that she will often "wait until the last minute" to void. There are no febrile UTIs, and urine cultures from her pediatrician's office reveal multiple organisms on 2 separate occasions in the last 3 months. A renal/bladder ultrasound demonstrates normal upper urinary tracts. Urinalysis in the office is negative and uroflow shows staccato waveform. You initiate behavioral modification and she returns 6 weeks later with improvement but remains wet during the day 1 time per week with urinary urgency and wets the bed 2 nights per week. The best next step is:

   a. anticholinergics.

   b. moisture alarm.

   c. alpha blockers.

   d. biofeedback.

   e. botulinum toxin.

7. Which of the following organ systems is implicated in the pathogenesis of enuresis?

   a. Bladder

   b. Brain

  c. Kidney

  d. All of the above

  e. None of the above

8. An 8-year-old boy presents to your office with his parents for consultation regarding treatment for primary nocturnal enuresis. Behavioral modification, desmopressin, and the enuresis alarm have failed. Which of the following parameters is the best predictor of response to treatment with desmopressin?

  a. Age of child

  b. Bladder capacity

  c. Motivation of family

  d. Nocturnal polyuria

  e. Poor arousal

ANSWERS

1 **b. Biofeedback.** Giggle incontinence (enuresis risoria) is an uncommon form of daytime incontinence and is classically seen in school-aged females. Typically, there is moderate to large amounts of urinary leakage triggered by laughing alone. The incontinence episodes are invariably significant, and often the entire bladder volume is drained. Daytime urinary incontinence in conjunction with laughter is also seen in children with OAB and is more common than true giggle incontinence. It is a diagnosis of exclusion and is usually established on history and is supplemented by the absence of other voiding symptoms and normal investigations. Currently, available treatment strategies include biofeedback or methylphenidate.

2 **d. Vaginal reflux.** Vaginal reflux (vaginal entrapment, vaginal voiding) is characterized by incontinence following normal voiding in the absence of other LUT symptoms. It is commonly seen in prepubertal girls, and the typical history is that of wetting of undergarments approximately 10 to 15 minutes following a normal void. It can often be associated with labial adhesions because of chronic irritation and inflammation from skin exposure to relatively caustic urine. Reassurance and postural modification to ensure complete vaginal emptying is the only treatment that is required.

3 **e. The child does not wake to void.** Pollakiuria is a disorder characterized by a very high daytime frequency of micturition (sometimes as high as 50 times per day). A key aspect of this syndrome, which differentiates it from OAB and can often clinch the diagnosis, is that the symptoms are limited to the daytime. It is seen in early childhood (4 to 6 years of age) in both genders and associated with a history of recent death or life-threatening event in the family. Usually, it runs a benign, self-limited course during a period of approximately 6 months.

4 **e. All of the above.** There are long-standing, clear associations between LUT dysfunction and bowel dysfunction, UTIs, VUR, and various psychiatric diagnoses. The incomplete bladder emptying that occurs in children with LUT dysfunction can lead to urinary stasis, with subsequent UTIs causing inflammatory changes in the bladder wall that stimulate hypertrophy and overactivity. It has been theorized that detrusor hypertrophy can alter the closure mechanism at the ureterovesical junction (UVJ), leading to reflux. It has also been shown that ongoing issues with bowel-bladder dysfunction can have a negative effect on VUR resolution rates, and that addressing bowel dysfunction alone can positively influence LUT function. Finally, clinicians should be cognizant of the association between neuropsychiatric diagnoses and daytime wetting, as the former is likely to interfere with treatment success of the latter.

5 **c. Paralysis of striated muscle of the external sphincter.** Botulinum-A toxin acts by inhibiting acetylcholine (ACh) release at the presynaptic neuromuscular junction. Inhibited ACh release results in regionally decreased muscle contractility and atrophy at the injection site, which in the case of dysfunctional voiding would be the striated muscle of the external urinary sphincter. The chemical denervation that ensues is a reversible process, and eventually the toxin is inactivated and removed. Clinical effects begin within 5 to 7 days of injection, with maximal effects reached within 4 to 6 weeks. The duration of induced paralysis varies depending on the type of muscle treated, with duration of treatment effect lasting between 3 and 12 months.

6 **d. Biofeedback.** All patients with lower urinary tract dysfunction (LUTD) should receive behavioral modification as treatment. A uroflow showing a staccato waveform along with incomplete emptying is consistent with dysfunctional voiding. Biofeedback is particularly valuable in the treatment of dysfunctional voiding and improves LUTD by coordinating the pelvic floor muscle activity and abdominal muscle activity to promote efficient bladder emptying.

7 **d. All of the above.** The three organ systems implicated in the pathogenesis of enuresis include the bladder (reduced nocturnal bladder capacity), the kidney (nocturnal polyuria), and the brain (e.g., a disorder affecting arousal from sleep). Enuresis is logically thought to result from a disruption or maturational lag in one or more of these critical domains.

8 **d. Nocturnal polyuria.** The nocturnal enuresis alarm and desmopressin are both valid treatment options. There exist patient, caregiver, and disease-related parameters that may aid in offering prognostic information in terms of which therapeutic modality should be first entertained. The enuresis alarm seems best fit for motivated patients and families and for children without polyuria but with low voided volume. Desmopressin seems best suited for children with nocturnal polyuria and normal bladder reservoir function, for those with infrequent wet episodes, and for families in whom alarm treatment has failed or who have refused alarm treatment.

CHAPTER REVIEW

1. Immature detrusor sphincter coordination manifested as detrusor hypercontractility and interrupted voiding commonly occurs in the first 2 years of life and results in functional bladder outflow obstruction.

2. Even in newborns, micturition does not occur during sleep, suggesting modulation of micturition by higher centers.

3. The association of constipation with urologic pathology is referred to as *bladder bowel dysfunction or BBD*. Abnormalities of bowel function are commonly present in young children with voiding dysfunction.

4. Giggle incontinence often results in complete emptying of the bladder.

5. In patients who develop acquired bladder sphincter dysfunction, a significant proportion also have bowel dysfunction.

6. There is a significant association of bladder dysfunction with nonresolution of high-grade vesicoureteral reflux.

7. Nocturnal urine output in many enuretic children is in excess of bladder reservoir capacity during sleep.

8. Many enuretic children have a marked reduction in functional bladder capacity when compared with age-matched controls and may have detrusor instability as well.

9. Overactive bladder is the most common lower urinary tract disorder in children, with a peak incidence between 5 and 7 years.

10. Behavioral and emotional disorders occur in 20% to 30% of children with lower urinary tract disorders.

11. Vaginal reflux (vaginal entrapment, vaginal voiding) is characterized by incontinence following normal voiding in the absence of other LUT symptoms. It is commonly seen in prepubertal girls, and the typical history is that of wetting of undergarments about 10 to 15 minutes following a normal void. It can often be associated with labial adhesions.

12. Pollakiuria is a disorder characterized by a very high daytime frequency of micturition (sometimes as high as 50 times per day). A key aspect of this syndrome, which differentiates it from OAB and can often clinch the diagnosis, is that the symptoms are limited to the daytime. It is seen in early childhood (4 to 6 years of age) in both genders and can be associated with stressors such as a history of recent death or life-threatening event in the family. Usually, it runs a benign, self-limited course over a period of approximately 6 months.

13. All children with LUTD should receive behavioral modification as treatment. Behavioral modification includes demystification, education, counseling, timed voiding, relaxation techniques, monitoring of stool consistency, and diary registration of bladder and bowel emptying patterns.

14. The use of an alarm in the treatment of enuresis seems best fit for motivated patients and families and for children without polyuria but with low voided volume. Desmopressin seems best suited for children with nocturnal polyuria and normal bladder reservoir function, for those with infrequent wet episodes, and for families for whom alarm treatment has failed or who have refused alarm treatment.

36 Management of Defecation Disorders

Martin A. Koyle and Armando J. Lorenzo

QUESTIONS

1. The Rome IV criteria evaluate the following aspects of bowel function EXCEPT:
   a. pain with bowel movements.
   b. production of large stools that can block the toilet.
   c. number of bowel movements per week.
   d. duration of symptoms.
   e. all of the above.

2. A 4-year-old girl presents with a 6-month history of urinary frequency and urgency. Parents report daily small bowel movements, which they attribute to poor diet ("picky eater"). Her physical exam is normal. There is no history of urinary tract infections. Which of the following interventions can lead to paradoxical worsening of her symptoms?
   a. Increase in fluid intake
   b. Polyethylene glycol (PEG)
   c. Oxybutynin
   d. Trimethoprim prophylaxis
   e. Biofeedback

3. Which one of the following aspects of a patient's history and physical examination should raise suspicion for an underlying organic pathology causing constipation?
   a. Early age of onset (before toilet training)
   b. Presence of a palpable mass in the left lower quadrant
   c. Onset after diet change
   d. Poor dietary habits ("picky eater")
   e. All of the above

4. Which part of the physical exam can be safely omitted during initial evaluation of a child with suspected functional constipation?
   a. Height and weight
   b. Inspection of the lower back
   c. Lower extremity muscle tone and reflexes
   d. Digital rectal exam
   e. Visual inspection of the perineum

5. Which of the following metabolic/endocrinologic pathologies is unlikely to cause constipation?
   a. Hypercalcemia
   b. Hypokalemia
   c. Hypothyroidism
   d. Diabetes insipidus
   e. Precocious puberty

6. Regarding the surgical management of refractory constipation, which of the following statements is TRUE?
   a. Access for antegrade irrigations should be limited to the cecum.
   b. Open surgical intervention carries a higher success rate than laparoscopic or percutaneous procedures.
   c. Malone antegrade continence enema (MACE) channels and C-tubes provide better procedural independence than retrograde enemas for patients with neuropathic bowel dysfunction.
   d. Similar success rates can be expected irrespective of the underlying pathology.
   e. All of the above.

7. The main principle behind daily antegrade enemas for continence is:
   a. washout with regular evacuation of the entire colon.
   b. direct softening of stools to facilitate passage during the day.
   c. improve hydration.
   d. decrease colon motility.
   e. decrease sphincter tone.

8. Initial workup of a child with constipation is most likely to benefit from:
   a. abdominal radiograph.
   b. anal manometry.
   c. colonic transit time studies.
   d. magnetic resonance imaging (MRI) of lumbosacral spine.
   e. contrast enema study.

9. Which of the following statements regarding creation of a MACE channel is TRUE?
   a. Previous surgical interventions are a contraindication for a laparoscopic approach.
   b. An aggressive bowel washout and mechanical preparation are always warranted before surgery.
   c. Presence of a ventriculoperitoneal shunt is a contraindication for laparoscopic approach.
   d. The appendix may be of sufficient length to be split in order to create a MACE and Mitrofanoff channel for neuropathic bowel and bladder management.
   e. An anti-reflux mechanism (cecal wrap) is always required in order to prevent stool leakage.

10. Which of the following statements regarding cecostomy tubes is most accurate?
    a. It is a good alternative for patients who have previously undergone an appendectomy.
    b. It avoids the need for regular instrumentation.
    c. It is difficult to remove or convert to a MACE channel.
    d. The most common problem is stenosis and difficulty accessing for fluid instillation.
    e. It is a great alternative for families who have problems with compliance.

11. Recommendations for antegrade enema regimens should include which of the following?
    a. Sterile saline is preferred versus tap water or "homemade" saline solution.
    b. Daily enemas are universally required to achieve continence.

c. Early morning irrigations are preferable as it allows the patients to enjoy better daytime continence.

d. Trial and error for more than 6 months may be warranted to reach a reliable enema routine.

e. All of the above.

12. What is the proposed mechanism of action of prucalopride?

a. Stool softener

b. Antispasmodic

c. Bulking agent

d. Prokinetic

e. Antiinflammatory

13. Which of the following agents is preferred (first-line) medication for maintenance management of constipation?

a. Milk of magnesia

b. Mineral oil

c. PEG

d. Prucalopride

e. Psyllium husk

14. Features of functional constipation include:

a. recurrence despite recommendations consistent with optimal medical management.

b. alternating constipation and diarrhea.

c. episodes of bowel obstruction.

d. bilious vomiting.

e. ribbon-like stools.

15. Which one of the following stool characteristics is NOT included in the Bristol scale?

a. Consistency

b. Shape

c. Difficulty having bowel movements

d. Odor

e. None of the above

16. Of the following, which one is the best diagnostic test to confirm Hirschsprung disease?

a. Barium enema

b. Computed tomography (CT) scan with oral and intravenous contrast

c. Rectal biopsy

d. Colonoscopy

e. Lumbosacral spine MRI

17. New onset of abdominal pain and distention after antegrade instillation of fluid in a child with a cecostomy tube in place for more than 6 months should alert the physician about:

a. spontaneous cecal perforation.

b. use of hypotonic fluid for irrigations.

c. presence of a large fecal load in the rectum and descending colon.

d. an incompetent ileocecal valve with retrograde irrigation into the terminal ileum.

e. irritable bowel syndrome.

18. Which of the following statements regarding abdominal plain film during initial assessment of a child with functional constipation is FALSE?

a. Amount and distribution of fecal material can predict likelihood of response and recurrence with medical therapy

b. Helps assess for fecal impaction

c. Helps assess response to bowel washout

d. Aids in demonstrating for parents or caretakers the presence of constipation

e. Detects bony abnormalities that may be associated with neuropathic bowel dysfunction

19. Which statement regarding diagnosis and management of functional constipation is TRUE?

a. Assessment during evaluation of a child with recurrent urinary tract infections is warranted.

b. It is an integral part of a program dealing with dysfunctional voiding.

c. It should be addressed before proceeding with surgical interventions for vesicoureteral reflux.

d. It can be managed by pediatric urologists and urology nurse practitioners.

e. All of the above.

IMAGING

1. The abdominal radiograph (left) and pelvic ultrasound (right) shown in Fig. 36.1 were obtained on a 5-year-old girl with recurrent abdominal pain and distention for the past year. She has a palpable soft, nontender mass in the left lower quadrant. Which one of the following interventions is LEAST likely to help with initial management?

a. Digital disimpaction under sedation

b. Enemas

c. "High-dose" PEG

d. Supplement fiber intake

e. Increase fluid intake

ANSWERS

1. **e. All of the above.** The Rome IV criteria requires symptoms to be present for at least 1 month, and takes into account developmental age and absence of an underlying organic pathology. Pain with defecation, history of large-diameter stools that may obstruct the toilet, and infrequent bowel movements (≤2 defecations per week) are all included in the diagnosis of functional constipation.

2. **c. Oxybutynin.** Constipation is a common side effect of medications used to deal with lower urinary tract symptoms (particularly antimuscarinics). Because of this common association, during the past few decades pediatric urologists have become comfortable with assessing and managing bowel problems. Development or worsening of constipation will sometimes coincide or worsen with precipitating factors, such as change in diet (for example, transitioning out of breastfeeding) and introduction of new medications (such as oxybutynin for management of urinary frequency). Increase in fecal load in the rectum, coupled with toilet avoidance due to lower abdominal pain and discomfort with defecation, may lead to paradoxical worsening of lower urinary tract symptoms. Increase in fluid intake and use of PEG is unlikely to worsen lower urinary tract symptoms and is part of initial recommendations for bowel retraining. Similarly, biofeedback may have a neutral or beneficial effect. Antibiotic prophylaxis, in the absence of recurrent infections, is not expected to influence symptomatology.

3. **a. Early age of onset (before toilet training).** The age of onset of symptoms is one of the easiest and most important pieces of information to obtain, as it can be an important indicator for underlying pathology, particularly if symptoms have been present since early in life (infancy). Other critical information to be actively gathered includes failure to toilet train within an age-appropriate and developmental timeframe, pain with

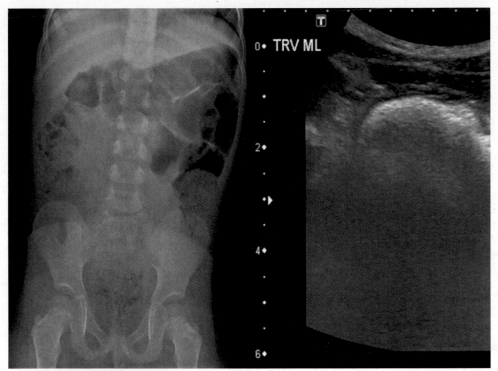

Fig. 36.1

defecation, bleeding per rectum, associated abdominal pain, fecal incontinence, holding behaviors, nausea or vomiting, weight loss, growth pattern (including height and weight), developmental delay, and failure to thrive. Patients with functional constipation often present or worsen after dietary changes. Not uncommonly, otherwise healthy children are described by parents as very selective (or "picky"). In the setting of significant fecal load or impaction in a child with constipation, a palpable mass in the left lower quadrant ("fecaloma") may be detected during examination.

4. **d. Digital rectal exam.** Physical exam should routinely include weight and height, and inspection of the perineum and genital and perianal regions (including anal position, stool present around the anus or on the underwear, signs of trauma, anal fissures, sensation). Although potentially considered to be an integral part of a complete physical exam, digital rectal examination should not be routinely conducted in children. It is reserved for difficult-to-treat cases and must be performed by health care professionals comfortable with interpreting features of anorectal anatomical abnormalities, to specifically evaluate for anal stenosis, a large fecal mass, or an empty rectum.

5. **e. Precocious puberty.** Endocrine disorders associated with chronic dehydration (such as diabetes insipidus), electrolyte disorders (most notably hypercalcemia and hypokalemia), hypothyroidism, and hypervitaminosis D are important potential organic etiologies. Precocious puberty presents with development of secondary sexual characteristics at an age before the expected onset during normal development. Constipation is not a presenting or common isolated feature of this condition.

6. **c. Malone antegrade continence enema (MACE) channels and C-tubes provide better procedural independence than retrograde enemas for patients with neuropathic bowel dysfunction.** In cases with severe constipation and a redundant colon, some have advocated the placement of conduits in the left colon rather than the cecum. By doing so, the length of bowel that has to be washed through is reduced and theoretically, so is the time taken for successful enema completion. Results with this approach have been encouraging. Both open and laparoscopic procedures are associated with similar success rates. Both C-tubes and MACE-type channels provide independence and allow patients greater ability to perform irrigations without assistance in comparison to self-administered retrograde enemas. The underlying diagnosis influences the success rate. Patients with a neuropathic bowel and anorectal malformations seem to fare better than those with chronic idiopathic constipation. Age at operation is also important, with failures more commonly seen in younger patients irrespective of the diagnosis.

7. **a. Washout with regular evacuation of the entire colon.** The success of antegrade enema regimens is based on two important principles: (1) complete colonic emptying can achieve bowel continence, and (2) antegrade colonic emptying is feasible. Regular complete emptying of the colon is the main mechanism associated with fecal continence.

8. **a. Abdominal radiograph.** Although of modest clinical value, abdominal radiographs are commonly used in the diagnosis and management of constipation. Proponents in favor of routine use argue that the study can clearly demonstrate the amount of fecal loading and delineate stool distribution throughout the colon and rectum, as well as help ascertain for the presence of fecal impaction. In addition, it may also reveal associated pathologies, such as bony abnormalities indicative of occult spinal dysraphism or sacral agenesis, and help provide a visual aid for family and patient recognition of stool retention despite a history of regular defecation. Colonic transit time studies are not recommended for routine diagnosis of functional constipation, being reserved for difficult-to-treat or unresponsive cases. Similarly, contrast enema series can be of value in selected cases, such as the evaluation of children with characteristics suggestive of Hirschsprung disease and repaired congenital anatomic abnormalities (i.e., anorectal malformation). Concern for a neuropathic process and/or lower spine stigmata should be evaluated with a spine ultrasound (if detected before calcification of the vertebral bodies in the first 3 to 6 months of life) or a lumbosacral MRI in older children. Anorectal manometry is useful only in very selected cases, such as suspected Hirschsprung disease and internal sphincter achalasia. In these conditions, the rectoanal relaxation reflex is absent. Nevertheless, in patients suspected of having functional constipation, manometry adds little to the diagnosis or therapeutic strategy.

9. **d. The appendix may be of sufficient length to be split to create a MACE and Mitrofanoff channel for neuropathic bowel and bladder management.** In children who require synchronous bladder reconstruction, a simultaneous MACE and Mitrofanoff urinary diversion offers the opportunity for dual fecal and urinary continence. If both a MACE and appendicovesicostomy are considered—and if the appendix is long enough with suitable, robust vascular anatomy—it is possible to split it. Previous surgical interventions are not an absolute contraindication for a laparoscopic approach, although the situation does demand for great care when entering the peritoneal cavity to avoid injuries related to adhesions or fibrosis. Although preoperative bowel preparation may facilitate the initiation of postoperative enemas, an aggressive cleanout is not necessary for the purpose of performing the procedure. Many patients with neuropathic bladder and bowel dysfunction have ventriculoperitoneal shunts. Although it is critical that appropriate use of prophylactic antibiotics and measures to minimize spillage be set in place, the presence of a shunt is not a contraindication for open or laparoscopic reconstruction involving bowel segments. Many descriptions of the MACE procedure propose an "anti-reflux" valve mechanism to prevent leakage of bowel contents via the cutaneous stoma. This is often achieved by wrapping the appendix with the cecal wall. However, recent reports have suggested that it is not always necessary to construct an anti-reflux mechanism. Thus far, data appear to support no increase in stomal bowel incontinence, based on retrospective reviews comparing MACE with and without cecal wrap.

10. **a. It is a good alternative for patients who have previously undergone an appendectomy.** Cecostomy tubes are favored when the appendix is known to be absent (i.e., postappendectomy), when the patient refuses to perform intermittent bowel catheterization, for patients who develop stomal complications such as stenosis (as an alternative to revision of the MACE channel), as a temporary therapeutic challenge to determine response to antegrade enemas, to determine if ideal placement of a permanent MACE should be in the right or left colon, and as a permanent option in cases in which a nonoperative access is favored. The main drawback is that the tube entry site can become unsightly, with granulation tissue and occasional fecal leakage. Stenosis is very rare, in contrast to issues related to MACE channels. In addition, regular instrumentation is needed in order to change the tube on a scheduled basis (i.e., every 6 to 12 months), or sooner if it dislodges or breaks. Patients may opt for subsequent formal conversion to a bowel-based MACE, which can be done either laparoscopically or open. Compliance with antegrade enema regimens is crucial for success, irrespective of how the bowel access has been achieved (C-tube or MACE).

11. **d. Trial and error for more than 6 months may be warranted to reach a reliable enema routine.** One of the most important points, especially in the early weeks and months after surgery, is to advise patients not to expect immediate success with the enema regimen, as early disappointment can lead to frustration and failure. In fact many children may not achieve a steady state or a reliable enema routine for a period of as long as 6 months. Enema protocols differ among centers, and patients and families will frequently modify them to suit their own particular needs. Initially, daily washouts with 20 mL/kg of solution are encouraged, but once the patient is comfortable with the process and a routine has been established, they may attempt to decrease frequency to alternate days. The time of day that the enema is administered is patient dependent, although most families prefer to give the enema during the early evening hours, after dinner. Purges can be done with large-volume tap or salt water, with the judicious mix of additives such as glycerin. The fluid does not have to be sterile.

12. **d. Prokinetic.** Prucalopride is a new oral, selective, high-affinity $5HT_4$ receptor antagonist with gastrointestinal prokinetic activities, which shows particular promise for management of difficult-to-treat constipation and may eventually represent a reasonable choice for children who fail to respond to more conservative measures. Its main mechanism of action does not influence stool consistency or bulk. As a prokinetic drug, it is likely to stimulate bowel smooth muscle contractions and not provide an antispasmodic effect.

13. **c. PEG.** With the introduction of PEG into routine clinical practice, tolerance of medical management has improved, and it is currently the preferred agent in many centers. PEG is better tolerated and easier to administer than alternative medications such as lactulose, mineral oil, and milk of magnesia (magnesium hydroxide). It is virtually tasteless and dissolves easily within seconds.

14. **a. Recurrence despite recommendations consistent with optimal medical management.** Functional constipation can be difficult to treat and a long-lasting problem for some children. Nevertheless, with adequate management close to 50% of patients monitored for 6 to 12 months can recover and successfully discontinue medications, whereas as many as 80% can be adequately controlled with routine interventions. Unfortunately, subsequent recurrences are fairly common, with as many as 50% of children experiencing one in the first 5 years after successful treatment. All the other listed factors (alternating constipation and diarrhea, episodes of bowel obstruction, bilious vomiting, and ribbon-like stools) are "warning signs and symptoms" that should raise suspicion for alternative diagnosis and an underlying process (i.e., not functional constipation).

15. **d. Odor.** Stool characteristics should be recorded with a validated scale. The most commonly used (Bristol scale) takes into account consistency and stool shape, capturing also the degree of difficulty passing the bowel movement. Smell (odor) is not part of the scale.

16. **c. Rectal biopsy.** If Hirschsprung disease or colon aganglionosis is suspected, a deep suction rectal biopsy (including submucosal) should be obtained, favoring a transanal approach and aiming at a location 2 to 3 cm from the dentate line. Diagnosis is supported by absence of ganglion cells, hypertrophied nerve fibers, and increase in acetylcholinesterase activity in the lamina propria and muscularis mucosa.

17. **c. Presence of a large fecal load in the rectum and descending colon.** Several difficulties can be experienced during enema infusion. The most common problem is pain or discomfort during instillation. In the majority of patients, this is a transient phenomenon that subsides during the first 3 months. It is always important to ensure that the pain is not due to distal fecal impaction, which can occur despite regular washouts. The presence of a large amount of fecal material in the distal colon and rectum can certainly lead to impaction in patients doing infrequent antegrade enemas through a cecostomy access or MACE channel. Attempts at clearing this fecal load with antegrade flushes can lead to abdominal pain, lack of tolerance, and poor response. Spontaneous colon perforation with antegrade enema regimens is exceedingly rare. The use of hypotonic fluids (such as tap water) is commonplace in many centers. Retrograde flow of fluid into the distal ileum is not a common cause of pain with antegrade enemas and is unlikely to develop suddenly in a patient who has been doing enemas for a period of 6 months.

18. **a. Amount and distribution of fecal material can predict likelihood of response and recurrence with medical therapy.** As discussed in question 8, there are some potential benefits to obtaining an abdominal radiograph during the evaluation of children with constipation. These include assessment for fecal impaction, to determine response to a bowel washout, to provide evidence for parents and caretakers, and to detect bony abnormalities suggestive of a possible neuropathic process. The distribution and amount of fecal material on one film have not been described to have any predictive value in terms of response to medical therapy or recurrence.

19. **e. All of the above.** Constipation is common and should be suspected in any patient who presents with lower urinary tract symptoms. Programs dealing with incontinence and dysfunctional voiding have successfully included this aspect of care into their protocols. Dysfunctional voiding and constipation should be addressed before proceeding with surgical correction and can be done by a pediatric urologist or urology nurse practitioner, assisted by the child's primary care physician.

IMAGING

1. **d. Supplement fiber intake.** The physical examination and imaging studies are suggestive of severe constipation and stool impaction. Decreasing fecal load in the colon and rectum is the first step toward establishing an optimal medical regimen. Impaction should be suspected when a mass is felt in the lower abdomen and/or left lower quadrant, or a dilated rectum filled with a large amount of stool is seen on pelvic ultrasound or abdominal radiography (as shown in **Fig. 36.1**). Approximately 30% of children with functional constipation present with fecal impaction. Disimpaction and bowel washout address the problem in a relatively short period of time, often with enemas or suppositories, in contrast to maintenance therapy. Popular regimens also include "high-dose" PEG with or without sodium chloride, sodium phosphate, or mineral oil enemas. In some circumstances clearance can only be achieved with digital disimpaction under sedation or anesthesia. The addition of fiber to the diet is bound to worsen the problem by increasing fecal load and is generally avoided during the initial management of fecal impaction.

CHAPTER REVIEW

1. Constipation may cause significant voiding dysfunction.
2. Functional constipation is a diagnosis of exclusion.
3. Organic conditions associated with elimination problems include cystic fibrosis, hypothyroidism, celiac disease, dietary allergies, Hirschsprung disease, anal stenosis, and trisomy 21. In the older child, mental health issues, eating disorders, sexual abuse, and irritable bowel syndrome should also be considered.
4. Initial medical management includes behavioral modification (regular defecation and nonsedentary activity), dietary changes (fluid and fiber intake), stool softeners and laxatives, and judicious use of enemas.
5. Antegrade continence enemas may be given through the cecum or left colon. It often requires that the child sit on the toilet for up to an hour before emptying is complete. The procedure is best employed in children 5–12 years of age who are motivated and is more successful in patients with neuropathic bowel or anorectal malformations.
6. Impaction should be suspected when a mass is felt in the lower abdomen and/or left lower quadrant, or a dilated rectum filled with a large amount of stool is seen on pelvic ultrasound or abdominal radiography.
7. In patients with fecal impaction, the addition of fiber to the diet is bound to worsen the problem by increasing fecal load and is generally avoided during the initial management.
8. The age of onset of symptoms is one of the easiest and most important pieces of information to obtain because it can be an important indicator for underlying pathology, particularly if it has been present since early in life (infancy).
9. Endocrine disorders associated with chronic dehydration (such as diabetes insipidus), electrolyte disorders (most notably hypercalcemia and hypokalemia), hypothyroidism, and hypervitaminosis D are important potential organic etiologies.
10. Although of modest clinical value, abdominal radiographs are commonly employed in the diagnosis and management of constipation. Proponents of routine use argue that the study can clearly demonstrate the amount of fecal loading and delineate stool distribution throughout the colon and rectum, as well as help ascertain the presence of fecal impaction. In addition, it may also reveal associated pathologies, such as bony abnormalities indicative of occult spinal dysraphism or sacral agenesis.
11. Polyethylene glycol is better tolerated and easier to administer than alternative medications such as lactulose, mineral oil, and milk of magnesia.
12. The most common problem with antegrade continence enemas is pain or discomfort during instillation. In the majority of patients, this is a transient phenomenon that subsides during the first 3 months. It is always important to ensure that the pain is not due to distal fecal impaction.

37 Lower Urinary Tract Reconstruction in Children

John C. Thomas, Douglass B. Clayton, and Mark C. Adams

QUESTIONS

1. Children with significant bladder or sphincter dysfunction requiring reconstructive surgery most likely have:
   a. bladder exstrophy or epispadias.
   b. posterior urethral valves.
   c. cloacal anomalies.
   d. prune-belly syndrome.
   e. spinal dysraphism.

2. The most important contribution to the field of pediatric reconstructive surgery has been:
   a. Mitrofanoff's description of a continent abdominal wall stoma using appendix.
   b. Lapides' introduction of clean intermittent catheterization (CIC).
   c. Goodwin's description of ileal reconfiguration.
   d. development of several effective means to increase bladder outlet resistance.
   e. recognition that a dilated ureter could be used for bladder augmentation.

3. Normal bladder compliance is based on:
   a. ample collagen type II.
   b. inverse relationship of bladder volume and bladder pressure.
   c. bladder unfolding, elasticity, and viscoelasticity.
   d. subepithelial matrix bridges associated with collagen.
   e. hypertrophic bladder bundles interspersed with collagen.

4. Chronically elevated bladder filling pressures may cause hydronephrosis, vesicoureteral reflux, and impaired renal function. The lowest pressure threshold most often reported to cause problems is:
   a. 20 cm H_2O.
   b. 30 cm H_2O.
   c. 40 cm H_2O.
   d. 50 cm H_2O.
   e. 60 cm H_2O.

5. Upper urinary tract changes associated with a poorly compliant, hyperreflexic bladder are initially treated by:
   a. autoaugmentation.
   b. pharmacologic management and intermittent catheterization.
   c. ileal augmentation.
   d. sigmoid augmentation.
   e. gastric augmentation.

6. Preoperative bladder capacity and compliance are best determined by urodynamics using:
   a. carbon dioxide as an irrigant at a slow fill rate (10% of capacity per minute).
   b. room-temperature saline at a slow fill rate (10% of capacity per minute).
   c. body-temperature saline at a fast fill rate (30% of capacity per minute).
   d. cooled saline at a slow fill rate (10% of capacity per minute).
   e. cooled saline at a fast fill rate (30% of capacity per minute).

7. Urinary tract reconstruction for urinary continence requires:
   a. confirmation of a normal upper urinary tract.
   b. identification of a highly compliant bladder.
   c. documentation of the presence or absence of vesicoureteral reflux.
   d. acceptance of and compliance with intermittent catheterization.
   e. documentation of a serum creatinine value less than 1.4 mg/dL.

8. Mechanical bowel preparation is performed in patients undergoing:
   a. ileocystoplasty.
   b. sigmoid cystoplasty.
   c. gastrocystoplasty.
   d. ureterocystoplasty.
   e. all of the above.

9. A urinary stricture after transureteroureterostomy is most likely due to:
   a. mobilization of the crossing ureter with periureteral tissue.
   b. mobilization of the crossing ureter without angulation beneath the inferior mesenteric artery.
   c. mobilization of the recipient ureter to meet the crossing one.
   d. wide anastomosis of the crossing ureter to the posteromedial aspect of the recipient.
   e. watertight anastomosis.

10. Creating an antireflux mechanism is most difficult with anastomosis to the:
    a. stomach.
    b. ileum.
    c. cecum.
    d. transverse colon.
    e. sigmoid colon.

11. The Young-Dees-Leadbetter bladder neck repair in children with neurogenic sphincter deficiency:
    a. results in limited success because of a lack of muscle tone and activity of the native bladder neck.
    b. can achieve successful continence results similar to those noted in children with bladder exstrophy.
    c. does not often require bladder augmentation or intermittent catheterization.
    d. is best performed in association with a Silastic sling.
    e. limits the necessity for intermittent catheterization in children who could empty by a Valsalva maneuver preoperatively.

12. An ambulatory 15-year-old girl with lumbosacral mye-lomeningocele voids to completion with a low-pressure detrusor contraction and the Valsalva maneuver. She remains incontinent because of bladder neck and intrinsic sphincter deficiency that is refractory to pharmacologic management. To limit the risk of intermittent catheterization, the next step is:
    a. Young-Dees-Leadbetter bladder neck repair.
    b. artificial urinary sphincter placement.
    c. fascial bladder neck sling placement.
    d. Kropp bladder neck repair.
    e. Pippi-Salle bladder neck repair.

13. One side effect associated with bladder neck repair that can be decreased with good preoperative evaluation is:
    a. recurrent urolithiasis.
    b. recurrent cystitis.
    c. inability to spontaneously void.
    d. associated need for augmentation cystoplasty.
    e. unmasking of detrusor hostility, resulting in upper urinary tract changes.

14. Fascial slings used for increasing outlet resistance in children with neurogenic sphincteric incompetence:
    a. are more effective in girls than in boys.
    b. are dependent on the type of fascial or cadaveric tissue used.
    c. are dependent on the configuration of the sling and wrap used.
    d. rarely result in the need for bladder augmentation and intermittent catheterization.
    e. frequently result in urethral erosion.

15. The least favorable indication for an artificial urinary sphincter is:
    a. neurogenic bladder dysfunction.
    b. bladder exstrophy or epispadias.
    c. inability to empty the bladder by spontaneous voiding.
    d. associated need for bladder augmentation.
    e. prepubertal age.

16. The most common limitation of a Kropp urethral lengthening for continence is:
    a. fistula from the urethra to the bladder, resulting in incontinence.
    b. inability to spontaneously void, resulting in urinary retention.
    c. difficulty with intermittent catheterization, particularly in boys.
    d. new vesicoureteral reflux.
    e. distal ureteral obstruction.

17. Urinary continence is most definitively achieved after:
    a. Young-Dees-Leadbetter bladder repair.
    b. placement of an artificial urinary sphincter.
    c. placement of a circumferential fascial wrap.
    d. urethral lengthening and reimplantation.
    e. bladder neck division.

18. To avoid uninhibited pressure contractions during an enterocystoplasty:
    a. large bowel should be used.
    b. the intestinal segment should be reconfigured.

c. the majority of the diseased bladder should be excised.
    d. a stellate incision into the bladder should be created to increase the circumference of the bowel anastomosis.
    e. small mesenteric windows are created in the bowel segment.

19. Potential ways to prevent reflux when using ileum for continent diversion include all of the following except:
    a. intussuscepted nipple valve.
    b. split nipple cuff of ureter.
    c. placement of the spatulated ureter into an incised mucosal trough.
    d. flap valve created beneath a taenia.
    e. placement of the ureter within a serosa-lined tunnel between two limbs of ileum.

20. The gastrointestinal segment that most often causes permanent gastrointestinal side effects when used in children with a neurogenic bladder is the:
    a. stomach.
    b. jejunum.
    c. ileum.
    d. ileocecal segment.
    e. sigmoid colon.

21. The most likely problem after gastrointestinal bladder augmentation is:
    a. early satiety.
    b. hyperchloremic metabolic acidosis.
    c. small bowel obstruction.
    d. chronic diarrhea.
    e. vitamin B_{12} deficiency with megaloblastic anemia.

22. The gastrointestinal segment resulting in the best long-term capacity and compliance after augmentation cystoplasty is the:
    a. gastric body.
    b. gastric antrum.
    c. ileum.
    d. cecum.
    e. sigmoid colon.

23. The risk of failure to achieve appropriate capacity and compliance after augmentation cystoplasty is:
    a. less than 5%.
    b. 5% to 10%.
    c. 11% to 15%.
    d. 16% to 20%.
    e. more than 20%.

24. The serum metabolic pattern that occurs most often after an ileocystoplasty or colocystoplasty is:
    a. hypochloremic metabolic acidosis.
    b. hyperchloremic metabolic acidosis.
    c. hypochloremic metabolic alkalosis.
    d. hyperchloremic metabolic alkalosis.
    e. hyponatremic metabolic acidosis.

25. The serum metabolic pattern that occurs most often after gastrocystoplasty is:
    a. hypochloremic metabolic acidosis.
    b. hyperchloremic metabolic acidosis.
    c. hypochloremic metabolic alkalosis.

d. hyperchloremic metabolic alkalosis.

e. hyponatremic metabolic acidosis.

26. The risk of intermittent hematuria and dysuria after gastrocystoplasty is most influenced by:

a. the gastric segment used.

b. persistent urinary incontinence.

c. decreased renal function.

d. diagnosis of bladder exstrophy.

e. neurogenic bladder dysfunction.

27. Bacteriuria should be treated after bladder augmentation when:

a. associated with CIC

b. urinalysis demonstrates microscopic hematuria.

c. there is increased mucus production.

d. etiology is posterior urethral valves.

e. urine culture reveals growth of a urea-splitting organism.

28. The gastrointestinal segment associated with the lowest incidence of stone formation is:

a. stomach.

b. jejunum.

c. ileum.

d. cecum.

e. sigmoid colon.

29. Adenocarcinoma of the bladder after augmentation cystoplasty can occur after:

a. 2 years.

b. 4 years.

c. 8 years.

d. 16 years.

e. 26 years.

30. The risk of perforation after bladder augmentation includes all but:

a. high outflow resistance.

b. persistent hyperreflexia or uninhibited bladder contractions.

c. use of sigmoid colon.

d. bladder exstrophy.

e. neurogenic bladder dysfunction.

31. The initial management of a spontaneous perforation of an augmented bladder in a child with a neurogenic bladder is:

a. placement of a large-bore urethral catheter for drainage.

b. placement of a large-bore suprapubic cystotomy tube for drainage.

c. immediate surgical exploration and repair.

d. serial abdominal examinations.

e. urine culture.

32. Pregnancy associated with urinary reconstruction:

a. is reasonable after urinary diversion but is contraindicated after augmentation cystoplasty.

b. results in the mesenteric pedicle positioned directly anterior to the uterus.

c. results in the mesenteric pedicle deflected laterally without vascular compromise to the augmented segment.

d. is avoided due to mechanical compression of the pedicle and ischemia with loss of the augmented segment.

e. is contraindicated because of increased risk of systemic sepsis complicating the hydronephrosis.

33. Ureterocystoplasty is limited because:

a. it requires an intraperitoneal approach.

b. complete mobilization of the ureter may result in vascular compromise.

c. a dilated ureter is not as compliant as a similar-sized bowel segment.

d. a dilated ureter is not available in many patients.

e. ureterocystoplasty precludes spontaneous voiding.

34. Autoaugmentation is contraindicated with:

a. serum creatinine value greater than 1.4 ng/dL.

b. CIC.

c. vesicoureteral reflux.

d. uninhibited bladder contractions.

e. small bladder capacity.

35. A ureterosigmoidostomy should not be undertaken in a patient with a history of:

a. dilated ureters.

b. anteriorly placed rectum associated with bladder exstrophy.

c. recurrent pyelonephritis.

d. fecal incontinence.

e. constipation.

36. The use of efferent nipple valves for continence in children:

a. has not approached the results achieved in adults.

b. has a higher complication and reoperation rate than a flap valve.

c. is equivalent to any other continence mechanism.

d. is often associated with difficulty in catheterization.

e. often results in stomal stenosis.

37. The least important factor when creating an appendicovesicostomy is:

a. taking a wide cecal cuff to decrease the risk of stomal stenosis.

b. creating a tunnel of 4 cm, at least greater than a 5:1 ratio of tunnel length to diameter, to achieve continence.

c. a small, uniform lumen allowing for easy catheterization.

d. mobilizing the right colon to adequately free the appendix.

e. tubularizing a small portion of the cecum in continuity with the appendix to increase length.

38. A frequent occurrence after an appendicovesicostomy is:

a. urinary incontinence due to inadequate length of the flap valve mechanism.

b. urinary incontinence due to persistently elevated reservoir pressure.

c. appendiceal perforation that often occurs due to catheterization.

d. appendiceal stricture or necrosis.

e. stomal stenosis.

39. A 12-year-old obese girl with spina bifida undergoes appendicocecostomy, bladder neck sling, bladder augmentation, and continent catheterizable bladder channel. The upper urinary tract is normal. The best source of tissue for the bladder channel is:

a. distal right ureter after right-to-left transureteroureterostomy.

b. tapered segment of small bowel of adequate length.

c. right fallopian tube.

d. gastric tube.

e. tubularized bladder flap.

40. In complex pediatric urinary undiversion procedures it is most difficult to:
    a. provide adequate outflow resistance.
    b. create a compliant urinary reservoir.
    c. achieve an effective antireflux mechanism without upper tract obstruction.
    d. provide a reliable access for intermittent catheterization.
    e. achieve urinary and fecal continence.

ANSWERS

1. **e. Spinal dysraphism.** Most pediatric reconstructive procedures are undertaken to correct a problem of the native urinary tract causing progressive hydronephrosis, urinary incontinence unresponsive to medical management, or temporary diversion. Children with bladder and sphincteric dysfunction are the most complex reconstructive cases seen in pediatric urology; children with the diagnoses of exstrophy, persistent cloaca and urogenital sinus, posterior urethral valves, bilateral single ectopic ureters, and prune-belly syndrome may be involved. However, children with a neurogenic bladder due to a myelomeningocele make up the vast majority of patients requiring this type of surgical intervention.

2. **b. Lapides' introduction of clean intermittent catheterization (CIC).** One of the most important contributions in the care of children with bladder dysfunction came with the acceptance of CIC described by Lapides and colleagues in 1972 and 1976, based on the work of Guttmann and Frankel. The effective use of CIC has allowed the application of augmentation and lower tract reconstruction to groups of patients who had not previously been candidates. The principle of intermittent catheterization allows the reconstructive surgeon to aggressively correct storage problems by providing an adequate reservoir and good outflow resistance. Spontaneous voiding, although a goal, is not imperative because catheterization can be used for emptying.

3. **c. Bladder unfolding, elasticity, and viscoelasticity.** Multiple factors contribute to the property of compliance. Initially the bladder is in a collapsed state, which allows for the storage of urine at low pressure by simply unfolding. While it expands, detrusor properties of elasticity and viscoelasticity take effect. Elasticity allows the detrusor muscle to stretch without an increase in tension until it reaches a critical volume. When filling is slow, as in a natural state, or stops, there is a rapid decay in this pressure known as stress relaxation. Normally, stress relaxation is in balance with the filling rate and prevents an increase in detrusor pressure.

4. **c. 40 cm H_2O.** Elevated passive filling pressure becomes clinically pathogenic when a pressure greater than 40 cm H_2O is chronically reached. Pressure at this level sustained during a prolonged period of time impairs ureteral drainage and can result in acquired vesicoureteral reflux, pyelocaliceal changes, hydroureteronephrosis, and decreased glomerular filtration rate.

5. **b. Pharmacologic management and intermittent catheterization.** Pharmacologic management can play a role in decreasing filling pressure, particularly when hyperreflexic detrusor contractions are present. A combination of medications and intermittent catheterization has a positive impact, particularly in children with neurogenic dysfunction.

6. **b. Room-temperature saline at a slow fill rate (10% of capacity per minute).** The testing medium and infusion rate can influence the results. Carbon dioxide is not as reliable as fluid infusion, particularly when evaluating bladder compliance and capacity. The most common fluids used for testing are saline and iodinated contrast material; both provide reproducible results. Use of testing media at body temperature is also appropriate, but room temperature has also been shown to be acceptable. End filling pressure and bladder compliance can be dramatically affected by simply changing the filling rate. The cystometrogram should be performed at a fill rate of 10% per minute of the predicted bladder capacity for age.

7. **d. Acceptance of and compliance with intermittent catheterization.** No test ensures that a patient will be able to void spontaneously and empty well after bladder augmentation or other reconstruction. Therefore, all patients must be prepared to perform CIC postoperatively. The native urethra should be examined for the ease of catheterization. Ideally, the patient should learn CIC and practice it preoperatively until the patient, family, and surgeon are comfortable that catheterization can and will be performed reliably. In spite of a technically perfect operation, failure to catheterize and empty the bladder after reconstruction can result in upper tract deterioration, urinary tract infection, or bladder perforation.

8. **e. All of the above.** Each patient undergoes preoperative bowel preparation to minimize the potential risk of surgery if the use of any bowel is contemplated. Even when ureterocystoplasty or other alternatives are planned, intraoperative findings may dictate the need for use of a bowel segment.

9. **c. Mobilization of the recipient ureter to meet the crossing one.** If the native urinary bladder is small and adequate for only a single ureteral tunnel, transureteroureterostomy and a single reimplant may be helpful. Typically, the better ureter should be implanted into the bladder. The contralateral ureter drains into the reimplanted ureter via a transureteroureterostomy. The crossing ureter should follow a smooth path and remain tension free. It should be carefully mobilized with all of its adventitia and as much periureteral tissue as possible to preserve blood supply. Care must be taken not to angulate the crossing ureter beneath the inferior mesenteric artery. The crossing ureter should be widely anastomosed to the posteromedial aspect of the recipient ureter. The recipient ureter should not be mobilized or brought medially to meet the contralateral ureter to minimize devascularization.

10. **b. Ileum.** The necessity of ureteral reimplantation into an intestinal segment may occasionally determine the segment to be used for bladder augmentation or replacement. Long-term experience with ureterosigmoidostomy and colon conduit diversion has established an effective means of creating a nonrefluxing ureteral implant. If a gastric segment is used for bladder augmentation or replacement, the ureters may be implanted into the stomach in a manner remarkably similar to that used in the native bladder. Creating an effective antireflux mechanism into an ileal segment is more difficult. The split nipple technique described by Griffith may prevent reflux at least at low reservoir pressure.

11. **a. Results in limited success because of a lack of muscle tone and activity of the native bladder neck.** Reports of success with the Young-Dees-Leadbetter bladder neck reconstruction in children with neurogenic sphincter dysfunction are limited, not only in the number of series but also in overall improvement of incontinence. Independent reviews of long-term results of this repair show minimal success in individuals with neurogenic dysfunction. These authors speculate that the lack of success was due to a lack of muscle tone and activity in the wrapped muscle related to the neurogenic problem.

12. **b. Artificial urinary sphincter placement.** The artificial urinary sphincter has been recognized as the only procedure that can result in prompt continence in selected children while preserving their ability to void spontaneously.

13. **e. Unmasking of detrusor hostility, resulting in upper urinary tract changes.** It is now recognized that occlusion of the bladder neck in children with neurogenic sphincter incompetence can result in the unmasking or development of detrusor hostility manifest by a decrease in bladder compliance or increase in detrusor hyperreflexia. Careful preoperative urodynamic assessment helps to identify some of the children who are at risk.

14. **a. Are more effective in girls than in boys.** Fascial slings have been used more extensively and with better results in girls with neurogenic sphincter incompetence, although recently some success has been reported in boys. Overall long-term success with fascial slings in the neurogenic population has varied greatly from 40% to 100%.

15. **c. Inability to empty the bladder by spontaneous voiding.** The ultimate benefits of the artificial urinary sphincter include its ability to achieve a high rate of continence while maintaining the potential for spontaneous voiding. For practical purposes, when intermittent catheterization is required along with augmentation cystoplasty, using native tissue for continence eliminates the long-term concern for infection/erosion and the risk of mechanical failure.

16. **c. Difficulty with intermittent catheterization, particularly in boys.** One study examined the results in 23 children, 22 of whom had neurogenic sphincter incompetence, and noted continence in more than 90% of the children. The most common complication was difficult catheterization, particularly in boys. Fewer than half of the boys in this series were catheterized through the native urethra; the majority were catheterized via an abdominal wall stoma.

17. **e. Bladder neck division.** The ultimate procedure to increase bladder outlet resistance is to divide the bladder neck so that it is no longer in continuity with the urethra. This must be accompanied by creation of a continent abdominal wall stoma and should be performed only in patients who will reliably be able to perform catheterization.

18. **b. The intestinal segment should be reconfigured.** Two studies demonstrated the advantages of opening a bowel segment on its antimesenteric border, which allows detubularization and reconfiguration of that intestinal segment. Reconfiguration into a spherical shape provides multiple advantages, including maximization of the volume achieved for any given surface area, blunting of bowel contractions, and improvement of overall capacity and compliance.

19. **d. Flap valve created beneath a taenia.** Small bowel does not have a taenia; this method is appropriate for large bowel. The split nipple technique described by Griffith may prevent reflux at least at low reservoir pressure. LeDuc and colleagues in 1987 described a technique in which the ureter is brought through a hiatus in the ileal wall. From that hiatus the ileal mucosa is incised and the edges are mobilized so as to create a trough for the ureter. It may also be possible to create antireflux mechanism using a serosal-lined tunnel created between two limbs of ileum as described by Abol-Enein and Ghoneim in 1999. Reinforced nipple valves of ileum have been used extensively to prevent reflux with the Kock pouch. Good long-term results have been achieved by Skinner after several modifications.

20. **d. Ileocecal segment.** Chronic diarrhea after bladder augmentation alone is rare. Diarrhea can occur after removal of large segments of ileum from the gastrointestinal tract, although the length of the segments typically used for augmentation is rarely problematic unless other problems coexist. Removal of the ileum and ileocecal valve from the gastrointestinal tract may cause diarrhea. One study noted that 10% of patients with neurogenic dysfunction have significant diarrhea after such displacement.

21. **b. Hyperchloremic metabolic acidosis.** Postoperative bowel obstruction is uncommon after augmentation cystoplasty, occurring in approximately 3% of patients after augmentation. The rate of obstruction is equivalent to that noted after conduit diversion or continent urinary diversion. Removal of the distal ileum from the gastrointestinal tract may result in vitamin B_{12} deficiency and megaloblastic anemia. The terminal 15 to 20 cm of ileum should not be used for augmentation, although problems may arise even if that segment is preserved. Early satiety may occur after gastrocystoplasty but usually resolves with time. Disorders of gastric emptying should be extremely rare, particularly when using the body of the stomach.

22. **c. Ileum.** Ileal reservoirs have been noted to have lower basal pressures and less motor activity when created for continent urinary diversion. Problems with pressure after augmentation cystoplasty usually occur from uninhibited contractions caused by the bowel segment. It is extremely rare not to achieve an adequate capacity or flat tonus limb unless a technical error has occurred with use of the bowel segment. Rhythmic contractions have been noted postoperatively with all bowel segments, particularly the stomach, although ileum is the least likely to demonstrate a remarkable urodynamic abnormality.

23. **b. 5% to 10%.** Hollensbe and associates at Indiana University reported on one of the largest experiences with pediatric bladder augmentation and found that approximately 5% of patients had significant uninhibited contractions causing clinical problems. Another study found that 6% required secondary augmentation of a previously augmented bladder for similar problems in long-term follow-up.

24. **b. Hyperchloremic metabolic acidosis.** The first recognized metabolic complication related to storage of urine within intestinal segments was the occasional development of hyperchloremic metabolic acidosis after ureterosigmoidostomy. Another study demonstrated the mechanisms by which acid is absorbed from urine in contact with intestinal mucosa. A later report noted that essentially every patient after augmentation with an intestinal segment had an increase in serum chloride and a decrease in serum bicarbonate levels, although clinically significant acidosis was rare if renal function was normal.

25. **c. Hypochloremic metabolic alkalosis.** Gastric mucosa is a barrier to chloride and acid resorption and, in fact, secretes hydrochloric acid. The secretory nature of gastric mucosa may at times be detrimental to the patient and can result in two unique complications of gastrocystoplasty. Severe episodes of hypokalemic hypochloremic metabolic alkalosis after acute gastrointestinal illnesses have been noted after gastrocystoplasty.

26. **e. Neurogenic bladder dysfunction.** Virtually all patients with normal sensation have occasional hematuria or dysuria with voiding or catheterization after gastrocystoplasty beyond that which is expected with other intestinal segments. All patients should be warned of this potential problem, although in most patients these symptoms are intermittent and mild and do not require treatment. The dysuria is less problematic in patients with limited sensation due to neurogenic dysfunction. Patients who are incontinent or have decreased renal function may be at increased risk. These problems occur less frequently after antral gastric cystoplasty in which there is a smaller load of parietal cells.

27. **e. Urine culture reveals growth of a urea-splitting organism.** It appears that the use of CIC is a prominent factor in the development of bacteriuria in patients after augmentation cystoplasty. Every episode of asymptomatic bacteriuria does not require treatment in patients performing CIC. Bacteriuria should be treated when significant symptoms occur, such as fever, suprapubic pain, incontinence, and gross hematuria. Bacteriuria should also be treated when the urine culture demonstrates growth of a urea-splitting organism that may lead to stone formation.

28. **a. Stomach.** Most bladder stones in the augmented child are of a struvite composition. Bacteriuria has been thought to be an important risk factor. Stones have been noted after the use of all intestinal segments with no significant difference appreciated between small and large intestine. Struvite stones are less likely after gastrocystoplasty.

29. **b. 4 years.** Patients undergoing augmentation cystoplasty should be made aware of a potential increased risk of tumor development. Yearly surveillance of the augmented bladder with endoscopy should eventually be performed; the latency period until such procedures are necessary is not well defined. The earliest reported tumor after augmentation was found only 4 years after cystoplasty.

30. **d. Bladder exstrophy.** The cause of delayed perforations after bladder augmentation is unknown. Perforations may occur in bladders with significant uninhibited contractions after augmentation. High outflow resistance may maintain bladder pressure rather than allowing urinary leakage and venting of the pressure, potentially increasing ischemia. The majority of patients suffering perforations after augmentation cystoplasty have a neurogenic etiology. At Indiana University, perforations were noted in 32 of 330 patients undergoing cystoplasty an average of 4.3 years after augmentation. Analysis of this experience suggested that the use of sigmoid colon was the only significant increased risk.

31. **c. Immediate surgical exploration and repair.** The standard treatment of spontaneous perforation of the augmented bladder is surgical repair, as it is for intraperitoneal rupture of the bladder after trauma. The majority of patients with perforations have myelodysplasia and present late in the course of the disease because of impaired sensation. Increasing sepsis and death of the patient may result from a delay in diagnosis or treatment.

32. **c. Results in the mesenteric pedicle deflected laterally without vascular compromise to the augmented segment.** Experience is limited regarding what is known about the changes to the pedicle of a bladder augmentation during pregnancy. It has been reported that the mesenteric pedicle to bladder augmentations is not stretched over the uterus at the time of cesarean section. The pedicle has been found to be deflected laterally. Urinary tract infections may be problematic in women who have undergone urinary reconstruction, including bladder augmentation. Ureteral dilatation, increased residual urine, and diminished tone to the upper tract may all be important risk factors.

33. **d. A dilated ureter is not available in many patients.** Several series have reported good results after ureteral augmentation with a follow-up as long as 8 years. The upper urinary tract has remained stable or improved in virtually all patients. Complications are uncommon. The main disadvantage to ureterocystoplasty is the limited patient population with a poorly functioning kidney drained by a megaureter.

34. **e. Small bladder capacity.** Although autoaugmentation can improve compliance, an increase in volume is "modest at best." In a report of 12 children who had undergone a detrusorotomy, five were considered to have excellent results, two had acceptable results, and one was lost to follow-up. The main disadvantage of autoaugmentation is a limited increase in bladder capacity such that adequate preoperative volume may be the most important predictor of success.

35. **d. Fecal incontinence.** Before ureterosigmoidostomy is considered, anal sphincter competence must be ensured. Tests used to assess sphincter integrity include manometry, electromyography, and practical evaluation of the ability to retain an oatmeal enema in the upright position for a time period without soilage. Incontinence of a mixture of stool and urine results in foul soilage and must be avoided.

36. **b. Has a higher complication and reoperation rate than a flap valve.** The greatest experience with nipple valves for achieving urinary continence has been with the Kock pouch. Skinner and associates made a series of modifications to aid in maintenance of the efferent nipple. Even with experience and these modifications, a failure rate of 15% or higher can be expected. Equivalent results with the nipple valve and a Kock pouch have been achieved in children.

37. **b. Creating a tunnel of 4 cm, at least greater than a 5:1 ratio of tunnel length to diameter, to achieve continence.** The appendix is an ideal natural tubular structure that can be safely removed from the gastrointestinal tract without significant morbidity. The small caliber of the appendix facilitates creation of a short functional tunnel with the bladder wall. Experience has shown that continence can be achieved with only a 2-cm appendiceal tunnel.

38. **e. Stomal stenosis.** Incontinence is rare with the Mitrofanoff procedure and may result from inadequate length of the flap valve mechanism or persistently elevated reservoir pressure. The most common complication has been stomal stenosis and occurs in 10% to 20% of patients. Stenosis resulting in difficult catheterization may occur early in the postoperative course and requires formal revision.

39. **b. Tapered segment of small bowel of adequate length.** When the appendix is unavailable for use, other tubular structures can provide a similar mechanism for catheterization and continence. Mitrofanoff, in 1980, described a similar technique using ureter. Woodhouse and MacNeily, in 1994, as well as others, have used the fallopian tube, which can accommodate catheterization. Monti and Yang have been credited with a novel modification of the tapered intestinal segment, which can be reimplanted according to the Mitrofanoff principle.

40. **c. Achieve an effective antireflux mechanism without upper tract obstruction.** The key to urinary undiversion is understanding the original pathologic condition that led to diversion. One report described a 26-year experience with urinary undiversion in 216 patients. In that series, management of the bladder was relatively straightforward and effective with bladder augmentation as necessary. Inadequate outflow resistance was usually treated with Young-Dees-Ledbetter bladder neck repair. Most complications were related to the ureters; 23 patients required reoperation for persistent reflux, whereas 10 did so for partial obstruction of the ureter. Those reoperation rates are indicative of the difficulty one faces in dealing with short, dilated, and scarred ureters, which may be present after urinary diversion.

CHAPTER REVIEW

1. Bladder volume (mL) in children is equal to 30 × (age in years + 2) or for infants, 7 × weight (kg).
2. Intermittent catheterization must be taught and accepted by the patient and caregiver before any urinary reconstruction is performed.
3. There is no test that ensures the patient will be able to void spontaneously and empty well after bladder augmentation or reconstruction.
4. Most patients prefer to catheterize an abdominal wall stoma rather than the native urethra.
5. Bladder neck bulking agents are not particularly effective in children.
6. When placing an artificial sphincter it should be placed at the bladder neck in females and in prepubertal males.
7. One-third of patients will require further surgery after augmentation cystoplasty because of various problems.
8. Bacteriuria is common after intestinal cystoplasty. After intestinal cystoplasty, routine bladder irrigation should be performed to evacuate inspissated mucus.
9. The use of stomach for bladder augmentation should be reserved for patients who have short-gut syndrome or who have received heavy pelvic irradiation.
10. Delayed spontaneous perforation of the bowel segment after intestinal cystoplasty occurs in approximately 5% of patients.
11. Most secondary vesicoureteral reflux will resolve after successful bladder reconstruction.
12. Nonfunctional bladders may need to be cycled to determine their true capacity.
13. Removing the ileal-cecal valve from the gastrointestinal tract in patients with neurogenic bladder and bowel dysfunction may result in intractable diarrhea.
14. It has been noted that there appears to be an increased incidence of malignant tumors in the gastric segment of patients who have had a gastrocystoplasty.
15. When the appendix is used to create a flap valve, the distance to the skin should be as short as possible to facilitate ease of catheterization.
16. The Young-Dees-Leadbetter bladder neck reconstruction in children with neurogenic sphincter dysfunction has had limited success.
17. Occlusion of the bladder neck in children with neurogenic sphincter incompetence can result in the unmasking or development of detrusor hostility manifest by a decrease in bladder compliance or increase in detrusor hyperreflexia.
18. Ileal reservoirs have been noted to have lower basal pressures and less motor activity when created for continent urinary diversion.
19. Essentially every patient after augmentation with an ileal or colonic intestinal segment has an increase in serum chloride and a decrease in serum bicarbonate levels, although severe acidosis is rare if renal function is normal.
20. Severe episodes of hypokalemic hypochloremic metabolic alkalosis after acute gastrointestinal illnesses have been noted after gastrocystoplasty.
21. The majority of patients suffering bladder perforations after augmentation cystoplasty have a neurogenic etiology.

38   Anomalies of the Upper Urinary Tract

Brian A. VanderBrink and Pramod P. Reddy

QUESTIONS

1. During a left inguinal herniorrhaphy, the vas deferens is absent and a 3-mm golden-yellow nodule is found along the spermatic cord. This boy may also have:
   a. a left appendage epididymis.
   b. left renal agenesis.
   c. malpositioned left adrenal gland.
   d. absent left head of epididymis.
   e. absent left testis.

2. A 14-year-old girl with abdominal pain undergoes an abdominal and pelvic ultrasound. A solitary right kidney is seen. Her abdominal pain is most likely associated with:
   a. skeletal anomalies.
   b. a unicornuate uterus.
   c. imperforate hymen.
   d. a didelphic uterus.
   e. an absent left ovary.

3. The most frequent renal fusion anomaly is:
   a. pancake kidney.
   b. crossed fused renal ectopia.
   c. horseshoe kidney.
   d. disc kidney.
   e. Sigmoid kidney.

4. The renal segment with the most variable blood supply is the:
   a. apex.
   b. upper.
   c. middle.
   d. lower.
   e. posterior.

5. A 22-year-old hypertensive woman is found to have a 2.7-cm renal artery aneurysm (RAA). Treatment is recommended:
   a. if the RAA rapidly decreases in size.
   b. when the woman is no longer of childbearing age.
   c. at this time.
   d. if there is no flank pain from emboli originating in the RAA.
   e. when the hypertension is well controlled.

6. A 5-year-old girl with a pelvic kidney has hydronephrosis most commonly due to:
   a. vesicoureteral reflux.
   b. malrotation.

   c. ureterovesical junction obstruction.
   d. ureteropelvic junction obstruction.
   e. ectopic ureter.

7. A newborn girl was noted prenatally to have coarctation of the aorta and a horseshoe kidney. After a renal bladder ultrasound, the next step is to obtain a(n):
   a. voiding cystourethrogram.
   b. magnetic resonance urography (MRU) with gadolinium.
   c. echocardiogram.
   d. karyotype.
   e. skeletal series.

8. Unilateral renal agenesis is commonly associated with:
   a. normal position of the splenic flexure.
   b. normal position of the adrenal gland.
   c. ipsilateral undescended testis.
   d. normal position of the hepatic flexure.
   e. rudimentary uterus.

9. A 2-month-old male is seen for prenatal ultrasound finding of left renal agenesis, and this is confirmed with postnatal ultrasound. The right kidney ultrasound findings show normal renal echogenicity and no renal collecting system or ureteral dilation. What testing/counseling would be advised?
   a. A voiding cystourethrogram (VCUG) must be performed.
   b. Serial renal ultrasounds annually for life even if asymptomatic.
   c. A confirmatory diuretic renal scan.
   d. Lifelong blood pressure check and urine analysis to monitor for evidence of chronic kidney disease.
   e. Nuclear glomerular filtration rate measurement.

10. Unilateral renal agenesis (URA) is best reliably diagnosed by finding:
   a. a single umbilical artery.
   b. preauricular skin tag(s).
   c. an imperforate hymen.
   d. absence of renal artery at L1-L2.
   e. specific radiographic evidence.

11. Male predominance of occurrence is most striking in:
   a. unilateral renal agenesis.
   b. bilateral renal agenesis.
   c. crossed fused renal ectopia.
   d. ectopic kidney.
   e. calyceal diverticulum.

12. The incidence of unilateral renal agenesis is:
    a. 1:2500.
    b. 1:4000.
    c. 1:1100.
    d. 1:5000.
    e. 1:500.

13. Unilateral renal agenesis and a unicornuate uterus will form when the embryologic insult occurs at which gestational time?
    a. Before the fourth week
    b. At the start of the fourth week
    c. At the end of the fourth week
    d. At the start of the fifth week
    e. At the end of the fifth week

14. In autopsy studies, unilateral renal agenesis was found in association with:
    a. absence of the gonad.
    b. a normally developed ureter.
    c. an ectopic ureteral orifice.
    d. adrenal agenesis.
    e. absence of the head of the epididymis.

15. Most ectopic kidneys are clinically asymptomatic EXCEPT:
    a. pelvic kidneys.
    b. thoracic kidneys.
    c. kidneys with ectopic ureters.
    d. lumbar kidneys.
    e. abdominal kidneys.

16. The isthmus of a horseshoe kidney is located adjacent to which vertebrae?
    a. T12 and L1
    b. L1 and L2
    c. L3 and L4
    d. L5 and S1
    e. S1 and S2

17. Between the sixth and ninth week, normal rotation of the kidney toward the midline to attain its orthotopic position involves:
    a. 60 degrees of lateral rotation.
    b. 90 degrees of lateral rotation.
    c. 180 degrees of lateral rotation.
    d. 90 degrees of medial rotation.
    e. 180 degrees of medial rotation.

18. Congenital renal arteriovenous fistulas are:
    a. usually congenital.
    b. cirsoid in configuration.
    c. symptomatic before the third decade.
    d. more common in males.
    e. usually located in the lower pole.

19. Bilateral megacalycosis:
    a. occurs more frequently in females.
    b. has an increased number of dilated calyces.
    c. is associated with ureteral dilation.
    d. is autosomal recessive in inheritance pattern.
    e. shows an obstructive pattern on renal scan.

ANSWERS

1. **b. Left renal agenesis.** The finding of a 3-mm golden-yellow nodule is indicative of ectopic adrenal. The adrenal develops just medial to the gonadal ridge. Their close proximity explains their location along the spermatic cord and their incidental identification at the time of herniorrhaphy or orchidopexy. Histologically, the nodules contain adrenal cortex but no medulla. In this case, the absent vas should raise a red flag for possible ipsilateral renal agenesis because the ureteral bud and vas are both derived from the wolffian duct. In one study, 79% of adult males with absence of the vas deferens have an absent ipsilateral kidney, with left-sided lesions predominating. The lower pole and mid-pole of the epididymis are wolffian duct derivatives. The head of the epididymis is derived from the mesonephric tubules, which link the mesonephric or wolffian duct with the gonad.

2. **d. A didelphic uterus.** Unilateral renal agenesis can be associated with didelphic uterus and obstruction of the ipsilateral vagina resulting in hematocolpos. This syndrome is referred to as OHVIRA (obstructed hemivagina ipsilateral renal agenesis). This would likely explain this girl's abdominal pain.

3. **c. Horseshoe kidney.** This anomaly represents the most frequently observed renal fusion anomaly.

4. **a. Apex.** The vessel to the apical segment has the greatest variation in origin; it arises from (1) the anterior division (43%), (2) the junction of the anterior and posterior divisions (23%), (3) the main-stem renal artery or aorta (23%), or (4) the posterior division of the main renal artery (10%).

5. **c. At this time.** Generally, treatment is recommended if patient presents with RAA rupture or deemed to be at high risk for rupture of the RAA. High risk for rupture is associated with rapidly expanding RAA or in pregnant females and those females who are considering pregnancy. Uncontrollable hypertension in association with renal artery stenosis and "shower" emboli from the RAA are additional indications.

6. **d. Ureteropelvic junction obstruction.** The renal pelvis is usually anterior (instead of medial) to the parenchyma because the kidney has incompletely rotated. As a result, 56% of ectopic kidneys have a hydronephrotic collecting system. Half of these cases are due to obstruction of the ureteropelvic or the ureterovesical junction (70% and 30%, respectively), 25% from reflux grade 3 or greater, and 25% from the malrotation alone.

7. **d. Karyotype.** Horseshoe kidney and coarctation of the aorta are seen in patients with Turner syndrome (45,XO). Therefore, a karyotype should be obtained. Other stigmata may include lymphedema, shield chest, low hairline, and webbed neck.

8. **b. Normal position of the adrenal gland.** Unilateral renal agenesis is commonly associated with an adrenal gland that is in a normal position, although it may be flattened. Regardless of sex, both gonads are usually normal. The most common müllerian duct anomalies are a true unicornuate uterus with complete absence of the ipsilateral horn and fallopian tube or a bicornuate uterus with rudimentary development of the horn on the affected side. A plain film of the abdomen (or other radiographic study such as magnetic resonance imaging) showing the gas pattern of the splenic flexure in the left renal fossa suggests left renal agenesis, ectopia, or crossed ectopia, whereas the gas pattern of the hepatic flexure positioned in the right renal fossa suggests congenital absence of the right kidney.

9. **d. Lifelong blood pressure check and urine analysis to monitor for evidence of chronic kidney disease.** Given the increased rate of chronic kidney disease seen in children with solitary functioning kidney, current suggestions include baseline and annual surveillance assessments of blood pressure and urine studies for proteinuria because hypertension and microalbuminuria are features of progressive decrease in glomerular filtration rate. A VCUG may reveal reflux at higher rate in unilateral renal agenesis

but it is not a mandatory test. Similarly, a well-performed renal ultrasound that does not reveal an ectopic kidney makes a renal scan to confirm the diagnosis an elective decision rather than mandatory one. There is no documented benefit to perpetual lifelong ultrasound screening in unilateral renal agenesis.

10. **e. Specific radiographic evidence.** Unilateral renal agenesis can be diagnosed reliably with radiographic examinations including abdominal and pelvic ultrasound, dimercaptosuccinic acid (DMSA) scan, and/or magnetic resonance angiography (MRA).

11. **b. Bilateral renal agenesis.** Male predominance is most striking in bilateral renal agenesis, with almost 75% of affected individuals being male. For unilateral renal agenesis, there is a male-to-female ratio of 1.8:1. Crossed fused ectopia has a slight male predominance (3:2), whereas ectopic kidneys have no significant difference in incidence between the sexes.

12. **c. 1:1100.** The incidence of unilateral renal agenesis is 1:1100.

13. **a. Before the fourth week.** Unilateral renal agenesis and a unicornuate uterus will form when the embryologic insult occurs before the fourth week. If the insult occurs early in the fourth week of gestation and affects both the wolffian duct and the ureteral bud, maldevelopment of the wolffian duct affects renal development, müllerian duct elongation, contact with the urogenital sinus, and subsequent fusion. Therefore, a didelphic uterus will form with obstruction of the horn and vagina on the side of the unilateral renal agenesis. If the insult occurs after the fourth week, the wolffian duct and müllerian duct elongation and differentiation proceed normally and only the ureteral bud and metanephric blastema are affected, thereby resulting in isolated unilateral renal agenesis.

14. **d. Adrenal agenesis.** In autopsy studies of unilateral renal agenesis, adrenal agenesis occurs in fewer than 10%, although the ipsilateral adrenal gland may be flattened or "lying down." The ureter is not normally developed, and the ipsilateral ureter is completely absent in approximately 60% of cases. The gonad is usually normal in both sexes. The head of the epididymis is normally formed because it is derived from the mesonephric tubules that link the mesonephric duct to the gonad.

15. **c. Kidneys with ectopic ureters.** Most ectopic kidneys are clinically asymptomatic except for the unusual cases of an ectopic kidney with an ectopic ureter.

16. **c. L3 and L4.** The isthmus of a horseshoe kidney is located adjacent to the third and fourth lumbar vertebrae.

17. **d. 90 degrees of medial rotation.** Between the sixth and ninth week, normal rotation of the kidney toward the midline to attain its orthotopic position involves 90 degrees of medial rotation.

18. **b. Cirsoid in configuration.** Fewer than 25% of all renal arteriovenous fistulas (AVFs) are congenital. They are identifiable by their cirsoid configuration and multiple communications between the main or segmental renal arteries and venous channels. Although congenital, they rarely present clinically before the third or fourth decade. Women are affected three times as often as men, and the right kidney is involved slightly more often than the left. The lesion is usually located in the upper pole (45% of cases), but not infrequently it may be found in the mid-portion (30%) or in the lower pole (25%) of the kidney.

19. **b. Has an increased number of dilated calyces.** Megacalycosis is defined as a nonobstructive enlargement of calyces resulting from malformation of the renal papillae. The calyces are generally dilated and malformed and may be increased in number. The renal pelvis is not dilated, nor is its wall thickened, and the ureteropelvic junction is normally funneled without evidence of obstruction. The ureter is usually normal. It occurs predominantly in males in a ratio of 6:1. Bilateral disease has been seen almost exclusively in males, whereas segmental unilateral involvement occurs only in females.

CHAPTER REVIEW

1. In bilateral renal agenesis, 40% of affected infants are stillborn. The ureters are almost always absent, and the bladder is either absent or hypoplastic. The adrenal glands, however, are usually in their normal anatomic position.
2. In patients with bilateral renal agenesis associated with oligohydramnios, Potter facies are pathognomonic of the process. Pulmonary hypoplasia is frequently present.
3. Ultrasound screening is recommended for parents and siblings of infants with unilateral or bilateral renal agenesis—there is a higher risk of renal agenesis in this population.
4. In unilateral renal agenesis, the ipsilateral ureter is completely absent in 60% of cases. Abnormalities of the contralateral ureter are not uncommon; reproductive tract anomalies in females are also common.
5. With unilateral renal agenesis, 25% of the contralateral ureters reflux.
6. There is an association of genital anomalies with renal ectopia. The upper pole of the ectopic kidney usually joins with the lower pole of the normal kidney.
7. In all types of fusion anomalies, the ureter from each kidney is usually orthotopic.
8. The highest incidence of associated anomalies occurs with solitary renal ectopia. Associated anomalies in the male include cryptorchidism, and vaginal atresia or unilateral uterine anomalies in the female.
9. In a horseshoe kidney, the isthmus is bulky and consists of parenchymatous tissue with its own blood supply. The blood supply to a horseshoe kidney is variable.
10. Ureteropelvic junction obstruction in horseshoe kidneys occurs one-third of the time.
11. The incidence of Wilms tumors and renal pelvic tumors in horseshoe kidneys is higher than would be expected in the general population. There is no increased risk of renal cell carcinoma.
12. Renal arteries are end arteries and, as such, have no collaterals.
13. Arteriovenous fistulas may result in hypertension in 50% of cases, due to relative ischemia beyond the fistula. It is renin-mediated hypertension.
14. Infundibulopelvic stenosis is usually bilateral and is commonly associated with vesicoureteral reflux.
15. Maternal diabetes is associated with a threefold increased risk of renal agenesis and dysplasia.
16. Patients born with renal agenesis may have decreased renal reserve in the remaining kidney, which results in a significant risk for end-stage renal disease.
17. Of adult males with absence of the vas deferens, 79% have an absent ipsilateral kidney.
18. Excision of a renal artery aneurysm is recommended if (1) the hypertension cannot be easily controlled; (2) incomplete ring-like calcification is present; (3) the aneurysm is larger than 2.5 cm; (4) the patient is female and of childbearing age, because rupture during pregnancy is a likely possibility; (5) the aneurysm increases in size on serial angiograms; or (6) an arteriovenous fistula is present.

39 Renal Dysgenesis and Cystic Disease of the Kidney

John C. Pope IV

QUESTIONS

1. Which of the following is a correct match regarding renal anomaly and associated finding?
   a. von Hippel-Lindau disease and adenoma sebaceum
   b. Tuberous sclerosis and angiomyolipoma
   c. Autosomal dominant polycystic kidney disease (ADPKD) and salt-losing nephropathy
   d. Congenital nephrosis (Finnish type) and medullary cysts
   e. Autosomal recessive polycystic kidney disease (ARPKD) and colonic diverticulosis

2. The primary feature(s) associated with Ask-Upmark kidney (segmental hypoplasia) is/are:
   a. hypertension.
   b. renal artery intimal disease.
   c. found in young men and boys.
   d. b and c.
   e. a and c.

3. The development of acquired renal cystic disease (ARCD) is most related to which factor?
   a. Age of the patient
   b. Duration of renal failure
   c. Recent initiation of hemodialysis
   d. *Escherichia coli* infection
   e. Genetic defect on chromosome 16

4. Which statement(s) about ARPKD is/are TRUE?
   a. The most severe forms develop in late childhood or adolescence.
   b. No matter the severity of the renal disease, all patients will have liver involvement in the form of congenital hepatic fibrosis.
   c. In newborns, ultrasound findings include very enlarged kidneys with increased parenchymal echogenicity.
   d. a and b.
   e. b and c.

5. Which of the following statements accurately describes a fundamental process essential for the development of renal cysts?
   a. Proliferation of epithelial cells in segments of the renal collecting system
   b. Accumulation of fluid within an expanding segment of the glomerulus
   c. An imbalance of the secretory and absorptive properties in proliferating tubular epithelial cells
   d. Hypertrophy of the basement membrane within the ascending loop of Henle
   e. Glomerular outpouching resulting from elevated glomerular hydrostatic pressure

6. Which of the following statement(s) is/are correct about ADPKD?
   a. The genetic defect is located on the short arm of chromosome 16.
   b. Most affected infants have congenital hepatic fibrosis.
   c. Renal cysts are infrequently seen on ultrasound in affected patients before 30 years of age.
   d. Glomerular cysts are never found in the kidneys of newborns diagnosed with ADPKD
   e. The incidence of renal cell carcinoma in ADPKD is twice that in the normal population.

7. All of the following are extrarenal manifestations of ADPKD EXCEPT:
   a. hepatic cysts.
   b. intracranial (berry) aneurysms.
   c. cerebellar hemangioblastomas.
   d. colonic diverticulosis.
   e. mitral valve prolapse.

8. Which of the following statements is FALSE regarding unilateral multicystic dysplastic kidneys?
   a. The majority of multicystic dysplastic kidneys become smaller or ultrasonographically undetectable with time.
   b. There is an absence of communication between cysts on ultrasonographic scans.
   c. Cysts are usually found in communication with each other when injected intracystically with contrast material.
   d. The sine qua non for histologic diagnosis of a multicystic dysplastic kidney is the presence of primitive ducts.
   e. Multicystic dysplastic kidneys appear more often in females and more often on the right side.

9. Flank pain is one of the most common presenting symptoms of ADPKD in adult patients. This is often caused by:
   a. bleeding into a cyst.
   b. renal cell carcinoma.
   c. cyst rupture.
   d. b and c.
   e. a and c.

10. Which gene is associated with clear cell renal cell carcinoma and a multiple malformation syndrome?
    a. PDK1
    b. PDK2
    c. TG737
    d. Wnt-2
    e. VHL

11. A benign multilocular cyst is seen most often:
    a. in males younger than 4 years and in females older than 30 years.
    b. in females younger than 4 years and in males older than 30 years.
    c. in males between 4 and 30 years.
    d. equally in both sexes before 4 years and in females after 30 years.

e. equally in both sexes before 4 years and in males after 30 years.

12. What is the primary distinguishing factor between juvenile nephronophthisis (NPH) and medullary cystic kidney disease (MCKD)?

a. NPH presents with polyuria and polydipsia, whereas MCKD does not.

b. NPH is an autosomal recessive disorder, whereas MCKD is an autosomal dominant disease.

c. NPH is diagnosed histologically with severe interstitial fibrosis, whereas MCKD is diagnosed by the presence of glomerulosclerosis.

d. Most patients with MCKD have extrarenal manifestations of the disease, whereas patients with NPH are usually affected only in the kidneys.

e. In patients with NPH, renal failure occurs in the third to fourth decade, whereas in patients with MCKD, renal failure typically occurs in adolescence.

13. A patient with which of the following entities has the highest likelihood of having a renal cell carcinoma develop?

a. ADPKD

b. Tuberous sclerosis

c. von Hippel-Lindau disease

d. Acquired renal cystic disease

e. Medullary sponge kidney

14. Which of the following is FALSE pertaining to MCDK?

a. MCDK is one of the most common causes of an abdominal mass in the newborn.

b. In patients with MCDK, the contralateral renal moiety is frequently affected by urologic disease.

c. MCDK is often difficult to differentiate from severe ureteropelvic junction obstruction.

d. Data from large series show that MCDK is associated with an increased risk for hypertension.

e. Roughly 40% of MCDKs will spontaneously involute over time.

15. Which of the following would confirm the diagnosis of tuberous sclerosis?

a. Renal angiomyolipoma and multiple renal cysts

b. Hamartomatous rectal polyps and facial adenoma sebaceum

c. Renal angiomyolipoma and cardiac rhabdomyoma

d. Multiple renal cysts, hepatic fibrosis, and pheochromocytoma

e. Mitral valve prolapse, renal angiolipoma, and gingival fibromas

16. The following are true of von Hippel-Lindau (VHL) disease EXCEPT:

a. VHL disease is an autosomal dominant syndrome.

b. VHL disease is caused by a mutation in the tumor suppressor gene, VHL, located on chromosome 3.

c. epididymal cysts are not infrequent in patients with VHL disease.

d. pheochromocytomas, cerebellar hemangioblastomas, and retinal angiomas are common extrarenal manifestations of VHL disease.

e. renal cell carcinomas, the most common manifestation, are seen in the vast majority of patients.

17. Renal sinus cysts are most likely derived from:

a. vascular elements.

b. renal parenchyma.

c. renal pelvis.

d. lymphatic system.

e. nephrogenic rests.

18. Most simple renal cysts that are identified in utero:

a. represent the first sign of a multicystic kidney.

b. represent the first sign of ARPKD.

c. represent the first sign of ADPKD.

d. represent a calyceal diverticulum.

e. resolve before birth.

19. Approximately what percentage of individuals older than 60 years will have an identifiable renal cyst on computed tomography (CT)?

a. 1% to 5%

b. 10%

c. 33%

d. 75%

e. 90%

20. Which of the following groups of antibiotics include the best choice for treating an infected renal cyst in a patient with ADPKD?

a. Trimethoprim-sulfamethoxazole, chloramphenicol, fluoroquinolones

b. Cephalosporins, trimethoprim-sulfamethoxazole, doxycycline

c. Gentamicin, cephalosporins, vancomycin

d. Fluoroquinolones, metronidazole, vancomycin

e. Doxycycline, amoxicillin, gentamicin

21. All of the following are reasonable treatment strategies for patients with ADPKD EXCEPT:

a. management of hypertension.

b. avoidance of surgical treatment for large or multiple cysts in patients with chronic flank pain.

c. surgical treatment of symptomatic urinary stone disease.

d. use of lipophilic antibiotics for treatment of a suspected renal cyst infection.

e. screening with magnetic resonance imaging (MRI) or CT for berry aneurysms in patients with a family history of subarachnoid hemorrhage.

22. In neonates with a unilateral multicystic kidney, what is the incidence of contralateral vesicoureteral reflux?

a. 0% to 7%

b. 18% to 43%

c. 50% to 67%

d. 75%

e. 7% to 15%

23. What is the most likely cause of flank pain and hematuria in a 50-year-old patient with end-stage renal disease who has been undergoing dialysis for 5 years?

a. Acute renal vein thrombosis

b. Acute renal artery thrombosis

c. Renal cell carcinoma

d. ARCD

e. Uric acid stones

24. Which group of three findings best describes the typical ultrasonographic image of a multicystic dysplastic kidney?

a. The cysts are organized around a central large cyst; there is no identifiable renal sinus; and there are communications between the cysts.

b. The cysts have a haphazard distribution; there is absence of a central or medial large cyst; and there are no obvious communications between the cysts.

c. The cysts have a haphazard distribution; there is no obvious renal sinus; and there is a large central cyst.

d. Connections exist between the cysts; a medial cyst is present; and a renal sinus is usually present.

e. The cysts are organized at the periphery; the largest is the central one; and there is an identifiable renal sinus.

25. Which one of the following conditions is most representative of a neoplastic growth?

a. Benign multilocular cyst

b. Oligomeganephronia

c. Multicystic dysplastic kidney

d. Calyceal diverticulum

e. Ask-Upmark kidney

26. Which of the following is the best match?

a. ARPKD and congenital hepatic fibrosis

b. Medullary sponge kidney and predominance of glomerular cysts

c. Juvenile nephronophthisis and cortical cysts

d. Ask-Upmark kidney and hypotension

e. von Hippel-Lindau disease and adenoma sebaceum

27. Which of the following matches is correct?

a. ARPKD and chromosome 2

b. ADPKD and chromosomes 4 and 16

c. Tuberous sclerosis and chromosomes 9 and 15

d. von Hippel-Lindau disease and chromosome 4

e. Juvenile nephronophthisis and chromosome 6

28. A renal cyst with increased number of septa and prominent calcification in a nonenhancing cyst wall does not require exploration, but requires timely follow-up. According to the Bosniak grading system, this cyst would be categorized as:

a. I.

b. II.

c. II F.

d. III.

e. IV.

29. Ultrasonography in neonates with ARPKD reveals kidneys that are hyperechogenic or "bright" in appearance. This finding is due to:

a. the presence of many small punctate calcifications within the renal papillae.

b. dysplastic, diseased renal parenchyma.

c. a vast increase in small fat deposits within the renal sinuses.

d. the presence of numerous microcysts created by tightly compacted, dilated collecting ducts that result in innumerable ultrasonographic interfaces.

e. the presence of renal hamartomas with increased cortical vascularity.

30. Ultrasound and/or CT criteria for the diagnosis of a simple renal cyst include all the following EXCEPT:

a. sharp, thin, distinct smooth walls and margins.

b. thickness of cyst wall less than or equal to 3 mm.

c. acoustic enhancement behind cyst (ultrasound).

d. spherical or ovoid shape.

e. homogeneous with absence of internal echoes.

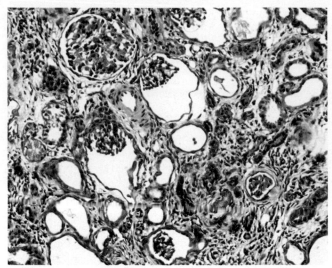

Fig. 39.1 (From Bostwick DG, Cheng L: *Urologic surgical pathology*, ed 3, St. Louis, 2014, Elsevier.)

31. A 50-year-old man with known von Hippel-Lindau disease presents with a single episode of gross hematuria. CT scan reveals a 3-cm enhancing mass in the upper pole of each kidney. Metastatic evaluation is negative. He is otherwise healthy. Appropriate treatment at this point would be:

a. bilateral radical nephrectomy with the placement of a peritoneal dialysis catheter.

b. bilateral upper pole partial nephrectomy.

c. right radical nephrectomy with left upper pole partial nephrectomy.

d. observation with serial CT every 4 months.

e. CT-guided needle biopsy of each lesion with surgical removal if diagnosis confirms renal cell carcinoma.

PATHOLOGY

1. A 2-year-old boy has a right nephrectomy following an automobile accident for a shattered kidney with uncontrollable bleeding. The histology depicted in Fig. 39.1 is reported as showing interstitial nephritis with cysts consistent with juvenile nephronophthisis. The next step in management is to:

a. have the pathologist reexamine the specimen for evidence of nephrogenic rests.

b. have the pathologist reexamine the specimen for an associated teratoma.

c. image the contralateral kidney for a renal mass.

d. image the liver for evidence of hepatic fibrosis.

e. inform the family that the child must be followed carefully for hypertension and decreased renal function.

ANSWERS

1. **b. Tuberous sclerosis and angiomyolipoma.** Angiomyolipomas occur in 40% to 80% of patients with tuberous sclerosis.

2. **a. Hypertension.** Hypertension and its sequelae (headache, hypertensive encephalopathy, retinopathy, etc.) are the hallmarks of Ask-Upmark kidney. Segmental vascular anomalies have been cited as a possible cause of the hypertension, but there is no evidence that renal artery intimal disease is associated. This disease is primarily found in young women and girls.

3. **b. Duration of renal failure.** At first, ARCD was thought to be confined to patients receiving hemodialysis. However, it

shortly became apparent that the disorder is almost as common in patients receiving peritoneal dialysis and that it may develop in patients with chronic renal failure who are being managed medically without any type of dialysis. Thus ARCD appears to be a feature of end-stage kidney disease, rather than a response to dialysis.

4. **e. b and c.** The most severe form of ARPKD appears earliest in life, in the newborn period. All patients with ARPKD have liver involvement in the form of hepatic fibrosis and vary in the degree of biliary ectasia and periportal fibrosis. In both fetus and newborn, ultrasonography identifies bilateral, very enlarged, diffusely echogenic kidneys, especially when compared with the echogenicity of the liver. The increased echogenicity is due to the presence of numerous microcysts (created by tightly compacted, dilated collecting ducts) that result in innumerable interfaces. Compared with normal newborn kidneys, in ARPKD the pyramids are hyperechogenic because they blend in with the rest of the kidney, and the kidneys typically have a homogeneous appearance.

5. **c. An imbalance of the secretory and absorptive properties in proliferating tubular epithelial cells.** The fundamental processes that are essential for the development and progressive enlargement of renal cysts include (1) proliferation of epithelial cells in segments of renal tubule, (2) accumulation of fluid within the expanding tubule segment, and (3) disturbed organization and metabolism of the extracellular matrix. An imbalance of the secretory and absorptive properties in proliferating epithelial cells leads to a net accumulation of fluid in otherwise normal renal tubules. Recent evidence indicates that, beyond the loop of Henle, tubule cells have the capacity to secrete solutes and fluid on stimulation with $3',5'$-cyclic adenosine monophosphate (cAMP). This secretory flux operates in competition with the more powerful mechanism by which sodium (Na^+) is reabsorbed through apical epithelial Na^+ channels (ENaC). Under conditions in which Na^+ reabsorption is diminished, the net secretion of sodium chloride (NaCl) and fluid occurs.

6. **a. The genetic defect is located on the short arm of chromosome 16.** Infants with ARPKD have hepatic fibrosis, and infants with ADPKD rarely have hepatic fibrosis but commonly have cysts in the liver. Renal cysts are frequently seen in individuals on ultrasonography by the age of 20 years. Glomerular cysts are sometimes found in the kidneys of newborns diagnosed with ADPKD. The risk of renal cell carcinoma in patients with ADPKD is no higher than that in the general population.

7. **c. Cerebellar hemangioblastomas.** All are extrarenal manifestations of ADPKD except cerebellar hemangioblastomas, which are seen in patients with von Hippel-Lindau disease.

8. **e. Multicystic dysplastic kidneys appear more often in females and more often on the right side.** At any age, the condition is more likely to be found on the left side. Males are more likely to have unilateral multicystic dysplastic kidneys (2.4:1).

9. **a. Bleeding into a cyst.** Pain (flank and/or abdominal) is the most common presenting symptom in adults. This results from a number of possible factors: mass effect (cysts impinging on abdominal wall or neighboring organs), bleeding into the cyst, urinary tract infection (including infected cysts), and nephrolithiasis.

10. **e. VHL.** The gene associated with the transmission of von Hippel-Lindau disease is located on chromosome 3. In non–von Hippel-Lindau patients with sporadic clear cell renal cell carcinoma, 50% of cell lines are associated with a mutational form of the VHL gene.

11. **a. In males younger than 4 years and in females older than 30 years.** The great majority of patients present before the age of 4 years or after the age of 30 years. Five percent present between 4 and 30 years. The patient is 2 times as likely to be male if younger than 4 years and 8 times as likely to be female if older than 30 years.

12. **b. NPH is an autosomal recessive disorder, whereas MCKD is an autosomal dominant disease.** Although either condition can occur sporadically, juvenile nephronophthisis usually is inherited as an autosomal recessive trait, whereas medullary cystic disease usually is inherited in an autosomal dominant fashion. Juvenile nephronophthisis and medullary cystic disease both cause polydipsia and polyuria in more than 80% of cases, but not to the extent observed in patients with diabetes insipidus. Pathologically, NPH and MCKD are similar. Histologically, there is a characteristic triad present that includes (1) irregular thickening and disintegration of the tubular basement membrane, (2) marked tubular atrophy with cyst development, and (3) interstitial cell infiltration with fibrosis. Twenty percent of juvenile nephronophthisis families have extrarenal manifestations, whereas MCKD usually affects only the kidneys. Another important difference between the two entities is that renal failure develops in patients with NPH at a mean age of 13 years and almost always before 25 years. MCKD is a milder disease when it presents in early adulthood, but it will manifest in all patients by 50 years (Bernstein and Gardner, 1979).[a] End-stage renal disease (ESRD) in patients with MCKD most often develops in the third or fourth decade of life.

13. **c. von Hippel-Lindau disease.** Tuberous sclerosis and von Hippel-Lindau disease are associated with epithelial hyperplasia (and adenomas as well) and have an increased incidence of renal cell carcinoma (tuberous sclerosis, 2%, and von Hippel-Lindau disease, 35% to 38%).

14. **d. Data from large series show that MCDK is associated with an increased risk for hypertension.** All statements are true of MCDK, except that large series indicate MCDK is NOT associated with an increased risk of hypertension.

15. **c. Renal angiomyolipoma and cardiac rhabdomyoma.** Definitive diagnosis of tuberous sclerosis (TSC) is dependent on the presence of certain major and minor clinical features. The diagnosis of TSC requires two major features (renal angiomyolipoma, facial angiofibromas or forehead plaques, nontraumatic ungual or periungual fibroma, three or more hypomelanotic macules, shagreen patch, multiple retinal nodular hamartomas, cortical tuber, subependymal nodule, subependymal giant cell astrocytoma, cardiac rhabdomyoma, lymphangioleiomyomatosis) or one major plus two minor features (multiple renal cysts, nonrenal hamartoma, hamartomatous rectal polyps, retinal achromic patch, cerebral white matter radial migration tracts, bone cysts, gingival fibromas, "confetti" skin lesions, multiple enamel pits).

16. **e. Renal cell carcinomas, the most common manifestation, are seen in the vast majority of patients.** All statements are true of VHL disease except that renal cysts, NOT *renal cell carcinoma*, are the most common and often earliest manifestation as seen in 76% of patients.

17. **d. Lymphatic system.** The predominant type of renal sinus cyst appears to be one derived from the lymphatics.

18. **e. Resolve before birth.** In 28 of 11,000 fetuses with renal cysts, 25 fetuses had the cysts resolve before birth. Of two cysts that remained postnatally, in one it was the first sign of a multicystic kidney.

19. **c. 33%.** In adults, the frequency of renal cyst occurrence increases with age. Using CT, one group demonstrated a 20% incidence of cysts by 40 years and approximately 33% incidence of cysts after 60 years.

20. **a. Trimethoprim-sulfamethoxazole, chloramphenicol, fluoroquinolones.** In the experience of one group of researchers, the only dependable antibiotics were those that were lipid soluble, namely, trimethoprim-sulfamethoxazole and chloramphenicol. Chloramphenicol produced better results. The fluoroquinolones, which are also lipid soluble, are

---

[a] Sources referenced can be found in *Campbell-Walsh-Wein Urology, 12th Edition*, on the Expert Consult website.

proving useful. If a patient with suspected pyelonephritis does not respond to an antibiotic, and if the antibiotic used is not lipid soluble, one must consider whether the infection may be present in a noncommunicating cyst.

21. **b. Avoidance of surgical treatment for large or multiple cysts in patients with chronic flank pain.** All are reasonable treatment strategies for a patient with ADPKD, except that when conservative measures of chronic pain treatment fail, surgical management must be considered. Ultrasonography- or CT-guided cyst aspiration is a straightforward procedure and may be both diagnostic and therapeutic. Surgical unroofing of multiple or very large cysts can potentially alleviate symptoms of pain and can be performed either laparoscopically or through open flank or dorsal lumbotomy incisions. Surgical intervention appears to only improve symptomatology and does not appear to either accelerate the decline of renal function or preserve declining renal function.

22. **b. 18% to 43%.** Contralateral vesicoureteral reflux is seen even more often than contralateral ureteropelvic junction obstruction, being identified in 18% to 43% of infants.

23. **d. ARCD.** The most common presentation of ARCD is loin pain, hematuria, or both. Bleeding occurs in as many as 50% of patients.

24. **b. The cysts have a haphazard distribution; there is absence of a central or medial large cyst; and there are no obvious communications between the cysts.** Renal masses in infants most often represent either multicystic kidney disease or hydronephrosis, and it is important to distinguish the two, especially if the surgeon wishes to remove a nonfunctioning hydronephrotic kidney or repair a ureteropelvic junction obstruction while leaving a multicystic organ in situ. In newborns, ultrasonography is generally the first study performed. In a few cases, it is difficult to distinguish multicystic kidney disease from severe hydronephrosis. In general, however, the multicystic kidney has a haphazard distribution of cysts of various sizes without a larger central or medial cyst and without visible communications between the cysts. Frequently, very small cysts appear in between the large cysts. By comparison, in ureteropelvic junction obstruction, the cysts or calyces are organized around the periphery of the kidney, connections can usually be demonstrated between the peripheral cysts and a central or medial cyst that represents the renal pelvis, and there is an absence of small cysts between the larger cysts. When there is an identifiable renal sinus, the diagnosis is more likely to be hydronephrosis than multicystic kidney.

25. **a. Benign multilocular cyst.** For the benign multilocular cystic lesion, certain authors prefer the term *cystic nephroma*, because this term implies a benign but neoplastic lesion.

26. **a. ARPKD and congenital hepatic fibrosis.** All patients with ARPKD have varying degrees of congenital hepatic fibrosis.

27. **b. ADPKD and chromosomes 4 and 16.** For the genetic cystic disease ADPKD, the chromosomal defect is on chromosome 16 for *PKD1* and 4 for *PKD2*; *PKD3* has not been mapped. Autosomal recessive polycystic kidney disease involves chromosome 6; tuberous sclerosis involves chromosomes 9 and 16; von Hippel-Lindau disease involves chromosome 3; and juvenile nephronophthisis involves chromosome 2.

28. **c. II F.** The Bosniak classification has recently been updated to include category II F. Bosniak I—simple cyst with imperceptible wall, rounded. Workup: none. Percentage malignant: ~0%. Bosniak II—minimally complex with a few thin <1 mm septa or thin calcifications (thickness not measurable); non-enhancing high-attenuation (due to proteinaceous or hemorrhagic contents) renal lesions <3 cm. These lesions are generally well marginated. Workup: none. Percentage malignant: ~0%. Bosniak IIF—minimally complex with increased number of septa, minimally thickened with nodular or thick calcifications. There may be perceived (but not measurable) enhancement of hairline-thin smooth septa, minimal thickening of the wall with perceivable enhancement, hyperdense cyst >3 cm diameter, mostly intrarenal (less than 25% of wall visible); no enhancement. Requires fol-

low-up (the "F" in 2F is for "follow"): needs ultrasound/CT/MRI follow-up—no strict rules on the time frame but reasonable at 6 months. Percentage malignant: ~5%. Bosniak III—indeterminate with thick, nodular multiple septa or wall with measurable enhancement. Treatment/workup: partial nephrectomy. Percentage malignant: ~55%. Bosniak IV—clearly malignant with solid mass with a large cystic or a necrotic component. Treatment: partial or total nephrectomy. Percentage malignant: ~100%

29. **d. The presence of numerous microcysts created by tightly compacted, dilated collecting ducts that result in innumerable ultrasonographic interfaces.** In both fetuses and newborns with ARPKD, ultrasonography identifies bilateral, very enlarged, diffusely echogenic kidneys, especially when compared with the echogenicity of the liver. The increased echogenicity is due to the presence of numerous microcysts (created by tightly compacted, dilated collecting ducts) that result in innumerable interfaces. Compared with normal newborn kidneys, in ARPKD the pyramids are hyperechogenic because they blend in with the rest of the kidney, and the kidneys typically have a homogeneous appearance.

30. **b. Thickness of cyst wall less than or equal to 3 mm.** One can safely make the diagnosis of a classic benign simple cyst by ultrasonography when the following criteria are met: (1) absence of internal echoes; (2) sharply defined, thin, distinct wall with a smooth and distinct margin; (3) good transmission of sound waves through the cyst with consequent acoustic enhancement behind the cyst; and (4) spherical or slightly ovoid shape. The CT criteria for a simple cyst are similar to those used in ultrasonography: (1) sharp, thin, distinct, smooth walls and margins; (2) spherical or ovoid shape; and (3) homogeneous content.

31. **b. Bilateral upper pole partial nephrectomy.** Because the tumors that characterize VHL disease are frequently multiple, bilateral, and recurrent, close surveillance and minimization of surgical procedures constitute the mainstay of treatment. For patients who have VHL disease and all patients who have hereditary cancer syndromes, the goal of treatment is cancer control, not cancer cure, and preservation of functional parenchyma to avoid the morbidity associated with renal loss. In patients who have VHL disease, surgical resection is performed with the understanding that microscopic disease probably is left behind. Currently, nephron-sparing surgery should be considered the standard of care for treating low-grade renal cell carcinoma in the setting of VHL disease. Patients with high-grade disease are still probably best served with bilateral nephrectomy. Despite having the objective of sparing as much renal parenchyma as possible and preventing metastasis of the lesions already present, it is not curative surgery (Reed, 2009). Although this approach does not reduce the risk of recurrence, reported to be 75% to 85%, the 10-year disease-specific survival rates are quite high (81% to 94%) (Malek, 1987; Steinbach, 1995; Roupret, 2003; Ploussard, 2007). Classically, the survival rate after nephrectomy has been only 50%. Because most of these tumors are low grade, a nephron-sparing approach provides very good survival rates while avoiding the diminished quality of life that comes with bilateral nephrectomy and subsequent dialysis/transplantation. Laparoscopic and percutaneous image-guided ablative techniques, such as radiofrequency ablation and cryoablation, have also been used and are currently under investigation.

PATHOLOGY

1. **e. Inform the family that the child must be followed carefully for hypertension and decreased renal function.** The histology is classic for juvenile nephronophthisis showing chronic interstitial nephritis-fibrosis, atrophic tubules, and glomerular microcysts. It is usually inherited as an autosomal recessive. These patients have a high likelihood of developing hypertension and eventually chronic renal failure. They may also develop retinitis pigmentosa.

CHAPTER REVIEW

1. Potter facies is manifested by hypertelorism, prominent inner canthal folds, and a recessive chin.
2. Dysplasia is histologically manifested by embryonic, immature mesenchyme, and primitive renal components; it is often associated with ureteric bud abnormalities and/or urinary obstruction.
3. Renal hypoplasia is manifested by less than the normal number of calyces and nephrons with absence of dysplasia.
4. Oligomeganephronia is a reduced number of nephrons with hypertrophy of the remaining nephrons. Many patients with the disorder develop renal failure.
5. The Ask-Upmark kidney (segmental hypoplasia) is often associated with reflux and patients develop severe hypertension.
6. Autosomal dominant polycystic kidney disease is associated with cysts of the liver, pancreas, spleen, and lungs, berry aneurysms; colonic diverticula; aortic aneurysms; and mitral valve prolapse. It usually becomes clinically manifest in the fourth and fifth decades.
7. Benign multilocular cyst and cystic nephroma fall into a spectrum of disease, with multilocular cyst on the one end being benign and, on the other end of the spectrum, cystic Wilms tumors being malignant. Multilocular cyst with nodules of Wilms tumor lies in the middle.
8. In the adult, there is a multilocular cystic renal cell carcinoma. Multilocular cystic lesions should therefore be removed.
9. One-third of patients with medullary sponge kidneys have hypercalciuria.
10. Congenital bilateral absence of the vas is associated with cystic fibrosis; unilateral absence of the vas may be associated with ipsilateral absence of the kidney.
11. Von Hippel-Lindau syndrome is inherited as an autosomal dominant and is manifested by cerebellar and retinal hemangioblastomas; cysts of the pancreas, kidney, and epididymis; epididymal cystadenoma, pheochromocytoma, and clear cell renal cell carcinoma.
12. Multicystic dysplastic kidney has no identifiable normal renal parenchyma; it is not associated with an increased risk of either hypertension or malignancy.
13. Medullary sponge kidney has dilated collecting ducts and is associated with hypercalciuria, hypocitraturia, and renal calculi.
14. All patients with autosomal recessive polycystic kidney disease (ARPKD) have liver involvement in the form of hepatic fibrosis and varying degrees of biliary ectasia and periportal fibrosis.
15. Juvenile nephronophthisis usually is inherited as an autosomal recessive trait, whereas medullary cystic disease usually is inherited in an autosomal dominant fashion. Juvenile nephronophthisis and medullary cystic disease both cause polydipsia and polyuria, and pathologically they are similar.

40 Pathophysiology of Urinary Tract Obstruction

Craig A. Peters and Kirstan K. Meldrum

QUESTIONS

1. Congenital obstruction differs from acquired obstruction in that it:
   a. causes renal atrophy.
   b. induces interstitial fibrosis.
   c. alters renal homeostasis.
   d. affects tubular function.
   e. affects glomerular development.

2. Renal dysplasia associated with obstruction is characterized by:
   a. renal atrophy.
   b. glomerular cysts.
   c. fibromuscular collars.
   d. heterotopic bone formation.
   e. excess production of afferent arteriole renin.

3. After relief of a unilateral obstructing lesion, decreasing relative uptake on radionuclide renal imaging is most likely due to:
   a. glomerular hyperfiltration.
   b. asymmetrical renal growth.
   c. established renal tubular fibrosis.
   d. neural imbalance.
   e. compensatory hypertrophy.

4. In the obstructed kidney, epidermal growth factor (EGF) has been shown to:
   a. reduce renal apoptosis.
   b. reduce glomerular sclerosis.
   c. accelerate interstitial fibrosis.
   d. improve collecting duct function.
   e. reduce renin recruitment in the afferent arteriole.

5. Epithelial to mesenchymal transformation in the developing kidney is:
   a. a one-way process.
   b. the basis for glomerular sclerosis.
   c. integral to glomerular development.
   d. seen only in the setting of obstruction.
   e. reflected in the presence of α-smooth muscle actin.

6. Regulation of the extracellular matrix in the kidney:
   a. depends on normal expression of EGF.
   b. depends entirely on collagen synthesis.
   c. is not related to angiotensin expression.
   d. depends on balanced synthesis and degradation.
   e. is independent of transforming growth factor-β (TGF-β) activity.

7. The principal effects of congenital renal obstruction are:
   a. glomerulosclerosis, interstitial fibrosis, and atrophy.
   b. hypoplasia and increased epithelial-mesenchymal transformation.
   c. altered growth regulation, renal differentiation, and functional integration.
   d. glomerulosclerosis, renin downregulation, and tubular hypertrophy.
   e. increased growth, fibrosis, and tubular atrophy.

8. In the fetal kidney, angiotensin activity:
   a. is tightly regulated by EGF.
   b. acts predominantly through the AT-1 receptor.
   c. affects epithelial-mesenchymal transformation.
   d. is an important regulator of renal growth.
   e. is unaffected by renal obstruction.

9. Inflammatory change in the congenitally obstructed kidney:
   a. is similar to those seen in postnatally obstructed kidneys.
   b. is mediated by the renin-angiotensin system.
   c. is minimal in the absence of overt infection.
   d. is the key element in glomerular damage.
   e. affects renal interstitial fibrosis.

ANSWERS

1. **e. Affects glomerular development.** Only congenital obstruction will change glomerular development, whereas acquired obstruction can produce all of the other changes indicated. Because it occurs during development, congenital obstruction can produce an altered developmental pattern, whereas acquired obstruction cannot change an already established pattern, only damage or distort it.

2. **c. Fibromuscular collars.** One of the histologic hallmarks of dysplasia is fibromuscular collars, so-called *primitive ducts* reflecting abnormal differentiation of the peritubular mesenchyme. Renal growth impairment is common with dysplasia; however, this is not atrophy but growth failure. Glomerular cysts are not characteristic of dysplasia. Heterotopic cartilage may be seen, but not bone. Excess renin expression may be seen in obstruction without dysplasia.

3. **b. Asymmetrical renal growth.** When renal function appears to decline after relief of obstruction, it is often due to different growth and functional development rates of the two kidneys, when the affected kidney cannot increase its absolute function as rapidly as the other intact kidney. This produces a progressive differential functional uptake on nuclear imaging that gives the impression of functional loss that is relative and not absolute.

4. **a. Reduce renal apoptosis.** Administration of EGF to the congenitally obstructed kidney can reduce renal apoptosis and reduce the effects of growth impairment. The other effects have not been reported.

5. **e. Reflected in the presence of α-smooth muscle actin.** Epithelial to mesenchymal transformations are an important part of renal development but have not been shown to be part of normal glomerular development. It is the presumed basis for the presence of α-smooth muscle actin in the obstructed kidney. It is bidirectional.

6. **d. Depends on balanced synthesis and degradation.** Extracellular membrane (ECM) regulation is due to collagen synthesis rates as well as to the rate of ECM breakdown. The latter is determined by the balanced activities of the tissue inhibitors of metalloproteinases (TIMPs) and matrix metalloproteinases (MMPs); these are regulated in part by TGF β and the renin-angiotensin system.

7. **c. Altered growth regulation, renal differentiation, and functional integration.** The key patterns defining congenital renal obstruction are altered growth regulation, renal differentiation, and functional integration, although interstitial fibrosis, tubular hypotrophy, and increased epithelial-mesenchymal transformation are components of these changes.

8. **d. Is an important regulator of renal growth.** In the developing kidney, angiotensin is an important growth regulator, as well as mediator of fibrosis, and is altered significantly by obstruction. Fetal angiotensin acts predominantly through the AT2 receptor until late in gestation, when the AT1 receptor begins to exert a greater role.

9. **c. Is minimal in the absence of overt infection.** In contrast to acquired obstruction, congenital obstruction is not characterized by a significant inflammatory infiltrate, except when complicated by infection.

CHAPTER REVIEW

1. A damaged kidney does not have the functional reserve to maintain normal renal function over time as the child grows. Thus, with time, the creatinine concentration will rise in patients who have no functional reserve in their nephron mass.
2. Obstructive processes may produce dysplasia.
3. In some cases, congenitally obstructed kidneys are smaller. This is not a result of atrophy but of hypoplasia.
4. A critical determinant of dysplasia in the kidney is complete obstruction early in gestation.
5. A universal characteristic of obstruction is renal fibrosis with infiltration of the interstitium with extracellular matrix.
6. The frequency with which a post-obstructed kidney has progressive deterioration in renal function is 20%–40%; it does not have the renal reserve of a normal kidney and may have a reduced number and function of nephrons. This results in hyperfiltration resulting in glomerulosclerosis and a progressive decline in renal function.
7. Measures of urinary sodium, chloride, osmolality, and calcium correlate with fetal renal function. When these measures approach serum levels, irreversible damage is suggested.
8. The distinctness of the calyx is helpful in determining the functionality of the obstruction. Thus, no caliectasis suggests a mild to minimal degree of functional obstruction.
9. ^{99m}Tc-Mercaptoacetyltriglycine is generally used for diuretic renography. It is taken up and excreted by the renal tubules relatively rapidly with little glomerular filtration.
10. Though other factors may play a role, if the diuretic renogram shows a T1/2 greater than 20 minutes, the kidney is

presumed to be obstructed; if it is less than 10 minutes, it is presumed normal; if it is between 10 and 20 minutes, it is considered indeterminate.
11. Obstruction can be very harmful to the developing kidney, far beyond that seen in the mature kidney. The effects of obstruction may not be reversible owing to alterations in structure and function in the developing kidney that do not occur in the mature kidney.
12. When obstruction results in a growth impairment, the results are fewer nephron units and delayed nephron maturation.
13. Angiotensin appears to be a key modulator of the inflammatory response in renal obstruction. It is also an important growth regulator, as well as mediator of fibrosis, and is altered significantly by obstruction.
14. Renal renin is increased in the obstructed kidney.
15. Inflammation with interstitial infiltration of lymphocytes is a common finding in postnatal acquired obstruction.
16. When renal function appears to decline after relief of obstruction, it is often due to differential growth and functional development rates of the two kidneys, when the affected kidney cannot increase its absolute function as rapidly as the contralateral intact kidney. This produces a progressive differential functional uptake on nuclear imaging that gives the impression of functional loss that is relative and not absolute.
17. In contrast to acquired obstruction, congenital obstruction is not characterized by a significant inflammatory infiltrate, except when complicated by infection.

41 Ectopic Ureter, Ureterocele, and Ureteral Anomalies

Irina Stanasel and Craig A. Peters

QUESTIONS

1. All of the following are possible drainage sites for an ectopic ureter in a female EXCEPT the:
   a. fallopian tube.
   b. uterus.
   c. ovary.
   d. vagina.
   e. urethra.

2. Inadequate interaction between the ureteral bud and metanephric blastema will most likely lead to which of the following conditions?
   a. Dysplasia
   b. Hydronephrosis
   c. Reflux
   d. Ureteral ectopia
   e. Multicystic dysplasia

3. The relationship between the upper and lower pole orifices in a complete ureteral duplication is best described by the upper pole:
   a. orifice being cephalad and lateral to the lower orifice.
   b. ureter joining the lower pole ureter just before entry into the bladder.
   c. orifice being caudal and medial to the lower pole orifice.
   d. orifice and lower pole orifice being located transversely side by side.
   e. ureter joining the bladder neck caudal to the lower pole orifice.

4. The most common site of drainage of an ectopic ureter in a male is:
   a. vas deferens.
   b. anterior urethra.
   c. seminal vesicle.
   d. posterior urethra.
   e. ampulla of the vas.

5. All of the following contribute to vesicoureteral reflux EXCEPT:
   a. lateral ureteral insertion.
   b. lax bladder neck.
   c. poorly developed trigone.
   d. gaping ureteral orifice.
   e. short intramural tunnel.

6. The voiding pattern most often seen in a girl with an ectopic ureter is:
   a. urge incontinence.
   b. stress incontinence.
   c. continuous incontinence.
   d. interrupted urinary stream.
   e. overflow incontinence.

7. Which of the following findings is most likely present on an ultrasound in a patient with an ectopic ureter in a duplicated system?
   a. Echogenic parenchyma of the lower pole of the kidney
   b. Medially displaced lower pole of the kidney
   c. Cystic structure in the bladder
   d. Tortuous lower pole ureter
   e. Cystic changes in the upper pole of the kidney

8. Ureteroceles can be associated with all of the following EXCEPT:
   a. smoking during pregnancy.
   b. vesicoureteral reflux.
   c. white race.
   d. female gender.
   e. duplicated kidneys.

9. All of the following can be caused by a ureterocele. Which is the LEAST likely to occur?
   a. Bladder outlet obstruction
   b. Upper pole obstruction
   c. Lower pole reflux
   d. Urinary incontinence
   e. Contralateral reflux

10. A child known to have a ureterocele based on ultrasound imaging undergoes cystography, but no filling defect is noted. The most likely explanation is:
    a. ureterocele eversion.
    b. lower pole reflux.
    c. ureterocele effacement.
    d. ureterocele prolapse.
    e. ureterocele disproportion.

11. A girl undergoes open resection of a large ectopic ureterocele. After removal of the catheter, she has high post-void residuals demonstrated on a sonogram. Which complication is most likely responsible?
    a. Persistent reflux
    b. Prolapsing residual ureterocele tissue
    c. Neurapraxia secondary to bladder retraction
    d. Excessive buttressing of deficient detrusor at the bladder neck
    e. Residual flap of the ureterocele in the urethra

12. What is the preferred method of endoscopic treatment of a ureterocele?
    a. Resection of the roof of the ureterocele
    b. Puncture of the distal urethral extension of the ureterocele
    c. Puncture of the roof of the ureterocele
    d. Transverse incision at the base of the ureterocele
    e. Resection of the base of the ureterocele only

13. An adult is evaluated as a possible kidney donor. An excretory urogram demonstrates a round contrast agent–filled area at the bladder base with a thin radiolucent rim around it. What is the most likely diagnosis?
    a. Single-system kidney with a ureterocele
    b. Marked opacification delay of the kidney
    c. Radio-opaque stone filling the ureterocele
    d. Extension of a ureterocele to the bladder neck and urethra
    e. Reflux

14. A white infant is found to have a smooth interlabial mass on the posterior aspect of the urethra. What would be the most appropriate initial management?
    a. Chemotherapy
    b. Puncture of the mass
    c. Topical estrogen cream
    d. Observation
    e. Resection of the mass

15. An 11-year-old child presents with flank pain and hematuria. There is left hydronephrosis to the ureteropelvic junction. There is no ureteral dilation. Diuretic renography shows symmetric uptake in both kidneys and a very delayed washout time with a half-life of 50 minutes. At the time of surgery, a retrograde pyelogram shows a proximal ureteral filling defect. The best course of action is:
    a. abandon the procedure and obtain computed tomography (CT) imaging with contrast.
    b. perform ureteroscopic biopsy.
    c. perform radical nephroureterectomy.
    d. perform ureteroscopic excision of the presumed fibroepithelial polyp.
    e. proceed with dismembered pyeloplasty and resect a fibroepithelial polyp.

16. An infant is seen with an intravesical ureterocele, no reflux, and an echogenic moderately dilated upper pole that has limited function. The washout curve of the upper pole moiety shows a T1/2 of 10 minutes. The most appropriate treatment option would be:
    a. observation with repeat ultrasound in 6 months.
    b. ureterocele excision and common sheath reimplantation.
    c. transureteral incision of the ureterocele.
    d. prophylactic antibiotics, observation, and repeat ultrasound in 4 months.
    e. upper pole partial nephrectomy.

17. Which of the following statements regarding duplex kidneys is TRUE?
    a. Duplex kidneys are the same size as single-system kidneys.
    b. The upper pole moiety is the more likely of the two to have a ureteropelvic junction obstruction.
    c. The duplex kidney arises as a consequence of two separate ureteric buds.
    d. A duplex kidney results from two separate metanephric blastemal entities arising near the mesonephric duct.
    e. The lower pole ureter is less likely to have vesicoureteral reflux.

18. In a child with a functioning nondilated upper pole segment associated with an ectopic ureter, the most efficient therapeutic option(s) (more than one answer may be correct) would be:
    a. common sheath ureteral reimplantation.
    b. upper to lower ureteropyelostomy.
    c. upper to lower distal ureteroureterostomy.

d. upper pole partial nephrectomy.
e. upper pole ureteral reimplantation.

19. Initial endoscopic incision of a ureterocele offers the following advantages EXCEPT:
    a. early relief of bladder outlet obstruction.
    b. potential for definitive therapy.
    c. possible improvement in trigonal deficiency.
    d. potential for improved function of the affected renal segment.
    e. decompression of a dilated upper pole ureter.

20. What is the most common form of ureteral triplication?
    a. All three ureters joining to terminate in a single bladder orifice
    b. Three ureters joining to form two ureteral orifices
    c. Three ureters draining as three separate orifices
    d. One of the three ureters terminating ectopically, the other two draining orthotopically
    e. Two ureters draining into three orifices

21. Failure of atrophy of which vessel leads to the formation of a preureteral vena cava?
    a. Posterior cardinal vein
    b. Subcardinal vein
    c. Supracardinal vein
    d. Umbilical artery
    e. Inferior vitelline vein

22. Which of the following types of ureterocele is associated with the lowest incidence of secondary procedures after transurethral decompression?
    a. Ectopic ureterocele
    b. Ureterocele in a female patient
    c. Intravesical ureterocele
    d. Ureterocele associated with a duplicated system
    e. Cecoureterocele

23. After the perinatal period, what is the most common method of presentation of a ureterocele?
    a. Incontinence
    b. Abdominal mass
    c. Failure to thrive
    d. Stranguria
    e. Urinary tract infection

24. A patient with a suspected ectopic ureter due to incontinence has no hydronephrosis on an ultrasonographic study and apparent single systems bilaterally. Which of the following tests is a sensitive method of determining if there is an ectopic ureter and associated renal moiety?
    a. Diethylenetriaminepentaacetic acid (DTPA) renal scanning
    b. Magnetic resonance imaging (MRI) of the abdomen and pelvis
    c. Nuclear voiding cystourethrography
    d. Positron emission tomography
    e. Intravenous pyelography

ANSWERS

1. **c. Ovary.** An ectopic ureter may drain into any of the structures related to the Wolffian duct and can rupture into the adjoining fallopian tube, uterus, upper vagina, or the urethra.

2. **a. Dysplasia.** Clinical and experimental observations combine to support the commonly held notion that dysplasia is the product of inadequate ureteric bud-to-blastema interaction. The other conditions may include such an abnormal interaction but are not specifically the result of that interaction.

3. **c. Orifice being caudal and medial to the lower pole orifice.** The upper pole orifice is caudal and medial to the lower pole orifice because of its later incorporation and migration into the trigonal structure. The lower pole orifice is more cranial and lateral to the caudad medial upper pole orifice.

4. **d. Posterior urethra.** In the male, the posterior urethra is the most common site of the termination of the ectopic ureter. All other sites except the anterior urethra are possible sites of ectopic ureteral insertion.

5. **b. Lax bladder neck.** It is owing to the combined effects of the lateral ureteral orifice position, the ureter's shortened submucosal course, the poorly developed trigone, and the abnormal morphology of the ureteral orifice that primary vesicoureteral reflux develops.

6. **c. Continuous incontinence.** Continuous incontinence in a girl with an otherwise normal voiding pattern after toilet training is the classic symptom of an ectopic ureteral orifice. This may not be obvious in a girl who has not yet been toilet trained, but can occasionally be seen as slow steady dribbling of urine on direct observation.

7. **d. Tortuous lower pole ureter.** The most obvious imaging sign on ultrasonography of an ectopic ureter is a tortuous dilated ureter due to distal obstruction. This is not always present, but when seen should direct further attention to the distal ureter and bladder to also assess for the presence of a ureterocele, which would appear as a cystic structure in the bladder. The upper pole may be dysplastic, but cystic changes are uncommon. The lower pole is usually normal, but may be hydronephrotic, yet uncommonly echogenic. The lower pole is displaced laterally, not medially.

8. **a. Smoking during pregnancy.** Ureteroceles occur most frequently in females (4:1 ratio) and almost exclusively in whites. Approximately 10% are bilateral. Eighty percent of all ureteroceles arise from the upper poles of duplicated systems, and approximately 50% will have associated vesicoureteral reflux.

9. **a. Bladder outlet obstruction.** Ultrasonographic study may show a dilated ureter emanating from a hydronephrotic upper pole. This finding should signal the examiner to image the bladder to determine whether a ureterocele is present. If the lower pole is associated with reflux, or if the ureterocele has caused delayed emptying from the ipsilateral lower pole, this lower pole may likewise be hydronephrotic. Similarly, the ureterocele may impinge on the contralateral ureteral orifice or obstruct the bladder neck and cause hydronephrosis in the opposite kidney, but the latter is uncommon. The upper pole parenchyma drained by the ureterocele will exhibit varying degrees of thickness and echogenicity. Increased echogenicity correlates with dysplastic changes. Reflux may also be seen in the contralateral system if the ureterocele is large enough to distort the trigone and the opposite ureteral submucosal tunnel. In one series, 28% of patients had reflux in the contralateral unit.

10. **c. Ureterocele effacement.** Voiding cystourethrography can usually demonstrate the size and laterality of the ureterocele as well as the presence or absence of vesicoureteral reflux. If early filling views are not obtained, the ureterocele may efface and the filling defect may not be visible. In some cases the ureterocele will evert and appear as a diverticulum.

11. **e. Residual flap of the ureterocele in the urethra.** The authors of one study emphasized the need for passing a large catheter antegrade through the bladder neck to ascertain that all mucosal lips that might act as obstructing valves have been removed. In some large ureteroceles, if repair of the maldeveloped trigone is not adequate, a posterior defect at the bladder neck can act as an obstructive valve during voiding.

12. **d. Transverse incision at the base of the ureterocele.** Our preferred method of incising the ureterocele is similar to that described by Rich and colleagues in 1990, a transverse incision through the full thickness of the ureterocele wall using the cutting current. The incision should be made as distally on the ureterocele and as close to the bladder floor as possible to lessen the chance of postoperative reflux into the ureterocele.

13. **a. Single-system kidney with a ureterocele.** Excretory urography often demonstrates the characteristic cobra head (or spring-onion) deformity: an area of increased density similar to the head of a cobra with a halo or less dense shadow around it. The halo represents a filling defect, which is the ureterocele wall, and the oval density is contrast material excreted into the ureterocele from the functioning kidney.

14. **b. Puncture of the mass.** A ureterocele that extends through the bladder neck and the urethra and presents as a vaginal mass in girls is termed a prolapsing ureterocele. This mass can be distinguished from other interlabial masses (e.g., rhabdomyosarcoma, urethral prolapse, hydrometrocolpos, and periurethral cysts) by virtue of its appearance and location. The prolapsed ureterocele has a smooth round wall, as compared with the grapelike cluster that typifies rhabdomyosarcoma. The color may vary from pink to bright red to the necrotic shades of blue, purple, or brown. The ureterocele usually slides down the posterior wall of the urethra, and, hence, the urethra can be demonstrated anterior to the mass and can be catheterized. The short-term goal is to decompress the ureterocele. The prolapsing ureterocele may be manually reduced back into the bladder; however, even if this is successful, the prolapse is likely to recur. Subsequent management is determined by further functional evaluation.

15. **e. Proceed with dismembered pyeloplasty and resect a fibroepithelial polyp.** This scenario most likely represents a fibroepithelial polyp of the ureteropelvic junction creating or associated with obstruction. The best approach is to proceed with the planned pyeloplasty and identify and resect the polyp thoroughly, followed by performing a conventional dismembered pyeloplasty. At times polyps may be multiple and complex, so this possibility should be looked for.

16. **d. Prophylactic antibiotics, observation, and repeat ultrasound in 4 months.** In the setting of no reflux and a draining upper pole associated with a ureterocele, the option of observation with prophylactic antibiotics has been seen to permit spontaneous resolution and no surgical intervention. Prophylactic antibiotics are recommended until resolution is demonstrated.

17. **c. The duplex kidney arises as a consequence of two separate ureteric buds.** Duplication anomalies arise as a consequence of two ureteral buds forming and inducing separate segments of the metanephric blastema. The duplex kidney may be completely normal, although it tends to be longer than normal, but if there is abnormal development, reflux and ureteropelvic junction obstruction occurs, most often in the lower pole, while ectopic ureteral insertion with or without a ureterocele is nearly always associated with the upper pole.

18. **b and c.** When the upper pole of a duplex system associated with an ectopic ureter demonstrates function, preservation is typically recommended. Two reasonable options exist for this, including proximal ureteropyelostomy, which excises most of the usually dilated upper pole ureter, or distal ureteroureterostomy, which permits drainage without any manipulation of the perirenal tissues. There are no data to support one over the other, and both are reasonable options. There is no evidence to indicate that the so-called *yo-yo phenomenon* of urine refluxing into more dilated segments of ureter is a clinically significant concern.

19. **c. Possible improvement in trigonal deficiency.** Transurethral puncture of a ureterocele offers all of the listed possible, but not certain, advantages, except to improve trigonal deficiency that can be associated with a severe ureterocele. This deficiency, which may lead to persisting reflux and bladder outlet obstruction, may require corrective surgery.

20. **a. All three ureters joining to terminate in a single bladder orifice.** In the classification used by most investigators, there are four varieties of triplicate ureter. In one variety, all three ureters unite and drain through a single orifice. This appears to be the most common form encountered, although all others have been reported.
21. **b. Subcardinal vein.** If the subcardinal vein in the lumbar portion fails to atrophy and becomes the primary right-sided vein, the ureter is trapped dorsal to it.
22. **c. Intravesical ureterocele.** Several studies have indicated that intravesical ureteroceles fared better than extravesical ureteroceles with regard to decompression, preservation of upper pole function, newly created reflux, and need for secondary procedures. Nonetheless, the clinical scenario will be the most important indicator of the appropriateness of endoscopic incision for a ureterocele in a particular patient.
23. **e. Urinary tract infection.** Many ureteroceles are still diagnosed clinically. The most common presentation is that of an infant who has a urinary tract infection or urosepsis. In the early perinatal period, prenatal identification of hydronephrosis is currently the most common means of diagnosis.
24. **b. Magnetic resonance imaging (MRI) of the abdomen and pelvis.** Occasionally, the renal parenchyma associated with an ectopic ureter is difficult to locate on ultrasound and may be identified only by alternative imaging studies. In such cases in which an ectopic ureter is strongly suspected because of incontinence yet no definite evidence of the upper pole renal segment is found, CT or MRI has demonstrated the small, poorly functioning upper pole segment.

CHAPTER REVIEW

1. An ectopic ureter in a duplex system inevitably drains the upper pole.
2. In females, the ectopic ureter may enter from the bladder neck to the perineum or into the vagina, uterus, or rectum.
3. In males, the ectopic ureter always enters the urogenital system above the external sphincter and may enter wolffian duct structures, such as the vas deferens, seminal vesicles, and ejaculatory duct.
4. The orifice of a cecoureterocele is within the bladder; however, the ureterocele may extend beyond the bladder neck into the urethra.
5. The ectopic ureter inserts into the wolffian duct structure and not directly into a müllerian structure. Therefore, in the female, for an ectopic ureter to enter the vagina, cervix, or uterus, it requires a rupture into those structures.
6. The Weigert-Meyer rule states that an ectopic ureter or ureterocele is associated with the upper pole and is located caudal and medial to the lower pole ureteral orifice.
7. A young boy presenting with epididymitis might have an ectopic ureter.
8. A toilet-trained girl with verified continuous urinary leakage should be evaluated for an ectopic ureter.
9. A ureterocele or ectopic ureter associated with a patulous bladder neck may be complicated by incontinence. Cecoureteroceles are at particular risk for this.
10. On endoscopy, ureteroceles vary in their appearance with bladder filling.
11. An obstructed ureterocele may be treated endoscopically by multiple punctures or by a transverse incision. Both techniques have similar rates of success in decompression. In a transurethral incision of the ureterocele, the incision is made transversely as close to the bladder floor as possible. This may prevent subsequent reflux.
12. In patients with an ectopic ureter who present with sepsis and have massive ureteral dilatation, a temporary end ureterostomy may be the best management.
13. When the upper pole of the kidney is removed for an ectopic ureter, the residual stump is rarely problematic.
14. The separation of duplex ureters distally in the intravesical dissection should be discouraged because it may injure the common blood supply.
15. Conditions that routinely affect the single-system kidney generally affect the lower pole of a duplex system, such as ureteropelvic junction obstruction and vesical ureteral reflux. Conditions that affect the upper pole are more likely due to abnormal ureteral formation, such as ectopia and ureterocele.
16. On a voiding cystourethrogram, if early filling views are not obtained, a ureterocele may efface and the filling defect may not be visible.
17. Fibroepithelial polyps most commonly occur at the ureteropelvic junction but may occur anywhere in the ureter.
18. Correction of the circumcaval ureter requires ureteral division and relocation ventral to the vena cava.
19. When the upper pole of a duplex system associated with an ectopic ureter demonstrates function, preservation of renal tissue is typically recommended. Two reasonable options exist for this, including proximal ureteropyelostomy, which excises most of the usually dilated upper pole ureter, or distal ureteroureterostomy, which permits drainage without any manipulation of the perirenal tissues. No data exist to support one versus the other, and both are reasonable options.

42 Surgery of the Ureter in Children: Ureteropelvic Junction, Megaureter, and Vesicoureteral Reflux

L. Henning Olsen and Yazan F.H. Rawashdeh

QUESTIONS

1. Which of the following is NOT correct concerning laparoscopic pyeloplasty?
   a. Discounted early as unacceptable due to degree of difficulty
   b. Can be performed after a failed previous pyeloplasty
   c. Has an overall higher success rate than endopyelotomy
   d. Should be performed in patients of all ages
   e. Many different techniques for laparoscopic approach have been described

2. In regard to closure of trocar sites:
   a. closing fascial wounds more than 3 mm is recommended.
   b. fascial closure devices facilitate closure in the obese patient.
   c. omentum is the most common herniated intra-abdominal structure.
   d. trocars should not be removed before the intra-abdominal pressure is close to normal
   e. all of the above are true.

3. Which is NOT true for transperitoneal procedures?
   a. Sutures may be passed through the anterior abdominal wall.
   b. For lower abdominal procedures, infants are best positioned across the foot of the bed.
   c. Laxity of the infant abdominal wall can limit exposure due to compression.
   d. Cannula fixation is a common problem in pediatric laparoscopy.
   e. Visibility is usually a problem.

4. A recognized risk of laparoscopy in all infants is:
   a. use of monopolar cautery.
   b. ventilatory compromise.
   c. abdominal adhesions.
   d. decreased renal perfusion.
   e. compartmental syndrome.

5. Which of the following is a relative contraindication to retroperitoneoscopic surgery in the pediatric population?
   a. Horseshoe kidneys
   b. Spinal deformity
   c. Previous abdominal surgery
   d. Weight
   e. Intestinal malrotation

6. Hypothermia during laparoscopy in all infants is caused by:
   a. Insufflation of large amount of CO_2 due to port leakage.
   b. High-frequency ventilation.
   c. Room-temperature insufflation.
   d. Evaporation.
   e. Cold room temperature.

7. Regarding pediatric minimally invasive surgery in obese patients:
   a. Suture can be placed from the skin at the entry site to the cannula to keep the cannula from sliding off if rapid desufflation is encountered.
   b. Hitch stitches are helpful.
   c. An insufflation needle works well in most children, because the abdominal wall is thin.
   d. Bladeless optical trocars or open access for the camera port might be helpful.
   e. Higher insufflation pressures are needed.

8. Which of the following is not found to be associated with higher success rate of endoscopic correction of vesicoureteral reflux?
   a. Volume of Dx/HA used
   b. Surgeon experience
   c. Volcano-shaped mound with no hydrodistention
   d. Negative intraoperative cystogram
   e. Utilization of the double hydrodistention-implantation technique

9. Regarding surgical correction of vesicoureteral reflux, which of the following is currently accepted?
   a. Extravesical ureteral reimplantation
   b. Intravesical ureteral reimplantation
   c. Endoscopic injection of bulking agent
   d. All of the above
   e. None of the above

10. Common to each type of open/laparoscopic/robotic repair for reflux is the creation of:
    a. a valvular mechanism that enables ureteral compression with bladder filling and contraction.
    b. a mucosal tunnel for reimplantation having adequate muscular backing.
    c. a tunnel length of three times the ureteral diameter.
    d. all of the above.
    e. none of the above.

11. Early postoperative obstruction can occur after a ureteral reimplant due to:
    a. edema.
    b. subtrigonal bleeding.
    c. twist or angulation of the ureter.
    d. blood clots.
    e. all of the above.

12. If early postoperative obstruction occurs after a ureteral reimplant, the next step is:
    a. immediate nephrostomy tube placement.
    b. immediate placement of a ureteral stent.
    c. initial observation and diversion for unabating symptoms.
    d. placement of both a nephrostomy tube and a ureteral stent.
    e. reoperation.

13. Which of the following is TRUE regarding persistent reflux after ureteral reimplantation?
    a. It may be due to unrecognized secondary causes of reflux such as neuropathic bladder and severe voiding dysfunction.
    b. It seldom results from a failure to provide adequate muscular backing for the ureter within its tunnel.
    c. It may be repaired surgically by using minor submucosal advancements.
    d. All of the above.
    e. None of the above.

14. Which of the following is TRUE regarding the treatment of vesicoureteral reflux?
    a. Since the widespread acceptance of endoscopic treatment, the indications for surgical correction differ between the open endoscopic and laparoscopic approaches.
    b. Long-term follow-up data support the durability of endoscopic injection therapy.
    c. All injection materials provide a similar success rate and are just as easily injected under similar circumstances.
    d. The accuracy of the needle entry point during endoscopic injection, as well as the needle placement, are important components for the success of the surgical procedure.
    e. The learning curve for endoscopic injection is similar to the learning curve for open surgical reimplantation.

15. Which of the following is TRUE regarding the laparoscopic/robotic approach for ureteral reimplantation?
    a. The advantages of this approach versus open surgery include smaller incisions, less discomfort, and quicker convalescence.
    b. As with other laparoscopic/robotic procedures, experience is essential to the success of this approach.
    c. Costs may be increased because of lengthier surgery and the expense of the equipment.
    d. All of the above.
    e. None of the above.

16. Which of the following is TRUE regarding primary obstructive megaureters?
    a. It is caused by a dysfunctional juxtavesical segment that is unable to propagate urine at acceptable rates of flow.
    b. It most commonly occurs with neurogenic and non-neurogenic voiding dysfunction or infravesical obstructions such as posterior urethral valves.
    c. It may be due to acute infections, nephropathies, and other medical conditions that cause significant increases in urinary output that overwhelm maximal peristalsis.
    d. It is diagnosed when reflux, obstruction, and secondary causes of dilatation are ruled out.
    e. None of the above.

17. Which of the following is TRUE regarding secondary obstructive megaureters?
    a. It is caused by an aperistaltic juxtavesical segment that is unable to propagate urine at acceptable rates of flow.

b. It most commonly occurs with neurogenic and non-neurogenic voiding dysfunction or infravesical obstruction such as posterior urethral valves.
    c. It may be due to acute infections, nephropathies, and other medical conditions that cause significant increases in urinary output that overwhelm maximal peristalsis.
    d. It is diagnosed once reflux, obstruction, and secondary causes of dilatation are ruled out.
    e. None of the above.

18. Which of the following is the most serious complication to ureteral tailoring?
    a. Gradual tapering can cause an abrupt change of the ureteral caliber and subsequently kinking.
    b. A too short intravesical tunnel can cause vesicoureteral reflux.
    c. Compromising of the distal vasculature of the ureter with subsequent fibrosis.
    d. Secondary stenosis of the ureteral orifice.
    e. Bladder dysfunction after intravesical dissection.

ANSWERS

1. **d. Should be performed in patients of all ages.** In newborns the access to the ureteropelvic junction only requires a very small incision. Laparoscopy is feasible in infants, but there is a lack of evidence of advantages for this age group.
2. **d. Trocars should not be removed before the intra-abdominal pressure is close to normal.** Lowering the pressure before removing the trocars will reveal that the hemostasis is under control and prevents intra-abdominal (bowel, omentum) content from entering the port holes.
3. **e. Visibility is usually a problem.** The peritoneal lining mirrors the light from the telescope giving a better visibility than in the retroperitoneal route.
4. **a. Use of monopolar cautery.** Monopolar cautery increases the risk of unrecognized lesions to intra-abdominal organs, particularly the bowel.
5. **a. Horseshoe kidneys.** The access to the UPJ from the posterior aspect is extremely difficult in horseshoe kidneys.
6. **a. Insufflation of large amount of CO_2 due to port leakage.** The large amount of gas exchange lowers the intra-abdominal temperature significantly.
7. **d. Bladeless optical trocars or open access for the camera port might be helpful.** Blind access to the peritoneal cavity imposes an inherent risk of organ damage.
8. **d. Negative intraoperative cystogram.** A negative intraoperative cystogram does not reveal the success rate of the treatment since the child is under anesthesia and unable to spontaneously void.
9. **d. All of the above.** Extravesical and intravesical ureteral reimplantation are all options for treatment of vesicoureteral reflux. In the past decade there has been widespread enthusiasm for endoscopic treatment, and different bulking agents have been used to correct vesicoureteral reflux by using minimally invasive techniques.
10. **a. A valvular mechanism that enables ureteral compression with bladder filling and contraction.** Common to each technique is the creation of a valvular mechanism that enables ureteral compression with bladder filling and contraction, thus reenacting normal anatomy and function. A successful ureteroneocystostomy provides a submucosal tunnel for reimplantation having sufficient length and adequate muscular backing. A tunnel length of five times the ureteral diameter is cited as necessary for eliminating reflux.
11. **e. All of the above.** Early after surgery, various degrees of obstruction can be expected of the reimplanted ureter. Edema,

subtrigonal bleeding, and bladder spasms all possibly contribute. Mucus plugs and blood clots are other causes. Most postoperative obstructions are mild and asymptomatic and resolve spontaneously. More significant obstructions are usually symptomatic. Affected children typically present 1 to 2 weeks after surgery with acute abdominal pain, nausea, and vomiting.

12. **c. Initial observation and diversion for unabating symptoms.** The large majority of perioperative obstructions subside spontaneously, but placement of a nephrostomy tube or ureteral stent sometimes becomes necessary for unabating symptoms.

13. **a. It may be due to unrecognized secondary causes of reflux such as neuropathic bladder and severe voiding dysfunction.** Other than technical errors, failure to identify and treat secondary causes of reflux is a common cause of the reappearance of reflux. Foremost among these secondary causes are unrecognized neuropathic bladder and severe voiding dysfunction.

14. **d. The accuracy of the needle entry point during endoscopic injection, as well as the needle placement, are important** components for the success of the surgical procedure. The learning curve for endoscopic injection is believed to be different from that of open surgical reimplantation.

15. **d. All of the above.** The advantages of this approach versus open surgery include smaller incisions, less discomfort, brief hospitalizations (although many centers now perform open reimplants on an outpatient basis), and quicker convalescence.

16. **a. It is caused by a dysfunctional juxtavesical segment that is unable to propagate urine at acceptable rates of flow.** Obstruction results from the presence of an abnormal adynamic segment at the terminal end of the ureter near or at the ureterovesical junction (UVJ).

17. **b. It most commonly occurs with neurogenic and non-neurogenic voiding dysfunction or infravesical obstruction such as posterior urethral valves.** High bladder pressure might result in secondary reflux.

18. **c. Compromising of the distal vasculature of the ureter with subsequent fibrosis.** Fibrosis can lead to recurrent obstruction and require redo surgery. However, when performed with care, the risk of vascular compromise should be minimal.

CHAPTER REVIEW

1. Ureteropelvic junction obstruction (UPJO) is typically due to either an intrinsic narrowing in which the ureteral segment has an interruption in the development of the circular musculature of the UPJ, an alteration in collagen fibers in and around the muscular cells, or an extrinsic obstruction that is seen in association with aberrant, accessory, or an early branching lower pole vessel that passes anteriorly to the UPJ or proximal ureter and contributes to mechanical obstruction.

2. Congenital renal malformations can be commonly seen in association with a UPJO, with a contralateral UPJO being the most common anomaly, followed by renal dysplasia and multicystic dysplastic kidney.

3. The surgical procedure favored in the repair of a UPJO is the dismembered pyeloplasty, which has been shown to be effective because of its broad applicability, means of allowing excision of the pathologic segment in question, and facilitation of a reduction pyeloplasty when necessary.

4. Laparoscopic pyeloplasty provides excellent visualization of the anatomy, enhances cosmesis, and duplicates the results of open pyeloplasty with short-term follow-up. The technical challenges of this approach have been facilitated by the use of a robotic-assisted procedure that improves the anastomotic repair.

5. Pyeloplasty complications include prolonged urinary drainage postoperatively, lack of improvement in renal function or improvement in washout, and occasionally, worsening hydronephrosis and diminished renal function postoperatively. Such a situation may lend itself to a repair using endoscopic procedures or preferably a repeat dismembered pyeloplasty.

43 Management of Pediatric Kidney Stone Disease

Gregory E. Tasian and Lawrence Copelovitch

QUESTIONS

1. A 5-year-old boy is seen in the office with complaints of intermittent right flank pain. There have been no episodes of nausea, vomiting, or fevers. He has 3+ blood on a urine dip. His physical exam reveals some mild right costovertebral angle (CVA) tenderness. Which imaging modality should be used first?
   a. Magnetic resonance imaging (MRI)
   b. Plain radiograph, kidney-ureter-bladder (KUB)
   c. Ultrasound
   d. Computed tomography (CT) scan
   e. Retrograde pyelogram

2. A 12-year-old girl presented to the emergency department with an acute episode of left flank pain and was diagnosed with 5-mm left distal ureteral stone. She responded well to conservative therapy (intravenous hydration and pain medication) and her pain subsides. The next step in management is:
   a. analgesics, trial of passage, and interval ultrasound imaging.
   b. analgesics, tamsulosin, trial of passage, and interval ultrasound imaging.
   c. ureteroscopy.
   d. shock wave lithotripsy (SWL).
   e. no further urologic management.

3. A 10-year-old male with spina bifida had an augmentation cystoplasty, bladder neck reconstruction, and bilateral Glenn-Anderson ureteral reimplantation for high-grade reflux at age 7 years. He now has a 1-cm lower pole stone. The therapy LEAST likely to yield an efficacious (stone-free) result is:
   a. SWL.
   b. ureteroscopy with laser lithotripsy.
   c. ureteral stenting and ureteroscopy with laser lithotripsy 6 weeks later.
   d. percutaneous nephrolithotomy (PCNL).
   e. open pyelolithotomy.

4. With regard to SWL in the treatment of pediatric nephrolithiasis, treatment failures are associated with:
   a. large stone burden (i.e., ≥2 cm).
   b. long infundibula.
   c. infundibulopelvic angle greater than 45 degrees.
   d. upper pole stone
   e. a, b, and c.

5. Complications that may occur during ureteroscopy while treating a ureteral stone include all EXCEPT:
   a. hyponatremia.
   b. hypertension.
   c. ureteral avulsion.
   d. hypothermia.
   e. ureteral false passage.

6. A 9-year-old female with cystinuria is found to have a right 2-cm renal pelvic stone. The treatment option that would provide the highest probability of stone clearance is:
   a. SWL.
   b. ureteroscopy with laser lithotripsy and stone basketing.
   c. PCNL.
   d. medical therapy with potassium citrate and tiopronin.
   e. anatrophic nephrolithotomy.

7. Which of the following urinary findings are the least commonly observed in children with renal calculi?
   a. High urine sodium content
   b. Hypocitraturia
   c. Hyperuricosuria
   d. Hypercalciuria
   e. Low urine volume

8. Which of the following interventions is NOT recommended for the treatment of cystinuria?
   a. D-penicillamine
   b. Potassium citrate
   c. Alpha-mercaptopropionylglycine
   d. High fluid intake
   e. Hydrochlorothiazide

9. Which of the following is generally NOT associated with normocalcemic hypercalciuria?
   a. Bartter syndrome
   b. Primary hyperparathyroidism
   c. Dent disease
   d. Distal renal tubular acidosis (DRTA)
   e. Idiopathic hypercalciuria

10. Which of the following medications are NOT typically associated with renal calculi or nephrocalcinosis?
    a. Levetiracetam
    b. Topiramate
    c. Indinavir
    d. Furosemide
    e. Acetazolamide

ANSWERS

1. **c. Ultrasound.** Ultrasound is the recommended initial diagnostic imaging study that should be obtained for suspected ureteral or renal stones.
2. **b. Analgesics, tamsulosin, trial of passage, and interval ultrasound imaging.** Given the size and location of the stone and the favorable clinical status of the patient, a trial of passage is indicated. Current evidence, although of low grade, supports use of medical expulsion therapy, namely tamsulosin 0.4 mg po daily. Interval ultrasound is indicated to ascertain stone passage. If the stone has not passed by 4 to 6 weeks, ureteroscopy is indicated.

3. **a. SWL.** Recent data suggest that stone-free rates in children with a history of urologic condition or urinary tract reconstruction are quite low (12.5%) and may be better served with ureterorenoscopy or PCNL.

4. **e. a, b, and c.** SWL failure and retreatment rates were associated with increased mean stone burden, increased infundibular length, and infundibulopelvic angle greater than 45 degrees.

5. **b. Hypertension.** Complications of ureteroscopy include unrecognized ureteral injury including mucosal flaps and tears, perforation, false passage, and partial to complete avulsion. Irrigating fluid, which may be used under pressure, should be isotonic and body temperature to avoid hypothermia and hyponatremia. Hypertension is not a recognized complication of ureteroscopy.

6. **c. PCNL.** Stone clearance for this 2-cm stone would be highest with a PCNL. Although ureteroscopy is an option, multiple sessions would most likely be required. Clearance of **cystine stones is poor for SWL**. Medical therapy helps to prevent cystine stones, not treat them. Anatrophic nephrolithotomy is not an appropriate surgical treatment for this stone.

7. **c. Hyperuricosuria.** Although uric acid nephrolithiasis and hyperuricosuria are relatively common in adults, they are relatively rare in childhood, accounting for < 5% of all renal calculi. Low urine volume, high urine sodium content, hypercalciuria, and hypocitraturia are commonly observed in pediatric stone formers.

8. **e. Hydrochlorothiazide.** D-penicillamine and alpha-mercaptopropionylglycine are thiol-containing medications that are used to treat cystinuria by increasing the urine solubility of cysteine. Potassium citrate is used to treat cystinuria by alkalizing the urine thereby increasing cysteine solubility if a pH of greater than 7.0 is maintained. High fluid intake is generally recommended to prevent urinary crystallization of all lithogenic substrates. Thiazide diuretics are generally used to treat hypercalciuria, which is not an expected feature in cystinuria.

9. **b. Primary hyperparathyroidism.** Primary hyperparathyroidism is generally, although not universally, associated with hypercalcemia and hypophosphatemia. Bartter syndrome, Dent disease, and dRTA are genetic conditions in which the serum calcium is normal. By definition, idiopathic hypercalciuria is always associated with normal serum calcium levels.

10. **a. Levetiracetam.** Topiramate and acetazolamide are both carbonic anhydrase inhibitors and are commonly associated with hypocitraturia and calcium phosphate stone formation. Loop diuretics such as furosemide promote hypercalciuria and chronic usage is frequently associated with nephrocalcinosis. Indinavir is a protease inhibitor with poor urinary solubility and has the ability to crystallize and form calculi. Levetiracetam is an antiepileptic medication which is not associated with renal calculi.

CHAPTER REVIEW

1. Although reference ranges for 24-h urine metabolites in children who form stones are not as well standardized as for adults, initial workup should include a 24-h urine for volume, calcium, citrate, oxalate, uric acid, sodium, pH, and creatinine.

2. A metabolic abnormality is often present in pediatric stone formers; hypercalciuria and hypocitraturia are the most common abnormalities.

3. A kidney and bladder ultrasound is the imaging modality of choice in a patient with a suspected stone or in a known stone former.

4. There has been a dramatic increase in pediatric nephrolithiasis, especially among adolescent females.

5. Children with either hypercalciuria or hypocitraturia have a markedly increased rate of stone recurrence as compared to those without an identifiable metabolic abnormality.

6. Renal/ureteral calculi smaller than 5 mm are likely to spontaneously pass; larger calculi are more likely to require surgical intervention.

7. SWL to the kidney has been associated with an increased risk of hypertension.

8. Perioperative antibiotics are indicated for those patients requiring urologic instrumentation.

9. Ureteroscopy (URS) and shockwave lithotripsy (SWL) are the recommended surgical intervention for ureteral stones and renal calculi smaller than 20 mm.

10. Ureteral stenting after a procedure should be considered in patients with solitary kidneys, staghorn calculi, large ureteral calculi, prior obstruction, or abnormal anatomy. It may also be used to dilate ureters too narrow to accommodate a ureteroscope.

11. Shock wave lithotripsy (SWL) has a poor success rate for stones with densities greater than 1000 Hounsfield units and those with previous urinary tract reconstruction.

12. Contraindications for ureteroscopic stone management include stone burdens greater than 20 mm and anatomic abnormalities precluding retrograde access.

13. Distal ureteral stones are best managed ureteroscopically.

14. Ureteroscopy should be performed under general anesthesia.

15. The most common intraoperative complication of ureteroscopy is ureteral injury.

16. Relative indications for PCNL include stone burden greater than 20 mm, lower pole calculi greater than 1 cm, and anatomic abnormalities that make stone clearance less likely.

17. Spinal deformities may alter the anatomic location of the kidney, increasing the risk of adjacent organ injury during percutaneous access.

18. Up to 50% of children with a reconstructed bladder will develop stones. Factors that play a role include stasis, bacterial colonization, retained mucus, or foreign body.

44 Management of Abnormalities of the External Genitalia in Boys

Lane S. Palmer and Jeffrey S. Palmer

QUESTIONS

1. In the male, which of the following stimulates the development of the external genitalia?
   a. Testosterone
   b. Human chorionic gonadotropin
   c. Dihydrotestosterone
   d. Luteinizing hormone (LH) and follicle-stimulating hormone (FSH)
   e. Maternal progesterone

2. What percentage of uncircumcised boys will have persistent phimosis by 17 years of age?
   a. Less than 1%
   b. 5%
   c. 10%
   d. 15%
   e. 20%

3. Circumcision should not be performed in neonates with which condition of the genitalia?
   a. Phimosis
   b. Undescended testis
   c. Inguinal hernia
   d. Penile curvature
   e. Testicular atrophy

4. What is the most common complication associated with circumcision?
   a. Trauma to the glans
   b. Bleeding
   c. Meatal stenosis
   d. Skin bridges
   e. Balanitis xerotica obliterans (BXO)

5. A 4-year-old boy presents with phimosis and BXO of the prepuce. What is the preferred treatment?
   a. Observation
   b. Topical corticosteroids
   c. Excision of BXO skin without circumcision
   d. Warm baths
   e. Circumcision

6. Penile agenesis is associated with all of the following malformations EXCEPT:
   a. cryptorchidism.
   b. vesicoureteral reflux.
   c. horseshoe kidney.
   d. ureteropelvic junction obstruction.
   e. renal agenesis.

7. The etiology of the buried penis includes all of the following EXCEPT:
   a. suprapubic fat pad.
   b. small penis.
   c. poor penopubic fixation of the penis.
   d. obesity.
   e. cicatrix scar after surgery.

8. A 9-month-old boy who was previously circumcised presents with a buried penis resulting from cicatricial scarring. What is the most appropriate initial treatment?
   a. Topical betamethasone and manual retraction
   b. Revision of circumcision
   c. Penopubic fixation of the penis
   d. Liposuction of the suprapubic fat pad
   e. Observation

9. What is the minimal normal stretched penile length of a full-term neonate?
   a. 1.2 cm
   b. 1.9 cm
   c. 2.5 cm
   d. 3.2 cm
   e. 4.5 cm

10. Which of the following statements is TRUE regarding a micropenis in a term male neonate?
    a. The testes are usually normal in size and not cryptorchid.
    b. It is best managed by gender reassignment.
    c. It has an abnormal ratio of the length of the penile shaft to circumference.
    d. It is unlikely to respond to testosterone stimulation until puberty.
    e. It is less than 1.9 cm in stretched length.

11. What is the most common cause of micropenis?
    a. Hypergonadotropic hypogonadism
    b. Hypogonadotropic hypogonadism
    c. Idiopathic
    d. Growth hormone deficiency
    e. Androgen insensitivity syndrome

12. Which of the following statements regarding penile masses is FALSE?
    a. The treatment of parameatal urethral cysts is complete excision of the cyst.
    b. The most common acquired cystic lesion of the penis is smegma under the unretractable prepuce.
    c. Congenital penile nevi tend to be malignant.
    d. The initial management of juvenile xanthogranulomas is expectant monitoring.
    e. Epidermal inclusion cysts may form after penile surgery.

13. A 13-year-old African American boy with sickle cell disease has a 6-hour painful erection. The initial management should include all of the following EXCEPT:
    a. alkalization.
    b. hydration.
    c. intracavernous injections of β-adrenergic sympathomimetic agents.
    d. analgesia.
    e. transfusion to reduce hemoglobin S concentration.

14. Which of the following statements is TRUE regarding high-flow priapism?
    a. It is usually a drug-induced etiology.
    b. The aspirated blood is similar to venous blood on blood gas analysis.
    c. Color Doppler ultrasonography commonly demonstrates the fistula.
    d. Surgical intervention is the initial management.
    e. Sickle cell disease is the most common cause

15. Penoscrotal transposition is associated with all of the following anomalies EXCEPT:
    a. sex chromosome abnormalities.
    b. distal shaft hypospadias with chordee.
    c. sex chromosome abnormalities.
    d. Aarskog syndrome.
    e. caudal regression.

16. All of the following are associated with patency of the processus vaginalis EXCEPT:
    a. transverse testicular ectopia.
    b. epididymal anomalies.
    c. cryptorchidism.
    d. spermatic cord torsion.
    e. polyorchidism.

17. Abdominoscrotal hydrocele is reported to be associated with all of the following features EXCEPT:
    a. a closed processus vaginalis.
    b. epididymal anomalies.
    c. testicular dysmorphism.
    d. hydronephrosis.
    e. increased pressure within the tunica vaginalis.

18. Irreversible ischemic injury of the testicular parenchyma may begin as early as how many hours after torsion of the spermatic cord?
    a. 1
    b. 2
    c. 4
    d. 6
    e. 8

19. Which of the following is most specific in diagnosing spermatic cord torsion?
    a. High-riding testis
    b. Absence of the cremasteric reflex
    c. Transverse lie of the testis
    d. Spermatic cord twist on high-resolution Doppler ultrasonography
    e. Acute severe pain

20. After manual detorsion of the spermatic cord, which of the following is appropriate management?
    a. Color Doppler ultrasonography
    b. Radionuclide scan
    c. Doppler examination of the testis and spermatic cord
    d. Discharge from the hospital and arrangement for an office reevaluation in 1 week
    e. Immediate scrotal exploration

21. An adolescent is evaluated for a history of self-limited, intermittent episodes of severe unilateral scrotal pain. Physical examination findings are normal. What is the most appropriate course of action?
    a. Color Doppler ultrasonography
    b. Reassessment in 6 months
    c. Elective scrotal exploration
    d. Radionuclide scrotal imaging
    e. Immediate scrotal exploration

22. When the diagnosis of torsion of the appendix epididymis is made, which of the following is optimal management?
    a. Observation
    b. Color Doppler ultrasonography
    c. Radionuclide scrotal imaging
    d. Immediate scrotal exploration
    e. Cord block and manual detorsion

23. Which of the following is the most likely diagnosis in an infant with sterile urine and epididymitis?
    a. Unilateral renal agenesis
    b. Large prostatic utricle
    c. Urethral stricture disease
    d. Persistent vasoureteral fusion
    e. Radiographically normal urinary tract

24. What is the most appropriate course of action in an otherwise healthy neonate with perinatal testicular torsion?
    a. Surgical exploration of the affected testis
    b. Surgical exploration of the affected testis with contralateral scrotal orchidopexy
    c. Color Doppler ultrasonography of the scrotum
    d. Radionuclide testicular scan
    e. Observation

25. Most adolescent varicoceles evaluated by urologists are:
    a. painful.
    b. of cosmetic concern.
    c. asymptomatic.
    d. associated with an ipsilateral hydrocele.
    e. bilateral.

26. Significant testicular volume differential in cases of varicocele is defined as greater than:
    a. 5%.
    b. 5% to 10%.
    c. 10% to 15%.
    d. 15% to 20%
    e. 25%.

27. Hydrocele formation after varicocele ligation is least likely to occur after which of the following procedures?
    a. Retroperitoneal ligation
    b. Subinguinal ligation
    c. Laparoscopic ligation
    d. Microscopic inguinal ligation
    e. Transvenous embolization

28. Which of the following is NOT a relative indication for elective varicocele repair?
    a. Pain
    b. Oligospermia
    c. Small testes
    d. Continuous spermatic venous reflux
    e. Testicular size discrepancy of greater than 20%

ANSWERS

1. **c. Dihydrotestosterone.** Influence of dihydrotestosterone on the androgen receptors results in the differentiation of the genital tubercle, genital (labioscrotal) folds, and genital swelling at between 9 and 13 weeks of gestation into the male structures of the glans penis, penile shaft, and scrotum, respectively.

2. **a. Less than 1%.** Preputial retractability increases with age with 90% of uncircumcised boys 3 years of age with completely retractable prepuces; less than 1% by 17 years of age have phimosis.

3. **d. Penile curvature.** Circumcision should not be performed in neonates with other penile conditions that require surgical correction. These conditions include hypospadias, penile curvature, dorsal hood deformity, buried penis, and webbed penis.

4. **b. Bleeding.** The risk of complications after circumcision is 0.2% to 5%. The most common complication is bleeding, which occurs in 0.1% and is more common in older children.

5. **e. Circumcision.** Treatment of BXO includes medical and surgical management. The use of topical corticosteroids has had limited benefit to treat mild BXO of the prepuce with minimal scar formation. Circumcision is the preferred treatment.

6. **d. Ureteropelvic junction obstruction.** Penile agenesis (aphallia) results from failure of development of the genital tubercle. The disorder is rare and has an estimated incidence of 1 in 10 to 30 million births. The karyotype almost always is 46,XY, and the usual appearance is that of a well-developed scrotum with descended testes and an absent penile shaft. The anus is usually displaced anteriorly. Associated malformations are common and include cryptorchidism, vesicoureteral reflux, horseshoe kidney, renal agenesis, imperforate anus, and musculoskeletal and cardiopulmonary abnormalities.

7. **b. Small penis.** A buried penis can be classified into three categories based on etiology for the concealment: (1) poor penopubic fixation of the skin at the base of the penis; (2) obesity; and (3) a trapped penis from a cicatrix scar after penile surgery, typically a circumcision.

8. **a. Topical betamethasone and manual retraction.** Young children with secondary cicatrix after penile surgery can undergo forceful dilation of the cicatrix with a fine hemostat in the office after the application or injection of local anesthesia. Another option is the combination of topical betamethasone and manual retraction.

9. **b. 1.9 cm.** Stretched penile length is determined by measuring the penis from its attachment to the pubic symphysis to the tip of the glans. One must be careful to depress the suprapubic fat pad completely to obtain an accurate measurement, especially in an obese infant or child. In general, the penis of a full-term neonate should be at least 1.9 cm long, which is 2.5 SD below the mean of 4.0 cm.

10. **e. It is less than 1.9 cm in stretched length.** Micropenis is a normally formed penis that is at least 2.5 SD below the mean size in stretched length for age. The ratio of the length of the penile shaft to its circumference is usually normal, but occasionally the corpora cavernosa are severely hypoplastic. The testes are usually small and frequently cryptorchid while the scrotum is usually fused and often diminutive. A stretched penile length less than 1.9 cm long is consistent with a micropenis.

11. **b. Hypogonadotropic hypogonadism.** The most common cause of micropenis is hypogonadotropic hypogonadism, which is the failure of the hypothalamus to produce an adequate amount of gonadotropin-releasing hormone (GnRH). This condition may result from hypothalamic dysfunction, which can occur in Prader-Willi syndrome, Kallmann syndrome (genital-olfactory dysplasia), Laurence-Moon-Biedl syndrome, and the CHARGE association.

12. **c. Congenital penile nevi tend to be malignant.** Congenital penile nevi tend to be superficial and benign. Congenital penile nevi are pigmented lesions that can form on the glans and penile shaft. They tend to be superficial and benign and should be excised.

13. **c. Intracavernous injections of β-adrenergic sympathomimetic agents.** The initial treatment of low-flow priapism resulting from sickle cell disease is conservative with hydration, oxygenation, alkalization, analgesia, and transfusion with the goal of reducing hemoglobin S concentration. Evacuation of blood and irrigation of the corpora cavernosa along with intracavernous injections of α-adrenergic sympathomimetic agents, such as phenylephrine or epinephrine solution, can be a concurrent therapy. Surgical intervention to allow corporeal drainage by shunt procedures is indicated if there is a lack of response to medical therapy.

14. **c. Color Doppler ultrasonography commonly demonstrates the fistula.** High-flow priapism is usually due to perineal trauma, such as a straddle injury. Corporeal irrigation is diagnostic and therapeutic. Typically, the aspirated blood is bright red and the aspirate is similar to arterial blood on blood gas analysis. Color Doppler ultrasonography often will demonstrate the fistula. The initial management is observation because spontaneous resolution may occur. Superselective embolization of cavernous and penile arteries is the next line of therapy. If not, angiographic embolization is indicated.

15. **b. Distal shaft hypospadias with chordee.** Frequently, penoscrotal transposition occurs in conjunction with perineal, scrotal, or penoscrotal hypospadias with chordee. Penoscrotal transposition has also been associated with caudal regression, sex chromosome abnormalities, and Aarskog syndrome. As many as 75% of patients with complete penoscrotal transposition and a normal scrotum have a significant urinary tract abnormality, including renal agenesis and dysplasia, and other nongenitourinary anomalies.

16. **d. Spermatic cord torsion.** Risk of torsion is associated with abnormal development of the tunica vaginalis but not patency of the processus vaginalis.

17. **b. Epididymal anomalies.** The processus vaginalis is closed in cases of abdominoscrotal hydrocele, and an elongated dysmorphic testis, increased pressure within the tunica vaginalis, and hydronephrosis have all been reported.

18. **c. 4.** Irreversible ischemic injury to the testicular parenchyma may begin as soon as 4 hours after occlusion of the cord.

19. **d. Spermatic cord twist on high-resolution Doppler ultra-**

sonography. Spermatic cord twist on high-resolution Doppler imaging is the most specific finding, that is, the least likely to be false positive, in spermatic cord torsion.

20. **e. Immediate scrotal exploration.** It should be remembered that manual detorsion may not totally correct the full rotation that has occurred and that prompt surgical exploration is still indicated. Further, studies have shown that while torsion of the cord generally occurs in a medial inward fashion (requiring detorsion in an outward "open book" fashion), one-third of cases show a torsion in the opposite direction. Thus the usual detorsion method may actually increase the torsion in some cases. Attempted detorsion should never delay a patient from going to the operating room.

21. **c. Elective scrotal exploration.** If the suspicion is strong that episodes of intermittent torsion and spontaneous detorsion have occurred, the author's experience has been that the finding of a bell-clapper deformity at exploration can be expected. Elective scrotal exploration should be performed, with scrotal fixation of both testes.

22. **a. Observation.** When the diagnosis of a torsed appendage is confirmed clinically or by imaging, nonoperative management will allow most cases to resolve spontaneously.

23. **e. Radiographically normal urinary tracts.** The majority of infants with epididymitis have sterile urine and apparently radiographically normal urinary tracts.

24. **b. Surgical exploration of the affected testis with contralateral scrotal orchidopexy.** Clearly, if the cause of scrotal swelling appears to be related to an acute postnatal event, all efforts should be made to pursue prompt surgical intervention.

If torsion is confirmed, contralateral scrotal exploration with testicular fixation should be performed.

25. **c. Asymptomatic.** Most adolescent varicoceles are asymptomatic.

26. **d. 15% to 20%.** In adults and adolescents, testicular size (volume) should be approximately equal bilaterally, with the normal differential not being more than 15% to 20% volume. Asynchronous testicular growth has been shown to occur normally throughout puberty.

27. **e. Transvenous embolization.** Hydrocele formation is related to failure to preserve lymphatic vessels associated with the spermatic cord and its vessels. Hydrocele formation seems most common after retroperitoneal ligation, especially when a mass ligation technique is used, and is least likely to occur after transvenous embolization.

28. **d. Continuous spermatic venous reflux.** Significant pain associated with varicocele (despite scrotal support), bilateral small testes (low total testicular volume), and oligospermia are reasonable indications to proceed with repair in an adolescent male. The standard indication is ipsilateral testicular volume loss, or hypotrophy, of at least 15% to 20%, although this should be documented on serial yearly testicular examinations, because variable growth of the testes may occur during puberty. Recent studies, however, have shown that differential testicular volume is a poor correlate of eventual total motile sperm count. Without attempted paternity history, the best indicator of testis health regarding fertility is a semen analysis. Continuous spermatic venous reflux may be documented on color Doppler imaging but is not a specific indication for surgery.

CHAPTER REVIEW

1. Primary phimosis resolves spontaneously in the vast majority of boys; fewer than 1% of 17-year-old boys have a phimotic prepuce.
2. Indications to facilitate preputial retractility include persistent primary phimosis, secondary phimosis, balanitis, posthitis, balanitis xerotica obliterans (BXO), and urinary tract infection (UTI).
3. The American Academy of Pediatrics acknowledges the potential health benefits of the circumcised penis thus warranting access to circumcision for families choosing it and endorse third-party payment for circumcision of male newborns.
4. Local or topical anesthetics should be administered routinely for circumcisions performed in the neonatal period.
5. Circumcisions should be deferred in the presence of other penile abnormalities detected in the newborn period that may require surgery.
6. Health benefits of circumcision include reduction in rates of penile cancer, sexually transmitted diseases including HIV, UTIs, balanitis, and phimosis.
7. Topical application of corticosteroids can relax the phimotic ring in 70%–80% of cases.
8. The risk of complications from circumcision is 0.2%–5% with bleeding being the most common.
9. Circumcision revisions require the child to be under general anesthesia.
10. Meatal stenosis occurs only in the circumcised penis.
11. Topical corticosteroids fail to resolve penile adhesions.
12. BXO is a chronic infiltrative and scarring (cicatrix) skin condition.
13. Micropenis is a normally formed penis that measures at least 2.5 SD below the mean size in the stretched length for age (<1.9 cm in neonates).
14. Buried penis is not synonymous with micropenis as the penis is of normal stretched length.
15. The most common causes of micropenis include hypogonadotropic hypogonadism, hypergonadotropic hypogonadism.
16. Patient evaluation includes karyotype, determination of serum LH and FSH concentrations; measurement of testosterone levels before and after hCG stimulation; serum studies of anterior pituitary function; and MRI of the brain to assess hypothalamus, anterior pituitary, and midbrain.
17. In adulthood, most men with micropenis have male gender identity and satisfactory sexual function.
18. Priapism can be ischemic (veno-occlusive, low flow), nonischemic (arterial, high flow), and stuttering (intermittent).
19. The most common cause for priapism in children is sickle cell disease.
20. The initial treatment of low-flow priapism due to sickle cell disease is conservative with hydration, oxygenation, alkalization, and transfusion. Evacuation of blood and irrigation of the corpora cavernosa along with intracavernous injection of alpha-adrenergic sympathomimetic agents can be done concurrently or after failure of conservative measures.
21. High-flow priapism is usually due to perineal trauma, such as a straddle injury. Angiographic embolization should be performed if spontaneous resolution fails to occur.
22. Transient but potentially prolonged periods (less than 2 h) of erection, stuttering priapism, can be treated with pseudoephedrine given at bedtime.
23. The prevalence of varicoceles in adolescent and adult men are similar, approximately 15%.
24. Tall thin males are more commonly noted to have varicoceles, implicating a genetic predisposition.
25. Varicoceles are commonly identified on examination and least commonly identified due to pain.
26. Testicular volume is most accurately measured using ultrasound.
27. Testicular hypotrophy of 15%–20% may arise in the presence of an ipsilateral varicocele that commonly resolves after varicocele repair but can resolve spontaneously as well.

28. Trends toward poorer sperm quality may be limited to a subset of affected males with varicocele, but grade and postoperative testicular catch-up growth do not reliably predict ultimate semen quality.

29. Surgical success rates are similar with retroperitoneal (open or laparoscopic) or subinguinal approaches. Lymphatic-sparing techniques offer the lowest rates of hydrocele formation. The majority of hydroceles require surgical intervention.

30. Inguinal hernias develop in 1%–5% of children, more commonly in boys and premature infants. The propensity for the right side (3:1) is attributed to the later descent of the right testicle. Female gender, prematurity, age younger than 1 year, and history of cryptorchidism are risk factors for bilaterality.

31. An intermittent bulge helps to distinguish a reducible inguinal hernia and communicating hydrocele from a scrotal hydrocele or hydrocele of the spermatic cord. If a bulge is not elicited at the time of examination, photographs of the bulge taken at home are diagnostically reliable.

32. Inguinal hernias should be repaired soon after diagnosis while hydroceles can often resolve spontaneously and warrant a period of observation.

33. Surgical repair can be performed through an inguinal, scrotal, or laparoscopic approach. The inguinal approach carries the highest success rates at this time.

34. The causes of recurrent hernias (0.5%–1%) include failure to properly identify or ligate the sac during the original procedure; a tear in the sac, leaving a strip of peritoneum along the cord; damage to the floor; a weal internal inguinal ring; or an unrecognized direct hernia at the original exploration.

35. Transperitoneal diagnostic laparoscopy offers a rapid, direct, and accurate inspection of the contralateral internal inguinal ring.

36. Delay in presentation for acute scrotal pain may stem from patient embarrassment or denial, but also from lack of public awareness regarding torsion and the possible consequences.

37. In cases where a reliable thorough history is taken and targeted physical examination is performed, a reliable diagnosis should be made in the majority of cases and adjunctive ultrasound serves to confirm a diagnosis.

38. Ultrasound features suggestive of torsion of the spermatic cord include absent blood flow, a "snail sign" (cord torsion), and heterogeneity of the parenchyma.

39. Testicular salvage rates from spermatic cord torsion are inversely related to duration and have some relationship to the degrees of torsion. Thus, in cases where torsion is highly suspected, emergent surgery should not be delayed by imaging studies.

40. Spermatic cord torsion occurring in the perinatal period is rarely salvageable when identified in the nursery and should be managed emergently when a change in physical examination has occurred.

41. Appendage torsion is the most common cause of acute scrotum in prepubertal children. A "blue dot sign," discoloration at the upper pole of the testis, may be seen through stretched scrotal skin. This is a self-limiting process requiring supportive care and analgesia management.

45 Hypospadias

Christopher J. Long, Mark R. Zaontz, and Douglas A. Canning

QUESTIONS

1. Hypospadias is typically made up of which of the following components?
   a. A high risk of associated anomalies outside of the genitourinary tract
   b. Ventral penile curvature with an orthotopic urethral meatus
   c. An intact prepuce
   d. An ectopic location to the urethral meatus below the center of the glans
   e. A bifid scrotum

2. The level of hypospadias is typically defined by what parameter?
   a. At the initial office visit by identifying the location of the urethral meatus
   b. By calculating the level of penile curvature in the office with a goniometer
   c. Based on the location of the meatus when inserting a feeding tube in the operating room
   d. After penile degloving, taking into account both the location of the urethral meatus and the degree of penile curvature
   e. In the operating room by determining the degree of separation of the glans wings

3. Which of the following is true about urethral development?
   a. The urethral groove forms between the urethral folds at an early stage in urethral development
   b. The urethral folds fuse between gestation weeks 8 to 16 to form the urethra
   c. Preputial skin folds fuse to complete the foreskin prior to fusion of the urethra
   d. a and b
   e. b and c

4. Which of the following support the disruption of androgen signaling as at least a partial cause of hypospadias?
   a. A shorter anogenital distance (AGD) and severity of hypospadias
   b. Increased rate of hypospadias development in boys conceived via in-vitro fertilization
   c. An increased risk of hypospadias development in monozygotic male twins compared to singleton live male births
   d. The concordance of rising rates of hypospadias, poor sperm quality, and cryptorchidism
   e. All of the above

5. An 8-month-old male presents for evaluation of subcoronal hypospadias. During physical examination, the left testicle is palpated in the groin but cannot be manipulated into the scrotum. The next step is to:
   a. reexamine in 6 months to allow for testicular descent.
   b. perform ultrasonography to rule out testicular retraction.
   c. obtain a karyotype.
   d. schedule hypospadias repair now, and orchiopexy in 6 months.
   e. schedule orchiopexy now, with hypospadias repair in 6 months.

6. At the beginning of a penoscrotal hypospadias repair, after degloving but prior to urethral tubularization, you pass a urethral catheter but are unable to enter the bladder. The most likely cause is:
   a. a false passage in the posterior urethra.
   b. an enlarged utricle.
   c. partial urethral duplication ending in a blind pouch.
   d. an elevated bladder neck.
   e. proximal urethral stricture.

7. A 6-month-old infant without other known medical problems is referred for proximal penile hypospadias. He is also found to have ventral penile curvature, a deep scrotal cleft, and penoscrotal transposition, but both testes are normally situated in the dependent scrotum. The next step is:
   a. proceed with surgery.
   b. obtain a karyotype.
   c. order a voiding cystourethrogram (VCUG) to rule out the presence of a utricle.
   d. obtain renal sonography to rule out a renal anomaly.
   e. delay surgery until 12 months of age to allow for interval penile growth.

8. Which of the following is true regarding penile innervation?
   a. The pattern of penile innervation does not have a significant impact on the choice of technique for correction of penile curvature.
   b. The nerve bundles remain as two well-defined structures on the dorsal aspect of the penis.
   c. In hypospadias surgery, a perineal nerve block may provide a better option than a caudal block in an 8-year-old boy.
   d. The pattern of innervation permits the safe use of dorsal plication techniques for orthoplasty, when the sutures are placed in the midline.
   e. b and d.
   f. b, c, and d.

9. Two years after a midshaft hypospadias repair a potty-trained 4-year-old boy presents with two febrile urinary tract infections (UTIs). Which of the following is the next step?
   a. Recommend that the boy sits to void
   b. A VCUG
   c. A daily cone enema
   d. Cystoscopy under general anesthesia
   e. Reassurance

10. A patient with penoscrotal hypospadias has 90 degrees of ventral curvature prior to making the initial incision. After the penis is fully degloved, artificial erection reveals residual curvature of 15 degrees. The best next step in correcting the curvature is:

    a. transection of the urethral plate.

    b. perform dermal grafting of the corpora cavernosa at the point of maximal curvature and complete with a 2-stage repair.

    c. proceed with urethroplasty.

    d. perform a midline dorsal plication.

    e. perform midline dorsal plication and ventral tunica vaginalis graft corporoplasty, then complete a single-stage urethroplasty repair.

11. A 6-month-old male is referred for hypospadias. On examination he is found to have a dorsally hooded prepuce, ventral penile curvature, a glanular meatus, and a normal scrotum. The parents should be informed that straightening the penile curvature most likely will require:

    a. skin degloving and ventral dartos dissection.

    b. multiple dorsal midline plications.

    c. ventral corporal grafting.

    d. transection of the urethra.

    e. single dorsal plication and ventral corporal graft.

12. A 6-month-old male is referred for hypospadias. On examination he is found to have a dorsally hooded prepuce, 90 degrees of ventral penile curvature, a coronal meatus, and significant penoscrotal webbing. The parents should be counseled as follows:

    a. Penile curvature will likely be corrected with skin degloving and ventral dartos dissection.

    b. The risk for hypospadias complication repair is 5%.

    c. Only one procedure should be required.

    d. A karyotype should be performed.

    e. A two-stage repair may be required.

13. A 6-week-old infant is evaluated after newborn circumcision. The primary care physician expresses concern for a "bad circumcision." On examination the meatus is coronal and the glans wings are separated. The meatus itself appears elongated with a deep groove. The parents report no excessive bleeding after the circumcision. There is no redundant shaft skin following the circumcision except in the ventral midline near the meatus. The family should be informed that:

    a. these findings indicate urethral injury during circumcision.

    b. urethroplasty will best be performed using a ventral preputial skin flap.

    c. circumcision most likely has affected vascularity to the redundant ventral skin, and so urethroplasty will best be done using the skin as a graft.

    d. following circumcision, urethroplasty will require buccal graft from the lower lip.

    e. their infant has a hypospadias variant.

14. The parents of a 6-month-old male with subcoronal hypospadias request foreskin reconstruction rather than circumcision. The parents should be informed that:

    a. preoperative testosterone therapy to enlarge the foreskin is recommended.

    b. complication rates are significantly greater with prepucioplasty.

    c. they should not retract the foreskin in the first 6 weeks after surgery.

    d. a gentle compression dressing should be used to minimize preputial edema after surgery.

    e. the foreskin most likely will be needed for urethroplasty and so circumcision will likely be necessary.

15. Each of the following is thought to reduce the likelihood for fistula development after hypospadias surgery EXCEPT:

    a. subepithelial suturing of the neourethra.

    b. 2-layer closure of the neourethra.

    c. use of monofilament sutures for urethroplasty.

    d. approximation of the corpus spongiosum over the neourethra.

    e. placement of a dartos flap over the neourethra.

16. A mother reports her 7-year-old child who had previously undergone a two-stage Byars flap hypospadias repair now has a prolonged urinary stream and significant dribbling from his meatus after voiding. All of the following are true EXCEPT:

    a. at the time of the repair local tissue can often be used to correct the problem.

    b. he will have erectile dysfunction as an adult.

    c. at the time of the repair the meatus should be calibrated to rule out a distal obstruction.

    d. the patient may note a bulging or ballooning of the ventral penile shaft when voiding.

    e. this complication can also occur in the setting of an island onlay flap repair.

17. An 8-year-old had distal hypospadias repair as an infant. Initially after surgery he was thought to have a normal urinary stream, although the parents only rarely observed urination because he used diapers. During the past year the parents think his stream has slowed and notice he seems to have to "push" to empty his bladder. Examination reveals a faint white discoloration around the meatus that seems to extend deeper into the urethra. The most effective course of action includes:

    a. intraoperative biopsy with frozen section.

    b. meatotomy for meatal stenosis.

    c. flip-flap reoperative urethroplasty.

    d. application of topical steroids for 6 weeks.

    e. excision of the distal urethra with two-stage buccal graft urethroplasty.

18. A 1-year-old boy had a subcoronal hypospadias repair 6 months ago but has a 2-mm fistula at the site of the original meatus. Distance from the fistula to the neomeatus is approximately 4 mm, and the glans wings still appear approximated. The meatus appears patent and the meatus is calibrated to 8Fr in the operating room. The best treatment of the fistula is:

    a. midline incision through the neomeatus to the fistula with reoperative distal urethroplasty.

    b. rotational skin flap fistula closure.

    c. primary fistula closure covered with a ventral dartos barrier flap.

    d. inlay buccal graft urethroplasty.

    e. insertion of urethral catheter to facilitate secondary closure.

19. A 10-year-old boy presents with midshaft hypospadias after seven prior operations on his penis. He appears to have ventral curvature greater than 30 degrees and has been circumcised. There is visible scarring between the meatus and the glans, and there appears to be significant penoscrotal webbing. The best surgical approach for him is:

    a. a redo tubularized incised plate (TIP) operation.

    b. flip-flap reoperative urethroplasty.

    c. island onlay flap reoperative urethroplasty.

    d. inlay buccal graft urethroplasty.

    e. two-stage buccal graft urethroplasty.

20. A 6-year-old boy who had a tubularized preputial flap hypospadias repair as an infant presents with a slow urinary stream and stranguria worsening over the past year. Physical examination is unremarkable, but the peak flow is 3 mL/s with a postvoid residual of 75 mL (estimated bladder capacity of 240 mL). At surgery cystoscopy shows a 5-mm stricture near the original meatus. This stricture is best corrected by:
    a. urethral dilation.
    b. direct vision internal urethrotomy (DVIU).
    c. DVIU with CIC for 3 months.
    d. inlay buccal urethroplasty.
    e. staged buccal graft reoperation.

21. A 9-year-old prepubertal boy has failed multiple prior operations for penoscrotal hypospadias. Examination shows a distal shaft meatus, persistent ventral curvature, and a flattened ventral glans. During planned two-stage buccal graft reoperation, it becomes apparent that the entire neourethra will have to be excised back to the penoscrotal junction. The best plan for first-stage grafting is to:
    a. use cheek buccal tissue on the penile shaft and maintain the current remnant prepuce within the glans.
    b. use cheek buccal tissue to graft the entire defect.
    c. use lower lip buccal tissue for the glans and cheek tissue on the penile shaft.
    d. use lip buccal tissue on the penile shaft and cheek tissue within the glans.
    e. use ventral penile shaft skin to graft the entire defect.

22. Preoperative androgen stimulation in patients with severe hypospadias has resulted in all of the following except:
    a. decreased penile size (compared to men without hypospadias) in adulthood.
    b. increase in penile size including length and glans width.
    c. hormonal levels that return to normal shortly after treatment is discontinued.
    d. nonappreciable long-lasting side effects of treatment.
    e. transient thin pubic hair.

23. Parents report that their 1-year-old boy seems to be having difficulty urinating 3 months after TIP repair for coronal hypospadias. They have observed the stream once or twice and thought it looked thin. On examination the glans looks normal, except that the meatus appears small. In the operating room you attempt to calibrate the meatus, and an 8-Fr sound will not pass. The most likely cause for this complication is:
    a. balanitis xerotica obliterans (BXO).
    b. ischemia of the neomeatus.
    c. postoperative edema of the meatus.
    d. suturing the urethral plate too far into the distal glans.
    e. prolonged urethral stent placement.

24. Parents report that their 1-year-old boy seems to be voiding without any problems 6 months after Thiersch-Duplay repair for coronal hypospadias, although they have not seen the actual urinary stream because he is still in diapers. On examination you observe that the meatus appears small. The next step is:
    a. calibrate the meatus.
    b. obtain VCUG.
    c. schedule examination under anesthesia and meatotomy.
    d. recommend reoperative urethroplasty, using either a ventral flip-flap if possible, or inlay buccal grafting from the lip.
    e. begin daily urethral dilations for 6 weeks.

25. If not repaired, an isolated glanular hypospadias with no penile curvature and a normal caliber to the meatus will result in which of the following long-term issues?
    a. Difficulty with micturition
    b. Inability to inseminate during sexual intercourse
    c. Clinically significant meatal stenosis
    d. Painful erections
    e. None of the above

26. A 19-month-old male presents for evaluation of scrotal hypospadias. The mother has noted that his pupils seem enlarged, and she is concerned he might have developmental delay. He is crying during examination, hindering inspection of his eyes. He has scrotal hypospadias with a deep scrotal cleft, but both testes are in the scrotum. His evaluation before surgery should include:
    a. renal sonogram.
    b. testicular sonogram.
    c. VCUG.
    d. assessment of testosterone/dihydrotestosterone (T/DHT) ratio.
    e. measurement of anti-Müllerian hormone (AMH).

27. A 12-year-old boy had hypospadias reoperation 1 year ago that included a tunica vaginalis barrier flap over the neourethra harvested from the right testicle. He reports no problems voiding, but with erection the penis is pulled to the right side. The next step is to:
    a. reassure him the tension on his penis will resolve at puberty.
    b. make a small scrotal incision and transect the tunica vaginalis flap.
    c. make a midline penile incision and excise the tunica vaginalis flap.
    d. create a tunica vaginalis flap from the left testis to evenly distribute the tension on the penis during erection.
    e. instruct the patient to pull the penis toward the left during erection to relax contracted tissues.

28. A 14-year-old undergoes a first-stage buccal graft reoperation that involves grafting along the entire penile shaft. The next morning he is found to have visible hematoma under the shaft skin. The next step is:
    a. return immediately to the operating room to evacuate the hematoma.
    b. apply a compression dressing over the penis and scrotum.
    c. check coagulation profiles for bleeding diathesis.
    d. observe with continued bed rest.
    e. evacuate the hematoma and regraft the penile shaft.

29. A 6-month-old boy has proximal hypospadias. In the operating room, there is 50 degrees of ventral penile curvature after penile degloving and division of the urethral plate. All of the following are viable repair options EXCEPT:
    a. corporal grafting with a dermal graft and 2-stage Byars flap repair.
    b. 2-stage STAG (staged tubularized autograft) repair with ventral corporotomies.
    c. single-stage repair with tunica vaginalis graft corporotomy followed by Duckett tube.
    d. single-stage repair with dorsal plication and island onlay urethroplasty.
    e. none of the above.

30. For hypospadias complication repairs, all of the following are true EXCEPT:

    a. a coronal fistula with a thin glans should be repaired with a redo urethroplasty and glansplasty.

    b. a small penoscrotal fistula identified 12 months after repair can be closed by placement of a urethral catheter and secondary closure.

    c. a urethral diverticulum can be closed using local tissue as a barrier layer.

    d. recurrent penile curvature should be assessed in the operating room to determine if penile skin scarring, corporal disproportion, or both are the cause.

    e. glans dehiscence may require buccal mucosa graft inlay in order to achieve a successful repair.

31. Regarding familial hypospadias:

    a. only hypospadias associated with malformation syndromes has familial recurrence.

    b. hypospadias will occur only if the mother was taking birth control pills containing progesterone shortly before she conceived.

    c. hypospadias will occur only if the father also has hypospadias.

    d. it will occur, because hypospadias is a Y-linked disorder.

    e. the odds are greatest that another son would not have hypospadias.

ANSWERS

1. **d. An ectopic location of the urethral meatus below the center of the glans.** The vast majority of boys with hypospadias do not have anomalies outside of the genitourinary tract or a bifid scrotum, the latter of which is typically seen in proximal hypospadias, which occurs 10% of the time. Some boys will have ventral curvature with an orthotopic urethral meatus, but they have chordee without hypospadias and can typically be corrected without repair of the urethra.

2. **d. After penile degloving, taking into account both the location of the urethral meatus and the degree of penile curvature.** The traditional method of diagnosis and risk stratification was based on the location of the urethral meatus at the time of diagnosis. Based on a number of different variants, the most accurate assessment of the degree of hypospadias is based upon the location of the urethral meatus after penile degloving combined with an assessment of the degree of penile curvature. Taking note of glans separation, although part of the assessment, is present in the majority of boys with hypospadias, and is not thought to correlate with the degree of hypospadias.

3. **d. a and b.** The urethral groove forms between the urethral folds and ultimately becomes the urethra. Preputial folds fuse as the urethra closes, in a dorsal to ventral fashion, hence the typical physical characteristics seen in hypospadias.

4. **e. All of the above.** A shorter AGD is thought to be secondary to exposure to environmental disrupting chemicals, currently theorized to inhibit the androgen cascade and penile development, resulting in hypospadias. The increased rate of hypospadias in twins and those boys conceived via in-vitro fertilization is thought, in part, to be secondary to hormone disruption. The testicular dysgenesis syndrome (TDS) includes several male reproductive developmental disorders, including poor sperm quality and rising rates of cryptorchidism and hypospadias, thought to be secondary to fetal exposure and resultant disruption of the normal androgen cascade during development, resulting in a life-long effect on these boys.

5. **c. Obtain a karyotype.** The combination of a penile anomaly with undescended testis may indicate a disorder of sex development. Although this is more commonly found with proximal hypospadias and a nonpalpable gonad, it is still advised to obtain a karyotype in any child with hypospadias and cryptorchidism.

6. **b. An enlarged utricle.** The most common reason for difficulty with catheter placement during hypospadias repair is an enlarged utricle, which occurs more frequently in boys with more severe hypospadias. Urethral duplication is rare in boys with hypospadias and a high bladder neck is encountered often in boys with posterior urethral valves, not hypospadias.

7. **a. Proceed with surgery.** Neither karyotyping nor urinary tract imaging is indicated for isolated hypospadias, even in patients with proximal defects. Associated renal anomalies are rare in nonsyndromic hypospadias. Karyotyping can be considered and offered to families with proximal hypospadias but is only strongly recommended in the setting of at least one undescended testicle. Delaying surgery will not significantly increase penile growth. If a utricle is encountered at the time of surgery maneuvers are taken to successfully place a catheter and removal at the time of primary hypospadias repair is not recommended.

8. **f. b, c, and d.** The pattern of penile nerve innervation plays a critical role in management of penile curvature and must be completely understood prior to correction. The nerve bundles are present at the 11 and 1 o'clock positions on the dorsal penile shaft and can be avoided with midline suture placement. Perineal nerve block can be attempted in older, ambulatory patients who would not otherwise tolerate the temporary lower extremity paralysis after caudal blockade.

9. **b. A VCUG.** Recurrent UTIs after a hypospadias repair are a relatively rare event. Anatomic concerns including distal stricture, new onset vesicoureteral reflux, or incomplete voiding must be explored. Constipation may be contributing to the UTIs, but a cone enema is not recommended at this point. If an anomaly is seen on VCUG a cystoscopy should be considered. Sitting to void will not help this issue.

10. **d. Perform a midline dorsal plication.** Persistent penile curvature of less than 30 degrees after penile degloving can be straightened by a single dorsal plication without clinically apparent shortening of the penis. Transection of the urethral plate and/or ventral corporal lengthening procedures are reserved for cases with curvature greater than 30 degrees after degloving and dartos dissection. In a boy with 15 degrees of ventral curvature, correction is recommended and proceeding with urethroplasty significantly increases the chance that an additional operation to correct curvature will be necessary in the future.

11. **a. Skin degloving and ventral dartos dissection.** Most often penile curvature noted in so-called chordee without hypospadias is due to shortened ventral skin and dartos and so corrects as the penis is degloved and ventral dartos dissected. Multiple plications should be avoided, ventral corporal grafting is reserved for curvature greater than 30 degrees after degloving and ventral dartos dissection, and urethral transection for a shortened urethra is only rarely indicated in this condition.

12. **e. A two-stage repair may be required.** Although difficult to fully assess in the office setting, a patient with significant curvature and penoscrotal webbing may be suggestive of a severely hypoplastic urethra with significant penile curvature that may require a 2-stage repair. Parent counseling at the time of the initial visit is a key component of setting expectations for surgical reconstruction. A patient with severe ventral curvature is unlikely to have a complication rate of 5% and most series suggest a total complication rate closer to 10% even for distal hypospadias. A karyotype is not necessary in isolated hypospadias.

13. **e. Their infant has a hypospadias variant.** The patient has megameatus intact prepuce (MIP) hypospadias variant, and urethroplasty is typically successful via tubularization of local skin flaps. Preputial skin flaps or buccal grafts are typically not necessary. This is not secondary to a circumcision injury.

14. **c. They should not retract the foreskin in the first 6 weeks after surgery.** Disruption of the reconstructed prepuce may result from attempts to retract the foreskin early after surgery, before edema subsides and the wound heals. Otherwise complication rates are similar between patients with distal hypospadias undergoing foreskin reconstruction versus circumcision. Dressings do not significantly affect postoperative edema. When a sufficient amount of redundant shaft skin is present preputioplasty can be performed, but the repair should not be compromised in order to achieve this. Tunica vaginalis can be considered for secondary layer closure in these patients.

15. **c. Use of monofilament sutures for urethroplasty.** No study demonstrates outcomes are influenced by suture type, but technical modifications such as subepithelial suturing of the neourethra and additional layers of vascularized tissue are beneficial.

16. **b. He will have erectile dysfunction as an adult.** The history of a 2-stage Byars flap and a prolonged voiding time with significant dribbling suggests a urethral diverticulum. It can be repaired using the redundant tissue present within the diverticulum itself, as some of the tissue can be de-epithelialized and used for additional layers of vascularized closure. They are thought to occur in preputial onlay flaps as well as 2-stage Byars flap repairs due to the dispensability of the preputial skin.

17. **e. Excision of the distal urethra with two-stage buccal graft urethroplasty.** The history and physical findings suggest BXO. A biopsy in the operating room (OR) can be performed at the time of the procedure, but this is not a definitive process. Office biopsy is not recommended. Meatotomy or skin flap repair of meatal stenosis most often fails in the presence of BXO, as residual BXO will progress into the reconstructed tissue. Given the extension of the suspected BXO into the urethra, a cystoscopy to determine proximal extent with subsequent excision of all tissues affected by BXO with staged buccal mucosa reconstruction is standard of care. Topical steroids may be initially effective, but stenosis recurs when therapy ends, and BXO may extend proximally along the urethra to a level not reached by topical applications. In spite of replacement with buccal mucosa, these patients will still be at risk for recurrence and must be monitored closely.

18. **c. Primary fistula closure covered with a ventral dartos barrier flap.** A fistula with good glans approximation usually can be primarily corrected with fistula closure followed by coverage with additional vascularized layers, in this case a Dartos barrier flap. In contrast, when the skin quality is thin and poor with separation of the glans wings in addition to a short distance between the neomeatus and the fistula, this is not recommended. Instead a reoperative distal urethroplasty/glansplasty should be performed, otherwise a high failure rate will follow. A rotational skin flap is not a good option in this case because it is necessary to dissect under the corona to completely free the fistula tract and advance a barrier flap. Although meatal stenosis has to be considered in any case with a fistula, appropriate therapy when it is present is reoperation, not dilations. Prolonged catheter insertion will not lead to fistula closure.

19. **e. Two-stage buccal graft urethroplasty.** Visible scarring is a relative contraindication to TIP or flip-flap reoperations, as there is likely significant compromise of the blood supply to these tissues, which will result in a high failure rate. The penoscrotal webbing and curvature suggests that there is a lack of shaft skin, particularly on the ventral portion of the penis, which will limit the ability to perform an onlay procedure The best plan is to excise scarred tissues and perform a staged buccal graft urethroplasty. The penile curvature must be assessed at the time of the repair to ensure that there is no residual curvature after the scar tissue is excised.

20. **d. Inlay buccal urethroplasty.** Distal urethral narrowing, particularly within the glans in which there is lack of normal expansion of the urethra, can lead to an elevated postvoid residual and slowed urinary stream. Direct vision internal urethrotomy (DVIU) has a long-term success less than 10% after TIP repairs, even when used in conjunction with clean intermittent catheterization (CIC). The best treatment in this case is inlay grafting into the stricture and either a buccal mucosa graft or a piece of redundant dorsal shaft skin or inner preputial skin can be used for a dorsal inlay graft repair. If an inlay graft repair fails, a staged buccal graft repair would be required.

21. **c. Use lower lip buccal tissue for the glans and cheek tissue on the penile shaft.** It is best to use lip tissue within the glans, because it is thinner than cheek tissue and results in less complications after glansplasty. Given the narrow and flat appearance of the glans and a history of multiple failed repairs, the skin with the glans is best excised to restore a deep groove that ultimately will result in a vertical meatus at the second stage. After multiple failed operations, redundant shaft skin sufficient for grafting and subsequent urethroplasty is not available.

22. **a. Decreased penile size (compared to men without hypospadias) in adulthood.** Preoperative androgen stimulation in prepubertal boys can transiently increase both the penile length and glans width. It is thought that a small glans width increases urethroplasty and glansplasty complications, therefore increasing the width of the glans at the time of closure is of some theoretical benefit. Several conflicting studies argue both sides of its use. Its side effects including increased frequency of erections, thin pubic hair, and increased aggression, all of which are transient after it is discontinued.

23. **d. Suturing the urethral plate too far into the distal glans.** The most common cause of meatal stenosis after TIP is suturing the urethral plate too far distally. The contour of the glans is such that this will narrow the distal portion of the meatus, causing stenosis and/or obstruction. BXO is unlikely early after surgery and often presents with white discoloration at the meatus. Ischemia is possible but unlikely, given the reliable vascularity of the urethral plate and glans tissues. Edema after surgery may slow the urinary stream, but at 3 months it should be resolved enough to not cause passage of a sound. Prolonged urethral stent placement does not cause obstruction.

24. **a. Calibrate the meatus.** The meatus may appear small after Thiersch-Duplay urethroplasty without indicating meatal stenosis. Passage of an 8- or 10-Fr sound would suffice to determine if the meatus is stenotic or not, although this is extremely difficult in the office setting. Passage of a sound without anesthesia is only possible in a small number of patients, and even insertion of an 8-Fr feeding tube may be difficult in this population. A small-appearing meatus in an asymptomatic (UTI, stranguria, prolonged urinary stream) patient should not prompt immediate concern that examination under anesthesia or reoperation is needed. If symptoms are present an examination under anesthesia is recommended. If repair is indicated, the intervention of choice would depend upon the length of narrowing, the quality of the glans closure, and the assessment of the remainder of the urethroplasty.

25. **e. None of the above.** In isolated hypospadias without any evidence of narrowing of the meatus, a glanular location, and no penile curvature, it is unlikely that significant morbidity would result for the patient. If penile curvature is noted, however, even with a mildly displaced meatus, surgical intervention would be warranted due to the potential for long-term sequelae.

26. **a. Renal sonogram.** The history suggests WAGR (Wilms tumor, Aniridia, Genital abnormalities, mental Retardation) syndrome, and so renal sonography is recommended because of the association with Wilms tumor.

27. **b. Make a small scrotal incision and transect the tunica vaginalis flap.** Failure to dissect the tunica vaginalis flap to the external ring can result in traction on the penis during erection, deviating it toward the base of the flap. The best therapy is to

make a small scrotal incision over the flap and transect it. As this has occurred several years after his initial repair, this should not compromise the blood supply to the urethroplasty.

28. **d. Observe with continued bed rest.** Hematoma formation under buccal mucosa graft can compromise the take rate of the graft. Technical modifications including graft quilting and the tie-over compression dressing prevent blood from accumulating under the graft. Hematoma under adjacent penile skin and within the scrotum as described here will resolve with minimal effect upon the graft itself. It is unlikely that a boy requiring a staged buccal graft repair has an undiagnosed coagulopathy following prior penile operations.

29. **d. Single-stage repair with dorsal plication and island onlay urethroplasty.** In a boy with severe ventral curvature after penile degloving and division of the urethral plate (50 degrees in this case), a two-stage repair should be performed. A corporal lengthening procedure should be performed, and dermal graft, corporotomies, and tunica vaginalis flap are all viable options.

Dorsal plication would put the boy at risk for recurrent penile curvature long term.

30. **b. A small penoscrotal fistula identified 12 months after repair can be closed by placement of a urethral catheter and secondary closure.** Fistulas rarely, if ever, close with catheter insertion. A coronal fistula with thin glans tissue will likely need a more aggressive repair. A urethral diverticulum can be de-epithelialized to add additional layers of closure. Recurrent curvature should be aggressively diagnosed and managed as there is a high rate of failure with plication alone.

31. **e. The odds are greatest that another son would not have hypospadias.** Sporadic and syndromic hypospadias can have familial recurrence, and the risk of a boy with a brother with hypospadias having hypospadias himself is as high as 15%. This rate would be higher in a twin pairing. Although the likelihood a sibling will have hypospadias is increased, the overall risk remains small.

CHAPTER REVIEW

1. Dihydrotestosterone at the 8- to 12-week gestational phase is a key mediator in the proper development of the penis.
2. There is an increased risk of hypospadias in births resulting from assisted reproduction and monozygotic twins.
3. The etiology of hypospadias is multifactorial, but placental disruption and androgen disruption, in part via environmental exposures, are potential culprits in what is thought to be an increasing rate of hypospadias development. Anogenital distance is a reflection of disruption of this cascade.
4. Parental discussion about the risk of hypospadias repair should include the risks of early anesthesia exposure versus the benefits of early surgery in infancy.
5. Preoperative androgen stimulation can transiently increase the penile length and size for surgery. Its impact on complication development is controversial.
6. Physical examination in a patient with hypospadias may reveal a ventral deficient prepuce, downward glans tilt, deviation of the median penile raphe, ventral curvature, scrotal encroachment onto the penile shaft, scrotal cleft, and penile scrotal transposition.
7. Eighty percent of urethroplasty complications occur within 1 year after surgery. Delayed complications, such as urethral stricture or penile curvature, can present in a delayed fashion. Thus boys, particularly those with proximal hypospadias, should be followed into puberty.
8. Risk factors for complications following urethroplasty include proximal meatus, reoperation, glans width less than 14 mm, and lack of a barrier flap over the neourethra.
9. Long-term follow-up of patients who have had a hypospadias repair indicates that they are more likely to have ejaculatory problems, are less satisfied with sexual function, and are more likely to be dissatisfied with the appearance of their penis than controls. Patient-reported outcomes are an underrepresented component of follow-up and must be a focus of future studies.
10. The combination of a penile anomaly with undescended testis may indicate a difference of sex development (DSD). Although more commonly found with proximal hypospadias and a nonpalpable gonad, it is still advised to obtain a karyotype in any child with hypospadias and cryptorchidism.
11. Curvature less than 30 degrees can be straightened by a single dorsal plication without clinically apparent shortening of the penis. Objective measurement of penile curvature, as identified by artificial erection after penile degloving, is an important part of the surgical procedure. Transection of the urethral plate and/or ventral corporal grafting are reserved for cases with curvature greater than 30 degrees after degloving and dartos dissection.
12. Meatotomy or skin flap repair of meatal stenosis most often fail in the presence of BXO, whereas excision of all tissues affected by BXO with staged buccal grafting is considered most likely to succeed without recurrent stenosis. These patients will have up to a 40% failure rate; therefore they must be closely monitored.
13. For buccal mucosal reconstruction, lip tissue placement is preferable within the glans, because it is thinner than cheek tissue and results in a lower complication rate.
14. Urethrocutaneous fistula is the most common complication after hypospadias repair. If there is supple tissue present, a primary closure can be attempted, but if thin glans tissue is present or located at the corona or distal, then redo urethroplasty and glans closure should be performed.

46 Etiology, Diagnosis, and Management of Undescended Testis

Julia Spencer Barthold and Jennifer A. Hagerty

QUESTIONS

1. What is the master gene responsible for male sexual differentiation?
   a. RSPO1
   b. SOX9
   c. WT1
   d. SRY
   e. WNT4

2. During male reproductive tract development, androgens mediate the differentiation of all of the following structures EXCEPT:
   a. seminal vesicles.
   b. ureter.
   c. epididymis.
   d. vas deferens.
   e. ejaculatory ducts.

3. Which of the following does not play a direct role in testicular descent?
   a. Testis
   b. Epididymis
   c. Genitofemoral nerve
   d. Gubernaculum
   e. Processus vaginalis

4. Peak levels of testosterone and insulin-like 3 occur in the male fetus at approximately what gestational week?
   a. 5
   b. 8
   c. 10
   d. 15
   e. 20

5. Cryptorchidism increases the risk of all of the following EXCEPT:
   a. spermatic cord torsion.
   b. clinical hernia.
   c. reactive hydrocele.
   d. infertility.
   e. testicular malignancy.

6. The risk of cryptorchidism is higher in all of the following syndromes EXCEPT:
   a. cerebral palsy.
   b. cystic fibrosis.
   c. arthrogryposis.
   d. prune belly syndrome.
   e. posterior urethral valves.

7. All of the following are associated with patency of the processus vaginalis EXCEPT:
   a. transverse testicular ectopia.
   b. epididymal anomalies.
   c. cryptorchidism.
   d. spermatic cord torsion.
   e. polyorchidism.

8. Histologic findings in cryptorchid testes may include all of the following EXCEPT:
   a. carcinoma in situ.
   b. absence of Ad spermatogonia.
   c. early disappearance of gonocytes.
   d. failure of Sertoli cell maturation.
   e. reduced germ cell counts.

9. What percentage of undescended testes are nonpalpable at presentation?
   a. 1%
   b. 3%
   c. 10%
   d. 20%
   e. 30%

10. During laparoscopy, spermatic cord structures exiting an open internal ring ipsilateral to a nonpalpable testis imply:
    a. vanishing testis, inguinal exploration unnecessary.
    b. vanishing testis, inguinal exploration necessary.
    c. intracanalicular atrophic testis, inguinal exploration unnecessary.
    d. intracanalicular testis, inguinal exploration necessary.
    e. further exploration unnecessary if contralateral testicular hypertrophy is present.

11. Advantages of laparoscopic management of an intraabdominal testis include all of the following EXCEPT:
    a. more accurately assesses the presence or absence, viability, and anatomy of the testis compared with radiographic imaging.
    b. reduces the risk of damage to the testis.
    c. enhances surgical exposure, lighting, and magnification.
    d. allows a greater degree of proximal dissection of the spermatic vessels.
    e. allows diagnosis of associated Müllerian ductal abnormalities if present.

12. Which statement is FALSE regarding Fowler-Stephens orchidopexy?
    a. It is less commonly associated with testicular atrophy than laparoscopic primary orchidopexy.
    b. It has a lower success rate in patients who have undergone previous inguinal surgery.

c. Blood supply is based on the deferential artery and collateral peritoneal vessels.

d. It should be performed at a similar age as a standard inguinal orchidopexy.

e. It should be considered if the testis is not near the internal ring.

13. Which of the following is least consistent with a diagnosis of vanishing testis?

a. Patent processus vaginalis

b. Contralateral testicular hypertrophy

c. Palpable nubbin in scrotum

d. Increased serum follicle-stimulating hormone

e. Micropenis

14. Lower than expected testicular volume has been associated with all of the following EXCEPT:

a. cryptorchid testes that have descended spontaneously.

b. solitary testes in boys with a vanishing testis.

c. Fowler-Stephens orchidopexy.

d. increased serum FSH.

e. surgery for congenital cryptorchidism at 3 years as compared to 9 months of age.

15. Regarding epididymal anatomy, which of the following is the most common finding in boys undergoing orchidopexy for acquired cryptorchidism?

a. Detachment of the cauda epididymis

b. Detachment of the caput epididymis

c. Looped epididymis

d. Long looping epididymis/vas

e. Normal anatomy

16. All of the following factors may influence the reliability of studies of the efficacy of hormone therapy for cryptorchidism EXCEPT:

a. treatment of boys with retractile testes.

b. initial position of the testis.

c. vanishing testis syndrome.

d. randomization protocol.

e. all of the above.

17. A healthy full-term newborn boy presents with a bilateral non-palpable testes. The next step in management should include:

a. karyotype analysis.

b. GnRH stimulation test.

c. abdominal ultrasound.

d. circumcision.

e. discharge home with MRI with gadolinium in four weeks.

18. Of the following, which is the LEAST reliable test in confirming the diagnosis of bilateral anorchia?

a. No change in serum testosterone following hCG stimulation

b. FSH level >2 IU/L at 1 year of age

c. Laparoscopy

d. Undetectable serum inhibin B

e. Undetectable serum anti-Müllerian hormone (AMH)

19. Which of the following is LEAST useful to the provider in determining the diagnosis of retractile vs. undescended testes?

a. Observation of testicular position with abduction of the patient's legs

b. History of prior testicular position provided by the primary care physician (PCP)

c. Failure of the testis to remain stable in the scrotum with sustained traction on the cord

d. Warm room and hands

e. Small ipsilateral testis

20. Which of the following is true regarding spontaneous descent of cryptorchid testes?

a. Spontaneous descent is independent of testicular position.

b. Reascent occurs in 40% of patients.

c. Early descent is more likely in premature boys.

d. Spontaneous descent is unlikely if the ipsilateral hemiscrotum is small.

e. The majority of testes that descend spontaneously do so in the first few months of life.

21. The risk of developing a testicular tumor in males with a history of cryptorchidism is:

a. 2 to 5 times the risk in normal boys.

b. minimal in boys who undergo orchidopexy in infancy.

c. determined by placental alkaline phosphatase (PLAP) staining in prepubertal testes.

d. similar in the contralateral descended testis.

e. increasing over time.

22. Each of the following is more common in association with cryptorchid testes, EXCEPT:

a. atrophy.

b. microlithiasis.

c. mature teratoma.

d. ectasia of the rete testis.

e. intratesticular varicocele.

23. The following are possible locations of an ectopic testis, EXCEPT:

a. peripenile.

b. perirenal.

c. perivesical.

d. perianal.

e. femoral.

24. Levels of all the following hormones peak after birth and remain low during childhood EXCEPT:

a. LH.

b. FSH.

c. AMH.

d. Inhibin B.

e. testosterone.

25. When in fetal development does the testicle pass into the inguinal canal?

a. 5 to 7 weeks gestation

b. 10 to 14 weeks gestation

c. 20 to 28 weeks gestation

d. 30 to 34 weeks gestation

e. None of the above

26. How commonly does cryptorchidism occur in full-term males?

a. <1%

b. 1% to 4%

c. 5% to 10%

d. 15%

e. None of the above

27. A 1-month-old full-term male presents with a unilateral non-palpable testicle. The next step after a confirmatory exam is:
    a. ultrasound to identify the position of the testicle.
    b. MRI with gadolinium.
    c. hormonal therapy to induce descent.
    d. surgical intervention.
    e. observation for spontaneous descent until 6 months of age.

ANSWERS

1. **d. SRY.** The SRY gene appears to be primarily responsible for male sexual differentiation through complex interactions involving both activation and repression of other male-specific genes.
2. **b. Ureter.** Androgens (testosterone, dihydrotestosterone) mediate the differentiation of the paired Wolffian ducts into the seminal vesicles, epididymis, vas deferens, and ejaculatory ducts.
3. **b. Epididymis.** Changes in the gubernaculum and processus vaginalis and their innervation by the genitofemoral nerve, and hormone secretion by the testis are all important in the process of testicular descent.
4. **d. 15.** Testosterone production peaks at 14 to 16 weeks and INSL3 peaks at 15 to 17 weeks.
5. **c. Reactive hydrocele.** All of the others are possible complications of cryptorchidism.
6. **b. Cystic fibrosis.** All the other syndromes are associated with a higher risk of cryptorchidism; mutations of the cystic fibrosis gene are associated with congenital absence of the vas deferens.
7. **d. Spermatic cord torsion.** Risk of torsion is associated with abnormal development of the tunica vaginalis but not patency of the processus vaginalis.
8. **c. Early disappearance of gonocytes.** Histological abnormalities that may be present in cryptorchid testes include delayed disappearance of gonocytes, reduced numbers of adult dark (Ad) spermatogonia, reduced number of germ cells per testicular tubule, and carcinoma in situ (CIS).
9. **d. 20%.** Approximately 20% of undescended testes are nonpalpable at presentation.
10. **d. Intracanalicular testis, inguinal exploration necessary.** While atretic spermatic vessels seen exiting the internal ring may be associated with a distal vanishing testis, the appearance of the spermatic vessels during laparoscopy is subjective and therefore exploration (inguinal or laparoscopic) is needed to rule out an intracanalicular viable or atrophic testis. Further exploration is unnecessary if blind-ending intraabdominal spermatic vessels are found. Hypertrophy of a normally descended contralateral testis is suggestive of monorchism.
11. **b. Reduces the risk of damage to the testis.** Laparoscopic orchidopexy still carries the risks of bleeding, infection, and damage to the testis and cord in addition to damage to intraabdominal structures such as bowel and the great vessels.
12. **a. It is less commonly associated with testicular atrophy than laparoscopic primary orchidopexy.** Fowler-Stephens orchidopexy, either one-or two-stage, has a higher reported testicular atrophy rate compared with laparoscopic orchidopexy. The other statements are true.
13. **a. Patent processus vaginalis.** Contralateral testicular hypertrophy and a palpable scrotal nubbin may present in boys with unilateral vanishing testis and increased serum FSH and micropenis may be seen in boys with bilateral vanishing testes. The processus vaginalis is closed in most cases of vanishing testis.
14. **b. Solitary testes in boys with a vanishing testis.** In vanishing testis syndrome, the contralateral testis may be larger than expected for age.
15. **e. Normal anatomy.** An abnormal epididymis was reported ipsilateral to 11% to 31% of acquired undescended testes at surgery.
16. **e. All of the above** are confounding factors that may affect the reliability of studies of the efficacy of hormone therapy for cryptorchidism.
17. **a. Karyotype analysis.** AUA Guidelines for cryptorchidism state that providers must immediately consult an appropriate specialist for all phenotypic male newborns with bilateral, nonpalpable testes for evaluation of a possible difference of sex development (DSD). A newborn with a male phallus and bilateral nonpalpable gonads is potentially a genetic female (46,XX) with congenital adrenal hyperplasia until proven otherwise. Circumcision should be avoided in the initial management. More than 70% of cryptorchid testes are palpable by physical examination and need no imaging. In the remaining 30% of cases with a nonpalpable testis, the challenge is to confirm absence or presence of the testis. At this time, there is no radiologic test that can conclude with 100% accuracy that a testis is absent.
18. **a. No change in serum testosterone following hCG stimulation.** Serum testosterone may not increase significantly in response to hCG stimulation in individuals with abnormal testes.
19. **b. History of prior testicular position provided by the PCP.** Testicular position can change over time and/or be difficult to ascertain in boys with retractile testes; therefore, a careful examination is necessary to differentiate between retractile and undescended testes.
20. **e. The majority of testes that descend spontaneously do so in the first few months of life.** For full-term boys of normal weight, spontaneous testicular descent typically occurs in the first months after birth and is rare after 6 months of age.
21. **a. 2 to 5 times the risk in normal boys.** Surgery may reduce but does not eliminate the risk of TGCT in boys with cryptorchidism and the risk exists in the contralateral testis as well, albeit lower. PLAP+ germ cells can be found in normal testes after birth.
22. **c. Mature teratoma.** The risk of benign testicular tumors is not increased in cryptorchidism.
23. **d. Perianal.** All the other answers reflect possible positions for ectopic testes that are possible although rare.
24. **c. AMH.** AMH levels remain high during childhood and are downregulated at puberty.
25. **c. 20 to 28 weeks gestation.** The testis passes into the inguinal canal at 20 to 28 weeks gestation during the fifth phase of testicular descent.
26. **b. 1% to 4%.** Cryptorchidism is one of the most common congenital anomalies occurring in 1% to 4% of full-term male infants.
27. **e. Observation until 6 months of age.** Descent may occur up until 6 months of age. If it hasn't occurred by this time, surgical treatment should be performed. Diagnostic imaging has not been shown to change the need for surgery. Hormonal therapy to induce descent is no longer supported given the lack of evidence that exists.

CHAPTER REVIEW

1. Gonadal determination involves separate genetic pathways for development of testis and ovary and *SRY* is a master switch in males that regulates downstream testis-determining genes.
2. Differentiation of gonocytes, Sertoli and Leydig cells occurs between 5 and 9 weeks' gestation and the gubernaculum, the guide for testicular descent, appears at 7 weeks.
3. Levels of the Leydig cell hormones testosterone and INSL3 peak between 14 and 17 weeks, and are critical for testicular descent.
4. Swelling of the gubernaculum, which starts in the second trimester, provides space for passage of the testis into the scrotum between 20 and 28 weeks.
5. Cryptorchidism occurs in 1%–4% of full-term males; both spontaneous descent (in the first few months of life, usually by 6 months) and reascent of testes may occur.
6. The causes of cryptorchidism are largely unknown, but birth weight, gestational age, and genetic and environmental risk factors likely contribute to disease risk.
7. Acquired cryptorchidism is not uncommon but is likely equivalent to cases diagnosed at birth. It may occur after scrotal testes are confirmed at birth, or after spontaneous descent of a cryptorchid testis, and may be more common in boys with retractile testes. Yearly testicular exams are recommended during childhood.
8. About 80% of undescended testes are palpable and 60%–70% are unilateral.
9. Epididymal anomalies and a patent processus vaginalis are common in cases of cryptorchidism.
10. Subsets of boys with cryptorchidism have subtle abnormalities of the hypothalamic-pituitary-gonadal axis during mini-puberty and/or reduced levels of hormones secreted by Sertoli cells, AMH, or inhibin B (INHB).
11. Orchidopexy is recommended for testes that remain undescended after 6 months of age; hormone therapy is not recommended.
12. Laparoscopy is the procedure of choice and imaging studies are rarely useful in the diagnosis and treatment of nonpalpable abdominal cryptorchidism.
13. Immediate urologic consultation is required for all phenotypic male newborns with bilateral, nonpalpable testes for evaluation of a possible DSD. A newborn with a male phallus and bilateral nonpalpable gonads is potentially a genetic female (46,XX) with congenital adrenal hyperplasia until proven otherwise.
14. Sperm counts are reduced in at least 25% of formerly unilateral and the majority of formerly bilateral cryptorchid men, but paternity rates in the unilateral group are similar to control men.
15. Ad spermatogonia counts may predict fertility potential in some males with cryptorchidism.
16. TGCT risk is 2–5 times higher in boys with cryptorchidism and is positively correlated with age at surgery.

47 Management of Abnormalities of the Genitalia in Girls

Martin Kaefer

QUESTIONS

1. Which of the following statements is TRUE regarding Mayer-Rokitansky Küster Hauser (MRKH) syndrome?
   a. Patients present most commonly with infertility.
   b. It is a homogeneous disorder entailing congenital absence of the uterus and vagina.
   c. It is associated with a spectrum of ovarian abnormalities.
   d. It has associated upper urinary tract anomalies, primarily with the atypical disorder.
   e. It is associated with persistent Wolffian duct structures.

2. What is the crucial period in embryogenesis for the formation of the terminal bowel, kidney, paramesonephric ductal system, and lumbosacral spine?
   a. 4 to 6 weeks
   b. 8 to 10 weeks
   c. 10 to 14 weeks
   d. 14 to 18 weeks
   e. After 18 weeks

3. Which of the following is FALSE regarding vaginal agenesis (Müllerian aplasia)?
   a. It occurs in approximately 1 in 5000 live female births.
   b. Serum follicle-stimulating hormone and luteinizing hormone levels can be expected to be abnormally high.
   c. Embryologically, it results from a failure of the sinovaginal bulbs to develop and form the vaginal plate.
   d. It is associated with renal abnormalities.
   e. It is associated with skeletal abnormalities.

4. Skeletal anomalies are found in what percentage of patients with Meyer-Rokitansky-Küster-Hauser syndrome?
   a. 10% to 20%
   b. 25% to 35%
   c. 40% to 60%
   d. 70% to 90%
   e. 0% (they are not seen in MRKH)

5. What is the most common cause of primary amenorrhea?
   a. Complete androgen insensitivity syndrome
   b. Vaginal agenesis
   c. Mixed gonadal dysgenesis
   d. Imperforate hymen
   e. Transverse vaginal septum

6. Which of the following statement is FALSE regarding the genitalia of women with Meyer-Rokitansky-Küster-Hauser syndrome?
   a. In approximately 10% of patients, a normal but obstructed uterus or rudimentary uterus with functional endometrium is present.
   b. Normal fallopian tubes are seen in approximately 35% of patients.
   c. The ovaries are not functional in the majority of patients.
   d. The hymenal ridge is usually present, along with a small vaginal pouch.
   e. The labia majora are typically normal in appearance.

7. Uterus didelphys with unilateral imperforate vagina is most commonly present with which condition?
   a. Primary amenorrhea
   b. Cyclic abdominal pain associated with normal cyclic menstruation.
   c. Renal anomalies contralateral to the side of the obstruction
   d. Anomalies of the axial skeleton
   e. Constipation

8. Urethral prolapse is most commonly seen in young females of which ethnic background?
   a. African American
   b. White
   c. Asian
   d. Hispanic
   e. Native American

9. In most cases of labial adhesions, which of the following is true?
   a. They are believed to occur because of a relative state of hyperestrogenism.
   b. They should be treated with surgical lysis.
   c. They require no treatment.
   d. They occur secondary to sexual abuse.
   e. They have associated renal anomalies.

10. What is the mean age of a child with vaginal rhabdomyosarcoma?
    a. Younger than 2 years
    b. 2 to 4 years
    c. 4 to 8 years
    d. 8 to 12 years
    e. Older than 12 years

11. All of the following statements are true of anogenital condyloma acuminatum EXCEPT:
    a. human papillomavirus is the etiologic agent.
    b. sexual abuse is the only means by which an infant can contract the disease.
    c. many cases in children resolve spontaneously.
    d. pediatric immunization should dramatically reduce the incidence of this disorder.
    e. carbon dioxide laser ablation is successful for anogenital lesions.

ANSWERS

1. **d. It has associated upper urinary tract anomalies, primarily with the atypical disorder.** Urinary tract anomalies occur more commonly in patients with the atypical form of the disorder than in patients with the typical syndrome.
2. **a. 4 to 6 weeks.** Laboratory data with teratogens support the concept of a key event occurring between the fourth and fifth weeks of gestation that results in an error in the simultaneous development of the terminal bowel, kidney, bladder, paramesonephric ductal system, and lumbosacral spine.
3. **b. Serum follicle-stimulating hormone and luteinizing hormone levels can be expected to be abnormally high.** Vaginal agenesis, which occurs in approximately 1 in 5000 live female births, is the congenital absence of the proximal portion of the vagina in an otherwise phenotypically (i.e., normal secondary sexual characteristics), chromosomally (i.e., 46,XX), and hormonally (i.e., normal luteinizing hormone and follicle-stimulating hormone levels) intact female. It results from a failure of the sinovaginal bulbs to develop and form the vaginal plate. Hauser brought further attention to the frequent association of renal and skeletal anomalies in these patients and stressed the differences between patients with these findings and those with complete androgen insensitivity syndrome (testicular feminization).
4. **a. 10% to 20%.** Associated congenital abnormalities of the skeletal system have been described in 10% to 20% of cases.
5. **c. Mixed gonadal dysgenesis.** Meyer-Rokitansky-Küster-Hauser syndrome is in fact secondary only to gonadal dysgenesis as a cause of primary amenorrhea.
6. **c. The ovaries are not functional in the majority of patients.** Although occasionally cystic, the ovaries are almost always present and functional.
7. **b. Cyclic abdominal pain associated with normal cyclic menstruation.** As with other obstructive disorders, the patient may present with cyclical or chronic abdominal pain. However, unlike other obstructive processes, duplication anomalies with unilateral obstruction are not associated with primary amenorrhea.
8. **a. African American.** This entity, which was first described by Solinger in 1732, occurs most often in prepubertal black girls and postmenopausal white women.
9. **c. They require no treatment.** Most children do not require treatment unless one of the aforementioned symptoms (urine pooling within the vagina, which may lead to postvoid dribbling; urinary tract infection; perineal irritation; physical findings of sexual abuse) occurs.
10. **a. Younger than 2 years.** The mean age of patients with primary vaginal tumors is younger than 2 years.
11. **b. Sexual abuse is the only means by which an infant can contract the disease.** Although a very high suspicion for sexual abuse is warranted, it should be kept in mind that perinatal transmission is also a possible mechanism. The ideal treatment depends on patient age and location and severity of the lesions.

CHAPTER REVIEW

1. Remnants of the prostatic ducts give rise to the Skene glands; remnants of the Wolffian ducts give rise to the Gartner ducts.
2. The Bartholin glands are homologues of the bulbourethral glands in the male.
3. The proximal portion of the vagina forms from the fused paired Müllerian ducts; the distal portion forms from the sinovaginal bulbs, which later canalize.
4. Clitoral hypertrophy in the newborn should suggest congenital adrenal hyperplasia; other etiologies include neurofibromatosis and an androgen-producing tumor in the mother.
5. A small clitoris may be seen in androgen insensitivity syndrome.
6. In planning treatment for a transverse vaginal septum, it is of critical importance to determine whether there is a cervix and, if present, its exact location relative to the septum.
7. Vaginal atresia differs from vaginal agenesis and testicular feminization in that the Müllerian structures are not affected. As a result, the uterus, cervix, and upper portion of the vagina are normal. In vaginal agenesis the uterus is generally absent or rudimentary; there are often associated renal and skeletal abnormalities.
8. A complication of the use of skin grafts to create a neovagina is the increased incidence of vaginal stenosis and the requirement for repeated vaginal dilatation.
9. Most anomalies of lateral fusion have no functional significance.
10. When an interlabial mass appears to be associated with the urethra, workup should always include renal pelvic ultrasonography.
11. Urethral prolapse appears as a doughnut-shaped mass with the urethral orifice in the center; a mass lateral to the orifice may be a paraurethral cyst, a prolapsed ureterocele, a urethral polyp, or an ectopic ureter.
12. An imperforate hymen at birth appears as a bulge in the perineum; it may present at puberty as cyclic abdominal pain and amenorrhea.

48

Disorders of Sexual Development: Etiology, Evaluation, and Medical Management

Richard Nithiphaisal Yu and David A. Diamond

QUESTIONS

1. Which of the following statements is TRUE about *SRY* (sex-determining region of the Y-chromosome gene)?

   a. It is synonymous with the H-Y antigen.

   b. SRY protein has a characteristic high-mobility group (HMG), DNA-binding domain.

   c. It is regulated by SOX9 expression.

   d. It was genetically mapped by the study of patients with Klinefelter and Turner syndromes.

   e. It is synonymous with Zfy in humans.

2. Which statement about steroidogenic factor 1 (SF1) is correct?

   a. The gene encodes a nuclear hormone transcription factor.

   b. It regulates the expression of anti-Müllerian hormone.

   c. It regulates the expression of enzymes involved in steroid production.

   d. Mutations in the gene are associated with undervirilization.

   e. All of the above are true.

3. Which of the following statements is TRUE regarding anti-Müllerian-hormone (AMH)?

   a. It acts systemically to produce Müllerian regression.

   b. It is secreted by the fetal Leydig cells.

   c. It functions normally in patients with hernia uteri inguinale.

   d. It is secreted at 7 to 8 weeks of gestation, representing the initial endocrine function of the fetal testis.

   e. It is secreted by the fetal testis at 10 weeks of gestation, after testosterone production has begun.

4. Which description of *WT1* is correct?

   a. Mutations in WT1 can result in either Denys-Drash or Frasier syndrome.

   b. Mutations in WT1 are associated with adrenocortical carcinoma.

   c. Loss of WT1 function has not been associated with genitourinary anomalies.

   d. Duplication of WT1 has been associated with dosage-sensitive sex reversal.

   e. The gene was originally isolated in cloning experiments and localized to the X chromosome.

5. Which of the following statements is TRUE regarding fetal testosterone?

   a. It causes regression of the Müllerian ducts.

   b. It is produced primarily by the adrenal gland.

   c. It acts locally to virilize the urogenital sinus and genital tubercle.

   d. It acts locally to virilize the internal Wolffian duct structures.

   e. It enters target tissue by active diffusion.

6. Which of the following statements is TRUE regarding dihydrotestosterone (DHT)?

   a. It produces virilization of Wolffian duct structures.

   b. It is converted by 5α-reductase to testosterone in the liver.

   c. It induces virilization of the urogenital sinus.

   d. It acts locally to produce regression of Müllerian structures.

   e. It is secreted in large quantities by the fetal testis.

7. Which of the following statements is TRUE regarding patients with Klinefelter syndrome?

   a. They have at least one X and two Y chromosomes.

   b. They are at increased risk for development of adenocarcinoma of the breast.

   c. They undergo replacement of Leydig cells with hyaline.

   d. They are normally fertile.

   e. They bear little resemblance to XX males.

8. The streak gonad of Turner syndrome:

   a. can descend to the scrotum.

   b. has a reduced number of oocytes.

   c. results in increased risk for development of seminoma since only one X chromosome is present.

   d. results in increased risk for development of gonadoblastoma when Y chromosome elements are present.

   e. is located in the round ligament.

9. Which of the following statements is TRUE regarding patients with 46, XY complete gonadal dysgenesis?

   a. They frequently have chromosomal anomalies.

   b. They are at significant risk for gonadal tumors.

   c. They have somatic defects similar to Turner syndrome.

   d. They have gonadal histology different from that of patients with Turner syndrome.

   e. They derive similar benefit from synthetic growth hormone as do patients with Turner syndrome.

10. What is the most common finding in ALL cases of Denys-Drash syndrome?

    a. Gonadoblastoma

    b. Nephropathy with early-onset proteinuria

    c. Wilms tumor

    d. Calyceal blunting

    e. Progressive renal failure

11. Which of the following statements is TRUE regarding patients with embryonic testicular regression or bilateral vanishing testes syndromes?

    a. They have normal testosterone and elevated estradiol levels.

    b. They have normal testosterone but decreased DHT levels.

c. They have castrate testosterone and elevated gonadotropin levels.

d. They have castrate testosterone and decreased gonadotropin levels.

e. They have normal follicle-stimulating hormone but decreased luteinizing hormone levels.

12. Which of the following statements is TRUE regarding the ovotestis in ovotesticular DSD?

a. It cannot descend from the retroperitoneum.

b. It is found in the minority of patients.

c. It can be unilateral or bilateral.

d. It has testicular and ovarian elements randomly distributed.

e. It is impossible to cleave surgically.

13. An important consideration for gender assignment in the ovotesticular DSD patient is:

a. the potential for fertility.

b. the impossibility of precisely dividing an ovotestis surgically.

c. the high incidence of gonadal tumors in 46, XX ovotesticular DSD.

d. the familial pattern of inheritance of the disorder.

e. androgen insensitivity.

14. Which of the following statements is TRUE regarding the 21-hydroxylase deficiency in congenital adrenal hyperplasia (CAH)?

a. It accounts for 50% of CAH cases.

b. It occurs as a result of *CYP21A* inactivation in the majority of cases.

c. It occurs with simple virilization in 75% of cases and salt wasting in 25% of cases.

d. It occurs with a predictable phenotype.

e. It is transmitted in an autosomal dominant pattern.

15. Prenatal treatment of fetuses with CAH using dexamethasone:

a. is appropriate therapy in the majority of at-risk fetuses.

b. can be initiated after a diagnosis of CAH is confirmed by amniocentesis.

c. is of no risk to the fetus.

d. has been demonstrated to be effective.

e. acts by suppressing maternal ACTH.

16. Which of the following statements is TRUE regarding enzymatic disorders of testosterone biosynthesis?

a. They are transmitted in an autosomal dominant pattern.

b. They are associated with persistent Müllerian structures.

c. They appear clinically with a predictable phenotype.

d. They may involve impaired glucocorticoid and mineralocorticoid synthesis.

e. They may be associated with fertility.

17. Which of the following statements is TRUE regarding patients with complete androgen insensitivity?

a. They are typically raised as female.

b. They have normal Wolffian duct structures.

c. They have persistent Müllerian duct structures.

d. They should undergo orchiectomy as early as possible.

e. They have a 2% incidence of inguinal hernia.

18. Partial androgen insensitivity syndrome is characterized as:

a. a group of defects in testosterone biosynthesis.

b. a form of 5α-reductase deficiency.

c. Y-chromosome mutations.

d. a disorder of androgen receptor quantity or function.

e. a disorder transmitted in an autosomal recessive manner

19. Which of the following statements is TRUE regarding patients with 5α-reductase deficiency?

a. Patients with a 46,XY karyotype are always infertile.

b. Isoenzymes 1 and 2 are abnormal.

c. Serum testosterone levels are normal, but there is a decreased testosterone/DHT ratio.

d. Masculinization occurs at puberty.

e. Prostatic enlargement occurs at puberty.

20. Which of the following statements is TRUE regarding patients with persistent Müllerian duct syndrome?

a. They have absent Wolffian duct structures.

b. They represent a homogeneous disorder of involving the AMH receptor.

c. They should undergo routine removal of Müllerian structures.

d. They experience a high incidence of transverse testicular ectopia.

e. They are uniformly infertile.

21. Which of the following statements is TRUE regarding Mayer-Rokitansky-Küster-Hauser (MRKH) syndrome?

a. It presents most commonly as infertility.

b. It is a homogeneous disorder entailing congenital absence of the uterus and vagina.

c. It is associated with a spectrum of ovarian abnormalities.

d. It has associated upper urinary tract anomalies, more frequently with the atypical disorder.

e. It is associated with persistent Wolffian duct structures.

22. In a neonate with hypospadias and a unilateral cryptorchid testis:

a. midshaft location of the urethral meatus is an important risk factor for DSD.

b. impalpability of the cryptorchid testis carries a 50% risk of a DSD.

c. palpability of the cryptorchid testis effectively rules out DSD.

d. perineal hypospadias is not a risk factor for a DSD.

e. difference in tissue texture of the poles of the cryptorchid gonad is suggestive of tumor.

23. Gender identity:

a. is synonymous with gender role.

b. is primarily determined by prenatal exposure to androgens.

c. is primarily determined by postnatal environmental influences.

d. is defined as the identification of self as either male or female.

e. does not play a role in gender dysphoria.

ANSWERS

1. **b. SRY protein has a characteristic high-mobility group (HMG), DNA-binding domain.** This domain can induce significant DNA bending when bound to the regulatory regions of target genes. *SRY* is not synonymous with H-Y antigen. The SRY gene is located on the short arm of the Y chromosome adjacent to the pseudoautosomal boundary. SRY regulates SOX9 expression during gonadal differentiation.

2. **e. All of the above are true.** The expressed SF1 protein is a nuclear hormone transcription factor that binds to DNA. Several studies have demonstrated that SF1 regulates the transcription

of AMH and multiple steroidogenic enzyme genes. Recent studies suggest that mutations in *SF1*, also known as *NR5A1*, have an additional role in DSD and are associated with varying levels of undervirilization, adrenal insufficiency, and gonadal dysgenesis.

3. **d. It is secreted at 7 to 8 weeks of gestation, representing the initial endocrine function of the fetal testis.** AMH is produced by the Sertoli cells and acts in a paracrine fashion to induce regression of Müllerian structures. Hernia uteri inguinale, also known as persistent Müllerian duct syndrome (PMDS), occurs in patients with a 46, XY karyotype and normal male external genitalia. These patients have persistent internal Müllerian duct structures that may herniate or be associated with an undescended testicle.

4. **a. Mutations in *WT1* can result in either Denys-Drash or Frasier syndrome.** Denys-Drash syndrome is characterized by a triad of Wilms tumor, congenital nephropathy, and genital atypia or Difference of Sex Development (DSD). Frasier syndrome is associated with gonadoblastoma, congenital nephropathy, and gonadal dysgenesis. Patients with Frasier syndrome do not have a known predisposition to Wilms tumor. The *WT1* gene is located on chromosome 11 and is not associated with dosage-sensitive sex reversal.

5. **d. It acts locally to virilize the internal Wolffian duct structures.** Androgens are essential for virilization of Wolffian duct structures, the urogenital sinus, and genital tubercle. Testosterone, the major androgen secreted by the testes, enters target tissues by passive diffusion. The local production and paracrine effect of androgen is important for Wolffian duct development, which does not occur if testosterone is supplied only via the peripheral circulation. Masculinization of the external genitalia results from systemic delivery of testosterone and local conversion to DHT.

6. **c. It induces virilization of the urogenital sinus.** In some cells, such as those in the urogenital sinus, testosterone is converted to DHT by intracellular 5α-reductase. Testosterone or DHT then binds to a high-affinity intracellular receptor protein, and this complex enters the nucleus, where it binds to acceptor sites on DNA, resulting in target gene activation and protein synthesis. Therefore, in tissues equipped with 5α-reductase at the time of sexual differentiation, such as prostate, urogenital sinus, and external genitalia, DHT is the active androgen.

7. **b. They are at increased risk for development of adenocarcinoma of the breast.** Gynecomastia, which can be quite marked, is a common pubertal development in patients with Klinefelter syndrome. As a result, these patients are at eight times the risk for developing breast carcinoma relative to normal males. Males with Klinefelter syndrome have one Y chromosome and at least two X chromosomes. The most common karyotype is 47, XXY. The cells lining the seminiferous tubules undergo replacement with hyaline during pubertal development.

8. **d. Results in increased risk for development of gonadoblastoma when Y chromosome elements are present.** In patients with occult Y chromosome material, the risk of gonadoblastoma, an *in situ* germ cell cancer, is approximately 30%. The streak gonad is usually abdominal in location, hypoplastic, and predominantly composed of fibrous tissue.

9. **b. They are at significant risk for gonadal tumors.** Up to 35% develop tumors by 30 years of age. Patients with 46,XX complete gonadal dysgenesis are closely related to those with Turner syndrome. But, they do not have somatic defects associated with Turner syndrome (e.g., broad chest, neck webbing, cardiac and renal anomalies, and short stature).

10. **b. Nephropathy with early-onset proteinuria.** The full triad of the syndrome includes nephropathy, characterized by the early onset of proteinuria, hypertension, and progressive renal failure in the majority, Wilms tumor, and DSD. Denys-Drash is caused by mutations in the Wilms tumor suppressor (*WT1*)

gene. Because incomplete forms of the syndrome may occur, the nephropathy aspect is regarded as the common denominator of the syndrome.

11. **c. They have castrate testosterone and elevated gonadotropin levels.** The diagnosis can be made on the basis of a 46,XY karyotype and castrate levels of testosterone, despite persistently elevated serum luteinizing hormone and follicle-stimulating hormone levels. This can be detected during "mini-puberty" from 2 to 6 months of age. Serum AMH is a useful marker to detect the presence of testicular tissue and is undetectable in these males.

12. **c. It can be unilateral or bilateral.** Ovotesticular DSD patients are individuals having both testicular tissue with well-developed seminiferous tubules and ovarian tissue with primordial follicles. The gonads may take the form of one ovary and one testis or, more commonly, one or two ovotestes. Histopathology of the ovotestis will typically demonstrate well-developed ovarian tissue and a dysgenetic testicular component. The ovotestis may be located at any point along the path of testicular descent. Ovotestes with bipolar distribution of tissue may often be surgically separated.

13. **a. The potential for fertility.** The most important aspect of management in ovotesticular DSD is gender assignment. An important factor to consider is the potential for fertility since individuals with ovotesticular DSD have the potential for fertility if raised as female with the appropriate ductal structures. Pregnancies have been reported in these women. Testicular tissue in an ovotestes is commonly dysgenetic. Approximately 3% of patients with 46, XY ovotesticular DSD develop gonadal tumors. Tumors are rare in patients with 46, XX ovotesticular DSD.

14. **b. It occurs as a result of *CYP21A2* inactivation in the majority of cases.** 21-Hydroxylase deficiency accounts for 95% of CAH cases, with 75% of patients presenting with salt wasting and 25% with simple virilization. Mutations leading to gene conversion of the active *CYP21A2* gene into the inactive gene occur in 65% to 90% of cases of the classic disorder (salt wasting and simple virilizing) and all cases of nonclassic 21-hydroxylase deficiency. 21-hydroxylase deficiency is transmitted in an autosomal recessive pattern.

15. **d. Has been demonstrated to be effective.** Treatment should be initiated before 9 weeks after the last menstrual period, once pregnancy is confirmed. A number of series have established the effectiveness of prenatal treatment of CAH with dexamethasone, which suppresses fetal secretion of adrenocorticotropic hormone. However, a diagnosis of CAH cannot be confirmed before therapy is initiated because the diagnosis is usually made by chorionic villus sampling (9 to 11 weeks gestation) or amniocentesis (16 to 17 weeks gestation). Therefore, if treatment is initiated for all at-risk fetuses, the majority (seven out of eight) may be treated unnecessarily before confirmatory diagnosis. Noninvasive prenatal diagnosis of CAH using cell-free fetal DNA obtained from maternal plasma is a promising new development that may allow identification of male fetuses, who would not benefit from treatment, well before 9 weeks gestation.

16. **d. They may involve impaired glucocorticoid and mineralocorticoid synthesis.** A defect in any of the five enzymes required for the conversion of cholesterol to testosterone can cause incomplete (or absent) virilization of the male fetus during embryogenesis. The first three enzymes (cholesterol side chain cleavage enzyme, 3β-hydroxysteroid dehydrogenase, and 17α-hydroxylase) are present in both the adrenals and the testes. Therefore, their deficiency results in impaired synthesis of glucocorticoids and mineralocorticoids in addition to testosterone. These enzymatic disorders are transmitted in an autosomal recessive pattern and appear clinically with a variable phenotype. Since testosterone biosynthesis is impacted, high concentration of testosterone within the testes is absent thus impacting spermatogenesis and fertility.

17. **a. They are typically raised as female.** It is of great interest that, currently, all studies of patients with complete androgen insensitivity support an unequivocal female gender identity, consistent with androgen resistance of brain tissue as well. To date there has been only one report of a patient raised as a female who needed gender reassignment to male.[a]

18. **d. A disorder of androgen receptor quantity or function.** Androgen receptor studies in cultured fibroblasts have demonstrated two forms of receptor defect in the partial androgen insensitivity syndrome. These include a reduced number of normally functioning androgen receptors and normal receptor number but decreased binding affinity. The androgen receptor gene is located on the long arm of the X chromosome, Xq12. Partial androgen resistance is, therefore, an X-linked disorder of incomplete masculinization.

19. **d. Masculinization occurs at puberty.** At puberty, partial masculinization occurs with an increase in muscle mass, development of male body habitus, increase in phallic size, and onset of erections. However, prostatic enlargement does not occur as this is dependent on DHT production. The type 2 isoenzyme is affected in patients with 5α-reductase deficiency, resulting in an increased testosterone/DHT ratio owing to a reduced testosterone-to-DHT conversion rate. There are reports of sperm production and fertility in some affected individuals.

20. **d. They experience a high incidence of transverse testicular ectopia.** Persistent Müllerian duct syndrome is thought to be etiologically important in transverse testicular ectopia, occurring in 30% to 50% of cases. Aberrant AMH function may be secondary to defects in the gene for AMH or for the AMH receptor. Individuals with a 46, XY karyotype develop Wolffian duct structures normally and may have impaired spermatogenesis associated with undescended testes.

21. **d. It has associated upper urinary tract anomalies, more frequently with the atypical disorder.** MRKH syndrome is a rare congenital disorder associated with absence of the uterus and vagina (typical variant). Patients commonly present with primary amenorrhea. The atypical form of MRKH syndrome (10% of cases) includes patients with uterine remnants and/or aplasia of one or both fallopian tubes. Urinary tract anomalies occur more commonly in patients with the atypical form of the disorder.

22. **b. Impalpability of the cryptorchid testis carries a 50% risk of a DSD.** With hypospadias and either unilateral or bilateral cryptorchidism, the incidence of a DSD is 30% overall, 15% if the undescended testis is palpable, and 50% if it is impalpable.

23. **d. Is defined as the identification of self as either male or female.** Gender role refers to aspects of behavior that distinguish males and females. The development of gender identity is poorly understood, but is influenced by prenatal and postnatal factors. Individual conflicts with gender identity are central to the concept of gender dysphoria.

---

[a]T'Sjoen G, De Cuypere, G, Monstrey S, et al: Male gender identity in complete androgen insensitivity syndrome. *Arch Sex Behav* 40:635—638, 2011.

CHAPTER REVIEW

1. *SRY* initiates testicular organogenesis. The *SRY* gene is located on the short arm of the Y chromosome.

2. The prostate, urogenital sinus, and external genitalia are all sensitive to DHT.

3. Estrogens are not required for normal female differentiation.

4. Patients with Klinefelter syndrome have eunuchoidism, gynecomastia, azoospermia, small testes, and are tall for their age. Muscle development is often poor.

5. Patients with Turner syndrome (XO) have sexual infantilism, webbed neck, and cubitus valgus; are of the female phenotype; are short in stature; and lack secondary sexual characteristics.

6. In patients with Turner syndrome, any Y-chromosome material increases the risk for the streak gonad developing a gonadoblastoma; these patients also have increased incidence of abnormalities of the kidney, including horseshoe kidney.

7. The diagnosis of the salt-wasting type of CAH is made by obtaining a serum 17-hydroxyprogesterone value 3 to 4 days after birth. If it is elevated, the patient has CAH.

8. In patients who have severe forms of CAH difficult to control medically, bilateral adrenalectomy may be the most effective approach.

9. A distinctly palpable gonad along the pathway of descent is highly suggestive of a testis or rarely of an ovotestis.

10. Patients with bilateral impalpable testes or a unilateral impalpable testis and hypospadias should be regarded as having a disorder of sexual development until proven otherwise whether or not the genitalia appear ambiguous. They should have a karyotype.

11. For normal ovarian development there must be two X chromosomes.

12. In the developing embryo, MIS and testosterone act locally and unilaterally.

13. Mixed gonadal dysgenesis is the second most common cause of DSD after CAH, and it is characterized by a unilateral testis, a contralateral streak gonad, and persistent Müllerian structures with varying degrees of inadequate masculinization.

14. The syndrome of complete androgen insensitivity is characterized by 46,XY karyotype, bilateral testes, female-appearing external genitalia, and absence of Müllerian structures; the testes are prone to tumors, which usually occur after puberty in 1% to 2% of affected individuals.

15. Persistent Müllerian duct syndrome is due to a defect in the gene for AMH or for the AMH type II receptor in patients with 46,XY karyotype. These patients have normal male external genitalia and internal Müllerian duct structures (fallopian tubes, uterus, and upper vagina).

16. The finding of a palpable gonad in a newborn with ambiguous genitalia effectively rules out overt masculinization of the female (CAH).

17. Patients with Klinefelter syndrome are at eight times the risk for breast carcinoma relative to normal males.

18. Serum MIS is a useful marker for the presence of testicular tissue in the newborn period.

19. Histopathology of the ovotestis will typically demonstrate well-developed ovarian tissue and a dysgenetic testicular component.

20. Patients with complete androgen insensitivity support an unequivocal female gender identity. However, there are a few case reports of patients with male gender identity. One patient required complete sex reassignment with both androgen treatment and phalloplasty.

49   Surgical Management of Differences of Sexual Differentiation and Cloacal and Anorectal Malformations

Richard C. Rink

QUESTIONS

1. Which of the following statements is FALSE regarding the construction of a neovagina utilizing bowel?
   a. Failure to develop an adequate space between the rectum and bladder can result in compromised blood flow to the segment used for vaginal construction.
   b. In general, colon is preferred versus ileum because of its lower incidence of associated postoperative stenosis.
   c. When compared with the McIndoe procedure, the bowel vagina suffers from a higher incidence of postoperative stenosis.
   d. An advantage of a bowel vagina versus the McIndoe procedure includes the lubricating properties of mucus (which may help facilitate intercourse).
   e. One specific indication for the use of ileum is a previous history of pelvic radiation.

2. Urogenital sinus anomalies in differences of sexual development states are most commonly seen in association with:
   a. congenital adrenal hyperplasia.
   b. mixed gonadal dysgenesis.
   c. ovotesticular disorder.
   d. cloacal anomalies.
   e. gonadal dysgenesis.

3. The most common finding in cloacal anomalies that have been diagnosed by antenatal ultrasonography is:
   a. ascites.
   b. distended rectum.
   c. distended bladder.
   d. distended vagina.
   e. distended bladder and rectum.

4. What is the most common vaginal anatomy in cloacal malformation?
   a. Single vagina, single uterus
   b. Single vagina, double uterus
   c. Two vaginas, two uteri
   d. Two vaginas, one uterus
   e. Single vagina, no uterus

5. Neonatal vaginoplasty combined with clitoroplasty and labiaplasty has all of the following advantages EXCEPT:
   a. it allows phallic skin for vaginal reconstruction.
   b. maternal estrogens increase vaginal thickness and vascularity.
   c. tissues are less scarred.
   d. vaginal stenosis is clearly less.
   e. clitoroplasty must retain normal clitoral innervation while providing excellent cosmesis.

6. The cut-back vaginoplasty is appropriate for:
   a. labial fusion.
   b. low vaginal confluence.
   c. high vaginal confluence.
   d. vaginal atresia.
   e. vaginal agenesis.

7. Surgical management of cloacal malformations involves all of the following steps EXCEPT:
   a. decompression of the gastrointestinal tract.
   b. decompression of the genitourinary tract.
   c. vaginostomy.
   d. definitive repair of the cloaca.
   e. correction of nephron destructive anomalies.

8. Fecal continence after cloacal reconstruction is most closely related to:
   a. the level of rectal confluence.
   b. associated urinary anomalies.
   c. neurologic status.
   d. the type of repair.
   e. the timing of the repair.

ANSWERS

1. **c. When compared with the McIndoe procedure, the bowel vagina suffers from a higher incidence of postoperative stenosis.** A high incidence of postoperative vaginal stenosis necessitates postoperative vaginal dilatation in the McIndoe procedure.
2. **a. Congenital adrenal hyperplasia.** Urogenital sinus abnormalities are most often seen in disorders of sexual differentiation states, most commonly in association with congenital adrenal hyperplasia, which has been noted to have an incidence as frequent as 1 in 500 in the nonclassic mild forms.
3. **d. Distended vagina.** The common finding in all reports has been a cystic pelvic mass between the bladder and rectum, representing a distended vagina.
4. **c. Two vaginas, two uteri.** In Hendren's report on 154 patients with cloacal anomalies, 66 patients had one vagina, 68 had two vaginas, and the vagina was absent in 20. The incidence of vaginal duplication is even higher in the author's own patient population. The uterus anomaly generally is similar to the vaginal anomaly, that is, two vaginas with two uteri.
5. **d. Vaginal stenosis is clearly less.** Other investigators, including the author's group, have thought that vaginoplasty, regardless of the vaginal location, is best combined with clitoroplasty in a single stage. This allows the redundant phallic skin to be used in the reconstruction, adding flexibility for the surgeon, which is compromised when the skin

has been previously mobilized. Furthermore, the authors and others have noted that maternal estrogen stimulation of the child's genitalia results in thicker vaginal tissue, which is better vascularized, making vaginal mobilization more easily performed.

6. **a. Labial fusion.** The cut-back vaginoplasty is rarely used and is appropriate only for simple labial fusion.

7. **c. Vaginostomy.** Surgical management now involves four basic steps: decompression of the gastrointestinal tract, decompression of the genitourinary tract, correction of nephron-destructive or potentially lethal urinary anomalies, and definitive repair of the cloaca.

8. **c. Neurologic status.** Fecal continence is directly related to neurologic status.

CHAPTER REVIEW

1. The communication of the vagina with the urinary tract usually occurs in the mid to distal urethra.
2. In patients with congenital adrenal hyperplasia, the location of the confluence of the vagina and the urethra is the critical determinant in the surgical management.
3. Hydrometrocolpos is frequently the initial sign of a urogenital sinus abnormality. It is caused by urine draining into the vagina with poor vaginal drainage.
4. Persistent clitoral hypertrophy may occur in premature infants without DSD.
5. A cervical impression in the dome of the vagina seen on genitography denotes normal female internal organs.
6. When gonads in the neonatal period require biopsy, a deep biopsy is appropriate because the ovarian component of an ovotestis may cover the testicular component.
7. Renal anomalies commonly occur in patients with a persistent cloaca.
8. Women with CAH are less satisfied as adults with their genitalia than are controls.
9. Genital reconstruction must address clitoroplasty, labiaplasty, and vaginoplasty.
10. When clitoroplasty is performed, the glans, tunics, and neurovascular bundles should be preserved. The neurovascular bundles should not be mobilized.
11. The timing of surgery for genital reconstruction is controversial: vaginoplasty is best combined with clitoroplasty and labiaplasty as a single procedure.
12. Vaginoplasty may be performed with a posterior-based perineal flap for low vaginal confluence, a pull-through vaginoplasty for a high confluence, and vaginal replacement for an absent or rudimentary vagina.
13. The flap in a "flap vaginoplasty" must reach the normal caliber of the vagina; that is, it must be placed cephalad to the narrowed area of the distal vagina.
14. A vaginoplasty performed in the neonatal period will usually require a secondary procedure after puberty.
15. In cloacal malformations, surgical management initially involves decompression of the gastrointestinal tract, generally with a colostomy, and decompression of the genitourinary tract. This is followed by correction of urinary collecting system abnormalities that impair urine flow. A single-stage repair of rectal, vaginal, and urethral abnormalities is performed at a later date when the child is stable.
16. Intermittent catheterization of the vagina may successfully decompress the genitourinary tract in cloacal malformations.
17. Spinal cord abnormalities are frequently found in patients with persistent cloaca.
18. In patients who have had corrective surgery for cloacal abnormalities, a high percentage have a neuropathic component to both urinary and fecal incontinence.
19. In planning treatment for a transverse vaginal septum, it is critical to determine whether there is a cervix and, if present, its exact location relative to the septum.
20. Vaginal atresia differs from vaginal agenesis and testicular feminization in that the Müllerian structures are not affected. As a result, the uterus, cervix, and upper portion of the vagina are normal.

50 Adolescent and Transitional Urology

Dan Wood

QUESTIONS

1. Patients with complex congenital urologic conditions:
   a. are unlikely to require surgery in adulthood.
   b. prefer to be looked after in a general urology clinic.
   c. generally do not work as adults.
   d. desire to be normal.
   e. can usually be discharged from care after 18 years of age.

2. Effective transition requires:
   a. a clear plan by the age of 14 years.
   b. a purposeful process to get a young adult to take responsibility for their health.
   c. preparation of the family.
   d. trust between pediatric and adolescent/adult teams.
   e. all of the above.

3. Adolescent urology training requires:
   a. a fellowship in plastic surgery.
   b. board certification (or equivalent) in urology.
   c. a fellowship in adolescent medicine.
   d. 1 year of training in psychology.
   e. all of the above.

4. Regarding young adults with congenital anomalies of the urogenital system:
   a. boys with posterior urethral valves commonly have a dorsal chordee.
   b. all young men with corrected hypospadias need lifelong follow-up.
   c. an augmentation cystoplasty can lead to a false-positive urinary pregnancy test.
   d. patients with spina bifida often die as a result of renal failure.
   e. in a boy with exstrophy, the testes are usually badly damaged.

5. In which of the following situations should elective cesarean section be performed for urologic indications?
   a. With an artificial urinary sphincter
   b. Women with exstrophy and an augmentation cystoplasty
   c. Women with a glomerular filtration rate (GFR) below 40 mL/min/m²
   d. Women with a neuropathic bladder
   e. Women with simple (nonsalt-wasting) congenital adrenal hyperplasia

6. In boys with posterior urethral valves:
   a. intervention in utero will prevent the need for renal transplant in adulthood.
   b. fertility will likely be normal.
   c. 60% will have urinary incontinence.
   d. there is no increased risk of proteinuria.
   e. bladder function will be normal if valves are incised in the first month of life.

ANSWERS

1. **d. Desire to be normal.** This a fundamental element of looking after patients with major congenital urologic anomalies. As they move into adulthood, they commonly express a desire to be normal and may exert their independence to try and appear more so—i.e., by not coming to a hospital or not catheterizing. Many will need lifelong care, many work, many prefer to be looked after in a clinic with an expertise in their (rare) condition, and a significant number will need surgery as adults.

2. **e. All of the above.** Planning and preparation definitely make life easier for patients, parents, and those looking after the patients as they move into adulthood. It appears to significantly reduce anxiety and improve engagement, and trust between the team who have looked after the patient in childhood and the adult team is important.

3. **b. Board certification (or equivalent) in urology.** This is the only requirement at present. A urology training program will offer most of the skills required. Important elements are training in complex pediatric urology and reconstructive urology. Psychology can be very important, hence it is important to have a trained member on the multidisciplinary team.

4. **c. An augmentation cystoplasty can lead to a false-positive urinary pregnancy test.** Data suggest this happens in 57% of augmentation cystoplasty cases. The testes are normal in exstrophy, valve boys would be expected to have a normal penis, mild forms of hypospadias do not usually need long-term follow-up—just information on who to contact if they do have problems. With aggressive early bladder management (clean intermittent catheterization [CIC] and antimuscarinics) deaths from renal failure have dramatically decreased in patients affected by spina bifida.

5. **b. Women with exstrophy and an augmentation cystoplasty.** A cystoplasty on its own is not an absolute indication for a caesarean section—if the pelvis is otherwise normal, a vaginal delivery may be possible (this is an obstetric decision). Fundamentally, it is important to avoid a caesarean section without appropriate urologic support—elective sections should be planned with such a urologist present, and unless such expertise is available 24 hours a day seven days a week, then an emergency caesarean section should be avoided.

6. **b. Fertility will likely be normal.** For many years this was not thought to be the case. More recent data suggest that fertility is likely to be normal.

CHAPTER REVIEW

1. Transition is the development of a young adult's understanding of and independence in their healthcare.
2. Preparation for transition can occur over a number of years.
3. A multidisciplinary team is essential in both pediatric and adult care.
4. There are a variety of models for delivering transition and adolescent care—these will vary depending on the healthcare system.
5. Those caring for adult patients with complex congenital anomalies must be trained in both pediatric and adult reconstructive urology.

6. Congenital lifelong urology requires a proactive approach and an understanding of complex congenital genitourinary conditions.
7. Regular follow up examining renal and urinary function are essential for many.
8. Sexual function and fertility must be proactively addressed and managed.
9. Pregnancy is likely to need preparation (for some) and combined urologic and obstetric care.
10. Collaboration with other specialties is essential for safe and appropriate care.

51 Urologic Considerations in Pediatric Renal Transplantation

Craig A. Peters and Armando J. Lorenzo

QUESTIONS

1. An indication for urodynamic evaluation of a child being prepared for renal transplant is:
   a. poststreptococcal glomerulonephritis-induced renal failure.
   b. ongoing grade III vesicoureteral reflux.
   c. end-stage renal disease (ESRD) in a child with nocturnal enuresis.
   d. prolonged anuria after focal segmental glomerulosclerosis (FSGS) renal failure.
   e. ESRD in a child with wetting but no urinary tract infection (UTIs).

2. Renal transplantation into a child with an augmented bladder is associated with:
   a. cyclosporine toxicity.
   b. hyperchloremic metabolic alkalosis.
   c. refractory rejection.
   d. recurrent infection and risk of sepsis.
   e. no significant change in graft survival.

3. In a 10-year-old boy with a 50-mL capacity bladder, a history of posterior urethral valves, ESRD, and anuria, optimal initial bladder management in preparation for renal transplantation is:
   a. ileocystoplasty at time of renal transplantation.
   b. gastrocystoplasty and continent catheterizable stoma.
   c. bladder cycling by intermittent catheterization.
   d. antimuscarinic medications and proceeding with transplantation.
   e. transplant into transverse colon loop and delayed augmentation.

4. Indications for pre-transplant native nephrectomy include all of the following EXCEPT:
   a. refractory two-drug hypertension.
   b. multicystic dysplastic kidney (MCDK).
   c. persisting grade III VUR in a 4-year-old.
   d. age under 12 months.
   e. ESRD associated with Denys-Drash syndrome.

5. A nonrefluxing transplant ureteroneocystostomy should be performed:
   a. in infants only.
   b. in any child undergoing renal transplantation.
   c. only in children on intermittent catheterization.
   d. in children at risk for UTI or bladder dysfunction.
   e. only in children with neurogenic bladder dysfunction.

6. Following a cadaveric renal transplant for FSGS, a 10-year-old boy is found to have distal ureteral obstruction from a 4-cm stricture that fails balloon dilation and stenting. The best option for management is:
   a. ileal interposition.
   b. Boari flap to graft pelvis.
   c. transplant nephrectomy.
   d. psoas hitch transplant ureteroneocystostomy.
   e. transplant ureter to native ureteroureterostomy.

7. Six months following an uncomplicated living related donor renal transplant for FSGS and prior native nephrectomies, a 7-year-old girl develops acute pyelonephritis of the graft with a rise in creatinine. There is no hydronephrosis on ultrasound. A voiding cystourethrogram (VCUG) demonstrates grade III reflux into the graft, but none in the native ureters. She has normal voiding patterns. The best option for management is:
   a. urodynamic evaluation and MR of the spine.
   b. transplant ureter to native ureteroureterostomy.
   c. endoscopic injection of subureteral bulking agent.
   d. 6 months of antibiotic prophylaxis and observation.
   e. continuous antibiotic prophylaxis and repeat studies in 18 months anticipating spontaneous resolution.

8. Eighteen months following an uncomplicated living related renal transplant, a 5-year-old boy with a history of posterior urethral valves develops a rising serum creatinine level, graft hydronephrosis, and two febrile UTIs. VCUG shows grade III reflux into the graft and moderate bladder trabeculation similar to his pre-transplant pattern. The next step in his care is:
   a. psoas hitch ureteral reimplantation.
   b. nontunneled ureteroneocystostomy.
   c. ileo-cystoplasty and appendicovesicostomy.
   d. transplant ureter to native ureteroureterostomy (U-U).
   e. urodynamic evaluation and likely antimuscarinics and intermittent catheterization.

9. Twenty-four hours after removal of a ureteral stent, an 8-year-old boy has minimal urine output and develops right lower quadrant tenderness. Two months prior, he had a living related renal transplant following bilateral nephrectomies, radiation, chemotherapy, and surveillance for stage 5 Wilms tumors. A Foley catheter was placed, draining 5 mL of clear urine in 2 hours. He underwent urgent ultrasound evaluation (Fig. 51.1). What is the next step in management?
   a. Replacement of ureteral stent
   b. Renal (allograft) biopsy
   c. Percutaneous nephrostomy placement
   d. Percutaneous drainage of fluid collection
   e. Treat for rejection with high-dose steroids

ANSWERS

1. **e. ESRD in a child with wetting but no urinary tract infections (UTIs).** The child with ongoing wetting is the most likely to have treatable voiding dysfunction that may put the renal graft at risk. Simple bladder defunctionalization with no history of underlying bladder dysfunction is unlikely to need urodynamic evaluation and often may not need bladder cycling. Reflux alone without recurrent UTI, wetting, or a neurogenic cause is not likely to benefit from urodynamics.

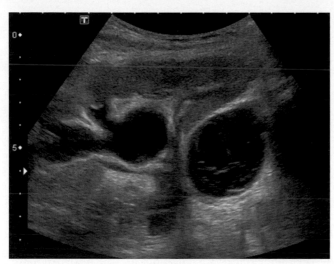

Fig. 51.1

Nocturnal enuresis is not an indication for invasive evaluation of bladder function.

2. **e. No significant change in graft survival.** Although early reports implied a high risk due to bladder augmentation in children undergoing renal transplant, modern series have demonstrated the safety, and indeed the benefits, of providing a low-pressure urinary reservoir on graft function. The incidence of positive urine cultures can be increased, but clinically significant infections are not markedly increased.

3. **c. Bladder cycling by intermittent catheterization.** In the child with anuria, bladder function cannot be easily assessed until the bladder has been cycled. While this child may require augmentation, that cannot be determined until after a trial of cycling is attempted. Transplanting into a diversion is not an acceptable alternative in a child who has the potential for adequate bladder function with medical management and intermittent catheterization.

4. **b. Multicystic dysplastic kidney (MCDK).** All of these clinical situations can justify native nephrectomy except for the presence of a MCDK. There is minimal to no risk of leaving the dysplastic kidney in place. Persisting reflux may be a relative indication, and some practitioners may choose to reimplant the native ureter or simply leave it alone if there is no significant history of infection. Denys-Drash kidneys are at increased risk for Wilms tumor formation. Children under 12 months in some centers do not routinely have native nephrectomy, although there is a slightly higher risk of graft loss without this.

5. **d. In children at risk for UTI or bladder dysfunction.** Any child with a risk for UTI or who has bladder dysfunction and may therefore develop a UTI, particularly if immunosuppressed, should have a nonrefluxing ureteroneocystostomy. Some centers perform a nonrefluxing ureteral implantation in all children, although this is probably not essential. Older children, those with no history of bladder dysfunction, recurrent infections, or a structural abnormality, can be effectively transplanted with a refluxing ureteroneocystostomy.

6. **d. Psoas hitch transplant ureteroneocystostomy.** Several options are available for salvage of the graft in this situation, but the most effective is a psoas hitch when there is still some graft ureter available. A transplant to native ureteroureterostomy is effective but may require nephrectomy in some cases. Boari flaps may be useful for cases in which the entire ureter is lost or if there is no native ureter remaining. Even with loss of the entire ureter, a renal pelvis to native ureter anastomosis is effective. Ileal interposition and graft nephrectomy are not viable options.

7. **b. Transplant ureter to native ureteroureterostomy.** The best option in this situation is redo open reimplantation to create an effective antireflux tunnel or transplant to native ureteroureterostomy if there is sufficient native ureter. In the absence of a prior urologic history, urodynamic evaluation and investigation for an occult spinal dysraphism is unlikely to be of value. Spontaneous resolution is highly unlikely, and simply waiting for another episode of pyelonephritis risks graft injury. Endoscopic injection has a limited success rate in published series and the durability is undefined. In the setting where another episode of pyelonephritis is associated with significant risk to the graft, such an approach does not seem prudent.

8. **e. Urodynamic evaluation and likely antimuscarinics and intermittent catheterization.** This boy is best served by a formal assessment of his bladder function with likely use of antimuscarinics to improve capacity and compliance and intermittent catheterization to provide for emptying. One can start this therapy empirically, but having a baseline permits assessment of the treatment effect. Moving directly to augmentation without knowing if medical management can be effective is not appropriate. Simply reimplanting the ureter or performing a U-U without treating the likely bladder dysfunction is also not appropriate.

9. **d. Percutaneous drainage of fluid collection.** This boy has a large fluid collection and associated hydronephrosis. The most likely cause of his oligo-anuria is extrinsic ureteral compression due to a lymphocele. Other causes need to be considered, including urinoma formation (and active perinephric urine leak). The next step is to drain the fluid collection and send the fluid for analysis and culture. This will determine the best course of action. Stent replacement and percutaneous nephrostomy placement will help with urine drainage yet fail to secure a diagnosis. A renal biopsy is unlikely to add to the diagnosis, except in the unlikely case that this represents rejection. Similarly, high-dose steroids will not address the most likely etiology, and can be harmful in less likely but important complications in the differential, most notably a perinephric abscess.

CHAPTER REVIEW

1. Goals of urologic evaluation and management are (1) normal urinary drainage from the kidney into a reservoir; (2) a urinary reservoir that permits low-pressure storage for a socially acceptable time; (3) volitional emptying of the reservoir, with continence; (4) absence of infection; and (5) the fewest surgical procedures and patient trauma.
2. A large fraction of children in need of renal replacement will have some type of uropathy, either congenital obstruction, vesicoureteral reflux, or neuropathic bladder dysfunction.
3. Pre-transplant assessment is directed by the underlying condition and the status of the bladder and kidneys
4. Urodynamic testing aims to assess bladder capacity, compliance, and emptying, as well as sphincter function.
5. Indications for urodynamics include a known neuropathic bladder, history of posterior urethral valves, and children with ongoing voiding dysfunction, high-grade hydronephrosis, or recurrent UTIs.
6. The most common bladder abnormality associated with uropathy and ESRD is a low-capacity, hypertonic bladder with poor compliance.
7. There is no evidence that bladder augmentation increases the risk of transplant.
8. Recurrent pyelonephritis is a potential hazard for the transplant and is associated with graft loss.
9. Initiating clean intermittent catheterization (CIC) in preparation for transplantation serves an assessment purpose as well as facilitating bladder emptying.
10. Bladder re-functionalization is often best accomplished by bladder cycling to increase capacity, determine bladder wall compliance, and assess the family's ability to perform CIC.
11. The ability to empty spontaneously will also impact the decision regarding the need for a continent catheterizable stoma.
12. Indications for augmentation prior to transplantation include capacity less than 75% of expected for age, with pressures above 30 cm H_2O, on catheterization every 3 h, and maximal antimuscarinic medications.
13. For patients on peritoneal dialysis, intraperitoneal surgery will likely require temporary transition to hemodialysis.
14. In general, any major urologic reconstruction should be undertaken well before anticipated transplantation.
15. Native nephrectomy is indicated for malignant hypertension, profound nephrotic syndrome with malnutrition due to protein loss, high risk for malignancy, recurrent upper tract infections, and massive reflux.
16. Extravesical ureteroneocystostomy is the preferred ureteral anastomosis.
17. Transplant to native ureteroureterostomy is an effective option.
18. There are no data to support routine ureteral stenting at the time of transplantation.
19. Common urologic complications for pediatric renal transplant include ureteral stenosis (6%), urinary leaks (3%), stones (2%), and clinically significant reflux (2%).
20. Urine leaks are typically identified in the early postoperative period with increasing fluid from the wound drains.
21. Urinary infection is a long-term and often delayed complication that largely reflects the status of bladder function.
22. Vesicoureteral reflux into the transplant is entirely distinct from routine reflux as the risk to renal function of acute pyelonephritis is greater.
23. In the setting of a rising creatinine level and hydronephrosis, obstruction and rejection may both be present.
24. The etiology of ureteral obstruction is usually in the distal ureter with stenosis at the reimplantation site.
25. Bladder dysfunction may produce infection, but may also create an obstructive process that impairs renal graft function.
26. Nephrolithiasis is uncommon, but may occur in up to 5% of patients.

52 Pediatric Genitourinary Trauma

Bruce J. Schlomer and Micah A. Jacobs

QUESTIONS

1. Which of the following is not an indication for renal trauma imaging in children?
   a. Significant deceleration injury
   b. Gunshot wound to upper abdomen
   c. Microscopic hematuria
   d. Stab wound to left flank
   e. Blunt trauma with rib fracture and flank bruising

2. Which of the following is an absolute indication for operative intervention for renal trauma?
   a. Grade 4 renal laceration
   b. Hypotension that initially responds to fluid resuscitation
   c. Renal artery occlusion from blunt trauma
   d. Pulsating hematoma at time of exploration for gunshot wound to abdomen
   e. Continued gross hematuria after superselective embolization

3. Which of the following is the preferred initial option for managing urine extravasation from a renal laceration?
   a. Observation
   b. Ureteral stent
   c. Percutaneous drain
   d. Nephrostomy tube
   e. Open exploration and repair

4. What is the appropriate management for a patient with renal arterial avulsion, hemodynamic instability, and a normal contralateral kidney?
   a. Vascular surgery consult
   b. Angiography with stenting
   c. Observation
   d. Nephrectomy
   e. Repair of renal artery injury

5. What is the appropriate management for a stable patient with isolated ureteropelvic junction (UPJ) disruption?
   a. Attempt at ureteral stent
   b. Percutaneous nephrostomy tube
   c. Nephrectomy
   d. Dismembered pyeloplasty
   e. Percutaneous drain into urinoma

6. Which of the following is not a reported high-risk criterion for undergoing intervention in renal trauma?
   a. Medial extravasation of contrast on delayed CT phase
   b. Lack of contrast in ipsilateral ureter on delayed CT phase
   c. Greater than 10% of kidney parenchyma devitalized
   d. Hematoma >2.2 cm in children
   e. Extravasation of contrast during arterial phase

7. Which of the following is not part of optimal open surgical management for a renal injury?
   a. Attempt at renal salvage
   b. Closure of the collecting system with permanent sutures
   c. Control of main renal vessels
   d. Debridement of nonviable parenchyma
   e. Closure of parenchymal defect

8. Should a patient who lost a kidney due to renal injury be allowed to participate in sports?
   a. Yes, but only noncontact sports
   b. Yes, no restrictions
   c. Yes, but use of protective equipment is recommended for contact sports
   d. Yes, but need a signed waiver releasing the physician of liability
   e. No sports activities should be allowed

9. Which of the following is not typically part of a nonoperative management plan for a grade 3 renal injury?
   a. Bed rest until gross hematuria resolves
   b. Routine monitoring of vital signs and blood counts
   c. Routine physical exams
   d. Routine repeat CT scan at 48 hours if stable
   e. Angiography with superselective embolization for continued transfusion requirement from renal bleeding

10. Which of the following is the best option for a complete upper ureteral laceration?
    a. Transureteroureterostomy
    b. Ureteral reimplantation with Boari flap
    c. Ureterocalicostomy
    d. Ureteroureterostomy
    e. Ureteral stent placement

11. In what type of patient should endourologic management not be attempted as a primary treatment?
    a. Ureteral contusion
    b. Partial ureteral laceration recognized intraoperatively
    c. Complete ureteral laceration recognized 10 days after injury
    d. Partial ureteral laceration recognized 5 days after injury
    e. High-velocity gunshot wound to abdomen with injuries near ureter but no apparent ureteral injury

12. Which of the following is not an indication to evaluate for bladder injury?
    a. Gross hematuria with pelvic fracture
    b. Microscopic hematuria with pelvic fracture
    c. Pelvic fracture and inability to void
    d. Abdominal trauma to lower abdomen with low urine output and ascites
    e. Microscopic hematuria after penetrating injury with knife over pubic bone

13. Which of the following is not an indication for open repair of bladder rupture?
    a. Extraperitoneal bladder rupture with gross hematuria
    b. Extraperitoneal bladder rupture undergoing exploratory laparotomy for unrelated injuries
    c. Extraperitoneal bladder rupture with bladder neck injury

d. Stable patient with intraperitoneal bladder rupture and normal serum creatinine

e. Extraperitoneal bladder rupture with vaginal laceration

14. Which of the following is not an acceptable option for initial management of urethral disruption?

a. Gentle attempt at blind catheter placement in suspected partial urethral disruption by retrograde urethrogram

b. Suprapubic tube placement in complete urethral disruption

c. Cystoscopy per urethra in emergency room (ER) for catheter placement in complete urethral disruption

d. Dual cystoscopy in operating room (OR) retrograde from urethra and antegrade from bladder in complete urethral disruption

e. Suprapubic tube placement in partial urethral disruption after failure to place urethra catheter

15. Which of the following is FALSE regarding management of testis injuries?

a. Testis injuries are more common in post pubertal patients.

b. One sign of testis rupture is irregular contour of the tunica albuginea on scrotal ultrasound.

c. Most experts agree that a testis rupture should be repaired surgically.

d. Hematocele on scrotal ultrasound is associated with testis rupture.

e. Homogeneous parenchyma on testis ultrasound is a sign of testis rupture.

ANSWERS

1. **c. Microscopic hematuria.** Microscopic hematuria alone is not an indication for renal trauma imaging. Mechanism of injury (a, b, d, e) is an important indication for renal trauma imaging.

2. **d. Pulsating hematoma at time of exploration for gunshot wound to abdomen.** A pulsating hematoma at time of exploration implies life-threatening ongoing renal bleedings. This is an absolute indication for renal exploration. All of the other options are not absolute indications for operative intervention.

3. **a. Observation.** Many cases of urinary extravasation will resolve with only observation. The other options are reserved for causes that do not resolve or develop complications such as fever, ileus, flank pain, expanding urinoma, or infection.

4. **d. Nephrectomy.** An emergent lifesaving operation (nephrectomy) is needed in this scenario. There is no time for vascular surgery consultation, and repair of renal artery injury will likely not be possible and is not indicated in the setting of a normal contralateral kidney.

5. **d. Dismembered pyeloplasty.** In a stable patient with UPJ disruption the preferred treatment is dismembered pyeloplasty. The majority of these patients, however, are not stable due to associated injuries, and other treatments such as nephrostomy tube and percutaneous drains are appropriate with delayed pyeloplasty or nephrectomy.

6. **c. Greater than 10% of kidney parenchyma devitalized.** High-risk criteria include a, b, d, and e. Another high-risk criteria for undergoing intervention in renal trauma is >25% of kidney parenchyma devitalized, not >10%.

7. **b. Closure of the collecting system with permanent sutures.** Absorbable sutures should be used for any collecting system repairs or closures to prevent urolithiasis formation.

8. **c. Yes, but use of protective equipment is recommended for contact sports.** Protective equipment is recommended for contact sports in children with solitary kidneys, according to American Academy of Pediatrics.

9. **d. Routine repeat CT scan at 48 hours if stable.** A repeat CT scan at 48 hours is recommended for higher-grade renal injuries according to AUA guidelines but is controversial for high-grade injuries if they are clinically doing well as it will unlikely change management. All of the other options are typically part of all nonoperative management plans.

10. **d. Ureteroureterostomy.** For an upper ureteral laceration, typically a ureteroureterostomy is the preferred surgical treatment. There is generally enough ureter that can be freed up for an anastomosis, and the injury is far from the bladder, making a Boari flap more difficult.

11. **b. Partial ureteral laceration recognized intraoperatively.** A ureteral laceration, partial or complete, recognized intraoperatively should be repaired.

12. **b. Microscopic hematuria with pelvic fracture.** Pelvic fracture with only microscopic hematuria is not an indication for cystogram.

13. **a. Extraperitoneal bladder rupture with gross hematuria.** An uncomplicated extraperitoneal bladder rupture with gross hematuria can often be managed with indwelling Foley and observation. If the gross hematuria cannot be managed with Foley due to clots, then open repair would be indicated.

14. **c. Cystoscopy per urethra in emergency room (ER) for catheter placement in complete urethral disruption.** If an attempt is going to be made at endoscopic realignment in complete urethral disruption, this should be performed in the operating room so retrograde and antegrade endoscopy can be performed.

15. **e. Homogeneous parenchyma on testis ultrasound is a sign of testis rupture.** Heterogeneous parenchyma on testis ultrasound is a sign of testis rupture, not homogeneous parenchyma.

1. The majority of renal trauma can be managed nonoperatively. Grade 4–5 injuries can be managed nonoperatively but have higher risk of undergoing intervention.
2. Around 25% of patients with grade 3–5 injuries being managed nonoperatively will have persistent or delayed bleeding. Superselective angioembolization of bleeding vessels is very successful and is the preferred method for management. Repeat angioembolization can also be successful if initial attempt fails.
3. Around 15% of patients with a urine leak being managed nonoperatively will have indication for intervention such as ureteral stent placement and/or percutaneous drain placement.
4. Repeat CT imaging 48–72 h after injury is not needed for patients with grade 1–3 injuries who are recovering without complication. Repeat CT imaging in 48–72 h may be obtained in patients with grade 4–5 injuries but is of unclear utility if the patient is stable and recovering without apparent complication.
5. Indications for operative intervention include hemodynamic instability due to renal bleeding, pulsatile or expanding retroperitoneal hematoma at time of laparotomy without prior renal imaging, and failure of angioembolization to control renal bleeding.
6. Control of renal vascular should be performed immediately after opening Gerota fascia or prior to opening Gerota fascia.
7. Operative intervention should include attempts to salvage kidney if possible.
8. UPJ disruptions should be repaired in acute phase if patient is stable; otherwise drainage with nephrostomy tube and possible percutaneous perirenal drain with delayed repair should be performed.
9. Renal pelvis ruptures may require operative intervention but have been managed successfully with endoscopic and percutaneous urinary drainage.
10. The risk of renal scarring is negligible in grade 1–2 injuries, approximately 50% in grade 3 injuries, and 100% in grade 4–5 injuries.
11. Follow-up imaging for grade 3–5 injuries should be considered. Starting with a renal ultrasound and obtaining CT, MRI, or DMSA scan if necessary is a common approach.
12. Hypertension is a rare occurrence after renal trauma in children and typically is only seen after grade 3–5 injuries.
13. The development of chronic kidney disease or end-stage renal disease is very rare after renal trauma even when nephrectomy is performed.
14. Patients with a normal solitary kidney can participate in sports, but protective equipment is recommended for contact sports. High-risk activities include dirt bike riding, cycling, and all-terrain vehicle riding.
15. Ureteral injuries are rare with any type of trauma but are most commonly seen with penetrating trauma.
16. A contrast-enhanced CT scan with delayed phase or a retrograde pyelogram is the preferred methods to diagnose a ureteral injury.
17. Ureteral injuries are often associated with other organ injuries in trauma cases and can be missed at initial laparotomy for trauma.
18. If a ureteral injury is diagnosed <1 week from injury, immediate repair can be performed and may be preferable if patient is stable.
19. If a ureteral injury is diagnosed >1 week from injury, an attempt at ureteral stent placement can be made, but often a nephrostomy tube with delayed open repair is needed.
20. Ureteral injuries in children are repaired similar to adults.
21. A history of pelvic trauma with gross hematuria or inability to void, and pelvic fracture necessitate urologic evaluation with retrograde urethrogram and/or cystogram.
22. Indications to repair an extraperitoneal bladder rupture include need for placement of orthopedic hardware in the field, bony pelvis fragments protruding into the bladder, involvement of the bladder neck in the injury, and concurrent abdominal surgery.
23. Intraperitoneal bladder ruptures are managed with surgical repair.
24. Bladder neck injuries are more common in children and best served with early repair.
25. Genital injury in children should raise suspicion for abuse, and if abuse is suspected, concomitant injury to the rectum and anus should be ruled out.
26. Most circumcision injuries can probably be avoided by ensuring that adhesions are properly reduced at the beginning of the procedure.
27. Findings on ultrasound consistent with testicular rupture should prompt surgical exploration.
28. Straddle injuries make up the majority of vaginal injuries. Injuries to bladder, urethra, anus, rectum, hymen, and internal vaginal structures are suggestive of penetrative injury and should prompt evaluation for abuse.

53   Pediatric Urologic Oncology: Renal and Adrenal

Michael L. Ritchey, Nicholas G. Cost, and Robert C. Shamberger

QUESTIONS

1. A chromosomal abnormality associated with an adverse prognosis in neuroblastoma is:
   a. mutation of chromosome 11p15.
   b. absence of the MDR gene.
   c. mutation of the TP53 gene.
   d. deletion of the short arm of chromosome 1.
   e. loss of heterozygosity (LOH) for chromosome 11p13.

2. In situ neuroblastoma:
   a. invariably progresses to clinical neuroblastoma.
   b. usually regresses spontaneously.
   c. is associated with deletion of chromosome 11.
   d. is usually detected on newborn screening.
   e. is frequently associated with amplification of the MYCN oncogene.

3. Ganglioneuroma is:
   a. a stroma-rich tumor by the Shimada classification.
   b. most commonly located in the adrenal gland.
   c. often found secondary to symptoms from metastatic disease.
   d. associated with acute myoclonic encephalopathy.
   e. associated with an unfavorable prognosis.

4. Screening for neuroblastoma:
   a. has improved survival in patients with neuroblastoma.
   b. has decreased the number of children older than 1 year of age with advanced stage disease.
   c. has identified more tumors with amplified *MYCN* oncogene expression.
   d. discovers tumors with a favorable prognosis.
   e. is widely performed in the United States.

5. A clinical feature associated with a favorable prognosis in neuroblastoma is:
   a. age >2 years.
   b. thoracic location of the primary tumor.
   c. *MYCN* amplification.
   d. chromosome 1p deletion.
   e. stroma-poor histology.

6. A 1-month-old girl has a right 4-cm suprarenal mass on abdominal ultrasound. Imaging evaluation detects liver metastases. A skeletal survey is normal. Physical examination reveals multiple subcutaneous skin nodules. The mass is removed, confirmed to be neuroblastoma, and analysis reveals no MYCN amplification. The next step is:
   a. observation.
   b. irradiation to the tumor bed.
   c. vincristine, cyclophosphamide, and doxorubicin.
   d. vincristine, cyclophosphamide, and irradiation to the tumor bed.
   e. autologous bone marrow transplantation after chemotherapy and total-body irradiation.

7. The WAGR (*Wilms tumor, Anirida, Genitourinary anomalies, mental Retardation*) syndrome is most frequently associated with:
   a. deletion of chromosome 15.
   b. advanced stage Wilms tumor.
   c. neonatal presentation of Wilms tumor.
   d. renal insufficiency.
   e. familial predisposition to Wilms tumor.

8. A 3-year-old boy had a hypospadias repair and orchiopexy as an infant and now develops renal insufficiency. Renal biopsy is consistent with a membranoproliferative glomerulonephritis. Appropriate management before renal transplantation is:
   a. voiding cystourethrogram.
   b. gonadal biopsy.
   c. observation.
   d. bilateral nephrectomy.
   e. serial renal ultrasounds.

9. A 2-year-old boy has a palpable right-sided abdominal mass, which on CT scan is a solid lesion. On physical examination the patient's right arm and leg are noted to be slightly longer in length. His diagnosis is most probably:
   a. Wilms tumor.
   b. neuroblastoma.
   c. angiomyolipoma.
   d. nephroblastomatosis.
   e. renal cell carcinoma.

10. A newborn is identified with Beckwith-Wiedemann syndrome (BWS). A renal ultrasound is obtained. The clinical finding that best predicts the risk of subsequent Wilms tumor development is:
    a. hepatomegaly.
    b. hemihypertrophy.
    c. nephromegaly.
    d. mutation at chromosome 1p.
    e. family history of Wilms tumor.

11. A 6-month-old girl is diagnosed with aniridia. Ultrasounds are done every 3 months. This will result in:
    a. increased survival.
    b. detection of lower-stage renal tumor.
    c. decreased incidence of bilateral tumors.
    d. decreased surgical morbidity.
    e. detection of tumors smaller than 3 cm in diameter.

12. A deletion of chromosome 11 has been found most frequently in Wilms tumor patients with:
    a. aniridia.
    b. bilateral tumors.
    c. hemihypertrophy.
    d. Denys-Drash syndrome (DDS).
    e. BWS.

13. A 5-year-old boy undergoes nephrectomy for a solid renal mass. Pathology reveals stage 1 favorable histology Wilms tumor. An increased risk for tumor relapse is associated with:
    a. tumor aneuploidy on flow cytometry.
    b. deletion of chromosome 11p13.
    c. duplication of chromosome 1.
    d. LOH for chromosome 16q.
    e. elevated serum ferritin level.

14. A 2-year-old girl undergoes left nephrectomy for Wilms tumor. A solitary left pulmonary lesion is noted on chest CT. The pathology shows negative nodes and favorable histology but with capsular penetration. The most important prognostic feature is:
    a. capsular presentation.
    b. histologic subtype.
    c. absence of lymph node involvement.
    d. age at presentation.
    e. presence of pulmonary metastasis.

15. The feature associated with the worst survival in children with Wilms tumor is:
    a. diffuse anaplasia.
    b. diffuse tumor spill.
    c. incomplete tumor resection.
    d. tumor spread to periaortic lymph nodes.
    e. lung metastasis.

16. An increased risk for metachronous Wilms tumor is associated with:
    a. anaplastic histology.
    b. clear cell sarcoma.
    c. blastemal predominant pattern.
    d. renal sinus invasion.
    e. nephrogenic rests.

17. A 1-year-old boy undergoes nephrectomy for Wilms tumor. The finding that has the most adverse impact on survival is:
    a. hilar lymph node involvement.
    b. renal sinus invasion.
    c. capsular penetration.
    d. ureteral extension of tumor.
    e. renal vein thrombus.

18. The factor associated with the lowest risk of local tumor relapse in children with Wilms tumor is:
    a. local tumor spill.
    b. unfavorable histology.
    c. incomplete tumor removal.
    d. absence of lymph node sampling.
    e. capsular penetration.

19. A 4-year-old girl undergoes nephrectomy for a favorable histology Wilms tumor. Imaging reveals multiple pulmonary metastases. Treatment should include vincristine, dactinomycin, and:
    a. observation.
    b. resection of the pulmonary lesions.
    c. doxorubicin and chest irradiation.
    d. doxorubicin, cyclophosphamide, and irradiation.
    e. doxorubicin and etoposide.

20. A 3-month-old boy undergoes removal of a 300 g Wilms tumor of the right kidney. The pathology shows diffuse anaplasia and tumor confined to the kidney. Lymph nodes were negative. The next step is:
    a. observation.
    b. vincristine and dactinomycin.
    c. vincristine, dactinomycin, and irradiation of the tumor bed.
    d. doxorubicin, vincristine, dactinomycin, and irradiation of the tumor bed.
    e. ifosfamide, etoposide, and doxorubicin.

21. A 5-year-old girl presents with hematuria. CT reveals a right abdominal mass with extension of tumor thrombus into the suprahepatic vena cava. The best next step is:
    a. chemotherapy.
    b. irradiation.
    c. open biopsy followed by chemotherapy.
    d. preoperative chemotherapy and radiation therapy.
    e. primary surgical removal of the kidney and tumor thrombus.

22. A 2-year-old boy is found to have bilateral Wilms tumor. There is a tumor occupying more than 50% of the left kidney and a 4.0-cm tumor in the upper pole of the right kidney. The best next step is:
    a. left nephrectomy and right renal biopsy.
    b. bilateral partial nephrectomy.
    c. right partial nephrectomy and left renal biopsy.
    d. bilateral nephrectomies.
    e. chemotherapy.

23. A 1-year-old girl has a stage III Wilms tumor. During the course of chemotherapy she develops an enlarged heart and evidence of congestive heart failure. The drug responsible for these findings is most likely:
    a. dactinomycin.
    b. etoposide.
    c. vincristine.
    d. cyclophosphamide.
    e. doxorubicin.

24. A 1-year-old boy undergoes left radical nephrectomy for a large renal mass. The pathologic features associated with the worst prognosis are:
    a. diffuse anaplasia stage I.
    b. focal anaplasia stage III.
    c. rhabdoid tumor of the kidney stage III.
    d. clear cell sarcoma of the kidney stage III.
    e. favorable histology stage IV.

25. A newborn boy was noted to have a left renal mass on prenatal ultrasound. Postnatal evaluation confirms a 5-cm solid mass in the lower pole of the left kidney. The right kidney is normal. Chest radiography and CT of the chest are negative for metastatic disease. The mass was completely removed by a radical nephrectomy. The tumor was confined to the kidney and weighed 300 g. The next step in treatment is:

    a. 1200-cGy abdominal irradiation to the left flank.

    b. observation only.

    c. dactinomycin and vincristine for 10 weeks.

    d. dactinomycin and vincristine for 18 weeks.

    e. 2000-cGy abdominal irradiation plus dactinomycin and vincristine for 18 weeks.

26. The tuberous sclerosis complex is associated with the development of angiomyolipoma and cystic renal disease. These patients have been found to have an abnormality of chromosome:

    a. 1.

    b. 7.

    c. 9.

    d. 12.

    e. 14.

ANSWERS

1. **d. Deletion of the short arm of chromosome 1.** Deletion of the short arm of chromosome 1 is found in 25% to 35% of neuroblastomas and is an adverse prognostic marker. The deletions are of different size, but in a series of eight cases a consensus deletion included the segment 1p36.1-2, suggesting that genetic information related to neuroblastoma tumorigenesis is located in this segment.

2. **b. Usually regresses spontaneously.** In 1963, Beckwith and Perrin coined the term *in-situ* neuroblastoma for small nodules of neuroblastoma cells found incidentally within the adrenal gland, which are histologically indistinguishable from neuroblastoma. In infants younger than 3 months of age undergoing postmortem examination, neuroblastoma *in-situ* was found in 1 of 224 infants. This represents an incidence of *in-situ* neuroblastoma 40 to 45 times greater than the incidence of clinical tumors, suggesting that these small tumors regress spontaneously in most cases. However, more recent studies have shown that these neuroblastic nodules are found in all fetuses studied and generally regress.

3. **a. A stroma-rich tumor by the Shimada classification.** The Shimada classification is an age-linked histopathologic classification. One of the important aspects of the Shimada classification is determining whether the tumor is stroma poor or stroma rich. Patients with stroma-poor tumors with unfavorable histopathologic features have a very poor prognosis (<10% survival). Stroma-rich tumors can be separated into three subgroups: nodular, intermixed, and well differentiated. Tumors in the last two categories more closely resemble ganglioneuroblastoma or immature ganglioneuroma and have a higher rate of survival.

4. **d. Discovers tumors with a favorable prognosis.** The goal of screening programs is to detect disease at an earlier stage and decrease the number of older children with advanced stage disease and thus improve survival. An increased number of infants younger than 1 year of age have been diagnosed with the mass screening program, and most of these patients have lower-stage tumors. Regrettably, the number of children older than 1 year of age with advanced-stage disease has not decreased.

5. **b. Thoracic location of the primary tumor.** The site of origin is of significance, with a better survival rate noted for nonadrenal primary tumors. Most children with thoracic neuroblastoma present at a younger age with localized disease and have improved survival even when corrected for age and stage.

6. **a. Observation.** The generally favorable behavior of stage IV-S disease has been explained with the identification of biologic markers. The vast majority of these infants have tumors with entirely favorable markers explaining their nonmalignant behavior. A small percentage, however, have adverse markers, and it is these children who have progressive disease to which they often succumb. Resection of the primary tumor is not mandatory. Although excellent survival has been reported after surgery, information regarding histologic prognostic factors was not available for all of these patients. A more recent review was performed of a large cohort of 110 infants with stage IV-S disease. The entire cohort of infants had an estimated 3-year survival rate of 85% ± 4%. This survival rate was significantly decreased, however, to 68% ± 12% for infants who were diploid, 44% ± 33% for those who were *MYCN* amplified, and 33% ± 19% for those with unfavorable histology tumors. Of note, there was no statistical difference in survival rate for infants who underwent complete resection of their primary tumor compared with those with partial resection or only biopsy. Patients with extensive metastatic disease who are *MYCN*–positive represent a high-risk group. These patients should be considered for a more aggressive treatment with multimodal therapy as per the risk group classification.

7. **d. Renal insufficiency.** Patients with the WAGR syndrome have a germline deletion at 11p13. WT1 mutations and deletions predispose patients to renal insufficiency. Both the Denys-Drash and WAGR syndrome are associated with an increased risk of renal failure. This occurs later in the WAGR syndrome, often in the second decade of life after treatment of the Wilms tumor.

8. **d. Bilateral nephrectomy.** One specific association of male pseudohermaphroditism, renal mesangial sclerosis, and nephroblastoma is the Denys-Drash syndrome. The majority of these patients progress to end-stage renal disease. A specific mutation of the 11p13 Wilms tumor gene has been identified in these children. Although XY individuals have been reported most often, the syndrome has been reported in genotypic/phenotypic females. One should have a high index of suspicion for the development of renal failure and Wilms tumor in patients with male pseudohermaphroditism.

9. **a. Wilms tumor.** BWS is characterized by excess growth at the cellular, organ (macroglossia, nephromegaly, hepatomegaly), or body segment (hemihypertrophy) levels. Most cases of BWS are sporadic, but up to 15% exhibit heritable characteristics with apparent autosomal dominant inheritance. The risk of nephroblastoma in children with BWS and hemihypertrophy is 4% to 10%.

10. **c. Nephromegaly.** Children with BWS found to have nephromegaly (kidneys at or above the 95th percentile of age-adjusted renal length) are at the greatest risk for the development of Wilms tumor.

11. **b. Detection of lower stage renal tumor.** Screening with serial renal ultrasonographic scans has been recommended in children with aniridia, hemihypertrophy, and BWS. Review of most studies suggests that 3 to 4 months is the appropriate screening interval. Tumors detected by screening will generally be at a lower stage.

12. **a. Aniridia.** Approximately 50% of patients with WAGR syndrome and a constitutional deletion on chromosome 11 will develop Wilms' tumor.

13. **d. LOH for chromosome 16q.** LOH for a portion of chromosome 16q has been noted in 20% of Wilms tumors. A study of 232 patients registered on the National Wilms Tumor Study Group (NWTSG) found LOH for 16q in 17% of the tumors. Patients with tumor-specific LOH for chromosome 16q had a statistically significantly poorer 2-year relapse-free and overall survival rate than did those patients without LOH for chromosome 16q.

14. **b. Histologic subtype.** Markers associated with unfavorable outcome include nuclear atypia (anaplasia), focal or diffuse, and sarcomatous tumors (rhabdoid and clear cell type). The latter two tumor types, however, are tumor categories distinct from Wilms tumor. These unfavorable features occurred in approximately 10% of patients but accounted for almost half of the tumor deaths in early NWTSG studies.

15. **a. Diffuse anaplasia.** Anaplasia is associated with resistance to chemotherapy. This is evidenced by the similar incidence of anaplasia (5%) in the NWTSG and International Society of Paediatric Oncology studies. Although the presence of anaplasia has clearly been demonstrated to carry a poor prognosis, patients with stage I anaplastic Wilms tumor as well as those with higher stages and focal rather than diffuse anaplasia seem to have a more favorable outcome. This confirms the observation that anaplasia is more a marker of chemoresistance than inherent aggressiveness of the tumor.

16. **e. Nephrogenic rests.** NWTSG investigators demonstrated the clinical importance of nephrogenic rests. Multiple rests in one kidney usually imply that nephrogenic rests are present in the other kidney. Children younger than 12 months of age diagnosed with Wilms tumor who also have nephrogenic rests, in particular perilobar nephrogenic rests, have a markedly increased risk of developing contralateral disease, and require frequent and regular surveillance for several years.

17. **a. Hilar lymph node involvement.** The most important determinants of outcome in children with Wilms tumor are histopathology and tumor stage. Accurate staging of Wilms tumor allows treatment results to be evaluated and enables universal comparisons of outcomes. The staging system used by the NWTSG is based primarily on the surgical and histopathologic findings. Examination for extension through the capsule, residual disease, vascular involvement, and lymph node involvement is essential to properly assess the extent of the tumor.

18. **e. Capsular penetration.** One study identified risk factors for local tumor recurrence as tumor spillage, unfavorable histology, incomplete tumor removal, and absence of any lymph node sampling. The 2-year survival rate after abdominal recurrence was 43%, emphasizing the importance of the surgeon in performing careful and complete tumor resection.

19. **c. Doxorubicin and chest irradiation.** Patients with stage III favorable histologic type tumors and stage II to III focal anaplasia are treated with dactinomycin, vincristine, and doxorubicin and 10.8-Gy abdominal irradiation. Patients with stage IV favorable histologic type tumors receive abdominal irradiation based on the local tumor stage and 12 Gy to both lungs.

20. **d. Doxorubicin, vincristine, dactinomycin, and irradiation of the tumor bed.** Anaplasia tumors are resistant to chemotherapy. However, if the tumor is confined to the kidney and completely resected the prognosis is good. They do require more intense treatment than children with stage I, favorable histology tumors.

21. **c. Open biopsy followed by chemotherapy.** The current recommendations from the NWTSG are that preoperative chemotherapy is of benefit in patients with bilateral involvement, inoperable at surgical exploration, and IVC extension above the hepatic veins. All other patients should undergo primary nephrectomy.

22. **e. Chemotherapy.** Patients with bilateral Wilms tumor have an increased risk for renal failure. These patients should receive preoperative chemotherapy without attempts at initial surgery. Repeat imaging after 6 weeks of chemotherapy can assess response to treatment.

23. **e. Doxorubicin.** In recent years, there has been increasing concern regarding the risk of congestive heart failure in children who receive treatment with anthracyclines such as doxorubicin. In addition to the acute cardiotoxicity, cardiac failure can develop many years after treatment.

24. **c. Rhabdoid tumor of the kidney stage III.** Typical clinical features include early age at diagnosis (median age of <16 months), resistance to chemotherapy, and high mortality rate. Unlike Wilms tumor, which typically metastasizes to the lungs, abdomen/flank, and liver, rhabdoid tumor of the kidney, which also metastasizes to these sites, is distinguished by its propensity to metastasize to the brain.

25. **b. Observation only.** The most common renal tumor in a newborn is congenital mesoblastic nephroma. The important aspect of the recognition of these tumors as a separate entity is the usually excellent outcome with radical surgery only. Wilms tumors do occur rarely in neonates, but these patients are eligible for observation only on current protocols.

26. **c. 9.** Two genes have been identified in the tuberous sclerosis complex on chromosome 9 (TSC1) and chromosome 16 (TSC2). It has been postulated that these genes act as tumor suppressor genes and that the LOH of TSC1 or TSC2 may explain the progressive growth pattern of renal lesions seen in these patients.

CHAPTER REVIEW

1. Neuroblastoma is the most common extracranial solid neoplasm in children.
2. Children 18 months of age or younger have a better survival rate than older children. This may be attributed to more favorable biologic parameters in tumors diagnosed at this age.
3. Complete surgical resection is curative for low-stage disease.
4. *MYCN* amplification, found in 20% of patients with primary tumors, is associated with tumor progression. This poor prognosis is independent of patient age and tumor stage. Additional biologic markers of poor prognosis have been defined and treatment protocols are currently based on these factors.
5. Deletions of *WT1*, located on chromosome 11p, are found in patients with aniridia and Wilms tumor. Mutations of *WT1* occur in DDS.
6. Local recurrence is increased in Wilms tumor patients with local tumor spillage, and this is now classified as stage III disease. The 2-year survival rate after local recurrence is 43%.
7. Patients with bilateral Wilms tumor should be treated with preoperative chemotherapy. This will allow more patients to undergo renal sparing surgery in an attempt to decrease the risk of renal failure.
8. Congenital mesoblastic nephroma (CMN) is the most common renal tumor in infants.

54 Pediatric Urologic Oncology: Bladder and Testis

Fernando A. Ferrer

QUESTIONS

1. A 3-year-old girl has vaginal rhabdomyosarcoma (RMS). Her mother has a history of breast cancer. This patient most likely has:

   a. Beckwith-Wiedemann syndrome (BWS).

   b. Li-Fraumeni syndrome.

   c. Perlman syndrome.

   d. Fragile X syndrome.

   e. Sotos syndrome.

2. A 3-year-old boy has RMS of the prostate. An unfavorable prognostic feature of this tumor is:

   a. alveolar histologic type.

   b. embryonal histology.

   c. LOH for chromosome 11p15.

   d. botryoid pattern.

   e. spindle cell variant.

3. A 1-year-old girl previously had a partial cystectomy for RMS of the bladder. After completion of vincristine, dactinomycin, and cyclophosphamide (VAC) chemotherapy and radiotherapy, biopsy of the bladder reveals rhabdomyoblasts. Abdominal and chest computed tomography (CT) are negative. The next step is:

   a. radiation therapy.

   b. continue chemotherapy.

   c. cystectomy with diversion.

   d. observation.

   e. a change in chemotherapy regimen.

4. A 4-year-old boy has paratesticular RMS noted on biopsy of a spermatic cord lesion. The next step is radical orchiectomy and:

   a. vincristine, dactinomycin, and cyclophosphamide.

   b. retroperitoneal lymph node dissection.

   c. retroperitoneal lymph node sampling.

   d. radiation therapy to the retroperitoneum.

   e. cisplatin, etoposide, and vincristine.

5. A 2-year-old boy undergoes left orchiectomy. Pathology reveals a yolk sac tumor confined to the testis. CT findings of the chest and abdomen are negative. No preoperative tumor markers were obtained. At 4 weeks after surgery, tumor markers are negative. The next step is:

   a. lymph node dissection.

   b. observation.

   c. chemotherapy.

   d. staining of the tumor for α-fetoprotein.

   e. retroperitoneal lymph node sampling.

6. A 6-year-old, phenotypic boy with hypospadias and bilateral cryptorchidism has a 3-cm lower abdominal mass. His karyotype is XO/XY. At exploration, a left inguinal testis is noted, a tumor is found in the right abdominal gonad, and gonadectomy is performed. Frozen section reveals gonadoblastoma. The next step is:

   a. left orchiopexy.

   b. retroperitoneal lymphadenectomy node sampling.

   c. left orchiectomy.

   d. chemotherapy.

   e. observation.

7. A 2-year-old boy has a left upper pole testicular mass that is cystic on ultrasonography. Excision of the lesion is performed by an inguinal approach leaving the lower half of the testis. Frozen section demonstrates clear margins. Final pathology reveals teratoma, and the margins are negative for tumor. Serum α-fetoprotein and β-hCG are negative. Chest and abdominal CT are negative. The next step is:

   a. radical orchiectomy and modified retroperitoneal lymph node dissection.

   b. observation.

   c. radical orchiectomy and combination chemotherapy.

   d. radical orchiectomy.

   e. radical orchiectomy and abdominal irradiation.

8. A 3-month-old boy undergoes removal of a solid yolk sac tumor. The margins of resection are negative for tumor. Chest and abdominal CT results show no signs of metastatic disease. Two weeks postoperatively, the serum α-fetoprotein value is 35 ng/dL. The next step is:

   a. chemotherapy.

   b. retroperitoneal lymph node dissection.

   c. observation.

   d. retroperitoneal lymph node sampling.

   e. abdominal irradiation.

9. A 10-year-old boy presents with an episode of gross hematuria. Ultrasound of the bladder demonstrates small, less than 1-cm lesion at the bladder base; cystoscopy reveals a small papillary lesion which is completely resected. Pathology reveals superficial low-grade transitional cell carcinoma. Appropriate next steps include:

   a. a course of BCG therapy in an attempt to prevent recurrence.

   b. routine cystoscopic surveillance for 5 years.

   c. surveillance by bladder sonography without further treatment.

   d. mitomycin C bladder instillation.

   e. staging abdominal-pelvic CT scan and chest x-ray.

10. A 5-year-old boy presents with hematuria. A 5-cm prostatic mass is biopsied and consistent with embryonal RMS. He undergoes therapy according to COG intermediate risk protocol (chemotherapy and radiation). At the completion of treatment, the child has a residual 0.5-cm mass, which is biopsied and confirmed to consist of mature rhabdomyoblasts. Future treatment should consist of:

    a. cystoprostatectomy and external beam radiotherapy.

    b. salvage chemotherapy.

    c. observation only.

    d. cystoprostatectomy followed by adjuvant chemotherapy.

    e. implantation of radiotherapy beads.

11. An 11-year-old male presents with a right paratesticular mass. An inguinal orchiectomy is performed. The pathologic diagnosis is RMS completely excised (clinical group 1). A CT scan of the retroperitoneum is negative. The next step is:

a. observation.

b. right staging ipsilateral RPLND.

c. right staging ipsilateral RPLND + inguinal lymph node dissection.

d. right inguinal lymph node dissection.

e. chemotherapy.

12. A 4-month-old male is noted to have a right testicular mass. Ultrasound reveals a well circumscribed, heterogenous, cystic mass with calcifications. Serum hCG is normal. Serum AFP is elevated at 90 ng/mL. The most likely appropriate treatment is:

a. radical inguinal orchiectomy.

b. transscrotal exploration and biopsy.

c. inguinal exploration, cord control, biopsy, and partial orchiectomy.

d. transscrotal partial orchiectomy.

e. staging CT scan.

13. A 5-year-old male presents with difficulty voiding and gross hematuria as well as right flank discomfort. US demonstrates a 5-cm mass at the level of the trigone with moderate-severe right hydronephrosis. A pelvic CT scan confirms these findings and does not show pelvic adenopathy. The next steps would be:

a. open resection and right ureteral reimplantation.

b. endoscopic biopsy followed by right internal stent placement if possible.

c. to attempt a complete endoscopic resection.

d. percutaneous nephrostomy tube placement followed by open biopsy.

e. transrectal sonography-guided needle biopsy.

ANSWERS

1. **b. Li-Fraumeni syndrome.** Subgroups of children with a genetic predisposition to the development of RMS have been identified. The Li-Fraumeni syndrome associates childhood sarcomas with mothers who have an excess of premenopausal breast cancer and with siblings who have an increased risk of cancer. A mutation of the *TP53* tumor suppressor gene was found in the tumors in all patients with this syndrome.

2. **a. Alveolar histologic type.** The second most common form is alveolar, which occurs more commonly in the trunk and extremities than in genitourinary sites and has a worse prognosis. Alveolar RMS also has a higher rate of local recurrence and spread to regional lymph nodes, bone marrow, and distant sites.

3. **d. Observation.** If tumor is shrinking during chemotherapy, and another biopsy after completing radiotherapy shows maturing rhabdomyoblasts without frank tumor cells (i.e., mitotic figures), total cystectomy can be postponed or possibly avoided altogether. The finding of rhabdomyoblasts requires close follow-up and possibly further surveillance biopsies.

4. **a. Vincristine, dactinomycin, and cyclophosphamide.** Before effective chemotherapy, surgery alone produced a 50% 2-year relapse-free survival rate. With current multimodal treatment, survival rates of 90% are expected. Currently, the Intergroup Rhabdomyosarcoma Study Group recommends that children 10 years of age and older undergo ipsilateral retroperitoneal lymph node dissection before chemotherapy.

5. **b. Observation.** It is important to note that an elevated α-fetoprotein level after orchiectomy for yolk sac tumor in an infant (<12 months) does not always represent persistent disease. Normal adult reference laboratory values for α-fetoprotein cannot be used in young children, because α-fetoprotein synthesis continues after birth. Normal adult levels (<10 mg/mL) are not reached until 8 to 12 months of age.

6. **a. Left orchiopexy.** In patients with mixed gonadal dysgenesis (MGD) who are reared as males, all streak gonads should be removed, and undescended testes, which are also at high risk of tumor formation, need to be relocated to the scrotum. If the testis is unable to be well palpated in the scrotum, then orchiectomy is indicated. Some advocate early orchiectomy of any undescended testis in MGD because tumors have been reported in children younger than 5 years of age. Scrotal testes can be preserved, because they are less prone to tumor development.

7. **b. Observation.** Prepubertal mature teratomas have a benign clinical course, which contrasts with the clinical behavior of teratomas in postpubertal adolescents and adults, which have the propensity to metastasize. This benign behavior has led to the consideration of testicular-sparing procedures rather than radical orchiectomy.

8. **c. Observation.** The initial treatment for yolk sac tumor is radical inguinal orchiectomy. This treatment is curative in most children. Routine retroperitoneal lymph node dissection and adjuvant chemotherapy are not indicated. Normal adult reference laboratory values for α-fetoprotein cannot be used in young children, because α-fetoprotein synthesis continues after birth. Normal adult levels (<10 mg/mL) are not reached until 8 to 12 months of age.

9. **c. Surveillance by bladder sonography without further treatment.** TCC in children is uncommon and the lesions are unifocal, typically low grade, and not prone to recurrence therefore treatment consisting of resection only is adequate. US is remarkably accurate and is an adequate surveillance strategy.

10. **c. Observation only.** Mature rhabdomyoblasts found after treatment for RMS do not require further treatment if confirmed by an experienced pathologist. Furthermore, prior studies have demonstrated that some residual mass does not necessarily mean active residual disease exists. In the case presented, further aggressive therapy is not warranted. Serial radiographic evaluation is indicated.

11. **b. Right staging ipsilateral RPLND.** Prior studies have shown that children over age 10 should always undergo staging ipsilateral RPLND and not observation due to a high occurrence of retroperitoneal failure. Paratesticular RMS rarely involves the inguinal nodes.

12. **c. Inguinal exploration, cord control, biopsy, and partial orchiectomy.** Teratoma is a common benign prepubertal tumor that can be treated by partial orchiectomy. Although not always accurate, the US features of this tumor are suggestive of teratoma. AFP levels do not reach normal adult levels until close to 1 year of life therefore this elevation is not necessarily reflective of a continued yolk sac tumor. In fact, yolk sac tumors typically have AFP elevations above 100 ng/mL. The likelihood of a benign etiology warrants attempt at partial orchiectomy.

13. **b. Endoscopic biopsy followed by right internal stent placement if possible.** This presentation is concerning for bladder RMS. In this case organ preservation strategies should be pursued and endoscopic biopsy is the correct answer. Chemotherapy for RMS can be deleterious to renal function so stenting to prevent any renal deterioration during treatment should be performed. Internal stent placement is typically more comfortable than percutaneous nephrostomy.

CHAPTER REVIEW

1. Embryonal is the most common histology for bladder/prostate lesions.
2. Alveolar histology is uncommon in the bladder or prostate. New studies indicated two distinct types, PAX-FOXO1 fusion positive and negative. Fusion-positive tumors carry a worse prognosis.
3. Bladder/prostate tumors typically present with symptoms of obstruction, retention, or hematuria.
4. Organ preservation is a principle goal of treatment; therefore, most patients treated in COG protocols undergo endoscopic/open biopsy as the initial step.
5. Pretreatment TNM staging and a surgical pathologic group classification contribute to the patient's final risk group assignment, which in turn determines therapy. New to the current study is the use of fusion status for therapeutic group assignment.
6. Bladder/prostate tumors arise from an unfavorable site and gross residual tumor usually remains after biopsy, therefore most patients are assigned into the intermediate risk group.
7. A residual mass after chemo/radiotherapy does not necessarily mean viable tumor remains.
8. Rhabdomyoblasts are differentiated tumor cells (not active malignant tumor) that do not require further treatment but should be followed closely.
9. Vaginal RMS is the most common female genital site. The majority are embryonal histology, and organ preservation strategies have resulted in excellent overall survival.
10. Ovarian tumors comprise 1% of all childhood cancers. Ovarian tumors are histologically classified as germ cell, sex cord, or epithelial tumors.
11. A large percentage of prepubertal testis tumors are benign; therefore testicular preservation approaches are often indicated.
12. Ultrasonography cannot reliably distinguish benign from malignant lesions.
13. AFP is the relevant biomarker in prepubertal testis tumors, and elevation is associated with yolk sac tumors.
14. AFP levels must be interpreted with caution as physiologic elevation above normal values is common in children less than age 1 year.
15. Paratesticular RMS arises from the testicular tunics, epididymis, or the spermatic cord.
16. In general, patients with paratesticular RMS enjoy a favorable prognosis in part due to the following: (1) upward of 80% are stage I at presentation; (2) greater than 90% are embryonal histology; (3) better than expected outcomes for patients with alveolar histology.
17. Patients suspected of having a paratesticular tumor should always be explored through an inguinal incision.
18. Tumors in children greater than age 10 require staging RPLND in COG protocols because of a higher retroperitoneal failure rate.

55   Infections of the Urinary Tract

Kimberly L. Cooper, Gina M. Badalato, and Matthew P. Rutman

QUESTIONS

1. Acute pyelonephritis is the most likely diagnosis in a patient with:
   a. chills, fever, and flank pain.
   b. bacteria and pyuria.
   c. focal scar in renal cortex.
   d. delayed renal function.
   e. vesicoureteral reflux.

2. Bacteriuria without pyuria is indicative of:
   a. infection.
   b. colonization.
   c. tuberculosis.
   d. contamination.
   e. stones.

3. Nosocomial urinary tract infections (UTIs):
   a. occur in patients who are hospitalized or institutionalized.
   b. are caused by common bowel bacteria.
   c. can be suppressed by low-dose antimicrobial therapy.
   d. are due to reinfection.
   e. are due to bacterial persistence.

4. Most recurrent infections in female patients are:
   a. complicated.
   b. reinfections.
   c. due to bacterial resistance.
   d. due to hereditary susceptibility factors.
   e. composed of multiple organisms.

5. Rates of reinfection (i.e., time to recurrence) are influenced by:
   a. bladder dysfunction.
   b. renal scarring.
   c. vesicoureteral reflux.
   d. antimicrobial treatment.
   e. age.

6. The long-term effect of uncomplicated recurrent UTIs is:
   a. renal scarring.
   b. hypertension.
   c. azotemia.
   d. ureteral vesical reflux.
   e. minimal.

7. The ascending route of infection is least enhanced by:
   a. catheterization.
   b. spermicidal agents.
   c. indwelling catheter.
   d. fecal soilage of perineum.
   e. frequent voiding.

8. Approximately 10% of symptomatic lower UTIs in young, sexually active female patients are caused by:
   a. *Escherichia coli (E. coli)*.
   b. *Staphylococcus saprophyticus*.
   c. *Pseudomonas*.
   d. *Proteus mirabilis*.
   e. *Staphylococcus epidermidis*.

9. The virulence factor that is most important for adherence is:
   a. hemolysin.
   b. K antigen.
   c. pili.
   d. colicin production.
   e. O serogroup.

10. Phase variation of bacterial pili:
    a. occurs only in vitro.
    b. affects bacterial virulence.
    c. is characteristic of pyelonephritic *E. coli*.
    d. is irreversible.
    e. refers to change in pilus length.

11. The finding that first suggested a biologic difference in women susceptible to UTIs is:
    a. increased adherence of bacteria to vaginal cells.
    b. decreased estrogen concentration in vaginal cells.
    c. elevated vaginal pH.
    d. nonsecretor status.
    e. postmenopausal status.

12. The primary bladder defense is:
    a. low urine pH.
    b. low urine osmolarity.
    c. voiding.
    d. Tamm-Horsfall protein (uromucoid).
    e. vaginal mucus.

13. The most significant sequela of renal papillary necrosis is renal:
    a. failure.
    b. abscess.
    c. obstruction.
    d. stone.
    e. cancer.

14. Severity and morbidity of bacteriuria is most morbid in patients with:
    a. spinal cord injuries.

b. pregnancy.

c. reflux.

d. diabetes mellitus.

e. human immunodeficiency virus (HIV) infection.

15. The validity of a midstream urine specimen should be questioned if microscopy reveals:

a. squamous epithelial cells.

b. red blood cells.

c. bacteria.

d. white blood cells.

e. casts.

16. Urinary tract imaging is NOT usually indicated for recurrent UTIs in:

a. women.

b. girls.

c. men.

d. boys.

e. spinal cord–injured patients.

17. The most sensitive imaging modality for diagnosing renal abscess is:

a. ultrasonography.

b. indium scanning.

c. gallium scanning.

d. excretory urography.

e. CT.

18. Treatment of UTIs depends most on an antimicrobial agent's:

a. serum half-life.

b. serum level.

c. urine level.

d. duration of therapy.

e. frequency of therapy.

19. An ideal class of drugs for the treatment of uncomplicated symptomatic UTIs in women is:

a. aminopenicillins.

b. aminoglycosides.

c. fluoroquinolones.

d. cephalosporins.

e. nitrofurantoins.

20. The host factor least likely to be associated with an increased risk of infection is:

a. advanced age.

b. a history of previous infection in the site/organ of interest.

c. residence in a chronic care facility.

d. indwelling orthopedic pins.

e. coexistent infection.

21. The optimal duration of antimicrobial therapy with Bactrim for symptomatic acute uncomplicated cystitis in women is:

a. 1 day.

b. 3 days.

c. 7 days.

d. 14 days.

e. 21 days.

22. Treatment of asymptomatic bacteriuria is most indicated in patients who are:

a. elderly.

b. catheterized.

c. pregnant.

d. confused.

e. incontinent.

23. Screening for bacteriuria is beneficial in:

a. pregnant women.

b. elderly patients.

c. men.

d. children.

e. spinal cord–injured patients.

24. The most common cause of unresolved bacteriuria during antimicrobial therapy is:

a. development of bacterial resistance.

b. rapid reinfections.

c. azotemia.

d. staghorn calculi.

e. initial bacterial resistance.

25. Nitrofurantoin is effective because of the concentration of the drug in the:

a. urine.

b. vaginal mucus.

c. bowel.

d. serum.

e. bladder.

26. The most common cause of acute pyelonephritis in young women is:

a. vesicoureteral reflux.

b. P-piliated bacteria.

c. type 1 piliated bacteria.

d. recurrent UTIs.

e. bacterial endotoxin.

27. An optimal oral antibiotic agent for the treatment of acute uncomplicated pyelonephritis in a pregnant women is:

a. TMP-SMX

b. Cephalexin

c. Amoxicillin

d. Levofloxacin

e. Macrobid

28. A patient with acute pyelonephritis, persistent fever, and flank pain for 24 hours warrants:

a. observation.

b. CT.

c. change in antimicrobial therapy.

d. ultrasonography.

e. blood cultures.

29. Emphysematous pyelonephritis usually occurs in:

a. children

b. adults with a history of renal transplant

c. women with a history of recurrent uncomplicated UTIs

d. diabetic adults

e. adults on clean intermittent catheterization

30. The primary treatment for a small perirenal abscess in a functioning kidney is:

a. nephrectomy.

b. partial nephrectomy.

c. open surgical drainage.

d. percutaneous drainage.

e. retrograde ureteral drainage.

31. Most patients with chronic pyelonephritis present with:

a. hypertension.

b. renal failure.

c. chronic infection.

d. flank pain.

e. no symptoms.

32. The most common bacterial cause of xanthogranulomatous pyelonephritis is:

a. *E. coli.*

b. *Pseudomonas.*

c. *Klebsiella.*

d. *Proteus mirabilis.*

e. *Staphylococcus.*

33. Michaelis-Gutmann bodies are associated with the following disease process:

a. Xanthogranulomatous pyelonephritis

b. Malacoplakia

c. Renal echinococcosis

d. Chronic pyelonephritis

e. Acute focal bacterial nephritis

34. Treatment of renal echinococcosis involves which of the following:

a. treatment with antibiotics and follow-up imaging to confirm regression of the hydatid cyst

b. observation

c. aspiration of cyst contents

d. surgical removal of the hydatid cyst

e. injection of the hydatid cyst with targeted antibiotics

35. The most reliable early clinical indicator of septicemia is:

a. chills.

b. fever.

c. hyperventilation.

d. lethargy.

e. change in mental status.

36. Compared with non-pregnant women, pregnant women have a higher prevalence of:

a. asymptomatic bacteriuria.

b. acute cystitis.

c. acute pyelonephritis.

d. recurrent cystitis.

e. bacterial persistence.

37. Clinical pyelonephritis during pregnancy is most commonly linked to:

a. maternal sepsis.

b. maternal anemia.

c. maternal hypertension.

d. eclampsia.

e. congenital malformations.

38. The drug thought to be safe in any phase of pregnancy is:

a. a fluoroquinolone.

b. nitrofurantoin.

c. a sulfonamide.

d. penicillin.

e. tetracycline.

39. The majority of elderly patients with bacteriuria are:

a. asymptomatic.

b. febrile.

c. incontinent.

d. confused.

e. dysuric.

40. In the absence of obstruction, treatment of asymptomatic bacteriuria in the elderly:

a. is cost effective.

b. prevents renal failure.

c. reduces mortality.

d. reduces morbidity.

e. is unnecessary.

41. Prophylaxis for endocarditis should be administered in patients with:

a. a history of childhood heart murmurs.

b. heart valves inserted more than 5 years ago.

c. calcified heart valves associated with a murmur.

d. all synthetic heart valves.

e. cadaveric heart valves.

f. none of the above.

42. The most common predisposing factor for hospital-acquired UTIs is:

a. surgery.

b. antimicrobial therapy.

c. age.

d. catheterization.

e. diabetes mellitus.

43. The most effective measure for reducing catheter-associated UTI is:

a. closed drainage.

b. antimicrobial prophylaxis.

c. catheter irrigation.

d. intermittent catheterization.

e. daily meatal care.

44. In spinal cord–injured patients the bladder drainage technique with the lowest complication rate is:

a. clean intermittent catheterization (CIC).

b. suprapubic drainage.

c. indwelling catheter.

d. condom catheter.

e. suprapubic pressure.

45. All of the following conditions are predisposing factors to the development of Fournier gangrene EXCEPT:

a. obesity

b. paraphimosis

c. diabetes mellitus

d. perirectal infections

e. urethral strictures

46. Which of the following is true of vaginal estrogen preparations and recurrent urinary tract infections in postmenopausal women?

a. The use of vaginal estrogen has been associated with an increased risk of breast cancer.

b. Vaginal estrogen use can confer an increased risk of thrombotic events in women.

c. Vaginal estrogen preparations can help with vaginal pain symptoms that can be conflated for UTI but do not modulate UTI risk independently.

d. Vaginal estrogen can prevent recurrent UTIs and these effects are immediate.

e. The effects of vaginal estrogen on recurrent UTI risk are related to modulation of local pH and vaginal microflora.

47. Which of the following is not a risk factor for UTI in a renal transplant recipient?

a. Cadaveric graft

b. Diabetes

c. Prolonged hemodialysis prior to transplant

d. Female gender

e. Polycystic native kidneys

48. Prophylaxis for endocarditis should be administered in patients with:

a. a history of childhood heart murmurs.

b. heart valves inserted more than 5 years ago.

c. calcified heart valves associated with a murmur.

d. all synthetic heart valves.

e. cadaveric heart valves.

f. none of the above.

49. Antimicrobial prophylaxis is characterized as:

a. administration of an antimicrobial agent within 4 to 6 hours of the procedure.

b. administration of an antimicrobial agent for a period of time covering the first 48 hours after the procedure.

c. administration of an antimicrobial agent within 30 minutes of the initiation of a procedure and for a period of time covering the first 48 hours after the procedure.

d. administration of an antimicrobial agent within 60 to 120 minutes of the initiation of a procedure and for a period of time that covers the duration of the procedure.

e. administration of an antimicrobial agent the night before the initiation of a procedure and for a period of time that covers the duration of the procedure.

50. Which of the following organisms is NOT associated with positive nitrites on urine analysis?

a. *Enterococcus*

b. *E. coli*

c. *Proteus mirabilis*

d. *Klebsiella pneumoniae*

51. All of the following are important factors to consider in a patient's ability to give a noncontaminated midstream urine sample except:

a. Vaginal atrophy

b. Poor manual dexterity

c. History of human papilloma virus (HPV)

d. Inability to weight beat

e. Presence of a vaginal pessary

52. Which of the following is least relevant to history-taking when interviewing a patient with recurrent UTIs?

a. Family history of postmenopausal UTIs

b. Spermicide use

c. Childhood voiding dysfunction

d. History of urologic surgery

e. Past urinary pathogens and antibiotics

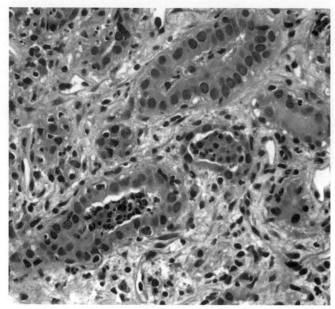

Fig. 55.1

PATHOLOGY

1. See Fig. 55.1. A 65-year-old woman has the acute onset of right flank pain, fever, and an enlarged kidney on imaging. Blood cultures and urine cultures are obtained and broad-spectrum antibiotics administered. The patient improves, but the kidney on imaging remains enlarged. A needle biopsy of the kidney is obtained. The pathology report is acute pyelonephritis with numerous neutrophils within the interstitium and the renal tubules. The biopsy:

a. provides information as to the length of time antibiotics should be administered.

b. suggests that the antibiotics should be changed.

c. is unnecessary.

d. suggests the need for a percutaneous drain.

e. suggests that an abscess is likely to develop.

2. A 65-year-old man has fever and malaise. A CT scan reveals an 8-cm solid mass in his left kidney with marked thickening of the retroperitoneum around the kidney and pancreas. The kidney is poorly functioning and there is a 1-cm stone in the renal pelvis. A biopsy is done and reveals xanthogranulomatous pyelonephritis, which is depicted in Fig. 55.2. The next step in management is:

a. extracorporeal shockwave lithotripsy.

b. biopsy of the retroperitoneum.

c. left nephrectomy.

d. urine culture and treatment according to sensitivities.

e. partial left nephrectomy

3. A 45-year-old woman is found to have a raised bladder lesion on cystoscopy. The biopsy shown in Fig. 55.3 reveals malakoplakia. The next step in management is:

a. intravesical bacille Calmette-Guérin.

b. fulguration of the lesions.

c. intravesical mitomycin C.

d. treat with a sulfonamide for several months.

e. a 3-day course of ciprofloxacin.

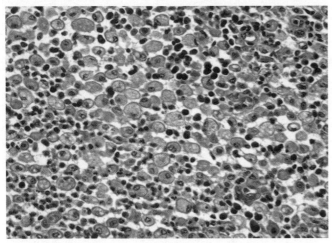

Fig. 55.2

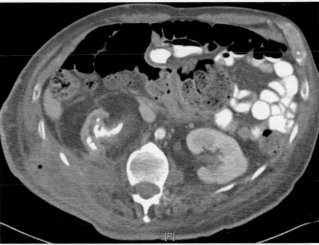

Fig. 55.4

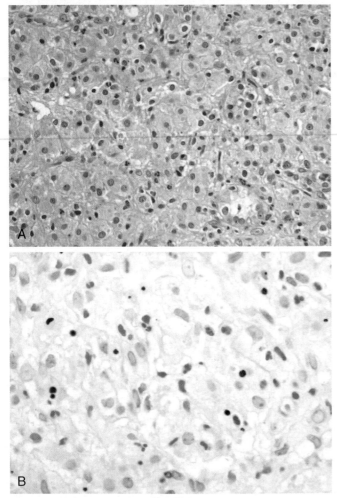

Fig. 55.3

IMAGING

1. A 72-year-old man presents with right flank pain and fever. A contrast-enhanced CT scan is shown in Fig. 55.4. The most likely diagnosis is:

   a. acute right renal obstruction.

   b. delayed excretion in left kidney.

   c. cellulitis in right flank.

   d. right perinephric abscess.

   e. xanthogranulomatous pyelonephritis.

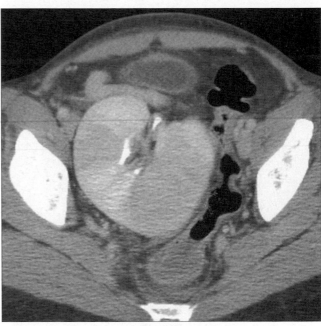

Fig. 55.5

2. A 40-year-old woman presents with pelvic pain and fever. A contrast-enhanced CT scan is shown in Fig. 55.5. The most likely diagnosis is:

   a. renal infarct.

   b. renal artery occlusion.

   c. chronic pyelonephritis.

   d. acute urinary obstruction.

   e. acute pyelonephritis.

3. A 22-year-old woman presents with shaking chills and fever. An enhanced CT image is shown in Fig. 55.6. The next step in management is:

   a. percutaneous drainage.

   b. nephrectomy.

   c. partial nephrectomy.

   d. open surgical drainage.

   e. cystoscopy and retrograde urography.

4. A 68-year-old diabetic woman presents to the emergency room with the chief complaint of abdominal pain. CT scan findings of her

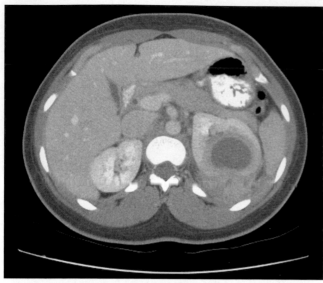

Fig. 55.6

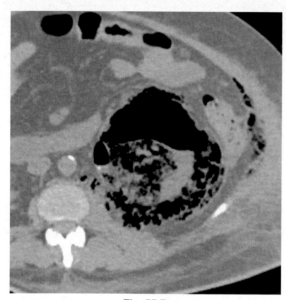

Fig. 55.7

pelvis are shown in Fig. 55.7. The next step in her management is:

a. inpatient antibiotics, Foley catheter placement, and glucose management
b. collection of a urine sample and discharge home with empiric antibiotic coverage
c. emergent exploration and surgical debridement with placement of a suprapubic tube
d. obtain an ultrasound to assess the upper urinary tract
e. reassurance

ANSWERS

1. **a. Chills, fever, and flank pain.** Acute pyelonephritis is a clinical syndrome of chills, fever, and flank pain that is accompanied by bacteriuria and pyuria, a combination that is reasonably specific for an acute bacterial infection of the kidney.
2. **b. Colonization.** Bacteriuria without pyuria is generally indicative of bacterial colonization without infection of the urinary tract.
3. **a. Occur in patients who are hospitalized or institutionalized.** Nosocomial or health care–associated UTIs occur in patients who are hospitalized or institutionalized and may be caused by *Pseudomonas* and other more antimicrobial-resistant strains.

4. **b. Reinfections.** Recurrent infections are hypothesized to be secondary to either bacterial persistence within the urinary tract or, more commonly, novel reinfection. Persistence, caused by the same bacterial strain, usually leads to recurrent infections in a short time frame, whereas reinfections generally occur over a more remote period. Reinfection is likely secondary to ascent of uropathogens from fecal flora into the urinary tract or from reemergence of bacteria from uroepithelial intracellular colonies.
5. **d. Antimicrobial treatment.** Whether a patient receives no treatment or short-term, long-term, or prophylactic antimicrobial treatment, the risk of recurrent bacteriuria remains the same; antimicrobial treatment appears to alter only the time until recurrence.
6. **e. Minimal.** The long-term effects of uncomplicated recurrent UTIs are not completely known, but so far, **no association between recurrent infections and renal scarring, hypertension, or progressive renal azotemia** has been established.
7. **e. Frequent voiding.** This route is further enhanced in individuals with significant soilage of the perineum with feces, women using spermicidal agents, and patients with intermittent or indwelling catheters.
8. **b. *Staphylococcus saprophyticus*.** *S. saprophyticus* is recognized as causing frequent symptomatic UTIs in young, sexually active females, whereas it rarely causes infection in males and elderly individuals.
9. **c. Pili.** Studies have demonstrated that interactions between FimH and receptors expressed on the luminal surface of the bladder epithelium are critical to the ability of many uropathogenic *E. coli* strains to colonize the bladder and cause disease.
10. **b. Affects bacterial virulence.** This process is called *phase variation* and has obvious biologic and clinical implications. For example, the presence of type 1 pili may be advantageous to the bacteria for adhering to and colonizing the bladder mucosa but disadvantageous because the pili enhance phagocytosis and killing by neutrophils.
11. **a. Increased adherence of bacteria to vaginal cells.** These studies established increased adherence of pathogenic bacteria to vaginal epithelial cells as the first demonstrable biologic difference that could be shown in women susceptible to UTI.
12. **c. Voiding.** Bacteria presumably make their way into the bladder fairly often. Whether small inocula of bacteria persist, multiply, and infect the host depends in part on the ability of the bladder to empty.
13. **c. Obstruction.** A patient who suffers from an acute ureteral obstruction caused by a sloughed papilla and who has a concomitant UTI should have the condition treated as a urologic emergency.
14. **a. Spinal cord injuries.** Of all patients with bacteriuria, no group compares in severity and morbidity with those who have spinal cord injury.
15. **a. Squamous epithelial cells.** The validation of the midstream urine specimen can be questioned if numerous squamous epithelial cells (indicative of preputial, vaginal, or urethral contaminants) are present.
16. **a. Women.** Imaging and cystoscopic evaluation are not warranted in all women with recurrent UTIs. Indeed, the yield of imaging in women without suspected complicated UTI is low and is not recommended by the American College of Radiology, the Canadian Urological Association Guidelines, or the European Association of Urology Guidelines. However, in women with risk factors for a complicated UTI the evaluation should include imaging and cystoscopy.
17. **e. CT.** CT and magnetic resonance imaging are more sensitive than excretory urography or ultrasonography in the diagnosis of acute focal bacterial nephritis, renal and perirenal abscesses, and radiolucent calculi.
18. **c. Urine level.** Efficacy of the antimicrobial therapy is critically dependent on the antimicrobial levels in the urine and the length of time that this level remains above the minimum inhibitory concentration of the infecting organism. Thus resolution of infection is closely associated with the susceptibility of the bacteria to the concentration of the antimicrobial agent achieved in the urine.

19. **e. Nitrofurantoin.** According to the Infectious Diseases Society of America 2010 update, nitrofurantoin 100 mg twice daily for 5 days or Bactrim DS twice daily for 3 days should be preferential regimens for the treatment of uncomplicated UTIs in women. Sensitivity to these agents should be confirmed on urine culture, especially if the patient does not report a resolution of symptoms at the end of their course.

20. **d. Indwelling orthopedic pins.** Bacterial seeding of implanted orthopedic hardware is a rare but morbid event. A joint commission of the American Urological Association, the American Academy of Orthopaedic Surgeons, and infectious disease specialists convened in 2003 and released an advisory statement on antibiotic prophylaxis for urologic patients with total joint replacement. In general, antimicrobial prophylaxis for urologic patients with total joint replacements, pins, plates, or screws is not indicated. Prophylaxis is advised for individuals at higher risk of seeding a prosthetic joint and include those with recently inserted implants (within 2 years).

21. **b. 3 days.** According to IDSA guidelines, a 3-day therapy is the preferred regimen for uncomplicated cystitis in women.

22. **c. Pregnant.** In populations other than those for whom treatment has been documented to be beneficial (e.g., pregnant women and patients undergoing urologic interventions), screening for or treatment of asymptomatic bacteriuria is not appropriate and should be strongly discouraged.

23. **a. Pregnant women.** In populations other than those for whom treatment has been documented to be beneficial (e.g., pregnant women and patients undergoing urologic interventions), screening for or treatment of asymptomatic bacteriuria is not appropriate and should be discouraged.

24. **e. Initial bacterial resistance.** Most commonly, the bacteria are resistant to the antimicrobial agent selected to treat the infection.

25. **a. Urine.** Nitrofurantoin, which does not alter the bowel flora, is present for brief periods at high concentrations in the urine and leads to repeated elimination of bacteria from the urine, presumably by interfering with bacterial initiation of infection.

26. **b. P-piliated bacteria.** If vesicourethral reflux is absent, a patient bearing the P blood group phenotype may have special susceptibility to recurrent pyelonephritis caused by *E. coli* that have P pili and bind to the P blood group antigen receptors.

27. **b. Cephalexin.** Macrobid is concentrated in the urine and cannot treat blood-borne infections. Amoxicillin has been used to treat cystitis in pregnancy but does not have broad enough gram-negative coverage for the treatment of pyelonephritis. Levofloxacin is contraindicated in pregnancy due to possible damage to fetal cartilage, and trimethoprim should be avoided in pregnancy because it may cause fetal megaloblastic anemia, and, in the first trimester, neural tube and cardiovascular defects by inhibiting folic acid metabolism.

28. **a. Observation.** Even though the urine usually becomes sterile within a few hours of starting antimicrobial therapy, patients with acute uncomplicated pyelonephritis may continue to have fever, chills, and flank pain for several more days after initiation of successful antimicrobial therapy. They should be observed.

29. **d. Diabetic adults.** Emphysematous pyelonephritis predominantly affects female diabetics and can occur in insulin-dependent and non-insulin-dependent patients in the absence of ureteral obstruction. Nondiabetic patients can also develop this form of pyelonephritis but often have ureteric obstruction and do not seem to develop extensive disease

30. **d. Percutaneous drainage.** Although surgical drainage, or nephrectomy if the kidney is nonfunctioning or severely infected, is the classic treatment for perinephric abscesses, renal ultrasonography and CT make percutaneous aspiration and drainage of small perirenal collections possible.

31. **e. No symptoms.** There are no symptoms of chronic pyelonephritis until it produces renal insufficiency, and then the symptoms are similar to those of any other form of chronic renal failure.

32. **d. *Proteus mirabilis*.** Although review of the literature shows *Proteus* to be the most common organism involved with xanthogranulomatous pyelonephritis, *E. coli* is also common.

33. **b. Malacoplakia.** Malacoplakia, from the Greek word meaning "soft plaque," is an unusual inflammatory disease that was originally described to affect the bladder. It is an inflammatory lesion described originally by Michaelis and Gutmann 1902. It was characterized by von Hansemann 1903 as soft, yellow-brown plaques with granulomatous lesions in which the histiocytes contain distinct basophilic lysosomal inclusion bodies or Michaelis-Gutmann bodies. Although its exact pathogenesis is unknown, malacoplakia probably results from abnormal macrophage function in response to a bacterial infection, which is most often E. coli.

34. **d. Surgical removal of the hydatid cyst.** Surgery remains the mainstay of treatment of renal echinococcosis. The cyst should be removed without rupture to reduce the chance of seeding, antigen reaction, and recurrence. If the cyst ruptures or cannot be removed and marsupialization is required, the contents of the cyst initially should be aspirated and filled with a scolicidal agent.

35. **c. Hyperventilation.** Even before temperature extremes and the onset of chills, bacteremic patients often begin to hyperventilate. Thus the earliest metabolic change in septicemia is a resultant respiratory alkalosis.

36. **c. Acute pyelonephritis.** Pyelonephritis develops in 1% to 4% of all pregnant women and in 20% to 40% of pregnant women with untreated bacteriuria.

37. **a. Maternal sepsis.** Pregnant women with asymptomatic bacteriuria are at higher risk for developing a symptomatic UTI that results in adverse fetal sequelae, complications associated with bacteriuria during pregnancy, and pyelonephritis and its possible sequelae, such as sepsis in the mother. Therefore all women with asymptomatic bacteriuria should be treated.

38. **d. Penicillin.** The aminopenicillins and cephalosporins are considered safe and generally effective throughout pregnancy. In patients with penicillin allergy, nitrofurantoin is a reasonable alternative.

39. **a. Asymptomatic.** Most elderly patients with bacteriuria are asymptomatic.

40. **e. Is unnecessary.** Prospective randomized comparative trials of antimicrobial or no therapy in elderly male and female nursing home residents with asymptomatic bacteriuria consistently document no benefit of antimicrobial therapy. There was no decrease in symptomatic episodes and no improvement in survival. In fact, treatment with antimicrobial therapy increases the occurrence of adverse drug effects and reinfection with resistant organisms and increases the cost of treatment. Therefore asymptomatic bacteriuria in elderly residents of long-term care facilities should not be treated with antimicrobial agents.

41. **f. None of the above.** The American Heart Association's recommendations on the prevention of bacterial endocarditis are based on the patient's risk of developing endocarditis and the likelihood that a procedure will cause bacteremia with an organism that can cause endocarditis. Antibiotic prophylaxis solely for the prevention of infectious endocarditis is not recommended for GU procedures, even in the setting of high-risk patients including individuals with prosthetic heart valves, previous bacterial endocarditis, cyanotic congenital heart disease, and systemic-pulmonary shunts or conduits.

42. **d. Catheterization.** Catheter-associated bacteriuria is the most common hospital acquired infection.

43. **a. Closed drainage.** Careful aseptic insertion of the catheter and maintenance of a closed dependent drainage system are essential to minimize development of bacteriuria.

44. **a. Clean intermittent catheterization (CIC).** Although never rigorously compared with indwelling urethral catheterization, CIC has been shown to decrease lower urinary tract complications by maintaining low intravesical pressure and reducing the incidence of stones.

45. **a. Obesity.** An association between Fournier gangrene and urethral obstruction associated with strictures and extravasation and instrumentation has been well documented. Predisposing factors include diabetes mellitus, local trauma, paraphimosis,

periurethral extravasation of urine, perirectal or perianal infections, and surgery such as circumcision or herniorrhaphy.

46. **e. The effects of vaginal estrogen on recurrent UTI risk are related to modulation of local pH and vaginal microflora.** Randomized controlled trials of vaginal estrogen use have not been designed to analyze outcomes such as cancer or cardiovascular disease. However, observational studies have found no increased risk of fracture or breast cancer in women who used vaginal estrogen. Vaginal estrogen is effective in preventing recurrent UTIs in postmenopausal women through lowering the vaginal pH and restoring the normal microenvironment such as lactobacilli. The beneficial effect from vaginal estrogen use can take at least 12 weeks to manifest.

47. **e. Polycystic native kidneys.** Transplant recipients are at higher risk for vesicoureteral reflux. Risk factors for infection include cadaveric graft, diabetes, prolonged hemodialysis prior to transplantation, two episodes of asymptomatic bacteriuria, and female gender.

48. **f. None of the above.** The American Heart Association's recommendations on the prevention of bacterial endocarditis are based on the patient's risk of developing endocarditis and the likelihood that a procedure will cause bacteremia with an organism that can cause endocarditis. Antibiotic prophylaxis solely for the prevention of infectious endocarditis is not recommended for GU procedures, even in the setting of high-risk patients including individuals with prosthetic heart valves, previous bacterial endocarditis, cyanotic congenital heart disease, and systemic-pulmonary shunts or conduits.

49. **d. Administration of an antimicrobial agent within 60 to 120 minutes of the initiation of a procedure and for a period of time that covers the duration of the procedure.** Surgical antimicrobial prophylaxis entails treatment with an antimicrobial agent before and for a limited time after a procedure to prevent local or systemic postprocedural infections.

50. **a. *Enterococcus.*** Most gram-negative bacteria are capable of producing positive results on a nitrite test. Pseudomonas aeruginosa and most gram-positive organisms do not produce nitrites.

51. **c. History of human papilloma virus (HPV).** HPV history does not impact ability to provide an adequate sample; the other variables are important influencing factors and a catheterized urine sample should be considered in these situations.

52. **a. Family history of postmenopausal UTIs.** Family history of postmenopausal UTIs is least relevant to the patient's immediate evaluation; the other variables list individual behaviors, infection history, and anatomic factors that can have a direct impact on the patient's ongoing UTI diathesis. Family history of UTIs in childhood or young adulthood bears more relevance regarding structural issues (such as vesicoureteral reflux) or genetic risk factors for recurrent infections.

PATHOLOGY

1. **c. Is unnecessary.** The figure shows numerous neutrophils within the interstitium and the renal tubules. The neutrophils in the tubules become white blood cell casts. The pathologic findings including an enlarged kidney may persist for several weeks despite appropriate treatment. There is no indication for a biopsy in this patient.

2. **c. Left nephrectomy.** The figure shows the foamy macrophages with neutrophils and cellular debris characteristic of xanthogranulomatous pyelonephritis. It may be associated with renal calculi and *Proteus* infection. *E. coli* is also a common organism found in this disease. Although partial nephrectomy

has been performed for a small localized mass in a functioning kidney, a left nephrectomy in this situation is likely required and is necessary to rid the patient of the infection. An associated retroperitoneal inflammatory process with thickening is not uncommon.

3. **d. Treat with a sulfonamide for several months.** Fig. 55.3A shows von Hansemann histiocytes, and Fig. 55.3B demonstrates the Michaelis-Gutmann bodies, both of which are characteristic of malakoplakia. It is thought to be infectious in origin, and therefore the treatment is an extended course of an antibiotic that achieves a high intracellular concentration.

IMAGING

1. **d. Right perinephric abscess.** The CT scan is obtained in the late arterial to nephrographic phase of the examination (the aorta is still opacified with contrast agent), before the excretion of the contrast agent. Thus option b is incorrect. There are multiple calculi in the right kidney, which is small and atrophic, indicating a chronic process (thus option a is incorrect). There is thickening of the perinephric fascia, and gas bubbles are seen in the posterior paranephric space, extending to the right flank. In addition, there are fluid collections in the posterior paranephric space and in the soft tissues of the right flank, making option d the most likely diagnosis. Xanthogranulomatous pyelonephritis is a chronic inflammatory condition associated with staghorn calculi. The affected kidney is usually enlarged rather than shrunken, as is the case here (making option e unlikely).

2. **e. Acute pyelonephritis.** The image demonstrates a pelvic kidney with wedge-shaped area of decreased enhancement, characteristic of acute pyelonephritis. Renal infarcts cause areas of poor perfusion that are more sharply defined and more poorly enhancing than in the present case (making option a unlikely). The clinical history of fever also supports an infection. With renal artery occlusion (option b) the kidney would demonstrate no enhancement. Chronic pyelonephritis causes scarring in the kidney, and the nephrogram is usually normal. The renal contour in the present case is smooth, making option c unlikely. Acute urinary obstruction (option d) is ruled out because the visualized collecting system does not appear dilated.

3. **a. Percutaneous drainage.** The image demonstrates a low-attenuation area in the posterior interpolar region of the left kidney, with perinephric fascial thickening, consistent with a renal abscess. Intravenous antimicrobial therapy with percutaneous drainage of renal abscesses is highly effective and is the treatment of choice. Antimicrobial therapy alone is unlikely to be effective, given the size of the abscess. Nephrectomy, partial nephrectomy, and surgical drainage are rarely indicated in young patients with normally functioning kidneys. Cystoscopy is not warranted.

4. **a. Inpatient antibiotics, Foley catheter placement, and glucose management.** The figure is an example of emphysematous pyelonephritis. The majority (90%) of these patients are treated with medical therapy alone, which consists of antibiotics (often parenteral), bladder drainage, and treatment of comorbid conditions such as poorly controlled diabetes. The need for surgical intervention is rare and is reserved for those cases that respond poorly to initial medical management or severe necrotizing infections.

1. Bacteriuria and pyuria are not synonymous with a UTI.
2. UTIs are classified based on their presumed site of origin.
3. UTIs can be uncomplicated (occurring in healthy patients with normal urinary tracts) or complicated (associated with factors that increase the likelihood of bacteriuria and decrease the efficacy of therapy).
4. UTIs are the most common bacterial infection, and, as such, make a significant impact on healthcare costs.
5. The incidence of bacteriuria increases with institutionalization/hospitalization as well as with pregnancy and certain comorbidities that alter lower urinary tract function or cause immunosuppression.
6. To date, no clear association has been described between recurrent uncomplicated UTIs and renal sequelae such as scarring, hypertension, or progressive renal insufficiency.
7. Most UTIs are caused by bacteria, usually originating from the bowel flora.
8. Bacterial virulence factors, including adhesin, play a role in determining which bacteria invade and the extent of infection.
9. Increased epithelial cell receptivity predisposes patients to recurrent UTIs and is a genotypic trait.
10. Obstruction to urine flow is a key factor in increasing host susceptibility to UTIs.
11. Clinical presentation is critically important in considering diagnosis; results of urine testing cannot be analyzed without knowledge of signs and symptoms.
12. Urine must be collected in a manner that minimizes contamination.
13. Formal urinalysis is preferred over dipstick testing.
14. Urine culture results provide bacterial sensitivities.
15. Urine is not sterile.
16. The female urinary microbiome has been identified using RNA sequencing techniques, and knowledge of these microbiota should inform UTI management and interpretation of novel culture techniques such as the expanded quantitative urine culture (EQUC) protocol.
17. The prevalence of asymptomatic bacteriuria varies with age, sex, and comorbid conditions.
18. Untreated asymptomatic bacteriuria is not associated with hypertension or renal insufficiency.
19. Several guidelines recommend not screening for or treating asymptomatic bacteriuria except in specific patient populations.
20. Treatment of asymptomatic bacteriuria contributes to development of multi-drug resistant symptomatic UTIs.
21. Antimicrobial resistance is increasing because of excessive utilization.
22. Antimicrobial selection should be influenced by efficacy, safety, cost, and compliance.
23. Both the choice of the agent as well as the duration of therapy are critical in preventing the perpetuation of antimicrobial resistance as well as adverse events related to treatment.
24. Obtaining a thorough history, with emphasis on prior symptoms, urinalysis and culture results, and triggers for infections, is critical.
25. Sources of possible bacterial persistence must be identified and eradicated.
26. Imaging and cystoscopy are NOT recommended for recurrent uncomplicated UTIs.
27. Prevention of recurrence should focus on non-antibiotic interventions.
28. Acute pyelonephritis classically presents as the abrupt onset of chills, fever, and flank or costovertebral angle tenderness but can present as symptoms as mild as cystitis or as severe as sepsis.
29. Emphysematous pyelonephritis is a life-threatening infection diagnosed radiographically by the presence of gas in the parenchyma or collecting system and can be managed via percutaneous drainage or surgically.
30. Renal abscesses are well delineated by CT and are classically managed with IV antimicrobial agents and drainage. Smaller abscesses may be amenable to conservative treatment with medical management.
31. Pyonephrosis is a bacterial infection in a hydronephrotic kidney. Prompt diagnosis is critical; treatment entails intravenous antimicrobial agents and drainage of the obstructed renal unit.
32. XGP is a chronic renal infection that is often found in poorly functioning renal units obstructed secondary to nephrolithiasis. XGP can be mistaken for renal tumors.
33. Malacoplakia is an unusual inflammatory disease thought to result from abnormal macrophage function. Michaelis-Gutmann bodies are lysosomal inclusion bodies that characterize this disease microscopically.
34. Fournier gangrene is necrotizing fasciitis arising from the perineal skin, scrotum, urethra, or rectum.
35. Emergent surgical debridement and broad-spectrum antimicrobial agents are the essentials of treatment of Fournier gangrene.
36. Periurethral abscess can occur secondarily to urethral stricture or catheterization; treatment entails surgical debridement, suprapubic urinary drainage, and antimicrobial agents.
37. Sepsis is a clinical syndrome characterized by extremes of body temperature, heart rate, respiratory rate, and WBC count that occurs in response to an infection.
38. The principles of management of sepsis include resuscitation, supportive care, monitoring, administration of broad-spectrum antimicrobial agents, and drainage or elimination of infection.
39. The surviving sepsis campaign and early goal-directed therapy has been shown to improve outcomes in critically ill patients.
40. Screening for bacteriuria via urine culture should be performed in all pregnant women during the first trimester.
41. The prevalence of bacteriuria does not change with the occurrence of pregnancy; however, unlike in non-pregnant women, spontaneous resolution of bacteriuria in pregnant women is unlikely.
42. All pregnant women with bacteriuria should be treated.
43. Bacteriuria more commonly progresses to acute pyelonephritis during pregnancy.
44. Screening for bacteriuria is not recommended in elderly patients because there is no relationship between asymptomatic bacteriuria and uncomplicated UTIs and deteriorating renal function; asymptomatic bacteriuria should not be treated.
45. Infections of the urinary tract may present as subtle signs, and a high index of suspicion is often required for diagnosis.
46. Careful aseptic insertion of the catheter and maintenance of a closed, dependent drainage system are essential to minimize development of bacteriuria.
47. The development of catheter-associated bacteriuria is inevitable. Only symptomatic catheter-associated UTIs require treatment.
48. The majority of spinal cord–injured patients with bacteriuria are asymptomatic. Only symptomatic patients require therapy.
49. UTI in patients with spinal cord injury commonly presents as fever; flank, back, or abdominal discomfort; leakage between catheterizations; increased spasticity; malaise; lethargy; and/or cloudy, malodorous urine.
50. Urine culture before the initiation of empirical therapy is essential because spinal cord–injured patients often culture diverse flora with a high probability of bacterial resistance.
51. Clean intermittent catheterization places patients with spinal cord injury at the lowest risk for significant long-term urinary tract complications.
52. Antimicrobial prophylaxis entails treatment with an antimicrobial agent before and for a limited time after a procedure to prevent local or systemic postprocedural infections.
53. The type of procedure and competency of the host defenses determine the need for antimicrobial prophylaxis.
54. Special considerations for antimicrobial prophylaxis include patients undergoing TRUS-Bx, those with a risk of endocarditis and bacteriuria, and patients with indwelling orthopedic hardware.

56

Inflammatory and Pain Conditions of the Male Genitourinary Tract: Prostatitis and Related Pain Conditions, Orchitis, and Epididymitis

Michel Pontari

QUESTIONS

1. A man with chronic pelvic pain has a negative urine culture and no evidence of inflammation on expressed prostatic secretions (EPS) or VB3 or in his seminal plasma. What is his category of prostatitis in the NIH classification?
   a. Category I
   b. Category II
   c. Category IIIA
   d. Category IIIB
   e. Category IV

2. A 65-year-old male undergoes a transrectal ultrasound-guided biopsy for an elevated PSA. He has no pelvic pain. Biopsy shows no cancer, but he does have many areas of prostate inflammation. What is his NIH prostatitis category?
   a. Category I
   b. Category II
   c. Category IIIA
   d. Category IIIB
   e. Category IV

3. A 58-year-old male with a history of autoimmune pancreatitis presents urinary retention. He is refractory to medical therapy for benign prostatic hyperplasia (BPH), and a transurethral resection of the prostate (TURP) is planned. What type of histology may be expected from the prostate resection?
   a. No inflammation
   b. Granulomatous prostatitis
   c. Scant periglandular mononuclear infiltrate
   d. Heavy intraductal lymphocytic infiltrate
   e. Immunoglobulin G4 (IgG4)-positive plasma cells and fibrosis

4. What is the most common causative organism in patients with category I acute bacterial prostatitis that develops after lower urinary tract manipulation?
   a. *Escherichia coli*
   b. *Pseudomonas*
   c. *Proteus*
   d. *Klebsiella*
   e. *Enterococcus*

5. A man presents after transrectal prostate biopsy with a fever of 102°F, rigors, and many white blood cells and bacteria in the urine. Which antibiotic is the best choice for initial therapy until urine and blood culture results are available?
   a. Ciprofloxacin
   b. Levofloxacin
   c. Trimethoprim-sulfamethoxazole
   d. Cefpodoxime
   e. Meropenem

6. A 35-year-old human immunodeficiency virus (HIV)-positive man presents with fever, dysuria, and leukocytosis. Imaging reveals a 0.9-cm hypoechoic area in the prostate consistent with a prostate abscess. Initial management for this patient is:
   a. intravenous (IV) antibiotics
   b. prostate massage to help drain the abscess
   c. percutaneous aspiration
   d. transurethral resection
   e. open perineal drainage

7. A 41-year-old male presents with his second urinary tract infection in the past 4 months. He is growing the same *E. coli* as his previous culture. Evaluation should include:
   a. computed tomography (CT) urogram
   b. uroflow and postvoid residual urine to rule out retention
   c. cystoscopy
   d. four-glass urine test
   e. nuclear amplification test for gonorrhea and chlamydia

8. What is the relationship between inflammation (white blood cells [WBCs]) found in expressed prostatic fluid and symptoms in men with chronic pelvic pain syndrome?
   a. Greater WBCs in men with predominantly voiding symptoms plus pelvic pain
   b. Inverse correlation between WBCs and symptoms
   c. Direct correlation between WBCs and symptoms
   d. No correlation between WBCs and symptoms
   e. Greater WBCs only in men with prior history of acute prostatitis

9. What psychological factor is correlated with overall pain along with urinary symptoms and depression in men with chronic prostatitis/chronic pelvic pain syndrome (CP/CPPS)?
   a. Neuroticism **START**
   b. Obsessive compulsive disorder
   c. Anger
   d. Catastrophizing
   e. Insecurity

10. What is the most common overlapping pain condition (COPC) in men with CP/CPPS?
    a. Fibromyalgia
    b. Chronic fatigue syndrome
    c. Irritable bowel syndrome (IBS)
    d. Temporomandibular joint disorder
    e. Tinnitus

11. In a case-crossover study in the NIH Multidisciplinary Approach to Pelvic Pain (MAPP) study, what correlated with development of symptom flares?
    a. Psychological stress
    b. Caffeine
    c. Alcohol
    d. Recent sexual activity
    e. Physical activity

12. Compared with age-matched controls, men with CP/CPPS have a greater prevalence of which of the following?
    a. BPH
    b. Urinary incontinence
    c. Premature ejaculation
    d. Condyloma
    e. Phimosis

13. The NIH–Chronic Prostatitis Symptom Index (NIH-CPSI) score has been used in many trials as an outcome measure for treatment of CP/CPPS. It is also used for diagnosis and epidemiologic studies. The Genitourinary Problem Index (GUPI) is a modified version that better reflects what symptoms found in men with CP/CPPS but not part of the NIH-CPSI?
    a. Penile pain
    b. Epididymal pain
    c. Scrotal skin pain
    d. Back pain
    e. Pain with bladder filling

14. Which of the following is an optional study in the evaluation of men with CP/CPPS?
    a. Symptom assessment
    b. Midstream urine for urinalysis and culture
    c. Abdominal exam
    d. Examination of pelvic floor tender points
    e. Cystoscopy

15. On electromyography (EMG) study during urodynamics, a man with pelvic pain, poor stream, and pain with sitting has retained electrical activity of the external sphincter during voiding. He is grossly neurologically intact. What is his diagnosis?
    a. Detrusor underactivity
    b. Upper motor neuron lesion
    c. Pseudodyssynergy
    d. Urethralis fugax
    e. Detrusor overactivity

16. In meta-analyses of treatments for CP/CPPS, which combinations of therapy show the best results?
    a. Antiinflammatory medications and α-blockers
    b. Antibiotics and α-blockers
    c. 5α-reductase inhibitors and α-blockers
    d. Skeletal muscle relaxants and antiinflammatory medications
    e. Antibiotics and 5α-reductase inhibitors

17. A 38-year-old male presents with a 4-month history of pelvic pain. Urine cultures are negative. He has some generalized increase in anxiety. On exam, he has significant increase in tone of the pelvic floor muscles around the prostate, especially the obturator internus. Management should consist of stress reduction and which of the following?
    a. Referral to a psychiatrist
    b. Oral valium

c. Microwave thermotherapy
    d. Pelvic floor physical therapy
    e. Injection of onabotulinumtoxinA into the perineal body

18. A 65-year-old male undergoes prostate biopsy for an elevated PSA of 5.4. Pathology reveals extensive glandular and periglandular inflammation with both acute and chronic inflammation. The best next step is:
    a. 4-week course of antiinflammatory medications.
    b. start finasteride.
    c. 4-week course of antibiotics and then reassess.
    d. observation.
    e. repeat biopsy.

19. UPOINT is a phenotyping tool that captures multiple aspects of symptoms and finding in men with CPPS. What does the "N" stand for in UPOINT?
    a. Nonbacterial
    b. Noninflammatory
    c. Neurologic
    d. Normal prostate exam
    e. Normotensive

20. Autoimmune orchitis is characterized by the presence of:
    a. antisperm antibodies (ASAs)
    b. antisperm granulomas
    c. testicular microinfarcts
    d. microlithiasis
    e. antilipid antibodies

21. A 25-year-old male presents with the acute onset of left epididymal pain. The left epididymis is tender to palpation and swollen. There are 1 to 3 WBCs per high-power field on urinalysis. He is afebrile. He denies being sexually active. The most likely cause for his acute epididymitis is:
    a. E. coli
    b. Pseudomonas
    c. Proteus
    d. Brucellosis
    e. Chlamydia

22. A 39-year-old male has had chronic orchialgia for 1 year. He has failed a course of antibiotics and antiinflammatory medications. He has no other medical conditions and no back pain. On examination his right testis is mildly tender. On digital rectal exam he has minimal prostate tenderness but has tenderness to the right obturator internus muscle. The next best step in treatment is:
    a. gabapentin
    b. pregabalin
    c. pelvic floor physical therapy
    d. microsurgical denervation of the right spermatic cord
    e. referral to pain management

23. Which area is part of the so-called trifecta nerve complex that should be addressed in microsurgical denervation of the spermatic cord for chronic scrotal pain?
    a. Epididymal tail
    b. Cremasteric muscle fibers
    c. Rete testis
    d. Epididymal tail
    e. Testicular artery

24. What technique has been noted to increase the success rate of epididymectomy performed for post vasectomy pain syndrome?
    a. Ligation of surrounding lymphatics
    b. Ligation of the spermatic veins
    c. Preservation of surrounding lymphatics
    d. Incorporation of the distal portion of the vasectomy site
    e. Inguinal approach

25. What technique has been reported to increase the success rate of orchiectomy for chronic scrotal pain?
    a. Ligation of surrounding lymphatics
    b. Ligation of the spermatic veins
    c. Preservation of surrounding lymphatics
    d. Scrotal approach
    e. Inguinal approach

ANSWERS

1. **d. Category IIIB.** TheNIH classification is IIIB, chronic prostatitis chronic pelvic pain syndrome. He has no infection to suggest acute or chronic bacterial prostatitis, and he is symptomatic and therefore not category IV. The absence of inflammatory cells separates the subclasses of IIA and IIIB. He has no inflammation on EPS, VB3, or seminal plasma and therefore is category IIIB.
2. **e. Category IV.** Category IV is asymptomatic inflammatory prostatitis. Asymptomatic means no symptoms of pelvic pain. This usually diagnosed on specimens taken for treatment of other problems such as BPH, prostate cancer, or infertility.
3. **e. Immunoglobulin G4 (IgG4)-positive plasma cells and fibrosis.** IgG4-positive plasma cells and a characteristic pattern of fibrosis are seen in IgG4 disease. First described in autoimmune pancreatitis, multiple previously described disorders including Ormond disease (retroperitoneal fibrosis) are currently considered to fall within this category. One of the characteristics of IgG4 disease is a dramatic response to corticosteroids.
4. **a. *Escherichia coli*.** Although *E. coli* is still the most commonly found organism in patients with acute bacterial prostatitis (ABP) after lower urinary tract manipulation, *Pseudomonas* is far more common in cases from manipulation compared with spontaneous or after transrectal prostate biopsy.
5. **e. Meropenem.** The Update of the American Urological Association White Paper on the prevention and treatment of complications after prostate biopsy recommends that patients who present with a fever after prostate biopsy should not be offered fluoroquinolones or trimethoprim-sulfamethoxazole. Management should consist of aggressive resuscitation and broad-spectrum antibiotic coverage—carbapenems, amikacin, or second- and third-generation cephalosporin (after urine and blood cultures).
6. **a. Intravenous (IV) antibiotics.** In men with prostate abscess, smaller lesions less than 1 to 2 cm can be treated conservatively with antibiotics. Larger lesions or lesions that do not respond to antibiotics can be treated with percutaneous aspiration or transurethral unroofing.
7. **b. Uroflow and postvoid residual urine to rule out retention.** In a man younger than 45 years, imaging is not usually helpful. A cystoscopy could be done if he has an elevated residual to rule out stricture if he has a decreased uroflow and elevated postvoid residual urine. The four-glass test is no longer routinely used for cases of suspected chronic bacterial prostatitis. The nuclear amplification test would be indicated if he had a urethral discharge.
8. **d. No correlation between WBCs and symptoms.** No correlation between WBCs and symptoms. In the Chronic Prostatitis Collaborative Research Network (CPCRN) study, men with no symptoms had equal amounts of inflammation in EPS as those with pelvic pain.
9. **d. Catastrophizing.** Helplessness and catastrophizing predict overall pain along with urinary symptoms and depression in men with CP/CPPS.
10. **c. Irritable bowel syndrome (IBS).** The most COPC is IBS. Men should be queried about signs and symptoms of bowel dysfunction such as constipation, diarrhea, and the relationship to pelvic pain to bowel movements. Referral to a gastroenterologist should be made if indicated.
11. **d. Recent sexual activity.** Only recent sexual activity and urinary tract infection (UTI)-like symptoms were predictive of flare. Items that did not predict a flare included diet, physical activity or sedentary behavior, stress, and constipation.
12. **c. Premature ejaculation.** Men with CP/CPPS are more likely to have ejaculatory pain and premature ejaculation.
13. **e. Pain with bladder filling.** The GUPI is a modified version that contains questions about bladder pain. These symptoms were found in approximately 40% of men in the NIH-sponsored MAPP study.
14. **e. Cystoscopy.** Cystoscopy is an optional study. Cystoscopy can be used in men with decreased uroflow and/or elevated postvoid residual urine to evaluate for urethral stricture. Cystoscopy should also be used in men who give a history of pain with bladder emptying and/or relieved by bladder emptying, suggestive of interstitial cystitis/bladder pain syndrome (IC/BPS) because in a small set of these patients, a Hunner ulcer is present which responds to fulguration or intralesional injections.
15. **c. Pseudodyssynergy.** Pseudodyssynergy is retained electrical activity of the external sphincter during voiding in the absence of abdominal straining, and/or brief and intermittent closing of the membranous urethra during voiding detected by electromyography, or fluoroscopy in videourodynamics. These men are considered to have pelvic floor dysfunction.
16. **b. Antibiotics and α-blockers.** Meta-analyses have shown the best response for a combination of antibiotics and α-blockers.
17. **d. Pelvic floor physical therapy.** Although he has anxiety, the best treatment is addressing the increased pelvic floor tension by referral a physical therapist for pelvic floor physical therapy (PT).
18. **d. Observation.** No treatment for asymptomatic prostate inflammation (category IV) is necessary. Treatment with antibiotics is not indicated and should not be used to "treat" his elevated PSA to try to get it back to normal levels. He should be followed for his PSA elevation and have periodic repeat PSA and digital rectal examinations.
19. **c. Neurologic.** The N stands for Neurologic. This is for men with widespread pain conditions, with pain outside the pelvis, and overlapping conditions such as IBS, fibromyalgia, or chronic fatigue syndrome. They are thought to possibly have upregulation of the sensitivity of their central nervous system (centralization or central sensitization) and may respond to medications that treat neuropathic pain.
20. **a. Antisperm antibodies (ASAs).** Autoimmune orchitis is defined as an autoimmune aggression of the testes characterized by the presence of ASAs. Primary autoimmune orchitis is primarily a problem in the evaluation of male infertility. The main causes of secondary autoimmune orchitis are usually associated with a primary vasculitis, particularly Behçet disease, polyarteritis nodosa, and Henoch-Schönlein purpura.
21. **e. Chlamydia.** Sexually transmitted diseases and particularly chlamydia are the most common cause of acute epididymitis. Patient should be suspected of chlamydia even if they deny recent intercourse, because the infection does not always correlate with the reported sexual history.
22. **c. Pelvic floor physical therapy.** He has signs or history to suggest a centralized pain condition. Pelvic floor therapy is emerging as a treatment for chronic orchialgia. All conservative measures should be tried prior to undergoing surgery.

23. **b. Cremasteric muscle fibers.** Three areas identified by Parekatil et al. that had the highest areas of wallerian degeneration (WD) were the cremasteric muscle fibers, the perivasal sheath, and the posterior lipomatous tissue; these areas were called the trifecta nerve complex and is thought to form the anatomic basis for relief from the denervation procedure.

24. **d. Incorporation of the distal portion of the vasectomy site.** Better rates are reported in cases with incorporation of the distal portion of the vasectomy site with the epididymectomy specimen.

25. **e. Inguinal approach.** Better results have been reported with the inguinal approach to orchiectomy performed for chronic scrotal pain.

CHAPTER REVIEW

1. Men with category I acute prostatitis present with acute symptoms of dysuria and frequency and may have fever.
2. The most common causative organism is *E. coli*.
3. Types of bacteria and antibiotic sensitivities differ by etiology: spontaneous, after transurethral procedure, or after transrectal biopsy.
4. Men with acute prostatitis after transrectal biopsy should be treated with carbapenems, amikacin, or send and third-generation cephalosporins.
5. A suprapubic tube should be used if long-term drainage is needed.
6. Failure to respond to therapy should prompt imaging to look for a prostatic abscess.
7. Chronic bacterial prostatitis is characterized by recurrent urinary tract infections with the same organism
8. Unlike men with category III prostatitis/chronic pelvic pain syndrome, they are then relatively asymptomatic between episodes.
9. Urinary retention as a cause of recurrent UTI must be ruled out.
10. Men younger than 45 years do not need imaging but need assessment for a urethral stricture.
11. Treatment is with antibiotics that achieve adequate prostate concentrations
12. For refractory cases, daily suppressive antibiotics or TURP can be used.
13. Men with CP/CPPS have equal amounts of bacteria in urine, prostate fluid, and seminal plasma as men without pain.
14. There is evidence of central sensitization of the CNS in both afferent and efferent nerves.
15. In those with inflammation in VB3, EPS, or seminal plasma, the degree of inflammation does not correlate with symptoms.
16. Helplessness and catastrophizing predict overall pain along with urinary symptoms and depression.
17. Men with CPPS also have a lower baseline adrenocorticotropic hormone (ACTH) level and blunted ACTH rise in response to stress than men without symptoms.
18. Men CP/CPPS have increased pain sensitivity compared with controls.
19. CP/CPPS is a diagnosis of exclusion and should be made only after a thorough search for other causes of pelvic pain.
20. CP/CPPS has potential issues outside of the pelvis (and usual scope of urology) such as psychological issues and neurologic problems.
21. Patients with CP/CPPS must be assessed for other chronic pain syndrome such as IBS, fibromyalgia, and chronic fatigue syndrome.
22. Patients with tenderness on pelvis exam may benefit from pelvic floor physical therapy/myofascial release.
23. Therapy for CPPS is best done in a multimodal fashion; the symptom classification UPOINT can be helpful in directing evaluation and subsequently therapy.
24. Repeated courses of antibiotics in the absence of a positive urine culture are not indicated.
25. The best treatment combination from meta-analyses is antibiotics plus α-blockers.
26. Men with bladder pain should be considered for bladder-specific therapies.
27. Men with tenderness on pelvic floor exam should be referred for pelvic floor physical therapy.
28. Sacral neuromodulation can be used in men with pain who also have frequency and urgency.
29. Treatment is best undertaken as simultaneous multimodal therapy addressing all aspects of the patient's symptoms.
30. Viral orchitis is most commonly caused by the mumps virus.
31. For scrotal pain a duplex Doppler ultrasound should be performed to assess for anatomic or congenital abnormality, torsion, or mass.
32. Pelvic floor physical therapy should be considered in men with orchialgia and abnormal tone on digital rectal exam.
33. Acute epididymitis is more commonly caused by an STD in men younger than 35 years and enteric organism in men older than 35 years.
34. For microsurgical spermatic cord denervation (MSDC) three areas that should be addressed are the cremasteric muscle fibers, the perivasal sheath, and the posterior lipomatous tissue.
35. The distal vas deferens should be incorporated into the surgical specimen during an epididymectomy for postvasectomy pain syndrome.

57

Interstitial Cystitis/Bladder Pain Syndrome and Related Disorders

Robert M. Moldwin and Philip M. Hanno

QUESTIONS

1. Essential for the diagnosis of interstitial cystitis/bladder pain syndrome (IC/BPS) is the presence of:
   a. urinary urgency.
   b. pain or discomfort related to the bladder.
   c. glomerulations on cystoscopy.
   d. Hunner lesion (HL).
   e. urinary frequency.

2. The definition of IC proposed by the National Institute of Arthritis, Diabetes, Digestive and Kidney Diseases (NIDDK) is best considered a:
   a. de facto definition of the disease.
   b. diagnostic pathway.
   c. definition applicable mainly to clinical research studies.
   d. historic document of no current value.
   e. purely symptom-based description of IC/BPS.

3. A clinical factor that is more common in IC/BPS patients with HLs than in non-HL patients is:
   a. IC/BPS patients with HL typically present with a history of microscopic hematuria.
   b. IC/BPS patients with HL have a higher mean age.
   c. IC/BPS patients with HL present with higher visual analog scores (VAS) for pain than wnon-HL patients.
   d. Treatment pathways are identical for IC/BPS patients regardless of the presence or absence of HLs.
   e. IC/BPS patients with and without HLs are indistinguishable upon office cystoscopy.

4. IC/BPS symptom and problem indices have been validated to:
   a. monitor disease progression or regression with or without treatment.
   b. correctly choose who should undergo cystectomy and diversion.
   c. determine on whom to perform diagnostic testing.
   d. accurately diagnose IC/BPS.
   e. determine appropriate candidates for clinical research.

5. Which of the following statements best categorizes the natural history of IC/BPS?
   a. The onset is generally insidious and progressive, occurring gradually over many years.
   b. Loss of bladder capacity over time is the rule.
   c. Symptoms follow a culture-documented urinary tract infection.
   d. Symptom resolution regardless of treatment after 1 to 2 years.
   e. Although clinical presentation is usually subacute, many patients have prodromal symptoms that occur decades before a formal diagnosis.

6. Which statement best describes the relationship of IC/BPS to bladder cancer?
   a. IC/BPS is a premalignant lesion.
   b. IC/BPS is often associated with bladder cancer.
   c. A positive urine cytology can safely be ignored in patients with IC/BPS.
   d. The vast majority of reports fail to document an association of IC/BPS with subsequent development of bladder cancer.
   e. Dysplasia is a typical pathologic finding on bladder biopsy in IC/BPS patients.

7. American Urological Guidelines require the following for a diagnosis of IC/BPS:
   a. Pain or discomfort perceived to be related to the urinary bladder
   b. Age >18
   c. Urinary urgency
   d. Pelvic discomfort that worsens with bladder filling
   e. Presence of petechial submucosal hemorrhages upon short-duration low pressure (60 to 80 cm H_2O) hydrodistention

8. The antibiotic of choice for diagnosed IC/BPS is:
   a. doxycycline.
   b. none.
   c. gentamicin.
   d. ciprofloxacin.
   e. amoxicillin.

9. The cell *most likely* to play a central role in the pathogenesis of IC/BPS without HLs is the:
   a. granulocyte.
   b. lymphocyte.
   c. mast cell.
   d. platelet.
   e. eosinophil.

10. Which statement best categorizes the potassium chloride test?
    a. It is soothing and calming to the painful bladder.
    b. It has high sensitivity and specificity for diagnosing IC/BPS.
    c. It is an important element in choosing effective therapy.
    d. It provides proof of abnormal mucosal permeability.
    e. None of the above.

11. A circumscribed inflammatory bladder lesion:
    a. is required to make a diagnosis of IC/BPS.
    b. is generally found in less than 30% of IC/BPS patients.
    c. was not considered a part of the syndrome when it was initially described by Hunner.
    d. is synonymous with glomerulation.
    e. is pathognomonic of IC/BPS even in the absence of symptoms.

12. Exclusive use of the NIDDK criteria to diagnose IC/BPS would result in:
    a. an accurate depiction of the true prevalence of the condition.
    b. an improved treatment algorithm.
    c. increased diagnostic specificity.
    d. increased diagnostic sensitivity.
    e. a minimum of diagnostic testing and significant cost savings.

13. All but which of the following disorders have a much higher prevalence in the IC/BPS population than in the general population?
    a. Irritable bowel syndrome
    b. Diabetes
    c. Fibromyalgia
    d. Allergy
    e. Chronic fatigue syndrome

14. A 27-year-old female presents to you with a history consistent with IC/BPS, but she also reports gross hematuria, and cystoscopic exam shows severe inflammation of the bladder wall. Further evaluation needed includes:
    a. hydrodistention of bladder with fulguration of inflammatory disease.
    b. laparoscopy for diagnosis of endometrial implants.
    c. a history of recreational drug use.
    d. bladder biopsy for mast cell count.
    e. HgbA1C.

15. A 45-year-old female IC/BPS patient presents with deep dyspareunia, constipation dominant IBS, urinary hesitancy, and the need to strain with urination. Which therapy is the LEAST likely to be helpful?
    a. Physical therapy
    b. Behavioral modification
    c. Neuromodulation
    d. Chemodeinnervation of the bladder
    e. Skeletal muscle relaxants

16. The central role of histopathology in IC/BPS is to:
    a. determine whether or not the patient has an HL.
    b. help determine the most efficacious treatment modality.
    c. predict prognosis.
    d. rule out other disorders that might be responsible for the symptoms.
    e. confirm the diagnosis with pathologic criteria.

17. Which of the following has the least in common with IC/BPS?
    a. Vulvodynia
    b. Chronic bacterial prostatitis
    c. Orchialgia
    d. Penile pain
    e. Perineal and scrotal pain

18. Urodynamic findings typical of IC/BPS include:
    a. uninhibited detrusor contractions.
    b. obstructed flow patterns.
    c. abnormal bladder compliance.
    d. decreased capacity and hypersensitivity.
    e. increased volume at first urge to void.

19. The finding of glomerulations:
    a. should modify treatment only when cystoscopy is performed with the patient under anesthesia.
    b. is of no significance in an asymptomatic patient.
    c. indicates a likelihood of response to laser fulguration of the bladder.
    d. is present only in patients with IC/BPS.
    e. is sufficient to make a diagnosis of IC/BPS.

20. Amitriptyline's potential beneficial effects for the IC/BPS patient include all of the below EXCEPT:
    a. its ability to promote sleep
    b. its anticholinergic effect
    c. its antihistaminic effect
    d. its effect on neuropathic pain
    e. its antidepressant effect

21. Which test is potentially most helpful for prognosis and therapy?
    a. Potassium chloride test
    b. Intravesical heparin trial
    c. Cystoscopy and low-pressure bladder hydrodistention
    d. Bladder biopsy
    e. Urodynamics

22. Which of the following treatments is targeted to the glycosaminoglycan layer of the bladder?
    a. Sodium pentosan polysulfate
    b. Amitriptyline
    c. Hydroxyzine
    d. l-Arginine
    e. None of the above

23. Which of the following intravesical treatments has shown proven efficacy for IC/BPS in pivotal U.S. Food and Drug Administration trials?
    a. BCG (bacille Calmette-Guérin)
    b. 4% lidocaine
    c. Botulinum toxin
    d. Heparin
    e. None of the above

24. Which of the following statements is true of opioids in the management of the IC/BPS patient?
    a. They have no place in the treatment of a chronic, nonmalignant condition such as IC/BPS.
    b. Chronic use will usually produce physical dependency.
    c. They generally result in drug addiction when used for chronic pain.
    d. They tend to cause diarrhea and sleeplessness.
    e. All of the above.

25. Which of the following is a reasonable surgical procedure to relieve the pain of IC/BPS?
    a. Transurethral fulguration of HL
    b. Reduction cystoplasty
    c. Sympathectomy and intraspinal alcohol injections
    d. Cystolysis
    e. Transvesical infiltration of the pelvic plexuses with phenol

26. The most important early step in the management of IC/BPS is:
    a. initiating intravesical treatment.
    b. patient education.

c. starting oral pentosan polysulfate therapy.

d. physical therapy.

e. strict adherence to "IC" diet.

27. A finding of detrusor overactivity on urodynamics in a patient with bladder pain in the absence of urinary urgency indicates:

   a. the patient needs treatment with antimuscarinic medication.

   b. the patient does not have IC/BPS.

   c. a urinary tract infection is likely.

   d. neuromodulation would be the most effective treatment.

   e. none of the above.

28. Men with irritative voiding symptoms and pelvic pain should be evaluated for:

   a. bacterial cystitis

   b. bacterial prostatitis.

   c. BPS.

   d. bladder carcinoma in situ.

   e. all of the above.

29. An IC/BPS patient with HLs, unremitting pain, and an anesthetic bladder capacity of 75 cc wishes to proceed with supratrigonal cystectomy with bladder augmentation. The most important factor to consider before embarking upon this procedure is:

   a. urethral pain

   b. body image

   c. preoperative bowel function

   d. the presence of HLs on the trigone

   e. the presence of extravesical fat stranding

30. Emotional, sexual, or physical abuse can be categorized as:

   a. risk factors for BPS.

   b. behaviors often attributed to patients with IC/BPS.

   c. unequivocally unrelated to IC/BPS.

   d. rare adverse events caused by medications used to treat IC/BPS.

   e. conditions for which there are no data to allow any tentative conclusions with regard to the relationship to IC/BPS.

31. The only phenotype of IC/BPS currently shown to have a unique response to therapy and different natural history is:

   a. nocturia.

   b. daytime frequency.

   c. absence of bladder pain.

   d. glomerulation.

   e. HL.

32. Intravesical therapy for the IC/BPS patient will probably be LEAST effective to reduce pelvic pain in:

   a. the patient with provoked vestibulodynia and high-tone pelvic floor dysfunction.

   b. the patient with fibromyalgia.

   c. the patient with an HL.

   d. the patient with diabetic neuropathy.

   e. the patient with a small-capacity bladder.

ANSWERS

1. **b. Pain or discomfort related to the bladder.** Pain, pressure, or discomfort related to the bladder is necessary to make a diagnosis of BPS. Urgency, frequency, and the presence of glomerulations or Hunner ulcer on endoscopy are often associated with IC/BPS, but the presence of pain or discomfort is the primary component.

2. **c. Definition applicable mainly to clinical research studies.** The definition of IC proposed by the NIDDK is best considered a definition applicable for use in research studies. It was never meant to define the disease but rather was developed to ensure that patients included in basic and clinical research studies were homogeneous enough that experts could agree on the diagnosis.

3. **b. IC/BPS patients with HL have a higher mean age.** Otherwise, the two patient groups share remarkable similarities in clinical presentation. Treatment algorithms for the patient with HLs are similar; however, these HL patients are more likely to respond to "bladder-centric" interventions such as lesion fulguration.

4. **a. Monitor disease progression or regression with or without treatment.** Symptom and problem indices like the one developed by O'Leary and Sant are not intended to diagnose IC/BPS. Like the American Urologic Association Symptom Score for benign prostatic hypertrophy, these indices are designed to evaluate the severity of symptoms and to monitor disease progression or regression and response to treatment.

5. **e. Although clinical presentation is usually subacute, many patients have prodromal symptoms that occur decades before a formal diagnosis.** The subacute presentation of IC/BPS is one factor that often prompts empiric therapy for overactive bladder syndrome or bacterial cystitis. Further questioning often reveals LUTS or pelvic pain/discomfort that dates back decades or to childhood.

6. **d. The vast majority of reports fail to document an association of IC/BPS with subsequent development of bladder cancer.** Until recently, no relationship has ever been shown between BPS and the subsequent development of bladder carcinoma. In the 1970s, the Mayo Clinic documented bladder cancer in 12 of 53 men who had been treated for IC, but the association was the result of incorrect diagnosis rather than progression. Peters and others have noted that patients with bladder cancer can be misdiagnosed with IC/BPS. A study from Taiwan reported a 2.95 relative risk compared with controls.

7. **a. Pain or discomfort perceived to be related to the urinary bladder.** Pain or discomfort is the central symptom of IC/BPS and is what usually drives the urinary frequency. Although patients often describe pelvic discomfort with bladder filling, it is not an association that is needed for current diagnosis. Urinary urgency is a term that is frequently misinterpreted by patients (painful urgency or urgency related to fear of urine loss) and not necessary for diagnosis. Bladder hydrodistention, although possibly useful as a form of therapy, has not shown significant sensitivity and specificity for an IC/BPS diagnosis. On the other hand, factors such as the anesthetic bladder capacity measured at the time of hydrodistention may have prognostic significance.

8. **b. None.** Antibiotics are not indicated for the treatment of IC/BPS, nor have they been implicated as a causative factor. An empiric trial of doxycycline is reasonable in patients who have never had an antibiotic trial to treat the symptoms. Numerous studies have concluded that it is unlikely that active infection is involved in the ongoing pathologic process or that antibiotics have a role to play in treatment.

9. **c. Mast cell.** Mast cells are strategically localized in the urinary bladder close to blood vessels, lymphatics, nerves, and detrusor smooth muscle. IC/BPS appears to be a syndrome with neural, immune, and endocrine components in which activated mast cells may play a central, although not primary, role in many patients.

10. **e. None of the above.** As many as 25% of patients who meet the NIDDK criteria for IC/BPS will have a negative KCl test. It is positive in the majority of patients with radiation cystitis, urinary tract infection, or nonbacterial prostatitis and in

women with pelvic pain. It is neither sensitive nor specific for IC/BPS, is uncomfortable for patients, and does not help to guide therapeutic decisions.

11. **b. Is generally found in less than 30% of IC/BPS patients.** The HL (formerly termed "Hunner ulcer") is found in a minority of patients with symptoms of IC/BPS. Prevalence of these lesions may vary based upon the method to diagnose. The finding can usually be easily identified upon office cystoscopy. Some authorities suggest that hydrodistention is necessary to better identify the vulnerable mucosa. Most recently, narrow-band imaging has been used to better identify these focal regions.

12. **c. Increased diagnostic specificity.** Exclusive use of the NIDDK criteria to diagnose BPS would result in increased specificity and decreased sensitivity. Ninety percent of expert clinicians in the NIDDK database study agreed that patients diagnosed with IC by those criteria had IC. However, 60% of patients diagnosed by these clinicians as having IC/BPS did not fulfill the NIDDK criteria. Using the criteria as a basis for diagnosis would probably exclude the majority of patients with this symptom complex from the correct diagnosis.

13. **b. Diabetes.** Fibromyalgia, irritable bowel syndrome, chronic fatigue syndrome, and atopic allergic reactions are overrepresented in the IC/BPS population. Studies are ongoing to find out the reason for such relationships in the NIDDK MAPP (Multidisciplinary Approach to the Study of Chronic Pelvic Pain) Network.

14. **c. A history of recreational drug use.** Ketamine cystitis may present with signs and symptoms identical to IC/BPS and is often associated with lower and upper tract inflammatory disease. After excluding other pathologies, that is, bladder cancer, tuberculosis cystitis, and without knowing this past history, the clinician could easily move forward with IC/BPS-based therapies when other approaches would be indicated.

15. **d. Chemodenervation of the bladder.** Off-label use of botulinum toxin A (BTX-A) in the IC/BPS may be considered when more conservative therapies fail. The patient described has symptoms suggestive of high-tone pelvic floor dysfunction with some obstructive voiding symptoms. Physical examination of this patient might reveal hypertonicity of the pelvic floor musculature along with discrete muscular tender points. Caution should be exercised when considering the use of (BTX-A) in patients who complain of obstructive voiding difficulties.

16. **d. Rule out other disorders that might be responsible for the symptoms.** The primary value of histopathology in IC/BPS is to rule out other diseases that may account for the symptoms and would be most benefit if inflammatory disease is identified. There is no pathognomonic histologic finding for IC/BPS, nor can histology predict prognosis. Even a severely abnormal microscopic picture does not necessarily indicate a poor prognosis. At this time, no data suggest that the treatment algorithm can be rationally predicated on the basis of the histologic findings alone.

17. **b. Chronic bacterial prostatitis.** IC/BPS can be considered one of the pain syndromes of the urogenital and rectal area, all of which are well described but poorly understood. These include vulvodynia, orchialgia, perineal pain, penile pain, and rectal pain. Bacterial prostatitis is a well-understood entity with a known etiology and generally responds to treatment directed at the offending organism. NIH type 1 includes acute bacterial prostatitis and NIH type 2 denotes chronic bacterial prostatitis. Unlike NIH type 3 chronic pelvic pain syndrome/nonbacterial prostatitis, types 1 and 2 have no relationship to IC/BPS.

18. **d. Decreased capacity and hypersensitivity.** Cystometry in conscious IC/BPS patients generally demonstrates normal function, the exception being decreased bladder capacity and hypersensitivity. Pain on bladder filling, which reproduces the patient's symptoms, is very suggestive of IC. Bladder compliance in patients with IC is normal, as hypersensitivity would prevent the bladder from filling to the point of noncompliance.

19. **b. Is of no significance in an asymptomatic patient.** Glomerulations are not specific for IC/BPS, and seem to have little diagnostic or therapeutic value. Glomerulations can be seen after radiation therapy, in patients with bladder carcinoma, after exposure to toxic chemicals or chemotherapeutic agents, and in patients undergoing dialysis or after urinary diversion when the bladder has not filled for extended periods.

20. **e. Its antidepressant effect.** Amitriptyline may be of clinical benefit for all of its qualities listed a to d. Although the anticholinergic effect may improve symptoms in those patients with concomitant overactive bladder syndrome, negative effects may include a worsening of constipation and/or worsening of obstructive voiding symptoms. The doses to achieve clinical benefit for IC/BPS are generally lower than those used to treat major depressive illness.

21. **c. Cystoscopy and low-pressure bladder hydrodistention.** Bladder hydrodistention with the patient under anesthesia is a common therapeutic modality used for IC/BPS, frequently as part of the diagnostic evaluation. Its primary value is in diagnosis of an HL. Between 30% and 50% of patients experience some short-term relief in symptoms after the procedure. If an HL is present, therapeutic response to resection or fulguration is excellent in many patients. About 30% of patients will note a brief exacerbation in their symptoms following hydrodistention. A bladder capacity under anesthesia of less than 200 mL is a sign of poor prognosis.

22. **a. Sodium pentosan polysulfate.** The target of sodium pentosan polysulfate therapy is the glycosaminoglycan (GAG) layer of the urothelium. This agent is an oral analog of heparin. The proposed mechanism of action is the correction of a GAG dysfunction, thus presumably reversing the abnormal epithelial permeability. Chronic use has recently been associated with pigmentary maculopathy and visual disturbances in some patients.

23. **e. None of the above.** None of these treatments has been proven efficacious for IC/BPS in double-blind placebo-controlled trials.

24. **b. Chronic use will usually produce physical dependency.** Unlike other classes of analgesics, they have no therapeutic ceiling, dosing being limited by tolerance of side effects. They tend to cause constipation and can cause sedation. Opioids can be very useful in a subset of IC/BPS patients with severe disease and in the setting of "universal precautions."

25. **a. Transurethral fulguration of HL.** Transurethral fulguration and/or steroid injection of an HL can provide symptomatic relief. None of the other procedures listed have any place in the treatment of IC/BPS.

26. **b. Patient education.** Patient education is the most important step in the initial treatment of IC/BPS. This condition is chronic, the symptoms wax and wane, and remissions are not uncommon. It lends itself to practitioner abuse, and the uninformed, desperate patient is easy prey. Treatment is symptom-driven, and an informed patient makes the best decisions.

27. **e. None of the above.** Clinically insignificant detrusor overactivity may be seen in 15% of patients with IC/BPS, a rate of involuntary contractions that has been reported in normal patients undergoing ambulatory urodynamics. The finding does not rule out the diagnosis of IC/BPS, and treatment of this finding would be unlikely to result in improvement of the patient's bladder pain.

28. **e. All of the above.** IC/BPS should be considered in the differential diagnosis of voiding disorders in men accompanied by irritative symptoms and pelvic pain. A rigorous IC/BPS evaluation can be useful in differentiating IC/BPS from bladder carcinoma in situ, functional or anatomic bladder outlet obstruction, and bacterial prostatitis. Many men with IC/BPS have undergone what has proved to be unnecessary and ill-founded bladder neck surgery.

29. **a. Urethral pain.** Patients with preexisting urethral pain would be poor candidates for supravesical diversion with bladder augmentation as upwards of 30% of patients will need to

self-catheterize due to poor emptying. The presence of extravesical fat stranding is commonly seen on CT scan, is consistent with the panmural inflammatory process, and should have no bearing upon the indications for surgery. HLs are always identified in a supratrigonal position. Concern for other pathologies, that is, CIS, should be raised if trigonal lesions are identified.

30. **a. Risk factors for BPS.** Emotional, sexual, and physical abuse was shown to be a risk factor in the Boston Area Community Health Survey, and this has been borne out in other studies. A Michigan study compared a control group of 464 women with 215 IC/BPS patients and found that 22% of the control group had experienced abuse versus 37% of the patient group. Those with a history of sexual abuse may present with more pain and fewer voiding symptoms. How reliable these data are is not clear, and it would be wrong to jump to any conclusions about

abuse in an individual patient. However, practitioners need to have sensitivity for the possibility of an abusive relationship history in all pain patients, and IC/BPS patients in particular. When patients are found to have multiple diagnoses, the rate of previous abuse also increases, and these patients may need referral for further counseling.

31. **e. HL.** Patients with HLs form a distinct subset of those with BPS. They have identifiable endoscopic and pathologic findings, are less likely to have comorbid conditions, tend to be older, and respond clinically to bladder fulguration and local steroid injection into the lesions.

32. **a. The patient with provoked vestibulodynia and high-tone pelvic floor dysfunction.** In the "bladder-centric" patient, intravesical therapy may improve bladder symptoms, but if other pain generators go untreated, the reduction of pelvic pain may go unnoticed.

CHAPTER REVIEW

1. IC/BPS may be defined clinically as "an unpleasant sensation (pain, pressure, discomfort) perceived to be related to the urinary bladder, associated with lower urinary tract symptoms of more than six weeks duration, in the absence of infection or other identifiable causes. The pain or discomfort usually mounts with bladder filling and is the factor that typically prompts urinary frequency. The diagnosis of IC/BPS is one of exclusion because there is no specific test or marker that is diagnostic.

2. Prevalence studies for IC/BPS show wide variation with a general upsurge over time likely related to a more "liberalized" definition of the condition.

3. Current epidemiology suggests approximately 3 million females and 2 million males in the USA with IC/BPS symptoms. A female to male ratio of 5:1 is cited, based upon clinical practice.

4. Sexual dysfunction in female IC/BPS may have a profound effect upon their physical and mental QoL, underscoring the importance of identifying and ultimately treating this problem when present.

5. Common overlapping functional disorders such as high-tone pelvic floor dysfunction, overactive bladder syndrome, vulvodynia, and IBS may necessitate a multidisciplinary approach to achieve symptom relief.

6. The MAPP research network has demonstrated two distinct pain phenotypes in the IC/BPS patient: those with pelvic pain only and those with "pelvic pain and beyond," the latter group representing over 75% of patients. This suggests that many patients have pain derived from the central nervous system.

7. Fibromyalgia, irritable bowel syndrome, chronic fatigue syndrome, and atopic allergic reactions are overrepresented in the IC/BPS population.

8. High-tone pelvic floor dysfunction has been identified in 70% to 94% of IC/BPS patients either on the basis of urodynamically proven voiding dysfunction or reproduction of pelvic pain upon examination of the pelvic floor musculature.

9. The Hunner lesion (formerly termed "Hunner ulcer") is the pathognomonic finding for the "classical form" of IC and represents a minority of the IC/BPS population. HLs are easily identified during office cystoscopy, although bladder distention beyond functional capacity and other imaging strategies have been used to enhance identification. Mounting evidence suggests that BPS is indeed a syndrome and distinct from those patients presenting with HLs.

10. There are no reliable differences in clinical presentation between IC/BPS patients with or without HLs.

11. IC/BPS is chronic, the symptoms wax and wane, and remissions are common. Symptom flares are identified in the

vast majority of patients, most commonly lasting for days. Common triggers are dietary factors and physical activities, that is, sexual relations, exercises.

12. Some men diagnosed with chronic prostatitis/chronic pelvic pain syndrome, Category III, may also meet criteria for an IC/BPS diagnosis.

13. Prodromal symptoms related to pelvic pain and irritative voiding are often experienced decades before a formal diagnosis.

14. A childhood presentation for IC/BPS is extremely rare. The average age of onset is 40 years.

15. Adult female first-degree relatives of patients with IC/BPS may have a prevalence of IC/BPS 17 times that found in the general population.

16. Although ketamine abuse may be seen at any age, the clinician should be especially wary of the young patient who presents with a clinical picture of IC/BPS with or without visible inflammation of the bladder wall.

17. There is no histology pathognomonic of IC/BPS. While inflammatory features can be seen in 24% to 76% of patients, histological features are often bland. HLs show a dense, often panmural lymphoplasmacytic infiltrate. The current role of biopsy in the management of the IC/BPS patient is in the patient with HLs to rule out other pathology such as carcinoma in situ.

18. Antiproliferative factor (APF) is secreted by bladder epithelial cells, inhibits bladder epithelial cell proliferation, and is used as a marker of the disease. It may be the primary cause of syndrome in some patients. Urine APF appears to have the highest sensitivity and specificity of the markers studied for this disease.

19. Current studies suggest that the etiology of IC/BPS symptoms may vary. Local processes such as "leaky epithelium," mast cell activation, and neurogenic inflammation may produce symptoms for some patients; however, the presence of co-morbid widespread pain syndromes, regional pain syndromes, and immune-mediated pain in the majority of patients suggest that more global pathologies may also be responsible.

20. Cross-sensitization among pelvic structures, that is, bowel and bladder, may contribute to chronic pain syndromes because this may result in alteration in function of adjacent pelvic organs.

21. Bladder compliance in patients with IC is normal; however, capacity is often reduced and pain/discomfort is reproduced with filling.

22. Failure to diagnose other causes of pelvic pain, that is, high-tone pelvic floor dysfunction, vulvodynia, that may occur with or without IC/BPS is one of the most common reasons for a suboptimal therapeutic outcome.

Continued

23. Microscopic hematuria and/or pyuria are not reliable findings to predict the presence of an HL. Office cystoscopy should be considered if an HL is suspected or the patient is not responding to empiric therapy.

24. Although hydrodistention of the urinary bladder is not part of the standard diagnostic evaluation, recent findings suggest that a low bladder capacity at the time of hydrodistention (anesthetic bladder capacity) may represent a distinct clinical phenotype, having higher symptom scores and fewer reports of depression and irritable bowel syndrome, essentially a more bladder-centric patient picture. The presence of glomerulations (puntate submucosal hemorrhages identified during hydrodistention) is not necessary for diagnosis. The finding lacks sensitivity and specificity.

25. Conservative treatment strategies are recommended with progression to more aggressive care in the setting of poor symptom control and an unacceptable quality of life. Initial aggressive care may be indicated for patients who present with severe symptomatology that, in the clinician's opinion, is unlikely to have an adequate response to more conservative measures.

26. Patient education, dietary manipulation, nonprescription analgesics, and pelvic floor relaxation sensation techniques constitute the initial treatment of BPS.

27. Catastrophic thinking, the irrational, consuming fear of a disastrous outcome, appears to enhance the perception of pain, but may be modified with cognitive behavioral therapy.

28. Many patients find their symptoms adversely affected by certain food/beverage groups. A step-wise method to determine dietary sensitivities such as an elimination diet may play an important role in patient management.

29. Pentosan polysulfate sodium (an oral agent) and dimethylsulfoxide (an intravesical agent) are the only two FDA-approved medications for the treatment of IC/BPS symptoms.

30. Amitriptyline, a tricyclic antidepressant, is not FDA approved for the treatment of IC/BPS. Nevertheless, it remains a staple of oral treatment given its antihistaminic properties, its ability to promote sleep, and reduce neuropathic (central and peripheral) pain.

31. Intravesical agents may improve symptoms of IC/BPS but would have limited success in those patients with centralized pain. The frequency and duration of therapy, and the value of maintenance therapy have not been well studied.

32. Sacral neuromodulation and intradetrusor injection of botulinum toxin A are currently considered as fourth-line treatment strategies. Although urinary retention is a relatively rare event with BTX-A, caution should be exercised when considering its use in the patient with obstructive voiding symptoms.

33. Major reconstructive procedures may be considered when all conservative forms of management have failed. Diversion, and even cystectomy with diversion, cannot guarantee a pain-free result, and it is critical for the patient to factor this into their decision. Patients with a clear-cut source of bladder pain (such as HLs) with a small-capacity, poorly compliant bladder are most likely to have a favorable clinical outcome.

34. Substitution cystoplasty and continent diversion both fail in some IC/BPS patients because of the development of pain in the bowel segment used or contraction of the bowel segment.

58 Sexually Transmitted Diseases

Kristy McKiernan Borawski

QUESTIONS

1. The most commonly diagnosed bacterial sexually transmitted infection (STI) in the United States is:
   a. gonorrhea.
   b. ureaplasma.
   c. syphilis.
   d. chlamydia.
   e. chancroid.

2. The major health risk to untreated *Chlamydia* infection in men is:
   a. epididymitis.
   b. Reiter syndrome.
   c. orchitis.
   d. chronic prostatitis/chronic pelvic pain syndrome.
   e. transmission to a female partner resulting in pelvic inflammatory disease.

3. In addition to treatment for chlamydia, what other medication is recommended as a first-line treatment for gonorrhea?
   a. Ciprofloxacin
   b. Levofloxacin
   c. Ceftriaxone
   d. Cefixime
   e. Penicillin VK

4. Which subtypes of human papillomavirus (HPV) are responsible for development of malignancies including cervical, penile, and anal?
   a. 16 and 18
   b. 13 and 14
   c. 6 and 11
   d. 31 and 33
   e. 26 and 28

5. HPV vaccines are indicated for which groups?
   a. All sexually active women
   b. All sexually active men who have sex with men (MSMs)
   c. Men and women up to age 26 years
   d. Only women up to age 26 years
   e. Only women with a family history of cervical cancer

6. Which STI often has no visible genital lesion because it has usually resolved by the time of presentation and is associated with tender, often suppurative adenopathy?
   a. Chancroid
   b. Herpes simplex virus type 2 (HSV-2)
   c. Herpes simplex virus type 1 (HSV-1)
   d. Donovanosis
   e. Lymphogranuloma venereum (LGV)

7. Which of the following is not a reportable STI in every state?
   a. HSV
   b. Syphilis
   c. Chancroid
   d. Chlamydia
   e. Human immunodeficiency virus (HIV)

8. Which of the following tests should be used to monitor the clinical response to treatment in patients with syphilis?
   a. *Treponema pallidum* particle agglutination (TP-PA)
   b. Rapid plasma reagin (RPR)
   c. Fluorescent treponemal antibody absorption (FTA-ABS)
   d. Darkfield microscopy
   e. Tzanck test

9. What is the treatment of choice for primary, secondary, and early latent syphilis?
   a. Azithromycin
   b. Benzathine penicillin
   c. Probenecid penicillin
   d. Ceftriaxone
   e. Procaine penicillin

10. Which statement is true regarding the likelihood of recurrent genital lesions in patients with HSV-1 and HSV-2?
    a. No difference except in HIV patients in whom HSV-1 recurs more often
    b. No difference except in HIV patients in whom HSV-2 recurs more often
    c. HSV-1 recurs more often
    d. HSV-2 recurs more often
    e. No difference

11. What is the causative organism for LGV?
    a. *Calymmatobacterium*
    b. *Klebsiella*
    c. *Chlamydia*
    d. *Haemophilus ducreyi*
    e. *Trichomonas*

12. Gardasil in males is recommended:
    a. to prevent transmission of HPV to their partners.
    b. only for persons with documented HPV.
    c. to prevent anal cancer and genital warts.
    d. to prevent genital warts only.
    e. only in men older than 26 years.

13. Donovan bodies are seen on:
    a. Thayer-Martin medium in gonorrhea.
    b. ulcer scraping in primary syphilis.
    c. biopsy of condyloma acuminata.
    d. lymph node aspiration in LGV.
    e. biopsy of ulcer in granuloma inguinale.

14. Clue cells are diagnostic of:
    a. bacterial vaginosis (BV).
    b. *Trichomonas.*
    c. scabies.
    d. *Candida* vulvovaginitis.
    e. *Torulopsis glabrata* vulvovaginitis.

15. HIV is what type of virus?
    a. Single-stranded RNA
    b. Double-stranded RNA
    c. Single-stranded messenger RNA (mRNA)
    d. Single-stranded DNA
    e. Double-stranded DNA

16. The HIV envelope precursor protein gp160 is cleaved into what two envelope proteins?
    a. gp123 and gp33
    b. gp124 and gp40
    c. gp141 and gp20
    d. gp120 and gp41
    e. gp120 and gp6

17. HIV infects which immune cells?
    a. Macrophages
    b. B cells
    c. CD4 T cells
    d. CD8 T cells
    e. Natural killer (NK) cells

18. The initial screening test for HIV is:
    a. Western blot.
    b. indirect immunofluorescence assay.
    c. nucleoside amplification assay.
    d. rapid enzyme immunoassay (EIA).
    e. viral culture.

19. Antiretroviral therapy is recommended for:
    a. patients with CD4 count of <200 only.
    b. patients with CD4 count of <350 only.
    c. patients with CD4 count of <500 only.
    d. patients with CD4 count of <500 and symptoms.
    e. all patients with HIV.

20. What factor is not associated with increased risk of seroconversion with HIV after a needle stick?
    a. Recent infection by patient
    b. Deep exposure of needle
    c. Visible blood on injuring device
    d. Prior placement of injuring device in artery or vein
    e. Patient dying within 2 months of exposure

21. Polymorphisms of which gene are associated with development of HIV-associated nephropathy (HIVAN) in African American patients?
    a. Tyrosine kinase
    b. Antichymotrypsin-1
    c. Apolipoprotein-1
    d. Tumor necrosis alpha
    e. Interleukin-10

22. Which type of antiretroviral medications are associated with formation of urinary tract stones?
    a. Integrase inhibitors
    b. Fusion inhibitors
    c. Protease inhibitors
    d. Non-nucleoside reverse-transcriptase inhibitors (NNRTIs)
    e. CCR5 blockers

23. What is the best diagnostic test to detect HIV in the acute phase of infection?
    a. Indirect immunofluorescence assay
    b. Viral load assay
    c. Western blot
    d. HIV-1/HIV-2 serology assay
    e. Rapid EIA

24. What class of medication can have a prolonged half-life when used in association with protease inhibitors and NNRTI's for treatment of HIV?
    a. Alpha-blockers
    b. 5-Alpha reductase inhibitors
    c. Beta-3 agonists
    d. PDE5 inhibitors
    e. Fluoroquinolones

25. What type of genitourinary (GU) cancer is not increased in frequency in patients with HIV?
    a. Prostate cancer
    b. Kidney cancer
    c. Penile cancer
    d. Testis cancer
    e. Kaposi sarcoma

Pathology

1. A 32-year-old sexually active woman has the lesion in Fig. 58.1A and B excised from her vulva. The diagnosis is condyloma acuminata. The most appropriate next step is:
   a. acetic acid test.
   b. podophyllin to the base of the lesion.
   c. HPV vaccine.
   d. vaginoscopy.
   e. cystoscopy.

2. A 22-year-old sexually active man has a 2-mm raised red lesion in the suprapubic area. A biopsy is performed (depicted in Fig. 58.2) and read as molluscum contagiosum. The patient is concerned and desires treatment. The most appropriate treatment is:
   a. wide local excision.
   b. 5-fluorouracil cream.
   c. ciprofloxacin for 2 weeks.
   d. bactrim for 4 weeks.
   e. liquid nitrogen application.

ANSWERS

1. **d. Chlamydia.** Chlamydia is the most common bacterial STI in the United States. The 1,422,976 cases of *Chlamydia trachomatis* infection reported to the Centers for Disease Control and Prevention (CDC) in 2012 was the largest number ever reported to the CDC for any condition. The second most common bacterial STI is gonorrhea.

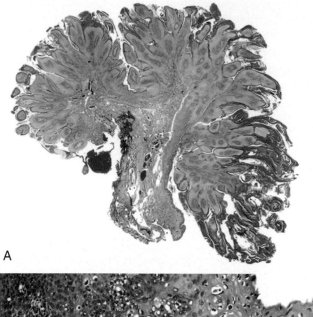

A

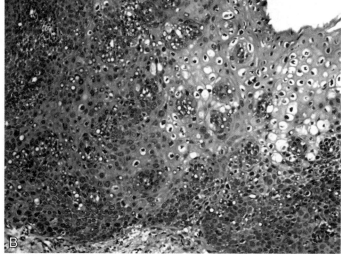

B

Fig. 58.1 A and B. (From Bostwick DG, Cheng L: *Urologic surgical pathology*, ed 3, St. Louis, 2014, Saunders.)

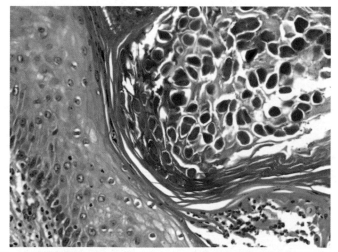

Fig. 58.2 (From Bostwick DG, Cheng L: *Urologic surgical pathology*, ed 3, St. Louis, 2014, Saunders.)

2. **e. Transmission to a female partner resulting in pelvic inflammatory disease.** Up to 75% of women with chlamydial infection can be asymptomatic. Ascending chlamydial infection can result in scarring of the fallopian tubes, pelvic inflammatory disease, risk for ectopic pregnancy, pelvic pain, and infertility. The risk of untreated chlamydial infection

producing pelvic inflammatory disease is estimated to be between 9.5% and 27% of cases.

3. **c. Ceftriaxone.** As of 2007, quinolones are no longer recommended in the United States for treatment of gonorrhea and associated conditions such as pelvic inflammatory disease. As of August 2012, because of high resistance, cefixime is no longer recommended as first-line therapy to treat gonorrhea. Current treatment of uncomplicated gonococcal infections of the cervix, urethra, and rectum is ceftriaxone, 250 mg IM, single-dose PLUS azithromycin, 1 g orally in single dose.

4. **a. 16 and 18.** Types 6 and 11 are nononcogenic and are responsible for about 90% of anogenital warts. Other subtypes, including 16 and 18, account for cervical cancer and other types of anogenital cancer including vulvar, vaginal, anal, and penile.

5. **c. Men and women up to age 26 years.** In June 2006, a quadrivalent HPV vaccine (Gardasil; Merck, Sharpe, and Dohme Corporation) was licensed for use in the United States in females aged 9 to 26 years. In October 2009, this vaccine also was licensed for use in males aged 9 to 26 years. This vaccine provides protection against HPV types 6, 11, 16, and 18. In October 2009, a bivalent HPV vaccine (Cervarix; Glaxo Smith-Kline Biologicals, Research Triangle Park, NC) that provides protection against types 16 and 18 was licensed for use in females aged 10 to 25 years.

6. **e. Lymphogranuloma venereum (LGV).** A self-limited genital ulcer or papule sometimes is present at the site of infection but usually has disappeared by the time of presentation. The secondary stage is the most common presentation in heterosexuals and is marked by tender inguinal and/or femoral lymphadenopathy, typically unilateral.

7. **a. HSV.** Diseases that must be reported to local health authorities: Syphilis, gonorrhea, chlamydia, chancroid, HIV infection, and acquired immunodeficiency syndrome (AIDS) are reportable diseases in every state.

8. **b. Rapid plasma reagin (RPR).** Nontreponemal tests (RPR or VDRL) are used to monitor disease activity. A fourfold change in titer equivalent to a change of two dilutions (e.g., from 1:16 to 1:4) is considered necessary to demonstrate a clinically significant difference.

9. **b. Benzathine penicillin.** Benzathine penicillin is the treatment of choice for all of the stages of syphilis. Treatment varies by dose and duration of therapy. Not considered appropriate treatments are combinations of benzathine and procaine penicillin (Bicillin C-R), or oral penicillin.

10. **d. HSV-2 recurs more often.** Genital HSV-1 recurs much less frequently (0.02 per month) than genital HSV-2 infections (0.23 per month), on the order of 10-fold less.

11. **c. *Chlamydia*.** LGV is an infection by *Chlamydia*, specifically serovars L1, L2, or L3.

12. **c. To prevent anal cancer and genital warts.** The quadrivalent vaccine is used in males to prevent genital warts and in both genders to prevent anal cancer. MSMs are particularly at risk for developing anal intraepithelial neoplasia and anal cancer. As in women, it is best started in males before the onset of sexual activity.

13. **e. Biopsy of ulcer in granuloma inguinale.** Granuloma inguinale (GI) is an infection by the intracellular gram-negative bacterium *Klebsiella granulomatis* (formerly called *Calymmatobacterium granulomatis*) that produces genital ulcers. The bacterium is a strict human pathogen, which makes culture difficult. Diagnosis requires visualization of dark-staining Donovan bodies on crush preparation or biopsy, described by Donovan in 1905. These are intracellular inclusions of the bacteria within the cytoplasm of macrophages and appear deep purple when stained with a Wright, Giemsa, or Leishman stain.

14. **a. Bacterial vaginosis (BV).** Characteristic findings for BV on microscopic exam are clue cells, which are vaginal epithelial cells covered with bacteria.

15. **a. Single-stranded RNA.** The genetic material in HIV is single-stranded RNA. After entry into the targeted cell, the RNA is reverse transcribed by a reverse transcriptase into a double-stranded DNA. This new DNA is assembled into complexes, which then associate with the target cell chromatin and integrate via the action of viral integrase. The cell then translates and transcribes the viral genes to produce proteins that will assemble new copies of the virus. Copies of the virus are called virions.

16. **d. gp120 and gp41.** The virus is shaped like a sphere. It is covered by an outer envelope that is a lipid bilayer derived from the host cell when it buds out of the cell. Embedded in the envelope is a complex of proteins known as Env. There is initially a precursor gp160 that is cleaved by a protease in the trans-Golgi network. It is cleaved into an outer subunit glycoprotein 120 (gp120) and a transmembrane subunit glycoprotein 41 (gp41). After proteolysis, the gp120 and gp41 remain coupled as noncovalent heterodimers.

17. **c. CD4 T cells.** Glycoprotein gp120 has a high-affinity binding site for the T lymphocyte receptor CD4.

18. **d. Rapid enzyme immunoassay (EIA).** Diagnosis of HIV includes the use of serologic tests that detect antibodies against HIV-1 (and HIV-2) and by virologic tests that detect HIV antigens RNA. The initial test is a screening test for antibodies, the conventional or rapid EIA. The initial result can be obtained in 30 minutes. Positive or reactive screening tests must be confirmed by a supplemental antibody test, Western blot, and indirect immunofluorescence assay (IFA) or by a virologic test, the HIV-1 RNA assay.

19. **e. All patients with HIV.** The benefit of treatment may depend on the starting CD4 count, but treatment guidelines recommend treatment for all patients regardless of CD4 count.

20. **a. Recent infection by patient.** A review of factors for increased risk of infection done by the CDC identified four that increased risk: deep as opposed to superficial exposure (odds ratio [OR] 15, 95% confidence index [CI] 6 to 41), visible blood on the injuring device (OR 6.2, 95% CI 2.2 to 21), prior placement of the injuring device in an artery or vein (OR 4.3, 95% CI 1.7 to 12), and patient dying within 2 months of the exposure (preterminal disease) (OR 5.6, 95% CI 2 to 16).

21. **c. Apolipoprotein-1.** African Americans carrying two variants of the APOL-1 gene are at very high risk for HIVAN. These genes encode a secreted lipid binding protein called apolipoprotein-1 (apoL1). The variants G1 and G2 are common in African chromosomes but absent in European chromosomes; these variants lyse trypanosomes, including *Trypanosoma brucei rhodesiense*, which causes African sleeping sickness. Thus, these loci are thought to be selected out in this population. The presence of these two genes together increases the risk 29-fold, resulting in a 50% risk of developing HIVAN in untreated individuals as compared with a 12% baseline risk. Focal segmental glomerulosclerosis (FSGS) found in individuals with the two risk genes also occurs at an earlier age and progresses much more rapidly.

22. **c. Protease inhibitors.** The protease inhibitors specifically have the possibility of stone formation. Indinavir can form crystals in the urine. Indinavir stones are typically radiolucent on both plain film and computed tomography scan but can also be mixed with calcium and appear radio-opaque. Newer inhibitors including lopinavir, atazanavir, amprenavir, and nelfinavir have also been associated with the development of stones, but with less frequency than reported for indinavir.

23. **b. Viral load assay.** During this initial 3-month period, the "window" period, antibody screening tests may be negative but the person is still infected. Virologic tests for HIV-1 RNA can be used to detect an acute infection in persons negative for HIV antibodies.

24. **d. PDE5 inhibitors.** PDE5 inhibitors depend on CYP3A for clearance, and all protease inhibitors and NNRTIs are inhibitors of CYP3A to some extent. This can lead to a significant increase in the serum dose of PDE5 inhibitors, and therefore they should be started at the lowest dose possible in patients on these antiretroviral medications.

25. **a. Prostate cancer.** The relative risk of prostate cancer in men with HIV compared to uninfected individuals has been reported as either no different or even less at 0.70.

Pathology

1. **d. Vaginoscopy.** The figure shows marked papillomatosis with koilocytic atypia. The patient should have a thorough genital examination, including vaginoscopy for other lesions.

2. **e. Liquid nitrogen application.** The biopsy shows an epidermal crater filled with molluscum bodies. This is usually a self-limited disease and requires no treatment. If treatment is desired, a local therapy is appropriate, such as curettage or liquid nitrogen application.

CHAPTER REVIEW

1. When exposed to STIs, women are more likely to become infected and less likely to be symptomatic.
2. Chlamydia is the most common sexually transmitted disease in the United States.
3. HSV-2 accounts for 90% of the genital herpes infections. HSV-1 accounts for the remainder and is the common cause of cold sores; silent infection is common in this disease. The diagnosis is made by viral culture and subtyping. HSV enters the nerve and remains latent in the nerve cell body. It may cause aseptic meningitis and autonomic dysfunction, which may lead to urinary retention.
4. Chancroid is caused by *Haemophilus ducreyi* and results in a painful, nonindurated ulcer covered by an exudate. Inguinal adenopathy occurs and may become suppurative.
5. Chancre of syphilis is single, painless, indurated, and clean. It is associated with nontender inguinal lymphadenopathy.
6. Latent syphilis is seropositive with no evidence of disease. Early latent syphilis occurs in less than 1 year. Late latent syphilis occurs beyond 1 year.
7. Primary syphilis is the acute infection. Secondary syphilis is manifested by mucocutaneous and constitutional signs and symptoms that are often associated with a maculopapular rash. Tertiary syphilis is a systemic disease involving the cardiovascular, skeletal, and central nervous system.
8. Treponemal tests for syphilis are generally positive for life and do not indicate treatment response. RPR, Venereal Disease Research Laboratory (VDRL), and the toluidine red unheated serum test (TRUST) are nontreponemal tests and correlate with disease activity. They usually become negative after treatment. Nontreponemal tests (RPR or VDRL) are used to monitor disease activity.
9. The Jarisch-Herxheimer reaction occurs when patients with syphilis are treated with penicillin, resulting in the release of toxic products when the treponemes are killed. The symptoms include headache, myalgia, fever, tachycardia, and increased respiratory rate.
10. LGV presents as a single painless ulcer and painful inguinal adenopathy. LGV is marked by tender inguinal and/or femoral lymphadenopathy, typically unilateral.
11. Polymerase chain reaction (PCR) assays are used for diagnosing chlamydial infection.
12. A strawberry rash on the vulva or strawberry cervix is seen in trichomoniasis.

13. More than 99% of cervical cancers and 84% of anal cancers are associated with HPV 16 or 18. The most common serotype associated with squamous cell carcinoma of the penis is HPV 16.

14. Biopsies of genital warts are not routinely indicated but should be performed when the wart is atypical, pigmented, indurated, or fixed and ulcerated.

15. HPV vaccine is recommended for females age 9 to 26 years and may also be given to males of the same age range.

16. The presence of STIs increases the risk for concurrent HIV.

17. Ulcerative STIs including herpes, syphilis, and chancroid enhance the susceptibility to HIV per sexual contact.

18. Antiviral therapy for HIV does not necessarily make the patient noninfectious.

19. Men who are circumcised are at lower risk for HIV infection.

20. There are two types of HIV viruses: HIV-1 and HIV-2. There are very few cases of HIV-2 in the developed world, and it is less easily transmitted and less virulent than HIV-1.

21. HIV is a retrovirus that infects T cells and dendritic cells.

22. Antiretroviral combination therapy delays the rate of progression of the disease and prolongs survival.

23. Overt AIDS is marked by a low CD4+ T-cell count.

24. Plasma HIV RNA load is the most accurate predictor of disease progression.

25. The diagnosis of HIV is made by screening for anti-HIV-1 and anti-HIV-2 antibodies. If this is positive, confirmation is made by using Western blot analysis. After treatment, the nadir of plasma HIV RNA predicts long-term outcome.

26. HIV testing is recommended for anyone diagnosed with a STI or at risk for STIs.

27. HSV increases HIV replication in persons infected with both viruses.

28. HPV infection increases the risk for carcinoma, especially in HIV-infected hosts.

29. The most common intrascrotal pathologic process in AIDS patients is testicular atrophy.

30. Voiding dysfunction is common in patients with advanced HIV infection.

31. Urinary calculi have been associated with, most notably, protease inhibitors such as indinavir. These stones are soluble at an acidic pH.

32. HIV-associated nephropathy is a glomerular disease that often presents as proteinuria.

33. Patients with HIV are at particular increased risk for Kaposi sarcoma and non-Hodgkin lymphoma. Kaposi sarcoma presents as a raised, firm, indurated purplish plaque, reflecting the presence of abundant blood vessels, extravasated erythrocytes, and siderophages.

34. Human herpesvirus 8 is essential for all forms of Kaposi sarcoma.

35. HIV protease inhibitors are also potent antiangiogenic molecules and are useful in treating Kaposi sarcoma. However, localized lesions may be treated by irradiation, laser, cryotherapy, or intralesional injections of antineoplastic drugs. Corticosteroids should not be used to treat the lesions.

36. There is an increased incidence of Kaposi sarcoma, non-Hodgkin lymphoma, and cervical cancer in patients with HIV infection. There also appears to be an increased incidence of the following GU tumors: testicular, renal, and penile.

37. The risk of untreated chlamydial infection producing pelvic inflammatory disease is estimated to be between 9.5% and 27% of cases.

38. Current treatment of uncomplicated gonococcal infections of the cervix, urethra, and rectum are ceftriaxone 250 mg IM single-dose PLUS azithromycin, 1 g orally in single dose or doxycycline, 100 mg orally twice per day for 7 days.

39. Donovan bodies noted in granuloma inguinale are intracellular inclusions of the bacteria within the cytoplasm of macrophages and appear deep purple when stained with a Wright, Giemsa, or Leishman stain.

40. Characteristic findings for bacterial vaginosis on microscopic exam are clue cells, which are vaginal epithelial cells covered with bacteria.

41. Factors that increase the risk for transmitting HIV include deep as opposed to superficial exposure (OR 15, 95% CI 6 to 41), visible blood on the injuring device (OR 6.2, 95% CI 2.2 to 21), prior placement of the injuring device in an artery or vein (OR 4.3, 95% CI 1.7 to 12), and patient dying within 2 months of the exposure (preterminal disease) (OR 5.6, 95% CI 2 to 16).

42. PDE5 inhibitors depend on CYP3A for clearance, and all protease inhibitors and NNRTIs are inhibitors of CYP3A to some extent. This can lead to a significant increase in the serum dose of PDE5 inhibitors, and therefore they should be started at the lowest possible dose in patients on these antiretroviral medications.

59 Cutaneous Diseases of the External Genitalia

Richard Edward Link and Nikki Tang

QUESTIONS

1. The periodic acid–Schiff stain is used to identify what organism in scraped or touched skin preparations?
   a. *Pseudomonas* sp.
   b. *Candida*
   c. *Corynebacterium minutissimum*
   d. Herpes simplex
   e. Molluscum contagiosum

2. Oral glucocorticosteroids are often used to treat dermatologic conditions and have a duration of effect lasting:
   a. 2 to 3 weeks.
   b. 30 to 90 minutes.
   c. 1 to 5 hours.
   d. 8 to 48 hours.
   e. 5 to 7 days.

3. The preferred dosage schedule for a short course of oral glucocorticosteroids used to treat a cutaneous disorder is:
   a. a single morning dose.
   b. a single evening dose.
   c. doses in the morning and evening.
   d. a dose every other day in the morning.
   e. redosing every 8 hours.

4. A 12-year-old boy has a long-standing history of asthma and occasional outbreaks of erythematous, pruritic papules on his scrotum and lower extremities. Which of the following options represents a rational approach to treating this condition?
   a. Long-term suppressive topical corticosteroids
   b. Frequent soaking in warm water to prevent the development of lesions
   c. Low-dose systemic corticosteroids
   d. The frequent application of emollients
   e. Application of a topical calcineurin inhibitor

5. Patch testing is a useful diagnostic test to identify:
   a. psoriasis.
   b. contact dermatitis.
   c. erythema gangrenosum.
   d. atopic dermatitis.
   e. Behçet disease.

6. The North American Contact Dermatitis Group identified a series of common allergens that were associated with contact dermatitis. Which allergen was the most common offending agent in contact dermatitis cases?
   a. Silver
   b. Textile dyes
   c. Ragweed
   d. Nickel sulfate
   e. Pet dander

7. A 35-year-old textile worker spills a small amount of green dye onto her left thigh. By the end of the workday, she is complaining of pain and burning over a 5-cm irregular patch of skin on her left thigh. What is the most likely diagnosis?
   a. Erysipelas
   b. Allergic contact dermatitis
   c. Hailey-Hailey disease
   d. Irritant contact dermatitis
   e. Koebner phenomenon

8. Following a recent exacerbation of genital herpes, a 22-year-old man notes the development of erythematous papules and targetoid lesions on his thighs, scrotum, and oral mucosa. The best next course of action is:
   a. oral antihistamines.
   b. systemic corticosteroids.
   c. observation.
   d. oral acyclovir.
   e. topical corticosteroids.

9. A 19-year-old woman is 2 days into a course of sulfonamides for an *Escherichia coli* urinary tract infection. She develops painful labial erosions that progress to a generalized rash with the formation of blisters. The most likely diagnosis is:
   a. erythema multiforme minor.
   b. Reiter syndrome.
   c. Stevens-Johnson syndrome.
   d. pyoderma gangrenosum.
   e. Sézary syndrome.

10. A 42-year-old circumcised man has a history of widely distributed erythematous plaques—most severe on his knees, elbows, inguinal folds, and glans penis. The condition has waxed and waned since he was in his early 20s. What is an appropriate therapy during an exacerbation?
    a. Topical 3% liquor carbonis detergens in 1% hydrocortisone cream
    b. Oral psoralen combined with ultraviolet radiation (PUVA)
    c. Systemic corticosteroids
    d. Topical 5-fluorouracil cream
    e. Oral azathioprine

11. A 21-year-old man presents with dysuria, blurred vision, oral ulcers, and erythematous plaques in his genitalia. He has mild soreness in his knees and ankles. He is negative for human immunodeficiency virus (HIV) and has no history of sexually transmitted disease. What is a likely risk factor for development of this disorder?
    a. Genital herpes simplex
    b. The human leukocyte antigen (HLA)-B27 haplotype
    c. A history of atopic dermatitis
    d. Exposure to benzene-containing chemicals
    e. Family history of psoriasis

12. Which of the following statements is true about the treatment of symptomatic genital lichen planus?
    a. Systemic corticosteroids can prevent the development of lesions.
    b. In clinical trials, the most effective agent for treating lichen planus is systemic acitretin.
    c. Systemic corticosteroids can shorten the time to clearance of existing lesions from 29 to 18 weeks.
    d. Phytotherapy is the therapeutic modality of choice for treating lichen planus.
    e. Metronidazole is an effective and well-established first-line agent in the treatment of lichen planus.

13. The late stage of lichen sclerosus involving the glans penis is termed:
    a. keratinizing balanoposthitis.
    b. pseudoepitheliomatous, keratotic, and micaceous balanitis.
    c. bowenoid papulosis.
    d. balanitis xerotica obliterans.
    e. Hailey-Hailey disease.

14. Which of the following cutaneous conditions has been associated with an increased risk of squamous cell carcinoma?
    a. Lichen sclerosus et atrophicus
    b. Lichen planus
    c. Psoriasis
    d. Bullous pemphigoid
    e. Lichen nitidus

15. An 18-year-old man has a history of seizures following an automobile accident 2 weeks ago. He was sexually active before the accident. Today, he presents with a solitary, painful erosion on the penis. What course of action is appropriate at this time?
    a. Perform a urethral swab for gonorrhea and chlamydia
    b. Consult with neurology to alter his antiseizure medication regimen
    c. Start oral acyclovir
    d. Perform a punch biopsy of the lesion
    e. Start oral doxycycline

16. A 35-year-old, previously healthy woman has noted the rapid development of sharply demarcated, pruritic, red-brown plaques over a large extent of her skin surface. The plaques are particularly dense in her nasolabial folds and perianal area, and the nails are spared. What is the next step?
    a. Systemic corticosteroids
    b. HIV test
    c. Skin culture for *Malassezia furfur*
    d. Examination of the lesions under ultraviolet (UV) light
    e. Biopsy of the lesions

17. In patients with pemphigus vulgaris, the characteristic clinical sign showing loss of epidermal cohesion is:
    a. the dimple sign.
    b. the Asboe-Hansen sign.
    c. the Leser-Trélat sign.
    d. the dimple sign.
    e. the bullous blanching sign.

18. Which of the following statements is FALSE concerning pemphigus vulgaris?
    a. The majority of pemphigus patients have painful oral mucosal erosions.
    b. Pemphigus appears to have an autoimmune pathogenesis.
    c. Blisters appear to form due to loss of keratinocyte cell-cell adhesion.

    d. Treatment of pemphigus relies on systemic corticosteroids.
    e. Given enough time, even advanced cases of pemphigus generally resolve spontaneously without sequelae.

19. Which of the following dermatoses has an association with celiac disease?
    a. Dermatitis herpetiformis
    b. Hailey-Hailey disease
    c. Behçet disease
    d. Bullous pemphigoid
    e. Psoriasis

20. Which of the following is not a vesicobullous dermatosis?
    a. Hailey-Hailey disease
    b. Pyoderma gangrenosum
    c. Pemphigus vulgaris
    d. Zoon balanitis
    e. Linear IgA bullous dermatoses

21. Which agent has been shown to be effective in treating linear IgA bullous dermatoses?
    a. Azathioprine
    b. Cyclosporine
    c. Dapsone
    d. Metronidazole
    e. Sulfonylurea

22. A 45-year-old woman has pruritic, foul-smelling blistering in the inframammary folds and groin. The skin findings are confluent areas of vesicles with fragile blisters. Which of the following statements is FALSE concerning this condition?
    a. The condition is usually worse during the summer months.
    b. Intralesional corticosteroids may be effective for treatment.
    c. Involvement of the vulva is common in women.
    d. Wide local excision may be necessary in refractory cases.
    e. Laser vaporization has been applied successfully to this condition.

23. A 35-year-old man presents with painful ulcerations in his mouth and on his penis, as well as blurred vision and a history of recurrent epididymitis. What is the likely diagnosis?
    a. Behçet disease
    b. Oculocutaneous aphthous ulcer syndrome
    c. Epidermolysis bullosa
    d. Fabry disease
    e. Pyoderma gangrenosum

24. Which of the following statements is FALSE concerning pyoderma gangrenosum?
    a. Pyoderma gangrenosum most likely has an autoimmune mechanism of pathogenesis.
    b. There is an association with collagen vascular disease.
    c. Corticosteroids may play a role in management.
    d. The presence of vacuolated keratinocytes in an inflammatory background is pathognomonic for this condition.

25. Which of the following cutaneous conditions has an association with borderline personality disorder?
    a. Factitial dermatitis
    b. "Innocent" traumatic dermatitis
    c. Sézary syndrome
    d. Munchausen syndrome by proxy
    e. Behçet disease

26. The most common organisms causing erysipelas are:
    a. dermatophytes.
    b. *Staphylococcus aureus.*
    c. *Streptococcus pyogenes.*
    d. *Escherichia coli.*
    e. *Pseudomonas* sp.

27. Which of the following statements is FALSE concerning Fournier gangrene?
    a. The mortality rate even with modern treatment may be greater than 15%.
    b. Most cases of Fournier gangrene are caused by *S. pyogenes.*
    c. Alcoholism is a significant risk factor for development of Fournier gangrene.
    d. In severe cases, debridement may need to extend into the chest wall.
    e. Fournier gangrene can be caused by a cutaneous, urethral, or perirectal source of infection.

28. An 18-year-old woman develops a pruritic rash over her thighs and buttocks after using a whirlpool spa. Her face and upper extremities are spared. What is the likely diagnosis?
    a. Candidal intertrigo
    b. Pseudomonal folliculitis
    c. Contact dermatitis
    d. Scabies infestation
    e. Herpes simplex

29. Which of the following conditions has an association with hyperhidrosis?
    a. Atopic dermatitis
    b. Trichomycosis axillaris
    c. Hidradenitis suppurativa
    d. Psoriasis
    e. Genital lichen planus

30. A patient being treated for tinea cruris has significant scrotal involvement. What alternative diagnosis does this suggest?
    a. Seborrheic dermatitis
    b. Erythrasma
    c. Cutaneous candidiasis
    d. Hidradenitis suppurativa
    e. Contact dermatitis

31. Which of the following is a treatment for scabies that is contraindicated in pediatric patients?
    a. Lindane
    b. Dapsone
    c. Permethrin
    d. Ivermectin
    e. Doxycycline

32. Which of the following statements concerning Bowen disease is FALSE?
    a. Bowen disease and squamous cell carcinoma in situ are the same condition.
    b. Bowen disease involving the glans penis is termed *erythroplasia of Queyrat.*
    c. Bowen disease may be treated with topical imiquimod.
    d. Bowen disease is associated with human papillomavirus types 6 and 11.
    e. Mohs microsurgery may play a role when tissue preservation is critical.

33. Which of the following statements concerning verrucous carcinoma is TRUE?
    a. Verrucous carcinoma has a high propensity to metastasize.
    b. Verrucous carcinoma should not be treated with primary radiotherapy because of the risk of anaplastic transformation.
    c. Verrucous carcinoma is an exceedingly rare malignancy of the genitalia.
    d. Verrucous carcinoma is associated with human papillomavirus types 16 and 18.
    e. Verrucous carcinoma may grow very rapidly and destroy local tissue.

34. What is the most common site of presentation for Kaposi sarcoma in immunocompetent individuals?
    a. Chest
    b. Face
    c. Lower extremities
    d. Genitalia
    e. Palms

35. The following malignancy has been found concurrently in lesions of pseudoepitheliomatous, keratotic, and micaceous balanitis:
    a. basal cell carcinoma
    b. cutaneous T-cell lymphoma
    c. squamous cell carcinoma
    d. verrucous carcinoma
    e. Kaposi sarcoma

36. Which of the following statements about extramammary Paget disease (EPD) is FALSE?
    a. EPD is an adenocarcinoma.
    b. EPD is associated with another underlying malignancy in more than 60% of cases.
    c. EPD has been associated with malignancies of the urethra and bladder.
    d. EPD lesions show vacuolated Paget cells on histopathologic exam.
    e. The vulva is the most common genital site involved in women.

37. Patients with cutaneous T-cell lymphoma who develop hematologic involvement are given the diagnosis of:
    a. lymphoid papulosis.
    b. mycosis fungoides.
    c. pagetoid reticulosis.
    d. Sézary syndrome.
    e. Fabry disease.

38. Which of the following conditions has the most in common histologically with pearly penile papules?
    a. Psoriasis
    b. Tuberous sclerosis
    c. Molluscum contagiosum
    d. Herpes simplex

39. The most effective treatment for Zoon balanitis is:
    a. topical 5-fluorouracil.
    b. topical corticosteroids.
    c. circumcision.
    d. laser therapy.
    e. topical calcineurin inhibitors.

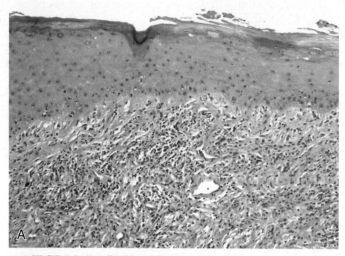

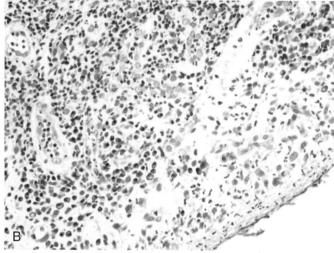

Fig. 59.1 (From Bostwick DG, Cheng L: *Urologic surgical pathology*, 3rd ed, St. Louis, 2014, Saunders.)

40. Skin tags are also termed:
    a. fibrofolliculomas.
    b. angiokeratomas.
    c. hamartomas.
    d. acrochordons.
    e. dermatofibromas.

41. The Leser-Trélat syndrome refers to:
    a. the rapid progression of lichen planus associated with the HLA-B27 haplotype.
    b. an abrupt increase in the size and number of seborrheic keratoses, suggesting internal malignancy.
    c. the combination of hand, foot, and genital psoriasis.
    d. the development of brown macules on the genitalia, unrelated to sun exposure.
    e. the combination of oral and genital ulcers often seen in Behçet disease.

42. A 70-year-old uncircumcised man has noted an erythematous macular lesion on his glans at the corona. The pathology report of the biopsy (Fig. 59.1) reads plasma cell infiltrate consistent with Zoon balanitis. The next step in management is:
    a. ask the pathologist if these are CD4 cells consistent with exposure to HIV.
    b. laser fulguration.
    c. ask the pathologist if he or she looked for an associated squamous cell carcinoma.
    d. circumcision.
    e. observation.

ANSWERS

1. **b. *Candida.*** To identify cutaneous fungi, such as dermatophytes and *Candida* species, periodic acid–Schiff (PAS) staining may be applied to scraped or touched skin specimens.
2. **d. 8 to 48 hours.** Oral glucocorticosteroids (GCS) are absorbed in the jejunum with peak plasma concentrations occurring in 30 to 90 minutes. Despite short plasma half-lives of 1 to 5 hours, the duration of effect of GCS is between 8 and 48 hours, depending on the agent.
3. **a. A single morning dose.** For short-term (≤3 weeks) treatment of dermatologic conditions such as allergic contact dermatitis, a single morning dose of oral glucocorticosteroids is given to minimize suppression of the hypothalamic-pituitary-adrenal axis.
4. **d. The frequent application of emollients.** The condition described is atopic dermatitis (AD or eczema), which is associated with susceptibility to irritants and proteins, as well as the tendency to develop asthma and allergic rhinitis. Intense pruritus is the hallmark of AD, and controlling the patient's urge to scratch is critical for successful treatment. Removal of various "trigger factors" from the environment (such as chemicals, detergents, and household dust mites) may be beneficial in some cases. The mainstay of treatment for AD includes gentle cleaning with nonalkali soaps and the frequent use of emollients.
5. **b. Contact dermatitis.** Patch testing is a simple technique of exposing an area of skin to a variety of potential allergens in a grid template. Generally performed by dermatologists, patch testing can help confirm the diagnosis of allergic contact dermatitis and the allergen involved.
6. **d. Nickel sulfate.** In 2003, the North American Contact Dermatitis Group (NACDG) reported a long list of common allergens implicated in allergic contact dermatitis based on patch testing results. The most common sensitizing allergen identified was nickel sulfate, which is a common component of costume jewelry and belt buckles.
7. **d. Irritant contact dermatitis.** Irritant contact dermatitis results from a direct cytotoxic effect of an irritant chemical touching the skin and is responsible for approximately 80% of contact dermatitis cases. Occupational exposure is also common. Examples of offending agents include soaps, metal salts, acid- or alkali-containing compounds, and industrial solvents.
8. **c. Observation.** Erythema multiforme (EM) minor is an acute, self-limited skin disease characterized by the abrupt onset of symmetrical fixed red papules that may evolve into target lesions. The majority of cases are precipitated by herpesvirus type I and II, with herpetic lesions usually preceding the development of target lesions by 10 to 14 days. Although continuous suppressive acyclovir may prevent EM episodes in patients with herpes infection, administration of the drug after development of target lesions is of no benefit. With observation alone, the natural history of EM minor is spontaneous resolution after several weeks without sequelae, although recurrences are common.
9. **c. Stevens-Johnson syndrome.** Stevens-Johnson syndrome (SJS) is a life-threatening severe allergic reaction with features similar to extensive skin burns. A vast array of inciting factors has been implicated in the development of SJS, with drug exposures being the most commonly identified. Nonsteroidal antiinflammatory agents are the most frequent offending agents, followed by sulfonamides, tetracycline, penicillin, doxycycline, and anticonvulsants.

10. **a. Topical 3% liquor carbonis detergens in 1% hydrocortisone cream.** Psoriasis is a papulosquamous disorder affecting up to 2% of the population with a relapsing and remitting course. For genital psoriasis, the mainstay of therapy is the use of low-potency topical corticosteroid creams for short courses. Photochemotherapy combining an ingested psoralen with ultraviolet radiation (PUVA) has been used extensively to treat psoriasis. However, a dose-dependent increase in the risk of genital squamous cell carcinoma has been associated with high-dose PUVA therapy for psoriasis elsewhere on the body. Genital shielding during PUVA therapy is strongly recommended; therefore, this modality is contraindicated for treating psoriatic lesions localized to genital skin.

11. **b. The human leukocyte antigen (HLA)-B27 haplotype.** Reiter syndrome is a syndrome composed of urethritis, arthritis, ocular findings, oral ulcers, and skin lesions. It is generally preceded by an episode of either urethritis (*Chlamydia, Gonococcus*) or gastrointestinal infection (*Yersinia, Salmonella, Shigella, Campylobacter, Neisseria,* or *Ureaplasma* species) and is more common in HIV-positive patients. **There is a strong genetic association with the HLA-B27 haplotype.**

12. **c. Systemic corticosteroids can shorten the time to clearance of existing lesions from 29 to 18 weeks.** Although bothersome pruritus is common with lichen planus (LP), asymptomatic lesions on the genitalia do not require treatment. The primary modality of treatment for symptomatic lesions is topical corticosteroids, although for severe cases, systemic corticosteroids have been shown to shorten the time course to clearance of LP lesions from 29 to 18 weeks.

13. **d. Balanitis xerotica obliterans.** Lichen sclerosus (LS) is a scarring disorder, with a predilection for the external genitalia of both sexes, characterized by tissue pallor, loss of architecture, and hyperkeratosis. The late stage of this disease is called *balanitis xerotica obliterans*, which can involve the penile urethra and result in troublesome urethral stricture disease.

14. **a. Lichen sclerosus et atrophicus.** Despite the similarities in name, LS shares little in common with lichen planus and lichen nitidus other than pruritus and a predilection for the genital region. Another critical distinction is that LS has been associated with squamous cell carcinoma of the penis, particularly those variants not associated with human papillomavirus, and may represent a premalignant condition. Biopsy is worthwhile both to confirm the diagnosis and to exclude malignant change.

15. **b. Consult with neurology to alter his antiseizure medication regimen.** The association of epileptic seizures and a solitary painful genital lesion is suspicious for a diagnosis of Behçet disease (BD). Other causes for genital ulceration, however, including aphthous ulcers, syphilis, herpes simplex, and chancroid, must be considered before a diagnosis of BD is made. In this case, the patient's neurologic issues should take priority over treatment for his genital ulcer.

16. **b. HIV test.** Seborrheic dermatitis (SD) is a common skin disease characterized by the presence of sharply demarcated, pink-yellow to red-brown plaques with a flaky scale. Particularly in immunosuppressed individuals, SD may involve a significant proportion of the body surface area. **Extensive and/or severe SD should raise concerns for possible underlying HIV infection.**

17. **b. The Asboe-Hansen sign.** The loss of epidermal cohesion seen in pemphigus vulgaris leads to the characteristic Asboe-Hansen sign: spreading of fluid under the adjacent normal-appearing skin away from the direction of pressure on a blister.

18. **e. Given enough time, even advanced cases of pemphigus generally resolve spontaneously without sequelae.** Severe cases of pemphigus vulgaris without appropriate treatment may be fatal because of the loss of the epidermal barrier function of large areas of affected skin. Treatment usually depends on systemic corticosteroids, although minimization of steroid dose is an important goal to limit side effects. The addition of immunosuppressive agents, such as azathioprine and cyclo-

phosphamide, may be beneficial because of their corticosteroid-sparing effect.

19. **a. Dermatitis herpetiformis.** Dermatitis herpetiformis (DH) is a cutaneous manifestation of celiac disease and is generally associated with gluten sensitivity. Diagnosis can be confirmed by biopsy and direct immunofluorescence, which shows a granular pattern of IgA deposition at the basement membrane. Treatment includes the use of dapsone and a strict gluten-restricted diet.

20. **b. Pyoderma gangrenosum.** Pyoderma gangrenosum (PG) is an ulcerative skin disease associated with systemic illnesses, including inflammatory bowel disease, arthritis, collagen vascular disease, and myeloproliferative disorders. The classic morphologic presentation of PG is painful cutaneous and mucous membrane ulceration, often with extensive loss of tissue and a purulent base.

21. **c. Dapsone.** Characteristic clinical features of linear IgA bullous dermatosis (LABD) include vesicles and bullae arranged in a combination of circumferential and linear orientations. Treatment with either sulfapyridine or dapsone is usually effective in controlling LABD, and long-term spontaneous remission rates of 30% to 60% have been described.

22. **c. Involvement of the vulva is common in women.** Hailey-Hailey disease (HH) is an autosomal dominant blistering dermatosis that has a predilection for the intertriginous areas, including the groin and perianal region. Symptoms include an unfortunate combination of pruritus, pain, and a foul odor. Because heat and sweating exacerbate the condition, HH tends to worsen during the summer months. In women, disease in the inframammary folds is common, although vulvar disease is unusual. For disease resistant to medical therapy, wide excision and skin grafting have been effective, as have local ablative techniques such as dermabrasion and laser vaporization.

23. **a. Behçet disease.** When oral and genital aphthous ulcers are coexistent, the clinician should consider the diagnosis of BD. BD is a generalized relapsing and remitting ulcerative mucocutaneous disease that likely involves a genetic predisposition and an autoimmune mode of pathogenesis. Affected individuals may also suffer from epididymitis, thrombophlebitis, aneurysms, and gastrointestinal, neurologic, and arthritic problems.

24. **d. The presence of vacuolated keratinocytes in an inflammatory background is pathognomonic for this condition.** Pyoderma gangrenosum (PG) is an ulcerative skin disease associated with systemic illnesses, including inflammatory bowel disease, arthritis, collagen vascular disease, and myeloproliferative disorders. It most commonly affects women between the second and fifth decade of life and likely has an autoimmune pathogenesis, given its association with other autoimmune diseases. As is the case in Behçet disease, no specific diagnostic laboratory test or histopathologic feature is pathognomonic for PG, although a history of underlying systemic disease may raise suspicion.

25. **a. Factitial dermatitis.** Factitial dermatitis is a psychocutaneous disorder in which the individual self-inflicts cutaneous lesions, usually for an unconscious motive. An association between factitial dermatitis and borderline personality disorder appears to exist.

26. **c. *Streptococcus pyogenes*.** Erysipelas is a superficial bacterial skin infection limited to the dermis with lymphatic involvement. In contrast to the cutaneous lesion of cellulitis, erysipelas generally has a raised and distinct border at the interface with normal skin. The causative organism is usually *S. pyogenes*.

27. **b. Most cases of Fournier gangrene are caused by *S. pyogenes*.** Fournier gangrene (FG) is a potentially life-threatening progressive infection of the perineum and genitalia. In the genital region, most cases of FG are caused by mixed bacterial flora, which include gram-positive, gram-negative, and anaerobic bacteria.

28. **b. Pseudomonal folliculitis.** Folliculitis is a common disorder characterized by perifollicular pustules on an erythematous

base. It occurs most frequently in heavily hair-bearing areas such as the scalp, beard, axilla, groin, and buttocks and can be exacerbated by local trauma from shaving, rubbing, or clothing irritation. Folliculitis has also been associated with the use of contaminated hot tubs and swimming pools, with the offending organism usually *Pseudomonas aeruginosa.*

29. **b. Trichomycosis axillaris.** Trichomycosis axillaris (TA) is a superficial bacterial infection of axillary and pubic hair caused by *Corynebacterium*, which is associated with hyperhidrosis. Shaving can provide immediate improvement, and antibacterial soaps may prevent further infection. For pubic TA, clindamycin gel, bacitracin, and oral erythromycin have also proven effective.

30. **c. Cutaneous candidiasis.** Tinea cruris is the term given to dermatophyte infection of the groin and genital area and is commonly known as "jock itch." The inner thighs and inguinal region are the most commonly affected areas, and the scrotum and penis are usually spared in men. Significant scrotal involvement should raise suspicion for cutaneous candidiasis as an alternative diagnosis.

31. **a. Lindane.** As in the case of pediculosis pubis, the treatment of choice for scabies is 5% permethrin cream applied to the entire body overnight, with a second application 1 week later. An alternative scabicide, lindane, is not favored because of both central nervous system (CNS) toxicity in children and a rising rate of resistance among mites.

32. **d. Bowen disease is associated with human papillomavirus (HPV) types 6 and 11.** Bowen disease occurring on the mucosal surfaces of the male genitalia is referred to as erythroplasia of Queyrat. In that location, coinfection with HPV type 8, 16, 39, and 51 has been identified. In contrast, the variant of squamous cell carcinoma termed "verrucous carcinoma" has been associated with HPV type 6 and 11 infection but not with the more classically oncogenic type 16 and 18.

33. **b. Verrucous carcinoma (VC) should not be treated with primary radiotherapy because of the risk of anaplastic transformation.** VC is a slow-growing, locally aggressive, exophytic, low-grade variant of squamous cell carcinoma that has little metastatic potential. It most commonly occurs in uncircumcised men on the glans or prepuce, although similar lesions can be found on the vulva, vagina cervix, or anus. Treatment is preferably by local excision. Primary radiotherapy is relatively contraindicated because of the potential for anaplastic transformation with a subsequent increase in metastatic potential.

34. **c. Lower extremities.** Kaposi sarcoma (KS) in immunocompetent individuals presents as slowly growing, blue-red pigmented macules on the lower extremities. Although oral and gastrointestinal lesions may occur, the genitalia are seldom involved. This is in contrast to the case with acquired immunodeficiency syndrome (AIDS), in which a solitary genital lesion may be the first manifestation of KS. The clinical features of KS in AIDS patients are diverse, ranging from a single lesion to disseminated cutaneous and visceral disease.

35. **d. Verrucous carcinoma.** Pseudoepitheliomatous, keratotic, and micaceous balanitis (PEKMB) is a rare entity characterized

by the development of a thick, hyperkeratotic plaque on the glans penis of older men. There remains controversy as to whether PEKMB is a premalignant condition. PEKMB was originally thought to be a purely benign process, although several case reports have documented the presence of concurrent verrucous carcinoma associated with this lesion.

36. **b. EPD is associated with another underlying malignancy in more than 60% of cases.** Extramammary Paget disease (EPD) is an uncommon intraepithelial adenocarcinoma of sites bearing apocrine glands. There is an important association between EPD and another underlying malignancy in 10% to 30% of cases. In the male, associations of urethral, bladder, rectal, and apocrine malignancies with EPD have been described.

37. **d. Sézary syndrome.** Cutaneous T-cell lymphoma (CTCL) represents a group of related neoplasms derived from T cells that home to the skin. CTCL generally presents with pruritus, which must be differentiated from a variety of benign dermatoses, including psoriasis, eczema, superficial fungal infections, and drug reactions. Patients may subsequently develop hematologic involvement (termed Sézary syndrome) and cutaneous plaques, erosions, ulcers, or frank skin tumors.

38. **b. Tuberous sclerosis.** Pearly penile papules (PPP) are white, dome-shaped, closely spaced, small papules located on the glans penis. Histologically, these lesions are angiofibromas similar to the lesions seen on the face in tuberous sclerosis.

39. **c. Circumcision.** Zoon balanitis, also called plasma cell balanitis, occurs in uncircumcised men from the third decade onward. Squamous cell carcinoma and extramammary Paget disease should be excluded, often by biopsy. Circumcision appears to be proof against development of the disease and can be performed to cure the majority of cases. For patients averse to circumcision, topical corticosteroids may provide symptomatic relief, and laser therapy may also have a role.

40. **d. Acrochordons.** Skin tags (acrochordons, fibroepithelial polyps) are soft, skin-colored, pedunculated lesions that can be present anywhere on the body. It is important to distinguish these lesions from the hamartomatous skin lesions (multiple fibrofolliculomas) associated with Birt-Hogg-Dubé syndrome, which are histologically distinct from common skin tags.

41. **b. An abrupt increase in the size and number of seborrheic keratoses, suggesting internal malignancy.** The presence of brown macules unrelated to sun exposure suggests a diagnosis of SK. This condition may commonly involve the genitalia but generally spares the mucous membranes, palms, and soles of the feet. An abrupt increase in the size and number of multiple SK has been termed Leser-Trélat syndrome and has been implicated as a cutaneous marker of internal malignancy. The HLA-B27 haplotype is associated with Reiter syndrome, not rapidly progressive lichen planus.

42. **d. Circumcision.** The patient has Zoon balanitis. The biopsy shows reactive epithelial changes with a plasma cell infiltrate into the dermis. Although the disease can be treated with immune modulators, these patients respond best to circumcision.

CHAPTER REVIEW

1. Topical application of steroids may result in systemic absorption resulting in significant side effects.
2. The majority of cases of erythema multiforme are precipitated by herpesvirus type I and II, with the herpetic lesions usually preceding the development of the target lesions by 2 weeks.
3. The major form of erythema multiforme is called Stevens-Johnson syndrome, which has a protracted course of 4 to 6 weeks and may have a mortality approaching 30%. Nonsteroidal antiinflammatory agents, sulfonamides, tetracyclines, penicillin, doxycycline, and anticonvulsants are the most common offending agents.
4. Reiter syndrome comprises urethritis, arthritis, ocular findings (conjunctivitis), oral ulcers, and skin lesions. It is generally preceded by an episode of urethritis or a gastrointestinal infection. It is more common in HIV-positive patients. It is associated with HLA-B27 haplotype.
5. The triad of clinical features in Behçet syndrome consists of mucocutaneous lesions of the oral cavity, genitalia, and uveitis. The ulcers are painful.
6. Hidradenitis suppurativa is an epithelial disorder of hair follicles that occurs in the apocrine gland–bearing skin, which results in a marked inflammatory response with formation of abscesses and sinus tracks. Bacterial infection does not appear to be the primary initiator. Rupture of the follicular contents—bacteria and keratin—into the dermis causes a marked inflammatory response.
7. Ecthyma gangrenosum is a result of pseudomonal septicemia and may result in gangrenous ulcers.
8. Dermatophytes are fungi of three genera: *Trichophyton, Microsporum,* and *Epidermophyton.* Tinea cruris, an infection of the groin and genital skin, may be caused by one of these fungi. Postinflammatory hyperpigmentation occurs with this disease and may not indicate an active infection.
9. Bowenoid papulosis consists of multiple small erythematous papules and is associated with HPV type 16.
10. Angiokeratomas of Fordyce are vascular ectasias of dermal blood vessels. They are 1- to 2-mm red or purple papules and may be the source of troublesome scrotal bleeding.
11. CIS of the penis rarely progresses to invasive disease.
12. Whether Kaposi sarcoma is a neoplastic or hyperplastic process is debated. When it is associated with organ transplantation, alteration of the immunosuppressive regimen may result in resolution.
13. Epidermoid cysts are commonly found in the scrotum.
14. Extensive and/or severe seborrheic dermatitis should raise concerns for possible underlying HIV infection.
15. Pyoderma gangrenosum is an ulcerative skin disease associated with systemic illnesses, including inflammatory bowel disease, arthritis, collagen vascular disease, and myeloproliferative disorders.
16. In tinea cruris, the inner thighs and inguinal region are the most commonly affected areas, and the scrotum and penis are usually spared in men.
17. Extramammary Paget disease (EPD) is an uncommon intraepithelial adenocarcinoma of sites bearing apocrine glands. There is an important association between EPD and another underlying malignancy in 10% to 30% of cases.

60 Tuberculosis and Parasitic Infections of the Genitourinary Tract

Alicia H. Chang, Brian G. Blackburn, and Michael Hsieh

QUESTIONS

Tuberculosis

1. All of the following mycobacteria cause tuberculosis (TB) EXCEPT:
   a. *Mycobacterium bovis.*
   b. *Mycobacterium avium-intracellulare.*
   c. *Mycobacterium africanum.*
   d. *Mycobacterium microti.*
   e. Bacille Calmette-Guérin (BCG).

2. Which of the following statements about the epidemiology of tuberculosis is FALSE?
   a. TB incidence and mortality have been decreasing worldwide since the year 2000.
   b. Tuberculosis incidence is higher in those who are born outside the United States than in those born in the United States.
   c. Prevalence of multidrug-resistant (MDR) tuberculosis cases is now approaching 12% in the United States.
   d. The lifetime risk of reactivation of TB is 5% to 10% in most people.
   e. Worldwide, tuberculosis is the cause of death in 25% of persons who test positive for human immunodeficiency virus (HIV).

3. Which of the following routes of infection is the most common in genitourinary tuberculosis?
   a. Hematogenous seeding
   b. Lymphatic spread
   c. Direct inoculation
   d. Sexual transmission
   e. Ascending or retrograde infection

4. Which of the following is a not a late complication of genitourinary tuberculosis?
   a. Infertility
   b. Scrotal fistula
   c. Autonephrectomy
   d. Thimble bladder
   e. Papulonecrotic tuberculid

5. Which of the following persons is LEAST likely to have tuberculosis infection?
   a. A patient with fibrosis on chest radiograph and a tuberculin skin test (TST) of 5 mm
   b. A patient with HIV infection and a TST of 3 mm
   c. A recent immigrant from Vietnam with a TST of 11 mm
   d. A BCG-vaccinated patient with a TST of 14 mm
   e. A healthy U.S.-born teacher with a TST of 11 mm

6. Which of the following results most specifically diagnoses genitourinary tuberculosis?
   a. A positive interferon γ release assay
   b. A positive urine polymerase chain reaction (PCR) for *Mycobacterium tuberculosis* complex
   c. A TST reaction of 25 mm
   d. A positive urine acid-fast bacilli (AFB) culture
   e. A renal biopsy showing AFB

7. Which of the following first-line antituberculosis agents does not cause hepatic toxicity?
   a. Isoniazid
   b. Rifampin
   c. Pyrazinamide
   d. Ethambutol
   e. Streptomycin

8. Which of the following drugs might have efficacy against extensively drug-resistant (XDR) tuberculosis?
   a. Isoniazid (INH)
   b. Rifampin
   c. Pyrazinamide
   d. Moxifloxacin
   e. Amikacin

9. Which of the urological interventions is emergently indicated?
   a. Nephrectomy of nonfunctional kidney in medically resistant hypertension
   b. Bladder augmentation of a contracted bladder in a patient with severe dysuria
   c. Percutaneous nephrostomy of obstructive hydronephrosis in acute renal failure
   d. Balloon dilatation and ureteral stenting of a proximal ureteral stricture
   e. Boari flap for a lower ureteral stricture that requires excision

10. Which of the following statements is FALSE about genitourinary (GU) TB patients?
    a. Magnetic resonance imaging (MRI) is often used to help diagnose patients with GU TB.
    b. Computed tomography (CT) is most useful in extensive TB disease when other organ systems might be involved.
    c. The most common finding of GU TB on plain film is calcification.
    d. Intravenous urography (IVU) is the best test to detect early renal changes due to TB.
    e. The most common finding on IVU is obstructive uropathy from scarring.

Schistosomiasis

1. Of the following drugs, the most effective to treat schistosomiasis is:
   a. albendazole.
   b. praziquantel.
   c. mebendazole.
   d. diethylcarbamazine.
   e. ivermectin.

2. The life cycle stage of *Schistosoma haematobium* that infects humans transdermally is:
   a. the worm.
   b. the schistosomule.
   c. the cercariae.
   d. the egg.
   e. the sporocyst.

3. *S. haematobium* infections are estimated to affect the following number of people:
   a. 1.1 billion
   b. 1.1 million
   c. 900,000
   d. 112 million
   e. 11 million

4. The life cycle stage of *S. haematobium* that induces the majority of human tissue pathology is:
   a. the worm.
   b. the schistosomule.
   c. the cercaria.
   d. the egg.
   e. the sporocyst.

5. The eponym for acute schistosomiasis is:
   a. Katayama fever.
   b. Bilharz syndrome.
   c. Barlow fever.
   d. Toshiro syndrome.
   e. Tan's triad.

6. The diagnostic, first-line gold standard for urogenital schistosomiasis is:
   a. polymerase chain reaction.
   b. serology.
   c. cystourethroscopy with bladder biopsy.
   d. rectal biopsy.
   e. urine egg counts.

7. Without treatment, *Schistosoma* worms can live in human hosts for an average of:
   a. 3 months.
   b. 9 months.
   c. 3 to 5 years.
   d. 5 decades.
   e. 5 weeks.

8. Surgical options for reconstruction of irreversible ureteral lesions caused by urogenital schistosomiasis include all of the following EXCEPT:
   a. renal autotransplantation.
   b. Boari flaps.
   c. ureteroureterostomies.
   d. ileal ureter.
   e. suprapubic intravesical ureterostomy.

9. Intermediate snail hosts for *S. haematobium* are members of the following genus:
   a. *Biomphalaria*.
   b. *Oncomelania*.
   c. *Bulinus*.
   d. *Helix*.
   e. *Achatina*.

Other Parasitic Infections

1. The rickettsia-like organism that is an endosymbiont of the parasites that cause lymphatic filariasis (LF) and onchocerciasis is:
   a. *Rickettsia rickettsii*.
   b. *Wuchereria bancrofti*.
   c. *Wolbachia* spp.
   d. *Brugia malayi*.
   e. *Brugia timori*.

2. The chronic manifestations of LF are mostly seen in:
   a. short-term missionaries to endemic areas.
   b. short-term aid workers to endemic areas.
   c. long-term (current) residents of endemic areas.
   d. short-term tourists to endemic areas.
   e. short-term visiting friends and relatives travelers (VFRs) to endemic areas.

3. Most patients infected with *Onchocerca volvulus* live in:
   a. Latin America.
   b. Oceania.
   c. Asia.
   d. Sub-Saharan Africa.
   e. the Middle East.

4. The majority of patients infected with *Wuchereria bancrofti* have:
   a. lymphedema.
   b. hydrocele.
   c. no clinical manifestations.
   d. acute adenolymphangitis (ADL).
   e. elephantiasis.

5. Which drug should not be given to patients infected with *O. volvulus* or to those infected with high-grade *Loa loa* microfilaremia?
   a. Diethylcarbamazine (DEC)
   b. Albendazole
   c. Doxycycline
   d. Azithromycin
   e. Amoxicillin

ANSWERS

Tuberculosis

1. **b. *Mycobacterium avium-intracellulare.*** *M. bovis, M. africanum,* and *M. microti* are members of the *M. tuberculosis* complex (MTBC) and can cause TB disease. BCG is derived from *M. bovis* and can cause TB in certain individuals. Of the mycobacteria listed, *M. avium-intracellulare* is one of the many nontuberculous mycobacteria.

TABLE 60.1 Guidelines for Determining a Positive Tuberculin Skin Test Reaction.

INDURATION ≥ 5 MM	INDURATION ≥ 10 MM	INDURATION > 15 MM
• HIV-positive persons • Silicosis • Fibrotic changes on chest radiograph consistent with old TB • Patients with organ transplants • Immunosuppressed therapy (receiving the equivalent of >15 mg/day prednisone for ≥1 month, or tumor necrosis factor α [TNF-α] antagonists) • Recent contacts of person with TB disease • Children <5 years of age	• Immigrants from high-prevalence countries (TB incidence >20/100,000) • Residents and employees[a] of high-risk congregate settings: prisons and jails, nursing homes and other health care facilities, residential facilities for AIDS patients, and homeless shelters • Mycobacteriology laboratory personnel • Persons with clinical conditions that make them high-risk: silicosis diabetes mellitus, chronic renal failure, some hematologic disorders (e.g., leukemias and lymphomas), other specific malignancies (e.g., carcinoma of the head or neck and lung), weight loss of >10% of ideal body weight, gastrectomy, jejunoileal bypass • Injection drug users	• Persons with no risk factors for TB

[a]For persons who are otherwise at low risk and are tested at entry into employment, a reaction of >15 mm induration is considered positive.
HIV, Human immunodeficiency virus; *TB*, tuberculosis.
From American Thoracic Society and Centers for Disease Control and Prevention: Diagnostic standards and classification of tuberculosis in adults and children. *Am J Respir Crit Care Med* 161(4 Pt. 1):1376–1395, 2000.

2. **c. Prevalence of multidrug-resistant (MDR) tuberculosis cases is now approaching 12% in the United States.** Although MDR TB is concerning because of the difficulty of treatment, in 2012, the proportion of TB cases caused by MDR TB was only 1.2% in the United States.
3. **a. Hematogenous seeding.** Each of the answers is a known route of infection for the development of GU TB. However, hematogenous seeding is by far the most common one.
4. **e. Papulonecrotic tuberculid.** Papulonecrotic tuberculid is the only manifestation listed that can present early in the course of TB disease. The tuberculids are hypersensitivity reactions to MTBC antigens that were disseminated to the skin from other infectious foci, and as such, they are culture negative and typically PCR negative.
5. **e. A healthy U.S.-born teacher with a TST of 11 mm.** Refer to Table 60.1 for the Centers for Disease Control and Prevention guidelines on TST interpretation. Patients (a), (b), and (c) are likely TB infected. A BCG-vaccinated person is likely from a country with high enough incidence of TB to warrant vaccination; hence a cutoff of 10 mm is likely to apply for this person. Patient (e) has no clear risk factors for TB; hence a cutoff of 15 mm would apply for this person. However, TST cutoffs may be set differently in local public health jurisdictions according to local epidemiology.
6. **d. A positive urine acid-fast bacilli (AFB) culture.**
7. **d. Ethambutol.** Ethambutol is rarely hepatotoxic. Its main toxicity is ocular, such as decreased visual acuity or red-green color blindness. Streptomycin is not considered hepatotoxic either, but it is also not considered a first-line agent in the United States.
8. **c. Pyrazinamide.** By definition, MDR TB is resistant to INH, rifampin, any quinolone, and at least an additional injectable aminoglycoside. Hence, of the choices, pyrazinamide is the most likely to have efficacy against XDR TB.
9. **c. Percutaneous nephrostomy of obstructive hydronephrosis in acute renal failure.** All of the choices are appropriate indications for urological intervention. However, only (c) is emergently indicated. For the other interventions, waiting at least 4 to 6 weeks after initiation of medical therapy is preferred.
10. **a. Magnetic resonance imaging (MRI) is often used to help diagnose patients with GU TB.** Although MRI has potential uses in the diagnosis of GU TB, it is not sufficiently superior to CT or IVU to warrant its frequent use.

Schistosomiasis
1. **b. Praziquantel.** Although all of the drugs listed are antiparasitic agents, only praziquantel is used to treat schistosomiasis. In fact, praziquantel is the only drug approved for schistosomiasis by the World Health Organization (WHO).
2. **c. The cercariae.** The worm and egg stages (Fig. 60.1) are found in chronically infected humans but are intravascular or deposited in tissues such as the bladder, respectively. Cercariae infect humans by burrowing through the skin, whereupon they transform into schistosomules.
3. **d. 112 million.** Although an estimated 1 billion people are at risk of contracting schistosomiasis because they live in endemic areas, only 112 million are actively infected with *S. haematobium*.
4. **d. The egg.** The majority of human tissue pathology caused by urogenital schistosomiasis is induced by the host immune response against *S. haematobium* eggs (see Fig. 60.1). In comparison to eggs, worms, schistosomules, and cercariae are much less immunogenic and are thought to correspondingly cause much less chronic tissue pathology.
5. **a. Katayama fever.** The syndrome associated with acute schistosomiasis is named after the Katayama valley in Japan, a formerly endemic region for *Schistosoma japonicum*.
6. **e. Urine egg counts.** Although PCR and serology are highly sensitive for detecting infection, they are not considered first-line diagnostic modalities. Cystourethroscopy (Fig. 60.2) with bladder biopsy and rectal biopsy are highly invasive and reserved for difficult-to-diagnose cases or suspected cancer. Microscopic enumeration of *S. haematobium* eggs shed in urine are the diagnostic, first-line gold standard (albeit slow and impractical in many field settings).
7. **c. 3 to 5 years.** Although there have been reports that some schistosome worms can live for several decades, on average they are believed to only live for 3 to 5 years.
8. **a. Renal autotransplantation.** Renal autotransplantation is reserved for reconstruction of the urinary tract in the setting of multiple and/or large renal tumors. There are much less morbid surgical options for reconstruction of schistosomiasis-associated ureteral lesions.
9. **c. Bulinus.** *Biomphalaria* and *Oncomelania* are host snails for *Schistosoma mansoni* and *S. japonicum*, respectively, but not *S. haematobium*. *Helix* and *Achatina* snails are terrestrial and not considered hosts for human-specific schistosomes.

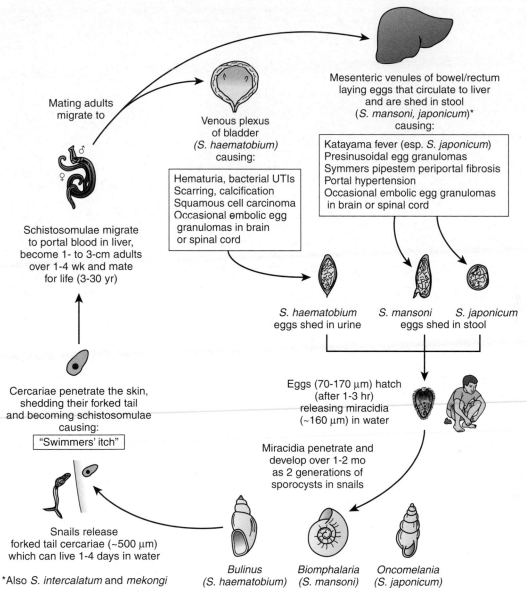

Mating adults
migrate to

Venous plexus
of bladder
(*S. haematobium*)
causing:

Mesenteric venules of bowel/rectum
laying eggs that circulate to liver
and are shed in stool
(*S. mansoni, japonicum*)*
causing:

Katayama fever (esp. *S. japonicum*)
Presinusoidal egg granulomas
Symmers pipestem periportal fibrosis
Portal hypertension
Occasional embolic egg granulomas
in brain or spinal cord

Hematuria, bacterial UTIs
Scarring, calcification
Squamous cell carcinoma
Occasional embolic egg
granulomas in brain
or spinal cord

Schistosomulae migrate
to portal blood in liver,
become 1- to 3-cm adults
over 1-4 wk and mate
for life (3-30 yr)

S. haematobium
eggs shed in urine

S. mansoni   *S. japonicum*
eggs shed in stool

Cercariae penetrate the skin,
shedding their forked tail
and becoming schistosomulae
causing:

"Swimmers' itch"

Eggs (70-170 μm) hatch
(after 1-3 hr)
releasing miracidia
(~160 μm) in water

Miracidia penetrate and
develop over 1-2 mo
as 2 generations of
sporocysts in snails

Snails release
forked tail cercariae (~500 μm)
which can live 1-4 days in water

*Also *S. intercalatum* and *mekongi*

Bulinus   *Biomphalaria*   *Oncomelania*
(*S. haematobium*) (*S. mansoni*)   (*S. japonicum*)

Fig. 60.1 Life cycle of a schistosome. *UTIs,* Urinary tract infections. From King CH. Schistosomiasis. In: Guerrant RL, Walker DH, Weller PF, editors. *Tropical infectious diseases, principles, pathogens, and practice.* 2nd ed. Philadelphia: Elsevier Churchill Livingstone; 2006.

Other Parasitic Infections

1. **c. *Wolbachia* spp.** *Wolbachia* endosymbionts infect *W. bancrofti, Brugia* spp., and *O. volvulus.* They appear to be involved in embryogenesis and, when killed with antimicrobial therapy (e.g., doxycycline), result in decreased microfilaria release and suppressed larval molting.
2. **c. Long-term (current) residents of endemic areas.** Because transmission is inefficient, long-term exposure to multiple infective bites appears to be necessary for transmission of LF and the development of chronic disease due to LF. Therefore, short-term visitors to endemic areas rarely develop LF, which is mostly seen in long-term residents of endemic areas.

3. **d. Sub-Saharan Africa.** Although endemic to Latin America and the Middle East as well, 99% of persons who have onchocerciasis live in sub-Saharan Africa.
4. **c. No clinical manifestations.** Although *W. bancrofti* infection can lead to all of these clinical manifestations, most infected persons remain asymptomatic.
5. **a. Diethylcarbamazine (DEC).** DEC can cause blindness in patients with onchocerciasis (due to the inflammatory response to parasites in the anterior chamber of the eye) and encephalopathy in patients with high-grade *L. loa* microfilaremia.

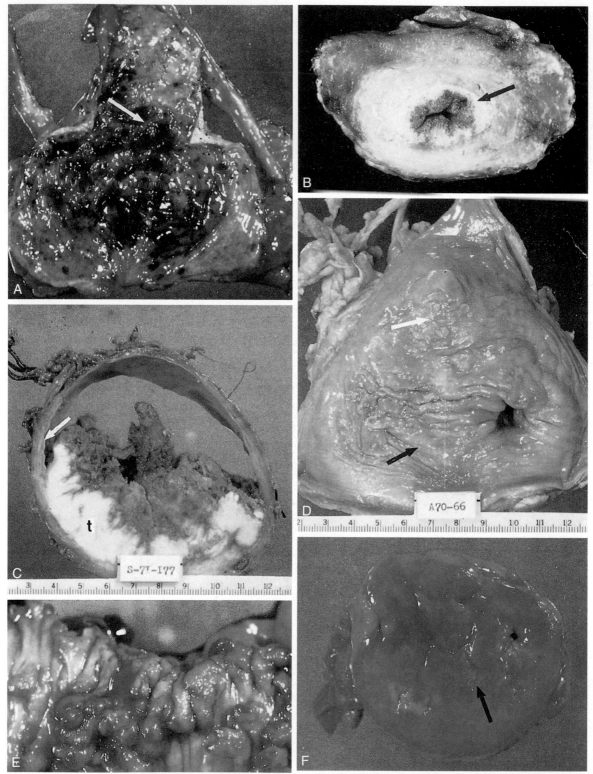

Fig. 60.2 Macroscopic appearance of human urinary schistosomiasis. (A) Urinary bladder opened with an anterior Y incision. The posterior and apical walls have many erythematous, granular, sessile, and pedunculated polyps *(arrow)*, characteristic of the early active stage of urinary schistosomiasis. (B) Coronal section through the apex of a formalin-fixed urinary bladder. The lamina propria has been expanded and is replaced by a yellow-tan, finely granular, sandy patch *(arrow)*, which is characteristic of chronic inactive foci. Small sandy patches are sprinkled through the fibrotic, atrophic detrusor muscle, even in perivesical fat. The more superficial erythematous portion of the lamina propria contains some viable eggs with granulomatous response (chronic active stage of urinary schistosomiasis). (C) Coronal section through the middle of a urinary bladder after formalin inflation and fixation. The lamina propria *(arrow)* has been replaced by a concentric sandy patch, most prominent at the margin of the exophytic, moderately differentiated squamous cell carcinoma. The bladder wall is attenuated except for the tumor *(t)*. No evidence of recent oviposition was found in the lower urinary tract (chronic inactive stage of urinary schistosomiasis, usually found with the bilharzial bladder cancer syndrome). (D) Urinary bladder opened with anterior Y incision shows several features of severe chronic inactive urinary schistosomiasis. The entire lamina propria has been replaced by a sandy patch. Foci of epidermization are seen at or near the white arrow. The left ureteral orifice *(right)* is markedly dilated (the so-called golf-hole ureter of schistosomal uropathy). The right ureteral orifice *(point of black arrow)* is markedly stenotic. (E) Rectosigmoid colon with polyposis. Numerous sessile and pedunculated polyps are seen. Many are erythematous, indicative of active oviposition with granuloma formation. Some have necrotic hemorrhagic tips. (F) Mucosal surface of partial cystectomy specimen (4- to 5-cm ellipse) from a patient with the chronic inactive stage of the disease. There is a stellate chronic schistosomal ulcer. Despite the inactivity of the disease, these ulcers may bleed profusely. Pale mucoid flecks at the margin of the ulcer *(arrow)* are areas of adenoid (goblet cell) metaplasia.

CHAPTER REVIEW

1. Untreated genitourinary TB can lead to irreparable tissue damage and extensive fibrosis, with serious consequences such as renal failure and infertility.
2. The principal route by which genitourinary TB develops is via hematogenous spread, localized to only the genitourinary tract or disseminated to multiple organ systems.
3. Genitourinary TB is associated with nonspecific symptoms and can be indolent, with fewer than 20% presenting with constitutional symptoms.
4. Eighty percent of genitourinary TB occurs in the kidney, and typical laboratory findings include sterile pyuria or hematuria.
5. Ureteral TB can lead to strictures throughout the ureter and impart a pipestem or beaded corkscrew appearance on imaging; bladder TB can lead to severe contracture and is a late complication more common in developing countries.
6. Another common presentation of genitourinary TB is chronic prostatitis that persists despite multiple course of antibiotics.
7. The gold standard for diagnosis of genitourinary TB is a positive AFB culture from urine or tissue biopsy. First void urine is the best sample for culture.
8. Genitourinary TB can also be made with alternate methods of diagnosis such as nucleic acid amplification of *M. tuberculosis* or the presence of granulomas on histopathology examination of tissue.
9. Genitourinary TB generates a wide spectrum of imaging findings. The test of choice depends on disease location. All patients should also have a chest x-ray to exclude concomitant infectious pulmonary TB.
10. Combination therapy with first-line antituberculous drugs achieves the best cure rates in the shortest time frame and should start with isoniazid, rifampin, pyrazinamide, and ethambutol.
11. Surgical interventions are performed to relieve urinary obstruction, to drain infected material, to remove nonworking infected kidneys in cases resisting cure, to improve medically resistant hypertension secondary to a functionally excluded kidney, or to reconstruct the urinary tract.
12. The optimal timing of surgery is 4 to 6 weeks after the initiation of therapy. This delay allows active inflammation to subside, the bacillary load to decrease, and lesions to stabilize.
13. Monitoring for relapse is important after treatment of genitourinary TB because it can occur in up to 22% of cases.
14. Rifampin resistance serves as a surrogate marker for MDR TB.
15. *S. haematobium* has a terminal spine and dwells principally in the perivesical venous plexuses.
16. Schistosomiasis may cause inflammatory polyps of the bladder, sandy spots in the bladder (which represent submucosal egg deposition), calcification of the entire outline of the bladder, and strictures of the ureter (usually in the distal portion) with hydronephrosis. It may be associated with bladder cancer.
17. Squamous cell carcinoma of the bladder is the most common histologic variant occurring as a result of schistosomiasis. These cancers are usually well differentiated or verrucous and therefore carry an overall good prognosis.
18. *W. bancrofti* accounts for 90% of human LF.
19. Obstructive lymphatic disease typically occurs in people who have multiple reinfections following the initial infection with filaria.
20. *W. bancrofti* results in chyluria and filarial hydrocele and occasional extensive scrotal and penile lymphedema.
21. Echinococcosis may result in cysts in the kidney; cyst rupture or spillage during surgical removal can cause anaphylaxis.

61

Basic Principles of Immunology and Immunotherapy in Urologic Oncology

Charles G. Drake

QUESTIONS

1. The immune system has two basic arms, designated "innate" and adaptive. Regarding these divisions, which of the following is true?
   a. The adaptive immune system is the more primitive of the two.
   b. The innate immune system includes long-lived "memory" cells that make secondary responses to pathogens more rapid and stronger.
   c. The adaptive immune system is the only part of the immune system involved in the immune response to cancer.
   d. The innate immune response is driven by recognition of repeated patterns in pathogens called pathogen associated molecular patterns (PAMPs).

2. Immunotherapy for non–muscle-invasive bladder cancer is based on intravesical administration of bacillus Calmette-Guérin (BCG). Initial contact between BCG and the immune system involves which cell type?
   a. Neutrophils, also known as polymorphonuclear cells (PMNs)
   b. CD4+ (helper) T cells
   c. Macrophages ("Big eaters")
   d. CD8+ (killer) T cells
   e. CD8+ regulatory T cells (Tregs)

3. Macrophages and neutrophils have the following feature(s) in common:
   a. they can both ingest pathogens.
   b. they can both present peptide antigens from pathogens on major histocompatibility complex (MHC) class II molecules.
   c. they can both kill pathogens via oxidative processes.
   d. they can both migrate along chemokine gradients to sites of infection.
   e. c and d.

4. Cytokines are chemical messengers that direct immune cell migration and differentiation. Which of the following is true regarding cytokines?
   a. Interleukin 8 (IL-8) is a Th1 cytokine that helps naive CD4+ T cells differentiate into cells that secrete IL-4.
   b. Interferon α is an adaptive cytokine that has no role in the response to BCG.
   c. Interferon γ is an innate cytokine mostly secreted by luminal epithelial cells in the bladder.
   d. Th1 cytokines include IL-4, IL-5, and IL-10.
   e. The primary Th1 cytokine is IL-12.

5. The most important adaptive immune cells are B and T cells. Which of the following is true?
   a. B cells are called B cells because they come from the bone marrow.
   b. CD4 (helper) T cells are mostly of a single phenotype.
   c. CD8 T cells are specialized for cytotoxicity; they evolved to destroy virally infected cells.
   d. Regulatory T cells (Tregs) are a subset of CD8 T cells.
   e. In non–muscle-invasive bladder cancer, a Th2 response involving IL-4, IL-5, and IL-10 is associated with a better outcome.

6. The major function of B cells is to:
   a. kill bacterially infected cells.
   b. generate antibodies which help macrophages to phagocytose and destroy pathogens.
   c. differentiate into memory cells that provide a secondary immune response about equal in magnitude to a primary response.
   d. ingest pathogens.
   e. augment the function of BCG by generating anti-BCG antibodies that lead to BCG persistence in the bladder.

7. CD4 T cell subsets include:
   a. Tregs that augment an antitumor immune response.
   b. Th1 T cells that secrete IL-1.
   c. Th2 T cells that secrete IL-4, IL-5, IL-10, and IL-13.
   d. Th9 T cells that are involved in CD8 T-cell killing.
   e. Th8 T cells that have a cytotoxic function.

8. The immune editing hypothesis explains how tumors evolve in an immunologically competent host. The three E's in the immune editing hypothesis (in order) include:
   a. elimination, equilibrium, and escape.
   b. escape, equilibrium, and elimination.
   c. elucidation, escape, and election.
   d. evolution, equilibrium, and elimination.

9. There is a clear epidemiologic link between chronic inflammation and certain genitourinary (GU) cancers. Which of the following best describes this relationship?
   a. Correlative data are strongest in kidney cancer, where chronic inflammation leads to clear cell cancer or renal cell carcinoma.
   b. Data for this link are absent in prostate cancer.
   c. In bladder cancer, chronic infection with *Schistosoma haematobium* (schistosomiasis) rarely leads to cancer with a squamous cell phenotype.
   d. In prostate cancer, inflammation has been associated with the consumption of charred meat and its associated toxins.

10. The presence of CD8 T cells is associated with:
    a. a better prognosis in all GU tumor types, since CD8 T cells are cancer-fighting cytotoxic cells.
    b. a better prognosis in bladder cancer and prostate cancer.
    c. A worse prognosis in kidney cancer.
    d. A better prognosis in prostate cancer. This is well documented, since prostate tumors are frequently highly infiltrated with CD8 T cells.

11. Immune checkpoint molecules are:
    a. a series of intracellular proteins that regulate progression of T cells through the cell cycle.
    b. a series of extracellular proteins that promote T-cell activation and effector function.
    c. a series of proteins on innate immune cells that inhibit their function.
    d. a series of cell-surface proteins that attenuate CD8 T-cell effector function when bound to their specific cognate ligands.

12. In non–muscle-invasive bladder cancer (NMIBC), the immunotherapeutic effects of BGC are mediated by all of the following EXCEPT which?
    a. The innate immune system, mostly through the activation of neutrophils and macrophages
    b. The release of chemokines from luminal epithelial cells in the bladder
    c. CD4 T cells of the Th2 phenotype
    d. CD8 T cells of the Tc1 phenotype that participate in the direct killing of tumor cells

13. Cancer vaccines are intended to raise an adaptive immune response to a target antigen expressed preferentially on tumor cells. Which of the following is a US Food and Drug Administration (FDA)–approved vaccine for a GU cancer type?
    a. ProstVac VF, which is used in prostate cancer
    b. IMA901, a multi-peptide vaccine for kidney cancer
    c. Gardasil, a vaccine against human papillomavirus
    d. Sipuleucel-T, a prostatic acid phosphatase (PAP)–directed vaccine for prostate cancer

14. The interaction between the immune checkpoint molecule PD-1 (on CD8 T cells) and its ligand PD-L1 (on tumor cells) does which of the following?
    a. Helps CD8 T cells to activate dendritic cells
    b. Drives CD8 T cells to secrete interferon γ, promoting antitumor responses
    c. Mediates an "exhausted" nonfunctional phenotype in the CD8 T cells that express PD-1
    d. Signals through PD-L1 back into the tumor cell to promote tumor cell destruction

15. In bladder cancer, blockage of the interaction between PD-1 and PD-L1 using monoclonal antibodies:
    a. provides a survival benefit but only when used with chemotherapy.
    b. improves both progression-free and overall survival as compared with second-line chemotherapy.
    c. improves survival but leads to tumor response (shrinkage) in less than 10% of treated patients.
    d. signals through PD-L1 back into the tumor cell to promote tumor cell destruction.
    e. frequently leads to complete responses.

16. PD-1 is not the only immune checkpoint molecule expressed on T cells in tumors; other checkpoint molecules include CTLA-4, LAG-4, and others. Simultaneously blocking *two* immune checkpoints (PD-1 and CTLA-4) in first-line kidney cancer:
    a. is less toxic than blocking a single immune checkpoint molecule.
    b. is more effective than first-line therapy with a vascular endothelial growth factor (VEGF) TKI (a tyrosine kinase inhibitor).
    c. never leads to complete responses.
    d. most likely functions by blocking both molecules on the same cell type.
    e. rarely leads to autoimmunity in endocrine organs.

ANSWERS

1. **d. The innate immune response is driven by recognition of repeated patterns in pathogens called pathogen associated molecular patterns (PAMPs).** The innate system is more primitive and does not contain cell types that can give rise to memory cells. In most immune responses, the innate and adaptive systems work together.
2. **c. Macrophages ("Big eaters").** Although BCG does bind directly to bladder epithelium, the first immune cell involved in BCG responses is the macrophage ("big eater").
3. **e. c and d.** Macrophages and PMNs are both innate immune cells involved in the early phases of an immune response. Although both have potent cytotoxic activity, only macrophages can ingest pathogens and present antigens in the context of MHC molecules.
4. **e. The primary Th1 cytokine is IL-12.** Th1 responses are characterized by IL-12, interferon γ (not α) and tumor necrosis factor (TNF) α. Th1 responses are involved in viral clearance and in antitumor immune responses. Th2 responses (IL4, 5, 10, and 13) are associated with chronic inflammation and infection and generally prevent an antitumor immune response. In bladder cancer, Th2 cytokines in the urine after BCG treatment portend a generally worse outcome.
5. **c. CD8 T cells are specialized for cytotoxicity; they evolved to destroy virally infected cells.** CD4 T cells are complex and include a number of phenotypes (Th1, Th2, Tregs, and others). CD8 T cells are cytotoxic and are capable of killing nearly any target cell (including cells resistant to chemotherapy). Although B cells DO come from the bone marrow, that is not how they got their name. They were discovered in chickens in an organ called the bursa of Fabricius. The B comes from the word *bursa*.
6. **b. Generate antibodies which help macrophages to phagocytose and destroy pathogens.** B cells secrete antibodies, which help to clear pathogens. They also differentiate into memory B cells, which drive a stronger and faster secondary response on reexposure to a pathogen. The generation of antibodies to BCG is probably a negative event; it would be expected to lead to a faster clearance and a less robust antitumor effect.
7. **c. Th2 T cells that secrete IL-4, IL-5, IL-10, and IL-13.** As earlier, Th2 cells secrete IL4, 5, 10, and 13, all of which generally inhibit a successful antitumor response.
8. **a. Elimination, equilibrium and escape.** See text for explanation.
9. **d. In prostate cancer, inflammation has been associated with the consumption of charred meat and its associated toxins.** In GU cancers, the strongest linkage between chronic inflammation and tumorigenesis is in bladder cancer, where chronic infection with schistosomiasis leads to squamous cell cancers. There are also strong data in prostate cancer, although the precise etiology of prostatic inflammation has yet to be fully defined.

10. **c. A worse prognosis in kidney cancer.** Although cytotoxic CD8 T cells are generally associated with a better prognosis, in kidney cancer the opposite relationship has been described. This is a puzzling finding, which is not well understood. In bladder cancer, a robust CD8 infiltrate is generally associated with an improved outcome.
11. **d. A series of cell-surface proteins that attenuate CD8 T-cell effector function when bound to their specific cognate ligands.** Immune checkpoint molecules are cell-surface proteins that attenuate CD8 T cell function.
12. **c. CD4 T cells of the Th2 phenotype.** As earlier, Th2 CD4 T cells are associated with a worse outcome in bladder cancer.
13. **d. Sipuleucel-T, a prostatic acid phosphatase (PAP)–directed vaccine for prostate cancer.** Although many cancer vaccines have been tested in GU cancers, only Sipuleucel-T is approved. This vaccine targets the antigen PAP in men with asymptomatic or minimally symptomatic metastatic castration-resistant prostate cancer.
14. **c. Mediates an "exhausted" nonfunctional phenotype in the CD8 T cells that express PD-1.** Expression of PD-1 on tumor-infiltrating CD8 T cells is associated with a nonfunctional, exhausted phenotype. Blockage of the PD-1/PD-L1 interaction with monoclonal antibodies restores CD8 T-cell function, leading to tumor destruction (and shrinkage) in a minority of treated patients.
15. **b. Improves both progression-free and overall survival as compared with second-line chemotherapy.** Blockage of either PD-1 or PD-L1 is effective in bladder cancer in the second-line setting (as compared with chemotherapy). The overall response rate to these agents is in the range of 20% to 25%.
16. **b. Is more effective than first-line therapy with a vascular endothelial growth factor (VEGF) TKI (a tyrosine kinase inhibitor).** Combined immune checkpoint blockade with anti-PD-1 (nivolumab) and anti-CTLA-4 (ipilimumab) is an approved first-line therapy for clear-cell RCC. It is more effective than treatment with the TKI sunitinib, as evidence by improved overall survival and progression-free survival. However, it is also considerably more toxic, with endocrine-related adverse events being reasonably common.

CHAPTER REVIEW

1. An immune response begins with an innate response, which is rapid but relatively nonspecific. It then progresses to include the adaptive immune system, which is characterized by both specificity and memory.
2. For an antitumor immune response, a Th1 response dominated by interferon γ, IL-2, and TNF α is desired.
3. CD4+ regulatory T cells (Tregs) inhibit an adaptive immune response.
4. The immune editing hypothesis explains how early tumors can be recognized and eliminated by the immune system, whereas clinically evident tumors must escape immune recognition to evolve.
5. Bladder cancer is promoted by chronic inflammation initiated by infection or other stimuli.
6. In kidney cancer, there is good evidence for an ongoing adaptive, CD8 T-cell–mediated response, but paradoxically, an increased CD8 density is associated with a worse prognosis.
7. Prostate cancer may also be driven by chronic inflammation.
8. Expression of immune checkpoint molecules on tumor-infiltrating lymphocytes (TILs) attenuates the adaptive immune response to GU tumors.
9. BCG therapy for bladder cancer stimulates both the innate and adaptive immune systems and is a prototype for successful cancer immunotherapy.
10. Cancer vaccines have been evaluated in both kidney and prostate cancer. A single vaccine (Sipuleucel-T) is FDA-approved for metastatic prostate cancer.
11. Several other vaccine approaches in phase III trials in kidney and prostate cancer have failed.
12. BCG therapy for bladder cancer stimulates both the innate and adaptive immune systems and is a prototype for successful cancer immunotherapy.
13. Cancer vaccines have been evaluated in both kidney and prostate cancer.
14. A single vaccine (Sipuleucel-T) is FDA-approved for metastatic prostate cancer.
15. Cancer vaccines are generally well tolerated but result in few objective clinical responses.
16. Blocking the PD-1/PD-L1 interaction is effective in second-line bladder cancer and has activity in first-line patients who are cisplatin-ineligible.
17. PD-L1 expression may distinguish bladder cancer patients more likely to respond to anti-PD-1/anti-PD-L1 therapy.
18. Anti-PD-1 is effective in second-line kidney cancer.
19. Anti-PD-1/PD-L1 has not shown robust monotherapy activity in metastatic prostate cancer.

62 Molecular Genetics and Cancer Biology

Karen Sandell Sfanos and Mark L. Gonzalgo

QUESTIONS

1. Deoxyribonucleic acid (DNA) is composed of all of the following elements EXCEPT:
   a. a base, either a purine or a pyrimidine.
   b. a sugar, called ribose.
   c. a phosphate.
   d. two complementary strands.
   e. hydrogen bonds.

2. The physical chemistry of DNA bases requires:
   a. uracil to form hydrogen bonds with guanine.
   b. purine to form hydrogen bonds with another purine.
   c. pyrimidine to form hydrogen bonds with a purine.
   d. adenine to form hydrogen bonds with cytosine.
   e. thymine to form hydrogen bonds with guanine.

3. Which of the following does DNA gene expression require?
   a. Linear DNA to be converted into linear ribonucleic acid (RNA), a process called translation
   b. Conversion of linear RNA into a linear set of amino acids, a process called transcription
   c. Protein synthesis exclusively within the nucleus
   d. Mitosis
   e. A mechanism to bridge the gap between the genetic code and protein synthesis

4. Which of the following statements about transcriptional regulation is NOT true?
   a. Two general components involved in transcriptional regulation are specific sequences in the RNA and proteins that interact with those sequences.
   b. In addition to the genetic information carried within the nucleotide sequence of DNA, it provides specific docking sites for proteins that enhance the activity of the transcriptional machinery.
   c. Specific sequences within the promoter or enhancer region of a gene are called response elements.
   d. DNA sequences, often referred to as consensus sequences, are found in many genes and respond in a coordinated manner to a specific signal.
   e. It is an important mechanism to ensure coordinated gene expression.

5. What is alternative splicing?
   a. A form of protein modification occurring after a mature polypeptide is produced
   b. A modification to DNA during meiosis
   c. A process of including or excluding certain exons in an mRNA transcript
   d. A process in which novel RNA sequences are randomly inserted into a transcript
   e. A method of RNA degradation

6. Which of the following statements is TRUE regarding the nuclear matrix?
   a. It has the same protein composition in every tissue type.
   b. It is the site of mRNA transcription.
   c. It has the same protein composition whether a cell is proliferating or undergoing differentiation.
   d. It provides a mechanism to trace the cell type of origin for a cancer, because the nuclear matrix is identical within tissue types.
   e. It is a form of DNA.

7. What happens in the process of translation?
   a. The RNA message of four parts (the nucleotides A, U, C, and G) is converted into 20 amino acids by using a functional group of three adjacent nucleotides called a codon.
   b. Each amino acid is encoded by only one codon.
   c. Shifts in the reading frame are of no consequence in the production of the polypeptide chain because of the fidelity of template DNA.
   d. Single-base substitutions always encode for the identical amino acid, known as a polymorphism.
   e. Transfer of genetic information from the DNA to the RNA occurs.

8. Which of the following statements about ubiquitization is NOT true?
   a. Ubiquitization is an important regulatory mechanism of a cell, used in the efficient disposal of proteins.
   b. A small protein called ubiquitin is linked to a protein, tagging it for destruction.
   c. The proteosome is the site of protein-ubiquitin complex degradation.
   d. The proteosome has a cylindrical shape.
   e. The targeted inhibition of proteosome function appears to enhance cancer progression.

9. Which of the following statements about oncogenes is TRUE?
   a. They are mutated forms of abnormal genes, known as proto-oncogenes.
   b. They can be produced by an inactivating mutation of a proto-oncogene, resulting in the silencing of the gene.
   c. They can be produced by gene amplification, resulting in many copies of the gene, or by chromosomal rearrangement.
   d. They are always due to retroviruses, capable of inducing malignant transformation of normal cells.
   e. They are endogenous cancer-fighting genes.

10. Which of the following statements about *hyper*methylation is TRUE?
   a. It is a direct change to the DNA sequence, similar to a mutation that alters the normal base-pairing.
   b. It occurs exclusively on cytosine nucleotides in the dinucleotide sequence CG.

c. Somatic methylation of CpG dinucleotides in the regulatory regions of genes is very often associated with increased transcriptional activity, leading to increased expression of that gene.

d. In cancer, hypermethylation is associated with enhanced activity of oncogenes, and demethylation may be an effective strategy for the treatment of cancer.

e. It marks cells for ubiquitinization.

11. Von Hippel-Lindau disease predisposes patients to:
   a. epididymal carcinoma
   b. clear cell renal carcinoma
   c. papillary renal cell carcinoma
   d. adrenocortical carcinoma
   e. all of the above

12. Hereditary prostate cancer genes that have been proven to cause prostate carcinoma include:
   a. ELAC2 (elaC ribonuclease Z 2)
   b. MSR1 (macrophage scavenger receptor 1)
   c. RNASEL (ribonuclease L)
   d. none of the above
   e. all of the above

13. Which of the following hereditary tumor syndromes are associated with genitourinary tumors?
   a. Von-Hippel-Lindau syndrome
   b. Birt-Hogg-Dubé syndrome
   c. Beckwith-Wiedemann syndrome
   d. None of the above
   e. All of the above

14. Which of the following cancer-associated chromosomal abnormalities would be most likely to be associated with inactivation of a tumor suppressor gene?
   a. Inversion
   b. Tetraploidy
   c. Amplification
   d. Deletion
   e. Double Minutes

15. The two main points of control in the cell cycle are:
   a. S and G_0
   b. S and the G_2M boundary
   c. M and the G_1S boundary
   d. G_1S and G_2M boundaries
   e. G_2 and M

16. The TP53 tumor suppressor gene plays a critical role in which of the following processes?
   a. Apoptosis
   b. Angiogenesis
   c. DNA replication
   d. Signal transduction
   e. All of the above

17. INK4 family members inhibit the activity of:
   a. cyclin D/cdk4.
   b. cyclin E/cdk2.
   c. cyclin A/cdk2.
   d. cyclin B/cdc2.
   e. all of the above.

18. Cyclin-cdk complexes primarily function at the G_1S boundary by:
   a. dephosphorylation of RB1.
   b. phosphorylation of MDM2.
   c. dephosphorylation of E2F.
   d. phosphorylation of E2F.
   e. phosphorylation of RB1.

19. The regulatory proteins at the G_2M checkpoint primarily respond to:
   a. hypoxia.
   b. nutrient poor environment.
   c. DNA damage.
   d. cytokines.
   e. all of the above.

20. Nucleotide excision repair (NER) primarily protects the cell from DNA damage caused by:
   a. reactive oxygen species.
   b. DNA polymerase errors.
   c. double-stranded breaks.
   d. ultraviolet light.
   e. all of the above.

21. Which of the following repair pathways is responsible for repairing double-strand DNA breaks?
   a. MSH2/MSH6
   b. homologous recombination (HR)
   c. NER
   d. mismatch repair (MMR)
   e. none of the above

22. Which of the following genes has been linked to double-strand break repair?
   a. TP53
   b. VHL (von Hippel-Lindau tumor suppressor)
   c. BRCA1 (breast cancer type 1 susceptibility protein)
   d. RB1 (retinoblastoma 1)
   e. PTEN (phosphatase and tensin homolog)

23. Procaspases are activated by which of the following?
   a. Phosphorylation
   b. Ubiquitination
   c. Dimerization
   d. Mitochondrial import
   e. Proteolytic cleavage

24. Ligand-dependent apoptosis is an attractive therapeutic target because activation is:
   a. independent of TP53.
   b. dependent on TP53.
   c. independent of caspases.
   d. dependent on caspases.
   e. dependent on RB1.

25. The TP53-induced apoptosis is mediated through:
   a. APAF-1/caspase 9.
   b. CD95 receptor.
   c. TRAIL.
   d. Bcl-2.
   e. CDKN1A (p21^{cip}).

26. How do proapoptotic bcl-2 family members function? By:
    a. digesting the mitochondria.
    b. increasing the cellular membrane permeability.
    c. increasing the mitochondrial membrane permeability.
    d. directly activating executioner caspases.
    e. increasing nuclear membrane permeability.

27. The enzyme telomerase immortalizes cells by:
    a. protecting the cells from DNA damage.
    b. stabilizing TP53.
    c. allowing the cell to grow in a nutrient poor environment.
    d. inhibiting apoptosis.
    e. maintaining chromosomal length.

28. Telomere loss can lead to all of the following EXCEPT:
    a. irreversible cell cycle exit termed senescence.
    b. apoptosis.
    c. DNA hypomethylation.
    d. chromosomal instability.
    e. increased tumor initiation.

29. Which of the following chromosomal rearrangements is not typically associated with a genitourinary malignancy?
    a. Fusion of BCR to ABL via chromosome translocation
    b. Fusion of TMPRSS2 to ERG via intra-chromosomal deletion
    c. Fusion of MiTF/TFE gene family members via chromosome translocation
    d. Isochromosome 8q
    e. Loss of chromosome 9

30. An isochromosome of 12p has been identified in which genitourinary carcinoma?
    a. Testis
    b. Prostate
    c. Renal
    d. Bladder
    e. Penile

31. Which of the following has been most consistently implicated in prostate cancer risk from GWAS studies?
    a. The 8q24 chromosomal region
    b. MSR1
    c. RNASEL
    d. TMPRSS2-ERG fusions
    e. None of the above

32. What type of genetic alteration in cancer could be identified using next-generation RNA sequencing (RNA-seq)?
    a. MicroRNAs associated with cancer
    b. Non-coding RNAs associated with cancer
    c. Gene fusions
    d. mRNA overexpression in cancer
    e. All of the above

33. An advantage of DNA sequencing-based technologies over standard clinical microbial culture for pathogen identification in body sites such as the urinary tract is:
    a. sequencing techniques can be used to define bacterial growth conditions
    b. sequencing technologies can identify the presence of organisms that cannot be grown in culture

    c. microbial culture cannot assist with the classification of bacterial species
    d. microbial culture cannot accurately identify pathogens
    e. none of the above

34. Which of the following medications has been shown to improve overall survival with fewer severe side effects among patients with clear cell renal cell carcinoma who received previous treatment?
    a. Atezolizumab
    b. Pembrolizumab
    c. Everolimus
    d. Nivolumab
    e. None of the above

ANSWERS

1. **b. A sugar, called ribose.** Ribose is an element of RNA, not DNA. In a rudimentary form, DNA is the fusion of three different elements: a base (either a pyrimidine or a purine), a sugar (in the case of DNA called 2-deoxyribose; for RNA called ribose), and a phosphate (which links individual nucleotides together). The repeating connections between the phosphates and the sugars provide the backbone from which the information-carrying bases protrude. In its "resting" or non-replicating form, this chain of elements forms a helix of two complementary strands; this double helix is held together by the hydrogen bonds.

2. **c. A pyrimidine to form hydrogen bonds with a purine.** The double helix is held together by the formation of hydrogen bonds between the pyrimidine on one strand and the purine base on the other. Uracil is in RNA not DNA. Purines do not form bases with purines. The purine adenine (A) always forms two hydrogen bonds to the pyrimidine thymine (T), and the purine guanine (G) always forms three hydrogen bonds to the pyrimidine cytosine (C), one consequence being that A-T bonding is weaker than G-C bonding.

3. **e. A mechanism to bridge the gap between the genetic code and protein synthesis.** The physical locations of DNA and its genetic code and protein synthesis and the manifestation of that code are separate: DNA is in the nucleus, and protein synthesis is cytoplasmic. The DNA message must be converted into mRNA by a process called transcription in the nucleus. The mRNA is transferred into the cytoplasm where the mRNA is converted into a protein by a process called translation.

4. **a. Two general components involved in transcriptional regulation are specific sequences in the RNA and proteins that interact with those sequences.** Specific sequences in the DNA called response elements bind to the nuclear proteins that control transcription. Importantly, this provides a mechanism to coordinate gene expression by providing similar docking sites for genes that need to be expressed at specific time points. Whereas mRNA transcription, stability, transport, and translation are all highly regulated, they are not controlled by the transcriptional machinery binding to specific mRNA sequences.

5. **c. A process of including or excluding certain exons in an mRNA transcript.** A specific gene may have multiple similar (not identical) forms (isoforms). This is accomplished by having specific exons included or excluded from the final mRNA transcript. This allows one DNA sequence to produce several protein products that have different functions. It is not a random process but is very tightly regulated to ensure that the correct mRNA transcript is produced in the correct cell at the correct point in time.

6. **b. It is the site of mRNA transcription.**

7. **a. The RNA message of four parts (the nucleotides A, U, C, and G) is converted into 20 amino acids by using a functional group of three adjacent nucleotides called a codon.** There is significant redundancy with several codons encoding for each amino acid. As a result, the RNA sequence between individuals can be different and yet still encode the same amino acid sequence (a polymorphism). However, some polymorphisms do result in amino acid changes. Shifts in reading frame are the most deleterious mutations because they result in a change in all the codons after the insertion/deletion and as a result a dramatic change in the amino acid sequence.

8. **e. The targeted inhibition of proteosome function appears to enhance cancer progression.** Degradation of proteins in the cell is an active, not passive, process. Ubiquitinization is the process by which proteins are tagged for transport to the proteosome for destruction. Perturbation of this process is often found in cancer, and therefore inhibition of ubiquitinization is a promising therapy for cancer.

9. **c. They can be produced by gene amplification, resulting in many copies of the gene, or by chromosomal rearrangement.** There are at least three ways a proto-oncogene can be converted into an oncogene. First, a mutation can occur within the coding sequence, producing a permanently activated form of the gene. A second mechanism converting a proto-oncogene into an oncogene is through gene amplification. A third mechanism of oncogene formation is through chromosomal rearrangement.

10. **b. It occurs exclusively on cytosine nucleotides in the dinucleotide sequence CG.** Hypermethylation is a normal process by which DNA is modified by the addition of a methyl group to a cytosine nucleotide in a CpG DNA sequence. There is no change in DNA sequence. Methylation results in gene silencing, that is, decreased expression of the gene. As a result, hypermethylation in cancer is associated with decreased transcription and, therefore, reduces expression of tumor suppressor genes. Ubiquitinization decreases levels of proteins but does so by increasing the degradation of the protein. Whereas alterations in ubiquitinization occur in cancer, they are not directly related to methylation.

11. **b. Clear cell renal carcinoma.** VHL is a hereditary tumor syndrome that predisposes patients to clear cell renal carcinoma, retinal angiomas, pheochromocytomas, hemangiomas of the CNS, epididymal cystadenomas, and pancreatic islet cell tumors. It is not associated with epididymal, papillary renal cell, or adrenocortical carcinomas.

12. **d. None of the above.** All of the genes above have been linked to prostate cancer by both linkage studies examining families with a strong predisposition to prostate cancer and in some cases by case control studies examining polymorphisms within these genes. However, no data have conclusively demonstrated that these genes cause prostate cancer.

13. **e. All of the above.** Each of these syndromes includes increased risk of specific genitourinary malignancies among their spectra of pathologies.

14. **d. Deletion.** A common mechanism of tumor suppressor gene inactivation is through deletion of the gene or a chromosomal region containing the gene. The other abnormalities listed produce either no net loss of genetic material or lead to a gain of genetic material, a finding often associated with increased oncogene activity due to increased copy number of the oncogene.

15. **d. G_1S and G_2M boundaries.**

16. **a. Apoptosis.** Active TP53 binds to the promoter region of TP53-responsive genes and stimulates the transcription of genes responsible for cell cycle arrest, repair of DNA damage, and apoptosis. TP53 responds to DNA damage by inducing cell cycle arrest through CDKN1A (p21cip1) and then transcriptionally activating DNA repair enzymes. If the cell cannot arrest growth and/or repair the DNA, TP53 induces apoptosis. Whereas angiogenesis, DNA replication, and signal transduction are all critical cellular processes, TP53 does not directly influence any of them.

17. **a. Cyclin D/cdk4.** The INK4 family of cdk inhibitors directly inhibits the assembly of cyclin D with cdk4 and cdk6 by blocking the phosphorylation of the cyclin D-cdk4/6 complex. This phosphorylation is necessary for activation of the complex.

18. **e. Phosphorylation of RB1.** Phosphorylation is the attachment of a phosphate to a protein. It alters the conformation of the protein and therefore is an excellent method of regulating gene function. Cyclin-cdk complexes phosphorylate RB1 or its family members, p107 and p130. Phosphorylated RB1 can no longer bind to members of the E2F family of transcription factors. Free E2F heterodimerizes with DP1 or DP2 and transcriptionally activates genes important in DNA replication, such as DNA polymerase-A and the cell cycle, such as E2F-1. Dephosphorylation of RB has the opposite effect. E2F regulation does not occur directly though phosphorylation or dephosphorylation. MDM2 regulates TP53 and is not directly affected by cyclin-cdk complexes.

19. **c. DNA damage.** Hypoxia, nutrient-poor environment, and cytokines are all signals to the cell that it is not in an environment that is conducive to cellular division. These signals influence the cell BEFORE it invests its energy in replicating the DNA, that is, it is a G1S checkpoint. If DNA damage occurs, it is critical the errors are repaired before cellular division. Therefore, DNA damage can lead to cell cycle arrest at both the G_1S and G_2M checkpoints.

20. **d. Ultraviolet light.** Nucleotide excision repair (NER) is a major defense against DNA damage caused by ultraviolet radiation and chemical exposure. NER acts on a wide range of alterations that result in large local distortions in DNA by recognizing distortions in the DNA helix, excising the damaged DNA, and replacing it with the correct sequence. Base excision repair (BER) is the primary mechanism for repairing damage caused by reactive oxygen species. MMR is the primary mechanism for polymerase errors. Double-strand break repair is the primary mechanism for repairing double-strand breaks.

21. **b. Homologous recombination (HR).** HR is one of two mechanisms for repairing DNA double-strand breaks, the other being non-homologous end joining (NHEJ). In HR, the normal undamaged sister chromatid is used as a template to repair the damaged segment of DNA.

22. **c. BRCA1 (breast cancer type 1 susceptibility protein).** BRCA1 is associated with familial breast and ovarian cancer. It is believed that the breast cancer susceptibility gene BRCA1 (as well as BRCA2) plays an important role in HR as well as sensing DNA damage. Both BRCA1 and BRCA2 are part of an enzymatic complex with RAD51- and BRCA1-associated RING domain 1 (BARD1). This complex is recruited by proliferating cell nuclear antigen (PCNA) to regions that have undergone DNA damage to repair DNA breaks.

23. **e. Proteolytic cleavage.** Procaspases are the larger, inactive precursor forms of the caspase proteins. Specific proteolytic cleavage is required for their activation. The caspases themselves are proteases and, once activated, proceed to cleave and activate other caspases, thus facilitating a proteolytic cascade that serves to amplify the initial apoptotic signal.

24. **a. Independent of TP53.** The identification of ligand-dependent apoptosis receptors may have a profound impact on therapy. Most cancer therapies (e.g., chemotherapy and external beam radiotherapy) depend on TP53 to induce apoptosis in the cancer cell. Because TP53 is mutated in more than half of malignancies, TP53-independent pathways for apoptosis are of great clinical interest. Because ligand-dependent apoptosis is independent of TP53, these receptors and ligands are attractive and novel treatment targets.

25. **a. APAF-1/caspase 9.** The TP53-induced apoptosis is dependent on the APAF-1/caspase 9 activation pathway.

26. **c. Increasing the mitochondrial membrane permeability.** Although each proapoptotic bcl-2 family member responds to different stimuli, the principal mechanism by which these family members induce cell death is by increasing mitochondrial membrane permeability.

27. **e. Maintaining chromosomal length.** Telomerase immortalizes cells by maintaining the ends of the chromosomes, or telomeres, which normally shorten with each cell division.
28. **c. DNA hypomethylation.** Normal cells closely monitor their telomere lengths and, should they fall below a critical threshold length, will initiate either cell senescence or apoptosis. If key players in these responses (e.g., TP53) are mutated, then chromosomal instability may result contributing to cancer initiation. To date, there is not a strong connection known for telomere loss and loss of DNA methylation.
29. **a. Fusion of BCR to ABL via chromosome translocation.** This particular chromosomal abnormality is typically found in chronic myelogenous leukemia patients, not in solid tumors. TMPRSS2-ERG gene fusions are found in ~50% of prostate cancer cases, MiTF/TFE gene family translocations have been associated with a subset of renal cell carcinomas, isochromosome 8q is found in a subset of prostate cancers and is often associated with the loss of 8p, loss of chromosome 9 is observed in a subset of urothelial cancers and enumeration of this chromosome by FISH is one of the components of a molecular test used for detecting bladder cancer.
30. **a. Testis.** The urologic malignancy most closely linked to a karyotypic abnormality is a testis tumor. A 12p isochromosome was first identified in a testis tumor in the 1980s, and experimentally this cytogenetic hallmark of testicular tumors has diagnostic and prognostic value.
31. **a. The 8q24 chromosomal region.** Systematic review of GWAS studies in prostate cancer indicate that the 8q24 region continues to be the most implicated in prostate cancer risk, and among different racial cohorts.
32. **e. All of the above.** RNA-seq technologies can unbiasedly sequence all RNA species in a sample, with an analysis that is not limited to "annotated" sequences.
33. **b. Sequencing technologies can identify the presence of organisms that cannot be grown in culture.** This serves as an advantage over standard microbial culture because many microorganisms that are present as members of the human microbiome are not readily culturable with standard clinical microbiology protocols.
34. **d. Nivolumab.** A randomized, open-label, phase 3 study comparing nivolumab with everolimus in patients with renal-cell carcinoma who received previous treatment demonstrated improved overall survival and fewer severe adverse events with nivolumab therapy (Motzer et al., 2015).

CHAPTER REVIEW

1. Mutations in DNA can lead to changes in protein function or expression that increase the potential for cancer initiation, progression, or metastasis.
2. Tumor suppressor genes normally negatively regulate and control cellular growth. Oncogenes normally promote cell growth.
3. Loss of tumor suppressor gene function can occur primarily by: (1) homozygous deletion, (2) loss of one allele and mutational inactivation of the second allele, (3) mutational events involving both alleles, and (4) loss of one allele and epigenetic inactivation of the second allele.
4. Certain tumor suppressor genes do not follow the "two-hit" hypothesis and may be inactivated via dominant negative mutations or haploinsufficiency.
5. Proto-oncogenes can be converted to oncogenes by: (1) mutation of the proto-oncogene resulting in an activated form of the gene, (2) gene amplification, and (3) chromosomal rearrangement.
6. The cell cycle consists of an ordered, unidirectional series of events, the main goal of which is to replicate the cell's genome and partition one copy into each of two resulting daughter cells.
7. The cell cycle is divided up into 4 phases; G1, S, G2, and M. The transition from G1 into S is critically dependent on phosphorylation of the RB1 tumor suppressor protein. Mutations in *RB1* are common in urologic malignancies.
8. Phase-specific phosphorylation of substrate proteins by cyclin-dependent kinases (cdks) orchestrates progression through the cycle.
9. The activities of cdks are dependent upon their association with specific cyclin proteins. Cyclins accumulate and are rapidly degraded in a phase-specific manner, thus assuring the proper sequencing and irreversibility of key events throughout the cell cycle.
10. Primary points of cell cycle control are the G1S and G2M checkpoints. Checkpoints employ cyclin-dependent kinase inhibitor (CDKI) proteins to pause the cell cycle in response to a variety of signals, including DNA damage, cell-cell contact, cytokine release, and hypoxia.
11. The TP53 tumor suppressor protein is a key player in cell cycle checkpoints, responding to DNA damage by signaling cell cycle arrest and repair of the DNA damage. If the DNA damage cannot be repaired, TP53 may trigger cell death (apoptosis).
12. *TP53* is the most commonly mutated gene in cancer and plays a prominent role in genitourinary malignancies.
13. Defects in cell cycle checkpoints lead to unregulated cell proliferation and genetic instability.
14. Methylation occurs specifically at CpG dinucleotides in the genome. The presence of 5-methylcytosine in DNA can result in spontaneous deamination to thymine and, therefore, the formation of C→T transition mutations.
15. DNA methylation can affect gene function by subsequent mutational events or epigenetic mechanisms. Methylation of CpG islands associated with the promoter region of genes may result in suppression of gene expression.
16. Loss of promoter methylation of normally methylated genes can lead to inappropriate gene expression; for example, expression of oncogenes.
17. DNA damage does not often lead to malignancy because the cell possesses multiple repair mechanisms.
18. Defects in DNA repair facilitate the accumulation of the mutations critical for tumor formation and progression.
19. NER is a major defense against DNA damage caused by ultraviolet radiation and chemical exposure.
20. BER repairs damage caused by spontaneous deamination of bases, radiation, oxidative stress, alkylating agents, and replication errors.
21. MMR removes nucleotides mispaired by DNA polymerase.
22. Double-stranded break repair (DSBR) is a major defense against DNA damage caused by ionizing radiation, free radicals, and chemicals.
23. Many syndromes involving inherited defects in DNA repair exhibit marked increases in cancer susceptibility, strongly linking genomic instability and cancer.
24. Large variations in chromosome numbers and complex structural rearrangements, as well as intra-tumoral variation in these aberrations, are hallmarks of most human solid tumors.
25. The extent of chromosomal abnormalities typically correlates with disease severity and aggressiveness.
26. Recurrent structural rearrangements occur in prostate (ETS gene fusions), renal (MiTF/TFE family translocation carcinomas), and testicular cancers (isochromosome 12p).

Continued

27. Copy number alterations in a particular gene, coupled with changes in the other allele, are evidence for that gene functioning as a disease-relevant oncogene or tumor suppressor gene.

28. Genes discovered to have germline mutations that cause familial forms of cancer may also be involved in the sporadic form of the disease (e.g., VHL in ccRCC).

29. High-density single nucleotide polymorphism (SNP) microarrays have been used in genome-wide association studies (GWAS) to identify DNA sequence variants associated with cancer risk.

30. Low-grade bladder cancers that progress are typically high-grade papillary tumors of the luminal molecular subtype, and high-grade bladder cancers that originate de novo are more consistent with basal-like expression.

31. Telomeres contain stretches of terminal, non-coding, repetitive DNA that cap the ends of each chromosome, thereby stabilizing them.

32. Telomere DNA repeats are progressively lost as cells divide and as a result of oxidative DNA damage at the telomeres.

33. Normal cells monitor their telomere lengths and permanently exit the cell cycle (cellular senescence) or commit suicide (apoptosis) in tumor-suppressive responses to telomere shortening. This telomere length checkpoint involves TP53 and RB1.

34. Loss of telomere length checkpoints leads to critical telomere shortening, which initiates chromosomal instability contributing to cancer initiation.

35. Most cancers and pre-malignant lesions have abnormally short telomeres.

36. Most cancers express the enzyme telomerase, which restabilizes the telomeres and allows unlimited cell division potential (immortalization); thus telomerase represents an attractive therapeutic target.

37. Apoptosis is a rapid, orderly programmed form of cell death that is utilized by multicellular organisms to eliminate unwanted cells.

38. Apoptosis is believed to play an important role in tumor suppression, as many of the signals that induce apoptosis arise from potentially tumorigenic cell stresses such as DNA damage.

39. Cancer is characterized by interruptions in the normal process of apoptosis, resulting in inappropriate cell survival.

40. Apoptosis is mediated by a conserved family of proteases known as caspases. Initiator caspases start caspase proteolytic cascades terminating in the activation of executioner caspases that target several cellular proteins.

41. Two main apoptotic pathways have been identified. In the intrinsic pathway, Bcl-2 family members modulate the release of cytochrome c from the mitochondria, which participates in the activation of initiator caspases. The extrinsic pathway activates caspases in response to signals from extracellular "death receptors."

42. In addition to its functions in cell cycle arrest and DNA repair, TP53 plays a key role in apoptosis.

43. Bcl-2 is a classic inhibitor of the mitochondrial pathway of apoptosis and is overexpressed in some genitourinary malignancies.

44. Therapeutic response is often dependent upon the integrity of apoptotic pathways in the cancer cells. Most testicular germ cell tumors (TGCT) retain intact DNA damage response (DDR), wild type TP53, and apoptotic responses, providing high cure rates with DNA damaging agents.

45. Novel agonists and antagonists of apoptosis, such as ceramide and clusterin, may successfully be controlled to combat cancer.

46. Stem cells are defined by their ability to differentiate along multiple lineages and their immortality.

47. Cancer is believed to be a stem cell disease in which a small population of cancer stem cells maintains the larger tumor.

48. Cancer may ultimately be eradicated by targeting only the cancer stem cell.

49. The PD-1 pathway limits immune activity resulting in decreased autoimmunity and cytokine.

50. Inhibition of the interaction between PD-1 and PD-L1 can enhance T-cell response and mediate antitumor activity.

51. PD-1/PD-L1 blockade for treatment of advanced or metastatic bladder cancer has demonstrated efficacy as first-line treatment for cisplatin-ineligible patients.

52. Nivolumab has been shown to improve overall survival with fewer adverse events compared to everolimus in patients with RCC who received previous treatment.

53. Loss-of-function mutations in PBRM1 were associated with clinical benefit among patients with metastatic clear cell RCC who received anti-PD-1 therapy.

54. The clinical dogma that urine is sterile has been challenged by studies describing distinct microbiota present in urine that are representative of species residing within the urinary tract. These microorganisms would have previously been under or unrecognized using standard clinical microbiology culture techniques.

55. Direct interactions between the urinary microbiome and genitourinary cancer development or progression is now an area of active study.

56. Indirect interactions between the microbiome, such as the GI microbiota, and genitourinary cancers is also an area of active research. The GI microbiota may have a strong influence on treatment response and/or related toxicities to cancer therapies.

63

Surgical, Radiographic, and Endoscopic Anatomy of the Male Reproductive System

Parviz K. Kavoussi

QUESTIONS

1. The route that sperm travel through from the seminiferous tubules to the epididymis, in order, is:
   a. straight tubules, efferent ductules, rete testis.
   b. rete testis, straight tubules, efferent ductules.
   c. efferent ductules, rete testis, straight tubules.
   d. straight tubules, rete testis, efferent ductules.
   e. rete testis, efferent ductules, straight tubules.

2. The testis is enveloped by a tough capsule composed from external to internal, in order, of the:
   a. visceral tunica vaginalis, tunica albuginea, tunica vasculosa.
   b. tunica vasculosa, tunica albuginea, visceral tunica vaginalis.
   c. tunica albuginea, tunica vasculosa, visceral tunica vaginalis.
   d. visceral tunica vaginalis, tunica vasculosa, tunica albuginea.
   e. tunica albuginea, visceral tunica vaginalis, tunica vasculosa.

3. What percentage of testicular volume is made up by interstitium?
   a. 10% to 20%
   b. 20% to 30%
   c. 30% to 40%
   d. 40% to 50%
   e. 50% to 60%

4. Which of the following is the main arterial supply to the testis?
   a. Testicular artery
   b. Superficial dorsal artery
   c. The artery of the vas deferens
   d. Cremasteric artery
   e. Deep dorsal artery

5. The lymphatic drainage from the testis drains to:
   a. superficial and deep inguinal nodes.
   b. external and internal iliac nodes.
   c. para-aortic and interaortocaval nodes.
   d. internal iliac and obturator nodes.
   e. external iliac and obturator nodes.

6. The cremaster muscle is innervated by the:
   a. ilioinguinal nerve.
   b. genital branch of the genitofemoral nerve.
   c. femoral branch of the genitofemoral nerve.
   d. terminal branches of the subcostal nerve (T12).
   e. iliohypogastric nerve.

7. The nerves thought to be the main contributors to pain in men with chronic orchialgia include:
   a. perivasal complex.
   b. posterior periarterial/lipomatous complex.
   c. intracremasteric complex.
   d. femoral branch of the genitofemoral nerve.
   e. a, b, and c.

8. The anatomic component of the blood-testis barrier is the:
   a. tight junctions between Sertoli cells.
   b. myoendothelial junctions.
   c. tunica albuginea.
   d. basement membrane of seminiferous tubules.
   e. centrifugal arteries.

9. The ducts of which of the following prostatic zones drain into the preprostatic urethra?
   a. Periurethral glands
   b. Central zone
   c. Transition zone
   d. Peripheral zone
   e. a and c

10. Benign prostatic hyperplasia (BPH) arises from the:
    a. periurethral glands.
    b. central zone.
    c. transition zone.
    d. peripheral zone.
    e. a and c.

11. Lymphatic drainage from the prostate drains to the:
    a. external iliac and common iliac nodes.
    b. internal iliac and obturator nodes.
    c. para-aortic nodes.
    d. internal iliac and inguinal nodes.
    e. perirectal and common iliac nodes.

12. The apex of the prostate is continuous with the:
    a. bladder neck.
    b. pubococcygeal portion of the of the levator ani.
    c. arcus tendineus fascia pelvis.
    d. bulbar urethra.
    e. striated urethral sphincter.

13. Lymphatic drainage from the bulbar urethra travels:
    a. through the perianal nodes to reach the pelvis.
    b. directly to the deep pelvic lymph nodes.

c. through the superficial and deep inguinal lymph nodes.

d. to the prepubic nodes.

e. to para-aortic lymph nodes along with testicular drainage.

14. The only segment of the urethra that does not have transitional epithelium is the:

a. prostatic urethra.

b. membranous urethra.

c. bulbar urethra.

d. bulbomembranous urethra.

e. fossa navicularis.

15. The glans penis is the most distal expansion of the:

a. corpus cavernosum.

b. corpus spongiosum.

c. prepuce.

d. urethra.

e. Buck's fascia.

16. The dartos layer of smooth muscle and fascia in the scrotum is continuous with:

a. the dartos layer of the penis.

b. Colles fascia.

c. Scarpa fascia.

d. Buck's fascia.

e. a, b, and c.

ANSWERS

1. **d. Straight tubules, rete testis, efferent ductules.** Septa form 200 to 300 cone-shaped lobules, each containing one or more convoluted seminiferous tubules. Each tubule is U-shaped and has a stretched length of nearly 1 m. Interstitial (Leydig) cells lie in the loose tissue surrounding the tubules and are responsible for testosterone production. Toward the apices of the lobules, the seminiferous tubules become straight (tubuli recti) and enter the mediastinum testis to form an anastomosing network of tubules lined by flattened epithelium. This network, known as the *rete testis*, forms 12 to 20 efferent ductules and passes into the largest portion of epididymis, the caput.

2. **a. Visceral tunica vaginalis, tunica albuginea, tunica vasculosa.** The testis is enveloped by a tough capsule composed, from external to internal, of the visceral tunica vaginalis, the tunica albuginea, and the tunica vasculosa, before reaching the parenchyma of the testis. The tunica albuginea is composed of smooth muscle cells that pass through collagenous tissue.

3. **b. 20% to 30%.** The testicular interstitial tissue includes Leydig cells, mast cells, macrophages, nerves, blood vessels, and lymphatic vessels. This interstitial tissue makes up 20% to 30% of the testicular volume.

4. **a. Testicular artery.** There are three arterial supplies to the testis: the testicular (internal spermatic) artery, the artery of the vas deferens (deferential artery), and the cremasteric (external spermatic) artery. The testicular artery is the main blood supply to the testis, and its diameter is greater than the deferential and cremasteric arteries combined.

5. **c. Para-aortic and interaortocaval nodes.** Lymphatic channels from the testis drain into the para-aortic and interaortocaval lymph nodes. These lymphatic channels ascend within the spermatic cord after leaving the testis.

6. **b. Genital branch of the genitofemoral nerve.** The genital branch of the genitofemoral nerve follows the spermatic cord through the inguinal canal, supplies the cremaster muscle, and supplies sensation to the anterior scrotum.

7. **e. a, b, and c.** Three distinct anatomic distributions of nerves have been isolated within the spermatic cord and are thought to be the primary contributors in men with chronic orchialgia. These include a perivasal complex, posterior periarterial/lipomatous complex, and intracremasteric complex.

8. **a. Tight junctions between Sertoli cells.** There are extremely strong tight junctions between Sertoli cells, which provide an intracellular barrier that allows for spermatogenesis in an immune-privileged site. This is the barrier known as the *blood-testis barrier*.

9. **a. Periurethral glands.** At its midpoint, the urethra turns approximately 35 degrees anteriorly, but this angulation can vary from 0 to 90 degrees. This angle divides the prostatic urethra into proximal (preprostatic) and distal (prostatic) segments, which are functionally and anatomically discrete. Small periurethral glands, lacking periglandular smooth muscle, extend between the fibers of the longitudinal smooth muscle to be enclosed by the preprostatic sphincter.

10. **e. a and c.** The periurethral glands can contribute significantly to prostatic volume in older men as one of the sites of origin of BPH. The transition zone commonly gives rise to BPH.

11. **b. Internal iliac and obturator nodes.** Lymphatic drainage is primarily to the obturator and internal iliac nodes.

12. **e. Striated urethral sphincter.** The prostate is enveloped by a collagen, elastin, and smooth muscle capsule. The capsule measures 0.5 mm in thickness posteriorly and laterally on average. There is no true prostatic capsule at the apex of the prostate, where normal prostate glands are seen blending into the striated muscle of the urethral sphincter.

13. **c. Through the superficial and deep inguinal lymph nodes.** The penis, scrotum, and perineum drain into the inguinal lymph nodes. These nodes can be divided into superficial groups and deep groups.

14. **e. Fossa navicularis.** Unlike the transitional epithelium of the remainder of the urethra, the urethral mucosa that traverses the glans penis is squamous epithelium. These cells become keratinized near the meatus.

15. **b. Corpus spongiosum.** The glans penis is an expansion of the corpus spongiosum.

16. **e. a, b, and c.** The dartos layer of smooth muscle is anatomically continuous with Colles fascia, Scarpa fascia, and the dartos fascia of the penis.

CHAPTER REVIEW

1. The normal testicle measures 2.5 × 3 × 4 cm and has a volume of 15 to 25 mL.
2. Both ends of the seminiferous tubules end in the rete testis.
3. Although there are three arteries that supply the testis, the testicular artery is the most important, and its ligation may result in testicular atrophy.
4. The testis, epididymis, vas, and seminal vesicles are innervated by the autonomic system, which is made up of afferent and efferent nerves.
5. The anatomic zones of the prostate include the transition zone, which is the site of benign prostatic hyperplasia; the central zone, which contains the ejaculatory ducts (glands arising in this zone are thought to be derived from the wolffian duct, unlike the glands in the rest of the prostate); the peripheral zone, which contains 70% of the glandular epithelium and where 70% of prostate cancers occur; and the anterior zone, which is made up of fibromuscular stroma.
6. Seventy percent of the prostate is made up of glandular tissue, and 30% is fibromuscular tissue.
7. A permeable septum separates the corpora cavernosa, one from the other, and allows for free communication between the vascular spaces of the corpora bodies.
8. Scrotal lymphatics do not cross the midline and drain into the ipsilateral groin, unlike the penis, where the lymphatics cross over, allowing drainage to either groin irrespective of the side of the lesion.
9. The rete testis forms 12 to 20 efferent ductules and passes into the largest portion of epididymis, the caput.
10. The tunica albuginea is composed of smooth muscle cells that pass through collagenous tissue.
11. The genital branch of the genitofemoral nerve follows the spermatic cord through the inguinal canal, supplies the cremaster muscle, and supplies sensation to the anterior scrotum.
12. There are extremely strong tight junctions between Sertoli cells, which provide an intracellular barrier that allows for spermatogenesis in an immune-privileged site.
13. There is no true prostatic capsule at the apex of the prostate.
14. The penis, scrotum, and perineum drain into the inguinal lymph nodes.
15. The urethral mucosa that traverses the glans penis is squamous epithelium.

64 Male Reproductive Physiology

Paul J. Turek

QUESTIONS

1. Embryologically, the vas deferens and body of the epididymis are derived from what developmental structure?
   a. Müllerian ducts
   b. Wolffian ducts
   c. Urogenital ridge
   d. Gubernaculum testis
   e. Metanephros

2. The proportion of testicular volume comprised of seminiferous tubules in the human testis is:
   a. 5%
   b. 10% to 20%
   c. 50% to 60%
   d. 70% to 80%
   e. 90% to 95%

3. Which hormones play a central role in regulation of Sertoli cell function?
   a. LH, follicle-stimulating hormone (FSH)
   b. FSH, estradiol
   c. Prolactin, LH
   d. FSH, testosterone
   e. Androgen-binding protein (ABP), testosterone

4. The vast majority of the fluid in the male ejaculate is derived from the:
   a. epididymides
   b. ejaculatory ducts
   c. seminal vesicles
   d. testicles
   e. vas deferens

5. Testicular blood supply is derived from all of the following sources EXCEPT:
   a. Internal spermatic artery
   b. Deferential artery
   c. External spermatic artery
   d. Cremasteric artery
   e. Pudendal artery

6. A 25-year old bodybuilder eschews the merits of "natural" bodybuilding and uses injectable anabolic steroids regularly to achieve muscle bulk. While on anabolic steroids, his fertility potential would be expected to be:
   a. normal, because exogenous testosterone does not impair production of endogenous testosterone.
   b. low, because exogenous testosterone stimulates pituitary production of FSH and LH
   c. low, because exogenous testosterone inhibits pituitary production of FSH and LH
   d. low, because exogenous testosterone is not as potent as endogenous testosterone at nurturing spermatogenesis.
   e. normal, because intratesticular testosterone concentrations are 50 times higher than serum levels, whether or not the blood contains exogenous testosterone.

7. Structural elements of the blood-testis barrier are observed in:
   a. Sertoli Sertoli cell junctions
   b. Leydig cells
   c. basement membranes
   d. desmosomes between spermatocytes
   e. spermatids

8. How do elevated levels of prolactin influence testosterone production?
   a. Inhibit gonadotropin-releasing hormone (GnRH) and LH
   b. Indirectly inhibit Sertoli cells
   c. Directly inhibit Leydig cells
   d. Upregulate inhibin
   e. Downregulate activin

9. What is the normal developmental pattern of spermatogenic cells within the seminiferous tubule?
   a. Sertoli, spermatogonia, spermatocyte
   b. Spermatocyte, spermatogonia, spermatid
   c. Spermatid, Sertoli, spermatocyte
   d. Spermatogonia, spermatid, spermatocyte
   e. Spermatogonia, spermatocyte, spermatid

10. What testicular hormone is the major feedback inhibitor of LH secretion?
    a. Testosterone
    b. Inhibin
    c. Activin
    d. Prolactin
    e. Sertolin

11. What is the normal size for adult human testes?
    a. 5 mL
    b. 10 mL
    c. 20 mL
    d. 30 mL
    e. 40 mL

12. Major components of the epididymis include:
    a. caput, corpus, cauda
    b. globus minor, ductus deferens, cauda
    c. rete testis, efferent ductules, caput
    d. efferent ductules, caput, cauda
    e. septa, efferent ductules, corpus

13. Which of the following is characteristic of meiosis?
    a. Cellular DNA content doubles during the first (meiotic) cell division.
    b. Chromosome number is maintained

c. Homologous chromosomes (non-sister) pair during the second cell division

d. Crossing over is present

e. Centromeres do not divide

14. When does a testosterone peak occur during a human male's life?

a. 2 months

b. 6 to 9 months

c. 30 to 40 years

d. 50 to 60 years

e. >70 years

15. With chronic vasal obstruction, the highest sperm motility is found in what region of the epididymis?

a. Rete testis

b. Efferent ducts

c. Proximal epididymis

d. Mid epididymis

e. Distal epididymis

16. Which of the following occurs during spermiogenesis?

a. Type B spermatogonia divide to form primary spermatocytes

b. Cellular remodeling within the basal compartment of the seminiferous tubule

c. DNA replication

d. Nuclear compaction

e. Cytokinesis

17. Changes to sperm during epididymal transit include:

a. increased positive charge.

b. sulfhydryl reduction.

c. decreased phospholipid content.

d. reduced membrane rigidity.

e. increased capacity for glycolysis.

18. Which of the following germ cell types is considered a true stem cell?

a. Elongating spermatids

b. Primary spermatocytes

c. Round spermatids

d. Secondary spermatocytes

e. Type A spermatogonia

19. During their development within the male reproductive tract prior to ejaculation, sperm spend the majority of time in which organ:

a. epididymis

b. ejaculatory ducts

c. seminal vesicle

d. testicle

e. vas deferens

20. The sperm region containing mitochondria is the:

a. tail.

b. head.

c. acrosome.

d. midpiece.

e. axoneme.

21. Which of the following statements about testosterone is most accurate?

a. It is produced by the exocrine testis

b. It exists mainly in the unbound or "free" form in the circulation

c. It is regulated by FSH

d. Its production is increased by excess prolactin

e. Its metabolite is dihydrotestosterone (DHT)

22. Spermiogenesis includes all of the following processes EXCEPT:

a. loss of cytoplasm

b. formation of the acrosome

c. flagellar formation

d. migration of cytoplasmic organelles

e. cell division

23. After ejaculation the contents of the vas deferens are:

a. returned to the seminal vesicles

b. maintained in the ampulla

c. released into the ejaculatory ducts

d. propelled back into the epididymis

e. released into the bladder

ANSWERS

1. **b. Wolffian ducts.** The müllerian ducts regress in the male. The indifferent gonad migrates to the urogenital ridge to become the testicle. The gubernaculum testis is responsible for pulling the testis into the scrotum during development.

2. **d. 70% to 80%.** In humans, interstitial tissue takes up 20% to 30% of the total testicular volume.

3. **d. FSH, testosterone.** FSH and testosterone play the most important role in the regulation of Sertoli cell function. The effect of prolactin and estradiol on Sertoli cells is not well defined. ABP is made by Sertoli cells.

4. **c. Seminal vesicles.** At least 65% to 70% of ejaculate volume is derived from the seminal vesicles, with the remainder from the vas deferens (with sperm) and prostatic secretions. Periurethral glands may also contribute a small amount of fluid to the normal ejaculate.

5. **e. Pudendal artery.** The arterial supply to the human testis and epididymis is derived from three sources: the internal spermatic artery, the deferential artery, and the external spermatic or cremasteric artery.

6. **c. Low, because exogenous testosterone inhibits pituitary production of FSH and LH.** Because of negative feedback inhibition that maintains homeostatic balance in the pituitary-gonadal axis, exogenous testosterone of any type will cause anterior pituitary production of LH and FSH to fall. This results in azoospermia in most of men on anabolic steroids, but the effect will vary based on the dose, frequency, and duration of the steroid regimen

7. **a. Sertoli-Sertoli cell junctions.** Sertoli-Sertoli tight junctions prevent the deep penetration of electron-opaque tracers into the seminiferous epithelium from the testicular interstitium. These junctions between Sertoli cells also segregate premeiotic germ cells (spermatogonia) from meiotic and postmeiotic germ cells and are the structural basis for the "blood-testis" barrier.

8. **a. Inhibits gonadotropin-releasing hormone (GnRH) and LH.** States of hyperprolactinemia act to inhibits GnRH pulses and also LH pulses, which is turn results in lower testosterone production.

9. **e. Spermatogonia, spermatocyte, spermatid.** Proceeding from the least to the most differentiated, they are named dark type A spermatogonia (Ad); pale type A spermatogonia (Ap); type B spermatogonia (B); preleptotene primary spermatocytes (R); leptotene primary spermatocytes (L); zygotene primary spermatocytes (z); pachytene primary spermatocytes (p); secondary spermatocytes (II); and Sa, Sb1, Sb2, Sc, Sd1, and Sd2 spermatids.

10. **a. Testosterone.** Inhibin and activin feedback on FSH secretion. Prolactin in excess can downregulate LH secretion.

11. **c. 20 mL.** Although ethnic and racial variations exist, 18 to 22 mL is considered normal testis volume for adult human males.

12. **a. Caput, corpus, cauda.** Anatomically, the epididymis is divided into three regions: the caput or head, the corpus or body, and the cauda or tail of the epididymis. On the basis of histologic criteria, each region can be subdivided into distinct zones separated by transition segments.

13. **d. Crossing over is present.** Crossing over of sister chromatids and exchange of genetic material is the hallmark of chromosomal recombination during meiosis. This does not occur in mitosis. Two other unique characteristics of meiosis are that homologous chromosomes pair during meiosis I, the first cell division, and chromosome numbers in daughter cells are half (haploid) that of mitotic cells.

14. **a. 2 months.** A testosterone peak occurs at approximately 2 months of age. Another peak occurs earlier, during the first trimester of gestation and a third peak occurs later at puberty.

15. **c. Proximal epididymis.** Studies in men with congenital absence of the vas deferens or epididymal obstruction from vasectomy frequently report poor motility in sperm aspirated from the distal epididymis, with optimal sperm quality and motility in the proximal epididymis.

16. **d. Nuclear compaction.** In spermiogenesis, cell division or cytokinesis does not occur. In addition, spermiogenesis occurs in the adluminal compartment and not the basal compartment. Spermatids and not spermatogonia are the cell types undergoing the metamorphosis characteristic of spermiogenesis.

17. **e. Increased capacity for glycolysis.** Sperm undergo numerous metabolic changes during epididymal transit. Animal studies describe the acquisition of an increased capacity for glycolysis, changes in intracellular pH and calcium content, modification of adenylate cyclase activity, and alterations in cellular phospholipid and phospholipid-like fatty acid content.

18. **e. Type A spermatogonia.** Type A spermatogonia are the only true stem cell in the testis as they can either self renew or differentiate down the spermatogenic pathway.

19. **d. Testicle.** Sperm spend 45 to 60 days developing in the testis and 2 to 12 days in the epididymis. Depending on ejaculation frequency, they can also be stored in the cauda epididymis from for days to several weeks.

20. **d. Midpiece.** The middle piece of the sperm is a highly organized segment consisting of helically arranged mitochondria surrounding a set of outer dense fibers and the characteristic 9 + 2 microtubular structure of the axoneme.

21. **e. Its metabolite is dihydrotestosterone (DHT).** Testosterone is converted to DHT in target tissue by 5α-reductase. Testosterone is produced by the endocrine testis, exists mainly in bound forms in plasma, and is mainly regulated by LH, not FSH. Excess prolactin decreases testosterone production.

22. **e. Cell division.** During spermiogenesis, the products of meiosis, the round Sa spermatids, metamorphose into mature spermatids. During this process, extensive changes occur in both the spermatid cytoplasm and the nucleus, but cell division is not required. These changes include loss of cytoplasm, formation of the acrosome, formation of the flagellum, and migration of cytoplasmic organelles to positions characteristic of the mature sperm.

23. **d. Propelled back into the epididymis.** Studies have shown that after sexual stimulation or ejaculation, the contents of the vas deferens are propelled back toward the cauda epididymis, because the distal portion of the vas deferens contracts with greater amplitude, frequency, and duration than does the proximal portion.

CHAPTER REVIEW

1. Normal testosterone and sperm production depends on the pulsatile secretion of hypothalamic GnRH and LH and FSH from the anterior pituitary gland.

2. Regulation of hypothalamic-pituitary-gonadal (HPG) axis hormones occurs primarily through negative feedback.

3. The determination of maleness is derived from the *SRY* gene on the Y chromosome. However, developmental genes such as *WNT4* and *DAX1* are considered antitestis genes and can proactively induce female gonadal development.

4. Changes to the HPG axis with paternal age include lower testosterone levels, blunted axis feedback, and irregular hormone pulsatility.

5. The testis contains 250 m of seminiferous tubules and 700 million Leydig cells in the young adult.

6. Spermatogenesis occurs in stages, cycles, and waves to ensure constant sperm production.

7. Genes on the X as well as the Y chromosome govern spermatogenesis and contribute to male infertility.

8. With paternal age, there are increases in sperm structural chromosomal abnormalities, autosomal dominant mutations, and epigenetic alterations leading to disease in offspring.

9. The epididymis consists of principal cells with absorptive and secretory function, basal cells derived from macrophages, and contractile cells that facilitate sperm transport.

10. During epididymal passage, sperm mature by gaining progressive motility and the ability to bind to and penetrate the egg zona pellucida.

11. Epididymal function is temperature and androgen (mainly DHT) dependent, important considerations for cryptorchidism, varicocele, and 5α-reductase use.

12. The vas deferens is of wolffian (mesonephric) duct origin and serves to transport sperm from the cauda epididymis to the ejaculatory duct during seminal emission.

13. The seminal vesicle and ejaculatory duct unit is analogous to the bladder and urethra and is subject to both physical blockage and functional disorders that result in infertility.

14. Sperm are ciliated cells that possess a "9 + 2" axonemal structure that allows motility.

15. It is estimated that 200 to 300 genes regulate sperm motility.

16. Sperm motility defects, termed ciliary dyskinesias, are common and can be either correctable (nonspecific flagellar anomalies) or genetic (dysplasia of the fibrous sheath).

17. Human sperm mtDNA is a circular, histone- and intron-free DNA ring that encodes for respiratory-chain–complex proteins and is very susceptible to mutations.

65 Integrated Men's Health: Androgen Deficiency, Cardiovascular Risk, and Metabolic Syndrome

Neil Fleshner, Miran Kenk, and Steven Kaplan

QUESTIONS

1. While present throughout the world, the region showing the largest gap in life expectancy between genders is:
   a. North America
   b. Southeast Asia
   c. Western Europe
   d. Eastern Europe
   e. sub-Saharan Africa

2. All of the following are proposed as factors contributing to the gender gap in life expectancy, EXCEPT:
   a. Increased exposure of males to physical and environmental harm in the workplace
   b. Higher propensity for risk-taking behaviors in males
   c. Masculinity-defined norms of health behavior
   d. Improved postpartum care
   e. Lower compliance with treatment in male patients

3. All of the following factors are classical components of metabolic syndrome, EXCEPT:
   a. Hypertension
   b. Abdominal obesity
   c. Insulin resistance/hyperglycemia
   d. Dyslipidemia
   e. Lower urinary tract symptoms

4. Which of the following statements regarding the physiology of metabolic syndrome is TRUE?
   a. Obesity, adipocyte hypertrophy, and adipocyte hyperplasia lead to systemic suppression of inflammatory processes
   b. Insulin resistance results in the suppression of pancreatic beta cells, leading to diminished insulin secretion and reduced circulating insulin levels
   c. Insulin resistance results in decreased very-low-density lipoprotein (VLDL) production and increased VLDL clearance
   d. Insulin resistance and hyperinsulinemia lead to sympathetic nervous system hyperactivity
   e. Genetics play a major role in the etiology of metabolic syndrome.

5. The following urological conditions are linked with metabolic syndrome, EXCEPT:
   a. Kidney stones
   b. Bladder cancer
   c. Overactive bladder
   d. Priapism
   e. Prostate cancer

6. Which of the following statements regarding metabolic syndrome is TRUE?
   a. Obesity is defined as BMI >20 kg/m^2 in adults.
   b. Dietary or lifestyle modifications such as physical fitness may impact both incidence and outcomes of urological diseases.

   c. Exercise decreases insulin-mediated glucose uptake and stimulates inflammation.
   d. Dietary change, weight loss, and exercise exacerbate erectile dysfunction in majority of patients.
   e. There is no clinical evidence showing that exercise programs improve quality-of-life factors.

7. Which of the following statements is FALSE?
   a. Reduction of circulating testosterone levels occurs as part of normal aging.
   b. Testosterone supplementation is available in formulations for oral, intramuscular, transdermal, sublingual, or transnasal routes.
   c. Clinical data suggest a modest impact of testosterone supplementation on physical functioning.
   d. Globally, testosterone prescribing has been decreasing over the past decades.
   e. Large-scale placebo-controlled prospective trials following patients over decades are needed to establish the safety and benefits of testosterone supplementation.

8. In making decisions regarding testosterone replacement therapy, the clinician should do all of the following, EXCEPT:
   a. Limit diagnosis of testosterone deficiency to symptomatic males with unequivocally low testosterone levels.
   b. Evaluate the patient's history and risk of cardiovascular events.
   c. Discuss potential risks of testosterone replacement therapy.
   d. Evaluate patient's history or risk of prostate cancer.
   e. Recommend testosterone supplementation in men who are planning fertility in the near term.

9. Testosterone replacement should not be recommended in:
   a. men planning fertility in the near term.
   b. men with breast or prostate cancer, or at significant risk of prostate cancer.
   c. men with elevated hematocrit.
   d. men with uncontrolled heart failure, myocardial infarction, or stroke within the last 6 months.
   e. all of the above.

10. The following predisposing risk factors and pathological processes apply to both cardiovascular disease and erectile dysfunction, EXCEPT:
    a. Dyslipidemia
    b. Inflammation
    c. Atherosclerosis
    d. Hypotension
    e. Type 2 diabetes mellitus

11. Which of the following is FALSE of the relationship between erectile dysfunction and cardiovascular disease?
    a. Erectile dysfunction could be an early warning of elevated risk of sudden cardiovascular events.

b. Severity and duration of erectile dysfunction has been correlated with the magnitude of coronary disease.

c. There is a clear and defined temporal relationship between erectile dysfunction and cardiovascular disease.

d. Coronary artery calcium score can serve as a marker of atherosclerosis in arteries, including penile arteries.

e. Erectile dysfunction and cardiovascular disorders are increasingly considered to be independent predictors of each other.

12. Which of the following statements about mental health is FALSE?

a. Suicide rate in women is four times higher than in men.

b. An equal number of men and women develop bipolar disorder.

c. Ninety percent of people diagnosed with schizophrenia before the age of 30 are men.

d. Men predisposed to suicide are those that are middle-aged and of lower socioeconomic class.

e. Over 6 million men in the United States suffer from depression.

13. Which of the following is TRUE of opioid abuse?

a. Prevalence of opioid abuse has been decreasing in recent years.

b. Physicians prescribing opioids are encouraged to initially prescribe the lowest effective dose.

c. Chronic opioid use stimulates hypothalamic-pituitary-gonadal axis.

d. Opioid-related endocrine dysfunction could drive some chronic opioid users to seek formal treatment.

e. b and d.

14. General categories of a comprehensive approach to integrative men's health should include all of the following, EXCEPT:

a. Conditions that are unique to men.

b. Diseases or illnesses that are more prevalent in men compared to women.

c. Health issues that are not covered by other specialties (e.g., cardiology, endocrinology).

d. Health issues for which risk factors and adverse outcomes are different in men.

e. Health issues for which different interventions to achieve improvements are required for men.

ANSWERS

1. **d. Eastern Europe.** Globally, average life expectancy is longer in women compared to men. While this difference in longevity is observed in all regions of the world (regardless of the level of industrial development), it is most pronounced in Eastern Europe. Women in this region tend to live approximately 7 years longer than men.

2. **d. Improved postpartum care.** A series of factors have been identified that place men at higher risk of death and disease. These include increased exposure to physical and environmental harm in the workplace, propensity for risk-taking behaviors, and masculinity defined norms of health behavior that may negatively impact both acute and chronic illness-related outcomes.

3. **e. Lower urinary tract symptoms.** The WHO, American Association of Clinical Endocrinologists (AACE), European Group for the Study of Insulin Resistance (EGIR), Adult Treatment Panel III (ATP III), and International Diabetes Federation definitions of metabolic syndrome comprise different criteria for defining metabolic syndrome. Classic definition includes hypertension, abdominal obesity, dyslipidemia, and insulin

resistance (or hyperglycemia). Lower urinary tract symptoms (LUTS) have been linked with metabolic syndrome by epidemiologic data but are not included in its definition.

4. **d. Insulin resistance and hyperinsulinemia lead to sympathetic nervous system hyperactivity.** Metabolic syndrome includes a number of physiological alterations, including abdominal obesity, insulin resistance, dyslipidemia, and hypertension. Insulin resistance and hyperglycemia are associated with increased stimulation of pancreatic beta cells to secrete more insulin, resulting in hyperinsulinemia. Insulin resistance and hyperinsulinemia lead to hyperactivation of the sympathetic nervous system and hypertension.

5. **d. Priapism.** Metabolic syndrome was classically associated with elevated risk of cardiovascular disease, diabetes, and stroke. Urological conditions are increasingly recognized to be highly prevalent among men with metastatic syndrome. Among these are renal conditions (such as renal insufficiency, urolithiasis, and renal tumors), bladder cancers, overactive bladder, lower urinary tract symptoms, prostate cancer, low testosterone levels, and erectile dysfunction.

6. **b. Dietary or lifestyle modifications such as physical fitness may impact both incidence and outcomes of urological diseases.** Frequent physical exercise reduces the risk of many chronic diseases. Exercise increases insulin-mediated glucose uptake and decreases inflammation by reducing circulating levels of insulin-like growth factor (IGF-1). In addition to the meta-analyses showing benefit of exercise for reducing prostate cancer, a growing body of data links inactivity with worse disease outcomes.

7. **d. Globally, testosterone prescribing has been decreasing over the past decades.** Testosterone has been approved and made available for treatment of hypogonadal males, including men with testicular trauma and those with rare bilateral tumors. While testosterone levels decrease as part of aging, the benefits and safety profile of exogenous testosterone supplementation have not been established. Despite the lack of conclusive data (requiring large-scale, placebo-controlled trials), use of testosterone supplements has increased significantly over the past years, with prescriptions for testosterone replacement therapy dramatically increasing in the UK and USA.

8. **e. Recommend testosterone supplementation in men who are planning fertility in the near term.** The lack of conclusive clinical trial data makes it essential that the practicing clinician understands the controversies and is able to communicate them to her/his patients. Endocrine Society guidelines published in 2018 (a) advised the clinicians to limit the diagnosis of testosterone deficiency to symptomatic males with unequivocally low testosterone levels; (b) recommend against testosterone replacement therapy in men planning fertility in the near term and those with conditions that could be exacerbated by testosterone; and (c) recommend discussing the potential risks (including cardiovascular) associated with testosterone-replacement therapy.

9. **e. All of the above.** According to the guidelines of the Endocrine Society, testosterone should not be prescribed to men with breast or prostate cancer, those planning fertility in the near term, or in those with significant prostate cancer risk, elevated hematocrit, untreated severe obstructive sleep apnea, severe lower urinary tract symptoms, uncontrolled heart failure, myocardial infarction, or stroke within the last 6 months, or thrombophilia.

10. **d. Hypotension.** There are a host of predisposing risk factors and underlying pathophysiologic processes for both cardiovascular disease (CVD) and erectile dysfunction (ED). These include, but are not limited to dyslipidemia, smoking, hypertension, and T2DM. The underlying mechanisms of both CVD and ED include inflammation, atherosclerosis, and endothelial dysfunction.

11. **c. There is a clear and defined temporal relationship between erectile dysfunction and cardiovascular disease.** There is emerging consensus that erectile dysfunction and cardiovascular disease are independent risk factors for each other. However, the temporal relationship between the two disorders is less clear. A landmark study, The Multi-Ethnic Study

of Atherosclerosis (MESA), demonstrated that subclinical cardiovascular disease is a predictor of erectile dysfunction and potentially of subsequent major adverse cardiac events. Earlier studies suggest that there is a 2- to 3-year interval between the onset of erectile dysfunction and cardiovascular symptoms. Since about 50% of men with sudden cardiovascular events may have had no previous symptoms, ED may be the single warning of the elevated risk of sudden cardiovascular events.

12. **a. Suicide rate in women is four times higher than in men.** Mental illnesses, including anxiety, depression, and suicide, are becoming increasingly prevalent, while concomitantly being underdiagnosed, in men. Specifically, over 6 million men suffer from depression including symptoms such as fatigue, irritability, and loss of interest in work or hobbies. High rates of mental illness have led to a significant increase in incidences of both suicide and substance abuse. Highest prevalence of suicide in the United States occurred in people between ages 45 and 54, with men exhibiting a suicide rate four times higher than women.

13. **b. Physicians prescribing opioid are encouraged to initially prescribe the lowest effective dose.** In recent years the emotional and economic consequences of opioid misuse on public health has increased dramatically and is now understood as a major source of morbidity and mortality in the United States. Despite a decrease in the number of total opioids prescribed in the U.S. from a peak in 2012, some 33,000 people died of opioid overdoses in 2015 (including 15,000 from prescription sources), and currently more than 115 Americans die daily after overdosing on opioids. There appears to be a high degree of variability in the dispensing of pain medications after surgery and there are some who routinely dispense above recommended safety thresholds. Urologists need to foster greater awareness of the potential harms associated with even a short course of opioids. Those prescribing should adopt responsible prescribing practices, such as initially prescribing the lowest effective dose and offering repeat assessments as needed.

14. **c. Health issues that are not covered by other specialties (e.g., cardiology, endocrinology).** A men's health center should be focused on conditions, diseases, and health issues that exhibit higher impact on men, or that require unique strategies in men. A men's health curriculum must include contributions from a host of medical specialties. Optimally, such a center should include partnerships with various subspecialists in cardiology, endocrinology, psychiatry, orthopedics, and dermatology.

CHAPTER REVIEW

1. Men throughout the world live shorter lives than women throughout the world.
2. The gender gap persists despite improvements in overall life expectancy at birth.
3. Men not only live shorter lives than women, they also live sicker lives.
4. Gender differences in illness-related outcomes reflect social, environmental, and physiological factors.
5. Innovative and coordinated programs targeting men are required to promote social and behavioral changes that would improve men's health.
6. Metabolic syndrome, defined as a combination of dyslipidemia, glucose insensitivity, and obesity is increasingly prevalent around the world.
7. In addition to its association with increased CVD risks, metabolic syndrome is linked with pelvic health issues, including lower urinary tract symptoms, ED, and hypogonadism, as well as genitourinary tumors (kidney, bladder, prostate).
8. Dietary or lifestyle modifications may improve outcomes in many of these urologic diseases, with clinical trials currently testing metabolic modulators statins and metformin.
9. Exercise-based interventions in men with advanced prostate cancer improve quality of life.
10. Dietary change, weight loss, and exercise may improve erectile function.
11. Men's health should include individualized and precision-based intervention programs to alter the arc of pelvic conditions.
12. Testosterone replacement therapy in countering low testosterone levels that occur as part of the aging process is controversial due to inadequately elucidated effectiveness and safety profile.
13. Recent large-scale randomized trials demonstrated some improvements in sexual and physical function and vitality.
14. Limited clinical trial evidence and retrospective cohort analyses suggest that testosterone replacement therapy increases the risk of cardiovascular events.
15. Practicing urologists should keep current with the recently updated guidelines and current research on testosterone-replacement therapy to be able to discuss the risks and benefits for individual patients.
16. There are a number of overlapping risk factors for both CVD and ED.
17. The temporal relationship between ED and subclinical CVD remains to be determined.
18. CAC score can serve as a "disease score" and a surrogate for accelerated atherosclerosis process in arteries, including penile arteries, with implications for vascular ED.
19. Mental health issues, including anxiety, depression, and suicide, are increasingly prevalent in men while concomitantly being under diagnosed.
20. Over 6 million men in the United States suffer from depression, including symptoms such as fatigue, irritability, and loss of interest in work or hobbies.
21. Men are at higher risk for suicide, with a rate approximately four times higher than that of women.
22. Opioid abuse is now a leading health care crisis, with significant morbidity and mortality.
23. The opioid epidemic is notable for the expansiveness of the problem in the United States, spanning divisions of gender, race, age, and income level.
24. Clinicians who treat hypogonadism should be cognizant of the relationship between chronic opioid and symptomatic hypogonadism.

66 Male Infertility

Craig S. Niederberger, Samuel J. Ohlander, and Rodrigo L. Pagani

QUESTIONS

1. For couples practicing optimal timing methods to conceive, the proportion who conceive after six cycles should be approximately:
   a. 1/2.
   b. 1/3.
   c. 1/5.
   d. 2/5.
   e. 4/5.

2. For couples desiring to conceive, around the time of ovulation, they should have intercourse:
   a. daily.
   b. twice daily.
   c. every other day.
   d. in the morning.
   e. near noon.

3. In the industrialized world, female fecundity typically declines most rapidly after:
   a. puberty.
   b. age 30 years.
   c. age 35 years.
   d. age 40 years.
   e. menopause.

4. All of the following medications are associated with male reproductive dysfunction EXCEPT:
   a. cimetidine.
   b. spironolactone.
   c. indinavir.
   d. prednisone.
   e. lisinopril.

5. A man with oligoasthenospermia has inflammatory bowel disease and is prescribed sulfasalazine. He should be counseled to:
   a. repeat a semen analysis.
   b. continue sulfasalazine.
   c. substitute sulfasalazine with colchicine.
   d. substitute sulfasalazine with mesalazine.
   e. discontinue all medications.

6. A 30-year-old man is attempting to conceive with his 28-year-old wife. She is diagnosed with premature ovarian failure, and hematoxylin and eosin microscopic staining of his sperm is consistent with the presence of *Escherichia coli*. His bulk seminal parameters are otherwise unremarkable. You recommend:
   a. swim up and intrauterine insemination (IUI).
   b. a 3-week course of ciprofloxacin, 500 mg twice daily.
   c. prostatic culture.
   d. seminal vesicle aspiration for culture.
   e. observation.

7. The effect of human immunodeficiency virus (HIV) infection on bulk seminal parameters is:
   a. none.
   b. decreased motility.
   c. increased number of morphologically abnormal forms.
   d. decreased concentration.
   e. decreased volume.

8. Direct exposure of the testis to ionizing radiation causes irreparable damage to spermatogenesis at doses at and above:
   a. 2.5 Gy.
   b. 5 Gy.
   c. 7.5 Gy.
   d. 10 Gy.
   e. 20 Gy.

9. The typical differential between core body and scrotal temperature is:
   a. 0.5°C.
   b. 0.5°F.
   c. 1°C to 2°C.
   d. 2°C to 4°C.
   e. 6°C.

10. An 18-year-old man has bilateral testes palpable at the external inguinal rings. He desires to father children in the future. Two centrifuged semen analyses reveal azoospermia. Serum testosterone is 410 ng/dL, and follicle-stimulating hormone is 22 IU/L. The best next step is:
    a. counsel that when he is ready, he and his partner should use donor sperm or adopt.
    b. clomiphene citrate, 50 mg every other day.
    c. testis biopsy.
    d. microsurgical testis sperm extraction with cryopreservation if sperm are found.
    e. bilateral orchidopexy.

11. The lubricant that does NOT affect sperm function or DNA integrity is:
    a. Astroglide.
    b. K-Y Jelly.
    c. Pre-Seed.
    d. Replens.
    e. saliva.

12. The serum hormonal pattern commonly observed in male obesity is:

	Testosterone	Sex Hormone–Binding Globulin (SHBG)	Estradiol
a.	↓	↓	↓
b.	↓	↓	↑
c.	↓	↑	↓
d.	↓	↑	↑
e.	↑	↑	↑

13. The finding most consistent with spermatogenic impairment is:
    a. a testis volume as measured by Prader orchidometer less than 30 mL.
    b. a testis volume as measured by scrotal ultrasonography less than 30 mL.
    c. a testis longitudinal axis as measured by caliper orchidometer less than 4.6 cm.
    d. an engorged epididymis.
    e. an absent vas deferens.

14. A man evaluated for azoospermia has absent vasa bilaterally. The next step is cystic fibrosis transmembrane conductance regulator (CFTR) gene sequence assay for him and his partner and:
    a. transrectal ultrasound.
    b. renal ultrasound.
    c. postejaculatory urinalysis.
    d. seminal vesicle aspiration.
    e. testis biopsy.

15. The following condition increases sex hormone–binding globulin (SHBG):
    a. aging
    b. diabetes mellitus
    c. hypothyroidism
    d. obesity
    e. testosterone therapy

16. A man is found to be azoospermic. The following most strongly suggests spermatogenic dysfunction as a cause rather than obstruction:
    a. testis long axis on physical examination 4.2 cm, FSH assay 4 IU/L
    b. testis long axis on physical examination 4.3 cm, FSH assay 10 IU/L
    c. bioavailable testosterone, 166 ng/dL, FSH assay 6 IU/L
    d. luteinizing hormone (LH), 2 IU/L, FSH 2 IU/L
    e. testosterone, 160 ng/dL, LH 9 IU/L

17. A reasonable threshold for sperm concentration above which a man can be considered fertile is:
    a. 15 million/mL.
    b. 20 million/mL.
    c. 48 million/mL.
    d. 80 million/mL.
    e. 200 million/mL.

18. Brown-hued semen is often associated with:
    a. ingested asparagus.
    b. ejaculatory ductal obstruction.
    c. sexual activity.
    d. spinal cord injury.
    e. urinary tract infection.

19. The optimal time in days of abstinence to wait after an ejaculate for a semen analysis is:
    a. 1.
    b. 2.
    c. 3.
    d. 5.
    e. 7.

20. A man who has been unsuccessful in impregnating his wife during the past year is identified to have azoospermia and semen volumes of 0.8 and 0.5 mL. The next step is:
    a. testis biopsy.
    b. scrotal ultrasound.
    c. postejaculatory urinalysis.
    d. clomiphene citrate, 50 mg every other day.
    e. transurethral resection of ejaculatory ducts.

21. A 32-year-old man presents for fertility evaluation. Physical exam and endocrine assessment are normal. Semen analysis demonstrates volume 2.5 mL, density 84 million/mL, motility 71%, and strict morphology 0% with a variety of abnormal forms. The next step is:
    a. vitamin E.
    b. reassurance.
    c. testis biopsy.
    d. scrotal ultrasound.
    e. antisperm antibody assay.

22. Two semen analyses from a man undergoing a reproductive evaluation include volumes of 2.5 and 1.8 mL, densities of 24 and 28 million/mL, and motility 0%. The next step is:
    a. vital stain.
    b. immunobead assay.
    c. repeat semen analysis.
    d. sperm chromatin structure assay (SCSA).
    e. computer-assisted semen analysis (CASA).

23. Semen observed under phase contrast light microscopy reveals abundant round cells similar in size and shape to leukocytes. The next step is:
    a. semen culture.
    b. Papanicolaou staining.
    c. transrectal ultrasound.
    d. ciprofloxacin, 1 g daily for 4 weeks.
    e. ibuprofen, 400 mg daily for 2 weeks.

24. A direct assay of sperm-head DNA fragmentation is the:
    a. terminal deoxynucleotidyl transferase dUTP nick end labeling (TUNEL) assay.
    b. acid comet assay.
    c. alkaline comet assay.
    d. sperm chromatin dispersion (SCD) assay.
    e. SCSA.

25. The assay that most closely models incubational in vitro fertilization is:
    a. reactive oxygen species-total antioxidant capacity (ROS-TAC).
    b. Penetrak assay.
    c. Tru-trax assay.
    d. sperm penetration assay.
    e. acrosomal assay.

26. A 26-year-old man presenting for fertility evaluation has two semen analyses, one with volume 2.1 mL and density 32 million/mL, and another with volume 2.3 mL and density 28 million/mL. No motile sperm are observed in either, and vital stain demonstrated greater than 80% metabolically active sperm in both. The next step is:
    a. immunobead assay.
    b. pyospermia stain.

c. electron microscopy.

d. SCSA.

e. repeat semen analysis.

27. A 30-year-old man has azoospermia. Physical examination reveals absent vasa bilaterally. CFTR analysis reveals a ΔF508 mutation. The next step is:

   a. repeat CFTR analysis of the man with a 1600-mutation screen.

   b. repeat semen analysis.

   c. CFTR analysis of his wife.

   d. testicular sperm extraction.

   e. testis biopsy.

28. A 28-year-old man desires a biological child. Physical examination is normal. Two semen analyses reveal azoospermia with volumes of 0.8 and 0.7 mL, and no sperm is identified in a postejaculatory urinalysis. FSH is 3.2 IU/L. Transrectal ultrasound reveals seminal vesicles of 0.9 and 1.1 cm in largest diameter, and no midline cyst is visualized. The next step is:

   a. reassurance.

   b. testis biopsy.

   c. repeat semen analysis.

   d. transurethral resection of ejaculatory ducts.

   e. testis sperm extraction and cryopreservation.

29. A 33-year-old man desires a biological child and is found to have azoospermia with semen volumes 2.2 and 2.4 mL on two analyses. Longitudinal axis of the left testis is 3.3 cm, and the right is 3.5 cm. Serum FSH is 9.3 IU/L, and testosterone is 440 ng/dL. The next step is:

   a. testis biopsy.

   b. epididymovasostomy.

   c. repeat semen analysis.

   d. microsurgical testis sperm extraction.

   e. clomiphene citrate, 50 mg every other day.

30. A 30-year-old man desires a biological child with his 28-year-old wife. Her evaluation is normal. Semen analysis reveals density 84 million/mL and globozoospermia. The next step is:

   a. repeat semen analysis.

   b. clomiphene citrate, 50 mg every other day.

   c. in vitro fertilization after incubation of sperm with pentoxifylline.

   d. intracytoplasmic sperm injection with ejaculated sperm.

   e. microsurgical testis sperm extraction.

31. The most common genetic cause of male infertility is:

   a. r(Y).

   b. 45,X0.

   c. 47,XXY.

   d. 47,XYY.

   e. 46,XY/47,XXY.

32. The biological system responsible for protecting haploid male germ cells from the immune system is:

   a. IgG.

   b. Prostate specific antigen (PSA).

   c. natural killer cells.

   d. reactive oxygen species.

   e. Sertoli cell tight junctions.

33. A man presents with azoospermia. Testis longitudinal axis is 3.0 cm bilaterally, and the testes are soft. Laboratory evaluation reveals testosterone 140 ng/dL, LH less than 1.0 IU/L, and FSH less than 1.0 IU/L. The next step is:

   a. repeat semen analysis.

   b. transrectal ultrasound.

   c. microsurgical testis sperm extraction.

   d. smell test.

   e. Y-chromosomal microdeletion assay.

34. A man presents with erectile dysfunction and azoospermia. Testis longitudinal axis is 5 cm bilaterally, and the testes are firm. Laboratory evaluation reveals bioavailable testosterone 150 ng/dL and prolactin 42 µg/L. The next step is:

   a. repeat prolactin.

   b. bromocriptine, 2.5 mg orally per day.

   c. cabergoline, 0.25 mg orally twice a week.

   d. clomiphene citrate, 50 mg orally every other day.

   e. cranial magnetic resonance imaging.

35. Laboratory values associated with androgen receptor insensitivity include:

   a. significantly elevated testosterone, LH, and FSH.

   b. mildly elevated testosterone, LH, and FSH.

   c. significantly elevated testosterone, mildly elevated LH, and normal FSH.

   d. decreased testosterone, and elevated LH and FSH.

   e. decreased testosterone, LH, and FSH.

36. The most common mutation in the cystic fibrosis transmembrane conductance region, or CFTR, is:

   a. R117H.

   b. R334W.

   c. R347P.

   d. ΔF508.

   e. G542X.

37. A man presents with a palpable right-sided varicocele of 3 months onset and no varicocele palpable on the left side. Testis longitudinal axis is 5 cm bilaterally, and a semen analysis reveals volume 2.0 mL, density 33 million/mL, and motility 38%. The next step is:

   a. semen analysis with strict morphology.

   b. renal ultrasound.

   c. CFTR testing.

   d. right varicocelectomy.

   e. bilateral varicocelectomy.

38. Electroejaculation is planned for a man with anejaculation due to spinal cord injury at T5. Treatment should include monitoring and therapy before the procedure with oral:

   a. lisinopril.

   b. nifedipine.

   c. pseudoephedrine.

   d. captopril.

   e. ciprofloxacin.

39. A couple desires children. Semen analysis reveals volume 2.2 mL, density 58 million/mL, and motility 18%, and all sperm have enlarged heads with multiple tails. The next step is:

   a. testis biopsy.

   b. scrotal ultrasound.

   c. repeat semen analysis.

   d. IUI with donor sperm.

   e. in vitro fertilization with intracytoplasmic sperm injection.

ANSWERS

1. **e. 4/5.** Cumulative pregnancy rates in a well-conducted study were 38% at one cycle, 68% at three cycles, 81% at six cycles, and 92% at 12 cycles (Gnoth et al., 2003).[a]

2. **a. Daily.** Although prior recommendations specified intercourse every other day to optimize the probability of conception, a recent study demonstrated that intercourse every day around the time of ovulation is likely the best strategy (Scarpa et al., 2007).

3. **c. Age 35 years.** Whereas women in developing nations may experience a rapid decline in fecundity at a younger age, in the industrialized world, female fecundity declines precipitously after age 35 years (Balasch and Gratacós, 2012).

4. **e. Lisinopril.** All agents listed are spermatotoxins except lisinopril, which may improve bulk seminal parameters (Mbah et al., 2012).

5. **d. Substitute sulfasalazine with mesalazine.** Sulfasalazine is associated with oligoasthenospermia (Stein and Hanauer, 2000). If sulfasalazine is substituted with mesalazine, adverse effects on sperm are generally reversible (Riley et al., 1987).

6. **e. Observation.** Limited seminal concentrations of the majority of bacteria including *E. coli* have minimal or no effects on sperm motility in vivo (Diemer et al., 2003; Lackner et al., 2006).

7. **a. None.** HIV does not appear to be correlated with a direct negative effect on sperm function (Garrido et al., 2005).

8. **c. 7.5 Gy.** The probability of future fatherhood is significantly decreased with radiation doses to the testes of 7.5 Gy and above (Green et al., 2010). The testis does not need to be directly exposed for adverse spermatogenic effects to occur.

9. **d. 2°C to 4°C.** Unlike female gonads, the testes are extracorporeal and subject to thermal regulation by a vascular heat exchange mechanism and muscular activity controlling proximity to the body, resulting in a scrotal temperature maintained between 2°C and 4°C below body core temperature (Setchell, 1998; Thonneau et al., 1998).

10. **e. Bilateral orchidopexy.** The most significant feature affecting this man's reproductive potential is bilateral cryptorchidism. Although the likelihood of improving fertility is hampered by his advanced age, no value will be derived from waiting. Testis biopsy is unnecessary, and his total testosterone is adequate. In this patient with distal cryptorchidism who does not desire offspring presently, removing the spermatotoxic insult of cryptorchidism is the most prudent course.

11. **c. Pre-Seed.** Nearly all lubricants are spermatotoxic, including saliva. In a study of a variety of lubricants, Pre-Seed did not result in a significant decrease in sperm motility or chromatin integrity (Agarwal et al., 2008).

12. **Row b.** In obese males, serum testosterone is decreased (Hammoud et al., 2006). SHBG is typically reduced, likely because of increased circulating insulin (Hammoud et al., 2006; 2008; Pauli et al., 2008; Teerds et al., 2011). Estradiol is increased because of peripheral conversion from testosterone by an overabundance of adipose cells containing the enzyme aromatase (Aggerholm et al., 2008; Chavarro et al., 2010; Hammoud et al., 2006, 2010; Hofny et al., 2010).

13. **c. A testis longitudinal axis as measured by caliper orchidometer less than 4.6 cm.** A measurement of the long axis of the testis of 4.6 cm or less is associated with spermatogenic impairment (Schoor et al., 2001).

14. **b. Renal ultrasound.** Renal agenesis is noted in 11% of men with congenital bilateral absence of the vas deferens (Schlegel et al., 1996).

15. **a. Aging.** Concentration of SHBG increases with age, resulting in decreased bioavailable testosterone (Bhasin et al., 2010).

16. **b. Testis long axis on physical examination 4.3 cm, FSH assay, 10 IU/L.** If the FSH assay result is 7.6 IU/L or less and the testis long axis is greater than 4.6 cm, the probability of obstruction is 96%; conversely, if the FSH values is greater than 7.6 IU/L and the testis long axis 4.6 cm or less, the probability that azoospermia is due to spermatogenic dysfunction is 89% (Schoor et al., 2001).

17. **c. 48 million/mL.** By classification and regression tree analysis, or CART, one large study demonstrated that for sperm concentration, 13.5 million/mL was found to be the lower parameter below which IUI success would be unlikely, and 48.0 million/mL was identified as the upper parameter above which IUI outcomes were favorable (Guzick et al., 2001).

18. **d. Spinal cord injury.** The ejaculate is normally white or light gray. A brown hue is often observed in spinal cord–injured men (Centola, 2011; World Health Organization, 2010).

19. **a. 1.** A single day of abstinence is optimal for assessing bulk seminal parameters (Elzanaty, 2008; Levitas et al., 2005).

20. **c. Postejaculatory urinalysis.** The differential diagnosis of seminal hypovolemia includes retrograde ejaculation, ejaculatory ductal obstruction, and accessory sex gland hypoplasia. The simplest and least invasive test to exclude a diagnosis of retrograde ejaculation is postejaculatory urinalysis, and this should be performed first.

21. **b. Reassurance.** This man's bulk seminal parameters are adequate with the exception of morphology. The variety of abnormal forms excludes rare genetic conditions such as failure of formation of the acrosomal cap. The assessing technician likely overread abnormal forms, and the patient should be reassured.

22. **a. Vital stain.** In cases of complete asthenospermia, assessment of antisperm antibodies with the immunobead assay is not possible, as it requires some motile sperm. The first diagnosis to exclude is necrospermia, which may be investigated with a vital stain.

23. **b. Papanicolaou staining.** Leukocytes and immature germ cells are not differentiated with light microscopy. A simple stain such as Papanicolaou allows the two to be distinguished (World Health Organization, 2010).

24. **a. Terminal deoxynucleotidyl transferase dUTP nick end labeling (TUNEL) assay.** Direct measures of sperm DNA fragmentation include the TUNEL assay and the comet assay at neutral pH. The other assays listed include denatured DNA (Sakkas and Alvarez, 2010).

25. **d. Sperm penetration assay.** To simulate incubational in vitro fertilization, human sperm are incubated with denuded hamster ova in the sperm penetration assay, or SPA (Margalioth et al., 1986; Yanagimachi et al., 1976).

26. **c. Electron microscopy.** Vital stain excluded necrospermia in this patient with complete asthenospermia. Electron microscopy will identify ultrastructural tail defects if present in the immotile cilia syndrome (Zini and Sigman, 2009).

27. **c. CFTR analysis of his wife.** Should the wife of this azoospermic man with a severe CFTR mutation harbor a severe mutation as well, a child born from surgically extracted sperm and intracytoplasmic sperm injection may be homozygous for a severe mutation and have clinical cystic fibrosis. In order to counsel the couple regarding the probability of that result, CFTR analysis of the wife is indicated.

28. **e. Testis sperm extraction and cryopreservation.** This man's normal physical examination and relatively low FSH indicates a high likelihood of adequate spermatogenesis and obstructive azoospermia. The lack of seminal vesicle dilation suggests that the probability of ejaculatory ductal obstruction is low. The next step is surgical sperm retrieval.

29. **d. Microsurgical testis sperm extraction.** With the FSH assay result greater than 7.6 IU/L and the testes long axis measurements of 4.6 cm or less, the probability that azoospermia is due to spermatogenic dysfunction is 89% (Schoor et al., 2001). The next step is microsurgical testis sperm extraction.

30. **d. Intracytoplasmic sperm injection with ejaculated sperm.** In globozoospermia, the sperm lack acrosomal caps, and sperm heads are rendered spheric rather than ovoid. Without

---

[a]Sources referenced can be found in *Campbell-Walsh-Wein Urology, 12th Edition,* on the Expert Consult website.

the acrosome, fertilization with sperm in the natural setting or with incubational in vitro fertilization will not be successful. Intracytoplasmic sperm injection is required. Ejaculated sperm is available in this patient, and surgical sperm extraction is consequently unnecessary.

31. **c. 47,XXY.** The presence of a supernumerary X chromosome in 47,XXY, or Klinefelter syndrome, is the most common genetic cause of male infertility (Groth et al., 2013; Oates and Lamb, 2009; Sigman, 2012).

32. **e. Sertoli cell tight junctions.** The haploid male gamete expresses different surface antigens than other diploid cells and is protected from the immune system by tight junctions between Sertoli cells (Walsh and Turek, 2009).

33. **d. Smell test.** Anosmia associated with hypogonadotropic hypogonadism is known as Kallmann syndrome (Kallmann and Schoenfeld, 1944). In a patient with significantly low gonadotropin assay results, the presence of the syndrome is confirmed by a smell test.

34. **a. Repeat prolactin.** Prolactin is a labile assay. Before continuing with further diagnostic assessment or therapy, moderately elevated assay results should first be confirmed with a second test.

35. **c. Significantly elevated testosterone, mildly elevated LH, and normal FSH.** Male infertility associated with androgen receptor insensitivity is characterized by increased testosterone, increased estradiol, increased LH to variable degrees, and typical FSH levels (Sokol, 2009).

36. **d. ΔF508.** The most common CFTR mutation is ΔF508, which is severe (Hampton and Stanton, 2010).

37. **b. Renal ultrasound.** Solitary right varicoceles are rare. Should one be of abrupt onset, renal pathology such as tumor should be considered (Masson and Brannigan, 2014).

38. **b. Nifedipine.** Ejaculatory stimulation for men with spinal cord injuries at a level of T6 or above may result in autonomic dysreflexia, which can be addressed before stimulation by treatment with nifedipine and during the procedure with monitoring of cardiac activity and blood pressure (Brackett et al., 2009; Phillips et al., 2014).

39. **d. IUI with donor sperm.** Because of the high rate of aneuploidy in sperm associated with macrocephaly and multiple tails, intracytoplasmic sperm injection with biological gametes is not recommended (Machev et al., 2005; Perrin et al., 2012; Sun et al., 2006).

CHAPTER REVIEW

1. Human spermatogenesis requires 64 days to complete and 5 to 10 days of epididymal transit time.
2. 5-α reductase inhibitors have a limited effect on spermatogenesis.
3. Cannabis decreases plasma testosterone; heavy alcohol use increases the conversion of testosterone to estradiol.
4. DNA damage can be detected up to 2 years following chemotherapy.
5. Following torsion of the testis, 11% of men develop antisperm antibodies.
6. Testis size correlates well with sperm production.
7. Patients with bilateral absence of the vas should be evaluated for a cystic fibrosis gene mutation.
8. Varicoceles are present in 15% of the adult population but occur in 30% to 50% of men presenting with fertility problems.
9. Normal semen volume is between 1 and 5 mL.
10. Progressive motility should be between 32% and 63%.
11. Antisperm antibodies are associated with vasectomy, testes trauma, orchitis, cryptorchidism, testis cancer, and varicocele.
12. Genetic testing should be considered in those with spermatogenic dysfunction causing azoospermia and in those with sperm densities of less than 5 million/mL.
13. The AZF factor is found on the long arm of the Y chromosome; the DAZ genes are located in the AZFc region. A microdeletion of the AZFc region may result in spermatogenic impairment but not necessarily absence of spermatogenesis, but a microdeletion of the AZFa and AZFb regions generally result in absence of spermatogenesis.
14. Spermatogenesis may be highly focal in men with azoospermia so that a random biopsy may miss areas of sperm production.
15. Cumulative pregnancy rates in a well-conducted study were 38% at one cycle, 68% at three cycles, 81% at six cycles, and 92% at 12 cycles.
16. Female fecundity declines precipitously after age 35 years.
17. Limited seminal concentrations of the majority of bacteria, including E. coli, have minimal or no effects on sperm motility in vivo.
18. If the FSH assay result is 7.6 IU/L or less and the testis long axis is greater than 4.6 cm, the probability of obstruction is 96%. Conversely, if the FSH value is greater than 7.6 IU/L and the testis long axis 4.6 cm or less, the probability that azoospermia is due to spermatogenic dysfunction is 89%.
19. A sperm concentration of 13.5 million/mL has been found to be the lower parameter below which IUI success is unlikely, and 48.0 million/mL is identified as the upper parameter above which IUI outcomes are favorable.
20. A single day of abstinence is optimal for assessing bulk seminal parameters.
21. The differential diagnosis of seminal hypovolemia includes retrograde ejaculation, ejaculatory ductal obstruction, and accessory sex gland hypoplasia.
22. Leukocytes and immature germ cells are not differentiable with light microscopy. A simple stain such as Papanicolaou allows the two to be distinguished.
23. Direct measures of sperm DNA fragmentation include the terminal deoxynucleotidyl transferase dUTP nick end labeling, or TUNEL.
24. To simulate incubational in vitro fertilization, human sperm are incubated with denuded hamster ova in the sperm penetration assay, or SPA.
25. In globozoospermia, the sperm lack acrosomal caps, and sperm heads are rendered spheric rather than ovoid. Without the acrosome, fertilization with sperm in the natural setting or with incubational in vitro fertilization will not be successful.
26. Klinefelter syndrome is the most common genetic cause of male infertility.
27. Male infertility associated with androgen receptor insensitivity is characterized by increased testosterone, increased estradiol, increased LH to variable degrees, and typical FSH levels.
28. Solitary right varicoceles are rare. Should one be of abrupt onset, renal pathology such as tumor should be considered.

67 Surgical Management of Male Infertility

Marc Goldstein

QUESTIONS

1. Which of the following venous structures are intentionally preserved during varicocelectomy?
   a. External spermatic veins
   b. Internal spermatic veins
   c. Gubernacular veins
   d. Deferential (vasal) veins
   e. Cremasteric veins

2. In the evaluation for vasectomy reversal, which clinical finding is suggestive of epididymal obstruction?
   a. Varicocele
   b. Hydrocele
   c. Sperm granuloma
   d. Normal serum follicle-stimulating hormone (FSH) level
   e. Vasal gap larger than 2 cm

3. Which of the following is NOT an indication for crossed vaso-vasostomy?
   a. Right: inguinal vas obstruction and normal testis; left: patent vas and atrophic testis
   b. Right: epididymal obstruction, patent vas, and normal testis; left: ejaculatory duct obstruction and normal testis
   c. Right: inguinal vas obstruction and normal testis; left: epididymal obstruction, patent vas, and normal testis
   d. Right: epididymal obstruction and patent right vas above vasectomy site; left: sperm in testicular end of vas and vasectomy site in convoluted vas
   e. Right: congenital absence of epididymis and normal patent vas; left: normal testis and partial absence of vas ending retroperitoneally

4. Compared with the other surgical options for varicocelectomy, the advantages of performing a subinguinal microsurgical varicocelectomy include all of the following EXCEPT:
   a. lower rate of arterial injury.
   b. lower rate of postoperative hydrocele.
   c. lower rate of varicocele recurrence.
   d. fewer veins ligated.
   e. lower overall complication rate.

5. Which maneuvers should be avoided when bridging a large vasal gap during vasovasostomy?
   a. Mobilization of the vas deferens toward the external inguinal ring
   b. Dissection of the sheath of the convoluted vas deferens off the epididymis and allowing the testis to drop upside-down
   c. Separation of the cauda and corpus epididymis from the testis
   d. Mobilization of the vas deferens toward the internal inguinal ring
   e. Unraveling of the convoluted vas deferens

6. In which of the following scenarios is a testis biopsy least helpful?
   a. Failure to retrieve motile sperm from the epididymis
   b. Sperm retrieval for nonobstructive azoospermia
   c. Diagnostic evaluation of men with congenital absence of vas and normal FSH levels
   d. Diagnostic evaluation in azoospermic men with normal findings on scrotal examination and normal serum testosterone and FSH levels
   e. Sperm retrieval for men diagnosed with Sertoli cell–only pattern in the testes

7. Which of the following scenarios has the lowest rate for sperm return to ejaculate after vasectomy reversal?
   a. Motile sperm in the vas and vasovasostomy
   b. Non-motile sperm in the vas and vasovasostomy
   c. Motile sperm in the vas and unilateral crossed vasovasostomy
   d. Thick, white vasal fluid devoid of sperm and vasovasostomy
   e. Copious clear vasal fluid but no sperm and vasovasostomy

8. In the evaluation for azoospermia, all of the following tests should be considered to confirm a diagnosis of obstructive azoospermia EXCEPT:
   a. transrectal ultrasonography.
   b. testicular biopsy.
   c. serum antisperm antibody assay.
   d. epididymal biopsy.
   e. serum testosterone and FSH assay.

9. Which of the following is TRUE regarding varicocele?
   a. Treatment in infertile men rarely results in improved semen parameters.
   b. Severity of testicular insult is related to the size of the varicoceles.
   c. Severity of testicular insult from varicocele is duration independent.
   d. Because of the severity of testicular insult, repair of large varicoceles is not warranted.
   e. Surgical treatment of subclinical varicoceles results in greater improvement in semen quality than treatment of large varicoceles.

10. After a bilateral vasoepididymostomy, a patient remained azoospermic in two semen analyses until 6 months postoperative, when the analysis revealed 8 million sperm/mL with 60% motility. What is the next management step?
    a. A plan for intrauterine insemination with ejaculated sperm
    b. A plan for assisted reproduction with intracytoplasmic sperm injection (ICSI) and ejaculated sperm
    c. Cryopreservation of semen
    d. No follow-up necessary
    e. Scrotal ultrasound

11. Which of the following is a disadvantage of the intussusception vasoepididymostomy?
    a. Inability to assess epididymal fluid for sperm before setting up for anastomosis
    b. Lower patency rate than end-to-side techniques
    c. Difficult hemostasis
    d. Placement of sutures into a collapsed epididymal tubule
    e. Transection of the epididymis required before anastomosis

12. All of the following situations are appropriate for assisted reproduction with ICSI as a first line of treatment EXCEPT:
    a. obstruction with multiple failures of reconstruction.
    b. mild oligoasthenospermia with varicoceles and a female partner of 29 years of age.
    c. Klinefelter syndrome.
    d. only a few viable sperm found in the ejaculate.
    e. post-chemotherapy azoospermia.

13. In which of the following settings are vasovasostomy and vasoepididymostomy contraindicated?
    a. Previous vasectomy more than 20 years ago
    b. Concomitant scrotal pain
    c. Concomitant hydrocele
    d. Concomitant varicoceles
    e. Nonobstructive azoospermia

14. In the presence of epididymal obstruction, which of the following statements is FALSE?
    a. The quality of sperm is better in caput than caudal tubules.
    b. Vasoepididymostomy to the caudal tubules has a better patency rate than to the caput tubules.
    c. Vasovasostomy can yield a satisfactory patency rate.
    d. A scrotal sonogram may demonstrate epididymal fullness and hydrocele.
    e. Intraoperative sperm cryopreservation is possible.

15. Which of the following statements is FALSE regarding microsurgical testicular sperm extraction (TESE)?
    a. Sertoli cell–only pattern is a contraindication for the procedure.
    b. Large seminiferous tubules typically give a higher sperm yield.
    c. It is best performed percutaneously.
    d. It can better preserve the blood supply to testis parenchyma than a non-microsurgical approach.
    e. It should be used in men with nonobstructive azoospermia.

16. All of the following are expected outcomes of varicocele repair EXCEPT:
    a. improved sperm motility.
    b. increased risk of multiple gestation.
    c. improved sperm counts.
    d. improved serum testosterone levels.
    e. return of sperm to the ejaculate in 40% to 50% of azoospermic men.

17. A 30-year-old man presenting with primary infertility was found to be azoospermic on two semen analyses. For which of the following findings is a diagnostic biopsy indicated?
    a. Ejaculate volume below 2 mL with negative fructose
    b. Semen pH less than 7.2
    c. Palpable vasa, normal serum FSH, normal testis volume, and negative antisperm antibodies

    d. Serum FSH of 25 IU/L and 12-mL soft testis
    e. Absence of vasa deferentia and normal serum FSH level

18. In which of the following scenarios is a vasogram indicated at the time of scrotal exploration/possible reconstruction?
    a. Azoospermia, Sertoli cell only on testis biopsy
    b. Azoospermia, testicular volume of 10 mL, FSH value 25 IU/L
    c. Azoospermia, normal testicular volume, biopsy revealing active spermatogenesis
    d. Azoospermia, no palpable vasa deferential
    e. Sperm count 5 million/mL, 5% motility, grade 2 varicoceles bilaterally

19. All of the following diagnoses can be made from a radiocontrast vasogram EXCEPT:
    a. inguinal vasal obstruction.
    b. ejaculatory duct obstruction.
    c. seminal vesicle agenesis.
    d. spermatogenic failure.
    e. partial agenesis of vasa deferentia.

20. All of the following are potential complications of transurethral resection of the ejaculatory ducts EXCEPT:
    a. urinary incontinence.
    b. retrograde ejaculation.
    c. recurrent epididymitis.
    d. testicular atrophy.
    e. contamination of semen with urine.

21. What is the pathogenesis of post-varicocelectomy hydrocele?
    a. Increased testicular venous pressure
    b. Lymphatic obstruction
    c. Soft tissue fibrosis
    d. Arterial injury
    e. Catch-up growth of testes

22. Which of the following is TRUE regarding the ejaculatory duct?
    a. It is a single midline duct formed by the confluence of the seminal vesicle ducts.
    b. It enters into the middle of the verumontanum.
    c. It joins with the prostatic ducts.
    d. It is a paired duct formed by the confluence of each seminal vesicle duct and vasa deferentia.
    e. It enters directly into the vesicle trigone.

23. All of the following are potential complications of vasography EXCEPT:
    a. vasal obstruction at the site of vasography.
    b. perivasal hematoma.
    c. sperm granuloma at the site of vasography.
    d. injury to the vasal artery.
    e. retrograde ejaculation.

24. What is the estimated percentage of men who develop antisperm antibodies after vasectomy?
    a. 0% to 20%
    b. 20% to 40%
    c. 40% to 60%
    d. 60% to 80%
    e. 80% to 100%

25. Intraoperatively during a vasectomy reversal, a sperm granuloma is found on the left side. What does this indicate?

a. Concomitant epididymal obstruction that requires a vasoepididymostomy

b. Infection requiring postoperative antibiotics

c. The need for genetic counseling

d. That sperm will be found at the testicular end of the vas

e. That the procedure should be abandoned and the patient should undergo re-exploration in 3 months

26. When is the best time to perform vasography?

a. At the time of diagnostic testis biopsy

b. At the time of reconstruction, if a prior testis biopsy result was normal

c. At the time of scrotal ultrasonography with color flow Doppler

d. At the time of transrectal ultrasonography revealing normal seminal vesicles

e. At the time of electroejaculation

27. Twelve years after vasectomy, a man was found on routine examination to have asymptomatic sperm granulomas bilaterally. All of the following scenarios are true EXCEPT:

a. Microrecanalization is possible with the appearance of rare sperm in the ejaculate.

b. If vasectomy reversal is performed, only bilateral vasovasostomy is likely to be necessary.

c. The epididymides are unlikely to be indurated.

d. The epididymides are likely to be obstructed.

e. No treatment is necessary for asymptomatic sperm granuloma.

28. A midline cyst compressing the ejaculatory duct is found on a transrectal ultrasonographic scan. What does the presence of sperm in the cyst aspirate suggest?

a. Congenital absence of vas on at least one side

b. Nonobstructive azoospermia

c. Bilateral epididymal obstruction

d. The possibility of XXY karyotype

e. Patency of a vas deferens and epididymis on at least one side

29. After transurethral resection of the ejaculatory ducts, the patient develops retrograde ejaculation. What is the next step of management?

a. Watchful waiting

b. Intrauterine insemination

c. ICSI

d. A trial of pseudoephedrine

e. Electroejaculation

30. One year after vasovasostomy, a progressive decline in sperm motility and sperm counts is noted. What does this indicate?

a. Progressive spermatogenic failure

b. Infection

c. Arterial injury to the testis and epididymis

d. Ejaculatory duct obstruction

e. Stricture of the vasovasostomy

31. In which of the following scenarios would a diagnostic testicular biopsy provide valuable clinical information?

a. Men with azoospermia, atrophic testes, and an FSH level of 25 IU/L

b. Men with a 47,XXY karyotype

c. Men with a fecundity history who seek vasectomy reversal

d. Men with primary infertility, azoospermia, normal physical examination findings, a normal serum FSH level, and a negative serum antisperm antibody assay

e. Men with anejaculation caused by high spinal cord injury

32. Which of the following is TRUE regarding retractile testes in adults?

a. As in the pediatric population, surgical repair is never indicated.

b. A dartos pouch operation is the treatment of choice.

c. Simple three-stitch orchiopexy of the tunica albuginea to the dartos, as for torsion prophylaxis, is effective in preventing retraction.

d. Bilateral orchiopexy is necessary for unilateral retractile testis.

e. Torsion of the testis is a common complication.

33. Which of the following is TRUE regarding vasoepididymostomy?

a. End-to-side anastomosis currently has the highest patency rate.

b. Microsurgical technique does not significantly improve the surgical outcome.

c. Assisted reproduction with ICSI is a more cost-effective option.

d. It should be reserved for azoospermia patients with spermatogenic arrest.

e. It should be performed only on an epididymal tubule containing sperm.

34. When a vasoepididymostomy is performed for fertility reasons, which of the following should be routinely done in the same setting?

a. Intraoperative epididymal sperm aspiration for sperm cryopreservation

b. Testicular biopsy for sperm cryopreservation

c. A touch preparation of testicular tissue

d. A squash preparation of testicular tissue

e. A radiocontrast vasogram

35. Which of the following is the most important factor in ensuring a high patency rate after a vasovasostomy?

a. Age of the patient

b. Time since vasectomy

c. Surgeon's technique and experience

d. Presence of motile sperm in the vasal fluid

e. Presence of a sperm granuloma at the vasectomy site

36. Which of the following surgical sperm retrieval techniques is inappropriate for the clinical situation indicated?

a. Percutaneous epididymal sperm aspiration (PESA) for congenital absence of vas

b. Percutaneous testicular sperm aspiration (PTSA) after failed vasoepididymostomy

c. Electroejaculation in a man with postretroperitoneal lymph node dissection for left testicular embryonal carcinoma

d. Microsurgical epididymal sperm aspiration (MESA) for spermatogenic maturation arrest

e. TESE in a man with azoospermia from chemotherapy

ANSWERS

1. **d. Deferential (vasal) veins.** All veins within the cord, with the exception of the vasal veins, are doubly ligated. Scrotal or gubernacular collateral veins have been demonstrated

radiographically to be the cause of 10% of recurrent varicoceles. All external spermatic veins are identified and doubly ligated with hemoclips and divided. The gubernaculum is inspected for the presence of veins exiting from the tunica vaginalis. These are either cauterized or doubly ligated.

2. **b. Hydrocele.** The presence of a hydrocele in the presence of excurrent ductal system obstruction is often associated with secondary epididymal obstruction. Surgeons attempting reconstruction should be aware of the possibility of the need for a vasoepididymostomy.

3. **d. Right: epididymal obstruction and patent right vas above vasectomy site; left: sperm in testicular end of vas and vasectomy site in convoluted vas.** Crossover is indicated in the following circumstances: (1) unilateral inguinal obstruction of the vas deferens associated with an atrophic testis on the contralateral side. A crossover vasovasostomy should be performed to connect a healthy testicle to the contralateral unobstructed vas. (2) Obstruction or aplasia of the inguinal vas or ejaculatory duct on one side and epididymal obstruction on the contralateral side. It is preferable to perform one anastomosis with a high probability of success (vasovasostomy) than two operations with a much lower chance of success such as unilateral vasoepididymostomy and contralateral transurethral resection of the ejaculatory ducts.

4. **d. Fewer veins ligated.** At the subinguinal level, significantly more veins are encountered, the artery is more often surrounded by a network of tiny veins that must be ligated, and the testicular artery has often divided into two or three branches, making arterial identification and preservation more difficult without using a microscope for the procedure.

5. **e. Unraveling of the convoluted vas deferens.** When large vasal gaps are present, a gauze-wrapped index finger is used to bluntly separate the cord structures from the vas. Blunt finger dissection through the external ring will free the vas to the internal ring if additional abdominal side length is necessary. These maneuvers will leave all the vasal vessels intact. When the vasal gap is extremely large, additional length can be achieved by dissecting the entire convoluted vas free of its attachments to the epididymal tunica, allowing the testis to drop upside-down. If the amount of the vas removed is so large that even these measures fail to allow a tension-free anastomosis, the incision can be extended to the internal inguinal ring, the floor of the inguinal canal cut, and the vas rerouted under the floor, as in a difficult orchiopexy. An additional 4 to 6 cm of length can be obtained by dissecting the epididymis off of the testis from the vasoepididymal junction to the caput epididymis. The superior epididymal vessels are left intact and provide adequate blood supply to the testicular end of the vas. With this combination of maneuvers, gaps up to 10 cm wide can be bridged. The convoluted vas should not be unraveled. This disturbs the blood supply at the anastomotic line.

6. **c. Diagnostic evaluation of men with congenital absence of vas and normal FSH levels.** Testis biopsy is indicated in azoospermic men with testes of normal size and consistency, palpable vasa deferentia, normal serum FSH levels, and a negative serum antisperm antibody assay. Under these circumstances, biopsy will distinguish obstructive azoospermia from primary seminiferous tubular failure. In the testes of men with congenital absence of vasa, biopsy always reveals normal or at least some spermatogenesis, and biopsy is not necessary before definitive sperm aspiration and in vitro fertilization (IVF) with ICSI.

7. **d. Thick, white vasal fluid devoid of sperm and vasovasostomy.** If the fluid expressed from the vas is found to be thick, white, water insoluble, and like toothpaste in quality, microscopic examination rarely reveals sperm. Under these circumstances, the tunica vaginalis is opened and the epididymis inspected. If clear evidence of obstruction is found (e.g., an epididymal sperm granuloma with dilated tubules above and collapsed tubules below), vasoepididymostomy is performed.

When the surgeon is in doubt or is not experienced with vasoepididymostomy, vasovasostomy should be performed. **However, only 15% of men with bilateral absence of sperm in the vasal fluid after barbotage and intensive search will have sperm return to the ejaculate after vasovasostomy.**

8. **d. Epididymal biopsy.** Before surgical reconstruction of the reproductive tract is attempted, spermatogenesis in the patient should be evident. A testicular biopsy may be indicated to confirm the presence of spermatogenesis. Men with a low semen volume should have a transrectal ultrasonographic scan to alert one to the possibility of an additional ejaculatory duct obstruction. For serum and antisperm antibody studies, the presence of serum antisperm antibodies corroborates the diagnosis of obstruction and the presence of active spermatogenesis. At present, this test is of unknown prognostic value and is optional. For serum FSH assay, men with small, soft testes should have serum FSH measured. An elevated FSH level suggests impaired spermatogenesis and potentially a poorer prognosis.

9. **b. Severity of testicular insult is related to the size of the varicoceles.** Larger varicoceles appear to cause more damage than small varicoceles; large varicoceles are associated with greater preoperative impairment in semen quality than are small varicoceles.

10. **c. Cryopreservation of semen.** With the older end-to-end or end-to-side vasoepididymostomy method, at 14 months after surgery 25% of initially patent anastomoses have shut down. For this reason, we recommend banking sperm both intraoperatively and as soon as sperm appear in the ejaculate postoperatively.

11. **a. Inability to assess epididymal fluid for sperm before setting up for anastomosis.** This method, also known as the *triangulation technique*, was introduced by Berger. There are several advantages of this method versus previous techniques. Two or three sutures placed in the epididymal tubule provide four and six points of fixation, and the anastomosis is virtually bloodless. However, one cannot assess tubular fluid for sperm before the anastomosis setup.

12. **b. Mild oligoasthenospermia with varicoceles and a female partner of 29 years of age.** Assisted reproduction can be offered to men with surgically unreconstructable obstruction such as congenital absence of the vas deferens; men with few viable sperm in the ejaculate; azoospermic men with varicoceles (half of these men will respond to varicocelectomy with return of enough sperm to ejaculate to achieve pregnancy using IVF with ICSI); and men with nonobstructive azoospermia.

13. **e. Nonobstructive azoospermia.** Before surgical reconstruction of the reproductive tract is attempted, spermatogenesis in the patient should be evident. A prior history of natural fertility pre-vasectomy is usually adequate. In other cases, a testicular biopsy may be indicated to confirm the presence of spermatogenesis.

14. **c. Vasovasostomy can yield a satisfactory patency rate.** If clear evidence of obstruction is found, vasoepididymostomy is performed. When there is doubt or the physician is not experienced with vasoepididymostomy, vasovasostomy should be performed. However, only 15% of men with bilateral absence of sperm in the vasal fluid after barbotage and an intensive search will have sperm return to the ejaculate after vasovasostomy.

15. **c. It is best performed percutaneously.** The use of an operating microscope for standard open diagnostic testes biopsy allows identification of an area in the tunica albuginea free of blood vessels, minimizing the risk of injury to the testicular blood supply and allowing a relatively blood-free biopsy specimen.

16. **b. Increased risk of multiple gestation.** Varicocelectomy results in significant improvement in the findings of semen analysis in 60% to 80% of men. Reported pregnancy rates after varicocelectomy vary from 20% to 60%. A randomized controlled trial of surgery versus no surgery in infertile men

with varicoceles revealed a pregnancy rate of 44% at 1 year in the surgery group versus 10% in the control group. In our series of 1500 microsurgical operations, 43% of couples were pregnant at 1 year and 69% at 2 years when couples with female factors were excluded. Microsurgical varicocelectomy results in return of sperm to the ejaculate in 50% of azoospermic men with palpable varicoceles. Repair of large varicoceles results in a significantly greater improvement in semen quality than repair of small varicoceles. In addition, large varicoceles are associated with greater preoperative impairment in semen quality than are small varicoceles, and consequently overall pregnancy rates are similar regardless of varicocele size. Some evidence suggests that the younger the patient is at the time of varicocele repair, the greater the improvement after repair and the more likely the testis is to recover from varicocele-induced injury. Varicocele recurrence, testicular artery ligation, and postvaricocelectomy hydrocele formation are often associated with poor postoperative results. In infertile men with low serum testosterone levels, microsurgical varicocelectomy alone results in substantial improvement in serum testosterone levels.

17. **c. Palpable vasa, normal serum FSH, normal testis volume, and negative antisperm antibodies.** Men with a positive antisperm antibody assay are always obstructed, and a biopsy is not necessary. Men with elevated FSH levels and small, soft testes always have nonobstructive azoospermia.

18. **c. Azoospermia, normal testicular volume, biopsy revealing active spermatogenesis.** The absolute indications for vasography are azoospermia, plus complete spermatogenesis with many mature spermatids on testis biopsy and at least one palpable vas. Relative indications for vasography are severe oligospermia with normal testis biopsy, a high level of sperm-bound antibodies that may be due to obstruction, low semen volume, and poor sperm motility (partial ejaculatory duct obstruction).

19. **d. Spermatogenic failure.** Vasography should answer the questions: Are there sperm in the vasal fluid? Is the vas obstructed? If the testis biopsy reveals many sperm, then the absence of sperm in vasal fluid indicates obstruction proximal to the vasal site examined, most likely an epididymal obstruction. Vasography is done in this case with saline or indigo carmine to confirm the patency of the seminal vesicle end of the vas before vasoepididymostomy. Copious vasal fluid containing many sperm indicates vasal or ejaculatory duct obstruction, and formal contrast vasography is performed to document the exact location of the obstruction. Copious thick, white fluid without sperm in a dilated vas indicates secondary epididymal obstruction in addition to potential vasal or ejaculatory duct obstruction.

20. **d. Testicular atrophy.** Reflux of urine into the ejaculatory ducts, vas, and seminal vesicles occurs after a majority of resections. This can be documented by voiding cystourethrography or by measuring semen creatinine levels. Reflux can lead to acute and chronic epididymitis. Recurrent epididymitis often results in epididymal obstruction. The incidence of epididymitis after transurethral resection is probably underestimated. Symptomatic chemical epididymitis may occur from refluxing urine. If epididymitis is chronic and recurrent, vasectomy or even epididymectomy may be necessary. Even when care has been taken to spare the bladder neck, retrograde ejaculation is common after transurethral resection. Transurethral instrumentation can increase the risk of urethral stricture.

21. **b. Lymphatic obstruction.** Analysis of the protein concentration of hydrocele fluid indicates that hydrocele formation after varicocelectomy is due to lymphatic obstruction.

22. **d. It is a paired duct formed by the confluence of each seminal vesicle duct and vasa deferentia.** The ejaculatory ducts course between the bladder neck and the verumontanum and exit at the level of and along the lateral aspect of the verumontanum.

23. **e. Retrograde ejaculation.** Complications of vasography include stricture, injury to the vasal blood supply, hematoma, and sperm granuloma. Multiple attempts at percutaneous vasography using sharp needles can result in stricture or obstruction at the vasography site. Careless or crude closure of a vasostomy can also result in stricture and obstruction. Non–water-soluble contrast agents may also result in stricture and should not be employed for vasography. If the vasal blood supply is injured at the site of vasography, vasovasostomy proximal to the vasography site may result in ischemia, necrosis, and obstruction of the intervening segment of vas. A bipolar cautery should be used for meticulous hemostasis at the time of vasostomy to prevent hematoma in the perivasal sheath. Leaky closure of a vasography site may lead to the development of a sperm granuloma, which can result in stricture or obstruction of the vas.

24. **d. 60% to 80%.** Systemic effects of vasectomy have been postulated. Vasectomy disrupts the blood-testis barrier, resulting in detectable levels of serum antisperm antibodies in 60% to 80% of men. Some studies suggest that the antibody titers diminish 2 or more years after vasectomy. Others suggest that these antibody titers persist. However, neither circulating immune complexes nor deposits are increased after vasectomy.

25. **d. That sperm will be found at the testicular end of the vas.** A sperm granuloma at the testicular end of the vas suggests that sperm have been leaking at the vasectomy site. This vents the high pressures away from the epididymis and is associated with a better prognosis for restored fertility regardless of the time interval since vasectomy.

26. **b. At the time of reconstruction, if a prior testis biopsy result was normal.** There is no need to perform vasography at the time of testis biopsy for azoospermia unless immediate reconstruction is planned and the touch or wet-preparation biopsy reveals mature sperm with tails. If performed carelessly, vasography can cause stricture or even obstruction at the vasography site, which can complicate subsequent reconstruction.

27. **d. The epididymides are likely to be obstructed.** Sperm granulomas form when sperm leak from the testicular end of the vas. Sperm are highly antigenic, and an intense inflammatory reaction occurs when sperm escape outside the reproductive epithelium. Sperm granulomas are rarely symptomatic. The presence or absence of a sperm granuloma at the vasectomy site seems to be of importance in modulating the local effects of chronic obstruction on the male reproductive tract. The sperm granuloma's complex network of epithelialized channels provides an additional absorptive surface that helps vent the high intraluminal pressure in the obstructed excurrent ducts. Numerous animal studies have correlated the presence or absence of sperm granuloma at the vasectomy site with the degree of epididymal and testicular damage. Species that always develop granulomas after vasectomy have minimal damage to the seminiferous tubules. Some studies of men undergoing vasectomy reversal have revealed somewhat higher success rates in men who have a sperm granuloma at the vasectomy site, whereas another large study has not. Although sperm granulomas at the vasectomy site are present microscopically in 10% to 30% of men undergoing reversal, it is likely that, given enough time, virtually all men develop sperm granulomas at the vasectomy site, the epididymis, or the rete testis. When chronic postvasectomy pain is localized to the granuloma, excision and occlusion of the vasa with intraluminal cautery usually relieve the pain and prevent recurrence. Men with postvasectomy congestive epididymitis may be relieved of pain by open-ended vasectomy designed to purposefully produce pressure, relieving sperm granuloma.

28. **e. Patency of a vas deferens and epididymis on at least one side.** The fine-needle aspirate is examined for sperm. If sperm are present, it means at least one vas and epididymis are patent.

29. **d. A trial of pseudoephedrine.** Pseudoephedrine (Sudafed), 120 mg orally, 90 minutes before ejaculation, may prevent retrograde ejaculation. If this is not successful, sperm can be retrieved from alkalinized urine and used for either intrauterine insemination or IVF with ICSI.

30. **e. Stricture of the vasovasostomy.** Late stricture and obstruction are disappointingly common. Progressive loss of sperm motility followed by decreasing counts indicates stricture. A trial of oral prednisone can sometimes prevent progression to azoospermia.

31. **d. Men with primary infertility, azoospermia, normal physical examination findings, and a normal serum FSH level, and a negative serum antisperm antibody assay.** Testis biopsy is indicated in azoospermic men with testis of normal size and consistency, palpable vasa deferentia, and normal serum FSH levels.

32. **b. A dartos pouch operation is the treatment of choice.** When scrotal orchiopexy is performed for retractile testis, a dartos pouch operation should be performed. Simple suture orchiopexy of the tunica albuginea of the testis to the dartos, such as is performed sometimes to prevent torsion, will not prevent retraction of these testes into the groin. Creation of a dartos pouch will keep the testis well down into the scrotum and permanently prevent retraction. This is also the most reliable and safest technique for the prevention of testicular torsion.

33. **e. It should be performed only on an epididymal tubule containing sperm.** Specific treatments for male factor infertility such as microsurgical reconstruction for obstructive azoospermia and varicocelectomy for impaired testes remain the safest and most cost-effective ways of managing infertile men. Microsurgical approaches allow accurate approximation of the vasal mucosa to that of a single epididymal tubule, resulting in marked improvement in the patency and pregnancy rates. If the level of obstruction is not clearly delineated, after the buttonhole opening is made in the tunica, a 70-μm diameter tapered needle from the 10 to 0 nylon microsuture is used to puncture the epididymal tubule, beginning as distal as possible, and fluid is sampled from the puncture site. When sperm are found, the puncture sites are sealed with microbipolar forceps, a new buttonhole is made in the epididymal tunica just proximally, and the tubule is prepared as described previously. Patency rates with the intussusception technique can exceed 80%. With the classic end-to-side or older end-to-end method, the patency rate is about 70%, and 43% of men with sperm will impregnate their wives after a minimum follow-up of 2 years.

34. **a. Intraoperative epididymal sperm aspiration for sperm cryopreservation.** Once sperm are identified, they are aspirated into glass capillary tubes and flushed into media for cryopreservation.

35. **c. Surgeon's technique and experience.** The responsibilities assumed by the surgeon demand the utmost in judgment and skill. Many of the procedures described in this chapter are among the most technically demanding in all of urology. Acquisition of the skills required to perform them demands intensive laboratory training in microsurgery and a thorough knowledge of the anatomy and physiology of the male reproductive system.

36. **d. Microsurgical epididymal sperm aspiration (MESA) for spermatogenic maturation arrest.** MESA is indicated for men with normal spermatogenesis and unreconstructable obstruction such as congenital bilateral absence of the vas deferens.

CHAPTER REVIEW

1. If the vas is transected at two different locations, the intervening segment will likely be fibrose because of lack of blood supply.
2. In repairing a hydrocele, the epididymis is often splayed, and one should leave a generous border around the epididymis to avoid injuring it.
3. When sperm are retrieved before any repair, it is prudent to cryopreserve some for future use, if necessary.
4. Following vasoepididymostomy, 50% to 85% of men will have sperm in the ejaculate; about half of these men will foster a pregnancy.
5. The indications for TESE are failure to find sperm in the epididymis and nonobstructive azoospermia.
6. During microsurgical TESE, larger tubules are more likely to yield sperm.
7. About 85% of patients following vasovasostomy will have sperm in their ejaculate; a little more than half will foster a pregnancy.
8. During vasovasostomy, repeated failure to identify sperm in the vasal fluid usually means epididymal obstruction; however, 15% of men with bilateral absence of sperm in the fluid will have sperm return in the ejaculate.
9. Testis biopsy is indicated in azoospermic men with testes of normal size and consistency, palpable vasa deferentia, and normal serum FSH level.
10. Varicocelectomy results in significant improvement in the findings of semen analysis in 60% to 80% of men. Reported pregnancy rates after varicocelectomy vary from 20% to 60%.
11. Men with a positive antisperm antibody assay are always obstructed, and a biopsy is not necessary.
12. A sperm granuloma at the testicular end of the vas predicts presence of sperm in the testicular vasal fluid.
13. Progressive loss of sperm motility followed by decreasing counts indicates stricture.

68

Physiology of Penile Erection and Pathophysiology of Erectile Dysfunction

Alan W. Shindel and Tom F. Lue

QUESTIONS

1. The thinnest portion of the tunica albuginea is the:
   a. lateral surface.
   b. ventral surface.
   c. crura.
   d. glans.
   e. dorsal surface.

2. The tunica albuginea of the corpora cavernosa consists of:
   a. concentric coats of nerves, arteries, and veins.
   b. an outer layer of circular fibers.
   c. type II collagen.
   d. valves to coapt emissary veins.
   e. a middle layer of obliquely oriented fibers.

3. Penile circulation is derived from both internal pudendal and accessory arteries in approximately what percentage of men?
   a. 5%
   b. 30%
   c. 50%
   d. 70%
   e. 90%

4. During the rigid phase of erection, all of the following are typically present except:
   a. arterial vasodilation.
   b. corporal sinusoid relaxation.
   c. corporal pressure increase.
   d. subtunical venous compression reducing venous outflow.
   e. relaxation of the ischiocavernosus muscles.

5. All of the following neurotransmitters are known to be highly relevant in male sexual function except:
   a. dopamine.
   b. oxytocin.
   c. vasoactive intestinal polypeptide (VIP).
   d. 5HT (serotonin).
   e. nitric oxide (NO).

6. All of the following statements are true except:
   a. NO stimulates the production of cyclic guanosine monophosphate (cGMP).
   b. NO released by endothelial nitric oxide synthase (eNOS) contained in the terminals of the cavernous nerve initiates the erection process, whereas nitric oxide released from neuronal nitric oxide synthase (nNOS) in the endothelium helps maintain erection.
   c. cGMP activates protein kinase G, which in turn opens potassium channels and closes calcium channels.

d. low cytosolic calcium favors smooth muscle relaxation.
   e. smooth muscle regains its tone when cGMP is degraded by phosphodiesterase.

7. According to Endocrine Society guidelines, testosterone therapy is indicated when:
   a. total testosterone levels are less than 300 ng/dL.
   b. the patient has low libido.
   c. the patient requests it.
   d. a dual-energy X-ray absorptiometry (DEXA) scan shows decreased bone mineral density.
   e. none of the above.

8. Which of the following antihypertensives is thought to potentially exert a beneficial effect on erectile function?
   a. Angiotensin-converting enzyme inhibitors
   b. Thiazide diuretics
   c. β blockers
   d. Calcium channel blockers
   e. None of the above

9. Erectile dysfunction (ED) in end-stage renal disease (ESRD) has been commonly associated with all of the following except:
   a. reduced bioavailability of NO
   b. autonomic neuropathy
   c. low serum prolactin
   d. endothelial dysfunction
   e. arterial calcification

10. Sonic hedgehog (SHH) protein has been shown to:
    a. inhibit normal penile development.
    b. reduce apoptosis in animal models of cavernous nerve injury.
    c. reduce expression of vascular endothelial growth factor (VEGF) and brain-derived neurotrophic factor (BDNF).
    d. enhance erectile responses in men after radical prostatectomy.
    e. increase penile tissues after cavernous nerve injury.

11. Rho kinase:
    a. phosphorylates the regulatory subunit of myosin light chain phosphatase.
    b. phosphorylates the regulatory subunit of myosin light chain kinase.
    c. inactivates RhoA.
    d. reduces smooth muscle contraction.
    e. activates soluble guanylate cyclase.

12. All of the following are **false** statements about nitric oxide synthase (NOS) except:
    a. synthesis of NO is catalyzed by NOS, which converts L-citrulline and oxygen to L-arginine and NO.

b. upregulation of nNOS expression has been found in the corpus cavernosum of aging and diabetic rats.

c. iNOS is a principle contributor to NO production in physiologic penile erection.

d. nNOS localizes to tyrosine hydroxylase containing nerve fibers.

e. NOS exists as three isoforms in mammalian cells.

13. All the following statements are true except:

a. C-type natriuretic peptide (CNP) is a potent natriuretic peptide; it relaxes isolated cavernous smooth muscle by binding to natriuretic peptide receptor-B (NPR-B)

b. protein kinase G-I (PKGI) may induce relaxation via activation of the plasma membrane Ca^{2+}-ATPase pump, inhibition of inositol trisphosphate (IP_3) generation, inhibition of Rho-kinase, stimulation of myosin light chain phosphatase (MLCP), and phosphorylation of heat shock proteins

c. reduced penile adenosine levels are associated with prolonged penile erection in animal models

d. calcitonin gene–related peptide is a potent vasodilator released from perivascular nerve fibers

e. the erectogenic effects of prostaglandin E_1 (PGE_1) as a pharmaceutic agent have been extensively documented

14. Relative to men without ED, psychogenic ED may be related to:

a. excessive sympathetic tone.

b. decreased activity of the "salience network."

c. increased activity of the "default mode network."

d. two of the above.

e. all of the above.

15. The temporal and parietal lobes

a. are activated during sexual arousal

b. govern introspection and self-reflection

c. trigger orgasmic response

d. are essential for cognitive evaluation of erotic stimuli

e. none of the above

16. All of the following statements about arteriogenic ED are **false** except:

a. carbon monoxide inhibits erectile responses by inhibiting heme oxygenase

b. protein kinase G inhibits myosin light chain phosphatase to induce penile erection

c. hyperpolarization of smooth muscle cells is associated with penile erection

d. prostaglandin PGI_2 induces penile erection

e. hydrogen sulfide induces penile erection and is produced by breakdown of arginine

17. Cavernous nerve injury is associated with

a. depletion of M_1 macrophages

b. upregulation of SHH

c. downregulation of RhoA/Rho-kinase

d. decreased oxidative stress

e. none of the above

ANSWERS

1. **b. Ventral surface.** Histological studies have indicated that the outer longitudinal layer of the tunica is absent between the 5 and 7 o'clock position on the penis. For this reason, erosion of penile prosthetics are more common through the ventral tunica toward the urethra.

2. **e. A middle layer of obliquely oriented fibers.** The tunica albuginea is a tough fibrous sheath containing type I and III collagen fibers (no type II). The outer layer of the tunica consists of longitudinally oriented fibers and the inner layer consists of circular fibers. A middle layer of obliquely oriented fibers connects the outer and inner layers. Penile erection does not require presence of valves to restrict blood flow; the emissary veins are compressed between the erectile tissue and the tough fibrous sheath of the tunica.

3. **d. 70%.** The majority of men have blood supply from both the internal pudendal and the accessory pudendal arteries. Vascular studies indicate that about 15% of men have corporal blood supply derived exclusively from either the internal pudendal or the accessory pudendal arteries. These men may be more vulnerable to vascular injury than men with redundant circulation from both arteries.

4. **e. Relaxation of the ischiocavernosus muscles.** The rigid erection phase corresponds to maximal sexual arousal and penile turgidity. Arterial vasodilation, sinusoid relaxation, increased corporal pressure, and venous occlusion are components of the full erection phase that continue into the rigid erection phase. Maximal engorgement of the entire penis requires contraction of the ischiocavernosus muscles to force blood into the distal corpora, glans, and corpus spongiosum.

5. **c. Vasoactive intestinal polypeptide (VIP).** Nitric oxide is critical for initiation of vasodilation. Dopamine, oxytocin, and serotonin play important roles regulating sexual responses (libido, erection, ejaculation) in the central nervous system. VIP containing nerves and peptides have been identified in the penis of experimental animals, but VIP administration does not produce substantive changes in penile erection and does not appear to be essential for erection response.

6. **b. NO released by endothelial nitric oxide synthase (eNOS) contained in the terminals of the cavernous nerve initiates the erection process, whereas nitric oxide released from neuronal nitric oxide synthase (nNOS) in the endothelium helps maintain erection.** NO activates guanylate cyclase, which in turn produces cGMP, which activates protein kinase G. Degradation of cGMP leads to reversal of smooth muscle tone. eNOS is activated in part due to shear stress from vasodilation and helps to maintain erection; the erection must be initiated by another process, typically release of nitric oxide from cavernous nerves and nNOS.

7. **e. None of the above.** It is recommended that testosterone therapy only be administered in the setting of biochemically low levels (less than approximately 300 ng/dL) AND symptoms potentially attributable to low testosterone (e.g., low libido, fatigue, loss of muscle mass, loss of bone density, depressed mood, weight gain). These symptoms are nonspecific and therefore do not in and of themselves merit T therapy but may improve with testosterone supplementation in the context of biochemically low levels.

8. **a. Angiotensin-converting enzyme inhibitors.** Thiazides and β blockers have been linked to ED. Angiotensin-converting enzyme (ACE) inhibitors do not have known effects that would interfere with erection, and there are data to suggest that there may be beneficial effects from ACE inhibition.

9. **c. Low serum prolactin.** Uremia and vascular changes are common in men with ESRD. There may be hormonal disruptions that contribute to ED in ESRD; however, it is typically elevated prolactin that plays a role in ED.

10. **b. Reduce apoptosis in animal models of cavernous nerve injury.** SHH is a trophic peptide that is essential in nervous system and musculoskeletal development. SHH enhances VEGF and BDNF expression; expression of SHH declines after cavernous nerve injury. While SHH has been associated with improvements in erectile function in animal models, it has not to date had proven efficacy in managing ED in human men who have undergone radical prostatectomy.

11. **a. Phosphorylates the regulatory subunit of myosin light chain phosphatase.** Rho kinase opposes penile erection by phosphorylating the regulatory subunit of MLCP, inhibiting it

and maintaining phosphorylation of the myosin light chain. This has the effect of stimulating smooth muscle contraction and vasoconstriction, opposing penile erection. Rho kinase does not directly act on guanylate cyclase. Dissociation of RhoA from the Rho-guanine dissociation inhibitor leads to activation of Rho kinase, not vice versa.

12. **e. NOS exists as three isoforms in mammalian cells.** Answer a is close but reversed, as it is conversion of arginine and oxygen to citrulline and NO that is facilitated by NOS. Upregulation of nNOS is associated with superior erectile function, which is counter to what is observed commonly in diabetic and aged animals. nNOS and eNOS are physiologically important whereas iNOS is activated in the setting of tissue stress. Tyrosine hydroxylase is an enzyme involved in production of catecholamines, which tend to favor sympathetic tone and oppose erectile processes. NOS does not co-localize with tyrosine hydroxylase in cavernous tissues and nerves.

13. **c. Reduced penile adenosine levels are associated with prolonged penile erection in animal models.** Adenosine can have either relaxant or constrictive effects on vascular tissue depending on the relative abundance of the various adenosine receptors in cells. Adenosine deaminase deficient mice and sickle cell transgenic mice experienced prolonged penile erections and are utilized as rodent models of the human condition of priapism. Accumulation of adenosine in these rodents is thought to be the mediator of these prolonged penile erections.

14. **d. Two of the above.** Sympathetic tone is associated with physiological and psychological stress and may contribute to impaired erectile response in psychogenic ED. The default mode network is the network of brain structures and connections thought to be involved with a state of "wakeful rest" and has been reported to exhibit decreased activity in men with ED thought to be psychogenic in origin. The salience network is involved in integrating and processing external stimuli and has been shown to be less active in men with psychogenic ED. Low-er-level activity of this network may hypothetically compromise self-recognition of autonomic and sexual responses and thus inhibit sexual response.

15. **b. Govern introspection and self-reflection.** The temporal and parietal lobes are involved in processes of introspection and self-reflection. It is thought that decreased activity of these brain regions plays a role in disinhibition, which may facilitate sexual responses. These regions are not thought to play a role in orgasmic response, which appears to primarily involve the mesodiencephalic transition zone (including the ventral tegmental area), the midbrain lateral central tegmental field, the zona incerta, the subparafascicular nucleus, and the thalamic nuclei.

16. **c. Hyperpolarization of smooth muscle cells is associated with penile erection.** Hyperpolarization is associated with reduction in intracellular calcium and subsequent inhibition of smooth muscle contraction; this has the net effect of facilitating penile erection. Carbon monoxide is produced by action of heme oxygenase and appears to facilitate erection response, possibly by binding to guanylate cyclase. Protein kinase G has the downstream effect of activating MLCP, which in turn works to deactivate the myosin light chain and oppose smooth muscle contraction. Prostaglandin E1 is associated with penile erection, but the PGI_2 isoform induces vasoconstriction, opposing erection response. Hydrogen sulfide induces penile erection but is produced by breakdown of L-cysteine.

17. **e. None of the above.** Cavernous nerve injury is associated with worsening of inflammation, tissue damage, and vascular response. All of the actions noted above would tend to facilitate penile erection response and/or preservation of penile tissues. M_1 macrophages are neurotoxic and are associated with tissue injury and remodeling. SHH is associated with nerve and smooth muscle trophism. RhoA/Rho-kinase enhance calcium sensitivity and vasoconstriction. Oxidative stress is associated with damage to penile tissues.

CHAPTER REVIEW

1. Penile erection is dependent on both increased arterial blood flow and coaptation of venous structures.
2. The structure of the corporal bodies of the penis is essential to the erectile process.
3. There is substantial variability in penile vascular anatomy between patients; this may have functional relevance in ED related to pelvic surgery.
4. Neuronal integrity at the brain, spinal cord, and peripheral level are essential to modulation of penile erections.
5. A wide range of neurotransmitters are involved in modulating sexual arousal and penile erection; key examples include dopamine, serotonin, oxytocin, nitric oxide, and norepinephrine.
6. Integration of erotic stimuli in the central nervous system is complex; magnetic resonance imaging (MRI) and positron emission tomography (PET) scanning has provided new insights on central mechanisms of sexual arousal in men.
7. Relaxation of the cavernous smooth muscle is the key to penile erection.
8. NO released by nNOS contained in the terminals of the cavernous nerve initiates the erection process whereas NO released from eNOS in the endothelium helps maintain erection.
9. On entering the smooth muscle cells, NO stimulates the production of cGMP by action on guanylate cyclase.
10. cGMP activates protein kinase G (PKG), which opens potassium channels and closes calcium channels.
11. Low cytosolic calcium favors smooth muscle relaxation.
12. Smooth muscle tone is restored when cGMP is degraded by phosphodiesterase (PDE) and intracellular calcium levels return to baseline levels.
13. Aging is an important contributing factor to ED. The aging process can affect the central regulation of erection, sensory mechanisms, hormonal and neural function, vascular flow, and penile structures.
14. ED is associated with a number of chronic health conditions and may be a sentinel event for serious disease.
15. Diabetes mellitus and metabolic syndrome are associated with particularly severe ED phenotypes. These disease processes may affect multiple organ systems and cause premature aging of central and peripheral structures and molecules that regulate erectile function.
16. Diseases that cause chronic renal failure are associated with ED; renal failure itself may contribute to ED, a condition that may persist despite successful renal transplantation.
17. Drugs most commonly associated with ED include antiandrogens, antidepressants, and antihypertensives.
18. Primary (lifelong) ED may be due to psychogenic causes, congenital arterial insufficiency, penile anomalies, and/or defects of penile vascular structures.

69 Evaluation and Management of Erectile Dysfunction

Arthur L. Burnett II and Ranjith Ramasamy

QUESTIONS

1. The best predictor for the development of erectile dysfunction (ED) is:
   a. young age.
   b. higher education.
   c. underweight status.
   d. passive cigarette smoke exposure.
   e. prediabetes.

2. "Shared decision making" is justified in the modern management of ED because of:
   a. availability of etiology-specific diagnostic testing.
   b. availability of increasingly invasive therapies.
   c. availability of irreversible therapies.
   d. central role of the clinician in directing proper treatment.
   e. acceptance of treatment preferences by patient and partner.

3. The risk association of ED with cardiovascular events:
   a. has not been established.
   b. is established unidirectionally to inform ED risk.
   c. is established unidirectionally to inform cardiovascular disease risk.
   d. is established bidirectionally to inform ED and cardiovascular disease risks.
   e. is established in conjunction with carcinogenesis risk.

4. Recommendations for lifestyle modification for the patient with ED require:
   a. stratification of cardiovascular risk.
   b. determination of high and moderate cardiovascular disease risk.
   c. cardiologic workup with diagnostic stress testing standardly.
   d. cardiologic medical treatment.
   e. basic medical assessment and health monitoring.

5. The characteristic that is typically associated with "organic" ED, in contrast with "psychogenic" ED, is:
   a. sudden loss of erections.
   b. situational erectile difficulty.
   c. erection responses on awakening.
   d. gradual decline in erectile ability.
   e. existence of an interpersonal relationship factor.

6. Self-administered ED questionnaires serve to:
   a. document responsiveness to treatment of ED.
   b. define the etiology of ED.
   c. indicate the objective severity of ED.
   d. distinguish the systemic type of ED (e.g., vascular, neurologic, endocrinologic).
   e. evaluate ED in research settings alone.

7. The best rationale for using specialized diagnostic testing is:
   a. to assess complex ED clinical presentations.
   b. as a requirement to direct ED treatment decisions.
   c. to ascertain a specific diagnosis underlying the ED presentation.
   d. to determine ED causation.
   e. to apply Grade A–level evidence-based ED diagnostic tools.

8. Duplex ultrasonography of the penis is a reliable diagnostic test when:
   a. combining pharmacostimulation.
   b. assessing intrapenile vascular communications.
   c. combining intracavernous pressure measurements.
   d. assessing penile and suprapubic penile flow velocities.
   e. indexing results to brachial systolic blood pressures.

9. A vascular test required for a patient under consideration for penile revascularization surgery is:
   a. combined intracavernosal injection and stimulation.
   b. duplex ultrasonography.
   c. dynamic infusion cavernosometry and cavernosography.
   d. penile angiography.
   e. radioisotopic penography.

10. Increased sex hormone–binding globulin (SHBG) is associated with:
    a. elevated bioavailable testosterone.
    b. lowered bioavailable testosterone.
    c. unaltered bioavailable testosterone.
    d. elevated total testosterone.
    e. lowered total testosterone.

11. The efficacy of testosterone therapy is best judged by:
    a. restored diurnal pattern of hormone levels.
    b. normal reference range serum testosterone level.
    c. midrange serum testosterone level.
    d. normal score using hypogonadism questionnaires.
    e. hypogonadism symptomatic improvement.

12. At the penile tissue level, a pharmacologic mechanism to promote penile erection is via the promoting actions of:
    a. cyclic nucleotides.
    b. phosphodiesterases.
    c. α_1 adrenergic agonists.
    d. dopaminergic D_2 receptor agonists.
    e. serotonergic receptor antagonists.

13. Intracavernosal pharmacotherapy is contraindicated for a patient with a clinical history of:
    a. neurological condition.
    b. cardiovascular disease.
    c. diabetes.
    d. priapism.
    e. anticoagulant use.

14. An advantage of alprostadil among pharmacologic agents for intracavernosal pharmacotherapy is:
    a. lower incidence of prolonged erection.
    b. lower incidence of painful erection.
    c. lower cost.
    d. long-term half-life once reconstituted.
    e. role in combination therapy.

15. The vacuum erection device is most advantageous for ED associated with:
    a. veno-occlusive dysfunction.
    b. glanular insufficiency.
    c. postpriapism.
    d. postexplantation of a penile prosthesis.
    e. Peyronie disease.

16. In patients with ED, the vascular lesion addressed by arterial revascularization surgery is:
    a. internal pudendal artery stenosis.
    b. penile dorsal artery stenosis.
    c. cavernosal artery stenosis.
    d. penile deep dorsal venous incompetence.
    e. internal pudendal venous incompetence.

ANSWERS

1. **d. Passive cigarette smoke exposure.** Predictors for the development of ED include older age, lower education, diabetes, cardiovascular disease (such as hypertension and stroke), cigarette smoke exposure (active and passive), and overweight condition.

2. **e. Acceptance of treatment preferences by patient and partner.** Shared decision making serves to allow the patient or couple to make an informed selection of the preferred therapy for sexual fulfillment on understanding all treatment options after completing a thorough discussion with the treating clinician.

3. **d. Is established bidirectionally to inform ED and cardiovascular disease risks.** Epidemiologic studies have documented a bidirectional risk relationship for ED and cardiovascular disease. This bidirectional paradigm carries ramifications with regard to overall male health status.

4. **e. Basic medical assessment and health monitoring.** All patients presenting for ED management carry some level of cardiovascular risk. Lifestyle modifications such as increased physical activity and improved weight control apply to all patients in accordance with a full medical assessment and regular health monitoring.

5. **d. Gradual decline in erectile ability.** "Organic" ED typically is characterized by a gradual onset of the problem, along with incremental progression, global dysfunction, and poor/absent erections on awakening.

6. **a. Document responsiveness to treatment of ED.** Self-administered ED questionnaires have served to document the presence, subjective severity, and responsiveness of treatment of ED in both clinical and research settings. They do not distinguish an etiologic basis for ED, differentiate among various causes of ED, or indicate an objective severity of ED.

7. **a. To assess complex ED clinical presentations.** Specialized diagnostic testing offers to improve diagnostic accuracy, but it is not a standard requirement to proceed therapeutically. Its best role at this time applies to the ED specialist who may elect certain tests to be done in settings of complex clinical presentations.

8. **a. Combining pharmacostimulation.** The combination of pharmacostimulation or combined intracavernosal injection and stimulation to duplex ultrasonography validates the imaging component of this test by establishing hemodynamic properties of a functionally relevant erection response. The quantification of blood flow in the penis applies to the main vascular tributaries and includes the entire penis from the crura in the perineum to the tip.

9. **d. Penile angiography.** Definition of the anatomy and radiographic appearance of the iliac, internal pudendal, and penile arteries by penile angiography is necessary in order to perform penile revascularization surgery.

10. **b. Lowered bioavailable testosterone.** Bioavailable testosterone can be affected to some extent by alterations in the SHBG fraction in serum associated with factors that increase SHBG, thereby accounting for a decrease in bioavailable testosterone.

11. **e. Hypogonadism symptomatic improvement.** The objective of testosterone therapy for hypogonadism is symptomatic improvement. The efficacy is not judged by a precise testosterone determination, although standard practice is to provide therapy at a normative serum testosterone level.

12. **a. Cyclic nucleotides.** Cyclic guanosine monophosphate and cyclic adenosine monophosphate act to promote proerectile molecular mechanisms resulting in corporal smooth muscle relaxation.

13. **d. Priapism.** Intracavernosal pharmacotherapy is contraindicated for men with psychological instability, a history or risk for priapism, histories of severe coagulopathy or unstable cardiovascular disease, reduced manual dexterity, and use of monoamine oxidase inhibitors.

14. **a. Lower incidence of prolonged erection.** Perceived advantages of alprostadil for intracavernosal pharmacotherapy relative to other agents are lower incidences of prolonged erection, systemic side effects, and penile fibrosis. Disadvantages include a higher incidence of painful erection, higher cost, and shortened half-life once reconstituted.

15. **b. Glanular insufficiency.** The effect of vacuum erection device therapy involves engorgement of the entire penis including the glans penis, such that it provides an advantage to patients experiencing glanular insufficiency. Special uses for this therapy such as preserving the elasticity of penile tissue after priapism or penile prosthesis explantation or after surgical correction of Peyronie disease have been suggested.

16. **a. Internal pudendal artery stenosis.** The penile arterial anatomic defect correctable by arterial revascularization commonly involves stenosis of the internal pudendal artery following perineal or pelvic trauma.

CHAPTER REVIEW

1. The prevalence of ED in the adult male is 20% and is correlated with age.
2. Men with ED are 45% more likely than men without ED to experience a cardiac event within 5 years of diagnosis.
3. The International Index of Erectile Function (IIEF) questionnaire has five domains: erectile function, orgasmic function, sexual desire, intercourse satisfaction, and overall satisfaction.
4. Erections observed with nocturnal penile tumescence monitoring do not necessarily equate with erections sufficient for sexual performance.
5. Cavernous arterial insufficiency is suggested when peak systolic velocity is less than 25 cm/s. A peak systolic velocity greater than 35 cm/s defines normal cavernous arterial inflow.
6. Testosterone circulates as free, bound to albumin, and bound to SHBG. Free testosterone and albumin-bound testosterone comprise the bioavailable testosterone.
7. Testosterone production is circadian, with the peak occurring in the morning. To evaluate testosterone status, blood should be drawn in the morning (between 7 AM and 11 AM).
8. Penile revascularization is reserved for patients in whom it is most likely to be successful: patients with a history of perineal trauma, age younger than 55 years, nondiabetic, nonsmoker, no venous leak, and a documented stenotic lesion in the internal pudendal artery on angiography.
9. Endocrine conditions that may be associated with erectile dysfunction include hypogonadism, hyperthyroidism, and diabetes.
10. Induction of a penile erection requires release of nitric oxide from penile nerve endings and vascular endothelium.
11. Nitrate use in any form is an absolute contraindication for the use of phosphodiesterase type 5 (PDE5) inhibitors.
12. Penile rehabilitation following radical prostatectomy using PDE5 inhibitors has not proved efficacious.
13. The vasoactive drugs commonly injected to produce an erection include prostaglandin E, papaverine, and phentolamine.
14. Predictors for the development of ED include older age, lower education, diabetes, cardiovascular disease (such as hypertension and stroke), cigarette smoke exposure (active and passive), and overweight condition.
15. Intracavernosal pharmacotherapy is contraindicated for men with psychological instability, a history or risk for priapism, histories of severe coagulopathy or unstable cardiovascular disease, reduced manual dexterity, and use of monoamine oxidase inhibitors.

70 Priapism

Gregory A. Broderick

QUESTIONS

1. Ischemic priapism is a persistent erection marked by each of the following clinical and pathophysiologic characteristics EXCEPT:
   a. rigidity of the corpora cavernosa.
   b. bright red corporal blood.
   c. hypoxic and acidotic corporal environment.
   d. painful rigidity.
   e. thrombus within the sinusoidal spaces.

2. Each of the following are etiologies typically associated with ischemic priapism EXCEPT:
   a. sickle cell disease (SCD).
   b. straddle injury.
   c. cocaine use.
   d. spider bite.
   e. pharmacologic erection therapy.

3. SCD is a risk factor for ischemic priapism; the pathophysiologic mechanisms include each of the following EXCEPT:
   a. decreased content of hemoglobin S (HgbS) in the plasma.
   b. the polymerization of HgbS when deoxygenated.
   c. scavenging of nitric oxide (NO).
   d. arginine catabolism removing substrate for NO synthesis.
   e. adhesive interactions among sickle cells, endothelial cells, and leukocytes.

4. Prolonged erection in males 40 years of age and older is usually attributed to:
   a. SCD.
   b. hematologic malignancy.
   c. erectile dysfunction (ED) pharmacotherapy.
   d. prostate cancer.
   e. testosterone supplementation.

5. Case reports have documented prolonged erections and, rarely, priapism in men by using phosphodiesterase type 5 (PDE5) inhibitor therapies. Associated risks for prolonged erection/priapism include each of the following EXCEPT:
   a. daily dosing.
   b. combination with intracavernous injection.
   c. history of penile trauma.
   d. psychotropic medications.
   e. narcotic use.

6. The associations and pathophysiology of high-flow priapism include each of the following EXCEPT:
   a. straddle injury.
   b. coital trauma.
   c. birth canal injury to the newborn male.
   d. cold-knife urethrotomy.
   e. hemodialysis.

7. The critical pathologic change occurring in the cavernosal tissue at 4 hours after the onset of ischemic priapism is:
   a. irreversible cavernous damage and ED.
   b. the beginning of glucopenia.
   c. the beginning of hypercoagulable thrombotic conditions.
   d. the deterioration of cavernous smooth muscle contractile responses.
   e. cavernous fibrosis.

8. The NO/cyclic guanosine monophosphate (cGMP) signaling pathway is implicated in the pathogenesis of priapism on the basis of scientific work showing:
   a. guanylate cyclase activity upregulation.
   b. guanylate cyclase activity downregulation.
   c. NO synthase activity upregulation.
   d. PDE5 activity upregulation.
   e. PDE5 activity downregulation.

9. An adolescent with SCD presents with a 6-hour erection. Initial cavernous blood gas results show Po_2 30 mm Hg, Pco_2 60 mm Hg, and pH 7.25. The first therapeutic step should be:
   a. oral terbutaline.
   b. oral pseudoephedrine.
   c. intracavernous aspiration.
   d. exchange transfusion.
   e. distal surgical shunt.

10. The characteristic blood flow defect of ischemic priapism found on color duplex ultrasonography is:
    a. normal cavernosal artery inflow.
    b. increased cavernosal artery inflow.
    c. decreased or absent cavernosal artery inflow.
    d. arteriovenous blush.
    e. sinusoidal fistula.

11. After initial intracavernous treatment for ischemic priapism, blood gas sampling produces an equivocal mixed-venous blood result. Priapism resolution is best confirmed by:
    a. color duplex ultrasonography.
    b. penile scintigraphy.
    c. corpus cavernosography.
    d. penile arteriography.
    e. pelvic computed tomography scan.

12. After a second session of intracavernous treatment consisting of aspiration/irrigation with phenylephrine administration, the priapic penis remains turgid. Cavernosal blood gas results are Po_2 40 mm Hg, Pco_2 50 mm Hg, and pH 7.35. The next step should be:
    a. observation.
    b. oral sympathomimetic.
    c. repeat intracavernous treatment.
    d. distal surgical shunt.
    e. proximal surgical shunt.

13. Phenylephrine is the preferred sympathomimetic used in the treatment of ischemic priapism because of its:

    a. α_1-selective activity.

    b. α_1 and α_2 activity.

    c. β_1-selective activity.

    d. β_2-selective activity.

    e. combined α and β activities.

14. The best indication for arterial embolization in the management of high-flow priapism is:

    a. unlikely spontaneous resolution.

    b. failure of sympathomimetic therapy.

    c. reduction of recurrent priapism risk.

    d. reduction of subsequent ED risk.

    e. patient preference to intervene.

15. Persistent penile rigidity after a technically successful proximal surgical shunt procedure in a patient with a 72-hour episode of ischemic priapism is an indication for:

    a. observation.

    b. gonadotropin-releasing hormone agonist therapy.

    c. pudendal artery ligation.

    d. distal surgical shunt.

    e. penile prosthesis surgery.

16. The mother of a child with SCD complains that her son has recently been awakening with erections lasting 3 to 4 hours. She is concerned that similar occurrences have been a warning sign for a major priapism. All of the following are appropriate management options EXCEPT:

    a. trial of nightly oral sympathomimetic drug.

    b. trial of low-dosage, daily PDE5 inhibitor.

    c. a gonadotropin-releasing hormone agonist or antiandrogen.

    d. intracavernous injection of phenylephrine in the morning.

17. Evidence-based studies of priapism therapies and outcomes are rare. A recent investigation of adult SCD patients presenting with ischemic priapism subjected all men to a standard protocol of aspiration and phenylephrine injections. Long-term sexual health function outcomes revealed complete ED in men with duration of priapism:

    a. less than 12 hours.

    b. 12 to 24 hours.

    c. longer than 36 hours.

    d. longer than 48 hours.

    e. longer than 72 hours.

18. An adult male presents with ischemic priapism of 8 hours duration. He fails to respond to serial aspiration and intracavernous injection after 4 hours in the emergency department. The recommended intervention at this time should be:

    a. hydration, nasal oxygen, and keeping the patient NPO for 8 hours to avoid risks of emergent intubation.

    b. a percutaneous distal penile shunt.

    c. an open distal shunt.

    d. an open proximal shunt.

    e. a saphenous vein shunt.

19. Radiographic imaging may be helpful in the diagnosis and management of priapism. Each of the following is correct EXCEPT:

    a. color Doppler ultrasound (CDU) in the evaluation of a persistent erection following treatments for ischemic priapism.

    b. penile arteriography to differentiate high-flow from ischemic priapism.

    c. magnetic resonance imaging (MRI) to diagnose corporal thrombus in men with refractory priapism or when there has been a significant delay in presentation.

    d. MRI in the differential diagnosis of corporal metastasis.

20. A 36-year-old tech entrepreneur is referred for a diagnosis of priapism after he slipped while climbing aboard his yacht. He initially had a saddle bruise on his perineum and pain; the next morning he awoke with persistent erection. The patient has a board of directors meeting at the end of the week and wants immediate treatment. The correct management strategy is:

    a. penile aspiration and α-adrenergic injection in the office or emergency department.

    b. penile arteriography.

    c. angio-embolization after a thorough discussion of chances for spontaneous resolution and risks of treatment-related ED.

    d. CDU-guided corporal exploration to ligate fistula.

    e. distal penile shunt.

21. Priapism associated with SCD is ischemic. The current pathophysiology is believed to be:

    a. obstruction of venous outflow by sickled erythrocytes.

    b. hemolysis and reduced NO.

    c. increased blood viscosity.

    d. a blood dyscrasia associated with reduced reticulocyte counts.

    e. dysregulated cavernous arterial inflow.

22. Ischemic priapism in boys and men with SCD should focus on correcting the hemoglobinopathy:

    a. with exchange transfusions.

    b. with hydration, alkalinization, and oxygen.

    c. with aspiration and pharmacologic detumescence.

    d. with hydroxyurea.

    e. with analgesia and expectant management.

23. A 27-year-old previously healthy white male is brought into the emergency department in the early morning hours by his girlfriend. She describes a night of partying with alcohol, energy drinks, and a small amount of cocaine. Her boyfriend has had a persistent erection for 6 to 8 hours. She says, "I've done all I can to help him—it won't go down!" The emergency department doctor calls the urologist to go over the case and initiate management. The best course of therapy would be:

    a. baclofen, 20 mg PO followed every 6 hours until erection subsides.

    b. pseudoephedrine, 60 mg PO.

    c. inhaled terbutaline, 4 mg.

    d. oral terbutaline, 4 mg.

    e. corporal aspiration and injection of phenylephrine, 200 µg.

24. PDE5 inhibitors are first-line therapy for ED, but like intracavernous therapy, PDE5 inhibitors have been associated with prolonged erection and priapism. Which agent is most likely to cause priapism?

    a. Sildenafil, 100 mg PRN sex

    b. Avanafil, 200 mg PRN sex

    c. Levitra, 20 mg PRN sex

    d. Cialis, 5 mg daily

    e. None of these agents is more likely to result in priapism

25. Early reviews concluded that the natural history of ischemic priapism is ED. Recent interventions have tracked sexual health function outcomes with evidence-based questionnaires such as the International Index of Erectile Function (IIEF-5). Improvements in medical and surgical management of ischemic priapism may preserve erectile function. Unfortunately, ED is likely to occur if reversal by medical or surgical means is not successful after how many hours?

a. 8 hours

b. 12 to 24 hours

c. 36 hours

d. 48 hours

e. 72 hours

ANSWERS

1. **b. Bright red corporal blood.** Ischemic priapism is a persistent erection marked by rigidity of the corpora cavernosa and little or no cavernous arterial inflow. In ischemic priapism there are time-dependent changes in the corporal metabolic environment with progressive hypoxia, hypercarbia, and acidosis. The patient typically complains of penile pain after 6 to 8 hours, and examination reveals a rigid erection. After 48 hours, thrombus can be found in the sinusoidal spaces and smooth muscle necrosis with fibroblast-like cell transformation is evident.

2. **b. Straddle injury.** Nonischemic priapism is much rarer than ischemic priapism, and the etiology is largely attributed to trauma. Forces may be blunt or penetrating, resulting in laceration of the cavernous artery or one of its branches within the corpora. The etiology most commonly reported is a straddle injury to the crura.

3. **a. Decreased content of hemoglobin S (HgbS) in the plasma.** The clinical features are seen in homozygous SCD patients: chronic hemolysis, vascular occlusion, tissue ischemia, and end-organ damage. HgbS polymerizes when deoxygenated, injuring the sickle erythrocyte, activating a cascade of hemolysis and vaso-occlusion. Membrane damage results in dense sickling of red cells, causing adhesive interactions among sickle cells, endothelial cells, and leukocytes. Hemolysis releases hemoglobin into the plasma. Free Hgb reacts with NO to produce methemoglobin and nitrate. This is a scavenging reaction; the vasodilator NO is oxidized to inert nitrate. Sickled erythrocytes release arginase-I into blood plasma, which converts L-arginine into ornithine, effectively removing substrate for NO synthesis. Oxidant radicals further reduce NO bioavailability. The combined effects of NO scavenging and arginine catabolism result in a state of NO resistance and insufficiency termed *hemolysis-associated endothelial dysfunction*. Therapeutic interventions include transfusion to decrease the relative concentrations of HgbS in the plasma.

4. **c. Erectile dysfunction (ED) pharmacotherapy.** The introduction of intracavernous pharmacotherapy approximately two decades ago led to a pronounced increase in the incidence of prolonged erection and true priapism. Prolonged erection is more commonly reported than is priapism, following therapeutic or diagnostic injection of intracavernous vasoactive medications. In many communities patients receiving intracavernous medications for ED will outnumber patients with SCD. The majority of men requiring treatment for ED are middle-aged to older men. In worldwide clinical trials of the Alprostadil Study Group, prolonged erection (defined as 4 to 6 hours) was 5%, and priapism (> 6 hours) was described in 1% of subjects. In papaverine/phentolamine/alprostadil intracavernous injection programs, prolonged erections have been reported in 5% to 35% of patients.

5. **a. Daily dosing.** Few cases reports have documented priapism following PDE5 inhibitor therapy. These reports suggest that men with the following conditions were at increased risk for priapism: SCD, spinal cord injury, men who used a PDE5 inhibitor recreationally, men who used a PDE5 inhibitor in combination with intracavernous injection, men with a history of penile trauma, men on psychotropic medications, and men abusing narcotics. Tadalafil, 5 mg daily dosing caused no priapism in a phase II clinical study of 281 men with history of lower urinary tract symptoms secondary to benign prostatic hyperplasia (BPH) for 6 weeks, followed by dosage escalation to 20 mg once daily for 6 weeks.

6. **e. Hemodialysis.** Nonischemic priapism is much rarer than ischemic priapism, and the etiology is largely attributed to trauma. Forces may be blunt or penetrating, resulting in laceration of the cavernous artery or one of its branches within the corpora. The etiology most commonly reported is a straddle injury to the crura. Other mechanisms include coital trauma, kicks to the penis or perineum, pelvic fractures, birth canal trauma to the newborn male, needle lacerations, complications of penile diagnostics, and vascular erosions complicating metastatic infiltration of the corpora. Although accidental blunt trauma is the most common etiology, high-flow priapism has been described following iatrogenic injury: cold-knife urethrotomy, Nesbitt corporoplasty, and deep dorsal vein arterialization. Any mechanism that lacerates a cavernous artery or arteriole can produce unregulated pooling of blood in sinusoidal space with consequent erection.

7. **d. The deterioration of cavernous smooth muscle contractile responses.** In ischemic priapism there are time-dependent changes in the corporal metabolic environment with progressive hypoxia, hypercarbia, and acidosis. In vitro studies have demonstrated that when corporal smooth muscle strips are exposed to a hypoxic condition, α-adrenergic stimulation fails to induce corporal smooth muscle contraction. Histologically, by 12 hours corporal specimens show interstitial edema, progressing to destruction of the sinusoidal endothelium, exposure of the basement membrane, and thrombocyte adherence at 24 hours.

8. **e. PDE5 activity downregulation.** Recent scientific advances have shown that priapism is associated with decreased PDE5 functional regulation in the penis. The relative lack of this molecular factor needed for controlling chemical signaling of penile erection accounts for stuttering and ischemic priapism in sickle cell patients. Experimental models of corpus cavernosum smooth muscle cells suggest that the cyclic nucleotide cGMP is produced in low steady-state amounts under the influence of priapism-related destruction of the vascular endothelium and thus reduced endothelial NO activity. This situation downregulates the set point of PDE5 function, secondary to altered cGMP-dependent feedback control mechanisms. When NO is neuronally produced in response to erectogenic stimulus or during sleep-related erectile activity, cGMP production surges in a manner that leads to excessive erectile tissue relaxation because of basally insufficient functional PDE5 to degrade the cyclic nucleotide.

9. **c. Intracavernous aspiration.** The history and blood gases define an ischemic priapism event, which warrants immediate attempts at decompression/aspiration of the corpora cavernosa. In SCD, concurrent systemic treatments may be offered, but relief of the penile ischemia should be pursued aggressively. Aspiration should be repeated until no more dark blood can be seen coming out of the corpora and bright red blood is obtained. This process decreases the intracavernous pressure, relieves pain, and resuscitates the corporal environment, removing anoxic, acidotic, and hypercarbic blood.

10. **c. Decreased or absent cavernosal artery inflow.** In presentations of ischemic priapism, minimal or absent blood flow in the cavernosal arteries is found using color Doppler ultrasonography. CDU is an adjunct to the corporal aspirate in

differentiating ischemic from nonischemic priapism. Patients with ischemic priapism will have no blood flow in the cavernous arteries; the return of the cavernous artery waveform will accompany successful detumescence. Patients with nonischemic priapism have normal to high blood-flow velocities in the cavernous arteries; an effort should be made to localize the characteristic blush of color emanating from flow signal of the disrupted cavernous artery or arteriolar-sinusoidal fistula.

11. **a. Color duplex ultrasonography.** This tool is the most reliable and least invasive imaging technique to differentiate ischemic from nonischemic priapism. CDU should always be considered in the evaluation of a full or partial erection after treatments for ischemic priapism. The differential diagnosis includes resolved ischemia with persistent tenderness and penile edema, persistent ischemia, or conversion to a high-flow state.

12. **a. Observation.** These blood gas results are consistent with normal mixed venous blood. The turgid penis may be due to tissue edema. Observation is appropriate at this time.

13. **a. α_1-Selective activity.** According to American Urological Association Guidelines, aspiration followed by intracavernous injection of sympathomimetic drugs is the standard of care in the medical treatment of ischemic priapism. Sympathomimetic pharmacotherapies (phenylephrine, etilefrine, ephedrine, epinephrine, norepinephrine, metaraminol) cause smooth muscle contraction in the corpora. Phenylephrine is a selective α_1-adrenergic receptor agonist, with minimal β-mediated inotropic and chronotropic cardiac effects. There are no comparative trials of sympathomimetic injectables in the management of priapism.

14. **e. Patient preference to intervene.** Nonischemic priapism should generally be managed by observation. Arterial priapism is not an emergency. Spontaneous resolution or response to conservative therapy has been reported in up to 62% of published series. Persistent partial erection from high-flow priapism may continue from months to years. There are no comparative outcome studies of intervention versus conservative management, but there are sufficient case descriptions in children to recommend initial watchful waiting. Adult patients demanding immediate relief can be offered selective arterial embolization.

15. **e. Penile prosthesis surgery.** Unfortunately, the natural history of untreated ischemic priapism or priapism refractory to interventions is severe fibrosis, penile length loss, and complete ED. The exact time point when penile prosthesis becomes a reasonable option is unclear, but most series describe complete ED in men who have had ischemic priapism for 36 to 72 hours. The advantages of early penile implantation in the acute management of ischemic priapism are preservation of penile length and a technically easier implantation; delayed implantation is technically challenging due to corporal fibrosis.

16. **c. A gonadotropin-releasing hormone agonist or antiandrogen.** The goals of managing stuttering ischemic priapism are prevention of future episodes, preservation of erectile function, and reducing the trauma to the patient from priapism management. A trial of daily oral sympathomimetic therapy, a trial of oral PDE5 inhibitor therapy, or intracavernous injection of phenylephrine should be considered in the management of children and adults with stuttering ischemic priapism associated with hemoglobinopathies. GnRH agonists or antiandrogens may be used in adults but should not be used in patients who have not achieved full sexual maturation and adult stature.

17. **c. Longer than 36 hours.** In those patients in whom priapism was reversed, spontaneous erection (with or without sildenafil) was reported in 100% of men when priapism was reversed in less than 12 hours; 78% when reversed by 12 to 24 hours; and 44% when reversed by 24 to 36 hours. No patient reported spontaneous erection after priapism duration of more than 36 hours.

18. **b. A percutaneous distal penile shunt.** The objective of shunt surgery is reoxygenation of the corpus cavernosum. The shared principle of all shunting procedures is to reestablish corporal inflow by relieving venous outflow obstruction. A distal cavernoglanular shunt should be the first choice of shunting procedures because it is technically easier to perform than proximal shunting. Percutaneous distal shunting is less invasive than open distal shunting and can be attempted in the emergency department with local anesthetic. Anesthesiologists must be educated that ischemic priapism is an emergency and sexual function outcomes are time dependent; appropriate airway precautions should be taken for emergent intubation as needed in the surgical management of priapism.

19. **b. Penile arteriography to differentiate high-flow from ischemic priapism.** CDU is an adjunct to the corporal aspirate in differentiating ischemic from nonischemic priapism. CDU imaging should include corporal shaft and transperineal assessment of the crural bodies when there is a history of penile trauma or straddle injury. CDU should always be considered in the evaluation of a persistent or partial erection after treatments for ischemic priapism. Penile arteriography is too invasive as a diagnostic procedure to differentiate ischemic from nonischemic priapism. Penile arteriography should be reserved for the management of high-flow priapism, when embolization is planned. There are three possible roles for MRI: (1) imaging of a well-established arteriolar-sinusoidal fistula, (2) identifying corporal thrombus, and (3) identifying corporal metastasis.

20. **c. Angio-embolization after a thorough discussion of chances for spontaneous resolution and risks of treatment-related ED.** Arterial priapism is not an emergency and may be managed expectantly. Diagnosis of high-flow priapism is best made by penile/perineal CDU. Penile aspiration and injection of α-adrenergic agents is not recommended for HFP. Angio-embolization should be preceded by a thorough discussion of chances for spontaneous resolution, risks of treatment-related ED, and lack of significant consequences expected from delaying interventions. Overall success rates with embolization are high, although a single treatment carries a recurrence rate of 30% to 40%. Where angio-embolization fails or is contraindicated, surgical ligation is reasonable. Formation of a pseudocapsule at the site of a sinusoidal fistula may take weeks to months following trauma. CDU guidance is recommended during exploration to locate the fistula.

21. **b. Hemolysis and reduced NO.** Contemporary science implicates hemolysis and reduced NO in the pathogenesis of pulmonary hypertension, leg ulcers, priapism, and stroke in SCD patients, whereas increased blood viscosity is believed to be responsible for painful crises, osteonecrosis, and acute chest syndrome. SCD patients with priapism have a fivefold greater risk of developing pulmonary hypertension. SCD priapism is also associated with reduced hemoglobin levels and increased hemolytic markers: reticulocyte count, bilirubin, lactate dehydrogenase, and aspartate aminotransferase.

22. **c. With aspiration and pharmacologic detumescence.** Classically, management of SCD-induced ischemic priapism involved analgesics, hydration, oxygen, bicarbonate, and exchange transfusion. It is very tempting, especially in boys, to defer management to pediatricians and hematologists. Hematologists have begun to question the emphasis on intravenous hydration, sodium bicarbonate for alkalinization, and exchange transfusion as first-line therapy for SCD-associated priapism. Unfortunately, acute neurologic complications may follow exchange transfusions. Hydroxycarbamide (hydroxyurea) is a hematologic agent used in the management of vaso-occlusive crises in SCD patients. The proposed mechanisms of action are increase in production of hemoglobin F, lowering of leukocytes–platelets–reticulocytes, and promoting release of NO. In the best interest of the patient, the urologist should seek hematologic consultation in the management of boys and men with SCD priapism, but remain assertive that hematolog-

ic therapy alone is not effective management of SCD priapism. One report suggested that blood transfusion may have no effective role in the treatment of sickle cell–induced priapism. Reports from hematology centers suggest high success rates using penile aspiration/injection/irrigation of intracavernous sympathomimetics for SCD priapism.

23. **e. Corporal aspiration and injection of phenylephrine 200 μg.** Oral agents are not recommended in the management of acute ischemic priapism (> 4 hours). Oral α-adrenergic agents may have a role in the management of stuttering priapism associated with prolonged nocturnal erections. The recommended initial treatment of ischemic priapism is the decompression of the corpora cavernosa by aspiration. Aspiration will immediately soften the erection and relieve pain. Aspiration alone may relieve priapism in 36% of cases. The AUA Guidelines Panel advised that there were not sufficient data to conclude that aspiration followed by saline intracorporal irrigation was any more effective than aspiration alone. Aspiration should be repeated until no more dark blood can be seen coming out from the corpora and fresh bright red blood is obtained. This process leads to a marked decrease in the intracavernous pressure, relieves pain, and resuscitates the corporal environment removing anoxic, acidotic, and hypercarbic blood. Corporal aspiration, if unsuccessful, should be followed by α-adrenergic injection.

24. **e. None of these agents is more likely to result in priapism.** The 2013 label for the most recently approved PDE5 inhibitor Stendra (avanafil 50 mg, 100 mg, 200 mg) contains precautionary wording virtually identical to that on prior labels for PRN oral dosing of sildenafil, vardenafil, and tadalafil: "There have been rare reports of prolonged erection greater than 4 hours and priapism (painful erections greater than 6 hours)." Once-daily tadalafil (2.5 mg and 5 mg) was approved for oral treatment of ED in 2008, and subsequently in 2011 tadalafil (2.5 mg and 5 mg) was approved for the signs and symptoms of BPH and treatment of ED and the signs and symptoms of BPH. Tadalafil 5 mg daily dosing caused no priapism in a phase II clinical study of 281 men with history of lower urinary tract symptoms secondary to BPH for 6 weeks.

25. **d. 48 hours.** Bennett and Mulhall in 2008 carefully documented 39 cases of SCD priapism presenting to their emergency department over 8 years; men were routinely interviewed for erectile function status within 4 weeks of priapism/interventions. Of the 39 African-American men followed, 73% acknowledged prior episodes of stuttering; 85% had previously been diagnosed with SCD; but only 5% had been counseled in SCD clinics or were aware that priapism was a complication of SCD. A standard protocol of aspiration and phenylephrine injection was performed; shunting for failure of medical management was performed in 28%. In those patients in whom priapism was reversed, spontaneous erections (with or without use of sildenafil) were reported in 100% of men when priapism was reversed by 12 hours; 78% when reversed by 12 to 24 hours; and 44% when reversed by 24 to 36 hours. In this contemporary series of SCD patients, no men reported the return of spontaneous erections after priapism lasting 36 hours or more. Ralph describes the efficacy and outcomes of combining the T-shunt with the corporal "snake" maneuver in 45 patients. All were refractory to medical reversal of ischemic priapism. The combined distal surgical technique was successful in resolving the acute priapism if duration was less than 24 hours but had limited efficacy in cases of priapism greater than 48 hours. Corporal needle biopsies were performed in each case and documented smooth muscle necrosis, worsening as a function of time and uniform in all men with more than 48 hours of ischemia. At 6 months erectile function outcomes were assessed by the erectile function domain score from the IIEF-5. T-shunt with corporal snake tunneling successfully reversed ischemic priapism in all patients with less than 24 hours' duration, but at 6 months ED was complained of by 50% of men. The authors conclude that the cutoff for irreversible restoration of erectile tissue is 48 hours; aggressive combined distal shunting may resolve priapism in a small cohort (30%), but all will have severe ED. They advise that management of refractory ischemic priapism greater than 48 hours should include discussion of immediate insertion of penile implant.

CHAPTER REVIEW

1. Ischemic priapism is the result of little or no cavernous arterial inflow.
2. Interventions 48 hours beyond the onset of ischemic priapism may relieve pain but will have little benefit in preserving potency.
3. Stuttering priapism is recurrent, unwanted, painful erections in men, usually with sickle cell disease.
4. Nonischemic or high-flow arterial priapism is usually the result of trauma, and the corpora are tumescent but not rigid.
5. The etiology of the majority of ischemic priapism is idiopathic; however, it may be associated with psychotropic medications, alcohol or drug abuse, hematologic dyscrasias, metastatic disease, perineal trauma, intracavernous injection of vasoactive drugs, and sickle cell disease.
6. Priapism following a PDE5 inhibitor usually occurs in men with other risk factors.
7. On rare occasions, following reversal of ischemic priapism, high-flow priapism may occur. Doppler ultrasound is useful in making this diagnosis.
8. Ischemic priapism and stuttering priapism are the result of NO imbalance.
9. In ischemic priapism, aspiration alone will be curative in a third of the patients.
10. Phenylephrine, 200 μg/mL given in 0.5-mL aliquots, not to exceed a total dose of 1 mg, is used to treat ischemic priapism. Corporal aspiration, if unsuccessful, should be followed by α-adrenergic injection.
11. Aspiration has no role in high-flow priapism other than for diagnosis; it plays no role in treatment.
12. PDE5 inhibitor therapy has been used to treat stuttering priapism in men with sickle cell disease.
13. When surgical therapy is indicated, a cavernosal glanular shunt should be the first choice.
14. Spontaneous resolution of high-flow arterial priapism generally occurs in two thirds of patients.
15. If a distal shunt fails, a proximal shunt should be considered.
16. In sickle cell disease, concurrent systemic treatments may be offered, but relief of the penile ischemia should be pursued aggressively. Aspiration should be repeated until no more dark blood can be seen coming out of the corpora and bright red blood is obtained.
17. Increased risk for priapism occurs in sickle cell disease, spinal cord injury, men who used a PDE5 inhibitor recreationally, men who used a PDE5 inhibitor in combination with intracavernous injection, men with a history of penile trauma, men on psychotropic medications, and men abusing narcotics.

71 Disorders of Male Orgasm and Ejaculation

Chris G. McMahon

QUESTIONS

1. The most important inhibitory neurotransmitter in the central neurochemical control of ejaculation is:
   a. dopamine
   b. serotonin
   c. noradrenalin
   d. oxytocin
   e. gamma aminobutyric acid (GABA)

2. Which of the following is incorrect?
   a. The ejaculatory process comprises three phases: emission, ejection, and orgasm.
   b. Emission is synergistic activation of both sympathetic and parasympathetic nerves (T10 to L2) but may also include a cholinergic excitatory mechanism.
   c. Ejection is mediated by somatic nerves (S2 to S4).
   d. Ejection involves a sympathetic spinal cord reflex upon which there is limited voluntary control.
   e. Closure of bladder neck, rhythmic contraction of the bulbocavernosus, bulbospongiosus, and other pelvic floor muscles, and relaxation of the internal urinary sphincter during emission prevents retrograde ejaculation.

3. The prevalence of intravaginal ejaculation latency times (IELT) of ≤1 minute in the general population is approximately
   a. <1%
   b. 2.5%
   c. 5.5%
   d. 11%
   e. 20%

4. Which of the following is incorrect?
   a. The *Diagnostic and Statistical Manual of Mental Disorders* (DSM-V) definition of premature ejaculation (PE) is an operationalized multivariate definition that captures the key dimensions of latency, control, and bother.
   b. Approximately 50% of heterosexual men seeking treatment for lifelong PE ejaculate within 1 minute after penetration.
   c. The consistent early ejaculations of lifelong PE suggest an underlying neurobiological functional disturbance.
   d. Acquired PE is most often due to psychological factors or comorbid erectile dysfunction (ED).
   e. Men with subjective PE complain of PE, often due to psychological and/or cultural factors, but have a normal or even extended IELT.

5. Which of the following is incorrect?
   a. The International Society for Sexual Medicine (ISSM) developed the first contemporary, evidence-based definition of lifelong and acquired PE.
   b. The main constructs in the ISSM definition of PE are time from penetration to ejaculation, inability to delay ejaculation, and the presence of negative personal consequences.

   c. Lifelong PE is, in part, defined by an IELT less than about 1 minute.
   d. Acquired PE is, in part, defined as a clinically significant and bothersome reduction in latency time, often to about 3 minutes or less.
   e. This definition is applicable to all men regardless of their sexual orientation or type of sexual contact.

6. The rationale for the ISSM definition of lifelong and acquired PE includes which of the following?
   a. Men with acquired PE tend to have lower IELT than men with lifelong PE
   b. Patient self-estimated IELT correlates poorly with stopwatch IELT
   c. Most men do not use cognitive or behavioral techniques to prolong intercourse and delay ejaculation
   d. Men with lifelong or acquired PE invariably experience a variety of negative psychological consequences such as bother, frustration, or the avoidance of sexual contact
   e. Men with PE had similar overall health-related quality of life, self-esteem, and confidence compared to non-PE groups

7. Which of the following is false?
   a. There is a substantial disparity between the incidence of PE in epidemiological studies that rely upon either patient self-report of PE and/or inconsistent and poorly validated definitions of PE.
   b. Community-based stopwatch IELT studies demonstrate that the distribution of the IELT is positively skewed, with a median IELT of 5.4 minutes (range, 0.55 to 44.1 minutes).
   c. Community-based stopwatch IELT studies demonstrate that IELT decreases with age and varies between countries.
   d. Some men may have a neurobiological and genetic predisposition toward early ejaculation.
   e. Subthyroidism is a common cause of PE.

8. In men with acquired PE and comorbid ED, which of the following is false?
   a. Intentionally "rushing" intercourse to prevent early detumescence of a partial erection is common
   b. PE is rarely compounded by the presence of high levels of performance anxiety related to their ED
   c. Limitation of arousal during foreplay to prevent early ejaculation may result in an incomplete erection
   d. The presence of vascular risk factors such as diabetes and hypertension is common
   e. Treatment with a PDE5 inhibitor alone or in combination with an SSRI is regarded as first-line treatment

9. In the evaluation of men with acquired PE, which of the following is false?
   a. A physical examination is mandatory in an effort to identify the etiology of the PE
   b. The presence of comorbid ED can be evaluated using a validated instrument such as the International Index of Erectile Function (IIEF) or the IIEF-5 Sexual Health Inventory for Men (SHIM)

c. The index of premature ejaculation (IPE) was developed specifically for use as a screening questionnaire

d. Laboratory or imaging investigations are occasionally required based upon the patient's medical history

e. A digital prostate examination, routine in an andrological setting for all men over 40, is useful in identifying possible evidence of prostatic inflammation or infection

10. In the management of PE, which of the following is false?

    a. All men seeking treatment for PE should receive basic psychosexual education or coaching.

    b. Present-day psychotherapy for PE is an integration of behavioral (e.g., the well-known start-stop and pause-squeeze methods) and cognitive approaches within a short-term psychotherapy model.

    c. Psychological-behavioral strategies for treating PE are moderately successful in the long term.

    d. Drawbacks to the psychological-behavioral approach are that it is time-consuming, requires substantial resources of both time and money, lacks immediacy, and requires the partner's cooperation.

    e. Combining PE pharmacotherapy and psychological approaches may be especially useful and potentially prevent symptom relapses.

11. In the pharmacotherapy management of PE, which of the following is false?

    a. Dapoxetine is a rapid-acting and short half-life SSRI taken 1 to 3 hours before sexual contact.

    b. Daily dosing of selective serotonin reuptake inhibitors (SSRIs) such as paroxetine, sertraline, fluoxetine, and citalopram are effective treatments for PE.

    c. SSRIs inhibit the postsynaptic 5-HT transporter system in the serotonergic neuron synapse.

    d. Dapoxetine can be combined with sildenafil as a treatment for PE in men with comorbid ED.

    e. The use of on-demand clomipramine taken 4 to 6 hours prior to sexual contact is limited by the occurrence of nausea and dizziness.

12. Which of the following is/are true?

    a. The DSM-IV-TR definition of delayed ejaculation is evidence-based on a small number of community-based IELT studies.

    b. Men with IELT greater than 2 standard deviations above the mean who report distress and/or cease sexual intercourse due to fatigue or irritation are regarded as suffering from delayed ejaculation.

    c. An IELT of 40 to 45 minutes represents an IELT in excess of 2 standard deviations above the mean.

    d. Many men with acquired DE can often masturbate to orgasm and may use idiosyncratic masturbation techniques that cannot be easily replicated during intercourse.

    e. Men with delayed ejaculation often have difficulty attaining or keeping their erections.

13. The causes of delayed ejaculation include which of the following? (Select all that apply.)

    a. Hyperthyroidism

    b. Hypogonadism

    c. Hyperprolactinemia

    d. Multiple sclerosis

    e. Antidepressant drugs such as SSRIs

14. In men with a spinal cord injury (SCI), which of the following is false? (Select all that apply.)

    a. The ability to ejaculate increases with descending levels of spinal injury.

    b. Less than 5% of patients with complete upper motor neuron lesions retain the ability to ejaculate.

    c. The ability to achieve an erection increases with descending levels of spinal injury.

    d. Semen harvesting with electroejaculation or vibratory stimulation is associated with a significant risk of autonomic dysreflexia.

    e. Pre-treatment of SCI men undergoing semen harvesting via vibratory stimulation with an α-adrenergic blocking drug such as tamsulosin minimizes the risk of severe hypertension.

15. Which of the following is true in men with retrograde ejaculation? (Select all that apply.)

    a. Retrograde ejaculation can be confirmed by the presence of spermatozoa in post-masturbation first-void urine.

    b. Retrograde ejaculation is more common following a bladder neck incision than transurethral resection of the prostate (TURP).

    c. Retrograde ejaculation may occur in men with diabetic autonomic neuropathy.

    d. Retrograde ejaculation in men with diabetic autonomic neuropathy is usually associated with hypogonadism.

    e. SSRIs are effective treatments for retrograde ejaculation.

ANSWERS

1. **b. Serotonin.** Many neurotransmitters are involved in the control of ejaculation, including dopamine, norepinephrine, serotonin, acetylcholine, oxytocin, GABA, and nitric oxide (NO). Of the many studies conducted to investigate the role of the brain in the development and mediation of sexual functioning, dopamine and serotonin have emerged as essential neurochemical factors. Whereas dopamine promotes seminal emission/ejaculation via D2 receptors, serotonin is inhibitory.

2. **e. Closure of bladder neck, rhythmic contraction of the bulbocavernosus, bulbospongiosus, and other pelvic floor muscles, and relaxation of the internal urinary sphincter during emission prevents retrograde ejaculation.** Based on functional, central, and peripheral mediation, the ejaculatory process is typically subdivided into three phases: emission, ejection (or penile expulsion), and orgasm. Emission consists of contractions of seminal vesicles (SV) and the prostate, with expulsion of sperm and seminal fluid into the posterior urethra, and is mediated by synergistic activation of both sympathetic and parasympathetic nerves (T10 to L2) but may also include a cholinergic excitatory mechanism. Ejection is mediated by somatic nerves (S2 to S4) within the pudendal nerve, and involves pulsatile contractions of the bulbocavernosus and pelvic floor muscles together with contraction of the internal urinary sphincter to prevent retrograde ejaculation. Ejection also involves a sympathetic spinal cord reflex upon which there is limited voluntary control. The bladder neck closes to prevent retrograde flow; the bulbocavernosus, bulbospongiosus, and other pelvic floor muscles contract rhythmically, and the internal urinary sphincter contracts. The external urinary sphincter exhibits intense contractions interrupted by silence periods during ejection of semen.

3. **b. 2.5%.** Community-based normative IELT research and observational studies of men with PE demonstrate that IELTs of less than 1 minute have a low prevalence of about 2.5% in the general population, although a substantially higher percentage of men with normal IELT complain of PE.

4. **b. Approximately 50% of heterosexual men seeking treatment for lifelong PE ejaculate within 1 minute after pen-**

etration. The medical literature contains several univariate and multivariate operational definitions of PE. Each of these definitions characterize men with PE using all or most of the accepted dimensions of this condition: ejaculatory latency, perceived ability to control ejaculation, reduced sexual satisfaction, personal distress, partner distress, and interpersonal or relationship distress. The first official definition of PE was established in 1980 by the American Psychiatric Association (APA) in the DSM-III. The current APA DSM-V definition of PE is largely based upon the unified PE definition of the ISSM and captures the key dimensions of latency, control, and bother. Earlier DSM definitions did not include latency.

Several observational studies in cohorts of heterosexual men with lifelong PE with prospective stopwatch IELT measurement showed that about 90% of men seeking treatment for lifelong PE ejaculated within 1 minute after penetration, and about 10% ejaculated between 1 and 2 minutes. These data support the proposal that lifelong PE is characterized by an IELT of less than or about 1 minute after vaginal penetration.

Recent studies have suggested that in some men neurobiological and genetic variations could contribute to the pathophysiology of lifelong premature ejaculation (L-PE), as defined by the ISSM criteria and that the condition may be maintained and heightened by psychological/environmental factors. Acquired PE is commonly due to sexual performance anxiety, psychological or relationship problems, ED, and occasionally prostatitis, hyperthyroidism, or during withdrawal/detoxification from prescribed or recreational drugs.

Four PE subtypes are distinguished on the basis of the duration of the IELT, frequency of complaints, and course in life. In addition to lifelong PE and acquired PE, this classification includes natural variable PE (or variable PE) and premature-like ejaculatory dysfunction (or subjective PE). Men with subjective PE complain of PE, while actually having a normal or even extended ejaculation time. The complaint of PE in these men is probably related to psychological and/or cultural factors.

5. **e. This definition is applicable to all men regardless of their sexual orientation or type of sexual contact.** In October 2007, the ISSM convened an initial meeting of the first Ad Hoc ISSM Committee for the Definition of Premature Ejaculation to develop the first contemporary, evidence-based definition of lifelong PE. Evidence-based definitions seek to limit errors of classification and thereby increase the likelihood that existing and newly developed therapeutic strategies are truly effective in carefully selected dysfunctional populations.

The committee unanimously agreed that the constructs that are necessary to define lifelong PE are time from penetration to ejaculation, inability to delay ejaculation, and negative personal consequences from PE, and they recommended the following definition. *"Lifelong PE is a male sexual dysfunction characterized by the presence of all of these criteria: (1) ejaculation that always or nearly always occurs prior to or within about 1 minute of vaginal penetration; (2) the inability to delay ejaculation on all or nearly all vaginal penetrations; and (3) negative personal consequences such as distress, bother, frustration, and/or the avoidance of sexual intimacy."*

In April 2013, a second Ad Hoc ISSM Committee for the Definition of Premature Ejaculation agreed that although lifelong and acquired PE are distinct and different demographic and etiological populations, they can be jointly defined, in part, by the constructs of time from penetration to ejaculation, inability to delay ejaculation, and negative personal consequences from PE. The committee determined that the presence of a clinically significant and bothersome reduction in latency time, often to about 3 minutes or less, was an additional key defining dimension of acquired PE. This definition is limited to men engaging in vaginal intercourse as there are few studies available on PE research in homosexual men or during other forms of sexual expression.

6. **d. Men with lifelong or acquired PE invariably experience a variety of negative psychological consequences such as bother, frustration, or the avoidance of sexual contact.** Waldinger et al. (1998) reported IELTs less than 30 seconds in 77% and

less than 60 seconds in 90% of 110 men with lifelong PE with only 10% ejaculating between 1 and 2 minutes. These data are consistent with normative community IELT data, support the notion that IELTs of less than 1 minute are statistically abnormal, and confirm that an IELT cut-off of 1 minute will capture 80% to 90% of treatment-seeking men with lifelong PE. A post hoc analysis of the dapoxetine Phase 3 COUPLE trial data confirms a statistically significant higher IELT in men with acquired PE and comorbid compared to men with lifelong PE with comorbid ED. Additional recent studies support this report and confirm that self-estimated IELT was lower in men with lifelong PE compared to acquired PE and highest in men with subjective PE. These data suggest 3 minutes as a valid cut-off for either self-estimated or stopwatch IELT for the diagnosis of acquired PE.

Several authors report that estimated and stopwatch IELT correlate reasonably well or are interchangeable in assigning PE status when estimated IELT is combined with patient-reported outcomes (PROs). Since patient self-report is the determining factor in treatment seeking and satisfaction, it is recommended that self-estimation by the patient and partner of ejaculatory latency is accepted as the method for determining IELT in clinical practice.

The ability to prolong sexual intercourse by delaying ejaculation and the subjective feelings of ejaculatory control comprise the complex construct of ejaculatory control. Virtually all men report using at least one cognitive or behavioral technique to prolong intercourse and delay ejaculation, with varying degrees of success, and many young men reported using multiple different techniques. Voluntary delay of ejaculation is most likely exerted either prior to or in the early stages of the emission phase of the reflex but progressively decreases until the point of ejaculatory inevitability.

Several authors have reported an association between lifelong or acquired PE and negative psychological outcomes in men with lifelong or acquired PE and their female partners. This personal distress has discriminative validity in diagnosing men with and without PE. The personal and/or interpersonal distress, bother, frustration, and annoyance that result from PE may affect men's quality of life and partner relationships, their self-esteem and self-confidence, and can act as an obstacle to single men forming new partner relationships.

7. **e. Subthyroidism is a common cause of PE.** Reliable information on the prevalence of lifelong and A-PE in the general male population is lacking. PE has been estimated to occur in 4% to 39% of men in the general community. Prevalence data derived from patient self-report is appreciably higher than prevalence estimates based on clinician diagnosis utilizing the more conservative ISSM definition of PE. As a result, there is a substantial disparity between the incidence of PE in epidemiological studies that rely upon either patient self-report of PE and/or inconsistent and poorly validated definitions of PE.

Community-based stopwatch studies of the IELT, the time interval between penetration and ejaculation, demonstrate that the distribution of the IELT is positively skewed, with a median IELT of 5.4 minutes (range, 0.55 to 44.1 minutes), decreases with age and varies between countries, and supports the notion that IELTs of less than 1 minute are statistically abnormal compared to men in the general western population.

Early ejaculation in humans has been explained by either hyposensitivity of the 5-HT2C and/or hypersensitivity of the 5-HT1A receptor. Recent studies have suggested that in some men neurobiological and genetic variations could contribute to the pathophysiology of L-PE, as defined by the ISSM criteria and that the condition may be maintained and heightened by psychological/environmental factors.

The majority of patients with thyroid hormone disorders experience sexual dysfunction. Studies suggest a significant correlation between PE and suppressed thyroid-stimulating hormone (TSH) values in a selected population of andrological and sexological patients. One author reports that the 50% prevalence of PE in men with hyperthyroidism fell to 15% after treatment with thyroid hormone normalization. Although occult thyroid disease has been reported in the elderly hospitalized population, it is uncommon in the population who present for treatment of PE, and routine TSH screening is not indicated unless clinically indicated.

8. **b. PE is rarely compounded by the presence of high levels of performance anxiety related to their ED.** Recent data demonstrates that as many as half of subjects with ED also experience PE. Subjects with ED may either require higher levels of stimulation to achieve an erection or intentionally "rush" intercourse to prevent early detumescence of a partial erection, resulting in ejaculation with a brief latency. This may be compounded by the presence of high levels of performance anxiety related to their ED, which serves to only worsen their prematurity.

ED is often associated with endothelial dysfunction and atherosclerosis of the internal pudendal and cavernous arteries due to the presence of vascular risk factors such as diabetes mellitus, hypertension, hyperlipidemia, and cigarette smoking.

Off-label on-demand or daily dosing of PDE-5 inhibitors is not recommended for the treatment of L-PE in men with normal erectile function. However, ED pharmacotherapy alone or in combination with PE pharmacotherapy is recommended for the treatment of L-PE or A-PE in men with co-morbid ED. Phosphodiesterase type-5 isoenzyme (PDE5) inhibitors, sildenafil, tadalafil, and vardenafil are effective treatments for ED. Several authors have reported experience with PDE-5 inhibitors alone or in combination with SSRIs as a treatment for PE.

9. **c. The index of premature ejaculation (IPE) was developed specifically for use as a screening questionnaire.** Men presenting with self-reported PE should be evaluated with a full medical/sexual history, a focused physical examination, inventory assessment of erectile function, and any investigations suggested by these findings. Current literature suggests that the diagnosis of L-PE is based purely on the medical history as there are no predictive physical findings or confirmatory investigations. However, in men with A-PE, a physical examination is mandatory in an effort to identify the etiology of the PE and to alleviate its possible cause. Laboratory or imaging investigations are occasionally required based upon the patient's medical history. A digital prostate examination, routine in an andrological setting for all men over 40, is useful in identifying possible evidence of prostatic inflammation or infection.

The presence of comorbid ED should be evaluated using a validated instrument such as the IIEF or the IIEF-5 (SHIM). The IIEF is not specifically validated in men with PE. Caution should be exercised in the IIEF diagnosis of comorbid ED in men with PE as 33.3% of potent men with PE confuse the ability to maintain erections prior to ejaculation and following ejaculation, record contradictory response/s to some/all questions of the SHIM especially Q3 and Q4, and receive a false positive IIEF/SHIM diagnosis of ED.

10. **c. Psychological-behavioral strategies for treating PE are moderately successful in the long term.** There are multiple psychosexual and pharmacological treatments for PE. Graded levels of patient and couple counseling, guidance, and/or relationship therapy, either alone or ideally in combination with PE pharmacotherapy, should be offered as a treatment option for most men with PE. All men seeking treatment for PE should receive basic psychosexual education or coaching.

Although the new and often more expedient pharmacological therapies are overshadowing traditional psychological-behavioral methods in the treatment of PE, the psychological-behavioral approach remains an attractive option but is time-consuming, requires substantial resources of both time and money, lacks immediacy, requires the partner's cooperation, and has mixed efficacy.

Psychological interventions are designed to achieve more than simply increasing the IELT. Targeted factors focus on the man, his partner, and their relationship. Psychotherapy and behavioral interventions improve ejaculatory control by helping men/couples to: (1) learn techniques to control and/or delay ejaculation, (2) gain confidence in their sexual performance, (3) lessen performance anxiety, (4) modify rigid sexual repertoires, (5) surmount barriers to intimacy, (6) resolve interpersonal issues that precipitate and maintain the dysfunction, and (7) increase communication.

Psychological-behavioral strategies for treating PE have been at least moderately successful in alleviating the dysfunction in the short term, but long-term outcome data are limited and suggest a significant relapse rate.

11. **c. SSRIs inhibit the postsynaptic 5-HT transporter system in the serotonergic neuron synapse.** Dapoxetine has received approval for the treatment of PE in over 50 countries worldwide. Dapoxetine has not received marketing approval for the United States by the Food and Drug Administration (FDA). It is a rapid-acting and short half-life SSRI with a pharmacokinetic profile supporting a role as an on-demand treatment for PE.

Several forms of pharmacotherapy have been used in the treatment of PE. These include the use of topical local anesthetics (LAs), SSRIs, tramadol, phosphodiesterase type 5 inhibitors (PDE5i), and alpha adrenergic blockers. The use of topical LA, such as lidocaine, prilocaine, or benzocaine, alone or in association, to diminish the sensitivity of the glans penis is the oldest known pharmacological treatment for PE. The introduction of the SSRIs—paroxetine, sertraline, fluoxetine, citalopram, and the tricyclic antidepressant (TCA) clomipramine—has revolutionized the treatment of PE. These drugs block pre-synaptic axonal reuptake of serotonin from the synaptic cleft of central serotonergic neurons by 5-HT transporters, resulting in enhanced 5-HT neurotransmission and stimulation of postsynaptic membrane 5-HT receptors.

On-demand administration of clomipramine, paroxetine, sertraline, and fluoxetine 3 to 6 hours before intercourse is modestly efficacious and well tolerated but is associated with substantially less ejaculatory delay than daily treatment in most studies.

12. **d. Many men with acquired DE can often masturbate to orgasm and may use idiosyncratic masturbation techniques that cannot be easily replicated during intercourse.** The DSM-IV-TR definition of delayed ejaculation contains no clear criteria as to when a man actually meets the conditions for DE, as operationalized criteria do not exist. As most sexually functional men ejaculate within about 4 to 10 minutes following intromission, a clinician might assume that men with latencies beyond 25 or 30 minutes (21 to 23 minutes represents about 2 standard deviations above the mean) who report distress or men who simply cease sexual activity due to exhaustion or irritation qualify for this diagnosis. Such symptoms, together with the fact that a man and/or his partner decide to seek help for the problem, are usually sufficient for a DE diagnosis.

Psychogenic DE, often described as inhibited ejaculation, is usually related to sexual performance anxiety, which may draw the man's attention away from erotic cues that normally serve to enhance arousal. It is occasionally characterized by the use of idiosyncratic and vigorous masturbation styles that cannot be replicated during intercourse with a partner, or an "autosexual" orientation where men derive greater arousal and enjoyment from masturbation than from intercourse. These men precondition themselves to possible difficulty attaining orgasm with a partner and, as a result, experience acquired DE. These men appear able to achieve erections sufficient for intercourse despite a relative absence of subjective arousal, and their erections are taken as erroneous evidence by both the man and his partner that he was ready for sex and capable of achieving orgasm.

13. **b. Hypogonadism, d. Multiple sclerosis, and e. Antidepressant drugs such as SSRIs.** Delayed ejaculation/anejaculation is associated with several differing pathophysiologies that include congenital disorders as well as ones caused by psychological factors, treatment of male pelvic cancers with surgery or radiotherapy, neurological disease, endocrinopathy, infection, and treatment for other disorders. When a medical history or symptomatology so indicates, investigation of such possible etiologies may be necessary. The most common causes of DE seen in clinical practice are psychogenic inhibited ejaculation, degeneration of penile afferent nerves and Pacinian corpuscles in the ageing male, hypogonadism, diabetic autonomic neuropathy, treatment with SSRI antidepressants and major tranquillizers, radical prostatectomy, or other major pelvic surgery or radiotherapy.

14. **c. The ability to achieve an erection increases with descending levels of spinal injury** and **e. Pre-treatment of SCI men undergoing semen harvesting via vibratory stimulation with an α-adrenergic blocking drug such as tamsulosin minimizes the risk of severe hypertension.** The ability to ejaculate is severely impaired by SCI. The level and completeness of SCI determine the post-SCI erectile and ejaculatory capacity. Unlike erectile capacity, the ability to ejaculate increases with descending levels of spinal injury. Less than 5% of patients with complete upper motor neuron lesions retain the ability to ejaculate. Ejaculation rates are higher (15%) in patients with both lower motor neuron lesions and an intact thoracolumbar sympathetic outflow. Approximately 22% of patients with an incomplete upper motor neuron lesion and almost all men with incomplete lower motor neuron lesions retain the ability to ejaculate. In those patients capable of successful ejaculation, the sensation of orgasm may be absent and retrograde ejaculation often occurs.

Several techniques for obtaining semen from SCI men with ejaculatory dysfunction have been reported. Vibratory stimulation is successful in obtaining semen in up to 70% of men with SCI. The use of electro-ejaculation to obtain semen by electrical stimulation of efferent sympathetic fibers of the hypogastric plexus is an effective and safe method of obtaining semen. Both vibratory stimulation and electro-ejaculation are associated with a significantly high risk of autonomic dysreflexia. Pre-treatment with a fast-acting vasodilator such as nifedipine minimizes the risk of severe hypertension, should autonomic dysreflexia occur with either form of treatment.

15. **a. Retrograde ejaculation can be confirmed by the presence of spermatozoa in post-masturbation first-void urine** and **c. Retrograde ejaculation may occur in men with diabetic autonomic neuropathy.** Antegrade (normal) ejaculation requires a closed bladder neck (and proximal urethra). Surgical procedures that compromise the bladder neck closure mechanism may result in retrograde ejaculation. The occurrence of orgasm in the absence of prograde ejaculation suggests retrograde ejaculation and can be confirmed by the presence of spermatozoa in post-masturbation first void urine.

Transurethral incision of the prostate (TUIP) results in retrograde ejaculation in 5% to 45% of patients and is probably related to whether one or two incisions are made and whether or not the incision includes primarily the bladder neck or extends to the level of the verumontanum. The importance of contraction of the urethral smooth muscle at the level of the verumontanum has been hypothesized to be important in preventing retrograde ejaculation. TURP carries a higher incidence of retrograde ejaculation than does TUIP. The reported incidence of retrograde ejaculation following TURP ranges from 42% to 100%.

Retrograde ejaculation is more common in diabetes mellitus (DM) than in age-matched controls ($P < .01$), has been reported in 30% of men with DM, and is not statistically associated with duration of DM, body mass index (BMI), waist circumference, or HgbA1c or total testosterone levels.

Several sympathomimetic amine agents have been described as useful with mixed results. These drugs include pseudoephedrine, ephedrine, midodrine, and phenylpropanolamine. These agents work by stimulating the release of noradrenaline from the nerve axon terminals but may also directly stimulate both α- and β-adrenergic receptors. The TCA imipramine, which blocks the reuptake of noradrenaline by the axon from the synaptic cleft, is also occasionally useful. The usual dose is 25 mg twice daily. The current feeling is that long-term treatment with imipramine is likely to be more effective. While medical treatment may not always produce normal ejaculation, it may result in some prograde ejaculation.

CHAPTER REVIEW

1. PE is a common sexual dysfunction.
2. PE is associated with negative psychological consequences including distress, bother, and frustration, which may affect quality of life, partner relationships, self-esteem, self-confidence, and can act as an obstacle to single men forming new partner relationships.
3. The evidence-based ISSM definition of lifelong and acquired PE should form the basis of the office diagnosis of lifelong PE.
4. There is limited evidence suggesting that lifelong PE has a genetic basis and acquired PE is most often due to sexual performance anxiety, psychological or relationship problems, and/or ED.
5. Oral SSRI drugs and topical anesthetic drugs are effective and safe treatments for PE.
6. Psychosexual cognitive behavioral therapy (CBT) has a limited role as a first-line treatment for PE but has an important role as an adjunct to pharmacotherapy, especially in men with acquired PE due to sexual performance anxiety.
7. Men with acquired PE most secondary to co-morbid ED, hyperthyroidism, chronic lower urogenital infection, prostatodynia, or chronic pelvic pain syndrome (CPPS) should receive appropriate etiology-specific treatment alone or in combination with an SSRI.
8. The causes of DE and anejaculation are manifold.
9. Failure of ejaculation can be a lifelong problem (25%) or an acquired problem (75%). It may be global and occur in every sexual encounter or be intermittent or situational.
10. Treatment of men with DE should be etiology-specific and address the issue of infertility in men of reproductive age.
11. Drug treatment of men with DE or anejaculation has limited success..
12. TURP and diabetic autonomic neuropathy are the most common causes of retrograde ejaculation.
13. RE and failure of emission can be distinguished by examination of a post masturbatory specimen of urine for the presence of spermatozoa and fructose.
14. Pharmacotherapy is associated with variable degrees of success and includes agents such as pseudoephedrine, midodrine, and imipramine.
15. The symptoms of post-orgasmic illness syndrome (POIS) occur following ejaculation and comprise severe myalgia, fatigue associated with a flu-like state, nasal congestion, and itching eyes.
16. POIS symptoms commence within 30 minutes of ejaculation in 87% of men and increase in intensity to a peak on day 2.
17. A type 1 hypersensitivity immunogenic reaction has been proposed as the underlying mechanism.
18. A prolonged hyposensitization program with multiple subcutaneous injections of autologous semen has been suggested as a possible treatment.

Surgery for Erectile Dysfunction

Matthew J. Mellon and John J. Mulcahy

QUESTIONS

1. A 27-year-old patient presented to the emergency room with 36 hours of a prolonged painful erection. Blood gas analysis shows this to be veno-occlusive priapism, and bilateral T-shunts with corporal dilation were performed. This was unsuccessful in reducing the erection, and 1 week later the erection detumesced. After counseling, the patient elects to have a penile implant placed at this time. The type of cylinder that should NOT be used in this circumstance would be:

   a. AMS 700 CX.
   b. AMS 700 LGX.
   c. Genesis.
   d. Titan.
   e. Tactra.

2. During dilation to place a cylinder into a scarred corporal body, a dilator enters the urethra in the fossa navicularis. All of the following would be acceptable approaches EXCEPT:

   a. abandon the case.
   b. proceed placing both cylinders.
   c. place a cylinder on the side without the perforation and return at a later date to place the other cylinder.
   d. create hypospadias, repair the perforation defect securely, and place both cylinders.

3. Select the TRUE statement:

   a. Repair of penile implants is currently in the range of 50% within 5 years.
   b. Satisfaction with penile implants among both patients and partners is in the 80% to 90% range.
   c. Infection rates with penile implant placement are comparable to those of other surgical procedures in the range of 5% to 7%.
   d. Semirigid rod prostheses are preferable to hydraulic implants in impotent spinal cord injury patients.
   e. The lock-out valves of the two vendors' three-piece inflatable penile implants designed to minimize autoinflation are in the same location.

4. A "salvage" or "rescue" procedure for an infected penile implant would likely be less successful in a patient with all of the following features EXCEPT:

   a. cellulitis around the incision and over prosthetic parts.
   b. purulent drainage from the incision.
   c. occurrence within 2 months of the implant placement.
   d. associated with an aggressive organism such as methicillin-resistant *Staphylococcus aureus* (MRSA) or *Pseudomonas aeruginosa*.
   e. diabetes mellitus as a comorbidity.

5. Which of the following is FALSE regarding informed consent for penile prosthesis surgery?

   a. The greatest disappointment after surgery is the size of the erection.
   b. Tissue problems such as pump migration, erosion, and extrusion of parts occur and require re-operation.
   c. Penile sensation and climax are not affected postoperatively.
   d. Alternative erectile dysfunction (ED) treatment options should be explained and offered prior to surgery.
   e. Unrealistic expectations for the results of penile implant surgery should be identified and discussed prior to surgery.

6. Advantages to the penoscrotal approach for penile implant placement include all of the following EXCEPT:

   a. secure placement of the pump in a subdartos pouch.
   b. cosmetic skin incision.
   c. avoidance of damaging the dorsal neurovascular bundle.
   d. easier placement of semirigid rod implants.
   e. allows placement of the two-piece inflatable implant.

7. Select the FALSE statement:

   a. A high electrocautery setting may damage the Bioflex cylinders but not silicone-covered cylinders.
   b. Both the Bioflex and triple-layer AMS 700 cylinders are very durable, but may form aneurysms when subjected to repeated high external pressure.
   c. Semirigid rod implant malfunction is very rare and is limited to central wire breakage.
   d. The Ambicor cylinders give less rigidity and flaccidity than three-piece inflatable cylinders.
   e. The AMS 700 LGX cylinders are superior to the AMS 700 CX and Titan cylinders for straightening a curved erection due to their ability to increase in length.

8. The following are features of crural crossover of penile implant cylinders EXCEPT:

   a. difficult cylinder insertion.
   b. cylinders not appearing to be symmetric on either side of a Foley catheter in the urethra.
   c. curved erection.
   d. lopsided appearing erection.
   e. total corporal length measurements significantly different on right and left sides.

9. The following are suitable locations for a penile implant reservoir EXCEPT:

   a. a scrotal cavity where the testis had been previously removed.
   b. below the rectus muscle above the transversalis fascia.
   c. the epigastrium through a subcostal incision.
   d. deep in the fat above the abdominal wall fascia in an obese patient.
   e. in the peritoneal cavity.

ANSWERS

1. **b. AMS 700 LGX.** The LGX is the only cylinder with distal expansion when inflated. Following a T-shunt, this cylinder may protrude through the defect at the end of the corporal body or create pressure on this weakened area when it is inflated.

2. **b. Proceed placing both cylinders.** Placing both cylinders would allow organisms to possibly enter the defect and contaminate the cylinder. In the other answers the cylinder is not exposed to possible infection.

3. **b. Satisfaction with penile implants among both patients and partners is in the 80% to 90% range.** Repair of penile implants is currently in the range of 15% at 5 years. Infection rates with penile implant placement are comparable to those of other surgical procedures in the range of 1% to 3%. Spinal cord injury patients have a high incidence of rod erosions (20% to 50%). Coloplast has the lock-out valve on the reservoir; BSci has the lock-out valve on the pump.

4. **e. Diabetes mellitus as a comorbidity.** Answers a through d are risk factors for failed salvage as noted in the chapter narrative. Diabetes mellitus, although a risk factor for implant infection, is not associated with a higher incidence of failed salvage.

5. **c. Penile sensation and climax are not affected postoperatively.** Penile sensation and ejaculation may both be diminished postoperatively.

6. **d. Easier placement of semirigid rod implants.** Semirigid rod cylinders are most easily placed through a subcoronal corporotomy.

7. **e. The AMS 700 LGX cylinders are superior to the AMS 700 CX and Titan cylinders for straightening a curved erection due to their ability to increase in length.** The LGX cylinders tend to exaggerate a curved erection.

8. **c. Curved erection.** Despite crossover, the erection is commonly straight.

9. **a. A scrotal cavity where the testis had been previously removed.** The Cloverleaf reservoirs contain lockout valves that could be manipulated through the scrotum, resulting in cylinder autoinflation. The Conceal reservoir is too large for scrotal placement, and the AMS spherical reservoir might fit with underfilling but would be subject to manipulation and wear in a scrotal location.

CHAPTER REVIEW

1. The size of the erect penis after surgery will likely be shorter and thinner than preoperatively.
2. The implant provides only a firm penis suitable for intercourse.
3. Penile sensation and ejaculation may both be diminished postoperatively.
4. There will be varying degrees of postoperative pain.
5. Reoperation for a mechanical problem with the implant may be necessary.
6. Tissue problems such as infection may necessitate another surgery.
7. There are other treatments of ED such as pills, penile inserts and injections, and vacuum erection devices (VEDs).
8. There is a variety of implants including three-piece and two-piece inflatables and semirigid rods.
9. The three-piece inflatable implants give the best rigidity and flaccidity and are by far the most popular among both patients and urologists.
10. A shorter size to the erection following penile implant placement is the major reason for disappointment after surgery, and should be stressed in the informed consent.
11. Patients with limited dexterity should be encouraged to choose a semirigid rod implant to avoid frustration, when trying to manipulate the pump of a hydraulic device.
12. Injuries between the corpus cavernosum and the exterior should always be closed securely before an implant cylinder is left in place.
13. Placing a cylinder that does not expand in length will usually adequately straighten a curved erection in patients with tunica albuginea scaring, i.e., Peyronie disease.
14. Always keep the distal end of scissors or dilating instruments pointing dorsolaterally and parallel to the penile shaft to avoid crural crossover and urethral injury.
15. In the presence of a penile implant infection, all foreign material should be removed from the wound, as remnant parts may harbor microbes that perpetuate the infection.
16. In patients at risk for reduced penile vascular perfusion, be aware that distal necrosis can occur. Limit or stage aggressive reconstructive procedures in such patients.
17. Place the implant reservoir in a capacious cavity to avoid injuring surrounding structures such as bladder or bowel when the balloon expands as it is filled with isotonic saline.

73 Diagnosis and Management of Peyronie's Disease

Allen D. Seftel and Hailiu Yang

QUESTIONS

1. Peyronie's disease (PD):
   a. is a wound healing disorder.
   b. is an autoimmune disease.
   c. is a transient disorder (30% to 50% of the time).
   d. may degenerate into cancer.
   e. is associated with Dupuytren contracture in 40% of men.

2. The fibrous plaques in PD originate in:
   a. Buck's fascia.
   b. corpora cavernosa.
   c. corpus spongiosum.
   d. the tunica albuginea surrounding the corpora cavernosa.
   e. the tunica albuginea surrounding the corpus spongiosum.

3. Based on recent natural history studies on PD, a 54-year-old man with a 60-degree dorsal curve 18 months after onset has:
   a. 40% chance of spontaneous improvement of deformity.
   b. 70% chance of getting worse.
   c. 10% chance of getting worse.
   d. 10% or less chance of spontaneous improvement of deformity.
   e. 80% chance of staying the same.

4. What is the prevalence of PD following radical prostatectomy?
   a. 4%
   b. 1% to 3%
   c. 11% to 16%
   d. >20%
   e. 0%

5. Plaque calcification:
   a. can be reliably identified on physical examination.
   b. can be found in 50% to 60% of men with PD.
   c. is not an indication of stable, mature disease.
   d. is associated with successful intralesional injection therapy.
   e. is a predictive factor for the need for surgical treatment.

6. Psychological distress in men with PD:
   a. is infrequent.
   b. is typically resolved by successful surgery.
   c. is frequently associated with penile shortening.
   d. correlates with degree of erect curvature.
   e. has no association with relationship issues with the patient's partner.

7. All of the following statements regarding the physical examination of a man presenting with PD are true EXCEPT that the examination:
   a. should include measurement of plaque size with calipers.
   b. should include direct assessment of curvature following injection of vasoactive agent.
   c. should include measurement of stretched penile length.
   d. can be supported with a picture of the erect penis by a smartphone.
   e. should include assessment of the patient's palms.

8. Penile duplex ultrasound provides information on all of the parameters below EXCEPT:
   a. penile deformity.
   b. erectile response to vasoactive penile injection.
   c. penile vascular flow parameters.
   d. penile sensory integrity.
   e. plaque calcification.

9. Pentoxifylline and the phosphodiesterase-5 (PDE5) inhibitors have been shown in an animal model of PD to reduce scarring by what proposed mechanism?
   a. Improved penile blood flow
   b. Antiinflammatory
   c. Elevated local levels of nitric oxide (NO)
   d. Anti–transforming growth factor-β (TGF-β)
   e. Mechanotransduction

10. Penile injection therapy (i.e., prostaglandin E1, TriMix-gel, etc.) for ED is not directly responsible for:
    a. cavernosal fibrosis.
    b. Peyronie's disease.
    c. penile pain.
    d. priapism.
    e. high success rate.

11. A 35-year-old man with PD is able to achieve an erection adequate for intercourse with minimal discomfort and reported dorsal erect penile curvature of 20 degrees. The initial treatment should be:
    a. reassurance.
    b. oral vitamin E.
    c. intralesional steroids.
    d. oral tamoxifen.
    e. intralesional collagenase.

12. A 66-year-old man presents with a 2-year history of PD and a 55-degree dorsal curvature. He also notes that his average-grade erection with sexual stimulation at home is a grade {5/10}, which would not be adequate for intromission even if the penis were straight. Duplex ultrasound analysis demonstrates arterial insufficiency and an inadequate erectile response to 90 mg of intracorporal papaverine. The most appropriate treatment option for this patient who wants to resume sexual activity would be:
    a. 16-dot plication.
    b. vacuum constriction device.
    c. penile prosthesis with penile straightening.
    d. intralesional verapamil injections.
    e. Plaque incision and grafting

13. Tunica plication is preferred for mild to moderate lateral curvature correction in a patient who is able to accomplish adequate erections with the assistance of PDE-5I because of:
    a. less shortening compared with grafting.
    b. better sensory protection.
    c. diminished risk of postoperative ED.
    d. greater potential for loss of erect length.
    e. less chance of recurrence

14. Postoperative rehabilitation is designed to aid in postoperative healing and outcomes in the following ways, EXCEPT:
    a. to prevent shortening and possibly recover some lost length.
    b. to encourage straight healing
    c. to enhance cicatrix contracture.
    d. to preserve vascular integrity.
    e. to encourage partner participation.

15. All of the following are true regarding penile traction therapy after surgical penile straightening, EXCEPT:
    a. increases or preserves postoperative length.
    b. encourages tissue remodeling.
    c. should be used for 3 or more hours/day for optimum results.
    d. increases the risk of sensory change.
    e. results appear dose-related.

16. What is the most dreaded complication occurring after manual modeling during placement of a penile prosthesis in a man with PD?
    a. Tunica tear proximal
    b. Urethral injury
    c. Sensory deficit
    d. Recurrent curvature
    e. Distal urethral perforation

17. Indications to perform a plaque incision or partial excision and grafting include all of the following, EXCEPT:
    a. severe curvature in excess of 70 degrees.
    b. indentation resulting in an unstable penis or hinge effect.
    c. a short penis (<9 cm) with severe curve and poor rigidity.
    d. a short penis with severe curvature and excellent rigidity.
    e. extensive plaque calcification associated with severe deformity.

18. The primary concern with a grafting procedure for PD is:
    a. postoperative erectile dysfunction (ED).
    b. incomplete correction of hinge effect.
    c. penile shortening.
    d. decreased penile sensation
    e. graft infection.

19. Which of the following is a candidate for plaque incision and grafting?
    a. 60-degree severe ventral curve
    b. 30-degree curvature with suboptimal rigidity even with PDE5 inhibitors
    c. 70 degrees with hinge effect
    d. 90-degree lateral curve presenting 5 months after onset
    e. 30-degree dorsal curvature in a patient who desires to gain length as a result of surgery

20. The ideal graft includes all of the following EXCEPT:
    a. thin, strong, and easy to suture.
    b. no rejection.
    c. resistant to infection.
    d. preserves erectile function.
    e. contracts during healing.

21. The IMPRESS trials for Clostridium Collagenase Histolyticum (CCH) with modeling found that which of the following patient group would benefit from CCH?
    a. Calcified plaques that have been present for less than 12 months
    b. Ventral plaques greater than 60 degrees
    c. Stable plaques between 30 and 90 degrees.
    d. Stable ventral plaques less than 60 degrees
    e. Hourglass deformities less than 45 degrees.

22. Which of the following is a significant concern with CCH?
    a. Cost and length of treatment
    b. Risk of ED
    c. Autoimmune reaction
    d. Penile bruising
    e. High risk of penile fracture

ANSWERS

1. **a. Is a wound healing disorder.** PD is currently recognized as a wound healing disorder of the tunica albuginea (Devine and Horton, 1988)[a] that results in the formation of an exuberant scar, occurring presumably after an injury to the penis, which activates an abnormal wound healing response (Ralph et al., 2010; Levine and Burnett 2013; Greenfield and Levine, 2005; Van De Water, 1997). PD is not a premalignant condition, spontaneous resolution is a rare event, and improvement likely does not take place in more than 13% of men over the first 12 to 18 months. Though an association with Dupuytren contracture has been described, studies vary widely on this association.

2. **d. The tunica albuginea surrounding the corpora cavernosa.** PD plaques originate in the tunica albuginea. Sixty percent to seventy percent of plaques are located on the dorsal aspect of the tunica albuginea and are usually associated with the septum (Pryor and Ralph, 2002). It is possible that pressures on the penis during intercourse result in a delamination between the two layers, activating the abnormal wound-healing process, which is trapped within the tunic, fostering the progressive scarring.

3. **d. 10% or less chance of spontaneous improvement of deformity.** Spontaneous regression has been looked at in several contemporary natural history studies, which have suggested that no more than 13% will experience improvement of deformity. Full spontaneous resolution is extremely rare. If no treatment is offered, up to 50% will experience worsening of their deformity (Mulhall et al., 2006).

4. **c. 11% to 16%.** Tal and associates (2010) demonstrated an incidence of PD of 15.9% with a mean time to development of disease of 13.9 months. Ciancio and Kim (2000) also examined the effects of prostatectomy on penile fibrosis and sexual dysfunction. Eleven percent of all patients undergoing prostatectomy developed fibrotic changes in the penis. This fibrosis led to penile curvature in 93%, "waistband" deformity in 24%, and palpable plaques in 69%.

5. **c. Is not an indication of stable, mature disease.** Only recently has it been recognized that calcification may occur early after the onset of the scarring process, and therefore the previously held notion that calcification is an indication of chronic,

---

[a]Sources referenced can be found in *Campbell-Walsh-Wein Urology, 12 Edition,* on the Expert Consult website.

severe, and/or mature disease appears untrue (Levine et al., 2013). Several investigators have indicated that intralesional injection therapy of verapamil and interferon is less likely to be successful in men with significant calcification (Levine et al., 2002b; Hellstrom et al., 2006). A "rock-hard" plaque may be an indicator of calcification but will need to be confirmed with some form of imaging, preferably ultrasound. A calcified plaque is readily identified by ultrasound because of the hyperdensity of the plaque with shadowing behind it. Calcification itself does not predict the need for surgery. Approximately 34% of PD patients will have some degree of plaque calcification.

6. **c. Is frequently associated with penile shortening.** Penile shortening and inability to have intercourse are the two most common and consistent risk factors for emotional distress and relationship problems associated with PD (Smith et al., 2008; Rosen et al., 2008). Psychosocial stress is common and is reported by 77% to 94% of men with PD (Gelbard et al., 1990; Tal et al., 2012; Nelson and Mulhall, 2013). PD also commonly affects the patient's sexual partner, causing feelings of helplessness, as well as feeling personally responsible for the PD due to trauma during intercourse and sadness over loss of intimacy (Rosen et al., 2008). For some patients even a lesser degree of curvature may be highly bothersome or provoke distress (Hellstrom et al., 2013). Despite "successful treatment" that may allow the patient to be sexually functional again, there is often persistent psychological distress, presumably due to the residual changes compared with that man's pre-PD penis (Jones, 1997; Gelbard et al., 1990).

7. **a. Should include measurement of plaque size with calipers.** Measurement of the size of the plaque with any modality has been found to be inaccurate, as the plaque is rarely a discrete lesion (Bacal et al., 2009; Levine and Burnett, 2013; Ralph et al., 2010; Hatzimouratidis et al., 2012). Deformity assessment via ultrasound after injection of vasoactive agent has been shown to be the best method of assessing curvature as well as erectile response. Pictures taken from multiple vantage points may give a better idea of deformity during initial consultation. Because of the association with other collagen vascular disorders, the patient's palms should be examined.

8. **d. Penile sensory integrity.** The benefits of a complete duplex ultrasound assessment include identification of calcification during initial surveillance in the flaccid state, assessment of penile vascular flow parameters following intracavernosal injection of vasoactive agent, observing the erectile response to the vasoactive injection compared to the patient's sexually induced erection at home, and finally providing the best opportunity to objectively assess deformity. These parameters are absolutely critical to the decision process for the patient who is considering surgery. Penile sensation is best evaluated with biothesiometry.

9. **c. Elevated local levels of nitric oxide (NO).** Pentoxifylline is a nonspecific phosphodiesterase inhibitor with combined antiinflammatory and antifibrogenic properties. NO synthesized by inducible nitric oxide synthase (iNOS) reacts with reactive oxygen species (ROS), thus reducing ROS levels and presumably inhibiting fibrosis. The antifibrotic effects of NO may be mediated at least in part by the reduction of myofibroblast abundance and lead to a reduction in collagen I synthesis (Vernet et al., 2002).

10. **b. Peyronie's disease.** Injection therapy has no association with leading to PD. It may, however, lead to some degree of cavernosal fibrosis, pain, and priapism. When used in the appropriate population, intracavernosal injection therapy for ED does have a high success rate.

11. **a. Reassurance.** In this case, a young man presents with PD with a minimal curvature and minimal discomfort. Pursuing aggressive therapy is not indicated because the disease process may not worsen. Therefore, reassurance is the proper answer. This patient should also be counseled to follow up should he see any exacerbation of his symptoms. At this time, intralesional collagenase is not indicated for curvature less than 30 degrees,

the two noted oral therapies are not noted to be beneficial, and intralesional steroids are not recommended because of lack of objective evidence of benefit.

12. **c. Penile prosthesis with penile straightening.** This man presents with stable PD, a borderline moderate to severe curvature, but a poor-quality erection at home and an inadequate erectile response during duplex ultrasound with a high dose of vasoactive intracorporal drug injection. For the motivated patient who has both ED and PD, placement of a penile prosthesis with straightening maneuvers is the most likely treatment to address both problems. Plication or plaque incision with grafting would not fix this man's ED. Use of oral therapy had not been proven to be beneficial in this circumstance. Intralesional injection of any sort may potentially benefit his deformity, but given that he has inadequate erectile response, intralesional injections would not result in ability to resume sexual activity.

13. **c. Diminished risk of postoperative ED.** A tunica plication procedure is the preferred approach because it has the least likelihood of causing injury to the underlying cavernosal tissue, which presumably is responsible for postsurgical ED seen most commonly with a grafting procedure. There is indeed a greater potential for loss of erect length with a plication and less likelihood of damaging the penile sensory nerves, but the diminished risk of postoperative ED is the strongest reason to pursue a plication rather than grafting procedure, particularly in patients with less than severe curvature.

14. **c. To enhance cicatrix contracture.** Postoperative rehabilitation with massage and stretch, nightly use of a PDE5 inhibitor, and traction therapy are designed to enhance postoperative healing in all listed ways except for c, which is the correct answer because enhancing cicatrix contracture would not enhance healing or postoperative outcomes.

15. **d. Increases the risk of sensory change.** Penile traction therapy has emerged as an effective adjunct treatment option. Traction therapy has been shown to increase or preserve postoperative length and encourage tissue modeling, and it does appear to be dose-related. In addition, one study suggested that the minimum average time for daily use following surgery would be 3 hours or more per day. There is no evidence that traction therapy causes injury to the sensory nerves, nor is there evidence to suggest that it increases the risk of sensory change.

16. **b. Urethral injury.** Manual modeling was introduced in the mid-1990s as a straightening maneuver to correct residual curvature after placement of a penile prosthesis. In performing this procedure, the primary reported risk is injury to the urethra at the meatus, where the prosthetic cylinder tips may extrude through the meatus as a result of pressure placed on the distal shaft during the modeling process. Although sensory deficit, recurring curvature, and tunica tear are possible complications, they have not been reported, nor has a proximal urethral perforation.

17. **c. A short penis (<9 cm) with severe curve and poor rigidity.** This is the only option noted that would not be appropriately treated by a grafting procedure for PD, primarily because of the poor rigidity. One of the primary indications to perform a grafting procedure would be the patient having a strong erection preoperatively with severe curvature in excess of 70 degrees, having indentation causing an unstable penis or hinge effect, hourglass deformity, or a short penis. The key here is the poor rigidity, which would be an absolute contraindication to performing a grafting procedure; it is more likely to cause further ED in this circumstance.

18. **a. Postoperative erectile dysfunction (ED).** Although the other listed side effects have been reported, the primary concern with patients undergoing this procedure is postoperative ED. Therefore, proper patient selection preoperatively would include only those men who have excellent-quality rigidity with or without PDE5 inhibitor therapy and have a normal vascular response during duplex ultrasound assessment.

19. **c. 70 degrees with hinge effect.** Severe curve greater than 70 degrees and hinge effect are two indications to perform an

incision and grafting procedure. Ventral curvatures when repaired with grafting have a much higher rate of complete ED. Those with suboptimal rigidity tend to also develop more erectile problems post-grafting. A 90-degree curve may be an indication, but all surgical procedures should be delayed at least 1 year from the time of onset with 6 months of stable disease. Finally, it should be recognized that although a patient is more likely to recover some length after performing a grafting procedure, neither grafting nor plication operations should be expected to result in substantial gain of length; the primary goal is straightening.

20. **e. Contracts during healing.** Contraction during the healing process would not be included in the criteria for an ideal graft.

21. **c. Stable plaques between 30 and 90 degrees.** IMPRESS Phase 3 Randomized clinical trials (RCTs) showed that CCH resulted in an improvement of 17 degrees versus 9 degrees (control) in patients with stable dorsal plaques between 30 and 90 degrees. Those who had unstable hinges, calcified plaques, hourglass effect, severe ED, or ventral plaques were excluded from the study. Various quality of life parameters were also improved with CCH injection.

22. **a. Cost and length of treatment.** In the IMPRESS trial, patients were given four treatment courses consisting of two injections each. Each injection costs $3300. This leads to significant cost and numerous office visits, which may pose a significant burden to the patient. De novo ED has not been reported with CCH. Penile bruising is a common side effect but is almost always benign. Penile fracture is a dreaded complication but occurs in less than 1% in a pooled analysis. There are no reports of severe autoimmune reactions associated with CCH.

CHAPTER REVIEW

1. There are two phases in the natural history of PD: the acute phase, in which changes occur, and the stable chronic phase, which is typically marked by 12 months onset and 6 months of stable curvature.
2. The incidence of PD is between 3% and 9% with a peak age of 50 years.
3. There is a high association (33%) of diabetes with PD.
4. Preoperative erectile function correlates strongly with postoperative results.
5. Patients with poor-quality erections preoperatively who have grafting procedures are likely to have significant problems postoperatively with erectile function. These patients should be steered toward inflatable penile prosthesis (IPP) placement with or without adjunct procedures.
6. PD is currently recognized as a wound healing disorder of the tunica albuginea.
7. Sixty percent to seventy percent of plaques are located on the dorsal aspect of the tunica albuginea and are usually associated with the septum.
8. The natural history of PD studies suggest that no more than 13% of patients will experience improvement of deformity.
9. Eleven percent of all patients undergoing prostatectomy developed fibrotic changes in their penis.
10. Penile shortening and inability to have intercourse are the two most common and consistent risk factors for emotional distress and relationship problems associated with PD.
11. Primary indications to perform a grafting procedure in a patient with a strong erection are severe curvature in excess of 70 degrees, an indentation causing an unstable penis or hinge effect, and a short penis. Poor rigidity is an absolute contraindication to performing a grafting procedure.
12. Ventral curvatures, when repaired with grafting, have a much higher rate of complete ED.
13. IMPRESS Phase 3 RCTs showed that CCH resulted in an improvement of 17 degrees versus 9 degrees (control) in patients with stable dorsal plaques between 30 and 90 degrees. Those who had unstable hinges, calcified plaques, hourglass defects, severe ED, or ventral plaques were excluded from the study. However, cost of treatment presents a significant barrier.
14. Injection site pain and bruising are common and usually benign. However, one should always suspect the rare but dreaded complication of penile fracture in these patients.
15. While graft incision/partial excision do typically result in less penile length loss versus plication, a patient should not expect to increase his penile length with any procedure.

74 Sexual Function and Dysfunction in the Female

Ervin Kocjancic, Valerio Iacovelli, and Ömer Acar

QUESTIONS

1. Sexual health encompasses which of the following concepts?
   a. Absence of sexual dysfunction/problem
   b. Mental well-being
   c. Human development and maturation
   d. All of the above
   e. a and c

2. Which of these molecules is thought to play only a minor role in female genital sexual response?
   a. Vasoactive intestinal polypeptide
   b. Nitric oxide
   c. Acetylcholine
   d. Norepinephrine
   e. Aquaporins

3. The Female Sexual Function Index (FSFI) assesses all but which of the following aspects of sexuality?
   a. Sexual distress
   b. Sexual desire
   c. Sexual arousal
   d. Sexual pain
   e. Orgasm

4. Which of the following is NOT an essential part of the physical examination in a woman with sexual concerns?
   a. Vital signs
   b. Assessment of vaginal pH
   c. Palpation of the levator ani musculature
   d. Careful inspection of the vulva
   e. Biothesiometry

5. Which of the following statements is TRUE?
   a. Assessment of the patient's intimate relationship(s) is a key aspect of treating sexual problems.
   b. Women with spinal cord injury cannot experience orgasm.
   c. A linear pattern for sexual response is typical for all women.
   d. Survey instruments may take the place of history in evaluation of sexual concerns.
   e. All women who have sex with women identify as lesbian or bisexual.

6. Which of the following statements is FALSE?
   a. Hysterectomy may improve or worsen sexual function in women depending on the indication.
   b. Low serum testosterone levels have been clearly linked to worse sexual function in all women.
   c. Phosphodiesterase type 5 inhibitors are not currently approved for the management of problems with sexual arousal response in women.
   d. Sexual activity during routine pregnancy is safe.
   e. Women may have genital arousal responses to erotic materials that they find mentally or emotionally unappealing.

7. Which of the following are potential adverse events associated with supplemental testosterone in women?
   a. Hirsutism
   b. Acne
   c. Decreased high-density lipoprotein
   d. Vaginal bleeding
   e. All of the above

8. Decreased sexual interest/desire has been associated with which of the following conditions in women?
   a. Use of antidepressants
   b. Life stressors
   c. Hypoestrogenism
   d. Relationship problems
   e. All of the above

9. Education on sexuality is always indicated; which of the following women is likely to also benefit from medical and/or psychological treatment?
   a. 24-year-old woman who does not climax with vaginal penetration but does climax with clitoral stimulation
   b. 56-year-old woman with vaginal dryness that is well managed with sexual lubricant
   c. 35-year-old woman with bothersome decline in sexual desire
   d. All of the above
   e. None of the above

10. Which of the following diagnoses are included in the *Diagnostic and Statistical Manual of Mental Illness Fifth Edition (DSM-5)*?
    a. Female orgasmic disorder (FOD)
    b. Hypoactive sexual desire disorder
    c. Genitopelvic pain/penetration disorder
    d. a and c above
    e. All of the above

11. Which of the following conditions has been associated with lower bioavailable androgen levels in women?
    a. Hormonal contraceptives
    b. Surgical menopause
    c. Elevated prolactin levels
    d. All of the above
    e. None of the above

12. Which of the following has NOT been shown to be useful in the management of problems with sexual arousal in women?
    a. Topical prostaglandins
    b. Muscle relaxants
    c. Vaginal lubricants
    d. Hormonal supplementation with androgens and/or estrogens
    e. Psychosocial counseling

13. Which of the following has been definitively linked to sexual dysfunction in women?
    a. Postmenopausal estrogen replacement
    b. Obesity
    c. High educational achievement
    d. Depression
    e. Metabolic syndrome

14. Which of the following has the least evidence for efficacy in management of antidepressant-associated sexual dysfunction in women?
    a. Use of an adjunctive antidepressant
    b. Reassurance
    c. Drug cessation
    d. Drug holiday
    e. Sildenafil

15. What is the most commonly purported etiology for the sexual problems that occur in some women using hormonal contraception?
    a. Reduction of bioavailable testosterone
    b. Reduction of bioavailable estrogen
    c. Psychological distress
    d. Partner dissatisfaction
    e. Alteration of vascular response

16. Which of the following is the possible anatomic location of the Grafenberg spot (G-spot), which is particularly sensitive to tactile stimulation in some women?
    a. Anterior wall of the vagina at the level of midurethra
    b. Cervical canal
    c. Clitoral surface
    d. Posterior vaginal wall
    e. Perianal ring

17. Choose the correct statement regarding the laboratory evaluation for female sexual dysfunction.
    a. It is mandatory in all cases
    b. Normal range of testosterone levels have been established in women
    c. It is rarely indicated unless there is suspicion for an underlying contributory medical condition
    d. Thyroid dysfunction is the most commonly encountered hormonal abnormality in female patients with sexual dysfunction
    e. Abnormalities in hormone levels provide extensive diagnostic and prognostic utility in female sexual dysfunction

18. Choose the correct statement regarding FSFI.
    a. Contains 29 items
    b. Has an abbreviated version that can be used for screening pre- and postmenopausal women
    c. It is not validated for use in patients with cancer
    d. Maximum total score is 30
    e. It is not validated for use in research

19. Which of the following is the most widely studied, most validated physiological test used in the assessment of female sexual function?
    a. Laser Doppler imaging
    b. Magnetic resonance imaging
    c. Thermistor clip
    d. Vaginal photoplethysmography
    e. Doppler ultrasonography

20. Choose the correct statement regarding the DSM-5 definitions of sexual dysfunctions in women:
    a. All disorders, including genitopelvic pain/penetration disorder, require that the symptoms meet the DSM-5 definitions of that condition.
    b. Symptoms should be present for 3 months
    c. Symptoms should occur on at least half of the sexual occasions
    d. Symptoms should cause clinically significant distress
    e. Symptoms can be a consequence of a severe relationship distress

21. Which of the following is the most prevalent type of female sexual dysfunction?
    a. Hypoactive sexual desire disorder
    b. Arousal disorder
    c. Orgasmic disorder
    d. Genitopelvic pain/penetration disorder
    e. Vaginismus

22. Choose the correct statement about the mechanism of action of Flibanserin, which is currently the only FDA-approved treatment for acquired, generalized hypoactive sexual desire disorder.
    a. Phosphodiesterase type 5 inhibitor
    b. α-adrenergic antagonist
    c. 5-HT1A receptor agonist and 5-HT 2A receptor antagonist
    d. 5-HT1A receptor partial agonist
    e. Estrogen receptor modulator

23. Choose the correct statement regarding FOD:
    a. Orgasmic disorder almost always occurs as an isolated form of female sexual dysfunction
    b. Selective serotonin reuptake inhibitors (SSRIs) are used to treat FOD
    c. The information gathered by the questionnaires about female sexual function is sufficient to arrive at the diagnosis of FOD
    d. DSM-5 definition of FOD does not contain the criterion that requires orgasmic difficulty to occur despite a normal excitement phase
    e. Systemic testosterone treatment (either alone or in combination with systemic/local estrogen treatment) has been approved by the FDA for the treatment for FOD

24. Which of the following is one of the criteria that have been suggested by Leiblum and Nathan and used in the diagnosis of persistent genital arousal disorder in women?
    a. Physiologic sexual arousal can be brief and remit on its own
    b. Symptoms of sexual arousal can be triggered by no stimulus at all
    c. Symptoms of sexual arousal are not distressing
    d. The signs of physiologic sexual arousal remit with ordinary orgasmic experience
    e. The signs of physiologic sexual arousal are experienced in the presence of subjective feelings of sexual desire and arousal

25. Choose the correct statement regarding provoked vestibulodynia (PVD):
    a. Patients with primary PVD appear to have greater nerve fiber density and thicker vulvar vestibule compared to the secondary group
    b. Pelvic floor muscles are usually hypotonic in both primary and secondary PVD

c. Positive family history and an association with enuresis is more commonly encountered in secondary PVD

d. Primary PVD is more common than its secondary counterpart

e. Local signs of inflammation are a common part of the clinical picture in primary vestibulodynia

ANSWERS

1. **d. All of the above.** Sexual wellness incorporates many aspects of human experience.
2. **c. Acetylcholine.** Acetylcholine is thought to play a relatively minor role in sexual response in women.
3. **a. Sexual distress.** The FSFI does not include a metric to quantify or measure sexuality-related distress.
4. **e. Biothesiometry.** Biothesiometry may be indicated in some cases of genital neuropathy, but much of the same information can be gleaned from careful history and physical examination (with or without basic sensory testing).
5. **a. Assessment of the patient's intimate relationship(s) is a key aspect of treating sexual problems.** Women with spinal cord injury may experience orgasm, and women may endorse a circular or linear sexual response. A history is critical to evaluation of sexual wellness, and up to half of women who have had sex with another woman do not identify as lesbian or bisexual.
6. **b. Low serum testosterone levels have been clearly linked to worse sexual function in all women.** There are data to support a role for testosterone in sexual function in some women, but this is the least well supported of the statements in this question.
7. **e. All of the above.** These are well-established potential effects of testosterone. There are substantial concerns about the potential for cardiovascular disease or neoplasia, but robust data on risk are scant.
8. **e. All of the above.** There are numerous potential causes of low sexual desire.
9. **c. 35-year-old woman with bothersome decline in sexual desire.** Many sexually healthy women do not climax with vaginal penetration. Use of vaginal lubricant is an effective and safe management option for vaginal dryness.
10. **d. a and c above.** The DSM V combined hypoactive sexual desire disorder and female sexual arousal disorder into female sexual interest/arousal disorder. Similarly, dyspareunia and vaginismus were combined into genitopelvic pain/penetration disorder. FOD was carried over from DSM IV TR.
11. **d. All of the above.** Hormonal contraception, prolactin, and surgical menopause all tend to decrease bioavailable testosterone.
12. **b. Muscle relaxants.** Muscle relaxants have been used with good efficacy for issues of sexual pain but have not been shown to directly aid sexual arousal response in women.
13. **d. Depression.** Depression is unambiguously linked to sexual dysfunction in women; the other entities have been linked to sexual dysfunction in some but not all studies.
14. **b. Reassurance.** There are peer-reviewed, published data to support all but answer b. Reassurance may be indicated for some women but may be viewed by others as a dismissal of their concerns related to antidepressant treatment.
15. **a. Reduction of bioavailable testosterone.** Hormonal contraception has been clearly linked to lower bioavailable serum testosterone. Other etiologies may contribute.
16. **a. Anterior wall of the vagina at the level of midurethra.** A region of the anterior wall of the vagina overlying the midurethra has been identified as the Grafenberg spot (or G-spot), an area that, in some women, is particularly sensitive to tactile stimulation. Grafenberg's original article identified the erogenous area as arising from the urethra. Controversy still exists over the possible anatomic structure and site of the G-spot.
17. **c. It is rarely indicated unless there is suspicion for an underlying contributory medical condition.** Laboratory evaluation for female sexual dysfunction (FSD) is rarely indicated unless there is a suspicion for a specific medical condition that might explain patient's sexual problems. Therefore, random testosterone measurement is worthless in the evaluation of FSD. Furthermore, there are no data to justify serum testosterone measurement for FSD unless there is a concern about hyper/hypoandrogenic state. Normal range of testosterone levels have not been established in women, and testosterone levels do not correlate with libido in females. Likewise, progesterone, measured either alone or in combination with estrogen, has very limited diagnostic/prognostic utility in FSD. If a hormonal abnormality is suspected based on the systemic evaluation of the patient, then a screening blood workup can be done to rule out prolactinoma, thyroid dysfunction, and adrenal disorders. If adrenal insufficiency is suspected, measurement of dehydroepiandrosterone sulfate (DHEA-S) is useful because of isolated adrenal production.
18. **b. Has an abbreviated version that can be used for screening pre- and postmenopausal women.** FSFI is a brief, 19-item, multidimensional self-report instrument that assesses six domains of sexual function: desire, arousal, lubrication, orgasm, satisfaction, and pain. Target population consists of hetero- and homosexual women. It is available for pre- and postmenopausal women and women with medical and sexual disorders. It refers to the past 4 weeks and administration time varies between 10 and 15 minutes. Each domain of FSFI is scored on a scale of 0 to 6 points with the exception of the desire domain (scored from 1.2 to 6) and the satisfaction domain (scored from 0.8 to 6). The instrument thus has a range of 2 to 36, with 36 representing a "perfect" score. The maximum total score is 36 and higher scores indicate better sexual functioning. A total FSFI score of less than 26.55 is considered at risk for sexual dysfunction. Although it is validated for use in research, it is not yet used in clinical practice. An abbreviated version (six items) also has been validated in pre- and postmenopausal women and has been proposed as a tool for screening women likely to have FSD. The FSFI also has been validated for use in patients with cancer, in whom strong psychometric properties have been reported in addition to women with chronic pelvic pain.
19. **d. Vaginal photoplethysmography.** There are many physiological monitoring parameters of sexual arousal, which could potentially assist in the diagnosis of organic diseases contributing to sexual dysfunctions. Genital blood flow can be measured with vaginal photoplethysmography, which is the most widely studied and most validated physiological test used in assessment of female sexual function. This method uses a vaginal light source on an acrylic tampon to illuminate the vaginal microcirculation and determine the level of vaginal engorgement. Most studies comparing genital responses of women with and without sexual dysfunction have used vaginal photoplethysmography that measures vaginal pulse amplitude (VPA).
20. **d. Symptoms should cause clinically significant distress.** Regarding the DSM-5 definitions and criteria for sexual dysfunctions in women, all disorders except genitopelvic pain-penetration disorder require that the symptoms meet the DSM-5 definition of that condition, have been present for 6 months on at least 75% of sexual occasions, cause clinically significant distress, are not a consequence of a nonsexual mental disorder or of a severe relationship distress or other significant stressors, and are not attributable to the effect of a medication or illness.
21. **b. Arousal disorder.** Shifren et al. (Prevalence of Female Sexual Problems Associated with Distress and Determinants of Treatment Seeking [PRESIDE] study) reported the overall prevalence of FSD associated with low desire to be 37.7% in a study involving 50,001 US women and 31,531 respondents aged 18 to 102 years who were evaluated by validated questionnaires. In this study, 8.9% of women aged 18 to 44 years, 12.3% of women aged 45 to 64 years, and 7.4% of women older than 65 years exhibited low desire accompanied by clinically significant distress (HSDD).

22. **c. 5-HT1A receptor agonist and 5-HT 2A receptor antagonist.** Flibanserin is currently the only US Food and Drug Administration (FDA)-approved medication that can be used for the management of premenopausal women with low sexual desire. All of the other medical treatment options that can be applied in patients diagnosed with HSDD are used off-label. Flibanserin (Valeant Pharmaceuticals North America LLC, Bridgewater, NJ), dosed at 100 mg PO once daily at bedtime, is a nonhormonal, centrally acting, postsynaptic 5-HT1A receptor agonist and 5-HT2A receptor antagonist that results in a decrease in serotonin activity and an increase in dopamine and norepinephrine activity.

23. **d. DSM-5 definition of FOD does not contain the criterion that requires orgasmic difficulty to occur despite a normal excitement phase.** FOD can be diagnosed concurrently with at least one other sexual dysfunction. It has been estimated that among women with FOD, 31% also report difficulties with sexual arousal, 18% with lubrication, 14% with desire, 12% with pain, and 0.9% with vaginismus. The DSM-5 definition of FOD does not contain the DSM-IV-TR criterion requiring that difficulty with orgasm occur despite "a normal excitement phase." This revision was based on the fact that FOD can occur despite intact arousal. A comprehensive sexual history is essential to diagnose and characterize FOD. Nature and onset of the problem should be carefully assessed as well as the other aspects of female sexual function, since FOD often accompanies problems with interest and arousal. Questionnaires alone are not sufficient to diagnose FOD. However, they can be used to track progress of the orgasmic function and monitor treatment response. Systemic testosterone treatment (either alone or in combination with systemic/intravaginal estrogens) and tibolone (a synthetic steroid available in Europe, which provides a mixture of estrogenic, progestonic, and androgenic actions) have a positive influence on all aspects of female sexual response (desire, arousal, and orgasm) in postmenopausal women with low testosterone/low estrogen levels. However, more research is warranted about the safety and efficacy of hormonal treatment in women with FOD as the primary complaint. SSRIs, which represent the cornerstone of pharmacotherapy of depression, have the potential to adversely affect various aspects of female sexual response cycle, including desire, arousal, and/or orgasm with estimates of 30% to 70% of patients on SSRIs reporting some degree of sexual dysfunction.

24. **b. Symptoms of sexual arousal can be triggered by no stimulus at all.** The International Consultation on Sexual Medicine (ICSM) definition for persistent genital arousal disorder in women is a spontaneous, intrusive, and unwanted genital arousal (i.e., tingling, throbbing, pulsating) in the absence of sexual interest and desire. Any awareness of subjective arousal is typically, but not invariably, unpleasant. The arousal is unrelieved by at least one orgasm, and the feeling of arousal persists for hours or days. In 2001, Leiblum and Nathan defined this syndrome according to the following criteria.
    - Physiologic sexual arousal (genital and breast vasocongestion and sensitivity) persists for an extended period (from hours to days) and does not remit on its own.
    - The signs of physiologic sexual arousal do not remit with ordinary orgasmic experience.
    - The signs of physiologic sexual arousal are experienced in the absence of subjective feelings of sexual desire and arousal.
    - The symptoms of sexual arousal can be triggered by sexual-related stimulus but also by nonsexual cues or no stimulus at all.
    - These symptoms are perceived as intrusive and unwanted, leading at least to some degree of distress.

25. **a. Patients with primary PVD appear to have greater nerve fiber density and thicker vulvar vestibule compared to the secondary group.**
    - An important difference between primary and secondary PVD is in the nerve fiber density and the presence of inflammation. Respectively, primary PVD patients appear to have greater nerve fiber density and thicker vulvar vestibule compared to the secondary group. Moreover, hypertonicity of pelvic floor muscles appears to be highly prevalent in patients with PVD. Pelvic muscles dysfunction in patients with PVD can present with decreased muscular strength, reduced speed of contraction, coordination, and reduced endurance.
    - Primary PVD: Pain experienced since the first attempt of any type of vaginal penetration (i.e., tampons or sexual activities.) This condition has an early onset, the duration of the pain is longer, and the women are less likely to have had children. They also have a positive family history of the same condition. Frequently there is also an association with enuresis and dysmenorrhea. The presence of local signs of inflammation is less common.
    - Secondary PVD: Pain experienced after a certain period of time pertaining to vaginal penetrative activities that previously were pain free. This condition is typically acquired and has a late onset. Larger areas of vestibule are involved in the pain process. The clitoral hood is the area with the most severe pain. Secondary PVD appears to be more frequent than the primary one (65% vs. 35%) and the primary PVD appears to be more frequent in Hispanic women.

CHAPTER REVIEW

1. The vagina is acidic, with a pH between 4 and 5, and is colonized by microorganisms that produce lactic acid.
2. Testosterone production in women comes directly from the ovaries and adrenal glands. Unlike estrogen and progesterone levels, which fall abruptly with menopause, testosterone levels diminish gradually throughout life.
3. Sexual neutrality or being receptive to rather than initiating sexual activity is considered a normal variation of female sexual functioning.
4. Women with incontinence are up to three times more likely to experience decreased arousal, infrequent orgasms, and increased dyspareunia.
5. Lack of estrogen may not directly impair female arousal and desire, but it impairs sexual function by resulting in a decreased vasocongestion and lubrication and increased vaginal epithelial atrophy. Estrogens maintain female genital tissue integrity and thickness.
6. SSRIs have an inhibitory effect on sexual desire, arousal, and orgasm.
7. Optimal female sexual health requires physical, emotional, and mental well-being.
8. Hormonal contraception, prolactin, and elevated sex hormone–binding globulin (SHBG) all tend to decrease bioavailable testosterone.

75 Surgical, Radiographic, and Endoscopic Anatomy of the Retroperitoneum

Drew A. Palmer and Alireza Moinzadeh

QUESTIONS

1. Which of the following structures is NOT in the retroperitoneum?
   a. Kidney
   b. Second portion of the duodenum
   c. Ascending colon
   d. Adrenal
   e. Transverse colon

2. Which muscle's function is most similar to psoas major?
   a. Iliacus
   b. Quadratus lumborum
   c. Transversus abdominis
   d. External oblique
   e. Vastus lateralis

3. Which of the following statements is TRUE?
   a. The intercostal neurovascular bundle travels between the internal intercostal and innermost intercostal muscles.
   b. The 10th, 11th, and 12th ribs are floating ribs.
   c. Fracture of the lower ribs does not pose a risk to the retroperitoneal structures.
   d. Bony landmarks are not useful for planning surgical incisions.
   e. The intercostal neurovascular bundle travels within the costal groove on the cephalad aspect of the rib.

4. Which fascial layer is immediately deep to the transversus abdominis muscle?
   a. Lumbodorsal fascia
   b. Lateroconal fascia
   c. Internal oblique fascia
   d. External oblique fascia
   e. Transversalis fascia

5. Despite warnings from his friends and colleagues, a 32-year-old urologist purchases a motorcycle. He is involved in an accident and suffers grade 2 renal trauma. The hematoma would most likely travel in which direction if it continued to expand?
   a. Superior
   b. Lateral
   c. Medial
   d. Caudal
   e. Cephalad

6. The anterior and posterior laminae of Gerota fascia merge laterally to form:
   a. transversus abdominis.
   b. lumbodorsal fascia.
   c. lateral renal fascia.
   d. lateroconal fascia.
   e. perirenal fascia.

7. The kidneys are associated with which embryologic structure?
   a. Outer stratum
   b. Intermediate stratum
   c. Inner stratum
   d. Ectoderm
   e. Endoderm

8. Which of the following statements are TRUE?
   a. Small mesenteric defects have a lower risk of internal hernia compared to large defects.
   b. Based on current understanding, the mesentery is continuous.
   c. In addition to its gastrointestinal (GI) function, the mesentery has distinct immunologic, endocrine, and vascular functions.
   d. a and b.
   e. a and c.
   f. b and c.
   g. a, b, and c.

9. The blood supply to the adrenal gland may include branches from the:
   a. inferior phrenic artery.
   b. aorta.
   c. renal artery.
   d. a and b.
   e. a and c.
   f. a, b, and c.

10. Which of the following statements is TRUE?
    a. The superior mesenteric artery (SMA) may be sacrificed without causing bowel ischemia.
    b. Ligation of the inferior mesenteric artery (IMA) will cause ischemia to the large bowel but not the small bowel.
    c. The IMA may be sacrificed without colonic ischemia because of collateral circulation via the marginal artery and hemorrhoidal arteries.

d. The IMA may be sacrificed without colonic ischemia because of collateral circulation via the ileocolic artery.

e. Neither the superior nor the inferior mesenteric arteries may be sacrificed without causing bowel ischemia.

11. Following colon mobilization for right-sided transperitoneal retroperitoneal surgery, which plane should be developed prior to approaching the renal hilum?

a. Medial to the gonadal vein

b. Posterior to the gonadal vein

c. Lateral to the gonadal vein

d. Medial to the inferior vena cava (IVC)

12. Which of the following statements is FALSE?

a. The right testicular vein typically drains into the IVC.

b. The left testicular vein typically drains into the left renal vein.

c. Unilateral varicoceles are more common on the left side.

d. A sudden-onset unilateral right-sided varicocele should prompt retroperitoneal imaging.

e. The left ovarian vein typically drains into the IVC.

13. Which of the following statements is TRUE?

a. The proximal ureter receives its blood supply medially, and the distal ureter receives its blood supply medially.

b. The proximal ureter receives its blood supply medially, and the distal ureter receives its blood supply laterally.

c. The proximal ureter receives its blood supply laterally, and the distal ureter receives its blood supply medially.

d. The proximal ureter receives its blood supply laterally, and the distal ureter receives its blood supply laterally.

14. Which of the following is NOT a tributary of the splenic vein?

a. Inferior mesenteric vein

b. Short gastric vein

c. Left gastroepiploic vein

d. Right gastroepiploic vein

e. Pancreatic veins

15. What statement best describes the lymphatic drainage of the right testis?

a. Superficial then deep right inguinal nodes

b. Left para-aortic with some drainage to the interaortocaval nodes

c. Only to the interaortocaval nodes

d. Primarily to the interaortocaval nodes with some drainage to the right paracaval nodes

e. Interaortocaval nodes primarily with some drainage to the right paracaval nodes and a small but appreciable amount of drainage to the left para-aortic nodes

16. In addition to cranial nerves III, VII, IX, and X, parasympathetic nervous system outflow includes:

a. preganglionic fibers from L3 to L4.

b. preganglionic fibers from T1 to L2.

c. preganglionic fibers from S2 to S4.

d. a and c.

e. b and c.

f. a, b, and c.

17. Which of the following statements is FALSE about the genitofemoral nerve?

a. One branch provides sensation to the upper anterior thigh.

b. The motor component of one branch allows for contraction of muscle during the cremasteric reflex.

c. It may be injured during a psoas hitch procedure.

d. It originates from the L3 to L4 segments.

e. Sensation to the anterior scrotum in males and the mons pubic and labium majus in females.

18. Damage to the hypogastric plexuses during retroperitoneal dissection may result in:

a. stress incontinence.

b. erectile dysfunction.

c. retrograde ejaculation.

d. varicocele.

e. autonomic dysreflexia.

19. What is the major function of the muscles innervated by the obturator nerve?

a. Hip adduction

b. Hip abduction

c. Hip flexion

d. Hip extension

e. Knee flexion

ANSWERS

1. **e. Transverse colon.** The contents of the retroperitoneum include the kidneys, ureters, adrenals, pancreas, second and third portions of the duodenum, ascending colon, descending colon, arterial structures including the aorta and its branches, venous structures including the IVC and its tributaries, lymphatics, lymph nodes, sympathetic trunk, and lumbosacral plexus. The transverse colon is considered to be an intraperitoneal structure.

2. **a. Iliacus.** Psoas major functions in flexion of the thigh at the hip joint and is innervated by the anterior rami of L1, L2, and L3. Iliacus is the only muscle listed that also functions in flexion of the thigh at the hip joint.

3. **a. The intercostal neurovascular bundle travels between the internal intercostal and innermost intercostal muscles.** Fracture of the lower ribs should lead to a high clinical suspicion for injury to the retroperitoneal structures. The 11th and 12th ribs must be distinguished from the other ribs because they have no anterior connection with the sternum and are often referred to as floating ribs. The 10th rib is not a floating rib. These ribs are of clinical significance during palpation for the marking of a surgical incision. Bony landmarks are of critical importance for surgical incision planning, as they do not typically move. Landmarks like the umbilicus are less useful as they can change location depending on the positioning (e.g., an obese patient with a large pannus in flank position). The intercostal vessels and nerves travel between the internal intercostal and innermost intercostal muscles within the costal groove on the caudal margin of the superior rib.

4. **e. Transversalis fascia.** The transversalis fascia lies deep to the transversus abdominis muscle and superficial to the preperitoneal fat and peritoneum.

5. **d. Caudal.** The perirenal space around the kidney is cone-shaped and is open at its inferior extent in the extraperitoneal pelvis. If a hematoma were to form within the Gerota fascia, it would be able to travel in a caudal direction.

6. **d. Lateroconal fascia.** The anterior and posterior laminae of Gerota fascia merge laterally to form the lateroconal fascia, which functions to separate the anterior and posterior pararenal spaces. It can be visualized radiographically on computed tomographic (CT) scan and continues anterolaterally deep to the transversalis fascia.

7. **b. Intermediate stratum.** The kidneys arise from mesoderm. The outer stratum covers the epimysium of the abdominal wall muscles and becomes the transversalis fascia. The intermediate

stratum is associated with the urinary organs, and the inner stratum is associated with the gastrointestinal organs.

8. **f. b and c.** Knowledge of mesenteric anatomy and function is important for urologist. The mesentery is known to be continuous based on current understanding and it has GI, immunologic, endocrine, and vascular functions. Smaller mesenteric defects have a higher risk of internal hernia than large defects. As such, smaller defects should be closed primarily.

9. **f. a, b, and c.** The adrenal gland may receive branches from the superior adrenal artery off of the inferior phrenic artery, the middle adrenal artery off of the aorta, and the inferior adrenal artery off of the renal artery.

10. **c. The IMA may be sacrificed without colonic ischemia because of collateral circulation via the marginal artery and hemorrhoidal arteries.** The SMA supplies the pancreas (inferior pancreaticoduodenal artery), small intestine, and the majority of the large intestine (ileocolic, right colic, and middle colic). Ligation of the SMA will result in catastrophic bowel ischemia (without pancreatic ischemia because of collaterals from the celiac artery and the superior pancreaticoduodenal artery). The branches of the IMA are the left colic, sigmoid, and superior hemorrhoidal (rectal) arteries. The collateral circulation of the sigmoid artery via the marginal artery of Drummond and the inferior and middle hemorrhoidal arteries allows for the IMA to be sacrificed without colonic ischemia.

11. **c. Lateral to the gonadal vein.** The next major step following colon mobilization is identification of the ureter. During this step on the right, the plane is developed lateral to the gonadal which leaves the gonadal vein in a medial position. If the plane medial to the gonadal vein is developed, there is a risk of injury to the IVC, and with elevation of the kidney, avulsion of the gonadal may occur.

12. **e. The left ovarian vein typically drains into the IVC.** The venous drainage of the ovarian and testicular veins is similar. The right testicular and the right ovarian veins typically drain into the IVC while the left testicular and the left ovarian veins drain into the left renal vein. Unilateral varicoceles are more common on the left, which may be a result of the increased length and perpendicular entry of the left testicular vein into the left renal vein. Given the rarity of unilateral right-side varicocele, a sudden-onset right-side varicocele should increase suspicion for a renal or retroperitoneal malignancy, leading to poor outflow and warrants retroperitoneal imaging.

13. **b. The proximal ureter receives its blood supply medially and the distal ureter receives its blood supply laterally.** In general, the blood supply of the ureter is medial proximally and lateral for the distal ureter. The renal artery and aorta supply the proximal ureter while the internal iliac artery, superior vesical, and inferior vesical arteries supply the distal ureter.

14. **d. Right gastroepiploic vein.** The tributaries of the splenic vein are the inferior mesenteric, short gastric, left gastroepiploic, and pancreatic veins. The right gastroepiploic vein is a tributary of the superior mesenteric vein.

15. **e. Interaortocaval nodes primarily with some drainage to the right paracaval nodes and a small but appreciable amount of drainage to the left para-aortic nodes.** The right testis drains primarily to the interaortocaval nodes, with some drainage to the right paracaval nodes. The left para-aortic region does receive a small but appreciable amount of lymphatic drainage from the right testis. This drainage pattern is consistent with the global lymphatic flow from right to left.

16. **c. Preganglionic fibers from S2 to S4.** The parasympathetic nervous system has craniosacral outflow with preganglionic fibers originating from cranial nerves III, VII, IX, and X, as well as the ventral rami of the second, third, and fourth sacral nerves.

17. **d. It originates from the L3 to L4 segments.** Each statement is true except for D. The genitofemoral nerve originates at the L1 to L2 segments.

18. **c. Retrograde ejaculation.** Much of the sympathetic innervation to the pelvic viscera travels through the superior and inferior hypogastric plexuses, which are contiguous. The superior hypogastric plexus originates at the caudal extent of the abdominal aorta and extends to the anterior surface of the fifth lumbar vertebra. Extensive retroperitoneal dissection that causes disruption of these plexuses may result in loss of seminal vesicle emission or failure of bladder neck closure, resulting in retrograde ejaculation.

19. **a. Hip adduction.** The obturator nerve innervates the muscles of the medial thigh compartment. These include the gracilis, adductor longus, adductor brevis, adductor magnus, and obturator externus muscles. The muscles function to adduct and rotate the thigh at the hip joint.

TABLE 75.1   Branches of the Abdominal Aorta

ARTERY	BRANCH	ORIGIN	SUPPLIES
Celiac trunk	Anterior	Immediately inferior to aortic hiatus of diaphragm	Abdominal foregut
Superior mesenteric artery	Anterior	Immediately inferior to celiac trunk	Abdominal midgut
Inferior mesenteric artery	Anterior	Inferior to renal arteries	Abdominal hindgut
Middle adrenal arteries	Lateral	Immediately superior to renal arteries	Adrenal glands
Renal arteries	Lateral	Immediately inferior to superior mesenteric artery	Kidneys
Testicular or ovarian arteries	Paired anterior	Inferior to renal arteries	Testes in male and ovaries in female
Inferior phrenic arteries	Paired lateral	Immediately inferior to aortic hiatus	Diaphragm
Lumbar arteries	Posterior	Usually four pairs	Posterior abdominal wall and spinal cord
Median sacral arteries	Posterior	Just superior to aortic bifurcation, pass inferiorly across lumbar vertebrae, sacrum, and coccyx	
Common iliac arteries	Terminal	Bifurcation usually occurs at the level of L4 vertebra	

Modified from Drake RL, Vogl W, Mitchell AWM: *Gray's anatomy for students,* Philadelphia, 2005, Elsevier, p 331.

TABLE 75.2   Branches of the Lumbosacral Plexus

BRANCH	ORIGIN	SPINAL SEGMENTS	MOTOR FUNCTION	SENSORY FUNCTION
Subcostal	Anterior ramus T12	T12	Muscles of the abdominal wall	Skin over the hip
Iliohypogastric	Anterior ramus L1	L1	Internal oblique and transversus abdominis	Posterolateral gluteal skin and skin in pubic region
Ilioinguinal	Anterior ramus L1	L1	Internal oblique and transversus abdominis	Skin in the upper medial thigh, and either the skin over the root of the penis and anterior scrotum or the mons pubis and labium majus
Genitofemoral	Anterior rami L1 and L2	L1, L2	Genital branch: male cremasteric muscle	Genital branch: skin of anterior scrotum or skin of mons pubis and labium majus. Femoral branch: skin of upper anterior thigh
Lateral cutaneous nerve of the thigh	Anterior rami L2 and L3	L2, L3	None	Skin on anterior and lateral thigh to the knee
Obturator	Anterior rami L2–L4	L2–L4	Obturator externus, pectineus, and muscles in medial compartment of thigh	Skin on medial aspect of the thigh
Femoral	Anterior rami L2–L4	L2–L4	Iliacus, pectineus, and muscles in anterior compartment of thigh	Skin on anterior thigh and medial surface of leg

Modified from Drake RL, Vogl W, Mitchell AWM: *Gray's anatomy for students,* Philadelphia, 2005, Elsevier, p 340.

CHAPTER REVIEW (SEE ALSO TABLES 75.1 AND 75.2)

RETROPERITONEUM AND POSTERIOR ABDOMINAL WALL

1. Retroperitoneal contents include the kidneys, ureters, adrenals, pancreas, portions of the duodenum, ascending colon, descending colon, mesentery, vasculature, lymphatics, and nervous structures.
2. The retroperitoneum is contained anteriorly by the posterior reflection of the peritoneum and posteriorly by the abdominal wall.
3. It is contained cranially and caudally by the diaphragm and the extraperitoneal pelvic structures, respectively.
4. The intercostal vessels and nerves travel between the internal intercostal and innermost intercostal muscles within the costal groove on the caudal margin of the superior rib.
5. The lumbodorsal fascia merges anterolaterally with the transversus abdominis muscle and is composed of three layers that cover the posterior abdominal wall musculature.

RETROPERITONEAL FASCIAE AND SPACES

1. The boundaries of the posterior pararenal space are the posterior lamina of Gerota fascia anteriorly and the transversalis fascia posteriorly and laterally.
2. The anterior and posterior laminae of Gerota fascia form the boundaries of the perirenal space which has a conelike shape that is open caudally in the extraperitoneal pelvis.
3. Perinephric fluids collections can expand caudally due to this opening in the perirenal space.
4. The white line of Toldt represents the lateral border of the fusion of the colonic mesentery with the posterior peritoneum.

VASCULATURE

1. The blood supply to the adrenal arises from the inferior phrenic, the aorta, and the renal artery.
2. The renal hila are at the level of L1, and the renal veins are anterior to the renal arteries.
3. The paired gonadal arteries typically arising anterolaterally from the aorta below the renal arteries
4. The SMA to IMA collateral circulation occurs via the marginal artery of Drummond, which allows the IMA to be sacrificed without colonic ischemia.
5. In general, the proximal ureter receives its blood supply medially, and the distal ureter receives its blood supply from a lateral direction.
6. The left gonadal vein enters left renal vein at a right angle and the right gonadal vein enters into the IVC directly; this anatomic distinction results in higher rates of varicoceles on the left.

LYMPHATIC SYSTEM

1. Testes are embryologically retroperitoneal and have retroperitoneal blood supply and primary lymphatic drainage.
2. The lymph of the left testis drains to the left para-aortic nodes with some drainage to the interaortocaval nodes.
3. The right testis drains primarily to the interaortocaval nodes with some to the right paracaval nodes and a small amount to the left para-aortic region.
4. The lymphatic drainage of the testicles is consistent with global lymphatic flow from right to left.

NERVOUS SYSTEM

1. The parasympathetic autonomic nervous system has craniosacral outflow and the postganglionic fibers are often contained within the walls of the innervated viscera.
2. The preganglionic sympathetic nervous system fibers exit from the spinal cord from T1 to L2 and may synapse within the sympathetic trunk or within the autonomic plexuses.
3. The somatic nervous system provides sensory and motor innervation to the pelvis and lower extremities through the lumbosacral plexus.

76 Neoplasms of the Testis

Andrew J. Stephenson and Timothy D. Gilligan

QUESTIONS

1. The following adult male germ cell tumor (GCT) subtypes arise from germ cell neoplasia in situ (GCNIS) EXCEPT:
   a. embryonal tumor.
   b. choriocarcinoma.
   c. classic seminoma.
   d. spermatocytic tumor.
   e. teratoma.

2. Which of the following statements is TRUE regarding spermatocytic tumor?
   a. Cryptorchidism is a risk factor.
   b. It may occur as a mixed GCT with other histologic GCT subtypes.
   c. It may contain i(12p) mutations.
   d. Bilateral testicular involvement may occur in 2% to 3% of cases.
   e. Metastatic spermatocytic tumor is rare.

3. Which of the following GCT subtypes is most likely to spread hematogenously?
   a. Choriocarcinoma
   b. Embryonal carcinoma
   c. Immature teratoma
   d. Teratoma with malignant transformation
   e. Seminoma

4. A 24-year-old man presents with a solid, painless, right intratesticular mass confirmed by scrotal ultrasonography. His left testis is normal. Serum tumor markers show a human chorionic gonadotropin (hCG) value of 96 mU/mL (upper limit: <5 mU/mL) and an α-fetoprotein (AFP) value of 58 ng/mL (upper limit: <11 ng/mL). The most likely histologic finding in the right testis is:
   a. pure teratoma.
   b. pure seminoma.
   c. pure embryonal carcinoma.
   d. pure yolk sac tumor.
   e. choriocarcinoma.

5. Which of the following is an acceptable indication for testis-sparing surgery?
   a. 1.3-cm solid intratesticular mass with a normal contralateral testis
   b. Suspected benign testicular lesion
   c. 2.4-cm solid mass in a solitary testis
   d. Hypogonadal male with 1.2-cm solid intratesticular mass in a solitary testis
   e. Small (<1 cm) hyperechoic lesion suggestive of a "burned out" primary tumor in a patient with disseminated nonseminomatous GCT (NSGCT) with serum-elevated AFP and hCG

6. A 37-year-old man presents with a 5-cm left testicular mass. Computed tomography (CT) reveals a 6-cm para-aortic mass but no evidence of distant metastases. Serum tumor markers show an AFP level of 1100 ng/mL (upper limit: <11 ng/mL) and an hCG level of 80 mU/mL (upper limit: <5 mU/mL). Left inguinal orchiectomy reveals a mixed GCT with 60% embryonal carcinoma, 30% yolk sac tumor, 5% seminoma, and 5% teratoma. The next best management step is:
   a. retroperitoneal lymph node dissection (RPLND).
   b. induction chemotherapy with three cycles of bleomycin-etoposide-cisplatin.
   c. induction chemotherapy with four cycles of bleomycin-etoposide-cisplatin.
   d. to obtain repeat serum tumor marker levels in 7 days.
   e. CT-guided biopsy of the para-aortic mass.

7. All of the following patients would be classified as "poor-risk" by International Germ Cell Cancer Collaborative Group (IGCCG) classification criteria EXCEPT those with:
   a. testicular seminoma with brain metastases.
   b. primary mediastinal NSGCT.
   c. testicular NSGCT with rising postorchiectomy AFP of 15,000 ng/mL (upper limit: <11 ng/mL).
   d. primary retroperitoneal NSGCT with liver metastases.
   e. testicular NSGCT with rising postorchiectomy hCG of 93,000 mU/mL (upper limit: <5 mU/mL).

8. A 34-year-old African American man with a left testicular mass undergoes inguinal orchiectomy that reveals a 1.2-cm pure seminoma that is confined to the testis with no evidence of lymphovascular invasion or rete testis invasion. His postorchiectomy serum tumor markers are within the normal range. CT of the chest-abdomen-pelvis reveals no evidence of retroperitoneal lymphadenopathy and no evidence of pulmonary metastases. However, on the chest images, there is evidence of bulky hilar adenopathy bilaterally. The next best management step is:
   a. induction chemotherapy with four cycles of bleomycin-etoposide-cisplatin.
   b. induction chemotherapy with four cycles of etoposide-cisplatin.
   c. mediastinoscopy and biopsy.
   d. close observation.
   e. bilateral thoracotomy and resection.

9. A 43-year-old man with clinical stage IIA left seminoma receives dog-leg radiation therapy to the retroperitoneum and ipsilateral pelvis with a boost to his solitary 2-cm para-aortic mass. Six months after completing treatment, surveillance CT reveals a persistent para-aortic mass that has now grown to 2.8 cm. The remainder of his metastatic evaluation is negative, and his serum tumor marker levels are all within normal limits. The next best management step is:
   a. RPLND.
   b. CT-guided biopsy of the retroperitoneal mass.
   c. close observation until the mass regresses or the patient develops distant metastases.
   d. induction chemotherapy with three cycles of bleomycin-etoposide-cisplatin.

e. salvage chemotherapy with four cycles of paclitaxel-ifosfa-mide-cisplatin.

10. A 41-year-old man has GCNIS discovered on biopsy of an atrophic right testis during investigations for infertility due to azoospermia. He has a history of left inguinal hernia repair. His left testis is normal in size and consistency, and there is evidence of normal spermatogenesis on testicular biopsy. His serum luteinizing hormone (LH), follicle-stimulating hormone (FSH), and testosterone levels are within the normal range. The most appropriate treatment for the GCNIS in the right testis now is:

a. inguinal orchiectomy.

b. low-dose radiation therapy.

c. carboplatin.

d. observation.

e. transscrotal orchiectomy.

11. Which of the following factors is NOT associated with the presence of occult metastases in clinical stage I NSGCT?

a. Lymphovascular invasion

b. Absence of yolk sac tumor in the primary tumor

c. Percentage of embryonal carcinoma in the primary tumor

d. Elevated preorchiectomy AFP level

e. Advanced primary tumor stage

12. A 27-year-old convict at a correctional facility presents for management of clinical stage I left NSGCT. He has a history of enlarging left testicular mass for 12 months that was discovered incidentally during a routine physical examination by the prison physician. Pathologic examination of the orchiectomy specimen revealed a 1.2-cm mixed GCT (40% seminoma, 40% embryonal carcinoma, 20% yolk sac tumor) confined to the testis without evidence of lymphovascular invasion. His postorchiectomy serum tumor markers are within normal limits. He has a history of multiple incarcerations in the past, and his viral serology is positive for hepatitis C. The most appropriate treatment is:

a. adjuvant radiation therapy to the retroperitoneum and ipsilateral pelvis.

b. surveillance.

c. chemotherapy with one cycle of bleomycin-etoposide-cisplatin.

d. chemotherapy with two cycles of carboplatin.

e. RPLND.

13. Which of the following factors is NOT associated with the presence of necrosis/fibrosis in residual masses after first-line chemotherapy?

a. Absence of teratoma in the primary tumor.

b. Residual mass size.

c. Percentage shrinkage of mass after chemotherapy.

d. Prechemotherapy mass size.

e. Lymphovascular invasion.

14. A 37-year-old man presents for treatment of a 1.2-cm left testicular mixed GCT (40% teratoma, 40% seminoma, 15% embryonal carcinoma, 5% yolk sac tumor) confined to the testis without evidence of lymphovascular invasion. His postorchiectomy serum tumor marker levels are within normal limits. Chest CT shows no evidence of metastatic disease. Abdominopelvic CT shows a 7-mm nodule in the paracaval location just inferior to the right renal hilum. The remainder of the CT study is unremarkable. His medical history is also unremarkable. The most appropriate management is:

a. CT-guided biopsy of the paracaval lesion.

b. RPLND.

c. two cycles of chemotherapy with bleomycin-etoposide-cisplatin.

d. observation.

e. three cycles of chemotherapy with bleomycin-etoposide-cisplatin.

15. The following factors are associated with the presence of occult distant metastases in patients with clinical stage IIA-B NSGCT EXCEPT:

a. elevated postorchiectomy hCG.

b. lymphovascular invasion.

c. retroperitoneal mass size.

d. large primary tumor with involvement of the scrotal skin.

e. retroperitoneal lymphadenopathy outside the primary landing zone.

16. The following are independent risk factors for relapse postchemotherapy RPLND EXCEPT:

a. evidence of viable malignancy in resected specimens.

b. incomplete resection.

c. rising pre-RPLND serum tumor markers.

d. poor-risk disease at diagnosis by IGCCCG criteria.

e. prior RPLND.

17. A 34-year-old man with right clinical stage III NSGCT (100% embryonal carcinoma) with good-risk features by IGCCCG criteria receives induction chemotherapy with three cycles of bleomycin-etoposide-cisplatin. At completion of chemotherapy, his serum tumor markers are within normal limits. On postchemotherapy CT studies he has a 1.7-cm mass (4.8 cm at diagnosis) in the interaortocaval region and a 0.8-cm mass in the para-aortic region (2.3 cm at diagnosis). He also has bilateral pulmonary nodules in the right lower lobe (0.6 cm; 1.4 cm at diagnosis) and left upper lobe (0.8 cm; 1.6 cm at diagnosis). The most appropriate management is:

a. four cycles of vinblastine-ifosfamide-cisplatin second-line chemotherapy.

b. resection of the interaortocaval mass.

c. bilateral postchemotherapy RPLND.

d. bilateral thoracotomy and resection of residual pulmonary masses.

e. CT-guided biopsy of the pulmonary mass(es).

18. Which of the following statements is FALSE concerning late relapse of NSGCT?

a. Surgical resection is the primary treatment modality.

b. Yolk sac tumor is the most common malignant histology.

c. The incidence is increasing.

d. The retroperitoneum is the most common site.

e. The outcome is poor relative to those with early NSGCT relapse.

19. A 35-year-old man with clinical stage IIC left mixed GCT (50% embryonal, 40% teratoma, 10% yolk sac) with good-risk features by IGCCCG criteria receives three cycles of bleomycin-etoposide-cisplatin chemotherapy. At the start of chemotherapy, his AFP was 380 ng/mL (upper limit: <11 ng/mL), and this has normalized at the end of chemotherapy. Restaging CT shows the solid para-aortic mass has increased from 5.3 cm to 8.9 cm with displacement of the aorta and left kidney as well as new lymphadenopathy in the left common iliac and left obturator region. The patient complains of recent onset of left-sided back pain. The most appropriate management is:

a. RPLND and pelvic lymph node dissection.

b. CT-guided biopsy of the para-aortic mass.

c. four cycles of paclitaxel-ifosfamide-cisplatin as second-line chemotherapy.

d. two cycles of bleomycin-etoposide-cisplatin followed by carboplatin-etoposide high-dose chemotherapy and autologous stem cell rescue.

e. bleomycin-etoposide-cisplatin plus radiation therapy.

20. The rationale for single-agent carboplatin as treatment for clinical stage I seminoma is based on all of the following factors EXCEPT:

a. absence of teratoma.

b. less neurotoxicity compared with cisplatin.

c. less nephrotoxicity compared with cisplatin.

d. less ototoxicity compared with cisplatin.

e. similar efficacy to cisplatin.

21. Late complications of infradiaphragmatic dog-leg radiotherapy include all the following EXCEPT:

a. peptic ulcer disease.

b. coronary artery disease.

c. secondary malignancy.

d. ejaculatory dysfunction.

e. impaired spermatogenesis.

22. The rationale for surveillance in clinical stage I seminoma is based on all of the following factors EXCEPT:

a. Utility of serum tumor markers to identify relapse at an early and curable stage.

b. Relapses are cured in virtually all cases by deferred dog-leg radiotherapy.

c. Lack of validated histopathologic prognostic factors to identify a high-risk subset.

d. Improved short- and long-term toxicity compared with primary radiotherapy and carboplatin.

e. 15% to 20% of patients are cured by orchiectomy.

23. A 44-year-old man with clinical stage III left testicular seminoma with IGCCCG good-risk features has a discrete 2.4-cm residual para-aortic mass (3.8 cm at diagnosis) after receiving three cycles of bleomycin-etoposide-cisplatin chemotherapy. His pulmonary nodules have regressed completely. His serum tumor markers are within the normal range. The most appropriate management is:

a. postchemotherapy radiation therapy to the residual mass.

b. fluorodeoxyglucose-labeled positron emission tomography (FDG-PET) at least 4 weeks after completing chemotherapy.

c. observation.

d. postchemotherapy surgical resection of the residual mass.

e. Four cycles of paclitaxel-ifosfamide-cisplatin as second-line chemotherapy.

24. A 42-year-old asymptomatic man presents for management of right NSGCT (80% embryonal carcinoma, 10% teratoma, 10% choriocarcinoma). His preorchiectomy hCG value was 15,000 mU/mL (upper limit: <5 mU/mL), and this has risen to 50,800 mU/mL after orchiectomy. Chest CT shows numerous pulmonary nodules. There is evidence of multiple masses in the inter-aortocaval region (largest, 4.8 cm) and masses in the para-aortic region (largest, 2.6 cm). The most appropriate management is:

a. three cycles of bleomycin-etoposide-cisplatin chemotherapy.

b. RPLND.

c. four cycles of bleomycin-etoposide-cisplatin chemotherapy.

d. CT of the head.

e. two cycles of bleomycin-etoposide-cisplatin followed by carboplatin-etoposide high-dose chemotherapy and autologous stem cell rescue.

25. Which of the following statements is FALSE regarding treatment-related toxicity?

a. Two cycles of platin-based chemotherapy do not increase one's risk of developing cardiovascular disease or secondary malignant neoplasm (SMN).

b. Frequent CT body imaging may increase the risk of SMN.

c. The risk of cardiovascular disease is highest among patients receiving mediastinal radiotherapy.

d. Exposure to cisplatin-based chemotherapy and history of cigarette smoking are associated with similar risks of cardiovascular disease and SMN.

e. Suprahilar dissection, vascular reconstruction, and hepatic resection are risk factors for chylous ascites after RPLND.

26. Which of the following are NOT similarities between Leydig cell tumors and GCT?

i. Both are associated with a history of cryptorchidism.

ii. Radical inguinal orchiectomy is the initial treatment of choice.

iii. Bilateral tumors occur in 2% to 3% of cases.

iv. Both may be associated with gynecomastia.

v. The retroperitoneum is the most common site of metastatic disease.

a. i, ii, and iii.

b. i and iii.

c. i, ii, iii, and iv.

d. v only.

e. All the above.

27. A 54-year-old man presents with an enlarging right inguinal mass. On examination, a palpable mass is noted in the right inguinal region that extends into the right hemiscrotum. The testis cannot be distinguished from this mass. Staging CT reveals a heterogeneous, infiltrative area of low-intensity mass (−20 Hounsfield units), 6 × 9 cm, involving the right spermatic cord and extending from the inguinal canal into the scrotum with displacement of the right testis. There is no evidence of retroperitoneal lymphadenopathy or distant metastases. The most appropriate management is:

a. inguinal orchiectomy followed by adjuvant radiotherapy.

b. inguinal orchiectomy alone.

c. transscrotal orchiectomy.

d. inguinal orchiectomy followed by ifosfamide-based adjuvant chemotherapy.

e. inguinal orchiectomy followed by RPLND.

PATHOLOGY

1. A 26-year-old man has a right radical orchiectomy for an embryonal carcinoma of the testis. At the time of surgery, a contralateral biopsy is performed and reveals intratubular germ cell neoplasia (Fig. 76.1). The patient should be advised that he:

a. should have a radical orchiectomy.

b. has a significant chance of developing a germ cell tumor in the left testis.

c. should not try to have a child.

d. should immediately receive radiation to the testis.

e. should receive salvage chemotherapy.

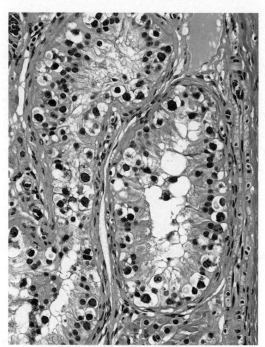

Fig. 76.1 (From Bostwick DG, Cheng L: *Urologic surgical pathology*, ed 2, Edinburgh, 2008, Mosby.)

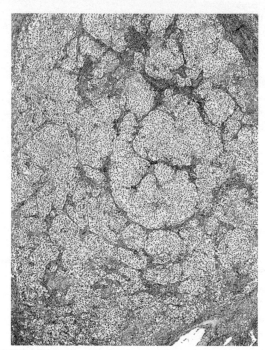

Fig. 76.2 (From Bostwick DG, Cheng L: *Urologic surgical pathology*, ed 2, Edinburgh, 2008, Mosby.)

2. A 35-year-old man has an asymptomatic right scrotal mass. Testicular ultrasonography reveals a 3-cm heterogeneous intratesticular mass. A right radical orchiectomy is performed. The histology is depicted in Fig. 76.2 and is reported as seminoma. Abdominal CT scan is normal. The patient should be advised to:

a. receive radiation to the contralateral testis.

b. receive at least four cycles of chemotherapy.

c. be advised that observation is not an option.

d. be advised to have radiation therapy to the retroperitoneum.

e. receive radiation to the abdomen and chest.

3. A 32-year-old man has a right radical orchiectomy for a testicular mass. Preoperatively, his AFP value was normal and his hCG level was elevated at 5000 units. The histology is depicted in Fig. 76.3 and is reported as seminoma with giant cells. The next step in management is:

a. follow markers and check half-life.

b. chemotherapy according to choriocarcinoma protocol.

c. RPLND.

d. radiation therapy to retroperitoneum.

e. three cycles of chemotherapy.

4. A 50-year-old man has a right radical orchiectomy for a testicular mass. The histology is depicted in Fig. 76.4 and is a spermatocytic tumor. Abdominal and chest CT are negative. Serum markers are normal. The patient should be advised to:

a. receive radiation to the retroperitoneum.

b. receive one cycle of chemotherapy.

c. have a biopsy of the contralateral testis.

d. not have any treatment.

e. have a PET-CT scan.

5. A 20-year-old man has a right radical orchiectomy. The pathology is depicted in Fig. 76.5 and is read as embryonal carcinoma. His hCG and AFP values are elevated and a CT of abdomen and chest reveals no evidence of metastatic disease. Three weeks later, repeat AFP and hCG testing show no change in either marker. The patient should be advised to:

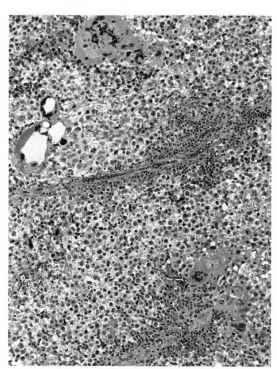

Fig. 76.3 (From Bostwick DG, Cheng L: *Urologic surgical pathology*, ed 2, Edinburgh, 2008, Mosby.)

a. have induction chemotherapy.

b. have an RPLND.

c. have a PET-CT.

d. receive radiotherapy below the diaphragm.

e. repeat the hCG and AFP tests in another month.

6. A 25-year-old man has a right radical orchiectomy. The histology is depicted in Fig. 76.6 and is reported as a mature teratoma. The patient's AFP is slightly elevated and bHCG is negative;

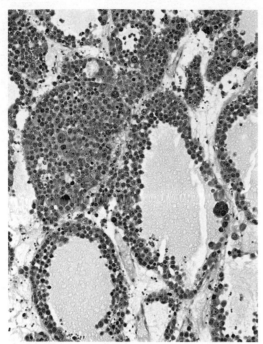

Fig. 76.4 (From Bostwick DG, Cheng L: *Urologic surgical pathology*, ed 2, Edinburgh, 2008, Mosby.)

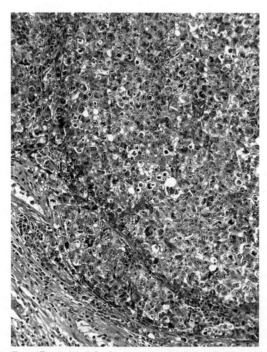

Fig. 76.5 (From Bostwick DG, Cheng L: *Urologic surgical pathology*, ed 2, Edinburgh, 2008, Mosby.)

however, there is a 3-cm mass in the retroperitoneum on CT. He is given chemotherapy and the mass shrinks to 1.8 cm. The patient should be advised to:

a. have a retroperitoneal lymphadenectomy dissection (RPLND).

b. have salvage chemotherapy.

c. get an FDG-PET scan.

d. receive radiation therapy.

e. be observed.

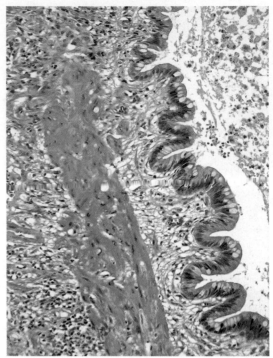

Fig. 76.6 (From Bostwick DG, Cheng L: *Urologic surgical pathology*, ed 2, Edinburgh, 2008, Mosby.)

IMAGING

1. A 36-year-old man noted a firm left scrotal mass. He was hit in the groin 1 month earlier with a tennis ball. Currently he has no pain, fever, or chills. The testicular ultrasound image is depicted in Fig. 76.7. The most likely diagnosis is:

   a. ruptured testis with peritesticular hematoma.

   b. testicular neoplasm.

   c. epidermoid cyst.

   d. dilated rete testis.

   e. testicular abscess.

2. A 32-year-old man had a left radical orchiectomy. Pathologic evaluation reveals a mixed GCT containing seminoma and embryonal cell carcinoma. Tumor markers are negative. The CT image depicted in Fig. 76.8 was obtained 1-day postoperation. Chest CT is negative. The next step in management is:

   a. biopsy.

   b. radiation therapy.

   c. chemotherapy.

   d. RPLND.

   e. repeat CT in 1 week to confirm a postsurgical inflammatory response.

ANSWERS

1. **d. Spermatocytic tumor.** GCNIS is the common precursor lesion for all types of adult male GCT with the exception of spermatocytic tumor. Pediatric GCTs do not typically arise from GCNIS.

2. **e. Metastatic spermatocytic tumor is rare.** Spermatocytic tumor differs from other GCT subtypes in that it does not arise from GCNIS, cryptorchidism is not a risk factor, bilaterality has not been reported, it does not express i(12p) or placental alkaline phosphatase, and it does not occur as a mixed GCT with

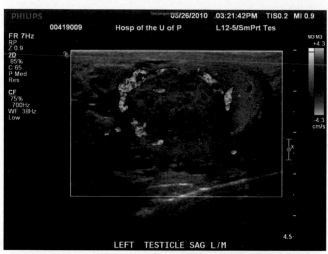

Fig. 76.7

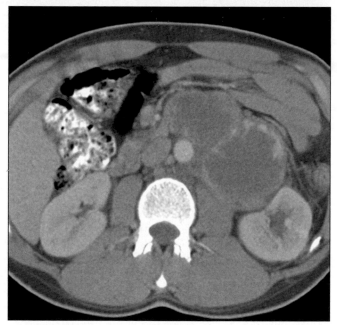

Fig. 76.8

other GCT subtypes. Only one documented case of metastasis has been reported, and these lesions are almost always cured by orchiectomy.

3. **a. Choriocarcinoma.** With the exception of choriocarcinoma, the most common route of disease dissemination is via lymphatic channels from the primary tumor to the retroperitoneal lymph nodes and subsequently to distant sites. Choriocarcinoma has a propensity for hematogenous dissemination. Yolk sac tumors in children are thought to spread hematogenously as well.

4. **c. Pure embryonal carcinoma.** Pure embryonal carcinoma may produce both AFP and hCG. Pure seminoma is associated with elevated serum hCG levels in 15% of cases but does not produce AFP. Pure teratoma typically is not associated with elevated serum tumor markers, although slightly elevated AFP levels may be observed. Choriocarcinoma is uniformly associated with elevated hCG levels but does not produce AFP. Most yolk sac tumors produce AFP, but they do not produce hCG.

5. **b. Suspected benign testicular lesion.** Testis-sparing surgery should be considered only in patients with suspected GCT who have normal testicular androgen production and who have a small (<2 cm) tumor either in a solitary testis or in the setting of bilateral synchronous testicular GCT. Testis-sparing surgery

should not be performed in patients with suspected GCT who have a normal contralateral testis. Testis-sparing surgery may also be considered in patients with suspected benign testicular lesions such as an epidermoid cyst or adenomatoid tumor arising from the tunica albuginea.

6. **d. To obtain repeat serum tumor marker levels in 7 days.** Patients with elevated serum tumor markers before orchiectomy should have these levels measured after orchiectomy to assess whether the levels are declining, stable, or rising. Management decisions should not be made based on serum tumor marker levels before orchiectomy. Patients with rising postorchiectomy serum tumor marker levels should receive chemotherapy. The IGCCCG classification of metastatic NSGCT is based on the postorchiectomy serum tumor marker levels.

7. **a. Testicular seminoma with brain metastases.** According to IGCCCG classification criteria, there is no "poor risk" category for metastatic seminoma. Patients with metastatic seminoma who have nonpulmonary visceral metastases (e.g., liver, bone, brain) are classified as at intermediate risk. Metastatic NSGCT patients with mediastinal primary tumor *or* nonpulmonary visceral metastases *or* postorchiectomy AFP >10,000 ng/mL, *or* postorchiectomy hCG of 50,000 mU/mL are classified as at poor risk.

8. **c. Mediastinoscopy and biopsy.** The presence of distant metastasis in the absence of retroperitoneal disease or elevated serum levels of tumor markers is uncommon, particularly for patients with testicular seminoma. Therefore, these patients should undergo biopsy and histologic confirmation of the suspected lesion before management decisions are made.

9. **b. CT-guided biopsy of the retroperitoneal mass.** The risk of teratoma at metastatic sites is less of a consideration for metastatic seminoma than for NSGCT. Although rare, seminoma may transform into NSGCT elements, and this should be considered in patients with metastatic seminoma who fail to respond to conventional therapy. These patients should undergo biopsy and histologic confirmation of the suspected lesion before management decisions are made. Either an open or a laparoscopic biopsy of the para-aortic mass is an acceptable approach if CT-guided biopsy is not feasible or the result is nondiagnostic. However, an RPLND should not be performed without histologic confirmation of NSGCT pathology.

10. **a. Inguinal orchiectomy.** Inguinal orchiectomy and low-dose radiation therapy are associated with the highest rates of local control of GCNIS. In a patient with a normal contralateral testis (particularly if future paternity is desired), inguinal orchiectomy is the preferred choice owing to the deleterious effects of radiation therapy on spermatogenesis within the contralateral testis.

11. **d. Elevated preorchiectomy AFP level.** Preorchiectomy serum tumor marker levels are not associated with the presence of occult metastases in clinical stage I NSGCT. The presence of postorchiectomy serum tumor marker levels in clinical stage I NSGCT indicates the presence of occult systemic disease.

12. **c. Chemotherapy with one cycle of bleomycin-etoposide-cisplatin.** Chemotherapy is associated with the lowest risk of recurrence and is thus preferred versus surveillance for patients who are anticipated to be noncompliant with surveillance imaging and testing (even for patients at low risk for occult metastases). Chemotherapy and RPLND are associated with similar rates of long-term cure, but the former may be preferable in patients with transmissible diseases. Adjuvant radiation therapy and carboplatin are standard treatment approaches for clinical stage I seminoma.

13. **e. Lymphovascular invasion.** Absence of teratoma in the primary tumor, prechemotherapy and postchemotherapy mass size, and percentage shrinkage of mass with chemotherapy are all associated with the presence of necrosis/fibrosis in residual masses after first-line chemotherapy. However, none of these factors (alone or together) is sufficiently accurate to exclude the presence of residual teratoma or viable malignancy in patients with residual masses greater than 1 cm. Lymphovascular invasion is associated with the presence of occult

metastases in patients with clinical stage I NSGCT and has no impact on the histology of residual masses after chemotherapy.

14. **d. Observation.** Patients at low risk for metastatic disease with indeterminate CT findings should be closely observed because small (<1 cm) retroperitoneal lesions may represent false-positive findings, particularly if they are located outside the primary landing zone. A CT-guided biopsy would be technically difficult to perform, given the lesion size and its proximity to the renal vessels.

15. **b. Lymphovascular invasion.** Lymphovascular invasion is associated with the presence of occult metastases in patients with clinical stage I NSGCT, but it has not been associated with an increased risk of distant metastases in patients with clinical or pathologic stage II disease. Elevated postorchiectomy serum tumor markers, bulky (>3 cm) retroperitoneal masses, or retroperitoneal lymphadenopathy outside the primary landing zone are associated with an increased risk of systemic relapse after RPLND. Thus, clinical stage IIA-B patients with these features are recommended to receive induction chemotherapy. Scrotal invasion by the primary tumor is associated with an increased risk of metastasis to the inguinal lymph nodes, which are considered nonregional lymph nodes.

16. **d. Poor-risk disease at diagnosis by IGCCCG criteria.** Although patients with poor-risk GCT have diminished survival and are more likely to have viable malignancy or incomplete resection at postchemotherapy RPLND, IGCCCG risk category is not a predictor of relapse independent of the histology of resected masses or completeness of resection. "Desperation" postchemotherapy RPLND in the setting of rising serum tumor markers after second- or third-line chemotherapy and reoperative RPLND are other conditions associated with an increased risk of relapse.

17. **c. Bilateral postchemotherapy RPLND.** Approximately one third of patients will have residual masses at multiple anatomic sites, and these patients should undergo resection of all sites of measurable residual disease because discordant histology between anatomic sites is reported in 22% to 46% of cases. However, the presence of necrosis in postchemotherapy RPLND specimens is highly predictive of necrosis at other sites. Thus, postchemotherapy RPLND should be performed before resection of residual masses at other sites. Observation of small residual masses at other sites is a reasonable option if the histology of the RPLND specimen is necrosis. Patients with viable malignancy discovered at postchemotherapy resection should have all residual masses resected and are usually treated with an additional two cycles of chemotherapy. A full course of second-line chemotherapy is reserved for patients with either serologic or radiographic progression during or after first-line chemotherapy.

18. **e. The outcome is poor relative to those with early NSGCT relapse.** Until recently, late relapse has been associated with a worse prognosis than early relapse, although more recent data suggest these patient groups have a similar probability of cure. Disease-free rates of 50% to 60% are reported after treatment of early and late relapse.

19. **b. CT-guided biopsy of the para-aortic mass.** Patients with good-risk metastatic NSGCT who have dramatic progression of their disease with first-line chemotherapy despite normalization of serum tumor marker levels should be considered to have either growing teratoma syndrome or teratoma with malignant transformation. The presence of an enlarging solid mass and new sites of disease suggest a malignant process. An enlarging mass only with cystic appearance is more suggestive of growing teratoma syndrome. A CT-guided biopsy to identify the presence of malignant transformation is indicated because this finding may influence the choice of chemotherapy.

20. **e. Similar efficacy to cisplatin.** All of the randomized trials in advanced GCT in which a cisplatin-based regimen has been compared with a carboplatin-based regimen have reported superior outcomes with cisplatin. The rationale for single-agent carboplatin is based on reduced toxicity compared with cisplatin and 65% to 90% response rates reported in studies of carboplatin in advanced seminoma.

21. **d. Ejaculatory dysfunction.** Dog-leg radiotherapy for clinical stage I seminoma is associated with infertility due to the direct effects of radiation on the germinal epithelium with resultant impaired spermatogenesis. Infertility related to ejaculatory dysfunction is not associated with radiation therapy and is most commonly associated with RPLND.

22. **a. Utility of serum tumor markers to identify relapse at an early and curable stage.** Only 15% of seminomas produce elevations in serum hCG, and serum tumor marker levels are uncommonly elevated in most patients with clinical stage I seminoma at diagnosis or at the time of relapse. This contrasts to clinical stage I NSGCT, in which serum tumor markers are commonly the first (and only) manifestation of disease relapse.

23. **c. Observation.** In contrast to advanced NSGCT, only 10% of residual masses in advanced seminoma after first-line chemotherapy contain viable malignancy (90% contain fibrosis/necrosis only), and residual teratoma is less of a consideration. Spontaneous resolution of these masses will occur in most cases. Approximately 30% of discrete residual masses greater than 3 cm will contain viable malignancy. FDG-PET is a useful adjunct to postchemotherapy staging CT to determine the need for postchemotherapy surgical resection. Residual masses larger than 3 cm that are PET negative and those less than 3 cm can be safely observed because of the high probability of necrosis/fibrosis. FDG-PET has no role in the characterization of residual masses less than 3 cm.

24. **d. CT of the head.** Choriocarcinoma spreads hematogenously and widely. Brain metastases should be suspected in any patient with a very high hCG level. Thus, patients with high hCG levels at diagnosis should have staging CT or magnetic resonance imaging (MRI) studies of the brain. Choriocarcinomas are highly vascular and tend to hemorrhage during chemotherapy, which may have catastrophic consequences in those patients with brain metastases. Brain metastases are also associated with a poor prognosis, and these patients should receive four cycles of bleomycin-etoposide-cisplatin as first-line chemotherapy, as should any patient with an hCG level over 5000 mU/mL at the time chemotherapy is initiated.

25. **a. Two cycles of platin-based chemotherapy do not increase one's risk of developing cardiovascular disease or secondary malignant neoplasm (SMN).** Although the risk of late complications of chemotherapy is dose dependent, there appears to be no safe lower limit. Thus, even patients receiving one to two cycles of platin-based chemotherapy may have an increased risk of late toxicity.

26. **b. i and iii.** Unlike GCT, Leydig cell tumors are not associated with a history of cryptorchidism, and bilateral tumors have not been reported.

27. **a. Inguinal orchiectomy followed by adjuvant radiotherapy.** A large infiltrative mass involving the spermatic cord in an adult man is a sarcoma until proved otherwise. The low-intensity signal on CT and patient age make liposarcoma the most common histology. Paratesticular liposarcomas rarely metastasize but tend to recur locally. Thus, adjuvant radiotherapy may be used to decrease the risk of local recurrence.

PATHOLOGY

1. **b. Has a significant chance of developing a germ cell tumor in the left testis.** The figure illustrates germ cell neoplasia in situ as evidenced by enlarged hyperchromatic nuclei and a lack of a spermatogenesis. This carries a 50% risk of developing a germ cell tumor.

2. **d. Be advised to have radiation therapy to the retroperitoneum.** Notice in the figure the sheathlike pattern of small cells interspersed with fibrous septa that contain lymphocytes, the hallmarks of seminoma. Although observation is an option, most would recommend radiation to the retroperitoneum, because seminoma is very sensitive to radiation and the morbidity

is low—although there is a risk for the development of secondary malignancies over the long term.

3. **a. Follow markers and check half-life.** The figure demonstrates seminoma with syncytiotrophoblasts. Approximately 15% of patients with seminoma have elevated hCG and will demonstrate syncytiotrophoblasts. Following orchiectomy, the hCG should decline according to its 24-hour half-life. This should be determined first before any treatment decisions are made.

4. **d. Not have any treatment.** The figure shows a spermatocytic tumor that has a very low malignant potential. Notice the small basophilic cells and the multinucleated tumor giant cell, which are characteristic for spermatocytic tumor.

5. **a. Have induction chemotherapy.** This patient has an embryonal carcinoma: notice the primitive, anaplastic epithelial cells. With persistently elevated serum markers, the patient should undergo induction chemotherapy. Surgery is not indicated, radiation therapy is inappropriate, and there is no reason to delay.

6. **a. Have an retroperitoneal lymphadenectomy dissection (RPLND).** The tumor depicted is a teratoma: notice the mature enteric epithelium. Because the specimen is in the primary tumor, there is a high likelihood that there is residual teratoma in the retroperitoneal mass. This tumor is chemoinsensitive and should be resected.

IMAGING

1. **b. Testicular neoplasm.** The ultrasound image shows an irregular vascular mass in the left testis that also has microlithiasis. This is most consistent with a testicular neoplasm. It is not unusual for patients to have a history of groin trauma before presentation.

2. **c. Chemotherapy.** The CT image shows a large (>5 cm) para-aortic mass that represents metastatic adenopathy. Because this represents bulky retroperitoneal disease (stage IIC), chemotherapy is the best option.

CHAPTER REVIEW

1. GCTs occur bilaterally approximately 2% of the time. The risk factors for developing GCTs include cryptorchidism, a family history of testicular cancer, a previous history of testicular cancer, and GCNIS.

2. In men with a history of GCTs, the finding of testicular microlithiasis on ultrasonography in the contralateral testis is associated with an increased risk of intratubular germ cell neoplasia; the significance of microlithiasis in the general population, however, is unclear.

3. One percent to five percent of GCTs are extragonadal; they are generally less sensitive to chemotherapy and are more likely to contain yolk sac tumor elements than tumors arising in the testis.

4. On rare occasion, teratomas may transform into somatic malignancies, such as rhabdomyosarcoma, adenocarcinoma, or neuroendocrine tumors.

5. Two-thirds of patients with GCTs have diminished fertility.

6. Choriocarcinomas and seminomas do not produce AFP.

7. The half-life of AFP is 5 to 7 days, hCG is 24 to 36 hours, and LDH is 24 hours.

8. The primary landing zone in the retroperitoneum for right testicular tumors is the interaortocaval lymph nodes; for left testicular tumors, it is the periaortic lymph nodes; the pattern of lymph drainage in the retroperitoneum is from right to left.

9. Patients with persistently elevated AFP and hCG after orchiectomy are given induction chemotherapy.

10. In clinical stage I disease, approximately 25% of patients will have metastases.

11. Lymphovascular invasion and a prominent component of embryonal carcinoma are risk factors for metastases in NSGCTs.

12. In seminomas, risk factors for metastases are rete testis involvement and tumor size greater than 4 cm.

13. Patients with bulky retroperitoneal lymph node disease greater than 3 cm should receive induction chemotherapy.

14. After initial treatment, patients with enlargement of a retroperitoneal mass or an increase in markers should undergo salvage chemotherapy. Consideration may be given to a CT-guided biopsy under selected circumstances.

15. Patients with an NSGCT, undetectable markers, and a residual mass greater than 1 cm after chemotherapy should undergo surgical resection.

16. Approximately half of those patients who have surgical resection of a retroperitoneal mass following chemotherapy will harbor teratoma or a viable malignancy. The remainder will have fibrosis.

17. Patients with viable malignancy in residual masses after salvage chemotherapy have a poor prognosis.

18. Predictors of relapse in patients with stage I seminoma on surveillance include rete testis invasion and size of tumor greater than 4 cm. Lymphovascular invasion is not predictive as it is in NSGCT.

19. In patients with seminomas who are treated with chemotherapy, the size of the residual mass is highly predictive of viable tumor. Masses less than 3 cm rarely have viable tumor in them, whereas about a third of residual masses greater than 3 cm contain viable malignancy. FDG-PET is a useful adjunct to postchemotherapy staging CT to determine the need for postchemotherapy surgical resection. Residual masses larger than 3 cm that are PET negative and those less than 3 cm can be safely observed because of the high probability of necrosis/fibrosis.

20. Late toxicity of chemotherapy includes peripheral neuropathy, Raynaud phenomenon, hearing loss, hypogonadism and infertility, secondary malignant neoplasms, and cardiovascular disease.

21. There is an increased number of copies of genetic material from the short arm of chromosome 12 in germ cell tumors.

22. There is no clinical distinction between immature and mature teratoma. Teratomas are resistant to chemotherapy. They also tend to be infiltrative when large and can be extremely difficult to resect.

23. Of patients with testicular tumors, 52% are oligospermic and 10% are azoospermic at presentation.

24. Of patients who receive radiation as treatment for intratubular germ cell neoplasia, 40% require testosterone supplementation.

25. The risk for a secondary malignancy after radiation therapy for seminoma is 18% at 25 years.

26. Ninety percent of Leydig cell tumors and Sertoli cell tumors are benign and 10% are malignant.

27. The most common testicular neoplasm in men older than 50 years is lymphoma.

28. Cystadenoma of the epididymis is associated with von Hippel-Lindau syndrome; adenomatoid tumor of the epididymis is benign.

29. Liposarcoma is the most common paratesticular tumor in the adult. Rhabdomyosarcoma is the most common paratesticular tumor in the child.

30. GCNIS is the common precursor lesion for all types of adult male GCT, with the exception of spermatocytic tumor.

CHAPTER REVIEW—cont'd

31. Choriocarcinoma has a propensity for hematogenous dissemination. Yolk sac tumors in children are thought to spread hematogenously as well.

32. Pure embryonal carcinoma may produce both AFP and hCG. Pure seminoma is associated with elevated serum hCG levels in 15% of cases but does not produce AFP. Pure teratoma typically is not associated with elevated serum tumor markers, although slightly elevated AFP levels may be observed. Choriocarcinoma is uniformly associated with elevated hCG levels but does not produce AFP. Most yolk sac tumors produce AFP, but they do not produce hCG.

33. Testis-sparing surgery should be considered only in patients with suspected GCT who have normal testicular androgen production and who have a small (<2 cm) tumor either in a solitary testis or in the setting of bilateral synchronous testicular GCT. Testis-sparing surgery should not be performed in patients with suspected GCT who have a normal contralateral testis. Testis-sparing surgery may also be considered in patients with suspected benign testicular lesions such as an epidermoid cyst or adenomatoid tumor arising from the tunica albuginea.

34. Absence of teratoma in the primary tumor, prechemotherapy and postchemotherapy mass size, and percentage shrinkage of mass with chemotherapy are all associated with the presence of necrosis/fibrosis in residual masses after first-line chemotherapy. However, none of these factors (alone or together) is sufficiently accurate to exclude the presence of residual teratoma or viable malignancy in patients with residual masses greater than 1 cm.

35. Approximately one-third of patients who have residual masses following chemotherapy will have residual masses at multiple anatomic sites (sites outside the retroperitoneum), and these patients should undergo resection of all sites of measurable residual disease because discordant histology between anatomic sites is reported in 22% to 46% of cases. However, the presence of necrosis in postchemotherapy RPLND specimens is highly predictive of necrosis at other sites outside the retroperitoneum.

77 Surgery of Testicular Tumors

Stephen Riggs, Kris E. Gaston, and Peter E. Clark

QUESTIONS

1. Which of the following nerves is at risk for injury during radical orchiectomy?
   a. Genitofemoral nerve
   b. Ilioinguinal nerve
   c. Obturator nerve
   d. Lateral femoral cutaneous nerve
   e. Pudendal nerve

2. Which of the following may be an indication to consider partial orchiectomy for a patient with a testicular mass?
   a. A polar tumor less than 2 cm in greatest dimension
   b. A normal contralateral testicle
   c. Hypogonadism
   d. Suspicion for benign tumor
   e. Infertility

3. Critical elements to clinically staging testicular cancer routinely include all of the following EXCEPT:
   a. radical orchiectomy
   b. chest radiograph
   c. whole-body positron emission tomography (PET) scan
   d. serum α-fetoprotein (AFP), human chorionic gonadotropin (hCG), and lactate dehydrogenase (LDH)
   e. contrasted computed tomography (CT) scan of the abdomen and pelvis

4. The incidence of perioperative acute respiratory distress syndrome (ARDS) in patients with prior receipt of bleomycin can be minimized by all of the following EXCEPT:
   a. avoidance of the Trendelenburg position
   b. keeping the FiO_2 as low as possible
   c. minimization of intraoperative fluid resuscitation
   d. minimization of postoperative fluid resuscitation
   e. three cycles of Bleomycin rather than four

5. Performing the aortic split-and-roll before that of the inferior vena cava (IVC):
   a. allows prospective identification of right accessory lower pole renal arteries not identified on preoperative imaging.
   b. facilitates identification of right-sided postganglionic sympathetic nerves as they cross over the aorta.
   c. minimizes risk of left ureteral injury.
   d. increases risk if injury to the inferior mesenteric artery.
   e. should never be performed.

6. The ureter is typically located:
   a. anterior to the ipsilateral renal artery.
   b. anterior to the ipsilateral retroperitoneal nodal packet.
   c. posterior to the ipsilateral gonadal vein adjacent to the lower pole of the ipsilateral kidney.
   d. anterior to the ipsilateral gonadal vein adjacent to the lower pole of the ipsilateral kidney.
   e. posterior to the ipsilateral common iliac artery.

7. Which of the following anatomic structures demonstrates the most predictable and constant anatomy?
   a. Postganglionic sympathetic nerve fibers
   b. Lumbar arteries
   c. Lumbar veins
   d. Number of nodes in each retroperitoneal packet
   e. Lymphatic vessels

8. The cisterna chylae is located:
   a. immediately posterolateral to the IVC, just cephalad to the right renal artery.
   b. immediately posterolateral to the IVC, just inferior to the right renal artery.
   c. immediately posterolateral to the aorta, just cephalad to the left renal artery.
   d. immediately posterolateral to the aorta, just inferior to the left renal artery.
   e. immediately posteromedial to the aorta, just cephalad to the right renal artery.

9. The most common auxiliary procedure required to ensure complete resection of residual tumor at postchemotherapy retroperitoneal lymph node dissection (PC)-RPLND is:
   a. IVC resection.
   b. retrocrural resection.
   c. nephrectomy.
   d. pelvic resection.
   e. aortic resection.

10. All of the following are associated with an increased risk of nephrectomy EXCEPT:
    a. Left-sided primary testicular tumor
    b. Prior receipt of salvage chemotherapy
    c. Larger retroperitoneal mass size
    d. Presence of ipsilateral accessory lower pole renal arteries
    e. Elevated serum tumor markers (STMs) at PC-RPLND

11. The histology encountered most often at resection of residual hepatic lesions after chemotherapy is:
    a. viable malignancy.
    b. teratoma.
    c. fibrosis/necrosis.
    d. somatic-type malignancy.
    e. hemangioma.

12. All of the following are associated with an increased risk of pelvic germ cell tumor (GCT) metastases EXCEPT:
    a. prior groin surgery.
    b. late relapse.
    c. require repeat RPLND.
    d. congenital absence of the vasa deferentia.
    e. prior chemotherapy.

13. All of the following are patient selection criteria for a unilateral modified template PC-RPLND (rather than full bilateral template) EXCEPT:
    a. normal STMs.
    b. International Germ Cell Cancer Collaborative Group (IGCCCG), good risk only.
    c. IGCCCG good or intermediate risk.
    d. residual mass less than 5 cm.
    e. well-defined mass confined to the primary landing zone before and after chemotherapy.

14. With regard to the use of postoperative adjuvant cisplatin-based chemotherapy in patients demonstrating pathologic stage IIA-B disease at primary RPLND, all of the following are true EXCEPT:
    a. it spares one to two cycles of chemotherapy for those patients destined to recur on postoperative observation.
    b. it nearly eliminates postoperative recurrences.
    c. it improves overall and cancer-specific survival.
    d. it results in overtreatment of 50% to 70% of patients if given to all patients.
    e. it is typically given in two cycles.

15. Which of the following characteristics has been associated with increased recurrence rate when teratoma is encountered at PC-RPLND?
    a. Extranodal extension
    b. Presence of somatic type malignancy
    c. Right-sided primary GCT
    d. Presence of immature teratoma
    e. Number of lymph nodes removed

16. All of the following factors have been associated with worse prognosis when viable GCT is encountered at PC-RPLND EXCEPT:
    a. incomplete resection.
    b. less than 10% viable GCT in resection specimen.
    c. IGCCCG intermediate or poor risk status.
    d. prior receipt of salvage chemotherapy.
    e. immature teratoma in the specimen.

17. Which of the following criteria is an accepted indication for two cycles of adjuvant chemotherapy after primary RPLND?
    a. Number of positive nodes relative to the number removed
    b. Teratoma only nodal metastases
    c. Extranodal extension of GCT
    d. pN1 disease or higher
    e. pN2 disease or higher

18. A patient has an isolated resectable residual retroperitoneal mass after induction chemotherapy without radiographic evidence of disease outside the retroperitoneum, but tumor markers have failed to normalize. All of the following are reasonable indications for the consideration of desperation RPLND EXCEPT:
    a. declining AFP after induction chemotherapy.
    b. slowly rising AFP after a complete serologic response to induction chemotherapy.
    c. all potentially curative chemotherapeutic options have been exhausted.
    d. persistently rising STMs through induction chemotherapy.
    e. plateauing AFP after induction chemotherapy.

19. Reoperative RPLND is thought to indicate a technical failure at prior RPLND. All of the following findings supportive of this hypothesis have been reported in the literature EXCEPT:

    a. the primary landing zone is the most common site of retroperitoneal recurrence.
    b. ipsilateral pelvic recurrences are common.
    c. incomplete ipsilateral lumbar vessel ligation encountered at reoperative RPLND has been associated with ipsilateral in-field recurrence.
    d. unresected ipsilateral gonadal vessels are frequently encountered at reoperative RPLND.
    e. the retroaortic and retrocaval regions are frequent sites of recurrence.

20. All of the following are true regarding late relapse of GCT EXCEPT:
    a. yolk sac tumor is the most common viable histology encountered.
    b. first-line treatment is generally systemic chemotherapy followed by consolidative PC-RPLND.
    c. patients who are chemotherapy-naïve demonstrate superior survival outcomes.
    d. GCT with somatic-type malignancy is seen with increased frequency in this population.
    e. the retroperitoneum is the most common site of late relapse.

21. What percentage of patients presenting with GCT have abnormal parameters on semen analysis?
    a. Less than 10%
    b. 20% to 60%
    c. 70% to 80%
    d. Greater than 90%

22. The processes required to ensure antegrade ejaculation of sperm-containing semen include all of the following EXCEPT:
    a. seminal emission through vasa deferentia.
    b. closure of the bladder neck.
    c. smooth muscle contraction of the prostate.
    d. penile erection.
    e. input from sympathetic fibers arising from L1 to L4.

23. All of the following interventions have demonstrated efficacy in managing chylous ascites EXCEPT:
    a. medium-chain triglyceride (MCT) diet.
    b. total parenteral nutrition.
    c. subcutaneous octreotide.
    d. limiting fat intake preoperatively.
    e. placement of peritoneovenous shunt.

24. Which of the following patients is at the greatest risk for neurologic compromise due to spinal ischemia?
    a. 32-year-old male undergoing resection of left para-aortic mass with apparent aortic invasion who will most likely require resection of the infrahilar aorta and tube graft reconstruction
    b. 29-year-old male with large-volume left para-aortic and interaortocaval masses that extend through the retrocrural region into the middle visceral mediastinum
    c. 27-year-old male with a completed occluded IVC due to large interaortocaval, retrocaval, and right paracaval masses with a tumor thrombus up the inferior border of the right renal vein
    d. 31-year-old male with a large infrarenal left para-aortic mass that is found to be invading the L2 vertebral foramina during resection

ANSWERS

1. **b. Ilioinguinal nerve.** The ilioinguinal nerve will be encountered immediately on opening the external oblique fascia and entering the inguinal canal. It courses parallel to the spermatic cord along the cephalad aspect of its anterior surface. Care should be taken to preserve this structure in order to prevent postoperative numbness and paresthesia of the ipsilateral medial thigh and scrotum.

2. **d. Suspicion for benign tumor.** For obvious reasons, patients who are suspected to have a benign tumor are prime candidates for partial orchiectomy. Patients with larger tumors in the setting of normal contralateral testicle should be managed with radical orchiectomy as they will not likely suffer permanent postoperative infertility or hypogonadism. In addition, the benefits of partial orchiectomy with the goal of saving poorly functioning testicular parenchyma in a patient with baseline infertility and/or hypogonadism are most likely outweighed by the potential for incomplete resection of tumor and/or ipsilateral testicular recurrence.

3. **c. Whole-body positron emission tomography (PET) scan.** Testicular GCT patients are clinically staged with radical orchiectomy (T stage), chest imaging such as a chest X-ray or Chest CT scan, a CT scan or magnetic resonance imaging (MRI) of the abdomen and pelvis (N and M stages), and postorchiectomy STMs (S stage). PET scans have no role in the initial clinical staging of seminomas or nonseminomas. PET scans do have a role in evaluating postchemotherapy residual masses in cases of pure seminoma that are over 3 cm in size.

4. **a. Avoidance of the Trendelenburg position.** Postoperative ARDS in patients with prior receipt of bleomycin is rare but most commonly encountered in patients having received four courses of bleomycin (rather than three) with significant pulmonary tumor burden. The two intraoperative/perioperative factors that have been associated with an increased risk of developing postoperative ARDS have been (1) exposure to high FiO_2 and (2) high-volume administration of intravenous fluids and blood products. Anesthesiologists should be made aware of these risk factors.

5. **a. Allows prospective identification of right accessory lower pole renal arteries not identified on preoperative imaging.** The advantage of splitting of the aorta before the IVC is that it allows for the prospective identification of right accessory lower pole renal arteries not identified on preoperative imaging. Such vessels may be inadvertently divided if the IVC split is performed first. This can lead to significant blood loss and renal parenchymal loss. The disadvantage of splitting of the aorta first is inadvertent division of postganglionic sympathetic fibers involved in ejaculation. This can be minimized by stopping the aortic split at the inferior mesenteric artery and prospectively identifying the sympathetic efferents before continuing the split caudally.

6. **c. Posterior to the ipsilateral gonadal vein adjacent to the lower pole of the ipsilateral kidney.** The ureters provide the anatomic landmark for the lateral border of dissection for the para-aortic and paracaval lymph node packets. However, the ureters are vulnerable to injury if not prospectively identified. The ureter can be easily found at the inferior border of the ipsilateral kidney where it typically passes behind the ipsilateral gonadal vein. The ureter passes anterior to the ipsilateral common iliac artery as it descends into the pelvis.

7. **b. Lumbar arteries.** There are three paired lumbar arteries located between the renal hilum and the aortic bifurcation in nearly all patients. The only subtle anomaly commonly encountered with aortic lumbars is that the paired lumbars may exit the aorta through a short common trunk before bifurcating, a variant that can result in significant blood loss if not identified before these structures are ligated and divided. Lumbar vein anatomy is high variable, with these structures varying widely in location and caliber. While the number of postganglionic

sympathetic roots in the field of RPLND tends to be relatively constant at four per side, the exact locations, paths, and patterns of fusion to adjacent roots is highly variable. Studies on lymph node counts have universally reported high standards of deviation and interquartile ranges.

8. **e. Immediately posteromedial to the aorta just cephalad to the right renal artery.** Failure to meticulously ligate large-caliber lymphatics in the region of the cisterna chylae can predispose patients to troublesome postoperative chylous ascites. Thus the use of clips and/or ties at the superior extent of the interaortocaval and para-aortic packets, as well as during retrocrural dissections, is advised.

9. **c. Nephrectomy.** The incidence of auxiliary procedures at the time of PC-RPLND ranges between 23% and 45% in the literature. The most common auxiliary procedure is nephrectomy followed by vascular interventions. The larger the volume of the residual retroperitoneal mass, the greater the need for possible auxiliary procedures.

10. **d. Presence of ipsilateral accessory lower pole renal arteries.** Reported nephrectomy rates at PC-RPLND have ranged from 5% to 31%. Increased nephrectomy rates have been reported for patients undergoing salvage RPLND, desperation RPLND, reoperative RPLND, and resection of late relapse. In addition, large retroperitoneal mass size and left-sided primary tumors are associated with increased rates of nephrectomy.

11. **c. Fibrosis/necrosis.** Approximately three quarters of residual hepatic lesions after chemotherapy will demonstrate fibrosis/necrosis only at resection. There is a 94% concordance between retroperitoneal and hepatic fibrosis/necrosis. Thus observation should be considered in patients with retroperitoneal necrosis and residual hepatic lesions that would require a potentially morbid resection.

12. **d. Congenital absence of the vasa deferentia.** Although the pelvis is the caudal extension of the retroperitoneum, it is not a common site of GCT metastases. Pelvic disease in metastatic testes cancer is rarely observed outside of prior groin surgery, repeat RPLND, or late relapsed disease. Data from Indiana University from 1990 to 2009 identified 2722 patients who underwent RPLND, of which 134 had pelvic disease—14% had prior groin surgery, 98% had prior chemotherapy, 19.4% underwent prior RPLND, and 24% had late stage relapse.

13. **b. International Germ Cell Cancer Collaborative Group (IGCCCG), good risk only.** The application of modified unilateral templates in the setting of PC-RPLND is critically reliant on proper patient selection. While no universal consensus exists, based on the reports to date patients who are potential candidates for modified template PC-RPLND should probably meet the following criteria. (1) Well-defined lesion measuring 5 cm or less confined to the primary landing zone of the primary tumor on imaging before and after chemotherapy (see Fig. 77.1 for representative CT examples). (2) Normal STMs. (3) IGCCCG good or intermediate risk. Following selection criteria similar to these has been reported in PC-RPLND with excellent local control, including in-field retroperitoneal recurrence rates of 0% to 1% and cancer specific survival rates of 98% to 100% at a follow-up of 2.6 to 10.4 years, while maintaining antegrade ejaculation in over 85% of men.

14. **c. Improves overall and cancer-specific survival.** Adjuvant chemotherapy for pathologic stage IIA-B disease encountered at primary RPLND consists of two cycles of bleomycin, etoposide, and cisplatin (BEP) or two cycles of etoposide and cisplatin (EP). This nearly eliminates the risk of recurrence but has no effect on cancer-specific survival, which approaches 100% whether chemotherapy is administered in the adjuvant setting or reserved for patients who experience relapse. Patients who relapse will require full induction chemotherapy consisting of BEP×3 or EP×4. When pathologic stage IIA-B patients are observed after primary RPLND, approximately 30% to 50% of patients relapse.

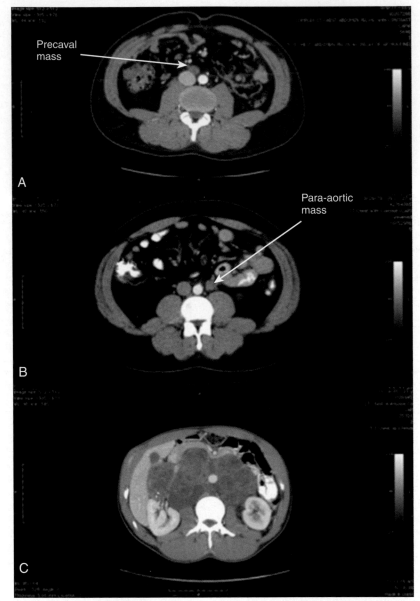

Precaval mass

Para-aortic mass

A

B

C

Fig. 77.1 Computed tomography images of postchemotherapy residual retroperitoneal masses. (A) This patient could be considered a candidate for modified right template postchemotherapy retroperitoneal lymph node dissection (PC-RPLND). (B) This patient could be considered a candidate for modified left template PC-RPLND. (C) This patient would require an extensive bilateral PC-RPLND.

15. **b. Presence of somatic type malignancy.** Patients with somatic-type malignancy and mediastinal primary GCT disease have a higher risk of postoperative recurrence. Although once thought to be a marker of more aggressive behavior, immature teratoma has demonstrated no decrement in survival outcomes compared with mature teratoma. Laterality, number of nodes removed, and extranodal extension have not been shown to have any relationship to the risk of relapse in the setting of teratoma only residual disease after PC-RPLND.

16. **e. Immature teratoma in the specimen.** In a large multicenter review by Fizazi and colleagues, incomplete resection, proportion of viable GCT in resection specimen, and IGCCCG risk status were used to classify patients into three risk categories that predicted survival outcomes. When evaluating patients with viable GCT at PC-RPLND, prior receipt of salvage chemotherapy has consistently been associated with significantly poorer survival outcomes. Although once thought to be a marker of more aggressive behavior, immature teratoma has demonstrated no decrement in survival outcomes.

17. **e. pN2 disease or higher.** There is relatively broad consensus that many patients with pN1 disease at primary RPLND who are reliable can be safely managed with observation. The

management of pN2 disease is more controversial with some centers advocating two cycles of adjuvant chemotherapy while others would manage many of these patients with observation. There have been a variety of other histologic variables tested for their prognostic ability to predict disease recurrence. These include such parameters as the number of positive nodes as a proportion of the number removed, the histologic type of GCT in the metastases, and the presence or absence of extranodal extension. None of these have proven reliable enough that they can accurately predict those who are at high risk for recurrence and warrant up front adjuvant therapy. The one exception is that the finding of only teratoma in the retroperitoneum is associated with very low relapse rates, and therefore observation is warranted.

18. **d. Persistently rising STMs through induction chemotherapy.** Investigators at Indiana University reported a 53.9% cancer-specific survival rate at a median follow-up of 6 years when the following criteria outlined were used to select patients to undergo desperation PC-RPLND. (1) Declining or Plateauing AFP after induction chemotherapy, a slowly rising AFP after a complete serologic response to induction chemotherapy, and all potentially curative chemotherapeutic options have been exhausted.

A patient with persistently rising STMs during chemotherapy should receive either standard or high-dose salvage chemotherapy.

19. **b. Ipsilateral pelvic recurrences are common.** Reoperative RPLND indicates a technical failure at prior RPLND in the majority of cases. Several reviews of reoperative experiences at high-volume centers have revealed that primary landing zone recurrence as well as signs of an inadequate prior resection (incomplete/absent lumbar vessel ligation, unresected ipsilateral gonadal vein, and recurrence posterior to the great vessels) are common in patients experiencing retroperitoneal recurrence after RPLND. Since pelvic lymph nodes are not routinely removed as part of a standard template RPLND disease relapse in this location does not necessarily reflect a technical failure of the any preceding RPLND.

20. **b. First-line treatment is generally systemic chemotherapy followed by consolidative PC-RPLND.** Late relapse in patients with prior receipt of chemotherapy is often composed of yolk sac tumor and tends to be relatively chemorefractory regardless of histology. Thus primary management of resectable disease at late relapse is surgical extirpation. Late relapse in chemotherapy-naïve patients has been associated with improved outcomes likely due to increased susceptibility to chemotherapy.

21. **b. 20% to 60%.** Infertility and subfertility are frequently present at GCT diagnosis. This can present challenges to pretreatment sperm banking. For unclear reasons, parameters occasionally improve after orchiectomy. However, this baseline infertility needs to be taken into account when evaluating fertility outcomes after treatment of GCT.

22. **d. Penile erection.** Antegrade ejaculation is reliant on the smooth muscle contraction of the vas deferentia, seminal vesicles, and prostate that results in seminal emission and prostate glandular secretion, as well as the subsequent closure of the bladder neck preventing retrograde ejaculation, are critically reliant on input from the postganglionic sympathetic fibers that emanate from L1 to L4. Penile erection is necessary for vaginal penetration, but not ejaculation. Notably, erection is a parasympathetic process.

23. **d. Limiting fat intake preoperatively.** Although it is a troublesome postoperative complication, chylous ascites tends to be transient, and management is usually directed at draining accumulated fluid and minimizing further production by instituting an MCT diet, progressing to total parenteral nutrition if the MCT diet fails, and possibly starting subcutaneous octreotide. A peritoneovenous shunt is an intervention of last resort. Limiting preoperative fat intake has not been shown to decrease the incidence of chylous ascites.

24. **b. 29-year-old male with large-volume left para-aortic and interaortocaval masses that extend through the retrocrural region into the middle visceral mediastinum.** Spinal ischemia leading to neurologic compromise is extremely rare. Patients at risk for this potentially devastating complication are those who will require resection of more than three sequential lumbar artery pairs. This tends to be in patients with high-volume para-aortic disease in the retroperitoneum, retrocrural region, and visceral mediastinum.

CHAPTER REVIEW

1. The proper performance of a radical inguinal orchiectomy includes mobilizing the cord 1 to 2 cm proximal to the internal inguinal ring and individually ligating the vas deferens and cord vessels with silk sutures so that the stump may be identified if an RPLND is performed.

2. When an orchiectomy has been performed through the scrotum in patients who have a low-stage seminoma, the radiation portals should be extended to include the ipsilateral groin and scrotum; for those with low-stage nonseminomatous germ cell tumor (NSGCT), the scrotal scar should be excised along with the spermatic cord remnant; and for those who have received a full cycle of platinum-based chemotherapy, only the cord stump need be removed at the time of RPLND.

3. The right testicular lymphatics drain to the interaortocaval lymph nodes followed by paracaval and pericaval nodes. The left testicular lymphatics drain to the periaortic and preaortic lymph nodes.

4. Contralateral lymphatic flow is more commonly seen in right-sided tumors than left-sided tumors.

5. There is a 20% to 30% incidence of positive nodes in clinical stage I disease and approximately a 25% relapse rate in such patients who are placed on a surveillance protocol.

6. Suprahilar metastases are rare in low-stage NSGCT. Three percent to 23% of patients with positive nodes at RPLND will have extra-template disease. The most common site of residual suprahilar disease is in the retrocrural space.

7. It is extremely important, when performing a primary RPLND, to secure all lymphatic vessels with either clips or ties, particularly in the region of the right renal artery and diaphragmatic crus, to minimize injury to the cisterna chyli, which could result in chylous ascites.

8. In the presence of documented or suspected metastatic disease, a full bilateral dissection should be performed. In selected cases, preservation of individual nerve fibers may be performed.

9. The anterior split over the vena cava is not likely to damage nerve fibers; however, the anterior split over the aorta risks injury to these fibers.

10. The most important nerves to preserve antegrade ejaculation are those arising from the L1 to L4 ganglia. To preserve nerve fibers, a dissection on the aorta should only be performed after the nerve fibers have been identified and isolated.

11. There is a sevenfold increase in cardiovascular complications in men treated with platinum-based chemotherapy.

12. All patients should be given the opportunity to bank sperm before RPLND.

13. In clinical stage I, NSGCT lymphovascular invasion; higher T stage; tumor involvement of the cord, capsule, or scrotum; and a high percentage of embryonal carcinoma are associated with an increased incidence of retroperitoneal relapse. Most relapses occur within the first 2 years and are rare after 5 years. The absence of teratoma in the primary tumor does not preclude its presence in the retroperitoneum.

14. Persistently elevated tumor marker levels after orchiectomy require systemic chemotherapy, as the next step is not RPLND.

15. Patients best suited for RPLND are those with clinical stage IIA and low-volume, less than 3-cm ipsilateral disease (stage IIB).

16. Sixty percent of patients with testicular cancer have subnormal pretreatment semen analyses. Sixty-five percent of men on surveillance can impregnate their partner after orchiectomy.

17. Bilateral RPLND is the standard template for patients with pathologic stage II NSGCT.

18. Bleomycin can cause restrictive pulmonary fibrosis with increased collagen deposition and makes the patient highly susceptible to fluid overload.

19. Increased serum concentration of AFP and hCG after primary platinum-based chemotherapy is usually characterized by unresectable viable tumor, and salvage chemotherapy rather than excision of the mass is recommended.

20. After chemotherapy, retroperitoneal masses are composed of necrosis/fibrosis in 40%, teratoma in 45%, and viable GCT in 15%. A residual mass after salvage chemotherapy is composed of viable GCT in 50%, teratoma in 40%, and fibrosis in 10%. The clinical behavior of a teratoma is unpredictable, and complete resection is required.

21. After chemotherapy, RPLND is indicated for NSGCT primary tumors in which the residual mass is larger than 1 cm. RPLND may be eliminated after chemotherapy if there was no evidence of the disease in the retroperitoneum before chemotherapy.

22. Late relapses occur in 2% to 4% of patients, and more than half of late relapses occur beyond 10 years, emphasizing the need for prolonged follow-up.

23. If the aortic wall is stripped of its adventitia, it should be replaced with a synthetic graft because delayed rupture may occur.

24. Tumor involvement of the superior mesenteric artery, celiac axis, or porta hepatis usually precludes resection. After chemotherapy, resection of residual masses should be accompanied by a complete RPLND. The standard bilateral dissection is the prudent approach.

25. After chemotherapy for seminoma, residual masses very rarely contain teratoma and are extremely difficult technically to remove. Thus a residual mass less than 3 cm should be observed, patients with masses larger than 3 cm should have PET, and if a viable seminoma is noted, then either additional chemotherapy or RPLND is indicated.

26. After chemotherapy, spermatogenesis may take 3 years to return to normal.

27. In the setting of complete or near-complete occlusion, routine reconstruction of the vena cava following resection is not required.

28. RPLND histology is a strong predictor of histology at thoracotomy: if necrosis is all that is found in the retroperitoneum, 89% of the time the chest lesions will be necrotic.

29. The ureters provide the anatomic landmark for the lateral border of dissection for the para-aortic and paracaval lymph node packets.

30. There are three paired lumbar arteries located between the renal hilum and the aortic bifurcation in nearly all patients.

31. Patients having received salvage chemotherapy who demonstrate viable GCT at PC-RPLND, those demonstrating teratoma only at PC-RPLND, and those demonstrating transformation to somatic-type malignancy have not been shown to benefit from adjuvant chemotherapy.

32. Late relapse in patients with prior receipt of chemotherapy is often composed of yolk sac tumor and tends to be relatively chemorefractory regardless of histology. Thus primary management of resectable disease at late relapse is surgical extirpation.

78 Laparoscopic and Robotic-Assisted Retroperitoneal Lymphadenectomy for Testicular Tumors

Mohamad E. Allaf and Louis R. Kavoussi

QUESTIONS

1. A 23-year old man presents after undergoing transscrotal orchiectomy for presumed hydrocele. Pathologic examination reveals embryonal carcinoma with vascular invasion. Serum levels of tumor markers and results of physical examination and computed tomography (CT) of the chest, abdomen, and pelvis were normal. Which of the following approaches is most appropriate?

   a. Observation

   b. Retroperitoneal lymph node dissection (RPLND)

   c. RPLND plus excision of scrotal scar and remnant cord

   d. RPLND plus scrotectomy and inguinal lymph node dissection

   e. RPLND plus scrotal and inguinal radiation

2. Late relapse is a feature most commonly associated with

   a. seminoma.

   b. yolk sac tumor.

   c. embryonal carcinoma.

   d. choriocarcinoma.

   e. teratoma.

3. A 25-year-old man with a stage IIC nonseminomatous germ cell tumor (NSGCT) has completed primary platinum-based chemotherapy. Tumor marker levels have normalized according to appropriate half-life, and he has undergone bilateral post-chemotherapy RPLND. Final pathologic analysis reveals a focus of yolk sac tumor. Appropriate therapy at this point is

   a. careful observation.

   b. radiation therapy.

   c. two additional cycles of platinum-based chemotherapy.

   d. four additional cycles of platinum-based chemotherapy.

   e. reexploration in 6 weeks.

4. A 20-year-old man with clinical stage I NSGCT undergoes laparoscopic RPLND. During surgery, a 2-cm lymph node is encountered. Which of the following is the most appropriate next step?

   a. Abort the procedure and administer chemotherapy.

   b. Convert to an open procedure.

   c. Perform a unilateral template dissection and administer chemotherapy.

   d. Continue the procedure and perform a full bilateral dissection.

   e. None of the above.

5. The most common cause of open conversion during laparoscopic RPLND is

   a. intraoperative discovery of bulky lymphadenopathy.

   b. failure to progress.

   c. bowel injury.

   d. hypercapnia.

   e. bleeding.

6. Two weeks after laparoscopic RPLND, a patient complains of abdominal distention and emesis. CT reveals ascites. Diagnostic paracentesis confirms the diagnosis of chylous ascites. The next best step is

   a. reassurance and discharge.

   b. reoperation to identify and treat the source of lymphatic leak.

   c. placement of a peritoneal drain and initiation of a low-fat diet.

   d. initiation of somatostatin.

   e. hydration and initiation of a low-fat diet.

7. A 20-year-old man undergoes laparoscopic RPLND after right radical orchiectomy for an NSGCT. All of the following regions should be dissected clear of all lymphatic tissue EXCEPT which?

   a. Right spermatic cord

   b. Paracaval region

   c. Interaortocaval region

   d. Retrocrural region

   e. Precaval region

8. Potential advantages to laparoscopic compared with open RPLND include all of the following EXCEPT which?

   a. Improved cosmesis

   b. Shorter convalescence

   c. Improved disease-free survival

   d. Shorter interval to chemotherapy when necessary

   e. Faster return to normal activities

ANSWERS

1. **c. RPLND plus excision of scrotal scar and remnant cord.** In the setting of scrotal contamination and clinical stage I disease, the patient is best managed with RPLND and wide excision of the scrotal scar. The remainder of the cord should also be removed. Observation is not optimal because of the presence of vascular invasion and scrotal contamination.

2. **e. Teratoma.** Late relapse of germ cell tumor (GCT) after definitive therapy is defined as recurrence more than 2 years after completion of therapy and occurring without evidence of disease. Teratoma is the most common histologic subtype involved in cases of late relapse. This is likely due to its combination of prolonged doubling time and chemotherapy resistance.

3. **c. Two additional cycles of platinum-based chemotherapy.** The patient's prognosis is related to serum tumor marker level at the time of RPLND, prior treatment burden, and the pathologic findings for the resected specimen. If viable GCT is present at any site but all disease is completely resected, two additional cycles provide survival benefit in this subset of patients. Einhorn reported only 2 long-term survivors of 22 patients (9%) with completely resected viable GCT after cisplatin, bleomycin, and vinblastine chemotherapy if additional postoperative chemotherapy was not given. Fox and colleagues reported that

70% of patients with completely resected viable GCT after primary chemotherapy followed by two cycles of postoperative chemotherapy remained disease free compared with none of 7 patients without additional chemotherapy.

4. **d. Continue the procedure and perform a full bilateral dissection.** Whenever a suspicious lymph node is identified, a full bilateral dissection should be performed. Chemotherapy will not compensate for an inadequate retroperitoneal dissection.

5. **e. Bleeding.** The most common reason for conversion to an open procedure is uncontrollable bleeding, and vascular injury is cited as the most common intraoperative complication. In experienced hands, this occurs less than 5% of the time.

6. **e. Hydration and initiation of a low-fat diet.** Chylous ascites is a devastating complication that occurs less than 2% of the time after primary laparoscopic (and open) RPLND. Initiation of a low-fat diet, hydration, and drainage of the fluid is usually the first step in management. Reoperation is considered only when all other options have been exhausted.

7. **d. Retrocrural region.** The superior boundary of a dissection template does not include lymph nodes superior to the renal hilum.

8. **c. Improved disease-free survival.** No study has demonstrated any difference in disease-free survival comparing open or laparoscopic approaches with node dissection.

79 Tumors of the Penis

Curtis A. Pettaway, Juanita M. Crook, and Lance C. Pagliaro

QUESTIONS

1. Which of the following penile lesions is not typically associated with viral infection?
   a. Balanitis xerotica obliterans
   b. Condylomata acuminatum
   c. Kaposi sarcoma
   d. Bowenoid papulosis
   e. Erythroplasia of Queyrat

2. Which of the following infections is associated with cervical dysplasia?
   a. Human immunodeficiency virus (HIV) infection
   b. Herpesvirus infection
   c. Gonorrhea
   d. Human papillomavirus (HPV) infection
   e. Lymphogranuloma venereum

3. What is the major difference between Bowen disease and erythroplasia of Queyrat?
   a. Loss of rete pegs
   b. Keratin staining
   c. Viral etiologic agents
   d. Location
   e. Treatment options

4. Kaposi sarcoma of the acquired immunodeficiency syndrome (AIDS)–related (epidemic) type is associated with which of the following etiologic agents?
   a. HPV type 16
   b. Human herpesvirus (HHV) type 8
   c. HPV type 32
   d. *Haemophilus ducreyi* (chancroid [soft chancre])
   e. Coxsackievirus type 23

5. Where do penile cancers most commonly arise?
   a. Glans
   b. Shaft
   c. Frenulum
   d. Coronal sulcus
   e. Scrotum

6. Which of the following is not considered a risk factor for the development of squamous cell carcinoma of the penis?
   a. Cigarette smoke
   b. HPV infection
   c. Phimosis
   d. Gonorrhea
   e. Chewing tobacco

7. All of the following are preventive strategies to decrease the incidence of penile cancer EXCEPT:
   a. circumcision after 21 years of age
   b. HPV vaccination
   c. daily genital hygiene
   d. avoiding tobacco products
   e. circumcision before puberty

8. Which of the following statements regarding penile cancer is FALSE?
   a. Cancer may develop anywhere on the penis.
   b. Because of the associated discomfort, patients usually present to physicians within the first month of noting the lesion.
   c. Phimosis may obscure the nature of the lesion.
   d. Penetration of the Buck fascia and the tunica albuginea by the tumor permits invasion of the vascular corpora.
   e. Cancer cells reach the contralateral inguinal region because of lymphatic cross-communications at the base of the penis.

9. Before a treatment plan for penile cancer is initiated, which of the following is TRUE?
   a. Adequate biopsies to determine stage are unimportant because all patients should be treated with amputation.
   b. Radiologic studies play no role in decision making.
   c. Tumor HPV status is critical for determining primary tumor therapy.
   d. Tumor stage, grade, and vascular invasion status all provide prognostically important information.
   e. No disfiguring therapy is indicated, because spontaneous remissions have been noted in approximately 10% of cases.

10. Which of the following statements is TRUE regarding the natural history of penile cancer?
    a. Metastases from the primary tumor often involve lung, liver, or bone as initial sites.
    b. Lymphatic drainage from the primary tumor is ipsilateral alone in most cases.
    c. Metastasis often initially involves spread from the corpora cavernosa to the pelvic lymph nodes.
    d. Metastasis initially involves inguinal lymph nodes beneath the fascia lata.
    e. Metastasis initially involves inguinal lymph nodes above the fascia lata.

11. Which of the following statements concerning hypercalcemia in patients with penile cancer is TRUE?
    a. It is more commonly due to massive bone metastases than bulky soft tissue metastases.
    b. It is often related to uremia due to ureteral obstruction.
    c. It may be due to the action of parathyroid hormone-like substances released from the tumor.
    d. It is related to the action of osteoblasts on bone formation.
    e. It is managed with aggressive diuretic administration as first-line therapy.

12. The following statements are true regarding imaging tests in patients with penile cancer EXCEPT:
    a. Both ultrasonography and MRI lack sensitivity for the detection of corpus cavernosum involvement.
    b. computed tomography (CT) is not an appropriate test for determining primary tumor stage.
    c. CT may be beneficial in detecting enlarged inguinal nodes in obese patients or those who have had prior inguinal therapy.
    d. lymphangiography can detect abnormal architecture in normal-sized lymph nodes.
    e. inguinal palpation is preferred to CT and lymphangiography for determining inguinal nodal status.

13. According to the eighth edition of the American Joint Committee on Cancer Staging System (i.e., tumor, node, metastases [TNM]) for penile cancer, which of the following statements is TRUE?
    a. Primary tumor stage is based on the size of the primary lesion.
    b. Lymph node stage is based in part on the size of an involved node.
    c. Stage T2 tumors invade the corpus spongiosum but not the cavernosum.
    d. Proven pelvic nodal metastases as well as bilateral inguinal metastases are both designated as stage pN3.
    e. Stage T1a tumors involve the dartos fascia and exhibit perineural invasion in less than 10% of the specimen.

14. What is the strongest prognostic factor for survival in penile cancer?
    a. The presence of lymph node metastasis
    b. The grade of the primary tumor
    c. The stage of the primary tumor
    d. Vascular invasion presence in the primary tumor
    e. The extent of lymph node metastasis

15. Criteria for curative surgical resection (>70% 5-year survival) in patients treated for lymph node metastasis include all of the following EXCEPT:
    a. no more than two positive inguinal lymph nodes.
    b. no positive pelvic lymph nodes.
    c. absence of extranodal extension of cancer.
    d. unilateral metastasis.
    e. a single metastasis of only 6 cm.

16. Surgical staging of the inguinal region is strongly considered under all of the following conditions EXCEPT:
    a. palpable adenopathy.
    b. stage T1b or greater primary tumor.
    c. presence of vascular invasion in primary tumor.
    d. presence of predominantly high-grade cancer in primary tumor.
    e. stage Ta tumors.

17. Strategies attempting to minimize the morbidity of inguinal staging in patients with no palpable adenopathy include all the following EXCEPT:
    a. superficial inguinal lymph node dissection.
    b. modified complete inguinal dissection.
    c. standard ilioinguinal dissection.
    d. laparoscopic and robotic inguinal node dissection.
    e. dynamic sentinel node biopsy.

18. Which of the following inguinal staging procedure(s) is/are considered standard for detecting microscopic metastases while limiting both morbidity and false-negative findings?
    a. Sentinel lymph node biopsy
    b. Superficial inguinal dissection
    c. Dynamic sentinel lymph node biopsy
    d. All of the above
    e. b and c only

19. For patients with proven unilateral metastasis involving two or more lymph nodes at presentation, all of the following surgical considerations are true EXCEPT:
    a. ipsilateral ilioinguinal lymphadenectomy should be performed
    b. a contralateral staging procedure is not indicated
    c. a contralateral staging procedure is indicated
    d. both a superficial dissection and a deep ipsilateral dissection are performed
    e. ipsilateral pelvic dissection provides useful prognostic information

20. Adjuvant or neoadjuvant chemotherapy should be considered in addition to surgery for all of the following EXCEPT:
    a. single pelvic nodal metastasis
    b. extranodal extension of cancer
    c. fixed inguinal masses
    d. two unilateral inguinal nodes with focal metastases
    e. single 6-cm inguinal lymph node

21. The majority of penile cancers are histologically:
    a. melanoma.
    b. bowenoid papulosis.
    c. squamous cell carcinoma.
    d. epidemic Kaposi sarcoma.
    e. verrucous carcinoma.

22. Which of the following chemotherapeutic agents used in combination therapy for penile cancer has been associated with significant pulmonary toxicity?
    a. Bleomycin
    b. Methotrexate
    c. Cisplatin
    d. 5-Fluorouracil (5-FU)
    e. Paclitaxel

23. Indications for radiation therapy as primary treatment for penile cancer include which of the following?
    a. Young, sexually active patient with a small lesion
    b. Patient refuses surgery
    c. Patient with distant or inoperable metastases who requires local control to the primary tumor
    d. None of the above
    e. a, b, and c

24. Primary penile melanoma is thought to be rare for what reason?
    a. Penile skin is protected from exposure to the sun.
    b. Keratin content in penile skin is decreased.
    c. Penile blood supply precludes such tumor development.
    d. Effective topical chemotherapy exists.
    e. None of the above.

25. Lymphomatous infiltration of the penis is most likely secondary to which condition?
    a. Autoimmune disorder
    b. Diffuse disease
    c. Metastasis from a distant primary tumor
    d. Chronic infection
    e. Previous venereal infection

26. What is the most frequently encountered sign of metastatic involvement of the penis?
    a. Pain
    b. Urethral discharge
    c. Ecchymoses
    d. Priapism
    e. Preputial swelling

27. Which of the following features of Buschke-Löwenstein tumor characterizes it as different from condyloma acuminatum?
    a. Propensity for early distant metastasis
    b. Disruption of the rete pegs
    c. Loss of pigmentation
    d. Autoamputation
    e. Invasion and destruction of adjacent tissues by compression

28. All of the following statements are true regarding the management of bulky inguinal metastases in patients with squamous penile carcinoma EXCEPT:
    a. cross-sectional imaging plays an important role in establishing the extent of disease.
    b. neoadjuvant chemotherapy with a cisplatin-containing regimen is recommended.
    c. post-chemotherapy surgical consolidation to achieve disease-free status is recommended following an objective response to chemotherapy.
    d. among patients who progress through chemotherapy, salvage surgery can often result in prolonged survival.
    e. chemo-radiation for tumor cytoreduction prior to surgical resection or as definitive treatment may play a role.

29. Small lesions of erythroplasia of Queyrat may be successfully treated with which of the following?
    a. Topical 5% 5-FU
    b. Neodymium:yttrium-aluminum-garnet (Nd:YAG) laser
    c. Local excision
    d. Imiquimod
    e. All of the above

ANSWERS

1. **a. Balanitis xerotica obliterans.** Also known as lichen sclerosus, manifests as a whitish patch on the prepuce or glans, often involving the meatus and sometimes extending into the fossa navicularis. The cause is unknown but has not been associated with known viruses. Condyloma, Bowenoid papulosis, and erythroplasia of Queyrat are associated with HPV infection while Kaposi sarcoma is associated with HPV 8 infection.
2. **d. Human papillomavirus (HPV) infection.** HPV is recognized as the principal etiologic agent in cervical dysplasia and cervical cancer.
3. **d. Location.** Carcinoma in situ of the penis is referred to by urologists and dermatologists as erythroplasia of Queyrat if it involves the glans penis or prepuce and as Bowen disease if it involves the remainder of the penile shaft skin, genitalia, or perineal region.

4. **b. Human herpesvirus (HHV) type 8.** HHV type 8—also known as Kaposi sarcoma-associated herpesvirus—is strongly suspected to be the etiologic agent of epidemic (AIDS-related) Kaposi sarcoma.
5. **a. Glans.** Penile tumors may present anywhere on the penis but occur most commonly on the glans (48%) and prepuce (21%).
6. **d. Gonorrhea.** No convincing evidence has been found linking penile cancer to other factors such as occupation, other venereal diseases (gonorrhea, syphilis, herpes), marijuana use, or alcohol intake.
7. **a. Circumcision after 21 years of age.** Adult circumcision appears to offer little or no protection from subsequent development of the disease. These data suggest that the crucial period of exposure to certain etiologic agents may have already occurred at puberty and certainly by adult age, rendering later circumcision relatively ineffective as a prophylactic tool for penile cancer.
8. **b. Because of the associated discomfort, patients usually present to physicians within the first month of noting the lesion.** Patients with cancer of the penis, more than patients with other types of cancer, seem to delay seeking medical attention. In large series, from 15% to 50% of patients have been noted to delay medical care for more than a year.
9. **d. Tumor stage, grade, and vascular invasion status all provide prognostically important information.** Confirmation of the diagnosis of carcinoma of the penis, an assessment of the structure(s) invaded, and tumor grade by the combination of an adequate biopsy, and complete clinical assessment are beneficial before the initiation of definitive therapy. Biopsy can be performed as a frozen section immediately before definitive therapy in some cases.
10. **e. Metastasis initially involves inguinal lymph nodes above the fascia lata.** The lymphatics of the prepuce form a connecting network that joins with the lymphatics from the skin of the shaft. These tributaries drain into the superficial inguinal nodes (the nodes external to the fascia lata).
11. **c. It may be due to the action of parathyroid hormone-like substances released from the tumor.** Parathyroid hormone and related substances may be produced by both tumor and metastases that activate osteoclastic bone resorption.
12. **a. Both ultrasonography and MRI lack sensitivity for the detection of corpus cavernosum involvement.** The sensitivity of ultrasonography for detecting cavernosum invasion was 100% in one study. This study confirmed the value of ultrasonography in assessing the primary tumor also reported by other investigators. For lesions suspected of invading the corpus cavernosum, both ultrasonography and contrast-enhanced MRI may provide unique information, especially when organ-sparing surgery is considered.
13. **c. Stage T2 tumors invade the corpus spongiosum but not the cavernosum** According to the 8th edition, staging system invasion of the corpus cavernosum is now designated T3, indicating a worse prognosis than tumors involving the spongiosum alone.
14. **e. The extent of lymph node metastasis.** The presence and extent of metastasis to the inguinal region are the most important prognostic factors for survival in patients with squamous penile cancer.
15. **e. A single metastasis of only 6 cm.** Pathologic criteria associated with long-term survival after attempted curative surgical resection of inguinal metastases (i.e., >70% 5-year survival) include (1) minimal nodal disease (up to two involved nodes in most series), (2) unilateral involvement, (3) no evidence of extranodal extension of cancer, and (4) the absence of pelvic nodal metastases. A lymph node larger than 4 cm is often associated with extranodal extension of cancer.
16. **e. Stage Ta tumors.** Tumor histologic type associated with little or no risk for metastasis includes those patients with primary tumors exhibiting (1) carcinoma in situ or (2) verrucous carcinoma.

17. **c. Standard ilioinguinal dissection.** In patients with no evidence of palpable adenopathy who are selected to undergo inguinal procedures by virtue of adverse prognostic factors within the primary tumor, the goal is to define whether metastases exist with minimal morbidity for the patient. A variety of treatment options for this purpose have been reported and include (1) dynamic sentinel node biopsy, (2) superficial dissection, (3) modified complete dissections, and (4) laparoscopic and robotic approaches.

18. **e. b and c only.** Both superficial inguinal lymph node dissection and dynamic sentinel lymph node biopsy (latter at experienced centers) are considered standard procedures for determining the presence of inguinal microscopic metastases. Biopsies directed to a specific anatomic area (i.e., sentinel lymph node biopsy) can be unreliable in identifying microscopic metastasis and are no longer recommended.

19. **b. A contralateral staging procedure is not indicated.** Support for a bilateral procedure is based on the finding of bilateral lymphatic drainage from the primary site in the majority of cases and contralateral metastases in more than 50% of patients so treated in some series, even if the contralateral nodal region was negative to palpation.

20. **d. Two unilateral inguinal nodes with focal metastases.** For patients requiring ilioinguinal lymphadenectomy because of the presence of metastases, adjuvant chemotherapy should be considered for those exhibiting more than two positive lymph nodes, extranodal extension of cancer, or pelvic nodal metastasis. Reports from one center further confirmed the value of adjuvant chemotherapy. Of 25 node-positive patients treated with adjuvant combination vincristine-bleomycin-methotrexate chemotherapy, 82% survived 5 years, compared with 37% of 31 patients treated with surgery alone.

21. **c. Squamous cell carcinoma.** The majority of tumors of the penis are squamous cell carcinomas demonstrating keratinization, epithelial pearl formation, and various degrees of mitotic activity.

22. **a. Bleomycin.** Response rates of bleomycin, whether as a single agent or in combination with other agents, has not been shown to be superior to cisplatin alone, but has been associated with significant pulmonary toxicity and death in several series of patients treated for metastatic penile cancer.

23. **e. a, b, and c.** Radiation therapy may be considered in a select group of patients: (1) young individuals presenting with small (2 to 4 cm), superficial, exophytic, noninvasive lesions on the glans or coronal sulcus; (2) patients who refuse surgery as an initial form of treatment; and (3) patients with distant or inoperable metastases who require local therapy and express a desire to retain the penis.

24. **a. Penile skin is protected from exposure to the sun.** Melanoma and basal cell carcinoma rarely occur on the penis, presumably because the organ's skin is protected from exposure to the sun.

25. **b. Diffuse disease.** When lymphomatous infiltration of the penis is diagnosed, a thorough search for systemic disease is necessary.

26. **d. Priapism.** The most frequent sign of penile metastasis is priapism; penile swelling, nodularity, and ulceration have also been reported.

27. **e. Invasion and destruction of adjacent tissues by compression.** The Buschke-Löwenstein tumor differs from condyloma acuminatum in that condylomata, regardless of size, always remain superficial and never invade adjacent tissue. Buschke-Löwenstein tumor displaces, invades, and destroys adjacent structures by compression. Aside from this unrestrained local growth, it demonstrates no signs of malignant change on histologic examination and does not metastasize.

28. **d. Among patients who progress through chemotherapy salvage surgery can often result in prolonged survival.** Surgery among patients who do not respond to chemotherapy is commonly associated with death due to either rapidly occurring locoregional recurrence or distant metastases

29. **e. All of the above.** When lesions are small and noninvasive, local excision, which spares penile anatomy and function, is satisfactory. Circumcision will adequately treat preputial lesions. Fulguration may be successful but often results in recurrences. Both Topical 5-FU as the 5% base and Imiquimod causes denudation of malignant and premalignant areas while preserving normal skin. There are also reports of successful treatment with Nd:YAG laser.

CHAPTER REVIEW

1. HPV infection among men is associated with penile carcinoma, as well as with cervical dysplasia and carcinoma among female partners.
2. Imiquimod cream is now the standard topical treatment of choice for condyloma.
3. Giant condyloma of Buschke Lowenstein are locally progressive HPV related tumors that are nonmetastatic but require complete excision and follow-up. The potential for coexisting or malignant degeneration to squamous carcinoma has been shown.
4. Penile carcinoma in situ (Tis) is an intraepithelial malignant process manifesting as three differing clinical entities including Bowenoid papulosis, Bowen disease, and erythroplasia of Queyrat.
5. Penile cancer is rare in developed countries and varies worldwide with age, circumcision, HPV exposure, and lifestyle/hygiene practices.
6. Recent epidemiologic data from the United States suggest a disparity in both incidence and outcome of penile cancer for Puerto Rican Hispanic men.
7. Risk factors for development of penile cancer include lack of neonatal circumcision, phimosis, HPV infection, exposure to tobacco products, penile lichen sclerosus, and potentially penile trauma.
8. Penile cancer represents a preventable disease in most cases via neonatal circumcision, HPV vaccination, and/or behavior modification.
9. Penile cancer often begins on the surface of the glans penis or in the preputial area, where it progressively enlarges.
10. Delay both in seeking medical attention and then in subsequent definitive biopsy is common.
11. Examination of both the penile primary tumor and the inguinal region is critical to treatment planning.
12. Metastasis occurs by embolization of tumor deposits from the penile tumor through penile lymphatics to the inguinal lymph nodes.
13. Distant metastases occur late in the history of the disease.
14. Adequate tumor biopsy is essential to diagnosis and treatment planning.
15. Squamous carcinoma histologic subtypes have recently been classified by into two major groups by their relationship to HPV and show distinct morphologic features and clinical behavior.
16. Pathologic description of anatomic structures invaded (i.e., stage), the grade, and the status of vascular and perineural invasion provide important information to assess the risk of metastasis.
17. Soft-tissue detail of penile tumors is best imaged by MRI.

CHAPTER REVIEW—cont'd

18. Physical examination provides the most reliable staging information for small distal lesions.
19. Penile MRI especially performed in combination with artificial erection may provide unique staging information when physical examination findings are equivocal.
20. Physical examination of the inguinal region remains the clinical gold standard for evaluating the presence of metastasis in the nonobese patient.
21. CT or MRI can be useful in evaluating the inguinal region of obese patients and in those who have had prior inguinal surgery.
22. Among patients with proven inguinal metastases, CT scan of the abdomen and pelvis may help determine those patients with poor prognostic features for cure with surgery alone.
23. Positron emission tomography (PET)/CT may be useful among patients with clinically detected inguinal metastases to define the presence of pelvic or distant metastasis.
24. Both clinical and pathologic factors related to the presence and extent of lymph node involvement determine survival and should be recorded.
25. The current, eighth edition unified TNM staging system represents a consensus document that includes both clinical and pathologic descriptors that provide important prognostic information.
26. Patients with small lesions of low grade and stage (Tis, Ta, T1; grade 1 and grade 2) are the optimal candidates for organ preservation to maintain sexual quality of life.
27. The goals of organ preservation are to maintain glanular tissue for sensory purposes when possible and/or to maintain penile length when glans penis preservation is not possible.
28. Surgical modalities include limited excision strategies, Mohs surgery, and laser ablation.
29. Local recurrence rates overall after organ preservation are higher than with traditional amputation; however, when local recurrences are detected and treated, early survival does not appear be adversely affected.
30. Amputation remains the standard for large or deeply invasive lesions, to gain rapid tumor control.
31. The presence and extent of inguinal metastases determine survival in penile cancer.
32. Patients with persistent palpable inguinal adenopathy should undergo an ultrasound or CT guided inguinal biopsy, followed by management appropriate for the clinical scenario.
33. On the basis of the histologic features of the primary tumor, the risk of lymph node metastases can be assessed in patients with no palpable adenopathy based upon the TMN staging system. Dynamic sentinel node biopsy (DSNB), superficial inguinal lymph node dissection (ILND), or close follow-up can be recommended based upon TMN stage and other histologic features.
34. Factors associated with a high cure in surgically treated patients include no more than two inguinal metastases, unilateral involvement, no extranodal extension (ENE) of cancer, and the absence of pelvic metastases. Patients with higher volumes of disease should be considered for adjuvant or neoadjuvant therapy.
35. Morbidity of lymphadenectomy is decreasing in contemporary series.
36. Superficial ILND reliably determines the presence of microscopic inguinal metastases without the need for specialized facilities but can have significant morbidity.
37. Modified DSNB techniques to determine microscopic inguinal disease exhibit low morbidity, have been validated externally in higher-volume centers, and are now a recommended procedure in such centers.
38. Laparoscopic and robotic ILND obtains lymph node yields that are comparable to those of open techniques when used in selected patients and are an appropriate staging procedure in clinically lymph node negative patients. Additional studies with larger patient numbers and longer follow-up are required before routine adoption into clinical practice among patients with clinically positive inguinal lymph nodes.
39. Pelvic lymph node dissection (PLND) is now recommended when more than one inguinal lymph node exhibits metastasis or when ENE of cancer is present.
40. Radiation provides an effective penile-preserving approach for T1 to T2 squamous cell carcinomas less than 4 cm using either external-beam radiotherapy or brachytherapy.
41. Since 20% of recurrences occur after 5 years, continued follow-up is required as salvage penectomy for persistent or recurrent disease may be curative.
42. The criteria for surgical staging of inguinal lymph nodes are the same whether patients undergo primary radiation or primary surgical management.
43. Unresectable lymph nodes may be rendered operable by neoadjuvant chemotherapy or chemo-radiation.
44. Integration of radiation, surgery, and chemotherapy in advanced disease is being investigated in a prospective international randomized trial (InPACT: EA 8134).
45. Palliative radiotherapy may be beneficial for metastatic disease.
46. Neoadjuvant chemotherapy with a cisplatin-containing regimen should be considered for patients with lymph node metastases, as responses in this setting may facilitate curative resection. In the absence of Level 1 evidence, the optimal or standard multimodal strategy remains undefined.
47. The use of bleomycin in the treatment of men with metastatic penile cancer was associated with an unacceptable level of toxicity and is discouraged.
48. Surgical consolidation to achieve disease-free status or palliation should be considered in fit patients with a proven objective response to systemic chemotherapy.
49. Among patients who progress through chemotherapy, surgery is not recommended.
50. Basal cell carcinoma represents a highly curable variant with a relatively low metastatic potential.
51. Sarcomas are prone to local recurrence; regional and distant metastases are rare. Superficial lesions can be treated with less radical procedures.
52. Melanoma is an aggressive form of cancer but can be cured if diagnosed and treated with the appropriate surgical procedure at an early stage. Novel immunotherapy strategies may improve survival in recurrent or advanced disease.
53. Extramammary Paget disease (EMPD) disseminates by intraepidermal spread initially. Wide local excision to achieve negative margins is the therapy of choice. Invasive EMPD can be lethal.
54. Penile metastases most often represent spread from a clinically obvious existing primary tumor. Prognosis is poor, and therapy should be directed toward the primary tumor site histology and local palliation.

80 Tumors of the Urethra

Christopher B. Anderson and James M. McKiernan

QUESTIONS

1. Which of the following is not a possible origin of female urethral adenocarcinoma?
   a. Müllerian tissue
   b. Cowper glands
   c. Glandular metaplasia
   d. Skene glands
   e. Urothelium

2. The most common histologic subtype of male anterior urethral cancer is:
   a. adenocarcinoma.
   b. squamous cell carcinoma.
   c. urothelial carcinoma.
   d. melanoma.
   e. sarcoma.

3. The histologic subtype of urethral cancer that is more common in women than in men is:
   a. adenocarcinoma.
   b. squamous cell carcinoma.
   c. urothelial carcinoma.
   d. melanoma.
   e. sarcoma.

4. In male pendulous urethral carcinoma:
   a. prognosis depends on histologic cell type.
   b. surgical excision alone is often curative.
   c. prognosis is worse than for bulbomembranous urethral cancer.
   d. a 2-cm margin is always required for penile preserving surgery.
   e. biopsy most commonly demonstrates transitional cell carcinoma.

5. A treatment that is NOT indicated in cT3N0M0 squamous cell carcinoma of the bulbar urethra is:
   a. radical cystectomy with urethrectomy.
   b. chemoradiotherapy.
   c. inguinal lymphadenectomy.
   d. pelvic MRI.
   e. neoadjuvant chemotherapy.

6. The strongest risk factor for male urethral recurrence after radical cystectomy is:
   a. carcinoma in situ.
   b. bladder tumor multifocality.
   c. prostatic urethral involvement.
   d. squamous cell histology.
   e. prior nonmuscle invasive bladder cancer.

7. Which of the following is FALSE about urethral recurrence after radical cystectomy and orthotopic neobladder?
   a. Urethral recurrences are more common after radical cystectomy and ileal conduit.

   b. Radical urethrectomy is always required.
   c. Transurethral resection and intraurethral bacille Calmette-Guérin (BCG) can be effective for noninvasive tumors.
   d. Bowel from the neobladder can be reconfigured for a cutaneous diversion.
   e. Patients with noninvasive recurrences have a good prognosis.

8. A 71-year-old man is diagnosed with a primary prostatic urothelial carcinoma. Transurethral biopsy demonstrates invasion into the prostatic stroma, and imaging is negative for metastasis. The best treatment option is:
   a. systemic immunotherapy.
   b. aggressive transurethral resection of the prostate followed by BCG.
   c. radical cystectomy and urethrectomy with neoadjuvant chemotherapy.
   d. whole pelvic radiation.
   e. radical prostatectomy.

9. When a delayed urethrectomy is performed after radical cystectomy in a male, the most important technical consideration to minimize the risk of a local recurrence is:
   a. removal of the entire distal urethra including the meatus.
   b. bilateral groin dissections.
   c. total penectomy.
   d. intraoperative ultrasound.
   e. neoadjuvant radiation.

10. A condition that does not increase the risk of female urethral carcinoma is:
    a. leukoplakia.
    b. bacterial vaginosis.
    c. urethral diverticulum.
    d. urethral stricture disease.
    e. human papillomavirus infection.

11. The strongest prognostic factor for survival in female urethral cancer is:
    a. tumor stage.
    b. age at presentation.
    c. histologic subtype.
    d. multimodal treatment.
    e. urinary retention.

12. A 68-year-old man presents with an anterior urethral tumor invasive into the corpora cavernosum. His tumor stage is:
    a. T1.
    b. T2a.
    c. T2b.
    d. T3.
    e. T4.

13. The best treatment for a small, exophytic cT2N0 female urethral carcinoma located near the urethral meatus is:
    a. excision of the distal 2/3 of the urethra.
    b. transvaginal biopsy followed by systemic chemotherapy.
    c. radical urethrectomy with bladder neck closure and ileovesicostomy.
    d. chemoradiation.
    e. inguinal lymphadenectomy.

14. A 76-year-old female presents with a locally invasive proximal urethral tumor abutting the pubic symphysis. The treatment that would be inappropriate is:
    a. radical cystectomy with pubectomy.
    b. external beam radiation with systemic chemotherapy.
    c. radical cystectomy with intraoperative radiation.
    d. radiation monotherapy.
    e. chemoradiation followed by surgical consolidation.

15. Two years after a radical cystectomy and ileal conduit in a male patient, a urethral wash cytology is positive for high-grade urothelial carcinoma. The next step is:
    a. repeat urethral wash cytology.
    b. urethroscopy with biopsy.
    c. radical urethrectomy.
    d. pelvic MRI.
    e. urine cytology.

16. All of the following are true about the male urethra EXCEPT:
    a. the anterior urethra drains into the inguinal lymph nodes.
    b. the glands of Littre line the anterior urethra.
    c. the posterior urethra consists of the prostatic and membranous urethra.
    d. the pseudostratified epithelium of the pendulous urethra transitions to glandular epithelium in the fossa navicularis.
    e. anterior urethral cancers are more common in the bulbar urethra.

17. A 56-year-old-man presents with an invasive pendulous urethral squamous cell carcinoma with palpable inguinal lymph nodes bilaterally. Imaging is negative for distant metastasis. The best treatment is:
    a. radiation monotherapy to the tumor and lymph nodes.
    b. chemoradiation to the penis and groins followed by surgical consolidation.
    c. radical penectomy.
    d. dynamic sentinel lymph node biopsy.
    e. distal urethrectomy with 6 weeks of oral antibiotics.

ANSWERS

1. **b. Cowper glands.** There are several proposed origins of female urethral adenocarcinoma, and more than one tissue may be involved. All of the listed tissue types are possible origins with the exception of Cowper glands, which are only present in men.
2. **b. Squamous cell carcinoma.** The male anterior urethra is lined by stratified and pseudostratified columnar epithelium, which transitions to squamous epithelium distally. The majority of male anterior urethral carcinomas are squamous cell carcinoma.
3. **a. Adenocarcinoma.** Gender is not independently associated with survival for urethral carcinoma; however, there are differences in the characteristics of male and female urethral carcinoma, including the distribution of histologic subtypes. Although squamous cell carcinoma is the predominant form in men, women are more likely to have adenocarcinoma compared to men.

4. **b. Surgical excision alone is often curative.** The prognosis of male pendulous anterior urethral cancer is strongly associated with stage, is more favorable than bulbomembranous urethral cancer, and is unrelated to histologic cell type. Most pendulous urethral tumors are squamous cell carcinomas. Low-stage pendulous anterior urethral cancers can often be cured with surgical excision alone, and penile preservation can often be achieved with margins as little as 5 mm.
5. **c. Inguinal lymphadenectomy.** Locally advanced bulbomembranous urethral carcinoma requires aggressive treatment. MRI is required to fully stage the disease, including the extent of local invasion and presence of pelvic nodal metastasis. Of the treatments listed, neoadjuvant chemotherapy, chemoradiation, and radical cystectomy with urethrectomy are all reasonable options. The role of inguinal lymphadenectomy for cN0 urethral cancer is controversial, but there is no role for this in bulbomembranous disease as these tumors are unlikely to drain into the inguinal lymph nodes.
6. **c. Prostatic urethral involvement.** Urethral recurrence after radical cystectomy occurs in 5% to 10% of patients. Of the multiple risk factors that have been studied, prostatic urethral involvement, a positive urethral margin, and cutaneous urinary diversions have the highest risk of urethral recurrence.
7. **b. Radical urethrectomy is always required.** Patients with large or invasive urethral recurrences after radical cystectomy require aggressive treatment, usually with radical urethrectomy. If a urethral recurrence occurs after an orthotopic neobladder, the bowel from the neobladder can be used for a cutaneous diversion in many cases. Patients with noninvasive urethral recurrences have a favorable prognosis and can often be managed with transurethral resection and topical BCG, thus avoiding radical urethrectomy in some cases. Prostatic urethral involvement, a positive urethral margin, and cutaneous diversions all increase the risk of urethral recurrences.
8. **c. Radical cystectomy and urethrectomy with neoadjuvant chemotherapy.** The prognosis of primary prostatic urethral carcinoma is strongly associated with depth of invasion into the prostate. Those with superficial or lamina propria invasion can often be managed with transurethral resection and BCG; however, those with tumors invasive into the stroma require aggressive treatment. Radical cystoprostatectomy with urethrectomy and preoperative chemotherapy is the best choice.
9. **a. Removal of the entire distal urethra including the meatus.** A delayed urethrectomy after radical cystectomy can be a challenging procedure. Critically, the entire urethra including the fossa navicularis and urethral meatus should be removed en bloc to eliminate the risk of a distal recurrence, even for proximal tumors. There is no role for routine inguinal lymphadenectomy, and penectomy is not required unless the urethral tumor is invasive into the deep structures of the penis.
10. **b. Bacterial vaginosis.** Urethral carcinoma is most likely caused by conditions that cause inflammation of the urethra, such as leukoplakia, urethral strictures, and HPV infection. Female urethral diverticula can increase the risk of urethral cancers, most commonly adenocarcinomas. Bacterial vaginosis has no known association with urethral cancer.
11. **a. Tumor stage.** The prognosis of female urethral cancer is strongly associated with stage at diagnosis. Tumors that arise from the proximal urethra tend to present at a more advanced stage. There is no known association between prognosis and histologic subtype, age at presentation, or presenting symptoms.
12. **d. T3.** Male anterior urethral cancer with invasion into the corpora cavernosum or anterior vagina are classified as T3 by the AJCC 8th Edition Staging System. Tumors invasive into the corpus spongiosum or periurethral tissue are classified as T2. The AJCC staging system does not have a T2a or T2b for urethral cancer.
13. **d. Chemoradiation.** Small exophytic distal female urethral cancers can be effectively treated with surgical excision or radiation with or without chemotherapy. Radical urethrectomy can usually be avoided for distal tumors. The distal 1/3 of the female urethra can be safely excised without compromising

urinary continence, but excision of the distal 2/3 will likely cause incontinence and is not a good option. There is currently no role for prophylactic inguinal lymphadenectomy for cN0 female distal urethral cancer. Most distal urethral tumors can be biopsied transurethrally.

14. **d. Radiation monotherapy.** Proximal female urethral cancer often presents at an advanced stage, tends to be aggressive, and can have a poor prognosis. Therefore, aggressive local therapy is required, often in a multidisciplinary setting. Of the listed options, radiation monotherapy is inadequate treatment.

15. **b. Urethroscopy with biopsy.** Urethral wash cytology may be beneficial for detecting early urethral recurrences after radical cystectomy. However, a positive cytology can be falsely positive and always requires confirmation with a biopsy prior to aggressive treatment or further imaging.

16. **d. The pseudostratified epithelium of the pendulous urethra transitions to glandular epithelium in the fossa navicularis.** All of the listed options are true except "d," as the urethral epithelium transitions to squamous, not glandular, in the fossa navicularis.

17. **b. Chemoradiation to the penis and groins followed by surgical consolidation.** Advanced staged urethral carcinoma requires aggressive multimodal treatment. Clinically positive inguinal lymph nodes with an invasive primary urethral cancer should be considered metastatic disease, therefore there is no role for antibiotics or sentinel lymph node biopsy. Radiation monotherapy and surgical monotherapy to the penis alone are both suboptimal treatment for invasive, cN+ penile cancers. Chemoradiation to the penis and groins with surgical consolidation is the best choice.

CHAPTER REVIEW

1. The prognosis of distal anterior male posterior urethral cancer (PUC) is better than that of proximal anterior PUC, which is often associated with local invasion and distant metastasis.
2. Multimodal therapy should be considered for advanced urethral tumors given the poor outcomes after surgery and radiation alone.
3. The benefit from prophylactic inguinal lymph node dissection has not been demonstrated in anterior urethral cancer.
4. Primary posterior urethral carcinoma is rare, and noninvasive tumors can be effectively managed with transurethral resection of the prostate and BCG.
5. The three most common histologies for female urethral cancer are urothelial carcinoma, squamous cell carcinoma, and adenocarcinoma.
6. Compared to anterior urethral cancers, posterior cancers present at a more advanced stage and are associated with worse survival.
7. Radiation and surgical excision are both options for low-stage anterior tumors, each with high cure rates.
8. Surgery and radiation therapy for proximal female urethral tumors have poor outcomes when used alone, therefore multimodal therapy is recommended.
9. Male urethral recurrence after radical cystectomy is rare, but more common with prostatic involvement, a positive urethral margin, and cutaneous diversions.
10. The primary risk factors for female urethral recurrences are bladder neck involvement and a positive urethral margin.
11. Most surgeons will proceed with orthotopic neobladder if an intraoperative frozen section of the urethral margin is negative.
12. After urethrectomy in patients with orthotopic neobladders, bowel from the neobladder can often be reconfigured and used for a cutaneous diversion.

81 Inguinal Node Dissection

Rene Sotelo, Luis G. Medina, and Marcos Tobias Machado

QUESTIONS

1. For lymphatic spread in penile cancer, which of the following statements is true?
   a. Penile carcinoma spreads initially to inguinal lymph nodes before the development of distant metastatic disease.
   b. There is significant crossover in the lymphatic drainage of the penis; hence bilateral inguinal lymph node dissection (ILND) is usually recommended.
   c. Lymph node metastases confers a poor prognosis overall when present for patients with penile carcinoma.
   d. Lymphovascular invasion or greater than 50% poorly differentiated tumors are at a higher risk for lymph node metastases.
   e. All of the above.

2. Preservation of the fatty layer within Camper fascia is directly associated with:
   a. infection rates after the surgery.
   b. lymphatic complications due to preservation of the lymphatics.
   c. blood supply of the overlying skin.
   d. preservation of the Innervation of the overlying skin.
   e. all of the above.

3. Which of the following imaging techniques are mandatory in the presurgery assessment of a patient with penile carcinoma for the inguinal region?
   a. Ultrasound with fine needle aspiration cytology (FNAC)
   b. Computed tomography (CT)
   c. Magnetic resonance imaging (MRI)
   d. MRI with nanotechnology
   e. Positron emission tomography (PET scan)
   f. None of the above

4. Which of the following statements are considered to be true for ILND?
   a. It is not useful because it overtreats around 80% of the patients that are at risk of surgical complications.
   b. It should be performed only when lymphatic affectation is clinically evidenced to avoid further spread of the disease.
   c. Has been substituted by the Sentinel Node biopsy proposed by Cabanas et al. because it decreases the complication rate, adding a good diagnostic assessment.
   d. It's useful for penile staging/treatment because 17% to 25% of patients with nonpalpable lymph nodes will have lymphatic metastases, but carries a high morbidity burden.

5. Which of the following statements is true regarding dynamic sentinel node biopsy (DSNB)?
   a. After a positive DSNB, patients should undergo strict active vigilance with PET scans and repeated biopsies every 6 months.
   b. DSNB has a relatively short learning curve that helped this procedure to be widely adopted in several centers around the world, avoiding unnecessary ILND.
   c. When properly done, DSNB can achieve more than 80% of sensitivity for lymph node metastases in patients with penile cancer.
   d. On the DSNB, there is only the use of technetium nanocolloid the day before the procedure described.
   e. All of the above.

6. Modifications of the original technique/template for inguinal lymph node dissection has been proposed, although no randomized clinical trials have been performed to compare them. Which of the following statements is the rationale for superficial inguinal node dissection and modified inguinal lymph node dissection (MILD)?
   a. All nodes affected in patients with penile cancer will be located within the reduced template whilst reducing morbidity.
   b. Frozen section is reliable for detection of lymph nodes affected.
   c. Preserving the saphenous vein decreases the complication rate.
   d. If nodes in the superficial compartment are negative, there should not be affectation of the deep package.

7. Based on the information gathered by previous series, what can be stated from the endoscopic inguinal lymph node dissection?
   a. It has to be performed in a two-staged fashion to perform both legs.
   b. It has been shown to have the same complication rate in most of the open series.
   c. Oncologically, it seems to be equivalent to open procedures.
   d. The limits of the triangle are the inguinal ligament, the abductor longus, and the fascia of the iliacus muscle.
   e. All of the above.

8. Which of the following statements is true regarding the robotic and laparoscopic ILND?
   a. Robotics have been proved to have less complications due to a more precise dissection.
   b. The 3D visualization that the robotic system offers allow the surgeon to identify more lymphatic nodes.
   c. The degrees of movements that the robotic system instruments have allows the surgeon to have easier control of the lymphatics with ultrasonic energy.
   d. The Xi platform allows repositioning without modifications from the operative room setting.
   e. None of the above.

9. During a radical ILND, sartorius muscle interposition is carried out in order to:
   a. improve the mobility of the lower limb after surgery.
   b. be used as an interposition tissue to avoid the formation of collections.
   c. protect the femoral vessels.
   d. none of the above.
   e. all of the above.

10. Which type of complication decreased in frequency as a result of the adoption of endoscopic/robotic techniques for ILND in penile cancer?

    a. Wound complications

    b. Lymphatic complications

    c. Bleeding complications

    d. Major complications that resulted in the death of the patient

    e. Deep venous thrombosis

11. What is the 5-year survival rate of a patient who, after ILND, was found to have 1 to 3 positive lymph nodes for malignancy?

    a. 5% to 15%

    b. 75% to 80%

    c. 90% to 95%

    d. 60% to 70%

    e. 30% to 50%

12. What is the overall 5-year survival rate of a patient with positive pelvic lymph nodes for malignancy?

    a. Less than 10%

    b. 25%

    c. 35%

    d. 45%

    e. 55%

ANSWERS

1. **e. All of the above.** Knowledge on the lymphatic anatomy and spread of the penile tumors is crucial to understand the rationale for its surgical management. In this question, some critical points are highlighted. First is the fact that penile cancer usually spreads in a stepwise manner going from the inguinal nodes (superficial package first, then deep package) and pelvic nodes before the appearance of the distant metastatic lesions. However, due to the crossover of the lymphatic channels in the symphyseal region, the ILND should be performed bilaterally independently of the side affected. Furthermore, positive lymph nodes have proved to be a prognostic survival factor in several studies, which underlines the importance of undertaking this procedure when indicated. One of the indications for ILND are high-risk tumors; these are defined as T1 with high-grade and/or lymphovascular invasion and/or >50% poorly undifferentiated. All T2 and T3 tumors are considered high risk.

2. **c. Blood supply of the overlying skin.** Irrigation of the skin flaps raised during the dissection depends on anastomotic vessels in the superficial fatty layer of Camper fascia. Because lymphatic drainage of the penis to the groin runs beneath Camper fascia, this layer can be preserved and left attached to the overlying skin when the working space is created.

3. **f. None of the above.** There are not imaging techniques formally recommended for the evaluation of the inguinal area in patients with penile cancer. Nonetheless, CT of abdomen, pelvis, and chest is recommended in patients with ILND involvement or in patients with clinically suspected pelvic lymph nodes.

4. **d. It's useful for penile staging/treatment because 17% to 25% of patients with nonpalpable lymph nodes will have lymphatic metastases, but carries a high morbidity burden.** ILND in patients with micrometastasis has shown to increase survival, 17% to 25% of the patients with clinically negative nodes will harbor micrometastasis. However, due to the morbidity burden that this represents for some patients, appropri-

ate patient selection is crucial to minimize morbidity without sacrificing oncological outcomes. Early ILND has shown to be beneficial concerning patients' survival, which is why it is not recommended to delay the surgery until lymphatic affectation is evidenced. Cabanas sentinel node has been disregarded due to lack of sensitivity in the diagnosis. However, dynamic sentinel node in expert hands could be an option for proper patient selection (see "Penile Cancer: Non-Palpable Inguinal Adenopathy").

5. **c. When properly done, DSNB can achieve more than 80% of sensitivity for lymph node metastases in patients with penile cancer.** After positive DSNB, patients should undergo ILND. This modality has shown to be effective in diagnosing patients with occult metastases. However, it has a long learning curve, which is why its worldwide adoption have been troublesome. In expert hands, it has shown to have an 80% sensitivity rate. One of the factors that this technique includes is the use of the nanocolloid and the blue dye, to improve results.

6. **d. If nodes in the superficial compartment are negative, there should not be affectation of the deep package.** Both templates share the fact that if nodes are negative in the superficial package, the chances of having positive deep lymph nodes are scarce. However, there has been reports of positive nodes in the superficial space outside the MILND template. The intraoperative frozen section can miss more than 25% of positive nodes, and definitive proof of diminishment of the morbidity with the preservation of the saphenous veins has not been given; reports on this regard are contradictory.

7. **c. Oncologically, it seems to be equivalent to open procedures.** Endoscopic ILND has been shown to be oncologically safe and equivalent by showing no differences in the number of positive nodes when comparing endoscopic versus open dissections. Endoscopic ILND can be performed in one time in both legs; it has shown a decreased complication rate (no randomized clinical trial has been done on this regard), and the limits are the inguinal ligament, the abductor longus, and the sartorius muscle.

8. **d. The Xi platform allows repositioning without modifications from the operative room setting.** Robotics has not shown superiority over the laparoscopic approach (not due to to the increased degrees of movements that allow for more precise dissection nor to the tridimensional view). However, Xi facilitates the repositioning of the robot when compared to other platforms such as the Si. This is possible in the Si system, but reaccommodation of the operative room is needed.

9. **c. Protect the femoral vessels.** Sartorius muscle had been used with the intention of protecting the femoral vessels. However, it has shown to be a predictor factor for complications in some series.

10. **a. Wound complications.** With a reduced incision size, decreased risk for skin/wound complications is posed on the patients when an endoscopic approach is used. This is the rationale for the endoscopic approach. Lymphatic complications are more related to the type of energy used in the lymph node management strategy used along with the postoperative care. Same for bleeding complications. Other complications should not have a difference between approaches. Although, no randomized clinical trial has been done on this regard.

11. **b. 75% to 80%.** Seventy-five percent to eighty percent is the 5-year survival rate of a patient who, after ILND, was found to have one to three positive lymph nodes for malignancy, which highlights the importance of a prompt ILND and the number of lymph nodes involved in patients with penile cancer.

12. **a. Less than 10%.** Less than 10% of patients with positive lymph pelvic nodes, bilaterally positive nodes, and/or extranodal extension survive after 5 years.

CHAPTER REVIEW

1. The most important independent prognostic factor related to cancer-specific survival in squamous cell carcinoma (SCC) of the penis is lymph node metastasis.
2. Immediate ILND is associated with improved survival compared to salvage surgery for clinically detectable disease.
3. For centers of excellence with expertise in penile cancer and ILND, DSNB can be performed with a false-negative rate of less than 5%.
4. Superficial and modified ILND are options in the initial management of inguinal region in patients with nonpalpable disease. These are techniques have less morbidity than radical ILND.
5. Endoscopic inguinal lymphadenectomy has been demonstrated to have less morbidity than open ILND and to remove comparable number of lymph nodes.
6. Radical ILND is indicated for palpable disease, with potential for cure in inguinal-only disease, and for palliation of pain, infection, or hemorrhage in selected patients.
7. Adjuvant chemotherapy can aid in better outcomes in patients with positive inguinal disease.
8. Pelvic metastasis do not occur in patients with negative inguinal nodes.

82

Surgery for Benign Disorders of the Penis and Urethra

Ramón Virasoro, Gerald H. Jordan, and Kurt A. McCammon

QUESTIONS

1. In terms of tissue transfer, which of the following statements concerning grafts is TRUE?

   a. The process of take is less than 48 hours.

   b. A graft is tissue that is excised from a donor site and reestablishes its blood supply by revascularization.

   c. During imbibition, the first phase of take, the graft exists above body temperature.

   d. Conditions of take are a reflection of only the graft host bed.

   e. Split-thickness skin grafts (STSGs) are less prone to contraction compared with full-thickness grafts.

2. With regard to the microanatomy of grafts, using skin as a model, which of the following statements is TRUE?

   a. The intradermal plexus is at the interface of the superficial and deep dermis.

   b. The subdermal plexus is carried at the juncture of the deep dermis and the underlying tissue.

   c. The lymphatics are most richly distributed in the adventitial dermis.

   d. The adventitial dermis, because of its collagen content, accounts for the majority of the physical characteristics.

   e. Genital and extragenital skin behave similarly when used in genitourinary reconstruction.

3. With regard to the grafts used most commonly in genitourinary reconstructive surgery, which of the following statements is TRUE?

   a. Full-thickness skin is an optimal replacement for the tunica albuginea of the corpora cavernosa.

   b. Bladder epithelial graft is fastidious because of the nature of the superficial lamina.

   c. Buccal mucosa graft is thought to have a panlaminar plexus.

   d. Tunica vaginalis graft has proved to be a very reliable one for single-stage urethral reconstruction.

   e. Buccal mucosa grafts should not be thinned because it will adversely affect the physical and vascular properties of the graft.

4. With regard to the anatomy of the penile shaft, which of the following statements is TRUE?

   a. Throughout most of the length of the penis, the septum is a true competent septum.

   b. The erectile tissues of the normal corpora cavernosa are separated from the tunica by the space of Smith.

   c. The dorsal arteries of the penis are carried in an envelope fashion in the dartos fascia.

   d. The Buck fascia is loosely areolar and lies immediately beneath the skin.

   e. The Buck fascia attenuates on the ventrum, lateral to the corpus spongiosum.

5. According to consensus, the urethra should be divided into six entities. Which of the following statements is most accurate?

   a. The fossa navicularis is that portion of the urethra that is most dorsally displaced with regard to the surrounding spongy erectile tissue.

   b. The bulbous urethral portion is invested by the thickest portion of the corpora spongiosum.

   c. The bulbous urethral at its proximal extent is part of the posterior urethra.

   d. The membranous urethra is invested by the most proximal aspect of the corpus spongiosum.

   e. The membranous urethra, throughout its length, is surrounded by the external rhabdosphincter.

6. With regard to the arterial vascularization of the deep structures of the penis, which of the following statements is TRUE?

   a. The circumflex cavernosal arteries are uniform in number and distribution.

   b. The arteries to the bulb arborize into the spongy erectile tissue of the glans.

   c. The common penile artery represents the end continuation of the superficial external pudendal artery.

   d. The common penile artery divides to become the cavernosal artery and the dorsal arteries, after branching off the circumflex cavernosal arteries.

   e. The blood supply of the deep structures of the penis is derived from the common penile artery, which is the continuation of the internal pudendal artery after it branches off its perineal branch and the posterior scrotal arteries.

7. With regard to the innervation to the penis, which of the following statements is TRUE?

   a. The cavernosal nerves are purely parasympathetic and are the extensions of the nervi erigentes.

   b. The pudendal nerves accompany the dorsal artery of the penis and the dorsal vein of the penis as they run through the obturator foramen.

   c. The dorsal nerve arises in the Alcock canal as a branch of the pudendal nerve.

   d. The dorsal nerves throughout their course are prominent, large nerve bundles.

   e. The skin of the shaft of the penis is innervated by a branch of the femoral nerve.

8. Which of the following statements regarding lichen sclerosus (LS) is FALSE?

   a. Lichen sclerosus is the preferred term for what was previously known as *balanitis xerotica obliterans*.

   b. LS is the most common cause of meatal stenosis.

   c. There is a strong association with an infectious etiology for the development of LS.

   d. Circumcision may be curative if only foreskin is involved with LS.

   e. Topical steroids may help stabilize the inflammatory process early in the disease course.

9. Each of the following statements regarding complications associated with LS are true, EXCEPT:

   a. Urethral stricture may develop secondary to iatrogenic injury from repeat instrumentation.

   b. Genital or extragenital skin may be used for urethral reconstruction for LS-associated urethral strictures.

   c. Meatal stenosis and high-pressure voiding with subsequent urinary extravasation into the glands of Littre may result in urethral stricture formation.

   d. Squamous cell carcinoma may develop in patients with a long history of LS.

   e. Patients under consideration for meatal reconstruction with LS must undergo retrograde urethrography to rule out proximal strictures before surgery.

10. Urethrocutaneous fistulae may develop secondary to all of the following, EXCEPT:

    a. Complication following hypospadias repair or other urethral surgery

    b. Recurrence following fistula repair as a result of distal obstruction and high-pressure voiding

    c. Extravasation of infected urine and periurethral abscess formation

    d. Complication of genital herpes simplex viral infection

    e. Early fistula following urethral surgery may result from hematoma, infection, or tension with the closure

11. With regard to urethral meatal stenosis in childhood, which of the following statements is TRUE?

    a. Meatal stenosis is a frequent complication of phimosis.

    b. Meatal stenosis is frequently associated with upper tract changes, and all patients should be evaluated with ultrasonography and voiding cystourethrography.

    c. When ammoniacal meatitis is noted, often a short course of meatal dilation and steroid cream application will resolve the problem.

    d. When meatal stenosis is present, usually a dorsally based YV advancement flap repair is preferred.

    e. Meatal stenosis in childhood is frequently associated with concomitant LS.

12. When treating a patient with penile amputation, which of the following statements is TRUE?

    a. Replantation is not a consideration in self-inflicted injury, because most of these patients are chronically psychotic and will eventually try to amputate the penis again.

    b. If the distal part of the penis is not available, even if the amputation involves mostly skin with much of the shaft preserved, it is recommended that the remaining shaft be buried in the scrotum.

    c. In the case of amputation associated with avulsion, debridement to undivided tissue must precede penile replantation.

    d. The classic technique for replantation involves coaptation of the dorsal nerve, the deep dorsal vein, and the cavernosal arteries.

    e. The McRoberts technique of macroreplantation is not the preferred method of management for these patients, but when the situation warrants it, it is very successful.

13. All of the following statements regarding circumcision are true, EXCEPT:

    a. Circumcision may be performed in the neonatal period in newborns born with a distal hypospadias, but not in those with proximal hypospadias.

    b. Young boys with recurrent urinary tract infections (UTIs) should be considered for circumcision.

    c. The most common complication following newborn circumcision is bleeding.

    d. Circumcision has been shown to reduce the risk of human immunodeficiency virus (HIV) transmission in heterosexual men.

    e. Small skin dehiscence following circumcision may be managed conservatively with local wound care and healing by secondary intention.

14. Concerning genital lymphedema, which of the following statements is TRUE?

    a. Reconstruction for lymphedema that is the consequence of the indirect effects of radiation is best accomplished with excision of the tissues and coverage with STSGs.

    b. In reconstruction for lymphedema, it is essential to maintain the parietal tunica vaginalis of the testes intact with grafting over that location.

    c. When considering reconstruction for lymphedema, full-thickness skin grafts (FTSGs) are preferable because of the distribution of the lymphatics in the superficial (adventitial) dermis.

    d. In the case of genital lymphedema, it is not unusual for the immune response of the tissues to be altered and for patients to have significant involvement with genital papillomas.

    e. Not unusually, in cases where the genital lymphedema is localized, the midline of the scrotum can be preserved for reconstruction.

15. Which of the following statements is MOST accurate concerning anterior urethral stricture disease?

    a. It causes limitation of the urethral lumen because of the bulk of the scar.

    b. It most often is limited to the urethral epithelium.

    c. It implies a scarring process, usually involving both the epithelium and the underlying spongy erectile tissue of the corpora cavernosa.

    d. It causes limitation of the urethral lumen because of contraction and noncompliance of the scar.

    e. It is a metaplastic process of the urethral epithelium.

16. Which of the following statements concerning pelvic fracture urethral injury (PFUI) is TRUE?

    a. It involves the tissues of the epithelium as well as the underlying erectile tissues of the corpora cavernosa.

    b. It involves the epithelium, as well as the underlying erectile tissue of the corpus spongiosum.

    c. It is not a true stricture but rather fibrosis that results from distraction of the urethra.

    d. The stricture process can often be occult because of the unpredictable involvement of the urethral tissues.

    e. The defect is usually predictably proximal to the external sphincter at the junction of the prostatic urethra with the membranous urethra.

17. In determining the anatomy of the stricture, all of the following provide useful information EXCEPT:

    a. Magnetic resonance imaging (MRI).

    b. High-resolution ultrasonography.

    c. Contrast studies.

    d. Urethroscopy.

    e. Calibration with bougie à boule.

18. With regard to planning of reconstruction for urethral stricture, which of the following statements is TRUE?

    a. Even if a patient does not have retention, placement of a suprapubic tube may help define strictured areas.

    b. Tightly stenotic areas should be dilated to pass endoscopes proximally.

    c. The effects of hydrodilation are manifested most immediately distal to the area of narrowest stenosis.

    d. Calibration of strictured areas to 16 Fr or greater reliably predicts the potential for segments to contract.

    e. Sonourethrogram by itself accurately predicts depth of spongiofibrosis.

19. With regard to direct visual internal urethrotomy, which of the following statements is TRUE?

    a. Strictures are best incised at the 12 o'clock position.

    b. Deep incision of the corpus spongiosum has been shown to optimize long-term results.

    c. In optimally selected patients, long-term success of internal urethrotomy is approximately 90%.

    d. Internal urethrotomy should be the first procedure considered for any stricture of the anterior urethra.

    e. It can be associated with erectile dysfunction (ED).

20. Concerning anterior urethral reconstruction, which of the following statements is TRUE?

    a. Excision and primary anastomosis reconstruction are severely limited and useful only for very proximal strictures 1 to 2 cm in length.

    b. Performance of the excision and primary anastomosis technique is facilitated by dissection of the corpus spongiosum to the level of the glans penis.

    c. Success requires total excision of the fibrosis with a widely spatulated anastomosis.

    d. Reconstruction is facilitated by development of the intracrural space with infrapubectomy.

    e. In cases of longer strictures, excision with partial anastomosis allowing one wall to granulate offers acceptable results.

21. With regard to genital skin flaps for anterior urethral reconstruction, which of the following statements is TRUE?

    a. Flap operations are best applied as individual techniques and require the surgeon to be intimately familiar with the individual steps of each technique.

    b. The operation can conceptually become one operation with multidimensional application.

    c. The operations are all based on mobilization of the extended Buck fascia.

    d. The operations require a comfortable understanding of the extended circumflex iliac superficial vascular pattern.

    e. They are of limited value in patients who have been previously circumcised.

22. With regard to continence after reconstruction for PFUIs, which of the following statements is TRUE?

    a. Location of the injury along the course of the membranous urethra is not associated with continence postoperatively.

    b. Continence can be accurately predicted by contrast studies.

    c. Continence is best predicted by the appearance of the bladder neck on endoscopy.

    d. Continence is best addressed after a procedure to reestablish urethral continuity is performed.

    e. Continence is best in patients with partial distraction injuries.

23. In dealing with the entity of chordee without hypospadias, which of the following statements is TRUE?

    a. Correction of curvature is often achieved with mobilization of the corpus spongiosum alone.

    b. It often can be corrected with maneuvers that lengthen the foreshortened ventral skin.

    c. It is best straightened by an incision and grafting operation.

    d. Division of the urethra/corpus spongiosum is virtually always indicated.

    e. It is usually present with either ventral curvature or ventral curvature associated with torsion.

24. With regard to acquired curvatures of the penis that are not Peyronie disease, which of the following statements is TRUE?

    a. Most are characterized by prominent dorsal scars.

    b. In most cases, global cavernosal veno-occlusive dysfunction (CVOD) is not a complicating factor.

    c. They are virtually never associated with "minimal" buckling trauma.

    d. Patients often have significant penile foreshortening.

    e. There is usually an association with either hypospadias or epispadias.

25. All of the following are true regarding PFUIs, EXCEPT:

    a. Pelvic fractures are associated with urethral injuries in about 10% of cases.

    b. PFUIs most commonly occur between the prostate and membranous urethra.

    c. In the prepubescent male, PFUI's are more likely to involve the prostatic urethra.

    d. A normal anterior urethral on retrograde urethrography nearly ensures an anastomotic repair of a PFUI is feasible.

    e. The appearance of the bladder neck on preoperative contrast studies does not accurately predict continence outcomes following anastomotic repair of PFUIs.

26. In PFUIs, after excision of the traumatic scar, the distance between the two ends of healthy urethra can be minimized by all of the following, EXCEPT:

    a. mobilizing the corpus spongiosum off the corpora cavernosa up to the corona of the glans.

    b. excision of Buck fascia from the corpus spongiosum.

    c. dissection of the intracrural space down to the pubis.

    d. periosteal elevation and infrapubectomy.

    e. rerouting of the spongiosum above the crura of the corpora cavernosa.

27. Which of the following patients should be considered for penile revascularization to prevent ischemic stenosis following PFUI repair?

    a. Men with ED following PFUI, but normal hemodynamics on penile duplex sonography

    b. Men with normal erectile function following PFUI

    c. Men following PFUI with ED and hemodynamics on penile duplex sonography suggesting venous leak

    d. Men with arteriogenic ED following PFUI who demonstrate bilateral occlusion of the internal pudendal arteries without reconstitution

    e. Men with arteriogenic ED following PFUI who demonstrate unilateral occlusion of the internal pudendal artery

28. Which of the following statements regarding total phallic construction is FALSE?
    a. Rigidity of the neophallus may be achieved by placement of a penile prosthesis before the return of tactile sensation of the phallus.
    b. Current techniques are accomplished with a variety of flap designs, which use microvascular free flap transfer.
    c. Urinary fistulae, although a common complication following phallic construction, are often resolved with conservative measures and do not routinely require operative repair.
    d. Complications following prosthesis placement into patients following total phallic construction are higher than those following placement into men with normal corporal anatomy.
    e. Penile tactile and erogenous sensation can be achieved following total phallic construction via coaptation of the flap cutaneous nerves to the dorsal penile/clitoral nerve, the pudendal nerve, or the ilioinguinal nerve.

29. All of the following may be repaired with excision and primary anastomotic urethroplasty, EXCEPT:
    a. PFUI with a 3-cm gap demonstrated on preoperative urethrography.
    b. straddle injury resulting in a 1-cm bulbar urethral stricture.
    c. iatrogenic urethral trauma during a transurethral resection resulting in a 1-cm bulbar urethral stricture.
    d. idiopathic proximal 1-cm bulbar urethral stricture in a patient with a history of a prior hypospadias repair.
    e. perineal trauma resulting in a 2-cm proximal bulbar urethral stricture.

30. Which of the following statements regarding vessel-sparing urethral reconstruction is FALSE?
    a. It preserves the vascularity of the bulbospongiosum.
    b. It requires a deep understanding of the anatomy and blood supply of the penile structures.
    c. It may be technically challenging in less experienced surgeons.
    d. By preserving the proximal blood supply of the urethra, it has better outcomes and less de novo erectile disfunction than a transecting excision and primary anastomosis.
    e. There are different applications of the technique, both for anterior urethral reconstruction and posterior urethral reconstruction.

31. Which of the following are the best candidates for vessel-sparing urethral reconstruction?
    a. Young man with less than 2-cm proximal bulbar urethral stricture
    b. Prior failed bulbar urethral reconstruction
    c. Proximal bulbar urethral stricture in previously reconstructed hypospadias
    d. a, b, and c
    e. b and c

ANSWERS

1. **b. A graft is tissue excised from a donor site that reestablishes its blood supply by revascularization.** The term *graft* implies that tissue has been excised and transferred to a graft host bed, where a new blood supply develops by a process termed *take*. Take requires approximately 96 hours and occurs in two phases. The initial phase, imbibition, requires about 48 hours. During that phase, the graft survives by "drinking" nutrients from the adjacent graft host bed, and the temperature of the graft is less than the core body temperature. The second phase, inosculation, also requires about 48 hours and is the phase in which true microcirculation is reestablished in the graft. During that phase, the temperature of the graft rises to core body temperature. The process of take is influenced by both the nature of the grafted tissue and the conditions of the graft host bed. Processes that interfere with the vascularity of the graft host bed thus interfere with graft take.

2. **b. The subdermal plexus is carried at the juncture of the deep dermis and the underlying tissue.** The epidermal, or epithelial layer, is a covering, the barrier to the "outside," and is adjacent to the superficial dermis, or superficial lamina. At approximately that interface is the superficial plexus. In the case of skin, the plexus is the intradermal plexus. There are some lymphatics in the superficial dermal or tunica layer. On the undersurface of the deep dermal layer or deep lamina is the deep plexus. In the case of skin, this is the subdermal plexus. The deep dermis contains most of the lymphatics and greater collagen content than found in the superficial dermal layer. The deep or reticular dermis is generally thought to account for the physical characteristics of the tissue. There is a difference between genital full-thickness skin (penile and preputial skin grafts) and extragenital full-thickness skin. This is probably a reflection of the increased mass of the graft in extragenital skin grafts. This increased mass makes the graft more fastidious, and the poor results reported with urethral reconstruction with extragenital FTSGs are probably due to poor or ischemic take.

3. **c. Buccal mucosa graft is thought to have a panlaminar plexus.** In the bladder epithelial graft, there is a superficial and a deep plexus; however, many more perforators connect the plexuses. Thus bladder epithelial grafts tend to have more favorable vascular characteristics. In the case of the oral mucosal grafts, there is a panlaminar plexus. Thus the oral mucosal graft can be thinned somewhat, provided a sufficient amount of deep lamina is carried to preserve the physical characteristics. The oral mucosal grafts are thought to have optimal vascular characteristics. The thinned graft diminishes the total graft mass while preserving the physical characteristics and not adversely affecting the vascular characteristics. Tunica vaginalis grafts have been tried for urethral reconstruction with uniformly poor results. The dermal graft (not full-thickness skin) has been used for years to augment the tunica albuginea of the corpora cavernosa.

4. **b. The erectile tissues of the normal corpora cavernosa are separated from the tunica by the space of Smith.** The corpora cavernosa are not separate structures but constitute a single space with free communication through an incompetent midline septum, composed of multiple strands of elastic tissue similar to that making up the tunica albuginea. The erectile tissue is separated from the tunica albuginea by a thin layer of areolar connective tissue that was described by Smith. The Buck fascia is directly abutted to the tunica albuginea of the corpora cavernosa. The Buck fascia surrounds the adventitia of the corpora spongiosum in envelope fashion, and the dorsal neurovascular structures are contained in envelope fashion between the superficial and deep laminar of the Buck fascia on the dorsum. The Buck fascia is thus "devoted" to the deep structures. The dartos fascia is loosely areolar and lies immediately beneath the skin. It is in that fascial layer that the arborizations of the superficial external pudendal vessels and the posterior scrotal vessels are carried.

5. **b. The bulbous urethral portion is invested by the thickest portion of the corpora spongiosum.** The fossa navicularis is contained within the spongy erectile tissue of the glans penis and terminates at the junction of the urethral epithelium with the skin of the glans. The bulbous urethra is covered by the midline fusion of the ischiocavernosus musculature and is invested by the bulbospongiosum of the proximal corpus spongiosum. It becomes larger and lies closer to the dorsal aspect of the corpus spongiosum, exiting from its dorsal sur-

face before the posterior attachment of the bulbospongiosum to the perineal body. The membranous urethra is the portion that traverses the perineal pouch and is partially surrounded by the external urethral sphincter. This segment of the urethra is unmatched to fixed structures, has the distinction of being the only portion of the male urethra that is not invested by another structure, and is lined with a delicate transitional epithelium.

6. e. **The blood supply of the deep structures of the penis is derived from the common penile artery, which is the continuation of the internal pudendal artery after it branches off its perineal branch and the posterior scrotal arteries.** The common penile artery is the continuation of the internal pudendal artery giving off perineal posterior scrotal branches. From that point onward, it is termed the *common penile artery.* As it nears the urethral bulb, the artery divides into its three terminal branches as follows: (1) the bulbourethral arteries, which enter the proximal corpus spongiosum; (2) the dorsal artery, which travels along the dorsum of the penis contained in envelope fashion between the superficial and deep lamina of the Buck fascia; and (3) the cavernosal arteries, usually a single artery, which arise and penetrate the corpora cavernosa at the hilum and run the length of the penile shaft. The circumflex cavernosal arteries are given off at varying locations along the dorsal artery, but their distribution is neither uniform nor dependable.

7. c. **The dorsal nerve arises in the Alcock canal as a branch of the pudendal nerve.** The cavernosal nerves are a combination of the parasympathetic and visceral afferent fibers that constitute the autonomic nerves of the penis. These provide the nerve supply to the erectile apparatus. The pudendal nerves enter the perineum with the internal pudendal vessels through the lesser sciatic notch at the posterior border of the ischiorectal fossa. They run in the fibrofascial pudendal canal of Alcock to the edge of the urogenital diaphragm. Each dorsal nerve of the penis arises on Alcock canal as the first branch of the pudendal nerve. On the shaft, their fascicles fan out to supply proprioceptive and sensory nerve terminals in the tunica of the corpora cavernosa and sensory terminals in the skin. The skin of the penis is innervated by branches of the genitofemoral nerve.

8. c. **There is a strong association with an infectious etiology for the development of LS.** The etiology of LS has not been well defined. Multiple potential infectious etiologies have been suggested, but recent studies have found no association. Other proposed etiologies include a Koebner phenomenon, autoimmune event, and genetic associations. The remaining answer choices are correct.

9. b. **Genital or extragenital skin may be used for urethral reconstruction for LS-associated urethral strictures.** Most surgeons now believe that LS is a disease of genital skin. For this reason, genital skin is not appropriate for reconstruction in patients with LS. Although it is technically possible to use extragenital skin for reconstruction, oral mucosal grafting has emerged as a better tissue in patients with LS associated urethral strictures. Patients with meatal stenosis from LS not infrequently also have more proximal strictures and need a complete workup prior to surgery. Patients with long-standing LS should be monitored for potential development of squamous cell carcinoma, because this has been reported.

10. d. **Complication of genital herpes simplex viral infection.** Genital HSV has not been reported to cause urethrocutaneous fistulae. Each of the remaining answers is a potential etiology for urethrocutaneous fistula formation.

11. c. **When ammoniacal meatitis is noted, often a short course of meatal dilation and steroid cream application will resolve the problem.** Meatal stenosis in the male child appears to be a consequence of circumcision, which allows for ammoniacal meatitis. Children seen with ammoniacal meatitis are usually started with meatal dilation using steroid cream. Within a

week, the process seems to settle down. Anecdotally, the fusion of the ventral meatus skin, which causes meatal stenosis, seems to be avoided. Because childhood meatal stenosis truly represents a fusion of the ventral urethral meatus, dividing the thin membrane of fusion is preferred. This leaves the child with a slit-shaped meatus.

12. e. **The McRoberts technique of macroreplantation is not the preferred method of management for these patients, but when the situation warrants it, it is very successful.** Often the amputation is self-inflicted, usually during an acute psychotic break. This should not preclude replantation unless the patient adamantly refuses such treatment. Even then, with a court order and the agreement of two or more surgeons, replantation may be undertaken. If possible, microreplantation should be carried out. This technique consists of an anatomic approximation of the tunica albuginea of the corporal bodies, a spatulated two-layer anastomosis of the urethra. The dorsal nerves are coapted using an epineural technique unless the injury is distal, at which point a vesicular coaptation may be required. The dorsal vein is anastomosed, and the dorsal arteries are anastomosed. Anastomosis of the cavernosal arteries is not possible and should not be attempted. If the situation is such that microreplantation cannot be undertaken, then the technique described by McRoberts can be carried out. His series and other series show that a high degree of success can be expected after replantation without microvascular reanastomosis. In most patients, however, they will have numbness distal to the replant site. With microreplantation, it is not at all unusual for patients to have excellent sensation distal to the area of injury and to have resumption of normal erectile function.

If the patient presents with the distal part having been disposed of or otherwise unavailable, then the wound should be closed. Often the penis will have been stretched during the amputation and an excess of skin will have been removed, leaving a good length intact with denuded penile shaft structures. In that case, the corporeal bodies would be closed, the urethral meatus must be spatulated, and the penis can be immediately covered with an STSG. If the injury occurs because of avulsion, replantation is not an option as the stretch injury to the spermatic vessels or vessels of the penis causes unpredictable damage to the endothelium.

13. a. **Circumcision may be performed in the neonatal period in newborns born with a distal hypospadias, but not in those with proximal hypospadias.** Newborns with any concern for hypospadias (distal or proximal) should NOT undergo circumcision. It is essential to preserve the foreskin so that it may be used for the hypospadias repair if necessary. Circumcision has consistently been shown in well-conducted randomized controlled trials to reduce the risk of HIV acquisition in heterosexual men by 50% to 60%. Circumcision will reduce the risk for UTI in infants and should be considered in those with recurrent infections. Most skin dehiscence following circumcision can be managed conservatively and does not require operative intervention.

14. a. **Reconstruction for lymphedema that is the consequence of the indirect effects of radiation is best accomplished with excision of the tissues and coverage with STSGs.** Patients with lymphedema can readily undergo reconstruction. When the lymphedematous tissue has been excised, the testes will be free and, as in a degloving injury, they must be fixed in the midline in an anatomically correct position. The shaft of the penis should be covered with a STSG. If the scrotum cannot be closed, a meshed STSG is used to cover the testes, as described. Not uncommonly, these patients have hydroceles, the parietal tunica vaginalis must be excised, and grafting can be done directly onto the visceral tunica vaginalis of the testicles. Unlike the full-thickness skin flap (FTSF), split-thickness skin carries little of the reticular dermis and hence few of the lymphatic channels. Reaccumulation of lymphedema will occur within a FTSG and can recur in a thick STSG. In many cases of lymphedema limited to the genitalia, the posterior scrotal

skin and the lateral scrotal skin are spared from the lymphe-dematous process. Thus, in some cases, primary closure after excision can be accomplished using these tissues. If grafting is required, using these tissues to blend the grafts into the groin and perineum technically is much easier. The lymphedema-tous process involves recurrent cellulitis, lymphedema, and the development of lymphangiectasia. Lymphangiectasia can look like genital papilloma; however, it is a very different process. If there is any question, biopsy can clarify the issue.

15. **d. It causes limitation of the urethral lumen because of contraction and noncompliance of the scar.** The term *urethral stricture* refers to anterior urethral disease. By virtue of the Consensus Conference, obliterative processes of the membranous urethra, such as those associated with pelvic fracture, would be referred to as PFUI, and other narrowing processes of the posterior urethra are correctly referred to as either contractures or stenosis. Thus the term *urethral stricture* describes a process that involves the urethral epithelium along with the spongy erectile tissue of the corpus spongiosum, and this is referred to as spongiofibrosis. In some cases, the scarring process can extend through the tissues of the corpus spongiosum and into the adjacent tissues. It is contraction of the scar that reduces the urethral lumen. Squamous metaplasia is often seen involving the urothelium of the urethra proximal to a narrow caliber urethral stricture.

16. **c. It is not a true stricture but rather fibrosis that results from distraction of the urethra.** By virtue of the Consensus Conference, narrowing of the posterior urethra is not referred to as a stricture. Those obliterative processes associated with pelvic fracture are termed PFUI. PFUI is an obliterative process of the posterior urethra that has resulted in fibrosis and is the defect of distraction of the urethra in that area. Although the distraction defect can be lengthy in some cases, the actual process involving the tissues of the urethra is usually confined.

17. **a. Magnetic resonance imaging (MRI).** To devise an appropriate treatment plan, it is important to determine the location, length, depth, and density of the stricture (spongiofibrosis). The length and location of the stricture can be determined using radiographs, urethroscopy, and ultrasonography. The depth and density of the scar in the spongy tissue can be deduced from the physical examination, the appearance of the urethra in contrast studies, the amount of elasticity noted on urethroscopy, and the depth and density of fibrosis as evidenced by ultrasonographic evaluation of the urethra, although the absolute length of spongiofibrosis may not be evident on ultrasonographic evaluation. MRI has been suggested as useful in patients with pelvic fracture urethral distraction, particularly in cases in which the anatomy of the pelvis has become significantly distorted. With regard to anterior urethral stricture, however, MRI has not been useful, with the exception of those cases in which there is urethral carcinoma. In those cases, MRI can provide invaluable information concerning the spread of the tumor. Bougie à boule calibration can be very helpful.

18. **a. Even if a patient does not have retention, placement of a suprapubic tube may help define strictured areas.** In selected patients, we have found it useful to place a suprapubic tube to defunctionalize the urethra. After 6 to 8 weeks, if there will be a constriction of an area that was hydrodilated with voiding, the tendency for that constriction to occur should become apparent. It is imperative, however, to completely evaluate the urethra proximal and distal to the stricture with endoscopy and bougienage during surgery, to ensure that all of the involved urethra is included in the reconstruction. Whereas hydraulic pressure generated by voiding may keep segments proximal to the stricture patent, unless these segments are included in the repair, they are at risk for contraction after obstruction of the narrow-caliber segment is relieved with reconstruction. For this reason, any abnormal areas of the urethra that are proximal to a narrow-caliber segment of the stricture must be treated with suspicion. If the lumen does not appear to demonstrate evidence of diminished compliance, then we

presume that area to be uninvolved in active stricture disease. However, coning down of the urethra suggests its involvement in the scar. Use of a sonourethrogram is thought by some to accurately establish length of stricture but not the extent of spongiofibrosis.

19. **e. It can be associated with ED.** Many surgeons have learned to perform internal urethrotomy by making a single incision at the 12-o'clock position. This location might be questioned, however, based on the location of the urethra within the corpus spongiosum. Distally, although the anterior aspect of the corpus spongiosum is thicker, a deep incision in the more distal aspects of the anterior urethra will certainly enter the corpora cavernosa, and these incisions have been associated with the creation of ED. The most common complication of internal urethrotomy is recurrence of stricture. Less commonly noted complications of internal urethrotomy include bleeding and extravasation of irrigation fluid into the perispongiosal tissues. One report that used the actuarial technique showed the curative success rate of internal urethrotomy to be 29% to 30% for all patients. Other evaluations have confirmed this success rate. However, a number of studies do show which strictures best respond to internal urethrotomy. These are strictures of the bulbous urethra that are less than 1.5 cm in length and are not associated with the dense or deep spongiofibrosis (i.e., straddle injuries). In those particular cases, long-term success has been shown to be 75% to 78%. For strictures outside the bulbous urethra, most studies do not show internal urethrotomy to have long-term success.

20. **c. Success requires total excision of the fibrosis with a widely spatulated anastomosis.** It has now been demonstrated with certainty that the most dependable technique of anterior urethral reconstruction is the complete excision of the area of fibrosis, with a primary reanastomosis of the normal ends of the anterior urethra. The best results are achieved when the following technical points are observed: (1) the area of the fibrosis is totally excised; (2) the urethral anastomosis is widely spatulated, creating a large ovoid anastomosis; (3) the anastomosis is tension free; (4) epithelial apposition is achieved. With vigorous mobilization, development of the intracrural space, and detachment of the bulbospongiosum from the perineal body, significant lengths of stricture can be excised and reanastomosed. For very proximal bulbous strictures, tension-free anastomosis can be facilitated by the dissection of the membranous urethra. As a rule, the closer the stricture is to the membranous urethra, the longer it can be and still be reconstructed by anastomotic techniques. The tenet that excision and primary anastomosis should be the goal for all bulbous strictures is one that is being further reinforced by current published series. Although guideline lengths of 1 to 2 cm are valuable for planning, most would agree that if excision and primary anastomosis is possible it should be done, and, with aggressive dissection and the maneuvers described earlier, often strictures much longer than the "guideline lengths" can be so reconstructed.

21. **b. The operation can conceptually become one operation with multidimensional application.** A number of applications of genital skin islands, mobilized on either the dartos fascia of the penis or the tunica dartos of the scrotum, have been proposed for repair of urethral stricture disease. In the past, these flap operations were considered to be separate procedures. We suggest that all of these procedures are really different applications of a single concept, proposed by the microinjection studies of Quartey. Skin islands, as mentioned, can be viewed as passengers on fascial flaps, and the design of flaps for urethral reconstruction can be done parallel to the design of flaps for reconstruction in general. These procedures that use skin islands oriented on the penile dartos fascia have been also useful for reconstruction of the fossa navicularis. There are three important considerations for the use of flaps in urethral reconstruction: (1) the nature of the flap tissue, (2) the vasculature of the flap, and (3) the mechanics of flap

transfer. The skin must be nonhirsute for urethral reconstruction. In addition, for donor site consideration, it is most convenient to use the areas of redundant nonhirsute genital skin. These skin islands can be reliably elevated even in patients who have been circumcised.

22. **d. Continence is best addressed after a procedure to reestablish urethral continuity is performed.** We have found, and others have reported, that the competence of the bladder neck is difficult to accurately assess before the reestablishment of urethral continuity. Even in cases in which an obvious scar is noted to involve the bladder neck, follow-up of these patients after urethral reconstruction has found many patients with more than adequate continence. Still other patients are believed to have incontinence due to scar incarceration of the bladder neck. In our experience, however, this is an infrequent occurrence, and the appearance of the bladder neck by any modality available is not predictive of continence. It is currently our practice to reestablish the continuity of the urethra and, in cases in which there are concerns about continence, to forewarn the patient before the urethral reconstruction. Colopinto and others have not shown an association of ultimate continence as related to the location of the distraction injury.

23. **e. It is usually present with either ventral curvature or ventral curvature associated with torsion.** In many cases, there are abnormalities of the ventral penile skin. In patients who have chordee without hypospadias, the photograph will reveal an erect penis commensurate with the size of the detumescent penis, whereas in the congenital curvature patient, the erect penis will be noticeably large. Because of their congenital anomaly, these patients often become relatively reclusive and have poor self and genital images and may benefit from sex therapy. Even in patients with obvious abnormalities of the corpus spongiosum (i.e., poor ventral fusion or frank bifid corpus spongiosum), wide mobilization usually reveals that it is not the corpus spongiosum that remains as the ventral limiting factor. In most patients, the penis will remain curved because of the inelasticity of the ventral aspect of the corpora cavernosa. If the epithelial tube has served as an adequate urethra (i.e., it is not stenotic), the morbidity of the urethral division and subsequent need for urethral reconstruction must be considered before undertaking such a procedure. In children, after mobilization and excision of the dysgenetic tissues, the residual chordee can usually be corrected by making a longitudinal incision with a sharp blade. If this maneuver is not sufficient, the dorsal neurovascular structures can be mobilized in concert with the Buck fascia and a small ellipse or ellipses of dorsal tunica albuginea excised and closed with watertight plicating sutures.

24. **b. In most cases, global cavernosal veno-occlusive dysfunction (CVOD) is not a complicating factor.** When a young man presents with an acquired curvature of the penis, one must always allow for the possibility of Peyronie disease. Occasionally, however, a patient or his initial-care physician will ignore the stigmata of the trauma (often described as "minimal" by patients), and the patient will present with a noticeable lateral scar that causes both indentation of the lateral aspect of the penis and, in some cases, curvature. Patients who had preexisting lateral curvature may actually notice that their penis has been straightened by the trauma, but they are disturbed by the concavity caused by the scar. The pathology of a subclinical fracture of the penis is believed to be due to either the disruption of the outer longitudinal layer of the tunica albuginea during the buckling trauma only or the disruption of both layers of the tunica albuginea during the buckling trauma but with preservation of Buck fascia. These patients usually have normal erectile function, and there is no association with concomitant global CVOD. However, the association of CVOD and trauma of the penis continues to be seen, and some patients, after fracture-type injuries of the penis, will have significant problems with ED. These injuries are not associated with shorten-

ing of the penis. It is the lack of ED and penile shortening that help distinguish these patients from those with Peyronie disease. Although foreshortening of the penis is not a characteristic of either the injury itself or the resulting scar in either of these injuries, these patients are not thought to be best treated by approaching the opposite aspect of the scar and excising an ellipse of the tunica. This would result in bilateral scars, which will cause bilateral indentation of the penis, and although the penis will have been straightened by the correction, most patients are upset by the cosmetic and functional result of a near-circumferential indentation of the penis. Curvatures associated with hypospadias or epispadias are not acquired curvatures.

25. **b. PFUIs most commonly occur between the prostate and membranous urethra.** Pelvic fracture distraction injuries of the membranous urethra have been compared with plucking an apple (prostate) off its stem (the membranous urethra). This analogy implies that the injury most frequently occurs at the apex of the prostate. Experience shows that this is not the case, however, and the most frequent point of distraction is at the departure of the bulbous urethra from the membranous urethra. The distraction can, however, involve all or any portion of the membranous urethra between the departure of the bulbous urethra and the apex of the prostate. The remaining answer choices are correct.

26. **a. Mobilizing the corpus spongiosum off the corpora cavernosa up to the corona of the glans.** Aggressive mobilization of the corpus spongiosum is performed with caution because it is thought to have possible ill effects on retrograde blood supply, which in the pelvic fracture patient may be tenuous. Meticulous detachment of the investment of Buck fascia from the corpus spongiosum increases the compliance of the corpus and limits the need for aggressive mobilization. It is important to try to avoid the creation of chordee during the repair of a distraction injury. To prevent chordee, the attachment cannot be carried beyond the area of the penoscrotal attachment. Development of the intracrural space, infrapubectomy, and, if needed, rerouting of the corpus spongiosum each shorten the course that the corpus spongiosum must traverse and allow reconstruction without attendant chordee.

27. **d. Men with arteriogenic ED following PFUI who demonstrate bilateral occlusion of the internal pudendal arteries without reconstitution.** Patients with an intact pudendal artery on one side are often potent and reliably cured with reconstruction. Patients with only reconstituted vessels, either unilateral or bilateral, are rarely potent but reliably reconstructed. Those patients at risk for ischemic stenosis are only those with bilateral complete obstruction of the internal pudendal vessels without reconstitution. In such a patient, we now perform penile arterial revascularization to augment the vascularity and, with that accomplished, then proceed to urethral reconstruction. Patients without ED by definition have normal penile hemodynamics and do not require further investigation before repair of a PFUI.

28. **a. Rigidity of the neophallus may be achieved by placement of a penile prosthesis before the return of tactile sensation of the phallus.** Rigidity for intercourse in the patient with phallic construction is usually achieved by either an externally applied or a permanently implanted prosthesis. Prosthetic implantation is never undertaken until 1 year after phallic construction, because protective sensibility must be demonstrated in the flap. When the flap is transferred, it is, by definition, rendered insensate. At about 3 to 4 months after reconstruction, however, as nerve regeneration occurs, sensation becomes noticeable. In addition, before prosthetic implantation is undertaken, the urethra must be patent and proved to be durable.

29. **d. Idiopathic proximal 1-cm bulbar urethral stricture in a patient with a history of a prior hypospadias repair.** Patients with a history of hypospadias can be expected to have altered or absent retrograde blood supply to the urethra through the normal arborization in the glans. In this situation, transecting techniques to repair urethral strictures should be avoided

unless performed in a "vessel-sparing" fashion to avoid the risk of ischemic urethral stenosis. Inlay or onlay graft or flap techniques may be used in these patients, as these do not disrupt the proximal blood supply to the urethra. The remaining scenarios can be reliably repaired with anastomotic urethroplasty.

30. **d. By preserving the proximal blood supply of the urethra, it has better outcomes and less de novo erectile disfunction a than transecting excision and primary anastomosis.** The vessel-sparing technique for anterior urethral reconstruction was first introduced by Jordan et al. in 2007 and later modified by Mundy et al. in 2010. It spares the bulbar urethral arteries but maintains the same principles of traditional excision and primary anastomosis (wide, spatulated, tension-free anastomosis). Originally intended to prevent potential future spongiosum atrophy in selected patients, it became part of the armamentarium in anterior urethral reconstruction for a variety of entities in some centers around the world, although

it may be reserved for experienced urethral reconstructive surgeons. To date, there is no evidence of benefit in terms of overall outcome or prevention of de novo ED. Since its introduction, the principle of vessel-sparing has been applied in a variety of techniques for repair of the anterior and even posterior urethra.

31. **e. b and c.** Despite that vessel-sparing urethral reconstruction has been embraced in several centers across the globe, there is no evidence that this technique is better than traditional excision and primary anastomosis. In cases where the proximal blood supply has already been compromised, such as stricture recurrence after prior transecting bulbar urethroplasty, or where the distal urethral blood supply of the urethra is poor, such in patients with hypospadias, especially after prior repairs, it makes sense to preserve the blood supply of the bulbospongiosum.

CHAPTER REVIEW

1. A meshed split-thickness graft that is applied to the genitalia should not be expanded but rather placed on the recipient site without expansion to allow collections from beneath the graft to escape.

2. Split-thickness grafts may contain some lymphatics; however, full-thickness grafts have a full complement of lymphatics.

3. Split-thickness grafts are more likely to take (become vascularized) but tend to contract and become brittle when mature, whereas full-thickness grafts have more difficulty becoming vascularized but are less likely to contract and are more durable when mature.

4. Tunica vaginalis grafts result in aneurysmal dilatation when they are used for large defects.

5. The superficial dorsal penile vein usually drains to the left saphenous vein; the deep dorsal and circumflex veins lying beneath the Buck fascia drain to the periprostatic plexus.

6. The Buck fascia is adjacent to the deep structures of the penis; the dartos fascia is next to the skin.

7. LS is a disease of the skin and may involve large portions of the genital skin; therefore, using the genital skin for reconstruction may result in recurrence of the disease. Oral mucosal grafting has emerged as a better tissue in patients with LS–associated urethral strictures.

8. LS may be a premalignant lesion and often results in meatal stenosis.

9. A spontaneous urethral fistula or unexplained periurethral abscess may be the harbinger of a urethral carcinoma.

10. Circumcision provides protection for heterosexual men in areas of endemic HIV; it reduces the risk of acquiring herpes simplex type 2, papillomavirus, and genital ulcer disease.

11. Cellulitis may be a problem in patients who have genital lymphedema.

12. As a general rule in the urethra, flaps are best suited for distal reconstruction, grafts for proximal reconstruction.

13. A urethral stricture involves the epithelium as well as the corpus spongiosum (spongiofibrosis).

14. For urethral distraction injuries (posterior urethral disruptions), an aligning catheter, at the very worst, facilitates subsequent reconstruction and, at best, may leave the patient with an endoscopically manageable urethra.

15. Because paraphimosis tends to recur, a dorsal slit or circumcision should be electively planned.

16. For urethral reconstruction an onlay graft or flap has a higher success rate than tabularized grafts.

17. Vesicourethrorectal fistulae are most successfully closed when normal tissue is interposed between the rectum and the bladder/urethra. The gracilis muscle interposition flap is an excellent tissue to interpose and, when used, has a high success rate.

18. Curvature of the penis in patients with Peyronie disease who require repair are best managed with corporal plication techniques and not grafting.

19. The corpora cavernosa are not separate structures but constitute a single space with free communication through an incompetent midline septum.

20. Meatal stenosis in the male child appears to be a consequence of circumcision.

21. It is imperative to completely evaluate the urethra proximal and distal to a stricture with endoscopy and bougienage during surgery, to ensure that all of the involved urethra is included in the reconstruction.

22. The curative success rate of internal urethrotomy is 29% to 30% for all patients. The strictures that respond best to internal urethrotomy are strictures of the bulbous urethra that are less than 1.5 cm in length and are not associated with the dense or deep spongiofibrosis.

23. The best results for primary reanastomosis are achieved when the following technical points are observed: (1) the area of the fibrosis is totally excised; (2) the urethral anastomosis is widely spatulated, creating a large ovoid anastomosis; (3) the anastomosis is tension free; and (4) epithelial apposition is achieved.

24. In complete membranous urethra disruption, the most frequent point of distraction is at the departure of the bulbous urethra from the membranous urethra. The distraction can, however, involve all or any portion of the membranous urethra between the departure of the bulbous urethra and the apex of the prostate.

25. Aggressive mobilization of the corpus spongiosum is performed with caution in patients with urethral disruptions because it is thought to have possible ill effects on retrograde blood supply to the urethra.

83 Surgery of the Scrotum and Seminal Vesicles

Dorota J. Hawksworth, Mohit Khera, and Amin S. Herati

QUESTIONS

1. Which of the following vessels has the least direct contribution to the arterial supply of the vas deferens?
   a. Deferential artery
   b. Internal spermatic artery
   c. Superior vesicle artery
   d. Inferior epigastric artery
   e. Inferior epididymal artery

2. The best reason for using the no-scalpel vasectomy technique is:
   a. it has a higher sterilization rate than standard vasectomy with incision.
   b. patients are rendered sterile in less time.
   c. it is easier to learn than the standard technique.
   d. it results in a lower rate of complications, including hematoma and infection.
   e. it results in a higher rate of reversibility.

3. The no-scalpel technique for vasectomy reduces the rate of:
   a. hematoma.
   b. vasectomy failures.
   c. recanalization.
   d. injury to testicular artery.
   e. chronic orchialgia.

4. Vasectomy failure rate when both the abdominal and testicular ends of the divided vas deferens are occluded with hemoclips is:
   a. less than 1%.
   b. 5% to 10%.
   c. 10% to 20%.
   d. 20% to 30%.
   e. 50% to 60%.

5. The technical aspect shown to decrease vasectomy failure rates the most is:
   a. no-scalpel technique.
   b. conventional technique.
   c. fascial interposition of dartos fascia between the divided ends of the vas deferens.
   d. occluding both ends of the divided vas deferens with hemoclips.
   e. occluding both ends of the divided vas deferens thermally with the use of intraluminal cautery.

6. The technical aspect when performing vasectomy to make vasectomy reversal easier in the future is:
   a. no-scalpel technique.
   b. not excising a long segment of vas deferens.
   c. dividing the vas deferens as close to the epididymis as possible.
   d. occluding both ends of the divided vas deferens with hemoclips.
   e. occluding both ends of the divided vas deferens thermally with the use of intraluminal cautery.

7. Vasectomy has been established as associated with:
   a. prostate cancer.
   b. dementia.
   c. cardiovascular disease.
   d. atherosclerosis.
   e. a 10% incidence of chronic scrotal pain.

8. What is the estimated percentage of men who develop antisperm antibodies after vasectomy?
   a. 0% to 20%
   b. 20% to 40%
   c. 40% to 60%
   d. 60% to 80%
   e. Greater than 80%

9. Which of the following is an indication for repeat vasectomy?
   a. Painless sperm granuloma
   b. Motile sperm found in semen analysis 3 months after vasectomy
   c. Nonmotile sperm found in semen analysis 3 months after vasectomy
   d. Persistent testicular pain 3 months after vasectomy
   e. All of the above

10. Pressure-induced injury following vasectomy occurs in:
    a. the testis.
    b. the ejaculatory duct.
    c. the epididymis.
    d. the vas deferens.
    e. the seminal vesicles.

11. In the management of chronic orchialgia, which of the following statements is TRUE?
    a. Imaging studies are not indicated.
    b. Varicocele is not a significant contributor of chronic scrotal pain.
    c. Orchiectomy usually relieves the pain.
    d. Denervation of the cord may offer relief in selected cases.
    e. Diagnostic epididymal puncture should be performed to rule out chronic bacterial epididymitis.

12. Which of the following statements is TRUE regarding hydrocelectomy?
    a. Hematoma is the least frequent complication.
    b. The Jaboulay bottleneck operation is associated with a high recurrence rate.
    c. The Lord plication is an ideal operation for long-standing postinfectious hydroceles.
    d. Sclerotherapy is often the treatment of choice for young men of reproductive age.
    e. The Jaboulay bottleneck operation is associated with a low recurrence rate.

13. A non-transilluminating, nontender mass is noted in the epididymis on physical examination and confirmed to be solid by sonography. What is the most likely diagnosis?
    a. Epididymal cyst
    b. Adenomatoid tumor
    c. Spermatocele
    d. Testicular tumor
    e. Hydrocele

14. Men who were treated with epididymectomy for chronic epididymitis responded the most favorably if:
    a. there was a palpable epididymal abnormality.
    b. there was no palpable abnormality, but there were sonographic changes of the epididymis.
    c. there were no palpable abnormalities and no sonographic changes of the epididymis.
    d. they had improvement of pain with spermatic cord block.
    e. none of the above apply.

15. Which of the following statements is TRUE regarding retractile testes in adults?
    a. As in children, surgical repair is never indicated.
    b. A dartos pouch orchidopexy is the treatment of choice.
    c. Simple three-stitch orchiopexy of the tunica albuginea to the dartos, as for torsion prophylaxis, is effective in preventing retraction.
    d. Bilateral orchiopexy is necessary for a unilateral retractile testis.
    e. Coexisting varicocele is common.

16. The most appropriate approach to a long-standing, thick-walled, loculated hydrocele is:
    a. excision of the hydrocele sac.
    b. the Jaboulay bottleneck technique.
    c. the Lord plication technique.
    d. the inguinal approach.
    e. sclerotherapy.

17. In men with chronic orchitis without an identifiable bacterial pathogen, antibiotics:
    a. decrease the length of symptoms.
    b. improve the severity of symptoms.
    c. decrease the length of time to full activity.
    d. are steadily being prescribed more frequently empirically.
    e. none of the above apply.

18. When a clinically palpable varicocele is encountered in a patient with orchialgia, varicocelectomy will resolve the pain:
    a. 10% of the time.
    b. 25% of the time.
    c. 50% of the time.
    d. 75% of the time.
    e. 90% of the time.

19. What is the embryologic origin of the seminal vesicles?
    a. Müllerian duct
    b. Ectodermal ridge
    c. Distal mesonephric duct
    d. Swelling of the distal paramesonephric duct
    e. Neural crest cells

20. What percentage of the ejaculate volume is made up of seminal vesicle secretions?
    a. 5% to 10%
    b. 20% to 30%
    c. 60% to 80%
    e. 90%
    e. The seminal vesicle does not contribute to the seminal plasma volume

21. What artery is the major blood supply to the seminal vesicle?
    a. Hypogastric
    b. Vesiculodeferential artery
    c. Inferior vesicle
    d. Internal iliac
    e. Deep dorsal penile

22. Decreased T1 signal intensity on MRI, along with increased T2 intensity of seminal vesicles, is indicative of which process?
    a. Inflammation of the seminal vesicles
    b. Hemorrhage within the seminal vesicles
    c. Seminal vesicle tumors
    d. Seminal vesicle cysts
    e. Normal seminal vesicles

23. Agenesis of the seminal vesicle is associated with significant ipsilateral renal anomalies. What is the embryologic reason for this?
    a. A genetic defect links seminal vesicle agenesis to renal agenesis.
    b. A mutation occurs in the cystic fibrosis transmembrane regulator gene.
    c. There was an insult to the mesonephric duct at approximately 12 weeks' gestation.
    d. There was an embryologic insult to the mesonephric duct earlier than 7 weeks' gestation.
    e. There is no association between agenesis of the seminal vesicle and ipsilateral renal anomalies.

24. What disorder is frequently associated with bilateral agenesis of the seminal vesicles?
    a. Cystic fibrosis
    b. Kartagener syndrome
    c. Young syndrome
    d. Kallmann syndrome
    e. Klinefelter syndrome

25. What causes the majority of seminal vesicle cysts?
    a. Ejaculatory duct stone
    b. Obstruction of the ejaculatory duct
    c. Inflammation
    d. Renal agenesis
    e. Trisomy 21

26. What is the most common type of malignant neoplasm found in seminal vesicles?
    a. Primary adenocarcinoma
    b. Sarcoma
    c. Cystosarcoma phyllodes
    d. Metastatic tumors
    e. Amyloidosis

27. What is the best initial test for a suspected seminal vesicle abnormality?
   a. Computed tomography (CT)
   b. Transrectal ultrasonography
   c. Magnetic resonance imaging (MRI)
   d. Fine-needle biopsy
   e. Vasography

28. What is the best method to differentiate a benign from malignant seminal vesicle mass?
   a. Biopsy of the lesion
   b. Contrast medium-enhanced CT
   c. Gadolinium enhanced MRI
   d. Transrectal ultrasonography
   e. Rectal examination

29. What is the best surgical approach to a congenital lesion of the seminal vesicle?
   a. The perineal route because this has the quickest recovery.
   b. The transcoccygeal route because these are usually large lesions.
   c. The laparoscopic route so that the ipsilateral kidney can be dealt with concomitantly and recovery may be shorter.
   d. The paravesical route because this has a lower incidence of postoperative erectile dysfunction.
   e. The transvesical route because rectal injury is much less likely.

30. What is the best indication for the transcoccygeal approach to the seminal vesicle?
   a. Need for exploration of the ipsilateral kidney
   b. Patient with previous suprapubic and/or perineal surgery
   c. Patient wishing to maintain potency
   d. Patient with bilateral large seminal vesicle lesions
   e. Patient with metastatic tumor to the seminal vesicle

31. In a patient with a seminal vesicle abscess, the treatment of choice is:
   a. laparoscopic unroofing.
   b. transvesical excision of the seminal vesicle.
   c. aspiration and antibiotic instillation.
   d. endoscopic unroofing by deep transurethral resection.
   e. retropubic approach to unroof the abscess.

ANSWERS

1. **c. Superior vesicle artery.** The superior vesicle artery does not supply the vas deferens, whereas all of the other arteries listed may have a branch to the vas deferens.
2. **d. It results in a lower rate of complications, including hematoma and infection.** This method eliminates the scalpel incision, results in fewer hematomas and infections, and leaves a much smaller wound than conventional methods of accessing the vas deferens for vasectomy.
3. **a. Hematoma.** The no-scalpel technique significantly decreases the rate of hematomas, infections, and pain during the procedure.
4. **a. Less than 1%.** Vasectomy failure rate when both the abdominal and testicular ends of the divided vas deferens are occluded with hemoclips is less than 1%.
5. **c. Fascial interposition of dartos fascia between the divided ends of the vas deferens.** Interposition of dartos fascia between the divided ends of the vas deferens is a technique for occlusion that has been reported to reduce the recanalization rate to nearly zero.

6. **b. Not excising a long segment of vas deferens.** The technical aspects when performing vasectomy to make vasectomy reversal easier in the future include not excising a long segment of vas deferens, dividing the vas deferens approximately 3 cm cephalad to the cauda of the epididymis in the straight portion of the vas deferens, and transecting the vas deferens, followed by low-voltage cautery occlusion and then by fascial interposition.
7. **e. A 10% incidence of chronic scrotal pain.** Vasectomy does not have an established association with prostate cancer, dementia, cardiovascular disease, or atherosclerosis, although it has been associated with a 10% incidence of chronic scrotal pain.
8. **d. 60% to 80%.** Vasectomy disrupts the blood–testis barrier, resulting in detectable levels of serum antisperm antibodies in 60% to 80% of men.
9. **b. Motile sperm found in semen analysis 3 months after vasectomy.** If any motile sperm are found in the ejaculate 3 months after vasectomy, consideration should be given to repeating the procedure.
10. **c. The epididymis.** The brunt of pressure-induced damage after vasectomy falls on the epididymis and efferent ductules.
11. **d. Denervation of the cord may offer relief in selected cases.** Microsurgical total denervation of the spermatic cord is a procedure used with reported success in several small series.
12. **e. The Jaboulay bottleneck operation is associated with a low recurrence rate.** The Jaboulay bottleneck operation, in which the sac edges are sewn together behind the cord, reduces the chance of recurrence caused by reapposition of the edges of the hydrocele sac.
13. **b. Adenomatoid tumor.** Most nontransilluminable solid epididymal masses are benign adenomatoid tumors.
14. **a. There was a palpable epididymal abnormality.** A retrospective review of men who underwent epididymectomy for chronic epididymitis showed that outcomes were best when the patient had a palpable epididymal abnormality on physical examination. Men in this study without a palpable abnormality, but with sonographic changes, had slightly worse outcomes, and those with neither a palpable abnormality nor a demonstrable ultrasonographic abnormality did not improve with epididymectomy.
15. **b. A dartos pouch orchidopexy is the treatment of choice.** Creation of a dartos pouch will keep the testis well down into the scrotum and permanently prevent retraction.
16. **a. Excision of the hydrocele sac.** Excising the hydrocele is recommended for long-standing, thick-walled, loculated hydroceles.
17. **d. Are steadily being prescribed more frequently empirically.** Despite evidence that up to 75% of patients with epididymitis/orchitis do not have an identifiable bacterial urinary tract infection concomitantly with their clinical epididymitis, antibiotics are routinely given. Empirical antibiotic administration in the absence of positive urine cultures has been steadily increasing, from 75% to 95% between the years of 1965 and 2005 and is not indicated.
18. **c. 50% of the time.** When a clinically palpable varicocele is encountered in a patient with orchialgia, varicocelectomy will resolve the pain 50% of the time.
19. **c. Distal mesonephric duct.** The seminal vesicle develops as a dorsolateral bulbous swelling of the distal mesonephric duct at approximately 12 fetal weeks.
20. **c. 60% to 80%.** The secretions from the seminal vesicle contribute 60% to 80% of the ejaculate volume.
21. **b. Vesiculodeferential artery.** The blood supply to the seminal vesicle is from the vesiculodeferential artery, a branch of the superior vesical artery.
22. **a. Inflammation of the seminal vesicles.** Seminal vesiculitis shows decreased signal intensity on the T1-weighted image, whereas the T2-weighted image intensity is higher than that of both fat and the normal seminal vesicle.

23. **d. There was an embryologic insult to the mesonephric duct earlier than at 7 weeks' gestation.** Unilateral agenesis of the seminal vesicles has an incidence of 0.6% to 1% and may be associated with unilateral absence of the vas deferens, as well as ipsilateral renal anomalies.

24. **a. Cystic fibrosis.** Of men with bilateral absence of the vas deferens or seminal vesicles, 70% to 80% carry the genetic mutation associated with cystic fibrosis. Conversely, 80% to 95% of men with cystic fibrosis have bilateral absence of the vas deferens or seminal vesicles.

25. **b. Obstruction of the ejaculatory duct.** Cysts of the seminal vesicles may be either congenital or acquired and are thought to be due to obstruction of the ejaculatory duct.

26. **d. Metastatic tumors.** Very few primary tumors of the seminal vesicles have been reported. It is more common for carcinoma of the bladder, prostate, or rectum, or lymphoma to secondarily involve the seminal vesicles.

27. **b. Transrectal ultrasonography.** Transrectal ultrasonography is the preferred initial test for seminal vesicle abnormality because of its low invasiveness, ease of performance, and ability to perform concomitant transrectal biopsies.

28. **a. Biopsy of the lesion.** Transrectal ultrasonography and biopsy of the seminal vesicle mass is accurate and easily accomplished.

29. **c. The laparoscopic route so that the ipsilateral kidney can be dealt with concomitantly and recovery may be shorter.** Although data are limited for laparoscopic excision of benign seminal vesicle disease alone, this approach appears to afford superb visualization with minimal postoperative morbidity and shorter hospitalization, compared with the open surgical alternatives.

30. **b. Patient with previous suprapubic and/or perineal surgery.** In individuals for whom the perineal or supine position may be difficult to maintain, or for those who have had multiple suprapubic or perineal surgeries, the transcoccygeal approach may be useful.

31. **d. Endoscopic unroofing by deep transurethral resection.** If the abscess is in the portion of the seminal vesicle adjacent to the prostate, a deep transurethral resection into the prostatic substance, just distal to the bladder neck at the 5-o'clock or 7-o'clock position, may be effective in relieving the problem. However, a CT-guided aspiration and drain placement is becoming the preferred least-traumatic option.

CHAPTER REVIEW

1. Because scrotal cases are considered clean rather than sterile, prophylactic antibiotics are recommended preoperatively. Hair removal should occur immediately before the procedure.

2. Fournier gangrene is a necrotizing fasciitis that involves the skin and subcutaneous tissue and is confined by the dartos fascia on the penis, Colles fascia in the perineum, and Scarpa fascia in the abdomen. Proper resuscitation requires broad-spectrum antibiotics, including a third-generation cephalosporin, an aminoglycoside, and metronidazole. These patients require fluid resuscitation and, when hemodynamically stable, debridement. Daily debridement in the operating room until all nonviable tissue is removed should be subsequently performed.

3. Ninety-seven percent of patients undergoing open-ended vasectomy develop sperm granulomas.

4. Division of the vas deferens during vasectomy should occur at least 3 cm from the epididymitis. There is no vasectomy technique that is 100% effective; more than 80% of the patients achieve azoospermia at 3 months following vasectomy.

5. When the testis is removed for orchialgia, pain relief is better achieved if the orchiectomy is performed through an inguinal incision rather than a transscrotal incision.

6. There is no level 1 evidence that orchiectomy is effective for the treatment of chronic orchialgia.

7. Any surgical manipulation of the epididymis results in azoospermia on that side.

8. Leaving a scrotal drain after scrotal procedures does not lessen the complication rate or the development of postoperative hematomas.

9. When repairing large hydroceles, the epididymis and spermatic vessels may be splayed by the hydrocele, and care must be taken to identify them to avoid injury.

10. Microsurgical denervation of the spermatic cord has been used for the treatment of orchialgia with reported success rates as high as two-thirds achieving pain relief. It should only be considered if a cord block is successful.

11. Seminal vesicle cysts are associated with ipsilateral renal agenesis or dysplasia in two-thirds of patients and have been associated with polycystic kidney disease.

12. *Mycobacterium tuberculosis* and *Schistosoma haematobium* may infect the seminal vesicles.

13. Vasectomy has not been established to be associated with prostate cancer, dementia, cardiovascular disease, or atherosclerosis, although it has been associated with a 10% incidence of chronic scrotal pain.

14. Vasectomy disrupts the blood-testis barrier, resulting in detectable levels of serum antisperm antibodies in 60% to 80% of men.

15. The Jaboulay operation, in which the sac edges are sewn together behind the cord, reduces the chance of recurrence caused by reapposition of the edges of the hydrocele sac.

16. Of men with bilateral absence of the vas deferens or seminal vesicles, 70% to 80% are carriers of the genetic mutation associated with cystic fibrosis. Conversely, 80% to 95% of men with cystic fibrosis have bilateral absence of the vas deferens or seminal vesicles.

17. Very few primary tumors of the seminal vesicles have been reported. It is more common for carcinoma of the bladder, prostate, or rectum or lymphoma to secondarily involve the seminal vesicles.

84 Surgical, Radiologic, and Endoscopic Anatomy of the Kidney and Ureter

Mohamed A. Elkoushy and Sero Andonian

QUESTIONS

1. The exact position of the kidney within the retroperitoneum varies during:
   a. different phases of respiration.
   b. presence of anatomic anomalies.
   c. body position.
   d. a, b, and c
   e. a and c

2. Gerota fascia envelops the kidney and the adrenal gland on all aspects but remains open:
   a. inferiorly.
   b. laterally.
   c. medially.
   d. inferiorly and laterally.
   e. inferiorly and medially.

3. The white line of Toldt is the lateral reflection of posterior parietal peritoneum that covers:
   a. the ascending colon.
   b. the descending colon.
   c. the transverse colon.
   d. the ascending and descending colons.
   e. the ascending and transverse colon.

4. What are the columns of Bertin?
   a. Extensions of renal medulla between the pyramids
   b. Extensions of renal cortex between the pyramids
   c. Cortical extensions between renal lobules
   d. The collecting ducts
   e. None of the above

5. Compared with the liver, the normal adult kidneys in gray-scale ultrasound appear:
   a. hyperechoic.
   b. isoechoic.
   c. hypoechoic.
   d. b and c.
   e. variable, depending on the renal function.

6. Occlusion or injury to a segmental renal artery will cause:
   a. no pathologic conditions.
   b. opening of the collateral circulation.
   c. segmental renal infarction.
   d. an effect that depends on the availability of collaterals.
   e. renal atrophy.

7. Ureteropelvic junction obstruction may be commonly caused by:
   a. the lower anterior segmental artery when it passes anterior to the ureter.
   b. crossing of the ureter by any of the renal segmental arteries.
   c. the posterior segmental artery when it passes posterior to the renal pelvis.
   d. the posterior segmental artery when it passes anterior to the ureter.
   e. the lower anterior segmental artery when it passes posterior to the ureter.

8. Occlusion of a segmental renal vein results in:
   a. segmental renal congestion.
   b. segmental renal atrophy.
   c. no pathologic conditions.
   d. an effect that depends on the availability of collaterals.
   e. gross hematuria.

9. The main renal vasculature can be accurately identified with 100% sensitivity by:
   a. Doppler ultrasonography.
   b. computed tomography angiography (CTA).
   c. intravenous urography.
   d. noncontrast computed tomography.
   e. all of the above.

10. Medial displacement of both pelvic ureteral segments might result from:
    a. pelvic lipomatosis.
    b. postabdominoperineal surgery.
    c. retroperitoneal fibrosis.
    d. all of the above.
    e. a and c.

11. If the small ureteral arteries that anastomose in the ureteral adventitia are disrupted, this may result in:
    a. ureteral ischemia.
    b. ureteral stricture.
    c. a and b.
    d. no impact on ureteral blood supply.
    e. gross hematuria.

12. The blood supply of the mid-ureter is mostly:
    a. anterior.
    b. posterior.
    c. medial.
    d. lateral.
    e. any of the above.

13. What is the Mercier bar?
    a. The intramural ureter
    b. The bladder trigone
    c. The interureteral ridge
    d. Intraureteral valves
    e. None of the above

14. The higher the grade of the ureteral orifice:
    a. the greater its tendency to be laterally located.
    b. the lesser its tendency to reflux.
    c. the greater its tendency to be associated with ureterocele.
    d. the greater its tendency to reflux.
    e. none of the above.

ANSWERS

1. **d. a, b, and c.** The exact position of the kidney within the retroperitoneum varies during different phases of respiration, body position, and presence of anatomic anomalies. For example, the kidneys move inferiorly about 3 cm (one vertebral body) during inspiration and during the changing of body position from supine to the erect position.

2. a. **Inferiorly.** Gerota fascia encasing the kidneys, adrenal glands, and abdominal ureters is closed superiorly and laterally and serves as an anatomic barrier to the spread of malignancy and a means of containing perinephric fluid collections. Superiorly, the Gerota fascia is continuous with the diaphragmatic fascia on the inferior surface of the diaphragm, whereas inferiorly, the anterior and posterior layers of Gerota fascia are loosely attached where perinephric fluid collections can track inferiorly into the pelvis without violating Gerota fascia.

3. **d. The ascending and descending colons.** To access the kidneys transperitoneally, the colon needs to be mobilized from the white line of Toldt, which is the lateral reflection of posterior parietal peritoneum over the ascending and descending colon.

4. **b. Extensions of renal cortex between the pyramids.** The renal cortex is about 1 cm in thickness and covers the base of each renal pyramid peripherally and extends downward between the individual pyramids to form the columns of Bertin.

5. **b. Isoechoic.** In adults, the normal kidneys have smooth margins and are isoechoic to the liver. However, both renal cortices and pyramids are usually hypoechoic to the liver, spleen, and renal sinus. Compared with renal parenchyma, renal sinus appears hyperechoic because of the presence of hilar adipose tissue, blood vessels, and lymphatics.

6. **c. Segmental renal infarction.** After entering the hilum, each artery divides into five segmental end arteries that do not anastomose significantly with other segmental arteries. Therefore, occlusion or injury to a segmental branch will cause segmental renal infarction. Nevertheless, the area supplied by each segmental artery could be independently surgically resected.

7. **d. The posterior segmental artery when it passes anterior to the ureter.** The posterior segmental artery from the posterior division **passes posterior to the renal pelvis** while the others pass anterior to the renal pelvis. If the posterior segmental branch passes anterior to the ureter, ureteropelvic junction obstruction may occur.

8. **c. No pathologic conditions.** The renal venous drainage correlates closely with the arterial supply with the exception that unlike the arterial supply, venous drainage has extensive collateral communication through the venous collars around minor calyceal infundibula. Furthermore, the interlobular veins that drain the post-glomerular capillaries also communicate freely with perinephric veins through the subcapsular venous plexus of stellate veins. Therefore, occlusion of a segmental venous branch has little effect on venous outflow.

9. **b. Computed tomography angiography (CTA).** Doppler ultrasonography clearly identifies renal arteries at their origin from the abdominal aorta. However, the main renal artery is often difficult to identify at baseline ultrasonography. Therefore, CTA is currently considered the gold standard to assess renal arteries with 100% sensitivity for identification of renal arteries and veins.

10. **d. All of the above.** Medial displacement of both pelvic ureteral segments might result from retroperitoneal fibrosis, pelvic lipomatosis, or postabdominoperineal surgery. However, medial displacement and concavity of **a single pelvic ureter** may result from enlarged hypogastric nodes, a bladder diverticulum, or aneurismal dilatation of the hypogastric artery. Nevertheless, this may be a normal finding in adult females if only the right ureter is affected because of the uterine tilt to the left.

11. **c. a and b.** The abdominal portion of the ureter is supplied mainly by arterial branches medially from the main renal artery or the aorta, which form a longitudinal anastomosis on the ureteral wall. Despite this anastomotic plexus, **ureteral ischemia is not uncommon** if these small and delicate ureteral branches are disrupted. Unnecessary lateral retraction and removal of the periureteral adventitial tissues containing the blood supply can result in ureteral ischemia and subsequent stricture.

12. **b. Posterior.** Although main renal arteries or the aorta supply the abdominal ureter medially, the blood supply to the distal ureter comes laterally from the superior vesical artery, a branch of the internal iliac artery, and the mid-ureter is supplied by branches **arising posteriorly** from the common iliac arteries. Therefore, the blood supply of the ureter is medial in the proximal part, posterior in the mid portion, and lateral in the distal portion.

13. **c. The interureteral ridge.** Once the cystoscope is inside the bladder neck, the trigone can be seen as a raised, smooth triangle. The apex of that triangle is situated at the bladder neck; its base is formed by the interureteral ridge or Mercier bar, extending between the two ureteral orifices.

14. **a. The greater its tendency to be laterally located.** The ureteral orifices are classified according to their position or configuration. They are normally located at the medial aspect of the trigone (position A). However, they may be located at the lateral wall of the bladder or at its junction with the trigone (position C) or in between positions A and C (position B). In terms of configuration, grade 0 indicates a normal ureteral orifice that looks like a cone or a volcano. Grades 1, 2, and 3 describe stadium, horseshoe, and golf-hole orifice, respectively. The higher the grade of the orifice, the greater its tendency to be laterally located and to reflux.

CHAPTER REVIEW

1. The medial aspect of each kidney is rotated anteriorly 30 degrees.
2. The 12th rib overlies the right kidney; the 11th and 12th ribs overlie the left kidney.
3. The columns of Bertin contain the interlobar arteries.
4. Renal hilar structures from anterior to posterior are renal vein, renal artery, and renal pelvis.
5. The line of Brodel is an avascular plane between the anterior and posterior segments. It is variable in location and must be defined for each individual kidney.
6. Lumbar veins may drain directly into the renal veins, which occurs more commonly on the left. They may be the source of troublesome bleeding when dissecting around the renal vein.
7. Gerota fascia encasing the kidneys, adrenal glands, and abdominal ureters is closed superiorly and laterally and serves as an anatomic barrier to the spread of malignancy as well as a means of containing perinephric fluid collections. Superiorly, the Gerota fascia is continuous with the diaphragmatic fascia on the inferior surface of the diaphragm, whereas inferiorly, the anterior and posterior layers of Gerota fascia are loosely attached where perinephric fluid collections can track inferiorly into the pelvis without violating Gerota fascia.
8. Each renal artery divides into five segmental end arteries that do not anastomose significantly with other segmental arteries. They are end arteries and, when occluded, cause renal tissue ischemia and tissue atrophy.
9. The renal venous drainage has extensive collateral communication, and occlusion of a segmental vein will not impair the venous drainage to that segment.
10. Removal of the periureteral adventitial tissues containing the blood supply can result in ureteral ischemia and subsequent stricture.
11. The blood supply of the ureter is medially in the proximal part, posteriorly in the mid portion, and laterally in the distal portion.

85

Physiology and Pharmacology of the Renal Pelvis and Ureter

Dana A. Weiss and Robert M. Weiss

QUESTIONS

1. During development, the ureteral lumen is obliterated and then recanalizes. Which of the following substances appears to be involved in this recanalization process?
   a. Prostaglandin E_2
   b. c-KIT
   c. Angiotensin
   d. Calcitonin gene-related peptide (CGRP)
   e. Acetylcholine

2. The resting membrane potential (RMP) is primarily determined by the distribution of which of the following ions across the cell membrane and the preferential permeability of the cell membrane to that ion?
   a. Potassium
   b. Sodium
   c. Calcium
   d. Chloride
   e. Barium

3. With excitation of the ureteral muscle cell, an action potential is formed. Which of the following pairs of ions are primarily responsible for the upstroke of the action potential?
   a. Potassium and calcium
   b. Sodium and chloride
   c. Calcium and sodium
   d. Potassium and sodium
   e. Calcium and chloride

4. Which of the following must be phosphorylated for smooth muscle contraction to occur?
   a. Actin
   b. Myosin
   c. Calmodulin
   d. Calcium
   e. Troponin

5. The primary site for intracellular storage of calcium is:
   a. mitochondria.
   b. caveolae.
   c. the nucleolus.
   d. actin.
   e. the endoplasmic reticulum.

6. The second messenger involved in β-adrenergic agonist-induced ureteral relaxation is:
   a. cyclic adenosine monophosphate (cAMP).
   b. cyclic guanosine monophosphate (cGMP).
   c. nitric oxide.
   d. inositol 1,4,5-triphosphate (IP_3).
   e. diacylglycerol (DG).

7. The enzyme that degrades cyclic GMP is:
   a. guanylyl cyclase.
   b. myosin light-chain kinase.
   c. phosphodiesterase.
   d. phospholipase C.
   e. nitric oxide synthase (NOS).

8. The enzyme that degrades cyclic AMP is:
   a. adenylyl cyclase.
   b. myosin light-chain kinase.
   c. phosphodiesterase.
   d. phospholipase C.
   e. NOS.

9. Nitric oxide causes smooth muscle relaxation. In doing so, it activates which of the following enzymes?
   a. Guanylyl cyclase
   b. Myosin light-chain kinase
   c. Phosphodiesterase
   d. Phospholipase C
   e. NOS

10. The substrate for NOS is:
    a. cyclic AMP.
    b. cyclic GMP.
    c. GTP.
    d. L-Arginine.
    e. L-Citrulline.

11. Inducible NOS (iNOS) is:
    a. nicotinamide adenine dinucleotide phosphate (NADPH) independent and calcium independent.
    b. NADPH independent and calcium dependent.
    c. NADPH dependent and calcium independent.
    d. NADPH dependent and calcium dependent.
    e. nitric oxide dependent and calcium dependent.

12. The enzyme involved in the formation of DG (diacylglycerol) is:
    a. adenylyl cyclase.
    b. guanylyl cyclase.
    c. phosphodiesterase.
    d. protein kinase C.
    e. phospholipase C.

13. DG increases the activity of which enzyme?
    a. Adenylyl cyclase
    b. Guanylyl cyclase
    c. Phosphodiesterase
    d. Protein kinase C
    e. Phospholipase C

14. An agent that prevents reuptake of norepinephrine in nerve terminals and thus potentiates and prolongs the activity of norepinephrine is:
    a. tyrosine.
    b. monoamine oxidase.
    c. imipramine.
    d. tetramethylammonium.
    e. tetraethylammonium.

15. Norepinephrine is synthesized from:
    a. tyrosine.
    b. arginine.
    c. choline.
    d. cocaine.
    e. imipramine.

16. Which of the following inhibits ureteral and renal pelvic contractile activity?
    a. Substance P
    b. Neurokinin A
    c. Neuropeptide K
    d. Neuropeptide Y
    e. CGRP

17. The enzyme involved in prostaglandin synthesis is:
    a. phospholipase C.
    b. cyclooxygenase.
    c. protein kinase C.
    d. phosphodiesterase.
    e. adenosine triphosphate.

18. Which of the following is a β-adrenergic agonist?
    a. Cromakalim
    b. Physostigmine
    c. Propranolol
    d. Phenoxybenzamine
    e. Isoproterenol

19. Which of the following conditions must be present for urine to pass efficiently from the ureter into the bladder?
    a. Intraluminal ureteral contractile pressure must be above 40 cm H_2O.
    b. The ureterovesical junction (UVJ) must relax.
    c. Intraluminal ureteral contractile pressures must be greater than intravesical baseline pressures.
    d. Intravesical contractile pressures must be less than 40 cm H_2O.
    e. The bladder must relax just before contraction of the ureter.

20. What is normal baseline or resting ureteral pressure?
    a. 0 to 5 cm H_2O
    b. 5 to 10 cm H_2O
    c. 10 to 15 cm H_2O
    d. 15 to 20 cm H_2O
    e. 20 to 25 cm H_2O

21. The Laplace equation expresses the relationship between the variables that affect intraluminal pressure. Which of the following conforms to the Laplace relationship?
    a. Tension = (radius × wall thickness)/pressure
    b. Tension = (radius × pressure)/wall thickness
    c. Tension = (wall thickness × pressure)/radius
    d. Pressure = (radius × wall thickness)/tension
    e. Pressure = (radius × tension)/wall thickness

22. Factors that facilitate ureteral stone passage include:
    a. increased hydrostatic pressures proximal to the calculus and relaxation of the ureter in the region of the stone.
    b. increased hydrostatic pressures proximal to the calculus and contraction of the ureter in the region of the stone.
    c. decreased hydrostatic pressures proximal to the calculus and relaxation of the ureter in the region of the stone.
    d. decreased hydrostatic pressures proximal to the calculus and contraction of the ureter in the region of the stone.
    e. decreased contractile pressures proximal to the calculus and contraction of the ureter in the region of the stone.

23. Which of the following hormones inhibits ureteral contractility?
    a. Bombesin
    b. Thyroxine
    c. Estrogen
    d. Aldosterone
    e. Progesterone

24. A drug that has efficacy in managing ureteral colic is:
    a. bethanechol.
    b. prostaglandin $F_{2\alpha}$.
    c. physostigmine.
    d. indomethacin.
    e. ephedrine.

25. Which of the following is a calcium-binding protein that plays a role in smooth muscle contraction?
    a. Connexin 43
    b. Calmodulin
    c. Cromakalim
    d. Survivin
    e. Myosin

26. In the ureter, the resting or the contractile force developed at any given length depends on the direction in which the change in length is occurring. This is referred to as:
    a. viscoelasticity.
    b. creep.
    c. hysteresis.
    d. stress relaxation.
    e. compensatory relaxation.

27. Which of the following is noted to be expressed before initiation of ureteral peristaltic activity?
    a. Prostanoids
    b. Nitric oxide
    c. c-KIT
    d. Myosin light chain
    e. Phosphodiesterase

28. Ureteral pacemaker activity is amplified by:
    a. prostanoids.
    b. norepinephrine.
    c. CGRP.
    d. cyclic GMP.
    e. potassium channel openers.

ANSWERS

1. **c. Angiotensin.** At a point during development, the ureteral lumen is obliterated and then recanalizes. It appears that angiotensin, acting through the AT2 receptor, is involved in the recanalization process. Knockout mice for the ATR2 gene have congenital anomalies of the kidney and urinary tract, which include multicystic dysplastic kidneys, megaureters, and ureteropelvic junction (UPJ) obstructions.

2. **a. Potassium.** When a ureteral muscle cell is in a nonexcited or resting state, the electrical potential difference across the cell membrane, the transmembrane potential, is referred to as the *resting membrane potential.* The RMP is determined primarily by the distribution of potassium ions (K^+) across the cell membrane and by the permeability of the membrane to potassium ions.

3. **c. Calcium and sodium.** When the ureteral cell is excited, its membrane loses its preferential permeability to K^+ and becomes more permeable to calcium ions (Ca^{2+}) that move inward across the cell membrane, primarily through L-type Ca^{2+} channels, and give rise to the upstroke of the action potential.

4. **b. Myosin.** The most widely accepted theory suggests that phosphorylation of myosin is involved in the contractile process.

5. **e. The endoplasmic reticulum.** Calcium release from tightly bound storage sites (i.e., the endoplasmic or sarcoplasmic reticulum) increases the Ca^{2+} concentration in the sarcoplasm.

6. **a. Cyclic adenosine monophosphate (cAMP).** Cyclic AMP is believed to mediate the relaxing effects of β-adrenergic agonists in a variety of smooth muscles.

7. **c. Phosphodiesterase.** Both cyclic AMP and cyclic GMP can cause smooth muscle relaxation. Cyclic GMP is synthesized from GTP by the enzyme guanylyl cyclase and is degraded to 5'-GMP by a phosphodiesterase.

8. **c. Phosphodiesterase.** Phosphodiesterases degrade both cyclic AMP and cyclic GMP. It has been demonstrated in the canine ureter that a variety of inhibitors can preferentially inhibit the breakdown of one or the other cyclic nucleotide.

9. **a. Guanylyl cyclase.** Nitric oxide released from the nerve activates the enzyme guanylyl cyclase in the smooth muscle cell, with the resultant conversion of guanosine triphosphate to cyclic GMP, with resultant smooth muscle relaxation.

10. **d. L-Arginine.** NOS converts L-arginine to nitric oxide and L-citrulline in a reaction that requires NADPH.

11. **c. NADPH dependent and calcium independent.** An inducible NOS isoform, iNOS, is NADPH dependent but Ca^{2+} independent and has been identified in ureteral smooth muscle.

12. **e. Phospholipase C.** Some actions of α_1-adrenergic and muscarinic cholinergic agonists and a number of other hormones, neurotransmitters, and biologic substances are associated with an increase in intracellular Ca^{2+} and are related to changes in inositol lipid metabolism. These agonists combine with a receptor on the cell membrane, and the agonist-receptor complex, in turn, activates an enzyme, phospholipase C, that leads to the hydrolysis of polyphosphatidylinositol 4,5-bisphosphate, with the formation of two second messengers: IP_3 and DG.

13. **d. Protein kinase C.** DG binds to an enzyme, protein kinase C, causes its translocation to the cell membrane, and, by reducing the concentration of Ca^{2+} required for protein kinase C activation, results in an increase in this enzyme's activity.

14. **c. Imipramine.** The greatest percentage of the norepinephrine is actively taken up (reuptake or neuronal uptake) into the neuron. Neuronal reuptake regulates the duration for which norepinephrine is in contact with the innervated tissue and thus regulates the magnitude and duration of the catecholamine-induced response. Agents such as cocaine and imipramine (Tofranil, Mallinckrodt, Inc., Hazelwood, MO), which inhibit neuronal uptake, potentiate the physiologic response to norepinephrine.

15. **a. Tyrosine.** Norepinephrine, the chemical mediator responsible for adrenergic transmission, is synthesized in the neuron from tyrosine.

16. **e. CGRP.** Tachykinins and CGRP are neurotransmitters released from peripheral endings of sensory nerves. Tachykinins stimulate contractile activity, and CGRP inhibits contractile activity.

17. **b. Cyclooxygenase.** The "primary" prostaglandins, PGE_1, PGE_2, and $PGF_{2\alpha}$, are synthesized from the fatty acid arachidonic acid by enzymatic reactions involving two cyclooxygenase (COX) isoforms, COX-1 and COX-2.

18. **e. Isoproterenol.** Isoproterenol, a β-adrenergic agonist, depresses smooth muscle contractility.

19. **c. Intraluminal ureteral contractile pressures must be greater than intravesical baseline pressures.** The theoretical aspects of the mechanics of urine transport within the ureter were described in detail by Griffiths and Notschaele in 1983.[a] At normal flow rates, while the renal pelvis fills, a rise in renal pelvic pressure occurs, and urine is extruded into the upper ureter, which is initially in a collapsed state. The contraction wave originates in the most proximal portion of the ureter and moves the urine in front of it in a distal direction. The urine that had previously entered the ureter is formed into a bolus. To propel the bolus of urine efficiently, the contraction wave must completely coapt the ureteral walls, and the pressure generated by this contraction wave provides the primary component of what is recorded by intraluminal pressure measurements. The bolus that is pushed in front of the contraction wave lies almost entirely in a passive, noncontracting part of the ureter.

20. **a. 0 to 5 cm H_2O.** Baseline or resting ureteral pressure is approximately 0 to 5 cm H_2O.

21. **b. Tension = (radius × pressure)/wall thickness.** The Laplace equation expresses the relationship between the variables that affect intraluminal pressure: pressure = (tension × wall thickness)/radius.

22. **a. Increased hydrostatic pressures proximal to the calculus and relaxation of the ureter in the region of the stone.** Two factors that appear to be most useful in facilitating stone passage are an increase in hydrostatic pressure proximal to a calculus and relaxation of the ureter in the region of the stone.

23. **e. Progesterone.** Several studies have shown an inhibitory effect of progesterone on ureteral function. Progesterone has been noted to increase the degree of ureteral dilatation during pregnancy and to retard the rate of disappearance of hydroureter in postpartum women.

24. **d. Indomethacin.** Indomethacin, by reducing pelviureteral pressure and thus pelviureteral wall tension, might eliminate some of the pain of renal colic that is dependent on distention of the upper urinary tract.

25. **b. Calmodulin.** With excitation, there is a transient increase in the sarcoplasmic Ca^{2+} concentration from its steady-state concentration of 10^{-8} to 10^{-7} M to a concentration of 10^{-6} M or higher. At this higher concentration, Ca^{2+} forms an active complex with the calcium-binding protein calmodulin. Calmodulin without Ca^{2+} is inactive. The calcium-calmodulin complex activates a calmodulin-dependent enzyme, myosin light-chain kinase. The activated myosin light-chain kinase, in turn, catalyzes the phosphorylation of the 20,000-dalton light chain of myosin. Phosphorylation of the myosin light chain allows activation by actin of myosin Mg^{2+}-ATPase activity, leading to hydrolysis of ATP and the development of smooth muscle tension or shortening.

26. **c. Hysteresis.** Because the ureter is a viscoelastic structure, the resting or contractile force developed at any given length depends on the direction in which change in length is occurring and on the rate of length change. This is referred to as

---

[a]Sources referenced can be found in *Campbell-Walsh-Wein Urology, ed 12,* on the Expert Consult website.

hysteresis; for the ureter, at any given length, the resting force is less and contractile force is greater when the ureter is allowed to shorten than when the ureter is being stretched.

27. **c. c-KIT.** This tyrosine kinase receptor is important in the development of pacemaker activity and peristalsis of the gut (Der-Silaphet et al., 1998). Pezzone and colleagues (2003) identified c-KIT-positive cells in the mouse ureter. The expression of c-KIT was noted to be upregulated in the embryonic murine ureter before its development of unidirectional peristaltic contractions (David et al., 2005). Incubation of isolated cultured embryonic murine ureters with antibodies that neutralize c-KIT activity alters ureteral morphology and inhibits unidirectional peristalsis. c-KIT-positive cells have been identified in the human ureter (Metzger et al., 2004).

28. **a. Prostanoids.** The ionic conduction underlying pacemaker activity in the upper urinary tract is due to the opening and slow closure of voltage-activated L-type Ca^{2+} channels, which are amplified by prostanoids (Santicioli et al., 1995a). This is opposed by the opening and closure of voltage and Ca^{2+}-dependent K^+ channels. It has been suggested that prostaglandins and excitatory tachykinins, released from sensory nerves, help maintain autorhythmicity in the upper urinary tract through maintenance of Ca^{2+} mobilization. Tetrodotoxin and blockers of the autonomic nervous system, both parasympathetic and sympathetic, have little effect on peristalsis, suggesting that autonomic neurotransmitters play little role in maintaining pyeloureteral motility.

CHAPTER REVIEW

1. Efficient propulsion of the urinary bolus depends on the ability of the walls of the ureter to coapt.
2. Autonomic neurotransmitters play little role in maintaining pyeloureteral motility even though the ureter is supplied by sympathetic and parasympathetic neurons.
3. Ureteral muscle fibers are arranged in a longitudinal, circumferential, and spiral configuration.
4. The ureter is a syncytial type of smooth muscle without discrete neuromuscular junctions.
5. Ureteral peristalsis can occur without innervation; however, the nervous system does play at least a modulating role in ureteral peristalsis, particularly the sympathetic nervous system.
6. α-adrenergic stimulation increases ureteral activity. β-adrenergic stimulation inhibits ureteral and renal pelvic activity.
7. Ureteral pressures can be as high as 20 to 80 cm of water during a contraction.
8. Pressure within the bladder during the storage phase is of paramount importance in determining the efficiency of urine transport across the UVJ.
9. Ureteral obstruction causes a gradual increase in ureteral length and diameter.
10. Infection impairs urine transport by reducing ureteral contractions; it also reduces compliance at the UVJ, which may permit reflux.
11. Progesterone has an inhibitory effect on ureteral function. Progesterone has been noted to increase the degree of ureteral dilatation during pregnancy and to retard the rate of disappearance of hydroureter in postpartum women. The obstruction of pregnancy is primarily due, however, to mechanical factors and secondarily due to the hormonal effects of progesterone.
12. Pacemaker cells have resting potentials less negative than non-pacemaker cells and are located near the pelvicalyceal border.
13. Phosphodiesterase inhibitors and α 1A antagonists cause ureteral smooth muscle relaxation.
14. UPJ obstruction may be anatomic or due to a disordered propagation of peristaltic activity. Some have suggested that the latter is due to an alteration in the configuration of the muscle fibers at the UPJ.
15. Ureteral decompensation will occur when there are sustained intravesicular pressures that exceed 40 cm H_2O.

86 Renal Physiology and Pathophysiology Including Renovascular Hypertension

Thomas Chi and Meyeon Park

QUESTIONS

1. Which of the following statements regarding erythropoiesis is FALSE?
   a. Reduced erythropoiesis and anemia are common in chronic renal disease.
   b. Erythropoiesis is inhibited by low circulating oxygen tension.
   c. During chronic inflammation, erythropoiesis is decreased.
   d. The kidney makes most of the erythropoietin in the body.
   e. There are erythropoietin receptors in many organs of the body.

2. Which of the following statements is TRUE about sodium and the kidney?
   a. By definition, hypernatremia is always associated with elevated total body sodium content.
   b. Normal compensation for hyponatremia is decreased antidiuretic hormone (ADH) secretion and thirst suppression.
   c. Abnormal elevation of serum lipids can lead to a false, elevated measurement of serum sodium.
   d. If asymptomatic hyponatremia does not improve within 24 hours, intravenous hypertonic saline should be started.
   e. In therapy for symptomatic hyponatremia, the goal should be a normal serum sodium value of 135 mEq/L within 48 hours.

3. Which of the following statements regarding therapy for hyponatremia is FALSE?
   a. Fluid overload as a result of hypertonic saline infusion should be treated with a loop diuretic such as furosemide.
   b. Too-rapid correction can lead to a cerebral demyelination syndrome.
   c. Aggressive therapy should be discontinued when the serum sodium concentration is raised 10% or symptoms subside.
   d. Intranasal desmopressin is a useful adjuvant therapy.
   e. For acute severe hyponatremia with symptoms, a typical infusion rate of hypertonic saline would be 1 mL/kg/h.

4. Which of the following statements regarding potassium is FALSE?
   a. Angiotensin-converting enzyme (ACE) inhibitors may be a cause of hypokalemia.
   b. Potassium is primarily an intracellular ion.
   c. Acidosis drives potassium out of the cell into the circulation.
   d. High-sodium load in the distal tubule promotes potassium excretion.
   e. The upper limit for safe intravenous potassium infusion is 40 mEq/h.

5. Which of the following statements regarding hyperkalemia is FALSE?
   a. Hemolysis of the blood sample may falsely elevate the measured potassium.
   b. Hyperkalemia can cause peaked T waves on the electrocardiogram (ECG).

   c. All patients with a serum potassium value greater than 5.5 mEq/L require immediate therapy.
   d. Nebulized albuterol can reduce serum potassium by promoting an intracellular shift of potassium.
   e. Intravenous calcium does not lower serum potassium but is given to protect the heart from the effects of hyperkalemia.

6. Which of the following statements regarding renal handling of acid is FALSE?
   a. Most bicarbonate is reabsorbed in the distal collecting tubule.
   b. Lungs can excrete volatile acid, but the kidneys must excrete fixed acid.
   c. Carbonic anhydrase catalyzes the production of H+ and HCO^-_3 from H_2O and CO_2.
   d. Chronic respiratory acidosis should lead to increased H+ in the kidney.
   e. Ammonium ion (NH+4) is produced from glutamine, primarily by proximal tubular cells.

7. Which of the following statements regarding renal tubular acidosis (RTA) is FALSE?
   a. The hallmark of RTA type I is a hyperchloremic metabolic acidosis with a high urinary pH (>5.5) in the presence of persistently low serum HCO^-_3.
   b. Type I RTA is also called distal RTA.
   c. Type II RTA is more common in children.
   d. The hallmark of type IV RTA is hypokalemia.
   e. The form of RTA most commonly associated with renal calculi is type I.

8. Which of the following statements is TRUE about vitamin D metabolism?
   a. Vitamin D deficiency is uncommon in chronic renal failure.
   b. Dermally synthesized cholecalciferol is the most potent form of vitamin D.
   c. Dermally synthesized cholecalciferol must be hydroxylated by both the liver and kidney for maximal potency.
   d. Vitamin D activity is mediated through membrane-bound vitamin D receptors.
   e. Vitamin D increases renal excretion of calcium.

9. Which of the following statements regarding parathyroid hormone (PTH) is FALSE?
   a. PTH secretion is increased by hypocalcemia.
   b. PTH secretion is increased by hyperphosphatemia.
   c. PTH receptors are found mainly in bone and kidney.
   d. PTH increases calcium and phosphorus reabsorption in the distal tubule.
   e. PTH helps regulate 1,25(OH)-vitamin D levels by increasing 1α-hydroxylase activity.

10. All of the following are important in GFR regulation EXCEPT:
    a. afferent arteriolar tone.
    b. distal tubule chloride concentrations.
    c. angiotensin II.
    d. nitric oxide.
    e. serum osmolality.

11. All of the following statements regarding GFR assessment are true EXCEPT:
    a. plasma creatinine is an accurate marker of early reductions in GFR.
    b. inulin clearance is an accurate but impractical measurement of GFR.
    c. twenty-four-hour creatinine clearance overestimates GFR by 10% to 20%.
    d. use of the four-variable modification of diet in renal disease (MDRD) formula improves the accuracy of the plasma creatinine.
    e. plasma urea is an unreliable estimate of GFR.

12. Which of the following statements about the proximal convoluted tubule is FALSE?
    a. It functions as a bulk transporter, rather than a fine-tuner of ultrafiltrate.
    b. It is able to increase or decrease reabsorption rates in response to changes in GFR.
    c. It has a minor role in sodium reabsorption.
    d. It reabsorbs 80% of filtered water, mainly through aquaporin-1 water channels.
    e. It is the major site of bicarbonate reabsorption.

13. All of the following statements are true regarding the loop of Henle EXCEPT:
    a. it is responsible for the generation of a hypertonic medullary interstitium, which is necessary for urinary concentration.
    b. it is able to increase or decrease reabsorption rates in response to changes in GFR.
    c. the descending limb is highly water permeable.
    d. the thin ascending limb actively reabsorbs sodium, chloride, and urea.
    e. the thick ascending limb is impermeable to water.

14. A 67-year-old male with stable renal function and a creatinine of approximately 3 mg/dL presents with peripheral vascular disease and a blood pressure of 160/70 mm Hg. He was a long-standing smoker but has recently stopped. He is referred for evaluation for treatment of "ischemic nephropathy." He has hyperlipidemia and had a myocardial infarction 3 years before presentation. His current medications are a calcium channel blocker, an adequate-dose diuretic, and a statin. Which of the following is the most appropriate next step?
    a. Refer the patient for magnetic resonance angiography (MRA) with gadolinium.
    b. Add an angiotensin-converting enzyme (ACE) inhibitor.
    c. Refer for an angiogram.
    d. Increase the diuretic.
    e. Observe for deterioration in renal function and then refer for an angiogram.

15. Which of the following is most similar to human renal vascular hypertension and is felt to be angiotensin dependent rather than volume dependent?
    a. The two-kidney, one-clip Goldblatt model
    b. The one-kidney, one-clip Goldblatt model
    c. The two-kidney, two-clip Goldblatt model

16. Since the results of the Coral trial have been published, which statement is true regarding progression to end-stage renal disease?
    a. Surgical intervention and/or percutaneous angioplasty with intervention is no longer ever indicated.
    b. Medical intervention is superior to surgical intervention.
    c. Medical intervention is superior to percutaneous angioplasty with stenting.
    d. Medical intervention is equal to percutaneous angioplasty with stenting.
    e. Percutaneous angioplasty with stenting is superior to medical intervention.

17. Which of the following statements is TRUE regarding surgical revascularization of a renal artery?
    a. A kidney less than 8 cm in length can be successfully revascularized.
    b. Retrograde filling of the distal renal artery by collateral circulation on radiographic or scintigraphic imaging studies is more likely to result in a successful surgical outcome.
    c. Patients who require renal vascular surgery do not have significant vascular disease elsewhere.
    d. Correction of a renal artery lesion and an aortic aneurysm need to be done simultaneously.
    e. A renal ostial lesion always requires surgical revascularization rather than percutaneous angioplasty and stenting.

18. Ischemic nephropathy results from:
    a. a reduction in renal blood flow and perfusion.
    b. proinflammatory cytokines and/or angiotensin II.
    c. an irreversible change in perfusion pressure.
    d. a failure of autoregulation alone.
    e. failure of development of collateral circulation.

ANSWERS

1. **b. Erythropoiesis is inhibited by low circulating oxygen tension.** Erythropoiesis is increased by low circulating oxygen tension.
2. **b. Normal compensation for hyponatremia is decreased antidiuretic hormone (ADH) secretion and thirst suppression.**
3. **d. Intranasal desmopressin is a useful adjuvant therapy.** Desmopressin is useful to treat hypernatremia caused by diabetes insipidus.
4. **a. Angiotensin-converting enzyme (ACE) inhibitors may be a cause of hypokalemia.**
5. **c. All patients with a serum potassium value greater than 5.5 mEq/L require immediate therapy.** Patients with mild elevation of potassium, especially when chronic and not associated with ECG changes, do not require emergent therapy.
6. **a. Most bicarbonate is reabsorbed in the distal collecting tubule.** Most bicarbonate reabsorption in the kidney occurs in the proximal tubule.
7. **d. The hallmark of type IV RTA is hypokalemia.** RTA type IV is most commonly associated with hyperkalemia. Aldosterone deficiency or resistance leads to decreased secretion of potassium in the distal tubule.
8. **c. Dermally synthesized cholecalciferol must be hydroxylated by both the liver and kidney for maximal potency.** Cholecalciferol is minimally active, but potency increases 100 times after it is hydroxylated at the 1- and 25-position to form calcitriol.
9. **d. PTH increases calcium and phosphorus reabsorption in the distal tubule.** PTH increases phosphorus excretion in the kidney.
10. **e. Serum osmolality.** GFR is not affected significantly by serum osmolality.

11. **a. Plasma creatinine is an accurate marker of early reductions in GFR.** Plasma creatinine is a very insensitive marker of early reductions in GFR, because increases in tubular secretion of creatinine keep plasma levels from rising until there has been a significant reduction in GFR.

12. **c. It has a minor role in sodium reabsorption.** The PCT accounts for 65% of sodium reabsorption, the most of any tubular segment.

13. **d. The thin ascending limb actively reabsorbs sodium, chloride, and urea.** Reabsorption of sodium, chloride, and urea occurs passively in the thin ascending limb.

14. **b. Add an angiotensin-converting enzyme (ACE) inhibitor.** According to the Coral trial, medical therapy consisted of an ACE inhibitor, a statin, and a diuretic. A calcium channel blocker was not necessarily part of the therapy unless blood pressure could not be controlled on an ACE inhibitor and a diuretic alone. With this combination, medical therapy proved to be as beneficial as more aggressive therapy with angiography and with stenting. The patient has significant renal failure, and gadolinium is relatively contraindicated because this may predispose to nephrogenic systemic fibrosis. In fact, further investigation at this point is not indicated because the patient's renal function is stable. Similarly, an angiogram is not indicated. Increasing the diuretic is not indicated because the diuretic is already on board and the presumption is that the dose is adequate. The final choice is not indicated unless there is rapid deterioration of renal function, and even then, there are no data to support that intervening with angiography and percutaneous angioplasty is helpful.

15. **a. The two-kidney, one-clip Goldblatt model.** The other choices do not allow for natriuresis/diuresis from the opposite unclipped kidney. Thus, those two models are volume-dependent causes of hypertension rather than angiotensin dependent.

16. **d. Medical intervention is equal to percutaneous angioplasty with stenting.** Surgical intervention and/or percutaneous angioplasty under certain circumstances may be indicated—specifically, if blood pressure cannot be well controlled medically or there is very rapid deterioration of renal function. The results of the trial are clearly outlined in the text and require no specific explanation.

17. **b. Retrograde filling of the distal renal artery by collateral circulation on radiographic or scintigraphic imaging studies is more likely to result in a successful surgical outcome.** As stated in the text, a kidney less than 8 cm in length cannot be successfully revascularized because it has reached end-stage. Most patients with renal vascular disease have significant vascular disease elsewhere. Renal artery correction and aortic aneurysm correction need not be done simultaneously. A renal ostial lesion may be corrected by percutaneous angioplasty and stenting depending on its radiologic appearance.

18. **b. Proinflammatory cytokines and/or angiotensin II.** Renal blood flow and perfusion may sometimes be maintained at baseline in patients with ischemic nephropathy. Ischemic nephropathy can reverse, and it is not secondary to a failure of autoregulation alone, as explained in the text. Many patients with progressive ischemic nephropathy have collateral circulation.

CHAPTER REVIEW

1. GFR reflects total renal function.
2. GFR can be approximated by creatinine clearance.
3. Formulas based on patient's age, weight, and serum creatinine can best estimate GFR.
4. The nephron has different functional segments that control homeostasis.
5. Most resorption of bicarbonate and ions occurs in the proximal tubule.
6. The architecture of the loop of Henle allows a highly hypertonic interstitium to develop, which is crucial to maximal urinary concentration.
7. Sodium imbalances should be evaluated in the context of fluid status.
8. The best tools to determine the cause of a sodium disorder are the history, volume status, and urinary sodium.
9. Severe sodium deficit or excess must be corrected slowly.
10. Potassium is primarily intracellular.
11. Serum potassium levels reflect total body potassium, as well as the equilibrium between intra- and extracellular potassium.
12. Symptomatic hyperkalemia requires urgent intervention to prevent cardiac dysfunction.
13. Water movement dictates solute concentrations, especially important for sodium balance.
14. Regulation of water movement is highly dependent on antidiuretic hormone.
15. Insertion of aquaporin channels facilitates water reabsorption.
16. Physiologic chemical reactions require a narrow range of serum pH.
17. Acid is excreted through the lungs and the kidney
18. Type 1 RTA (distal) is the only type associated with renal stones.
19. In acid-base disorders, first determine whether the kidney (HCO_3^-) or lungs (pCO_2) are responsible for the primary disorder, then determine whether the compensatory response is appropriate.
20. The renin-angiotensin system is one of multiple chemical mediators that act on renal vascular tone to control renal blood flow.
21. Endothelin is the most potent vasoconstrictor.
22. Nitric oxide and carbon monoxide are potent vasodilators.
23. Renal physiology influences bone metabolism through several hormonal actions.
24. In the kidney, vitamin D is hydroxylated into calcitriol which helps maintain systemic calcium and phosphate levels.
25. PTH influences the kidney to increase calcium reabsorption.
26. Renal artery stenosis is the most common cause of renovascular hypertension.
27. Atherosclerotic vascular disease accounts for 2/3 of cases of renal artery stenosis.
28. Four types of fibromuscular dysplasia can also cause renal artery stenosis. Of these types, medial fibroplasia is the most common and least likely to progress over time.
29. Suspect renovascular hypertension in patients with severe or abrupt-onset hypertension who otherwise have no risk factors for high blood pressure.
30. Two models of renovascular hypertension were established with classic dog model experiments—the two-kidney, one-clip and one-kidney, one-clip models.
31. Noninvasive diagnostic imaging, including MR angiography, CT angiography, and duplex ultrasonography, should be first-line screening to diagnosis renal artery stenosis.
32. Medical management for renovascular hypertension is the mainstay of therapy.
33. Percutaneous intervention to treat renal artery stenosis may be effective, but growing evidence calls into question its efficacy to control blood pressure or prevent renal failure long term.
34. While surgical treatment is no longer first-line therapy for renal artery stenosis, its role still exists for the appropriately selected patient.

87 Renal Insufficiency and Ischemic Nephropathy

Joshua J. Augustine, Alvin C. Wee, Venkatesh Krishnamurthi, and David A. Goldfarb

QUESTIONS

1. A 70-kg man will have the greatest change in glomerular filtration rate (GFR) when the creatinine changes from:
   a. 0.9 to 1.2 mg/dL.
   b. 1.8 to 1.9 mg/dL.
   c. 3.2 to 3.9 mg/dL.
   d. 4.1 to 4.7 mg/dL.
   e. 7.9 to 11 mg/dL.

2. In patients with occult renal artery stenosis, angiotensin-converting enzyme (ACE) inhibitors cause acute renal failure (ARF) due to:
   a. sodium retention.
   b. increased antidiuretic hormone.
   c. afferent arteriolar vasoconstriction.
   d. efferent arteriolar vasodilation.
   e. decreased sympathetic nervous system activity.

3. Six days after partial nephrectomy in a solitary kidney, the patient is oliguric. Large amounts of fluid are coming from the flank drain. The serum creatinine increases from 1.7 to 3.2 mg/dL. The next step in management is:
   a. renal angiography.
   b. computed tomography (CT) scan with intravenous contrast.
   c. renal scan.
   d. immediate surgical exploration.
   e. magnetic resonance imaging (MRI).

4. After a 7-hour-long, complex urethral reconstruction performed in the extended lithotomy position, a patient has severe thigh and buttock pain. The creatinine phosphokinase (CPK) is dramatically elevated. The next step is:
   a. dopamine infusion.
   b. plasmapheresis.
   c. dobutamine infusion.
   d. forced alkaline diuresis.
   e. dialysis.

5. The sentinel cellular change in renal ischemic injury is:
   a. loss of cell polarity.
   b. depletion of adenosine triphosphate (ATP).
   c. alteration of Na^+ metabolism.
   d. increased intracellular Ca^{2+}.
   e. increased oxidant stress.

6. The renal structure at greatest risk for ischemic injury is the:
   a. afferent arteriole.
   b. cortical collecting duct.
   c. juxtaglomerular apparatus.
   d. straight segment (S3) proximal tubule.
   e. distal convoluted tubule.

7. A patient with acute kidney injury (AKI) has a urinary sodium of 10 mEq/L, urinary osmolality of 650, and a renal failure index of < 1. Urinalysis shows 10 to 20 red blood cells (RBCs) per high-power field (HPF), 3 to 5 white blood cells per HPF, 2 + proteinuria, and RBC casts. The most likely diagnosis is:
   a. acute tubular necrosis (ATN).
   b. prerenal azotemia.
   c. acute glomerulonephritis.
   d. acute interstitial nephritis.
   e. obstruction.

8. When AKI is first recognized in a patient, the initial therapeutic intervention should be to:
   a. begin low-dose dopamine.
   b. administer a cardiac inotropic agent.
   c. restore adequate circulating blood volume.
   d. administer a loop diuretic.
   e. begin a mannitol infusion.

9. Loop diuretics are of benefit in the management of AKI due to:
   a. improved patient survival.
   b. decreased metabolic demand.
   c. decreased hypoxic cell swelling.
   d. free radical scavenging.
   e. increased renal vascular resistance.

10. The major risk of MRI with gadolinium in patients with advanced chronic kidney disease (CKD) is:
    a. nephrotoxicity.
    b. anaphylaxis.
    c. nephrogenic systemic fibrosis.
    d. seizures.
    e. hepatotoxicity.

11. Dopamine therapy in AKI:
    a. causes efferent arteriolar vasodilation.
    b. is recommended for routine use after renal transplantation.
    c. is effective due to improved cardiac function.
    d. is an unproven treatment.
    e. improves patient survival.

12. A patient with AKI after partial nephrectomy has a serum potassium of 6.9 mEq/L and widening of the QRS complex on electrocardiogram (ECG). The initial step in management should be:
    a. intravenous (IV) calcium.
    b. IV insulin and glucose.
    c. sodium polystyrene sulfonate resin (Kayexalate).
    d. IV furosemide.
    e. dialysis.

13. A patient with a serum creatinine level of 2.7 mg/dL requires renal angiography. The best way to protect renal function is:
    a. saline diuresis.
    b. pre-study mannitol.
    c. furosemide before study.
    d. dopamine throughout the study.
    e. atrial natriuretic factor before study.

14. In response to a reduction in renal mass, a number of events occur within the kidney that include all of the following except:
    a. activation of the sympathetic nervous system.
    b. hyperfiltration.
    c. glomerular hypertrophy.
    d. intrarenal vascular occlusion.
    e. interstitial fibrosis.

15. A 65-year-old man has a radical nephrectomy. The estimated GFR by the Modification of Diet in Renal Disease (MDRD) equation is 52 mL/min. Follow-up should include:
    a. low-protein diet.
    b. renal transplant evaluation.
    c. nephrology consult for stage 3 CKD.
    d. reassessment of kidney function every few months.
    e. loop diuretics.

16. A hypertensive patient with CKD should take an ACE inhibitor drug to:
    a. improve renal function.
    b. prevent progressive kidney disease.
    c. improve cardiac ejection fraction.
    d. enhance glycemic control.
    e. control blood lipids.

17. The most common cause for end-stage renal disease (ESRD) in the United States is:
    a. focal segmental glomerulosclerosis (FSGS).
    b. membranoproliferative glomerulonephritis (type 2).
    c. membranous glomerulonephritis.
    d. autosomal dominant polycystic kidney disease.
    e. diabetes mellitus.

18. The patient at lowest risk for progressive CKD is:
    a. diabetic, GFR = 86, albuminuria >300.
    b. postnephrectomy, GFR = 62 mL/min, albuminuria ≤30 mg/g.
    c. hypertensive, GFR = 75 mL/min, albuminuria = 80 mg/g.
    d. IgA nephropathy, GFR 42 mL/min, albuminuria = 70 mg/g.
    e. autosomal dominant polycystic kidney disease (ADPKD), GFR 28 mL/min, albuminuria ≤ 30 mg/g.

19. A hypertensive 38-year-old man has a serum creatinine of 2.4 mg/dL. The urinalysis has 10 to 20 RBCs/HPF, 3 + protein, and RBC casts. Ultrasound shows echogenic kidneys without hydronephrosis. The best way to achieve a diagnosis is:
    a. renal angiography.
    b. renal biopsy.
    c. retrograde pyelography.
    d. MRI.
    e. spiral CT scan.

20. All of the following promote fibrosis in the kidney except:
    a. angiotensin II.
    b. aldosterone.
    c. atrial natriuretic peptide.
    d. transforming growth factor–β.
    e. high-salt diet.

21. CKD patients treated with an ACE inhibitor may experience a decrease in residual renal function in the setting of:
    a. unilateral renal artery stenosis.
    b. concomitant treatment with an alpha-blocker.
    c. acquired renal cystic disease.
    d. left ventricular hypertrophy.
    e. ADPKD with cysts >10 cm.

22. The best renal replacement therapy for an otherwise healthy 37-year-old woman with chronic interstitial nephritis is:
    a. preemptive transplantation.
    b. stabilize with hemodialysis 1 year, then transplant.
    c. stabilize with peritoneal dialysis 1 year, then transplant.
    d. home hemodialysis.
    e. peritoneal dialysis with an automated cycler.

23. Hospitalization in ESRD patients on hemodialysis is most commonly due to:
    a. hypertension.
    b. ileus.
    c. diabetes.
    d. hyperkalemia.
    e. access catheter infection.

24. All the following have a direct toxic effect on the kidney except:
    a. iodinated contrast agent.
    b. myoglobin.
    c. gadolinium-based contrast agents.
    d. carboplatin.
    e. aminoglycoside antibiotics.

25. The strongest predictor of hospitalization in chronic dialysis patients is:
    a. African American race.
    b. hematocrit <30%.
    c. glomerulonephritis.
    d. poor nutritional status.
    e. age <30 years.

Imaging

1. See Fig. 87.1. A 55-year-old woman had this abdominal radiograph 1 day after a contrast-enhanced CT scan was done for abdominal pain. Her creatinine before the CT scan was 1.9 mg/dL. The most likely diagnosis is:
   a. normal film.
   b. ATN.
   c. renal artery occlusion.
   d. hypertensive kidneys.
   e. nephrocalcinosis.

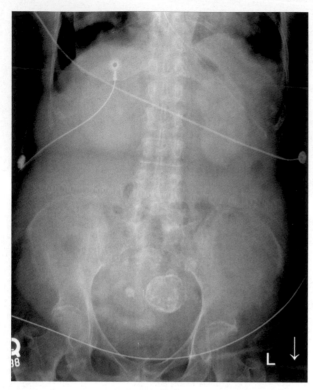

Fig. 87.1

ANSWERS

1. **a. 0.9 to 1.2 mg/dL.** The relationship between serum creatinine is not linear. Above a GFR of 60 mL/min, changes in serum creatinine are minimal. The change in serum creatinine from 0.9 to 1.2 may be associated with a large drop in GFR (120 to 60 mL/min). Below a GFR of 60, proportional increments in creatinine are associated with smaller changes in GFR. This is most notable at very high creatinine levels.

2. **d. Efferent arteriolar vasodilatation.** Angiotensin II has selectively greater vasoconstrictor effects on the efferent than on the afferent arteriole, whereas vasodilatory prostaglandins cause afferent arteriolar vasodilatation. Drugs that block angiotensin II synthesis (ACE inhibitors), block angiotensin II receptor binding (angiotensin II receptor antagonists), or inhibit vasodilatory prostaglandin synthesis (nonsteroidal anti-inflammatory drugs) may cause ARF in selected clinical settings.

3. **c. Renal scan.** There are several ways to confirm urinary extravasation. These include assessment of drain fluid for creatinine, intravenous administration of a vital dye excreted by the kidneys (such as indigo carmine or methylene blue), and radiographic demonstration of a fistula (isotope renography, retrograde pyelography, cystography, computed tomography). Renal scan can assess perfusion and also demonstrate extravasation.

4. **d. Forced alkaline diuresis.** The combination of renal hypoperfusion and the nephrotoxic insult of myoglobin or hemoglobin within the proximal tubule may result in ATN. Early recognition of this disorder is crucial, because a forced alkaline diuresis is indicated to minimize nephrotoxicity.

5. **b. Depletion of adenosine triphosphate (ATP).** The sentinel biochemical event in renal ischemia is the depletion of ATP, which is the major energy currency for cellular work.

6. **d. Straight segment (S3) proximal tubule.** The S3 segment of the proximal tubule is associated with the greatest ischemic damage. Other structures that sustain injury in this region include the medullary thick ascending limb, which is metabolically active and rich in the energy-requiring Na^+, K^+-ATPase.

7. **c. Acute glomerulonephritis.** A low fractional excretion of sodium (or renal failure index) may be associated with either prerenal azotemia or acute glomerulonephritis. These entities could be separated clinically by examination of the urinalysis results. Conditions associated with prerenal azotemia would have a bland urinalysis, whereas proteinuria, RBCs, and RBC casts would be seen with acute glomerulonephritis.

8. **c. Restore adequate circulating blood volume.** During the initial stages, a trial of parenteral hydration with isotonic fluids may correct ARF secondary to prerenal causes.

9. **b. Decreased metabolic demand.** Loop diuretics decrease active NaCl transport in the thick ascending limb of Henle and thereby limit energy requirements in the metabolically active segment, which often bears the greatest ischemic insult.

10. **c. Nephrogenic systemic fibrosis.** Recently, gadolinium-based contrast agents have been associated with the development of nephrogenic systemic fibrosis. At-risk patients include those with advanced CKD. It is important that these compounds be given to these patients only after careful consideration of the indication for the study.

11. **d. Is an unproven treatment.** Results of clinical studies have not conclusively proved that dopamine infusion improves ARF.

12. **a. Intravenous (IV) calcium.** Priorities for treatment of acute hyperkalemia with electrocardiographic changes include stabilizing the electrical membrane of the cardiac conduction system, which may be accomplished with the use of intravenous calcium salts. These have an immediate effect and a rather short duration of action.

13. **a. Saline diuresis.** A study by Solomon and coworkers confirmed that prestudy intravenous hydration with saline was crucial in limiting the nephrotoxic effect of radiocontrast agents in patients with preexisting azotemia. The addition of either a loop diuretic or mannitol did not improve outcome.

14. **d. Intrarenal vascular occlusion.** In response to reduced nephron mass, a mosaic of events occurs linking sympathetic nervous system activation, renal structural remodeling, altered gene expression and regulation, and several regulatory mechanisms for progression.

15. **c. Nephrology consult for stage 3 CKD.** According to the National Kidney Foundation (K/DOQI) guidelines, this patient indeed has stage 3 CKD. A nephrologist should be following this patient and appropriate preventive strategies instituted for preservation of kidney function and minimizing the impact of comorbidities.

16. **b. Prevent progressive kidney disease.** ACE inhibitors work by hemodynamic and nonhemodynamic mechanisms to slow the progression of renal disease.

17. **e. Diabetes mellitus.** Diabetes mellitus and hypertension account for the greatest percentage of cases, followed by glomerular diseases (e.g., FSGS, membranous glomerulonephritis), and then secondary glomerulonephritis associated with systemic diseases (e.g., systemic lupus erythematosus, Wegener granulomatosis).

18. **b. Postnephrectomy, GFR = 62 mL/min, albuminuria ≤ 30 mg/g.** The risk of progressive renal disease is based on the cause for renal function reduction, the GFR, and the albuminuria score. In a and c the GFR is higher, and there is cause for ongoing injury. One-time reduction in GFR with nephrectomy in the absence of ongoing injury (no albuminuria) should yield a more favorable prognosis.

19. **b. Renal biopsy.** For definitive diagnosis, a renal biopsy is required to aid prognosis and therapy decisions, especially in the setting of abnormal renal function.

20. **c. Atrial natriuretic peptide.** All choices promote renal fibrosis except atrial natriuretic peptide, which may have the opposite effect.

21. **e. ADPKD with cysts larger than 10 cm.** Individuals with bilateral renal artery stenosis and autosomal dominant PKD patients with cyst size greater than 10 cm may also experience a decrease in residual renal function while being given ACE inhibitor therapy.

22. **a. Preemptive transplantation.** A comparison of outcomes suggests that renal transplantation is the best overall treatment for ESRD patients.
23. **e. Access catheter infection.** The most recent USRDS data identify the most common reason for hospital admission in ESRD patients on hemodialysis is catheter infection.
24. **c. Gadolinium-based contrast agents.** Gadolinium is not toxic to the kidney. Its risk relates to the development of nephrogenic systemic fibrosis, which can carry a high mortality in patients with severely reduced GFR. All the others demonstrate direct toxicity to the kidney.
25. **d. Poor nutritional status.** The strongest predictors of the number of hospitalizations per year of patients at risk include low serum albumin, decreased activity level, diabetes mellitus as a primary cause of ESRD, peripheral vascular disease, white race, increasing age, and congestive heart failure. Both nutritional status (levels of serum albumin, creatinine, transferrin, and prealbumin, and lean body mass) and inflammatory response (e.g., C-reactive protein) are independent predictors of hospitalization in chronic hemodialysis patients.

Imaging

1. **b. ATN.** Both kidneys are diffusely dense 24 hours after contrast administration (persistent nephrogram), with no excretion into the collecting system, making ATN the best diagnosis. The process is likely related to contrast-induced nephropathy. Renal artery occlusion is usually a unilateral process, and the nephrogram is absent in the affected kidney because of the lack of perfusion. The kidneys are small in patients with severe hypertension, and the nephrogram would have washed out at 24 hours rather than be persistent. No calcifications are seen in the kidneys, making nephrocalcinosis an unlikely diagnosis.

CHAPTER REVIEW

1. ARF is divided into prerenal, intrarenal, and postrenal.
2. Prerenal failure is the result of decreased renal blood flow or increased nitrogen load. The serum blood urea nitrogen-to-creatinine ratio is greater than 10:1. Urine volume is generally low, osmolality high, and sodium content very low.
3. Intrarenal failure is due to parenchymal disease. It may involve the glomerulus as in acute glomerulonephritis, the tubule as in ATN, or the interstitium as in acute interstitial nephritis. The serum blood urea nitrogen-to-creatinine ratio is 10:1. Urine output is variable, and urinary sodium is generally above 20 mEq/L. If the cause is ATN, urinary sodium is generally greater than 40 mEq/L.
4. Postrenal failure is due to obstruction of the entire nephron mass. Patients who are anuric should be suspected of having complete urinary tract obstruction, acute cortical necrosis, or bilateral vascular occlusion. The serum blood urea nitrogen-to-creatinine ratio is 10:1.
5. In ATN, renal blood flow is reduced by 50% or more with the perfusion defect most marked in the outer medulla. Tubule permeability is also increased.
6. The use of mannitol before an ischemic insult has been shown to be of benefit.
7. Hyperkalemia, as evidenced on the electrocardiogram by peaked T-waves, a prolonged PR interval, and widening of the QRS complex is initially treated with IV calcium salts to stabilize the myocardium and then transiently lower serum potassium with IV glucose and insulin or IV sodium bicarbonate, as well as to permanently lower the potassium with either Kayexalate or dialysis. Administration of Kayexalate has been associated with colonic necrosis
8. The indications for initiation of dialysis include volume overload, severe hyperkalemia, severe metabolic acidosis, pericarditis, selected poisonings, and uremic symptomatology.
9. Peritoneal dialysis is less stressful hemodynamically.
10. The mortality rate for patients with ATN approximates 50%. Of those who survive ATN, 5% will require chronic dialysis.
11. Patients who are to receive IV contrast and are at risk for renal failure should be given IV hydration with saline before the use of nonionic IV contrast.
12. CKD is defined as a GFR less than 60 mL/min.
13. Hyperfiltration results when a decreased number of nephrons are called on to perform the entire workload. This results in elevated glomerular hydrostatic pressure, which is a major contributor to decreased renal function.
14. A family history of ESRD is a strong predictor of future risk for renal failure.
15. The Cockcroft Gault formula, MDRD equation, and CKD-EPI equation are all used to estimate GFR from serum creatinine. These equations are inaccurate for patients who have changing renal function, are at the extremes of age or body size, are obese, have decreased muscle mass, or are sick with moderately advanced renal failure.
16. Cystatin-C, a serum protein, may be more predictive of renal function than creatinine.
17. Mortality rates secondary to sepsis are one to several hundred times higher in dialysis patients.
18. Creatinine is secreted by the renal tubule and may overestimate renal function, particularly at low GFRs. Cimetidine and trimethoprim block this secretion.
19. Drugs that block angiotensin II production or action appear to decrease the rate of decline in renal function in patients with chronic renal disease.
20. In urology, rhabdomyolysis is associated with the protracted exaggerated lithotomy and lateral decubitus positions.
21. The sentinel event in renal ischemia is depletion of ATP.
22. The presence of albumen in the urine of patients with chronic renal failure is an important predictor of the rate of decline in renal function.
23. When the GFR falls below 50% of normal, progressive loss of renal function occurs even though the cause of the renal failure is inactive or no longer present.
24. The remaining lifetime for patients on dialysis is 15% to 25% of the general population.
25. Myoglobin can be nephrotoxic to the proximal tubule and may result in ATN. Early recognition of muscle necrosis with resultant myoglobinuria is crucial because a forced alkaline diuresis is indicated to minimize nephrotoxicity.
26. A low fractional excretion of sodium (or renal failure index) may be associated with either prerenal azotemia or acute glomerulonephritis.
27. Gadolinium-based contrast agents have been associated with the development of nephrogenic systemic fibrosis. Patients at risk are those with advanced CKD.
28. Individuals with bilateral renal artery stenosis and those with autosomal dominant PKD with cyst size greater than 10 cm may experience a decrease in residual renal function when receiving ACE inhibitor therapy.

88 Urological Complications of Renal Transplantation

Mohammed Shahait, Stephen V. Jackman, and Timothy D. Averch

QUESTIONS

1. In renal transplant recipients, all of the following are true EXCEPT:
   a. Recipients usually have classical symptoms of ureteral obstruction.
   b. Ureteral stricture is the most common cause of late ureteral obstruction.
   c. Ureteral obstruction should be suspected in any deterioration of renal function.
   d. Ureter ischemia is the main etiology for ureteral stricture formation.

2. The predominant type of stones in renal transplant patients is:
   a. calcium oxalate.
   b. calcium phosphate.
   c. struvite.
   d. uric acid.
   e. a and b.

3. Early stent removal is associated with:
   a. decrease in incidence of urinary tract infection (UTI).
   b. decrease in risk of stent colonization.
   c. increase in risk of UTI.
   d. increase in risk of developing urine leak.
   e. increase in risk of graft rejection.

4. All of the following have been related to the development of clinically significant vesicoureteral reflux (VUR) in renal transplant recipients EXCEPT:
   a. bladder outlet obstruction.
   b. neurogenic detrusor overactivity.
   c. reduced bladder capacity and compliance.
   d. ureterovesical anastomosis technique.
   e. use of ureteral stent.

5. The success rate of laparoscopic marsupialization of lymphocele in renal transplant recipients is:
   a. 30%.
   b. 41%.
   c. 69%.
   d. 92%.
   e. 84%.

6. The following statements regarding renal cell carcinoma in renal transplant recipients are true EXCEPT:
   a. Most of the kidney tumors develop in the native kidneys.
   b. Renal cell carcinoma incidence is higher in the transplant population compared to the general population.
   c. Renal cell carcinoma in renal transplant patients is aggressive and associated with worse oncological outcome.
   d. Partial nephrectomy is a feasible option to treat small renal masses in the allograft.
   e. Mass screening for renal cell carcinoma in renal transplant recipients is not recommended.

7. The following statements regarding the management of benign prostatic hypertrophy (BPH) in renal transplant recipients are FALSE EXCEPT:
   a. Transurethral resection of prostate (TURP) can be done in the first 3 weeks after transplant.
   b. TURP can be done in the presence of ureteral stent.
   c. TURP should be avoided in the first 3 weeks after transplant.
   d. Medical treatment of BPH should be avoided in renal transplant recipients.
   e. Renal transplant recipients are at increased risk of developing urethral stricture after TURP.

8. The following statements regarding the management of bladder cancer in renal transplant recipients are true EXCEPT:
   a. Intravesical bacillus Calmette-Guerin can be used in renal transplant patients.
   b. Muscle-invasive bladder cancer can be treated by chemoradiotherapy.
   c. Muscle-invasive bladder cancer can be treated by radical cystectomy and urinary diversion.
   d. Early cystectomy should be offered to patients with high-grade non–muscle-invasive bladder cancer.
   e. Bladder cancer in renal transplant recipients has indolent behavior.

9. All of the following are predisposing factors to the development of lymphocele EXCEPT:
   a. Extensive dissection of the lymphatic around the iliac vessels.
   b. Use of mammlian target of rapamycin (mTOR) inhibitors.
   c. Prolonged warm ischemia time.
   d. Delayed graft function.
   e. Atherosclerosis.

10. Initial management of a low-volume urine leak may include all of following EXCEPT:
    a. bladder catheter.
    b. JJ stent placement.
    c. percutaneous nephrostomy tube placement.
    d. percutaneous drainage of urinoma.
    e. fluid restriction.

11. Which of the following is a contraindication for surgical reconstruction of ureteral stricture?
    a. Strictures less than 3 cm in length.
    b. Late stricture recurrence after endourological treatment.
    c. Surgeon preference.
    d. All of above.
    e. None of above.

ANSWERS

1. **a. Recipients usually have classical symptoms of ureteral obstruction.** Due to renal allograft during the procurement process, kidney transplant recipients rarely manifest the classical symptoms of ureteral obstruction. As a result, usually recipients present with a progressive decline in renal function, a decrease in urine output, and recurrent UTIs. In a rare instance, patients may present with poorly characterized ache over the allograft due to irritation of peritoneum.

2. **e. a and b.** The most common stone composition in recipients is calcium-based stones (67%), followed by struvite stones (20%) and uric acid stones (13%).

3. **a. Decrease in incidence of urinary tract infection (UTI).** In a recent meta-analysis, early stent removal, defined by removal of the stent before the third postoperative week (< day 15), has been shown to reduce the incidence of UTI without increasing the incidence of urine leak and stenosis. On the other hand, 27% of the ureteral stents are colonized regardless of the indwelling time.

4. **d. Ureterovesical anastomosis technique.** VUR can be related to a technical error during the ureteroneocystostomy anastomosis, bladder outlet obstruction, or high-pressure urine storage secondary to either detrusor overactivity or reduced bladder compliance. However, VUR can develop regardless the ureterovesical anastomosis technique used.

5. **d. 92%.** The success rate for aspiration alone, sclerotherapy using different composite, drain placement, laparoscopic, and open surgery is 41%, 69%, 50%, 92%, and 84%, respectively.

6. **c. Renal cell carcinoma in renal transplant patients is aggressive and associated with worse oncological outcome.** Majority of kidney graft tumors has indolent behavior. In a recent analysis of allograft tumors, it was found that papillary carcinomas are reported in 56% of kidney graft tumors and low-grade tumors (Fuhrman grades 1 and 2) accounted for 65% of nonpapillary kidney graft tumors.

7. **c. TURP should be avoided in the first 3 weeks after transplant.** There is no contraindication for medical therapy in renal transplant recipients. TURP or Holmium enucleation of the prostate has been reported to be safe and effective in this subset of patients if performed at least 3 weeks post-transplant. It is crucial to avoid TURP in the first 2 weeks and in the presence of a ureteral stent after the transplant as it has been associated with devastating complications such as sepsis and death.

8. **e. Bladder cancer in renal transplant recipients has indolent behavior.** Bladder cancer in kidney transplant patients is aggressive and tends to be associated with higher recurrence rates, progression, and metastasis. For that reason, early cystectomy should be offered to patients with high-grade non–muscle-invasive bladder cancer. However, intravesical bacillus Calmette-Guerin can be used in selected patients with high-risk non–muscle-invasive bladder cancer. Muscle-invasive bladder cancer can be treated with chemoradiotherapy or radical cystoprostatectomy and urinary diversion.

9. **e. Atherosclerosis.** Lymphoceles occur mainly due to extensive dissection of the lymphatics around the iliac vessels of the recipient or renal vessels of the donor occurring during the time of organ procurement surgery or back table preparation. Other factors found to be associated with lymphocele formation include obesity, recipient age, duration of dialysis treatment, warm ischemia time, use of prophylaxis low-molecular-weight heparin, delayed graft function, acute rejection, redo transplant, and the use of mTOR inhibitors.

10. **e. Fluid restriction.** The initial treatment of urine leak is by diverting the urine from the leak site, and this can be achieved by a Foley catheter and a percutaneous nephrostomy tube. Retrograde stent placement has also been proposed when a double-J stent was not placed at the time of surgery. Percutaneous drainage is recommended if a substantial urinoma forms or causes ureteral obstruction or there is evidence of infection.

11. **e. None of above.** Open surgical repair for ureteral stricture remains the most effective treatment modality with superior long-term results when compared to endoscopic management. The only relative contraindication is very highly co-morbid patients with short life expectancy.

CHAPTER REVIEW

1. Majority of postoperative hematuria is self-limiting.
2. Consider duplex US for severe or persistent hematuria after renal biopsy to rule out arteriovenous (AV) fistula.
3. Ureteral stent decreases ureteral stricture and urinary leak.
4. Individualized stent removal can be after 3 weeks post-transplantation.
5. Strictures are the predominant cause of ureteral obstruction in patients greater than 3 months post-transplantation.
6. The primary etiology of ureteral stricture development is ischemia.
7. Stricture should be suspected in patients with hydronephrosis and decreased graft function.
8. A variety of endourological treatment options have been described to treat ureteral strictures, however, open reconstructive surgery offers superior long-term results.
9. Most of the kidney tumors develop in the native kidneys and are low-grade tumors.
10. Active surveillance, radiation, and surgery (open and minimally invasive) are reasonable options to treat prostate cancer in kidney transplant patients.
11. Kidney transplant recipients have a threefold risk of urothelial carcinoma (UC) compared with the general population, and it is biologically more aggressive.

89 Management of Upper Urinary Tract Obstruction

Stephen Y. Nakada and Sara L. Best

QUESTIONS

1. Ureteropelvic junction (UPJ) obstruction in the neonate is most frequently found as a result of:
   a. maternal-fetal ultrasonography.
   b. voiding cystourethrography.
   c. diuretic renography.
   d. abdominal radiography.
   e. physical examination.

2. Which study is diagnostic for functional obstruction at the UPJ?
   a. Retrograde pyelography
   b. Three-dimensional helical computed tomography (CT)
   c. Diuretic renography
   d. Renal ultrasound
   e. Renal angiography

3. A 62-year-old man presents with left flank pain. CT urography reveals delayed excretion and hydronephrosis to the level of a 2.5-cm calculus at the UPJ. Percutaneous stone extraction is accomplished without difficulty, but a postextraction nephrostogram reveals hydronephrosis to the level of the UPJ without residual stone. A follow-up nephrostogram 1 week later is unchanged. The best next step is:
   a. removal of the nephrostomy tube.
   b. diuretic renography.
   c. CT angiography.
   d. antegrade endopyelotomy.
   e. Whitaker pressure-perfusion test.

4. A 27-year-old woman has right flank pain, and her diuretic renography reveals UPJ obstruction and a differential renal function of 75:25 (L:R). The next best step is:
   a. CT angiography.
   b. stent placement.
   c. endopyelotomy.
   d. laparoscopic pyeloplasty.
   e. laparoscopic nephrectomy.

5. The highest failure rate in treating UPJ obstruction is associated with:
   a. antegrade endopyelotomy.
   b. retrograde ureteroscopic endopyelotomy.
   c. balloon dilation.
   d. pyeloplasty.
   e. cautery balloon incision.

6. The most appropriate location for endoscopic incision of a proximal ureteral stricture is:
   a. lateral.
   b. anterior.
   c. medial.
   d. posterior.
   e. anterolateral.

7. The best treatment option for a patient with a functional left ureteroenteric anastomotic stricture is:
   a. metallic stent.
   b. balloon dilation.
   c. laser endoureterotomy.
   d. cautery wire balloon incision.
   e. open repair.

8. The most common cause of retroperitoneal fibrosis is:
   a. methysergide.
   b. infection.
   c. lymphoma.
   d. breast cancer.
   e. immune-mediated aortitis.

9. Retrocaval ureter results from:
   a. persistence of posterior cardinal veins.
   b. persistence of anterior cardinal veins.
   c. duplication of inferior vena cava.
   d. aberrance of lumbar veins.
   e. retroaortic renal veins.

10. Transperitoneal laparoscopic pyeloplasty:
    a. is used rarely compared with the retroperitoneal approach.
    b. does not require water-tight, tension-free anastomosis.
    c. provides more working space than in the retroperitoneal approach.
    d. provides unfamiliar anatomy.
    e. does not require an external surgical drain.

11. Surgical repair of UPJ obstruction requires:
    a. a funnel-shaped transition between the renal pelvis and ureter.
    b. dependent drainage.
    c. water-tight anastomosis.
    d. tension-free anastomosis.
    e. all of the above.

12. Contraindications for transureteroureterostomy include a history of:
    a. retroperitoneal fibrosis.
    b. urothelial malignancy.
    c. nephrolithiasis.
    d. a, b, and c.
    e. b and c.

13. A 25-year-old man presents with right flank pain. He underwent a laparoscopic pyeloplasty, which failed within 1 year. Consequently, he underwent failed endopyelotomy. A CT scan shows a small, intrarenal pelvis and moderate cortical loss in the right kidney with a normal-appearing left kidney. A renogram reveals 35% differential function on the affected side, and a diuretic study demonstrates functional obstruction (>30 minutes). The next step is:
    a. chronic internal ureteral stent.
    b. ileal ureter.
    c. Davis intubated ureterotomy.
    d. ureterocalicostomy.
    e. renal autotransplantation.

14. Spiral flap procedures for UPJ obstruction are used:
    a. to bridge a shorter-length stenosis.
    b. to treat crossing vessels.
    c. to bridge a longer-length stenosis.
    d. for a small, intrarenal pelvis.
    e. only in the presence of greater than 30% ipsilateral renal function.

15. Foley Y-V-plasty is a suitable approach when encountering:
    a. high ureteral insertion.
    b. small intrarenal pelvis.
    c. anterior crossing vessel.
    d. duplication of collecting system.
    e. redundant renal pelvis.

16. Which type of pyeloplasty is suitable when there is an aberrant crossing vessel?
    a. Foley Y-V-plasty
    b. Culp-DeWeerd spiral flap
    c. Dismembered pyeloplasty
    d. Scardino-Prince vertical flap
    e. Ligation and transection of the crossing vessel

17. Ileal ureter can be performed when the patient has:
    a. renal insufficiency (serum creatinine > 2 mg/dL).
    b. inflammatory bowel disease.
    c. bladder dysfunction.
    d. radiation enteritis.
    e. small intrarenal pelvis.

18. A 55-year-old woman underwent left transperitoneal laparoscopic dismembered pyeloplasty over an internal ureteral stent. An abdominal drain was placed at surgery, and there was minimal drain output during the first 24 hours after surgery. Within 3 hours after Foley catheter removal, the patient's nurse noted a significant amount of fluid coming out of the drain site. The next step is to:
    a. change dressings frequently and continue observation.
    b. replace the urethral catheter.
    c. restrict fluid intake.
    d. remove the surgical drain.
    e. change the ureteral stent.

19. In performing a psoas hitch, additional bladder mobility can be achieved by transection of the:
    a. contralateral superior vesical artery.
    b. ipsilateral inferior vesical artery.
    c. contralateral inferior vesical artery.
    d. ipsilateral superior vesical artery.
    e. ipsilateral gonadal artery.

20. A 40-year-old woman with a history of hypertension and recurrent nephrolithiasis presents with a 5-cm proximal right ureteral stricture following an iatrogenic injury in a recent abdominal surgery. She has had an indwelling right nephrostomy tube for more than 6 months. Her baseline serum creatinine is 2.5 mg/dL. Renal scan shows split function of 65% in the right kidney. Her bladder capacity is found to be less than 300 mL. The next step is:
    a. ureteroureterostomy.
    b. Boari flap.
    c. transureteroureterostomy.
    d. ileal ureteral substitution.
    e. autotransplantation.

21. During a psoas hitch, the structure particularly susceptible to injury is the:
    a. obturator nerve.
    b. iliohypogastric nerve.
    c. ilioinguinal nerve.
    d. sacral nerve.
    e. genitofemoral nerve.

22. The technique that does not require normal bladder capacity, drainage, and function is the:
    a. ileal ureteral substitution.
    b. psoas hitch.
    c. ureteroneocystostomy.
    d. endoscopic incision of transmural ureter.
    e. Boari flap.

IMAGING

1. See Fig. 89.1. A 72-year-old man with malaise has this CT scan. The serum creatinine is mildly elevated. What is the best diagnosis?
    a. Retroperitoneal fibrosis
    b. Retroperitoneal hematoma

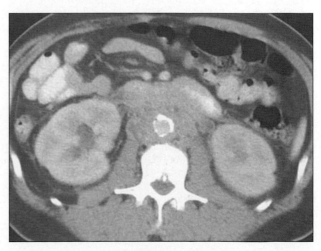

Fig. 89.1

c. Tuberculosis

d. Retroperitoneal sarcoma

e. Perianeurysmal fibrosis

ANSWERS

1. **a. Maternal-fetal ultrasonography.** The current widespread use of maternal ultrasonography has led to a dramatic increase in the number of asymptomatic newborns who are diagnosed with hydronephrosis, many of whom are subsequently found to have UPJ obstruction.

2. **c. Diuretic renography.** Provocative testing with a diuretic urogram may allow accurate diagnosis of UPJ obstruction. Renal ultrasound, CT scan, and retrograde pyelogram give anatomic assessments of the UPJ without quantitatively assessing urinary drainage and function.

3. **e. Whitaker pressure-perfusion test.** When doubt remains as to the clinical significance of a dilated collecting system, placement of percutaneous nephrostomy allows access for pressure perfusion studies. In the pressure perfusion test, first described by Whitaker in 1973 and then modified in 1978, the renal pelvis is perfused with normal saline or dilute radiographic contrast solution, and the pressure gradient across the presumed area of obstruction is determined. Renal pelvic pressures in excess of 15 to 22 cm H_2O are highly suggestive of a functional obstruction. Although diuretic renography is useful for diagnosis as well, the Whitaker test is ideal for this situation because a nephrostomy tube is already in situ.

4. **b. Laparoscopic pyeloplasty.** Evidence from several investigators indicates that crossing vessels lower the success rate of endopyelotomy. When such patients were culled from the pool of candidates available for treatment of UPJ obstruction, endopyelotomy success rates improved in most studies. A CT angiography would be necessary to assess this. However, laparoscopic pyeloplasty would be a straightforward minimally invasive option for this young patient. The kidney has too much function to remove at this stage.

5. **c. Balloon dilation.** McClinton reported long-term follow-up data on balloon dilation of the UPJ, finding a success rate of only 42%, which was significantly lower than the initial publications would indicate.

6. **a. Lateral.** Proximal ureteral strictures are incised laterally, similar to UPJ strictures. Posterior incision is offered to UPJ obstruction patients who have failed open pyeloplasty. Distal strictures are incised anteriorly, as are strictures of the middle ureter.

7. **e. Open repair.** Several studies have linked poor outcomes with endoscopic management of left ureteroenteric strictures. This may be a result of diminished blood flow to the ureter because the left ureter requires more mobilization than the right side at the time of diversion. Although metallic stents show promise in limited studies, using open repair, reports demonstrate an 80% success.

8. **e. Immune-mediated aortitis.** Growing evidence indicates that the majority of cases of retroperitoneal fibrosis are, in fact, immune-mediated aortitis. Regardless, the other conditions are relatively rare causes of retroperitoneal fibrosis.

9. **a. Persistence of posterior cardinal veins.** Retrocaval ureter results from the persistence of the posterior cardinal veins.

10. **c. Provides more working space than that in the retroperitoneal approach.** Transperitoneal laparoscopic pyeloplasty provides a larger working space relative to a retroperitoneoscopic approach. Together with more familiar anatomy, the transperitoneal approach is used most commonly in the laparoscopic urologic community to date.

11. **e. All of the above.** For any surgical repair of UPJ obstruction, the resultant anastomosis should be widely patent and completed in a watertight fashion without tension. In addition, the reconstructed UPJ should allow a funnel-shaped transition between the pelvis and the ureter that is in a position of dependent drainage.

12. **d. a, b, and c.** Relative contraindications include history of nephrolithiasis, retroperitoneal fibrosis, urothelial malignancy, chronic pyelonephritis, and abdominopelvic radiation.

13. **d. Ureterocalicostomy.** Direct anastomosis of the proximal ureter to the lower calyceal system is a well-accepted salvage technique for the failed pyeloplasty and small renal pelvis.

14. **c. To bridge a longer-length stenosis.** Flap procedures can be useful in situations involving a relatively long segment of ureteral narrowing or stricture. Of the various flap procedures, a spiral flap can bridge a strictured or narrow area of longer length. The flap procedures are not appropriate in the setting of crossing vessels.

15. **a. High ureteral insertion.** The Foley Y-V-plasty is designed for repair of a UPJ obstruction secondary to a high ureteral insertion. It is specifically contraindicated when transposition of lower pole vessels is necessary. In situations requiring concomitant reduction of redundant renal pelvis, this technique is also of little value.

16. **c. Dismembered pyeloplasty.** In the presence of crossing aberrant or accessory lower pole renal vessels associated with UPJ obstruction, a dismembered pyeloplasty is the only method to allow transposition of the UPJ in relation to these vessels.

17. **e. Small intrarenal pelvis.** In ileal segment usage, a small intrarenal pelvis is not contraindicated and an ileocalycostomy can be performed successfully.

18. **b. Replace the urethral catheter.** If the drain output increases following the removal of the Foley catheter, the catheter should be replaced for several days to avoid vesicoureteral reflux up the stent in the operated ureter and decrease urinary extravasation.

19. **a. Contralateral superior vesical artery.** In psoas hitch, transection of the contralateral superior vesical artery can be helpful to bridge the gap to the ipsilateral ureteral end, thereby achieving tension-free anastomosis.

20. **e. Autotransplantation.** Ureteroureterostomy is inappropriate for a 5-cm upper ureteral defect. Boari flap is inappropriate for a small bladder capacity. Transureteroureterostomy is contraindicated in the patient with a history of recurrent nephrolithiasis. Ileal ureter is contraindicated in the presence of elevated serum creatinine above 2 mg/dL. Autotransplant is appropriate for this particular patient.

21. **e. Genitofemoral nerve.** The genitofemoral nerve courses over the psoas muscle.

22. **d. Endoscopic incision of transmural ureter.** Normal bladder function without significant outlet obstruction is crucial to the success of ileal ureteral substitution, psoas hitch, Boari flap, and ureteroneocystostomy.

IMAGING

1. **a. Retroperitoneal fibrosis.** There is increased soft tissue in the retroperitoneum, which obscures and effaces the planes between the inferior vena cava and the aorta. Tuberculosis causes calcification and stricturing in the kidneys and collecting systems, and tuberculous iliopsoas abscess extends along the iliopsoas muscles. Retroperitoneal hematoma and sarcoma are not centered solely around the aorta and the inferior vena cava. In perianeurysmal fibrosis, a retroperitoneal fibrosis-like picture occurs in association with an abdominal aortic aneurysm; the aorta is of normal caliber in this case.

CHAPTER REVIEW

1. Intrinsic UPJ obstruction is a result of an aperistaltic segment in which the normal spiral arrangement of the muscle bundles is replaced by longitudinal muscle bundles and fibrous tissue.
2. A crossing vessel has the most detrimental effect on the success of an endopyelotomy.
3. UPJ obstruction may coexist with vesicoureteral reflux.
4. A multicystic kidney is distinguished from a UPJ obstruction on ultrasound by the "cyst" being connected in hydronephrosis as opposed to being distinct in a multicystic dysplastic kidney.
5. A Whittaker test is performed by perfusing the renal pelvis at 10 mL/min. Pressures less than 15 cm H_2O suggest a nonobstructed system. Pressures greater than 22 cm H_2O suggest an obstructed system, and pressures between the two are indeterminate.
6. The indications for repair of a UPJ include symptoms, impairment of renal function, stones, infection, and hypertension.
7. In neonates, unilateral hydronephrosis when carefully followed results in 7% of patients requiring a pyeloplasty.
8. Generally, kidneys with less than 15% function are not salvageable in adult patients.
9. A long segment stricture (>2 cm) is generally not successfully managed by the endopyelotomy method. An endopyelotomy cannot be performed safely by any route until access across the UPJ is established.
10. The majority of endopyelotomy failures occur within the first year. Success rates for endopyelotomy in properly selected patients range between 60% and 80%.
11. High-grade hydroureteronephrosis and crossing vessels have a detrimental effect on the success rate of endopyelotomy.
12. When bleeding occurs following an endopyelotomy, one should have a low threshold to proceed to angiography to thrombose the severed vessel.
13. Seventy percent of failures following laparoscopic pyeloplasty occur in the first 2 years.
14. When repairing a retrocaval ureter, the ureter is transected and relocated ventral to the vena cava.
15. Lower ureteral strictures are incised in an anterior medial direction; upper ureteral strictures are incised in a lateral or posterior lateral direction.
16. With ureteral strictures, one must always rule out malignancy.
17. There is no significant difference in preserving renal function in the adult when reimplanting the ureter into the bladder by either a refluxing or antirefluxing method.
18. Most patients with long-term urinary conduits will have an element of hydronephrosis that is not secondary to obstruction.
19. Retroperitoneal fibrosis secondary to malignancy is often indistinguishable from idiopathic retroperitoneal fibrosis and can be identified only with appropriate biopsy that identifies islands of tumor cells.
20. The initial management of retroperitoneal fibrosis is generally with steroids. Steroids are more likely to be beneficial if there is evidence of active inflammation as indicated by an elevated erythrocyte sedimentation rate, leukocytosis, and infiltration of lymphocytes on biopsy.
21. In addition to steroids, azathioprine, cyclophosphamide, cyclosporine, colchicine, and tamoxifen have been used to treat retroperitoneal fibrosis with some success.
22. Generally, 25% renal function is required to keep a repair of the UPJ or ureter open.
23. For any surgical repair of UPJ obstruction, the resultant anastomosis should be widely patent and completed in a watertight fashion without tension. In addition, the reconstructed UPJ should allow a funnel-shaped transition between the pelvis and the ureter that is in a position of dependent drainage.

QUESTIONS

1. Which of the following are mechanisms of injury or physical exam findings concerning for a potential blunt renal injury?
   a. Significant blow to the flank
   b. Lower rib fractures
   c. Significant flank ecchymoses
   d. A fall from a third-story window
   e. All of the above

2. What is the best option for repair of midureteral transection after a stab wound, in a stable patient?
   a. Ureteroureterostomy
   b. Transureteroureterostomy
   c. Boari flap
   d. Nephrectomy
   e. Cutaneous ureterostomy

3. When ureteroureterostomy is performed, which of the following is required?
   a. Postoperative interposition of omentum
   b. Postoperative nephrostomy tube
   c. Spatulated, watertight repair over a ureteral stent
   d. Nonabsorbable sutures
   e. Intraperitonealization of the ureteral anastomosis

4. Which maneuver is a common cause of ureteral injury during stone basketing?
   a. Ureteroscopy without dilating the ureteral orifice first
   b. Ureteroscopy in nondilated systems
   c. Use of the holmium laser
   d. Pulsatile saline irrigation to assist visualization
   e. Persistence in stone basketing attempts in the face of a ureteral tear

5. Which of the following is a contraindication to transureteroureterostomy for repair of significant lower ureter injury?
   a. History of urolithiasis
   b. History of ureteral trauma
   c. Morbid obesity
   d. Neurogenic bladder
   e. Thoracic spine fracture

6. What is the best treatment for a short, mid ureter ureteral contusion caused by a high-velocity bullet?
   a. Observation
   b. Ureteral stent placement
   c. Transureteroureterostomy
   d. Excision and ureteroureterostomy
   e. Oversew the contusion with healthy ureteral tissue

7. Which imaging technique is most useful for detecting ureteral injuries in the stable trauma patient?
   a. Computed tomography (CT) of the abdomen/pelvis without use of contrast material
   b. CT of the abdomen and pelvis with IV contrast with immediate images only
   c. CT of the abdomen and pelvis with IV contrast with immediate and delayed imaging (10 to 15 minutes)
   d. IVP
   e. Diuretic (Lasix) renography

8. Which of the following statements is TRUE about ureteral injuries during laparoscopy?
   a. The total number of injuries has stayed steady over the years.
   b. Surgery for endometriosis greatly increases the risk.
   c. Bipolar cautery use during tubal ligation eliminates risk.
   d. Most ureteral injuries are recognized immediately.
   e. Indigo carmine dye injection eliminates the risk of injury.

Imaging

1. A 22-year-old woman has a CT scan (Fig. 90.1) after a motor vehicle accident. Her vital signs are stable, and there are no other significant injuries.
   The next step is:
   a. open surgical repair of the kidney.
   b. delayed imaging to evaluate the collecting system.
   c. left nephrectomy to avoid future complications.
   d. renal artery embolization.
   e. intravenous urogram.

2. A 42-year-old man had a CT scan (Fig. 90.2) 36 hours after a motor vehicle accident. The most likely diagnosis is:
   a. ureteral injury.
   b. segmental renal artery transection.
   c. main renal artery occlusion.
   d. ureteropelvic junction disruption.
   e. traumatic renal vein occlusion.

ANSWERS

1. **e. All of the above.** CT of the abdomen and pelvis with IV contrast is warranted in blunt trauma patients with a rapid deceleration mechanism, significant blow to the flank, lower rib fractures, or significant flank ecchymosis. Kidney injuries should be suspect here, even if hematuria and shock are absent.

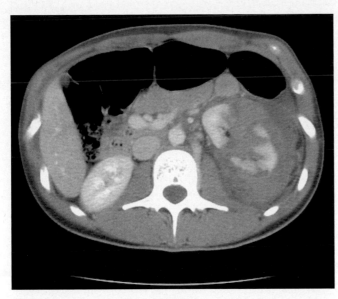

Fig. 90.1

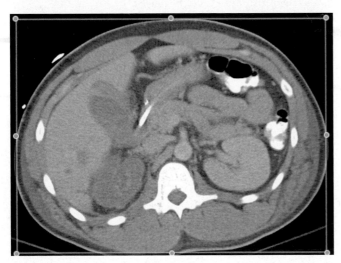

Fig. 90.2

2. **a. Ureteroureterostomy.** Ureteroureterostomy, so-called end-to-end repair in injuries to the upper two-thirds of the ureter, is common (up to 32% of one large series) and has a reported success rate as high as 90%.

3. **c. Spatulated, watertight repair over a ureteral stent.** A proper ureteral repair entails a spatulated, tension-free, stented, watertight anastomosis and a retroperitoneal closed suction drain.

4. **e. Persistence in stone basketing attempts in the face of a ureteral tear.** One factor cited as a cause of injury was the persistence in stone basketing attempts after recognition of a ureteral tear. Current recommendations are to stop and place a ureteral stent.

5. **a. History of urolithiasis.** TUU is contraindicated in patients with a history of kidney stones because a distal ureteral obstructing stone can put then put both kidneys at risk.

6. **d. Excision and ureteroureterostomy.** High-velocity gunshot wounds to the ureter result in blast injury and thus often heal with stricture or break down from ureteral necrosis. Such contusions should be treated with excision and ureteroureterostomy. Low-velocity bullet ureter contusions can be safely managed by ureteral stent placement.

7. **c. CT of the abdomen and pelvis with IV contrast with immediate and delayed imaging (10 to 15 minutes).** Because CT scanners can obtain early phase images before intravenous contrast dye is excreted in the urine, delayed images must be obtained (10 to 15 minutes after contrast material injection) to allow sufficient time for contrast to be excreted by the kidney and into the collecting system, renal pelvis, and down the ureter.

8. **b. Surgery for endometriosis greatly increases the risk.** A large percentage of ureteral injuries after gynecologic laparoscopy occur during electrosurgical or laser-assisted lysis of endometriosis.

Imaging

1. **b. Delayed imaging to evaluate the collecting system.** When blunt renal trauma results in deep parenchymal lacerations, delayed imaging at the time of the CT is essential to evaluate the collecting system for injury. In a stable patient with this type of injury, neither surgical repair nor angiographic embolization is indicated. Most renal injuries heal well with conservative and expectant management, making options a and c incorrect.

2. **c. Main renal artery occlusion.** There is complete absence of enhancement of the entire right kidney, which is caused by intimal injury and then main renal artery occlusion. Segmental occlusion would cause abnormality only in a portion of the right renal nephrogram. Ureteral injury and UPJ disruption may cause delay in the nephrogram but not complete absence of enhancement.

CHAPTER REVIEW

1. The best indication of significant urinary system injury is gross hematuria. However, the absence of hematuria does not exclude a significant GU injury.
2. Evaluation of urologic trauma in children differs from adults in that children: (1) are at greater risk for renal trauma, (2) often do not become hypotensive with major blood loss, and (3) have a higher propensity for renal anomalies.
3. Rapid deceleration from a fall from height or a high-velocity impact may result in injuries at points of fixation such as the ureteral pelvic junction and the renal hilum (renal artery intimal disruption).
4. The degree of hematuria and the severity of renal injury are not consistently correlated.
5. Criteria for radiologic imaging include (1) all penetrating trauma, (2) high-impact rapid deceleration trauma, (3) all blunt trauma with gross hematuria, (4) all blunt trauma with microhematuria and hypotension, and (5) pediatric patients with hematuria.
6. Adult patients with microscopic hematuria without shock may be observed without imaging studies.
7. Findings suggestive of a major renal injury on CT include medial laceration, perinephric hematoma size, intravascular contrast extravasation, medial urinary extravasation, and devitalized renal fragments.
8. Nonoperative management for renal injuries is preferred in the hemodynamically stable patient, particularly with grades I to III renal injuries.

9. Exploration of low-velocity renal gunshot wounds is not mandatory in selected cases. Such patients with isolated renal parenchymal lacerations with stable and contained hematomas who are hemodynamically stable, with no intra-abdominal organ injury, may be observed expectantly.

10. Absolute indications for renal exploration are (1) hemodynamic instability with shock, (2) expanding or pulsatile hematoma, (3) suspected renal pedicle avulsion, and (4) uncontained retroperitoneal hematoma.

11. For kidney trauma, perinephric hematoma size, intravascular contrast extravasation, devitalized renal fragments, arterial thrombosis, and collecting system contrast extravasation are relative indications for intervention.

12. "Damage control" is the management technique of immediate control of bleeding, and fecal and urinary leak only, in the unstable patient. Definitive reconstruction is deferred until the patient is stable and fully resuscitated. For ureter injuries this entails ligation and nephrostomy, externalizing, or stenting. At a staged/planned laparotomy, the ureter is later repaired.

13. Hypertension from renal parenchymal injury is usually short lived. Renal vascular injury or compression of the renal parenchyma by a subcapsular hematoma (Page kidney) can also cause high blood pressure.

14. When repairing ureteral injuries, the ureteral tissue should be debrided back to a bleeding edge to remove all traumatized microvascular damaged tissue.

15. Placement of vascular graft aneurysms in proximity of the ureter may cause a periureteral inflammatory reaction and ureteral injury/stenosis.

16. Ureteral injuries to the proximal and mid ureter can often be managed by uretroureterostomy. The gap being bridged is based on ureter mobilization and its elasticity.

17. In the stable trauma patient, distal ureteral injuries should be reimplanted into the bladder. In select cases, a ureteroureterostomy can be considered. If the gap is large, then psoas hitch or Boari bladder flap is the better management.

18. For delayed ureteral injury, the best diagnostic radiographic test (in the stable patient) to confirm injury, is a retrograde urogram.

19. Ureteral transections should be repaired within a week of the injury, or the repair should be delayed for 6 or more weeks.

20. It is prudent to isolate the ureteral repair from other injured organs (such as colon) with omentum or peritoneum.

21. Ureteral injury noted during ureteroscopy should be managed by ureteral stent placement. When a stent cannot be placed or inadequately diverts the urine, then a percutaneous nephrostomy should be placed.

22. Ureteral injury occurring during vascular surgery should be repaired and isolated from the graft with normal tissue such as omentum.

91 Urinary Lithiasis Etiology Epidemiology and Pathogenesis

Margaret S. Pearle, Jodi A. Antonelli, and Yair Lotan

QUESTIONS

1. The ethnic/racial group with the highest prevalence of stone disease is:
   a. African-American
   b. Hispanic
   c. White
   d. Asian
   e. American Indian

2. The geographic area in the United States associated with the highest incidence of calcium oxalate stone disease is the:
   a. northeast.
   b. southeast.
   c. southwest.
   d. west.
   e. northwest.

3. Which of the following conditions is associated with an increased risk of nephrolithiasis?
   a. Underweight
   b. Metabolic syndrome
   c. Rheumatoid arthritis
   d. Hypothyroidism
   e. Atopy

4. Which of the following occurs when the concentration product of urine is in the metastable range?
   a. Urine is supersaturated.
   b. Homogeneous nucleation occurs.
   c. Solubility product is reduced.
   d. Urinary inhibitors decrease the formation product.
   e. Nucleation never occurs.

5. The process by which nucleation occurs in pure solutions is:
   a. homogeneous nucleation.
   b. heterogeneous nucleation.
   c. epitaxy.
   d. aggregation.
   e. agglomeration.

6. The proteinaceous portion of stones is composed of:
   a. concentric lamination.
   b. protein-crystal complex.
   c. matrix.
   d. nephrocalcin.
   e. osteocalcin.

7. Stone-forming propensity is best described by:
   a. formation product.
   b. ionic activity.
   c. saturation index.
   d. solubility product.
   e. relative saturation ratio.

8. The most common abnormal urinary finding in patients undergoing Roux-en-Y gastric bypass surgery is:
   a. hypercalciuria.
   b. low urine pH.
   c. low urine volume.
   d. hypocitraturia.
   e. hyperoxaluria.

9. The vitamin D metabolite that stimulates intestinal calcium absorption is:
   a. 7-dehydrocholesterol.
   b. cholecalciferol.
   c. 25-dihydroxyvitamin D_3.
   d. 1,25-dihydroxyvitamin D_3.
   e. calcitonin.

10. Which of the following factors increases intestinal oxalate absorption?
    a. High dietary calcium intake.
    b. Low dietary calcium intake.
    c. *Oxalobacter formigenes* colonization in the colon.
    d. *Helicobacter pylori* colonization in the stomach.
    e. Irritable bowel syndrome.

11. The primary determinant of urinary citrate excretion is:
    a. acid–base status.
    b. urinary sodium excretion.
    c. citric acid intake.
    d. insulin sensitivity.
    e. urinary calcium excretion.

12. The underlying abnormality of renal hypercalciuria is:
    a. enhanced calcium filtration.
    b. enhanced calcium secretion.
    c. enhanced calcium reabsorption.
    d. primary renal wasting of calcium.
    e. primary renal storage of calcium.

13. Enteric hyperoxaluria occurs as a result of:
    a. excessive intake of oxalate.
    b. reduced excretion of oxalate.
    c. increased dietary fat.
    d. low calcium intake.
    e. fat malabsorption.

14. The most likely mechanism accounting for low urinary pH in uric acid stone formers with type 2 diabetes mellitus is:
    a. defective ammoniagenesis.
    b. impaired urinary bicarbonate excretion.
    c. lactic acidosis
    d. glucosuria.
    e. ketoacidosis.

15. In idiopathic calcium oxalate stone formers, Randall plaques originate in the:
    a. basement membrane of the thin loops of Henle.
    b. terminal collecting ducts.
    c. medullary interstitium.
    d. vasa recta.
    e. papillary tip.

16. In calcium oxalate stone formers, Randall plaques are composed of:
    a. calcium oxalate.
    b. brushite.
    c. calcium carbonate.
    d. calcium apatite.
    e. uric acid.

17. Urinary saturation of calcium oxalate is most strongly dependent on:
    a. urinary calcium concentration.
    b. urinary oxalate concentration.
    c. both urinary calcium and oxalate concentrations.
    d. urinary pH.
    e. urinary citrate concentration.

18. *O. formigenes* reduces urinary oxalate by:
    a. reducing intestinal calcium absorption, leading to decreased luminal free oxalate and reduced oxalate absorption.
    b. degrading urinary oxalate in infected urine.
    c. binding oxalate in the intestinal lumen and preventing its reabsorption.
    d. inhibiting the intestinal oxalate transporter.
    e. using oxalate as a substrate in the intestine, thereby reducing intestinal oxalate absorption.

19. Which of the following organisms is most likely to produce urease?
    a. *Staphylococcus aureus*
    b. *Escherichia coli*
    c. *Streptococcus pneumoniae*
    d. *Serratia marcescens*
    e. *Chlamydia*

20. The mechanism responsible for type 1 (distal) renal tubular acidosis (RTA) is:
    a. impaired bicarbonate reabsorption in the proximal tubule.
    b. defective H+-ATPase in the distal tubule that is unable to excrete excess acid.

c. defective ammoniagenesis.
d. impaired excretion of nontitratable acids.
e. hypoaldosteronism.

21. Patients with Lesch-Nyhan syndrome treated with high doses of allopurinol are at risk for formation of stones of which of the following compositions?
    a. Hypoxanthine
    b. Uric acid
    c. Xanthine
    d. 2,8-Dihydroxyadenine
    e. Calcium apatite

22. The etiology of ammonium acid urate stone formation in patients abusing laxatives is:
    a. recurrent infections with urease-producing bacteria.
    b. chronic dehydration and excessive uric acid excretion.
    c. increased ammoniagenesis.
    d. urinary phosphate deficiency and intracellular acidosis.
    e. chronic dehydration, intracellular acidosis, and low urinary sodium.

23. The primary mechanism of action of citrate in preventing stone formation is:
    a. reducing urinary calcium excretion.
    b. reducing urinary oxalate excretion.
    c. complexing calcium in urine.
    d. complexing oxalate in urine.
    e. complexing phosphate in urine.

24. Type 1 (distal) RTA is characterized by which abnormality?
    a. Hyperkalemia
    b. Hypochloremia
    c. Alkalosis
    d. Hypercitraturia
    e. Hypokalemia

25. The primary defect in type 2 (proximal) RTA is failure of bicarbonate reabsorption in the:
    a. glomerulus.
    b. proximal tubule.
    c. loop of Henle.
    d. distal tubule.
    e. collecting duct.

26. The most common abnormality identified in patients with uric acid stones is:
    a. acidic urine.
    b. alkaline urine.
    c. low uric acid concentration.
    d. high uric acid concentration.
    e. distal renal tubular acidosis.

27. Carbonic anhydrase inhibitors are associated with formation of stones composed of:
    a. calcium oxalate.
    b. calcium phosphate.
    c. struvite.
    d. cystine.
    e. uric acid.

28. Which of the following physiologic changes occurs in the kidney during pregnancy?
    a. Decreased uric acid excretion
    b. Decreased citrate excretion
    c. Increased calcium excretion
    d. Decreased glomerular filtration rate (GFR)
    e. Increased magnesium excretion

29. Which of the following substances acts as a promoter of calcium oxalate stone formation?
    a. Matrix-Gla protein
    b. Bikunin
    c. Citrate
    d. Pyrophosphate
    e. Uric acid

30. Which of the following amino acids is subject to impaired renal reabsorption in cystinuria?
    a. Arginine
    b. Glycine
    c. Alanine
    d. Leucine
    e. Methionine

ANSWERS

1. **c. White.** The highest prevalence of stone disease in both men and women occurs in whites. In men the lowest prevalence occurs in African-Americans, whereas Asian women have been found to have the lowest prevalence in one series.
2. **b. Southeast.** According to hospital discharge rates among U.S. veterans, calcium oxalate stone disease is most prevalent in the southeast.
3. **b. Metabolic syndrome.** Metabolic syndrome is characterized by obesity, hypertension, dyslipidemia, and insulin resistance, and is associated with an increased risk of kidney stone formation. Although impaired ammoniagenesis accounts for an increased risk of uric acid stones due to low urine pH, association with stone disease in general has been demonstrated. None of the other conditions has been associated with stone disease.
4. **a. Urine is supersaturated.** The solubility product refers to the point of saturation where dissolved and crystalline components in solution are in equilibrium. Addition of more crystals to the solution will result in precipitation of crystals. In this supersaturated urine (metastable state), crystallization can occur on preexisting crystals, but spontaneous crystallization occurs only when the concentration product exceeds the formation product. In the metastable state, the presence of inhibitors prevents or delays crystallization.
5. **a. Homogeneous nucleation.** The process by which nuclei form in pure solutions is called *homogeneous nucleation*. Heterogeneous nucleation occurs when microscopic impurities or other constituents in the urine promote nucleation by providing a surface on which the crystal components can grow.
6. **c. Matrix.** Depending on their type, kidney stones contain between 2.5% and 65% of noncrystalline material or matrix. Extensive investigations have characterized matrix as a derivative of several of the mucoproteins of urine and serum.
7. **c. Saturation index.** The state of saturation of the urine with respect to particular stone-forming salts indicates the stone-forming propensity of the urine. The state of saturation is determined by pH and the ionic strength of the major ions in solution. Relative saturation ratio, determined by the EQUIL 2 computer program, has been the standard for determining stone-forming propensity. However, the newer *JESS* computer

program takes into account several soluble complexes not recognized by the EQUIL 2 program and is likely a more accurate measure of stone-forming propensity, although it has not yet gained widespread use.
8. **e. Hyperoxaluria.** Hyperoxaluria has been described in both stone-forming and non-stone-forming patients who have undergone Roux-en-Y gastric bypass surgery, with urinary oxalate levels in some patients exceeding 100 mg/day. A mild decrease in urinary calcium compared with stone-forming control subjects has been described by some investigators but is a less consistent and severe finding.
9. **d. 1,25-dihydroxyvitamin D_3.** It is generally accepted that 1,25-dihydroxyvitamin D_3 is the vitamin D metabolite that is the most potent stimulator of intestinal calcium absorption. The other metabolites, except for calcitonin, are precursors of 1,25-dihydroxyvitamin D_3.
10. **b. Low dietary calcium intake.** Intestinal oxalate absorption is modulated by dietary oxalate and calcium intake and by the presence or absence of *O. formigenes*. In the setting of a high calcium intake, oxalate absorption decreases, and during calcium restriction, oxalate absorption increases because of reduced formation of a soluble calcium oxalate complex and increased availability of oxalate for absorption. *H. pylori*, which can colonize the stomach, has no effect on intestinal oxalate absorption. *O. formigenes*, an oxalate-degrading bacterium, uses oxalate as a substrate in the intestinal lumen, thereby reducing oxalate absorption. Irritable bowel syndrome, unless it is associated with chronic diarrhea, does not affect intestinal oxalate absorption.
11. **a. Acid–base status.** Acid-base status determines urinary citrate excretion. Metabolic acidosis reduces citrate excretion by augmenting citrate reabsorption and mitochondrial oxidation, whereas alkalosis enhances citrate excretion. Citric acid intake has a limited effect on urinary citrate excretion because only a small portion of dietary citrate is excreted into the urine unmetabolized. The majority of absorbed citrate is metabolized to bicarbonate, which is neutralized by the free proton from citric acid, thereby providing no net alkali load that would increase urinary citrate excretion.
12. **d. Primary renal wasting of calcium.** In this condition, the underlying abnormality is a primary renal leak of calcium due to impaired renal tubular calcium reabsorption.
13. **e. Fat malabsorption.** Malabsorption from any cause, including small bowel resection, intrinsic disease, or jejunoileal bypass, increases luminal fatty acids and bile salts. Calcium, which normally complexes with oxalate to form a soluble complex that is lost in the stool, instead binds to fatty acids, thereby increasing luminal oxalate available for absorption. In addition, poorly absorbed bile salts increase colonic permeability to oxalate, further increasing oxalate absorption.
14. **a. Defective ammoniagenesis.** Patients with type 2 diabetes mellitus typically exhibit characteristics of the metabolic syndrome, including insulin resistance. Although peripherally, insulin resistance leads to typical symptoms of diabetes, insulin resistance at the level of the kidney leads to impaired ammoniagenesis, by way of reduced production of ammonia from glutamine and reduced activity of the Na+/H+ exchanger in the proximal tubule that is responsible for either the direct transport or trapping of ammonium in the urine. The result is reduced urinary ammonium and low urine pH.
15. **a. Basement membrane of the thin loops of Henle.** In idiopathic calcium oxalate stone formers, Randall plaques have been found to originate in the basement membrane of the thin loops of Henle. From there, they extend through the medullary interstitium to a subepithelial location, where they serve as an anchoring site for calcium oxalate stone formation.
16. **d. Calcium apatite.** Randall plaques are invariably composed of calcium apatite, which serve as an anchoring site onto which calcium oxalate crystals can adhere and grow.
17. **c. Both urinary calcium and oxalate concentrations.** Urinary saturation of calcium oxalate is strongly, positively correlated

with urinary calcium and oxalate concentrations. Both contribute equally to urinary saturation of calcium oxalate.

18. **e. Using oxalate as a substrate in the intestine, thereby reducing intestinal oxalate absorption.** *O. formigenes* is an oxalate-degrading bacterium found in the intestinal lumen that uses oxalate as an energy source, thereby reducing luminal oxalate and intestinal oxalate absorption. *Oxalobacter* is not found in urine.

19. **a.** *Staphylococcus aureus.* Although *Proteus* species are most commonly associated with struvite stones, more than 90% of *S. aureus* organisms produce urease and are therefore associated with struvite stone formation.

20. **b. Defective H⁺-ATPase in the distal tubule that is unable to excrete excess acid.** A defective H^+-ATPase in the distal tubule has been implicated in the inability to excrete excess acid in the presence of an oral acid load among patients with distal RTA. Type 2, or proximal RTA, is characterized by impaired bicarbonate reabsorption in the proximal tubule, and type 4 RTA is common in diabetics with chronic renal damage who demonstrate aldosterone resistance.

21. **c. Xanthine.** Patients with Lesch-Nyhan syndrome suffer from an inherited deficiency of the purine salvage enzyme hypoxanthine-guanine phosphoribosyltransferase, which leads to the accumulation of hypoxanthine, which is ultimately converted to uric acid. Allopurinol inhibits xanthine oxidase, which is responsible for converting hypoxanthine to xanthine and xanthine to uric acid. High doses of allopurinol in these patients lead to the accumulation of hypoxanthine and xanthine, but because xanthine is less soluble in urine than is hypoxanthine, xanthine stones form.

22. **e. Chronic dehydration, intracellular acidosis, and low urinary sodium.** Subjects who abuse laxatives are chronically dehydrated, resulting in intracellular acidosis. In addition, urinary sodium is low from sodium loss as a result of the laxatives. In this environment, urate preferentially complexes with the abundant ammonium rather than sodium and produces ammonium acid urate stones.

23. **c. Complexing calcium in urine.** The primary mechanism of action of citrate is as a complexing agent for calcium, thereby reducing ionic calcium and urinary saturation of calcium oxalate.

24. **e. Hypokalemia.** Distal RTA is characterized by hypokalemic, hyperchloremic, nonanion gap metabolic acidosis and a urinary pH consistently above 6.0.

25. **b. Proximal tubule.** The primary defect in type 2 or proximal RTA is a failure of bicarbonate reabsorption in the proximal tubule, leading to excessive urinary bicarbonate excretion and metabolic acidosis.

26. **a. Acidic urine.** Patients with uric acid stones often have prolonged periods of acidity in the urine.

27. **b. Calcium phosphate.** Carbonic anhydrase inhibitors such as acetazolamide and topiramate block reabsorption of bicarbonate in the renal proximal and distal tubules, thereby preventing urinary acidification and inducing a metabolic acidosis. Similar to RTA, carbonic anhydrase inhibition results in the formation of calcium phosphate stones because of the high urine pH, hypercalciuria, and hypocitraturia.

28. **c. Increased calcium excretion.** During pregnancy, increased renal blood flow increases GFR, thereby increasing the filtered load of calcium, sodium, and uric acid. Placental production of 1,25-dihydroxyvitamin D_3 increases intestinal calcium absorption, further increasing urinary calcium.

29. **e. Uric acid.** Uric acid is thought to promote calcium oxalate stone formation by removing urinary inhibitors, by "salting out" calcium oxalate in solution and by heterogeneous nucleation, or epitaxy. The other substances are all natural inhibitors of stone formation.

30. **a. Arginine.** Renal reabsorption of the four dibasic amino acids—cystine, ornithine, lysine, and arginine—is affected by dysfunction of the heteromeric amino acid transporter located in the renal proximal tubule. Because of the poor solubility of cystine in urine, only cystine stones occur in this condition.

CHAPTER REVIEW

1. Renal calculi are two to three times more common in men than women, and in this country whites have the highest prevalence. They are uncommon before the age of 20 years, and the peak incidence occurs in the fourth to sixth decades of life.

2. The prevalence and incidence of stone disease is directly correlated with body mass index; patients with high body mass index excrete increased levels of oxalate, uric acid, sodium, and phosphorus, and are more likely to have urinary supersaturation for uric acid. The incidence and prevalence of stone disease has been increasing around the world.

3. Concentration product is the product of the concentrations of the chemical components.

4. Solubility product is the concentration at which precipitation of the components occurs.

5. A solution is saturated when the solubility product is exceeded.

6. When the solubility product is exceeded and precipitation does not occur, the solution is said to be metastable. When precipitation occurs, the concentration at that point is called *formation product.*

7. Magnesium and citrate inhibit crystal aggregation (the former complexes with oxalate and the latter with calcium); nephrocalcin inhibits nucleation, growth, and aggregation; Tamm-Horsfall glycoprotein inhibits aggregation; and osteopontin inhibits crystal growth, nucleation, and aggregation of calcium oxalate crystals.

8. Nanobacteria have been implicated in calcifying nanoparticles and serving as a nidus for stone formation.

9. Most stone-forming salts are found in the urine in a supersaturated state. Inhibitors keep them in solution.

10. The noncrystalline component of stones is called *matrix* and generally accounts for about 2.5% of the weight of the stone. It is composed of mucoproteins, carbohydrates, and urinary inhibitors.

11. Parathyroid hormone increases renal calcium reabsorption and enhances phosphate excretion.

12. Patients with small bowel disease or a history of intestinal resection and an intact colon have an increased oxalate absorption.

13. Calcium absorption occurs primarily in the small intestine at a rate that is dependent on calcium intake.

14. Calcium oxalate accounts for 60% of stones; mixed calcium oxalate and hydroxyapatite, 20%; brushite, 2%; uric acid, 10%; struvite, 10%; and cystine, 1%.

15. Hypercalciuria is the most common abnormality identified in calcium stone formation. Hypercalciuria is defined as a urinary excretion greater than 4 mg/kg/day.

16. Absorptive hypercalciuria is defined as an increased urinary calcium excretion after an oral calcium load and is due to increased intestinal absorption of calcium. Alteration of vitamin D receptors and/or sensitivity has been suggested as the etiology. Renal hypercalciuria is due to impaired renal tubular reabsorption of calcium and leads to secondary hyperparathyroidism.

17. Reabsorptive hypercalciuria is due to hyperparathyroidism. The administration of thiazides to patients with primary hyperparathyroidism exacerbates hypercalcemia.

CHAPTER REVIEW—cont'd

Parathormone-like hormone resulting in hypercalcemia is produced by lung, breast, renal, penile, and head and neck tumors; lymphoma; and myeloma.

18. Hyperoxaluria is defined as greater than 40 mg/day excreted in the urine. Foods that are oxalate rich include nuts, chocolate, brewed tea, spinach, broccoli, strawberries, and rhubarb.

19. Hyperuricosuria is defined as urinary uric acid excretion exceeding 600 mg/day.

20. Hyperuricosuria promotes sodium urate formation, which promotes calcium oxalate stone formation through heterogenous nucleation.

21. Citrate inhibits stone formation by complexing with calcium and thereby preventing spontaneous nucleation of calcium oxalate; it inhibits agglomeration and growth of the crystal, and it enhances the inhibitory effect of Tamm-Horsfall glycoprotein. It prevents heterogeneous nucleation of calcium oxalate by monosodium urate.

22. Hypocitraturia is defined as urinary citrate excretion of less than 320 mg/day.

23. Renal tubular acidosis, type 1 (distal tubular RTA) is characterized by calcium phosphate stone formation, hypercalciuria, hypocitraturia, and an increased urinary pH.

24. Low magnesium levels result in reduced inhibitory activity and are often associated with decreased urinary citrate levels.

25. Cystine stones form due to a defect in the transport of four amino acids: cystine, lysine, ornithine, and arginine. It is inherited as an autosomal recessive and accounts for up to 10% of stones in children. There are two genes involved in the inheritance of the disease. There are three types based on urine excretion amounts: types A, B, and AB.

26. Stones of infection (struvite stones) are composed of magnesium ammonium phosphate and may contain carbonate apatite; they occur in association with urea-splitting bacteria. Urease-producing pathogens include *Proteus*, *Klebsiella*, *Pseudomonas*, and *Staphylococcus*.

27. The cause of stones associated with horseshoe kidneys and ureteropelvic junction obstructions is due to both the anatomic abnormality resulting in stasis and an underlying metabolic abnormality.

28. Medullary sponge kidney is characterized by ectasia of the renal collecting ducts and leads to stones through renal acidifying defects, hypercalciuria, and hypocitraturia.

29. Most stones in pregnancy pass spontaneously.

30. The most important determinate of uric acid stone formation is low urinary pH. Low urinary pH in uric acid stone formers is likely due to impaired ammoniagenesis associated with insulin resistance.

31. Medications that may precipitate as stones include triamterene, silica, indinavir, ephedrine, and ciprofloxacin.

32. Heterogeneous nucleation occurs when microscopic impurities or other constituents in the urine promote nucleation by providing a surface on which the crystal components can grow.

33. Intestinal oxalate absorption is modulated by dietary oxalate and calcium intake and by the presence or absence of *O. formigenes*.

34. Acid–base status determines urinary citrate excretion. Metabolic acidosis reduces citrate excretion.

35. The sarcoid granuloma produces 1,25-dihydroxyvitamin D_3, causing increased intestinal calcium absorption, hypercalcemia, and hypercalciuria.

36. Malabsorption from any cause, including small bowel resection, intrinsic disease, or jejunoileal bypass, increases luminal fatty acids and bile salts. Calcium, which normally complexes with oxalate, forming a soluble complex that is lost in the stool, instead binds to fatty acids, thereby increasing luminal oxalate available for absorption. In addition, poorly absorbed bile salts increase colonic permeability to oxalate, further increasing oxalate absorption.

37. Type 1 or distal tubule RTA is characterized by an impairment in hydrogen ion secretion. Type 2, or proximal RTA, is characterized by impaired bicarbonate reabsorption in the proximal tubule. Type 4 RTA is common in diabetics with chronic renal damage who demonstrate aldosterone resistance.

92 Evaluation and Medical Management of Urinary Lithiasis

Nicole L. Miller and Michael S. Borofsky

QUESTIONS

1. Each of the following could be considered a high-risk feature for stone formation EXCEPT which?
   a. Diabetes
   b. Sarcoidosis
   c. Parkinson disease
   d. Family history of stones
   e. Inflammatory bowel disease

2. Each of the following is a medical condition associated with calcium nephrolithiasis EXCEPT which?
   a. Hyperparathyroidism
   b. Malignancy
   c. Primary hyperoxaluria
   d. Medullary sponge kidney
   e. Lesch-Nyhan syndrome

3. Standard 24-hour urine testing for stone disease should measure the following EXCEPT which?
   a. Sodium
   b. Oxalate
   c. pH
   d. Creatinine
   e. Glucose

4. A 45-year-old male with a history of recurrent calcium oxalate stones returns for counseling regarding a recent 24-hour urine test. A single 24-hour urine collection reveals abnormal elevations in calcium, oxalate, uric acid, sodium, and potassium. Urinary volume is 4.5 L, pH is 5.8, and 24-hour creatinine per kilogram is 47. These findings are most likely explained by:
   a. dietary indiscretion
   b. steroid administration
   c. overcollection
   d. undercollection
   e. contamination

5. Patients with enteric hyperoxaluria are most likely to form stones composed of:
   a. calcium phosphate.
   b. calcium oxalate.
   c. magnesium ammonium phosphate.
   d. uric acid.
   e. cystine.

6. The risk factor most associated with recurrent stone formation in patients with inflammatory bowel disease is:
   a. hyperabsorption of oxalate in the jejunum.
   b. hyperexcretion of calcium from the distal tubule.
   c. diminished citrate absorption in the terminal ileum.
   d. hyperabsorption of calcium in the small bowel.
   e. increased colonic absorption of free oxalate.

7. Hypocitraturia in patients with inflammatory bowel disease or chronic diarrhea syndrome is due to:
   a. persistent bicarbonate losses.
   b. hypokalemia.
   c. metabolic acidosis.
   d. intracellular acidosis.
   e. all of the above.

8. The optimal treatment for patients with enteric hyperoxaluria includes:
   a. calcium supplements, potassium citrate, and increased oral fluid intake.
   b. dietary restriction of oxalate.
   c. thiazides and potassium citrate.
   d. allopurinol.
   e. pyridoxine.

9. The most important factor predisposing patients to gouty diathesis is:
   a. hypercalciuria.
   b. low urinary pH.
   c. hypocitraturia.
   d. low urine volumes.
   e. hyperuricosuria.

10. The most appropriate medical treatment of a patient with uric acid calculi is:
    a. allopurinol.
    b. thiazides.
    c. increased fluids.
    d. dietary calcium restriction.
    e. potassium citrate.

11. A patient with recurrent uric acid calculi is placed on oral medical treatment and returns for follow-up 3 months later. He is noted to have significantly elevated urinary uric acid levels as compared with his first 24-hour urine collection. This finding is due to:
    a. increased production of endogenous uric acid.
    b. failure to avoid high-sodium foods.
    c. increased solubility of uric acid.
    d. increased consumption of red meat.
    e. inhibition of xanthine oxidase.

12. A patient with uric acid calculi is placed on alkali therapy but returns 1 year later having passed two calcium phosphate stones. A repeat 24-hour urine collection demonstrates a urine pH of 7.4, a urinary citrate of 450 mg/day, and a urinary uric acid of 875 mg/day. The most likely cause for recurrent stone formation is:
    a. cessation of potassium citrate.
    b. increase in oral purine intake.
    c. decrease in solubility of uric acid.
    d. excess alkalization.
    e. increase in saturation of oxalate.

13. A 58-year-old Hispanic woman with a history of recurrent urinary tract infections treated three to four times in the past 18 months is seen by her family physician. At present she is asymptomatic. She has no history of nephrolithiasis. Renal ultrasound demonstrates moderate left hydronephrosis and a large density within the renal pelvis with posterior shadowing. A kidney-ureter-bladder (KUB) view with tomography reveals a poorly opacified dendritic stone in the renal pelvis and lower pole calyces. Prior urine cultures have revealed *Proteus* and *Klebsiella* species. The stone composition of this patient is most likely:

    a. calcium oxalate.

    b. uric acid.

    c. magnesium ammonium phosphate.

    d. cystine.

    e. hydroxyapatite.

14. The most significant factor contributing to stone formation in patients with struvite calculi is:

    a. gouty diathesis.

    b. recurrent urinary tract infections.

    c. family history.

    d. hyperoxaluria.

    e. hypercalciuria.

15. Which of the following bacteria would be the least likely to contribute directly to struvite stone formation?

    a. *Proteus mirabilis*

    b. *Escherichia coli*

    c. *Staphylococcus aureus*

    d. *Klebsiella pneumoniae*

    e. *Pseudomonas aeruginosa*

16. Acetohydroxamic acid (AHA) contributes to reducing infectious stone formation by:

    a. reversing associated metabolic defects.

    b. preventing recurrent urinary tract infections.

    c. alkalization of the urine.

    d. irreversibly inhibiting urease.

    e. all of the above.

17. A 12-year-old boy is seen for the evaluation of recurrent nephrolithiasis. He has spontaneously passed three stones over the previous 4 years and has recently undergone shock-wave lithotripsy twice without success. He has been treated in the past with an unknown medication, but this was discontinued because the parents believed it to be of no benefit. Urinalysis demonstrates hexagonal crystals. The likely metabolic diagnosis contributing to this patient's recurrent stone formation is:

    a. hypocitraturia.

    b. hyperoxaluria.

    c. low urine volumes.

    d. gouty diathesis.

    e. cystinuria.

18. First-line medical treatment for the prevention of recurrent cystine stones would be aimed at:

    a. urinary acidification.

    b. increasing the solubility of cystine.

    c. decreasing urinary sodium.

    d. decreasing the solubility of cystine.

    e. binding of cystine within the intestines.

19. α-Mercaptopropionylglycine (α-MPG, Thiola Mission Pharmacal Company, San Antonio, TX) may be helpful in the management of cystinuria because it:

    a. acts as a diuretic, further decreasing urinary cystine concentration.

    b. is significantly more effective than D-penicillamine.

    c. can be used as both an oral and intrarenal chemolytic agent.

    d. has equivalent efficacy at increasing solubility with reduced toxicity compared with D-penicillamine.

    e. adequately alkalizes the urine, obviating the need for potassium citrate.

20. Three years after initiating treatment for cystine stones with α-MPG, 800 mg/day, a patient returns with a follow-up 24-hour urine collection demonstrating a significant reduction in cystine excretion from 740 to 250 mg/day. Urine volume is 775 mL/day. He has two additional stones. The reason for recurrent stone formation is:

    a. increased age, thereby exacerbating the disorder.

    b. decreased efficacy of α-MPG.

    c. continued supersaturation of urinary cystine.

    d. continued hypocitraturia.

    e. increased urine acidity.

21. A 19-year-old white woman with a 6-year history of recurrent stone disease is found to have multiple bilateral renal calculi by renal ultrasound during an evaluation for recurrent flank pain. She reports having passed more than 10 stones in the previous 2 years. Review of the renal ultrasound indicates no evidence of hydronephrosis. Her KUB film and tomograms demonstrate five stones on the left and eight stones on the right, all less than 4 mm. She has a strong family history of stones, having three first-degree relatives and two cousins with nephrolithiasis. Urine pH is consistently above 6.8. Stone composition has been mixed calcium phosphate and calcium oxalate. The most definitive test to identify this disorder would demonstrate:

    a. decreased serum parathyroid hormone (PTH) levels.

    b. persistently elevated urine calcium.

    c. inability to reduce the urine pH below 5.3.

    d. normalization of hypercalciuria.

    e. a marked increase in urinary uric acid levels with initiation of treatment.

22. The most appropriate treatment for patients with renal tubular acidosis is:

    a. thiazides.

    b. allopurinol.

    c. sodium alkali.

    d. AHA.

    e. potassium alkali.

23. Renal tubular acidosis may be associated with nephrolithiasis due to:

    a. hypercalciuria and hypocitraturia.

    b. hyperoxaluria and hypercalcemia.

    c. hyperuricosuria.

    d. hypocitraturia with normal urine magnesium.

    e. hypercitraturia and hypercalciuria.

24. Chronic metabolic acidosis may cause:

    a. increased PTH levels.

    b. significantly reduced bone density.

    c. hypercalcemia.

    d. increased intestinal calcium absorption.

    e. all of the above.

25. Which of the following findings would support the diagnosis of renal leak hypercalciuria?
    a. Hypocitraturia
    b. Low urinary pH
    c. Normocalciuria on a calcium-restricted diet
    d. Decreased urinary sodium with thiazide challenge
    e. Low or low-normal radial bone density

26. The primary abnormality in patients with renal leak hypercalciuria is considered to be:
    a. impairment of renal tubular reabsorption of calcium.
    b. excessive mobilization of calcium from bone.
    c. increased 1,25-$(OH)_2$ vitamin D levels.
    d. elevation of serum PTH levels.
    e. hyperabsorption of intestinal calcium.

27. In treating patients with renal leak hypercalciuria, thiazides are effective because they:
    a. bind calcium in the intestinal tract.
    b. cause intracellular volume depletion.
    c. augment calcium reabsorption in the proximal tubule.
    d. directly inhibit calcium absorption.
    e. restore normal serum 1,25-$(OH)_2$ vitamin D levels.

28. Which of the following are potential side effects of treatment with thiazides?
    a. Hypokalemia
    b. Hypocitraturia
    c. Hyperuricemia
    d. Hypomagnesuria
    e. All of the above

29. After 18 months of chlorthalidone treatment, a patient with hypercalciuria is doing well with no further stone formation. However, 8 months later, while still on thiazides, she passed a small stone. The most likely cause of her recurrent stone formation is:
    a. excessive intake of dietary calcium.
    b. inappropriate fluid management.
    c. excessive sodium intake.
    d. thiazide-induced hypocitraturia.
    e. cessation of medications.

30. A patient with hypercalciuria is continued on chlorthalidone and potassium citrate without problems for 18 months and then passes two stones spontaneously. She claims that she is still on her medications. The most likely cause of her continued stone formation is:
    a. excessive calcium intake.
    b. heterogeneous nucleation of calcium oxalate.
    c. high dietary sodium intake.
    d. bone mobilization of calcium.
    e. exacerbation of intestinal calcium absorption.

31. The metabolic abnormality most commonly seen after Roux-en-Y gastric bypass surgery is:
    a. hypercalciuria.
    b. gouty diathesis.
    c. hyperuricosuria.
    d. hyperoxaluria.
    e. hypomagnesemia.

ANSWERS

1. **c. Parkinson disease.** To date, there is no recognized direct association between neurologic disorders and stone formation. The remaining conditions are all potential risk factors for increased likelihood of stone formation and should prompt evaluation with 24-hour urine testing if a stone is diagnosed.

2. **e. Lesch-Nyhan syndrome.** Lesch-Nyhan syndrome is a rare inherited disorder that leads to hyperuricemia and hyperuricosuria with resulting uric acid stone formation. Hyperparathyroidism can lead to calcium stone formation through improper calcium regulation. Malignancy can cause calcium nephrolithiasis through hypercalciuria. Primary hyperoxaluria, though primarily an oxalate disorder, results in calcium oxalate stones most commonly. Medullary sponge kidney may lead to calcium stone formation through urinary stasis and pooling.

3. **e. Glucose.** Based on expert opinion of the guidelines panel, metabolic testing should consist of one or two 24-hour urine collections obtained on a random diet and analyzed at minimum for total volume, pH, calcium, oxalate, uric acid, citrate, sodium, potassium and creatinine (Pearle, 2014). Glucose in the urine may be indicative of diabetes, which can be a risk factor for stone formation; however, it is not routinely quantified or measured on 24-hour urine testing for stones.

4. **c. Overcollection.** Normal 24-hour creatinine per kilogram for a male is between 20 and 25. The high value, near 50 in the example, is indicative of excess creatinine in the specimen, most commonly caused by overcollection of urine beyond a 24-hour time period. This is a common occurrence and may happen if a patient does not follow the instructions and provides a 48-hour collection by mistake. The elevated levels of calcium, oxalate, uric acid, sodium, and potassium are thus unreliable, as their values are set based on normal values for a 24-hour time period, not the extended collection time that was likely followed in this study.

5. **b. Calcium oxalate.** Patients with enteric hyperoxaluria are more likely to form calcium oxalate stones owing to increased urinary excretion of oxalate and decreased inhibitory activity from hypocitraturia secondary to chronic metabolic acidosis and hypomagnesuria. In addition, fluid loss from persistent diarrhea from inflammatory bowel disease may cause an extremely concentrated environment that is suitable for stone formation.

6. **e. Increased colonic absorption of free oxalate.** Intestinal hyperabsorption of oxalate in patients with enteric hyperoxaluria is the most significant risk factor leading to recurrent calculus formation. Intestinal transport of oxalate is primarily increased because of the effects of bile salts and fatty acids on the permeability of colonic intestinal mucosa to oxalate. The total amount of oxalate absorbed may also be increased because of an enlarged intraluminal pool of oxalate available for absorption. Intestinal fat malabsorption characteristic of ileal disease will exaggerate calcium soap formation, limit the amount of "free" calcium to complex to oxalate, and thereby raise the oxalate pool available for absorption.

7. **e. All of the above.** Acid–base status is probably the most important factor in the renal handling of citrate. Hypokalemia with its induced intracellular acidosis (caused by bicarbonate loss from chronic diarrhea) will reduce urinary citrate by both enhancing renal tubular resorption and reducing the synthesis of citrate. Therefore, in patients with enteric hyperoxaluria in whom bicarbonate loss and hypokalemia both contribute to metabolic acidosis, the hypocitraturia is often profound.

8. **a. Calcium supplements, potassium citrate, and increased oral fluid intake.** The initial goals of medical management are to rehydrate and reverse metabolic acidosis. Hydration is sometimes difficult in some patients because an increase in oral fluids may exacerbate diarrhea. Hydration and potassium citrate will contribute to the reversal of the metabolic

acidosis as well as enhance the excretion of citrate to increase its inhibitory effects on stone formation. Calcium supplements will bind excess oxalate within the intestine, thereby reducing intestinal oxalate absorption. Calcium citrate may offer an ideal calcium supplement in this condition because it should reduce urinary oxalate and increase urinary citrate. Thiazides may worsen metabolic acidosis and hypokalemia through their diuretic effects and renal potassium losses. Colonic resection may be of benefit in those patients refractory to medical management because the primary site of intestinal absorption of oxalate is the large bowel.

9. **b. Low urinary pH.** Although low urine volumes and hyperuricosuria contribute to the possibility of uric acid stone formation, the most critical determinant of the crystallization of uric acid remains urinary pH. In addition, uric acid stones may be formed in patients with primary gout with associated severe hyperuricosuria and other secondary causes of purine overproduction, such as myeloproliferative states, glycogen storage disease, and malignancy. Patients with uric acid stones will characteristically have urinary pH lower than the dissociation constant for uric acid (5.5). In fact, many will have a urine pH consistently close to 5. Whereas serum and urine uric acid levels may be elevated in patients with uric acid calculi, the urine pH remains the most cost-effective means of screening for this condition and monitoring therapy.

10. **e. Potassium citrate.** Allopurinol will decrease the production of uric acid by inhibiting xanthine oxidase in the purine metabolic pathway, but it is most effective in patients with extremely elevated levels of uric acid (urinary uric acid >1500 mg/day). In addition, increasing total urine volume will decrease the concentration of uric acid to assist in preventing stone formation. However, raising the urinary pH above the dissociation constant of uric acid is the key to preventing recurrent uric acid stone formation and correcting gouty diathesis. The urine pH should be maintained between 6.0 and 6.5. Thiazides and calcium restriction have limited roles in the medical treatment of patients with uric acid stones.

11. **c. Increased solubility of uric acid.** With adequate alkali therapy, this patient has been able to raise the urine pH above the dissociation constant of uric acid. The solubility of uric acid is more than 10 times greater at a pH of 7 than at a pH of 5. Therefore patients may initially present with low/normal 24-hour urinary uric acid levels because the uric acid will precipitate out of solution in the acid urinary environment. Once the urine has been alkalized, all of the uric acid will come back into solution, causing a significant increase in the measured urinary uric acid.

12. **d. Excess alkalization.** Excessive alkalization with urinary pH values above 7.0 may result in calcium phosphate stone formation. Alkali therapy with potassium citrate should aim to keep the urinary pH between 6.5 and 7.0 when patients with gouty diathesis are being treated.

13. **c. Magnesium ammonium phosphate.** Ascending urinary tract infections with urea-splitting organisms such as *Proteus* species will metabolize urea to ammonia. Ammoniuria—in conjunction with a matrix composed of organic compounds, carbonate apatite, inflammatory cells, and bacteria—results in the rapid formation of an "infectious" calculus, eventually progressing into a mineralized, dense stone. Bacteria trapped within the stone perpetuate the recurrent urinary tract infections, and further stone formation eventually develops into the classic staghorn calculus.

14. **b. Recurrent urinary tract infections.** Etiologic factors involved with infection calculi include a history of recurrent urinary tract infections and potential anatomic or physiologic abnormalities. It is important to remember that these patients may also have underlying metabolic disorders such as hypercalciuria, which could contribute to the stone formation. These disorders are most commonly found in patients with mixed stone composition (i.e., struvite and calcium

calculi). A comprehensive metabolic evaluation is warranted in these patients.

15. **b. *Escherichia coli*.** Of the listed bacteria, *E. coli* is the only one that does not commonly express urease activity, the enzyme responsible for struvite stone formation in a majority of cases.

16. **d. Irreversibly inhibiting urease.** AHA, a competitive inhibitor of the bacterial enzyme urease, will reduce the urinary saturation of struvite and retard stone formation. When given at a dose of 250 mg orally three times a day, this medication can prevent the development of new stones and inhibit the growth of existing stones in patients with chronic urea-splitting infections. AHA can also cause dissolution of small stones. However, up to 30% of patients will experience minor side effects including headache, nausea, vomiting, anemia, rash, and alopecia. In addition, 15% of patients have developed deep venous thrombosis while on long-term treatment. Therefore careful monitoring is required when this medication us being used.

17. **e. Cystinuria.** Cystinuria is a complex autosomal recessive disorder of amino acid transport involving cystine, ornithine, lysine, and arginine (COLA). Supersaturation of the urine will occur in patients with the homozygous state. Therefore it is unusual to see a family history with cystine stones, and the age at onset is often in the first or second decade.

18. **b. Increasing the solubility of cystine.** Increasing the solubility of cystine is the mainstay of treating this disorder. Therefore medical therapy is aimed at dissociating cystine into cysteine, which is 200 times more soluble than cystine. Solubility increases dramatically when this disulfide exchange occurs, effectively preventing further stone formation.

19. **d. Has equivalent efficacy at increasing solubility with reduced toxicity compared with D-penicillamine.** D-Penicillamine and α-MPG are equally effective in their ability to decrease urinary cystine levels. However, studies have demonstrated that α-MPG is significantly less toxic than D-penicillamine. Moreover, the side effects that may occur with α-MPG are also less severe. However, if a patient has been doing well on D-penicillamine with no significant complications, there is no need to switch medications.

20. **c. Continued supersaturation of urinary cystine.** The primary goal of medical therapy is to reduce the urinary cystine concentration below the solubility limit of 200 to 250 mg/L of urine. Because many of these patients present at a young age, compliance may be difficult. Even though this patient's cystine excretion has been reduced to 250 mg/day by the α-MPG therapy, his cystine concentration remains greater than 300 mg/L. Therefore a combination of medication along with an increased urine output is essential to reduce the urinary cystine concentration. Long-term follow-up is necessary to ensure urinary cystine beneath the saturation concentration.

21. **c. Inability to reduce the urine pH below 5.3.** Renal tubular acidosis is a clinical syndrome of chronic metabolic acidosis resulting from renal tubular abnormalities while glomerular filtration is relatively well preserved. Although patients may present with many different symptoms and physical findings, renal stone formation is a well-recognized manifestation of distal renal tubular acidosis (dRTA). Patients with the incomplete form of dRTA are not persistently acidemic despite their inability to lower urinary pH with an acid load. These patients are able to compensate for their acidification defect and remain in acid–base balance by increasing ammonia synthesis and ammonium excretion as a buffering mechanism. The initial identification of incomplete dRTA is often a chance finding. Many of these patients will present with recurrent nephrolithiasis or may be referred for evaluation after the discovery of nephrocalcinosis after routine abdominal radiographs. Most patients will have normal serum electrolytes, yet they will have a high-normal urine pH along with significant hypocitraturia. The diagnosis of incomplete dRTA can be confirmed by

inadequate urinary acidification after an ammonium chloride loading test.

22. **e. Potassium alkali.** In the past, sodium alkali has been the treatment of choice for chronic therapy in patients with dRTA. It was given in the form of either sodium bicarbonate or Shohl solution (a combination of sodium citrate and citric acid). Although sodium alkali is beneficial in correcting the acidosis, excess sodium may be detrimental to calcium metabolism, especially with respect to nephrolithiasis. Sodium alkali therapy has been complicated by the development of calcium stones (calcium phosphate or calcium oxalate), especially when the urinary pH is above 7. Potassium citrate has been shown to reduce the excretion of urinary calcium, whereas sodium alkali has no effect on urinary calcium. Therefore potassium alkali, usually in the form of potassium citrate (POLYCITRA-K, ALVA Pharmaceuticals, Mountain View, CA; Urocit-K, Mission Pharmacal Company, Mountain View, CA), is the recommended first-line therapy.

23. **a. Hypercalciuria and hypocitraturia.** Hypocitraturia, commonly seen in patients with dRTA, promotes the formation of nephrolithiasis due to reduced inhibitory action of urinary citrate. In addition, hypercalciuria will occur due to mobilization of calcium from bone and impaired renal tubular absorption of calcium, both as a result of chronic acidosis.

24. **b. Significantly reduced bone density.** It is well established that metabolic acidosis may cause a negative calcium balance as a result of impaired renal tubular reabsorption of calcium in the proximal tubule, leading to excessive renal loss of calcium. In addition, intestinal calcium absorption is diminished in patients with persistent acidosis. Slow dissolution of bone mineral can also be identified as calcium and phosphate act as buffering mechanisms to correct the acidosis. Chronic acidosis has been cited as a major factor in the genesis of bone disease.

25. **e. Low or low-normal radial bone density.** Patients with renal hypercalciuria may display a low or low-normal radial bone density. The diminished bone density is a result of the secondary hyperparathyroidism, which causes stimulation of PTH and subsequent production of 1,25-$(OH)_2$ vitamin D. Both PTH and vitamin D will act on bone to mobilize calcium and cause a loss in bone density. Calcium restriction has no effect in managing renal hypercalciuria.

26. **a. Impairment of renal tubular reabsorption of calcium.** The primary abnormality in renal hypercalciuria is an impairment in proximal renal tubular calcium reabsorption. This urinary calcium wasting and subsequent reduction in serum calcium concentration stimulates the production of PTH. As a result, vitamin D synthesis in the kidney is stimulated. Both PTH and vitamin D will increase bone resorption and absorption of intestinal calcium, increasing the circulating concentration and filtered load of calcium. This often causes significant hypercalciuria. Unlike primary hyperparathyroidism, serum calcium is normal and the state of hyperparathyroidism is secondary.

27. **c. Augment calcium reabsorption in the proximal tubule.** Thiazide is the primary medical treatment of renal hypercalciuria and has been shown to correct the renal leak of calcium by augmenting calcium reabsorption in the distal tubule. In addition, thiazides cause extracellular volume depletion, thereby stimulating proximal tubular reabsorption of calcium. A positive calcium balance ensues, with correction of the secondary hyperparathyroidism.

28. **e. All of the above.** Thiazide diuretics can cause hypokalemia. Symptoms of hypokalemia include muscle cramps and weakness. Consideration should be given to starting patients concurrently on potassium supplementation with potassium citrate, as patients can also become hypocitraturic. It is reasonable to check a basic metabolic panel 1 to 2 weeks after initiating a thiazide to monitor potassium levels. Thiazides can also cause low urinary citrate and magnesium. In addition, they can lead to impaired carbohydrate metabolism and hyperuricemia. A small percentage of patients may also have sexual side effects including decreased libido or erectile dysfunction.

29. **d. Thiazide-induced hypocitraturia.** Intracellular acidosis resulting from thiazide-induced hypokalemia will augment renal tubular reabsorption of citrate with resultant hypocitraturia. The reduction in the inhibitory effects of hypocitraturia may promote further stone formation. Therefore potassium repletion is necessary if long-term thiazide treatment is anticipated. Our potassium supplement of choice is potassium citrate, in either pill or liquid preparations.

30. **c. High dietary sodium intake.** A high dietary sodium intake has two deleterious effects in this case. An excess sodium load will inhibit reabsorption of calcium in the proximal tubule, thereby causing hypercalciuria. Moreover, sodium will block the hypocalciuric action of thiazides. Therefore patients placed on thiazide diuretics for management of hypercalciuria should also be placed on a dietary sodium restriction.

31. **d. Hyperoxaluria.** Roux-en-Y gastric bypass has been shown to lead to significantly increased urinary oxalate. Other metabolic abnormalities seen in patients with Roux-en-Y gastric bypass include low urine volumes and hypocitraturia. In contrast, restrictive bariatric surgery—such as gastric band or sleeve—does not lead to hyperoxaluria. These patients have low urine volumes as their primary metabolic abnormality.

CHAPTER REVIEW

1. First-time stone formers are at a 50% risk for recurrence. Males have both a higher incidence of calculi and a higher recurrence rate.
2. Infectious calculi may contain large quantities of endotoxin.
3. A complete urine collection is confirmed by the 24-hour excretion of creatinine. On average 1 mg/kg per hour is excreted.
4. As the phosphate content of the stone increases from calcium oxalate to calcium oxalate-calcium apatite to calcium apatite, the incidence of renal tubular acidosis increases from 5% to 39% and the incidence of primary hyperthyroidism increases from 2% to 10%. Thus higher phosphate content in stones correlates with an increased incidence of renal tubular acidosis and primary hyperparathyroidism.
5. Obesity increases the risk of nephrolithiasis.
6. Hypercalciuria not associated with hypercalcemia may be subdivided into (1) excess gastrointestinal absorption, (2) renal tubular leak, or (3) normocalcemic hyperparathyroidism.
7. Patients with hyperuricosuria have increased calcium oxalate urolithiasis due to heterogeneous nucleation.
8. Increased protein intake increases the likelihood of renal stones due to increased urinary calcium, oxalate, and uric acid excretion. Moderate calcium ingestion and a reduced sodium diet, when combined with animal protein restriction, reduce calcium stone episodes by approximately 50%.
9. Thiazides may unmask primary hyperparathyroidism by causing a marked rise in serum calcium. They also cause hypocitraturia.
10. Indinavir stones may not be visible on CT.
11. Furosemide-induced nephrolithiasis should always be considered in neonates who develop nephrolithiasis.

Continued

CHAPTER REVIEW—cont'd

12. Children with stones should always be worked up because inborn errors of metabolism may be responsible for the stones in a significant number of patients. The inborn errors of metabolism most commonly found in this circumstance include cystinuria, renal tubular acidosis, and primary hyperoxaluria.

13. Patients with diabetes mellitus may have altered ammonium metabolism resulting in acidic urine that predisposes them to calcium oxalate and/or uric acid calculi.

14. Sulfate content in a 24-hour urine collection is an indication of the amount of protein intake. Protein intake increases calcium, oxalate, and uric acid excretion.

15. Intestinal fat malabsorption characteristic of ileal disease will exaggerate calcium soap formation, limit the amount of "free" calcium to complex to oxalate, and thereby raise the oxalate pool available for absorption.

16. Acid–base status is probably the most important factor in the renal handling of citrate.

17. The primary site of intestinal absorption of oxalate is the large bowel.

18. The solubility of uric acid is more than 10 times greater at a pH of 7 than at a pH of 5.

19. Sodium alkali therapy has been complicated by the development of calcium stones (calcium phosphate or calcium oxalate), especially when the urinary pH is above 7.

93

Strategies for Nonmedical Management of Upper Urinary Tract Calculi

David A. Leavitt, Jean J.M.C.H. de la Rosette, and David M. Hoenig

QUESTIONS

1. The best predictor of post–percutaneous nephrolithotomy (PNL) urosepsis is:
   a. preoperative bladder urine culture.
   b. intraoperative bladder urine culture.
   c. stone culture.
   d. preoperative blood culture.
   e. intraoperative blood culture.

2. What is the risk of mortality from an untreated struvite staghorn stone?
   a. Less than 10%
   b. 10% to 30%
   c. 30% to 50%
   d. 50% to 70%
   e. Greater than 70%

3. The increased risk of residual fragments after extracorporeal shockwave lithotripsy (SWL) of large-volume calculi is of particular importance for patients with stones composed of:
   a. brushite.
   b. uric acid.
   c. struvite.
   d. calcium oxalate monohydrate.
   e. calcium oxalate dihydrate.

4. What is the single most important factor when choosing among SWL, ureteroscopic stone removal, and PNL for renal calculi?
   a. Stone composition
   b. Stone location
   c. Anatomic abnormalities
   d. Stone burden
   e. Body habitus

5. What is the preferred treatment for a known brushite stone former harboring a lower pole renal calculus 25 mm in diameter?
   a. SWL
   b. SWL with ureteral stenting
   c. Flexible ureteroscopy with holmium laser lithotripsy
   d. PNL
   e. Laparoscopic pyelolithotomy

6. What is the preferred initial treatment for staghorn calculi?
   a. SWL with ureteral stenting
   b. Flexible ureteroscopy with holmium laser lithotripsy
   c. PNL
   d. Extended pyelolithotomy
   e. Anatrophic nephrolithotomy

7. Which of the following is the most difficult stone composition to fragment with SWL?
   a. Calcium oxalate dihydrate
   b. Calcium oxalate monohydrate
   c. Struvite
   d. Hydroxyapatite
   e. Uric acid

8. What is the preferred treatment approach for a symptomatic 1.5-cm stone in a lower pole calyceal diverticulum?
   a. SWL
   b. Flexible ureteroscopy
   c. PNL
   d. PNL with fulguration of the diverticulum
   e. Laparoscopic diverticulectomy

9. What is the preferred initial treatment for a 10-mm stone in the renal pelvis of a horseshoe kidney with minimal hydronephrosis?
   a. SWL
   b. Flexible ureteroscopy
   c. PNL
   d. Laparoscopic pyelolithotomy
   e. Symphysiotomy with pyelolithotomy

10. What is the preferred treatment approach for a 10-mm renal calculus in a patient who weighs 375 lb?
    a. SWL
    b. Flexible ureteroscopy
    c. PNL
    d. SWL using the "blast path" technique
    e. Open surgery

11. What is the preferred treatment option for a patient with a symptomatic 1.5-cm renal calculus and a coagulopathy?
    a. SWL
    b. SWL after administration of fresh-frozen plasma
    c. Indwelling ureteral stent
    d. Flexible ureteroscopy
    e. PNL

12. Residual fragments after SWL have been associated with which of the following?
    a. Hypertension
    b. An increased rate of recurrent stones
    c. A decreased rate of recurrent stones
    d. Perinephric hematomas
    e. Hematuria

13. What is the most sensitive test for identifying residual fragments after PNL?
    a. Nephrotomography
    b. Magnetic resonance imaging (MRI)
    c. Ultrasonography
    d. Noncontrast computed tomography (CT)
    e. Contrast-enhanced CT

14. Factors affecting the probability of spontaneous passage of ureteral calculi include all of the following EXCEPT:
    a. stone size.
    b. stone location at presentation.
    c. stone composition.
    d. degree of hydronephrosis.
    e. duration of symptoms.

15. Irreversible loss of renal function can occur within what time period when a completely obstructing ureteral stone is present?
    a. 1 week
    b. 2 to 4 weeks
    c. 4 to 6 weeks
    d. More than 6 weeks
    e. 3 months

16. A first-time stone former is diagnosed with a 4-mm proximal ureteral calculus. The best initial management is:
    a. ureteroscopic laser lithotripsy.
    b. ureteral stent placement.
    c. SWL.
    d. expectant management.
    e. SWL with ureteral stent placement.

17. Large-volume matrix calculi, which form as a consequence of urinary tract infection, are:
    a. effectively fragmented with SWL.
    b. best approached in a ureteroscopic fashion.
    c. generally sterile.
    d. radiopaque and well visualized on plain radiographic studies.
    e. most efficiently treated with PNL.

18. Ureteral stent placement when SWL is performed for ureteral stones is appropriate for all of the following reasons EXCEPT:
    a. solitary kidney.
    b. relief of severe symptoms.
    c. enhancement of stone fragmentation.
    d. relief of obstruction.
    e. aid in localization of difficult-to-visualize stones.

19. The preferred single agent for medical expulsive therapy for distal ureteral calculi is:
    a. nifedipine.
    b. tamsulosin.
    c. Solu-Medrol.
    d. ibuprofen.
    e. terazosin.

20. The treatment modality associated with the greatest stone-free rates and the least morbidity for patients with distal ureteral stones of any size is:
    a. PNL.
    b. SWL.

c. ureteroscopy.
d. open ureterolithotomy.
e. laparoscopic ureterolithotomy.

ANSWERS

1. **c. Stone culture.** The best predictor of post-PNL urosepsis is stone culture or renal pelvic urine culture results.
2. **b. 10% to 30%.** The 10-year mortality rate of untreated staghorn stones was 28%, versus 7.2% in patients treated with surgery.
3. **c. Struvite.** Struvite stones must be removed completely to minimize the risk of continued urea-splitting bacteriuria.
4. **d. Stone burden.** Stone burden (size and number) is perhaps the single most important factor in deciding the appropriate treatment modality for a patient with kidney calculi.
5. **d. PNL.** The Lower Pole Stone Study Group compared ureteroscopy and PNL for patients with 10- to 25-mm lower pole stones and found a significant difference in stone clearance, with only 40% of the ureteroscopic cohort stone free at 3 months versus 76% of the PNL cohort.
6. **c. PNL.** The management of staghorn stones with a combined approach must be viewed as primarily percutaneous, with SWL being used only as adjunct to minimize the number of accesses required.
7. **b. Calcium oxalate monohydrate.** Cystine and brushite are the stones most resistant to SWL, followed by calcium oxalate monohydrate. Next, in descending order, are hydroxyapatite, struvite, calcium oxalate dihydrate, and uric acid stones.
8. **d. PNL with fulguration of the diverticulum.** The percutaneous approach for the management of patients with calyceal diverticular stones provides the patient with the best chance of becoming stone and symptom free. Fulguration of the diverticulum will reduce the risk of recurrence of the diverticulum.
9. **a. SWL.** SWL can achieve satisfactory results in properly selected patients, such as those with small stones (<1.5 cm) in the presence of normal urinary drainage. For larger stones, or when there is evidence of poor urinary drainage, PNL should be used as the primary approach.
10. **b. Flexible ureteroscopy.** Retrograde ureteroscopic intrarenal surgery may be the preferred modality of treatment for morbidly obese patients when the stone burden is not excessively large.
11. **d. Flexible ureteroscopy.** When anticoagulation cannot be temporarily discontinued, the use of ureteroscopy in combination with holmium laser lithotripsy is preferred. One study reported that even when patients' coagulopathies were not fully corrected, the stones could be successfully treated with no increase in hemorrhagic complications.
12. **b. An increased rate of recurrent stones.** At follow-up (1.6 to 85.4 months), 43% of the patients with residual fragments had a significant symptomatic episode or required intervention.
13. **d. Noncontrast computed tomography (CT).** Although flexible nephroscopy is often considered the gold standard for assessing residual stones after PNL, the routine use of flexible nephroscopy has been challenged by studies showing the high sensitivity of noncontrast CT in detecting residual stones. Noncontrast CT had 100% sensitivity for detecting residual stones after PNL in 36 patients evaluated by both CT and flexible nephroscopy.
14. **c. Stone composition.** One study analyzed 75 patients with ureteral calculi and found that the interval to stone passage was highly variable and dependent on stone size, location, and side. Stones that were smaller, more distal, and on the right side were more likely to pass spontaneously. In another study, duration of symptoms before presentation was the most influential factor, followed by the degree of hydronephrosis.

15. **b. 2 to 4 weeks.** Even with complete ureteral obstruction, irreversible loss of renal function does not occur for more than 2 weeks but can progress to total renal unit loss at up to 6 weeks.
16. **d. Expectant management.** The majority of ureteral stones less than 5 mm will pass spontaneously and therefore can be treated with expectant management.
17. **e. Most efficiently treated with PNL.** Matrix stones are most effectively treated with PNL. SWL is usually ineffective because of the stone's gelatinous nature, and ureteroscopy may be compromised by the large volume of stone material present.
18. **c. Enhancement of stone fragmentation.** Although early reports supported the routine use of a ureteral stent to bypass ureteral stones before SWL, data analyzed by the American

Urological Association Ureteral Calculi Guidelines Panel showed no improvement in fragmentation with stenting, and therefore routine stent placement before SWL was discouraged. However, ureteral stent placement is appropriate for other indications, such as management of pain, relief of obstruction, and stones that are difficult to visualize, and is mandatory in a patient who has a solitary obstructed kidney.
19. **b. Tamsulosin.** Tamsulosin, a selective α-adrenergic blocker, is the preferred agent for medical expulsive therapy, owing to its reported efficacy and superior side effect profile.
20. **c. Ureteroscopy.** The stone-free rate for distal ureteral stones approached with ureteroscopy was 91% in the American Urological Association/European Association of Urology Ureteral Stones Guidelines document, an outcome superior to SWL.

CHAPTER REVIEW

1. Determinants of poor stone clearance rates after SWL include large renal calculi, lower pole or obstructed portions of the collecting system, very hard stones, and obesity.
2. Most calyceal stones in the absence of intervention are likely to increase in size and cause pain or infection.
3. If left untreated, staghorn calculi are likely to be associated with a progressive decrease in renal function.
4. Patients with cystinuria are more likely to have decreased renal function than other stone formers.
5. There is a linear correlation between Hounsfield units (density) and success of SWL.
6. Complete stone clearance from lower pole calyces is less likely than from other calyces for reasons that are not totally clear.
7. Spontaneous passage of a distal ureteral stone is more likely than that of a proximal ureteral stone.
8. For patients with proximal ureteral stones, there is no difference between treating the stone in situ or pushing it back into the renal pelvis when utilizing SWL.
9. In humans, there is no clear time threshold for irreversible damage in complete ureteral obstruction. It is clear, however, that patients with compromised vasculature, decreased renal reserve, poor nutrition, and other comorbid diseases such as diabetes tolerate obstruction less well than do patients with normal kidneys. Most agree that a significantly obstructing stone should not be allowed to persist beyond 2 to 4 weeks.
10. Untreated staghorn calculi are associated with recurrent urinary tract infections, urosepsis, renal function deterioration, and increased mortality.
11. Renal stones less than 1 cm are best treated with SWL or ureterorenoscopic extraction; stones between 1 and 2 cm that are not in the lower pole are best treated with SWL or PNL; stones greater than 2 cm are best treated with PNL.
12. Matrix renal stones are best removed with PNL.
13. Alpha blockers increase the rate of spontaneous passage of ureteral stones. Tamsulosin, a selective α-adrenergic blocker, is the preferred agent for medical expulsive therapy.
14. Bacteria may reside deep in the stone and may be impossible to eradicate without complete stone removal.
15. Medications responsible for producing stones include ephedrine, indinavir, triamterene, magnesium trisilicate, ciprofloxacin, and sulfa drugs.
16. The best predictor of post-PNL urosepsis is stone culture or renal pelvic urine culture results.
17. Stone burden (size and number) is perhaps the single most important factor in deciding the appropriate treatment modality for a patient with kidney calculi.
18. Cystine and brushite are the stones most resistant to SWL, followed by calcium oxalate monohydrate.
19. The percutaneous approach for the management of patients with calyceal diverticular stones provides the patient with the best chance of becoming stone and symptom free.
20. When anticoagulation cannot be temporarily discontinued, the use of ureteroscopy in combination with holmium laser lithotripsy is preferred.
21. The majority of ureteral stones less than 5 mm will pass spontaneously.
22. Pregnant women who require admission and require treatment for renal colic have a greater risk of preterm delivery.
23. Pregnancy induces a state of absorptive hypercalciuria and mild hyperuricosuria that is offset by increased excretion of urinary inhibitors such as citrate and magnesium, as well as increased urinary output.
24. SWL is now known to induce acute structural changes in the treated kidney in most, if not all, patients. The insult is primarily a vascular injury.
25. Uncorrected coagulopathy and an active, untreated urinary tract infection are two absolute contraindications to PNL.
26. Physiologic solutions should be used for irrigation during PNL to minimize the risk of dilutional hyponatremia in the event of large-volume extravasation.

94

Surgical Management for Upper Urinary Tract Calculi

Brian R. Matlaga and Amy E. Krambeck

QUESTIONS

1. The risk of ureteral perforation is greatest with which of the following intracorporeal lithotripsy technologies?
   a. Electrohydraulic lithotripsy (EHL)
   b. Holmium laser
   c. Pulsed-dye laser
   d. Ultrasonic lithotripsy
   e. Ballistic lithotripsy

2. The risk of retrograde stone propulsion is greatest with which of the following intracorporeal lithotripsy technologies?
   a. EHL
   b. Holmium laser
   c. Pulsed dye laser
   d. Ultrasonic lithotripsy
   e. Ballistic lithotripsy

3. What are the preferred initial power settings for holmium laser lithotripsy of ureteral stones?
   a. 0.6 J, 6 Hz
   b. 0.6 J, 10 Hz
   c. 1.0 J, 10 Hz
   d. 1.2 J, 10 Hz
   e. 1.0 J, 15 Hz

4. Which intracorporeal lithotripsy technology will most efficiently fragment and evacuate renal calculi?
   a. Ultrasonic lithotripsy
   b. Ballistic lithotripsy
   c. Combination ultrasonic/ballistic lithotripsy
   d. Holmium laser
   e. EHL

5. Which intracorporeal lithotripsy technology has the least risk of ureteral perforation?
   a. Ultrasound
   b. Ballistic
   c. Holmium laser
   d. EHL
   e. Erbium laser

6. Energy sources for shockwave lithotripsy (SWL) include all of the following EXCEPT:
   a. electrohydraulic.
   b. holmium laser.
   c. piezoelectric.
   d. electromagnetic.
   e. microexplosive.

7. What is a major disadvantage of ultrasound imaging for SWL?
   a. Inability to visualize ureteropelvic junction (UPJ) stones
   b. Exposure to ionizing radiation
   c. Inability to visualize radiolucent stones
   d. Expense of ultrasonography systems
   e. Inability to visualize ureteral stones

8. Factors influencing the amount of pain during SWL include all but which of the following?
   a. Power level applied
   b. Stone composition
   c. Type of shockwave generator
   d. Shockwave energy density at the point of skin penetration
   e. Stone location

9. Possible mechanisms producing stone fragmentation during SWL include all of the following EXCEPT:
   a. compression fracture.
   b. spallation.
   c. acoustic cavitation.
   d. dynamic fatigue.
   e. vaporization.

10. What percentage of kidneys experience trauma during SWL?
    a. 0% to 20%
    b. 20% to 40%
    c. 40% to 60%
    d. 60% to 80%
    e. 80% to 100%

11. Risk factors that will enhance the bioeffects of shockwaves include all of the following EXCEPT:
    a. patient age older than 60 years.
    b. pediatric age.
    c. stone burden.
    d. preexisting hypertension.
    e. reduced renal mass.

12. The primary insult to the kidney exposed to shockwaves occurs in which of the following tissues?
    a. Blood vessels
    b. Proximal tubule
    c. Renal papillae
    d. Glomerulus
    e. Renal capsule

13. Which anesthetic technique is associated with the greatest likelihood of a successful SWL treatment outcome?
    a. General endotracheal
    b. Intravenous sedation
    c. Epidural
    d. Sedation
    e. Topical anesthetic

14. Which of the following is an absolute contraindication to percutaneous nephrolithotomy (PNL)?
    a. Morbid obesity
    b. Uncorrected coagulopathy
    c. Neurogenic bladder
    d. Pelvic kidney
    e. Horseshoe kidney

15. Which treatment maneuver will reduce the likelihood of SWL-induced renal injury?
    a. Begin treatment at a high energy level
    b. Treat at a rate of 120 shocks per minute
    c. Treat with a topical local anesthetic
    d. Pretreat the targeted kidney at a low energy level and then ramp up treatment to a high energy level
    e. Pretreat the contralateral kidney at a high energy level and then ramp up treatment of the target kidney to a high energy level

16. What is the most common secondarily infecting organism after percutaneous stone removal?
    a. *Proteus mirabilis*
    b. *Klebsiella oxytoca*
    c. *Pseudomonas aeruginosa*
    d. *Staphylococcus epidermidis*
    e. *Enterococcus (Streptococcus) faecalis*

17. Which of the following is the antimicrobial of choice for ureteroscopy?
    a. First-generation cephalosporin
    b. Second-generation cephalosporin
    c. Aminoglycoside
    d. Fluoroquinolone
    e. Nitrofurantoin

18. What is the preferred site of puncture into the renal collecting system during access for PNL?
    a. Upper pole infundibulum
    b. Anterior lower pole calyx
    c. Posterior lower pole calyx
    d. Upper pole calyx
    e. Renal pelvis

19. Risk factors for colon injury during PNL include all of the following EXCEPT:
    a. horseshoe kidney.
    b. kyphoscoliosis.
    c. access lateral to the posterior axillary line.
    d. previous jejunoileal bypass for obesity.
    e. upper pole puncture.

20. To minimize the risk of lung and pleura injury during supracostal upper pole access for PNL:
    a. the puncture should be performed during full expiration.
    b. the puncture should be performed during full inspiration.
    c. CO_2 should be injected through the ureteral catheter to identify the upper pole calyx.
    d. the puncture should be done with local anesthesia.
    e. the puncture should be performed by a radiologist.

21. Indications for supracostal access during PNL include all of the following EXCEPT:
    a. predominant stone distribution in the upper pole.
    b. access to the UPJ or proximal ureter required.
    c. cystine stones.

    d. multiple lower pole infundibula and calyces containing stone material.
    e. horseshoe kidneys.

22. When performing PNL and endopyelotomy in the same setting, the optimal point of entry is:
    a. posterior upper pole calyx.
    b. posterior lower pole calyx.
    c. anterior upper pole calyx.
    d. anterior lower pole calyx.
    e. renal pelvis.

23. During access for PNL, what is the preferred initial wire?
    a. Amplatz Super-stiff
    b. Benson
    c. Hydrophilic glide
    d. Lunderquist
    e. J-tipped movable core

24. What is the most common serious error in PNL access?
    a. Not using an Amplatz sheath
    b. Overadvancement of the dilator/sheath
    c. Anterior calyceal puncture
    d. Ultrasonographically guided puncture
    e. The use of telescoping metal dilators

25. What is the appropriate irrigating solution for PNL?
    a. 3% sorbitol
    b. Sterile water
    c. Glycine
    d. Dilute contrast material
    e. 0.9% saline

26. Middle or upper pole access for PNL in horseshoe kidneys is preferred for all of the following reasons EXCEPT:
    a. a higher incidence of retrorenal colon.
    b. malrotation of the renal collecting system.
    c. incomplete ascent of horseshoe kidneys.
    d. anterior medial location of lower pole calyces.
    e. facilitated access to the UPJ or upper ureter.

27. What is the most significant complication of PNL?
    a. Hemorrhage
    b. Extravasation of irrigation fluid
    c. Incomplete stone removal
    d. Urinary tract infection
    e. Pleural effusion

28. What is the risk of arteriovenous fistula formation after PNL?
    a. 1 in 10
    b. 1 in 100
    c. 1 in 200
    d. 1 in 500
    e. 1 in 1000

29. If uncontrolled bleeding persists after nephrostomy tube placement after PNL, what would the preferred approach be?
    a. Insertion of a double-J stent
    b. Administration of furosemide (Lasix) to promote diuresis
    c. Surgical exploration
    d. Immediate angiography
    e. Insertion of a Kaye tamponade balloon

30. If a retroperitoneal injury to the colon is diagnosed after PNL, what is the preferred management?
    a. Surgical exploration and repair
    b. Diverting colostomy with later definitive repair
    c. Leaving the nephrostomy tube in for 2 weeks to allow the tract to mature
    d. Insertion of a double-J stent and withdrawal of the nephrostomy tube into the colon
    e. Immediate removal of the nephrostomy tube

31. The use of double-J stents to reduce the risk of steinstrasse after SWL has been demonstrated to be beneficial for what size of stones?
    a. Greater than 5 mm
    b. Greater than 10 mm
    c. Greater than 15 mm
    d. Greater than 20 mm
    e. Greater than 25 mm

32. Proper management of a stone trapped in a basket, with an avulsed ureter all in continuity and no safety guidewire in place, is:
    a. immediate surgical exploration and primary repair.
    b. cystoscopy to place a guidewire and ureteral stent.
    c. placement of a percutaneous nephrostomy drain.
    d. immediate ureteral reimplantation.
    e. immediate ileal ureter.

33. During the course of a ureteroscopic laser lithotripsy procedure for a 1-cm proximal ureteral stone, a ureteral perforation is noted after fragmentation and removal of the calculus. On inspection of the perforation, a stone fragment is noted outside the ureter in the retroperitoneum. The most appropriate management is to:
    a. terminate the procedure and place a ureteral stent.
    b. advance the ureteroscope into the retroperitoneum and remove the stone fragment with a basket device.
    c. place a nephrostomy tube.
    d. perform laparoscopic exploration and removal of the residual fragment.
    e. advance the ureteroscope into the retroperitoneum and fragment the stone with the holmium:YAG laser.

ANSWERS

1. **a. Electrohydraulic lithotripsy (EHL).** The major disadvantage of EHL is its propensity to damage the ureteral mucosa and its association with ureteral perforation.
2. **e. Ballistic lithotripsy.** Ballistic lithotripsy is accompanied by a relatively high rate of stone propulsion of between 2% and 17% when ureteral stones are treated. The holmium laser has been associated with a reduced potential for causing retropulsion owing to the weak shockwave that is typically induced during holmium laser lithotripsy.
3. **a. 0.6 J, 6 Hz.** It is recommended to begin treatment using low pulse energy (i.e., 0.6 J) with a pulse rate of 6 Hz and increase the pulse frequency (in preference to increasing the pulse energy) as needed to speed fragmentation.
4. **c. Combination ultrasonic/ballistic lithotripsy.** Combination ultrasonic and ballistic lithotrites have been reported to provide greater stone clearance rates than do conventional ultrasonic or ballistic lithotrites.
5. **b. Ballistic.** When compared with EHL or ultrasonic or laser lithotripsy, ballistic devices have a significantly lower risk of ureteral perforation.
6. **b. Holmium laser.** There are three primary types of shockwave generators: electrohydraulic (spark gap), electromagnetic,

and piezoelectric. Microexplosive generators have also been produced but have not gained mainstream acceptance.
7. **e. Inability to visualize ureteral stones.** Sonographic localization of a kidney stone requires a highly trained operator. Furthermore, localization of stones in the ureter is difficult or impossible.
8. **b. Stone composition.** The discomfort experienced during SWL is related directly to the energy density of the shockwave as it passes through the skin as well as the size of the focal point, parameters that are affected by all of the choices listed except for stone composition.
9. **e. Vaporization.** Several potential mechanisms for SWL stone breakage have been described: (1) spall fracture, (2) squeezing, (3) shear stress, (4) superfocusing, (5) acoustic cavitation, and (6) dynamic fatigue.
10. **e. 80% to 100%.** SWL is now known to induce acute structural changes in the treated kidney in most, if not all, patients. Morphologic studies using both MRI and quantitative radionuclide renography have suggested that 63% to 85% of all SWL patients treated with an unmodified Dornier HM3 lithotripter exhibit one or more forms of renal injury within 24 hours of treatment.
11. **c. Stone burden.** Patients with existing hypertension are at increased risk for the development of perinephric hematomas as a consequence of SWL. Age is a factor on both ends of the scale in that children and the elderly both appear to be at a greater risk for structural and functional changes after exposure to shockwaves. These responses are probably related to a reduction in the large renal reserve present in most healthy adult patients.
12. **a. Blood vessels.** Macroscopically, the acute changes noted in dog and pig kidneys treated with a clinical dose of shockwaves are strikingly similar to those described for patients. This lesion is predictable in size, is focal in location, and is unique in the types of injuries (primarily vascular insult) induced. Regions of damage reveal rupture of nearby thin-walled veins, walls of small arteries, and glomerular and peritubular capillaries, which correlates with the vasoconstriction measured in both treated and untreated kidneys. These observations show that both the microvasculature and the nephron are susceptible to shockwave damage; however, the primary injury appears to be a vascular insult.
13. **a. General endotracheal.** Patients undergoing SWL with general endotracheal anesthesia experience a significantly greater stone-free outcome than do patients undergoing SWL with alternative anesthetics.
14. **b. Uncorrected coagulopathy.** Uncorrected coagulopathy and an active, untreated urinary tract infection are two absolute contraindications to PNL.
15. **d. Pretreat the targeted kidney at a low energy level and then ramp up treatment to a high energy level.** A number of studies have demonstrated that pretreating the target kidney with low-energy shockwaves, followed by a full clinical treatment dose, will attenuate the renal injury associated with SWL.
16. **d. *Staphylococcus epidermidis*.** Cephalosporins are the most appropriately used antibiotics for prophylaxis of surgical procedures in noninfected stone cases, because the most common secondarily infecting organism is *S. epidermidis*.
17. **d. Fluoroquinolone.** The prophylactic antimicrobial agent of choice for ureteroscopy is a fluoroquinolone.
18. **c. Posterior lower pole calyx.** Because the posterior calyces are generally oriented so that the long axis points to the avascular area of the renal cortex, a posterolateral puncture directed at a posterior calyx would be expected to traverse through the avascular zone.
19. **e. Upper pole puncture.** A puncture placed too laterally may injure the colon. The position of the retroperitoneal colon is usually anterior or anterolateral to the lateral renal border. Therefore, risk of colon injury is usually only with a very lateral (lateral to the posterior axillary line) puncture. Posterior colonic displacement is more likely in thin female patients with very little retroperitoneal fat and/or elderly patients, as well as in patients with jejunoileal bypass resulting in an enlarged colon. Other factors increasing the risk of colon injury include anterior calyceal puncture, previous extensive renal

operation, horseshoe kidney, and kyphoscoliosis. A retrorenal colon is more frequently noted on the left side.

20. **a. The puncture should be performed during full expiration.** A supracostal puncture should be performed only during full expiration.

21. **c. Cystine stones.** A supracostal puncture is indicated when the predominant distribution of stone material is in the upper calyces, when there is an associated UPJ stricture requiring endopyelotomy, in cases of multiple lower pole infundibula and calyces containing stone material or an associated ureteral stone, in staghorn calculi with substantial upper pole stone burden, and in horseshoe kidneys.

22. **a. Posterior upper pole calyx.** A posterior upper pole calyx puncture, typically through a supracostal approach, aligns the axis of puncture with the UPJ. This allows the treating urologist to perform endopyelotomy with a rigid nephroscope, while exerting minimal torque on the instrument.

23. **c. Hydrophilic glide.** The hydrophilic glide wire is preferred for entering the collecting system because it is the most flexible and maneuverable wire available.

24. **b. Overadvancement of the dilator/sheath.** Overadvancement of the dilator/sheath is the most common serious error in access for PNL and may result in significant trauma to the renal collecting system and/or excessive hemorrhage.

25. **e. 0.9% saline.** Physiologic solutions should be used for irrigation during PNL to minimize the risk of dilutional hyponatremia in the event of large-volume extravasation.

26. **a. A higher incidence of retrorenal colon.** The optimal point of entry for a horseshoe kidney is through a posterior calyx, which is typically more medial than in the normal kidney because of the altered renal axis and rotation associated with the midline fusion. An upper pole collecting system puncture is often appealing, because the entire kidney is usually subcostal. In most cases the lower pole calyces are anterior and inaccessible percutaneously.

27. **a. Hemorrhage.** Bleeding is the most significant complication of PNL, with transfusion rates varying from less than 1% to 10%.

28. **c. 1 in 200.** Bleeding from an arteriovenous fistula or pseudoaneurysm requiring emergency embolization is seen in less than 0.5% of patients.

29. **e. Insertion of a Kaye tamponade balloon.** If bleeding is not controlled by nephrostomy tube placement and clamping, a Kaye nephrostomy tamponade balloon catheter should be placed (Cook Urological, Spencer, IN). The Kaye nephrostomy tube incorporates a low-pressure 12-mm balloon that may be left inflated for prolonged periods to tamponade bleeding from the nephrostomy tract.

30. **d. Insertion of a double-J stent and withdrawal of the nephrostomy tube into the colon.** Colonic injury is an unusual complication often diagnosed on a postoperative nephrostogram. Typically, the injury is retroperitoneal; thus signs and symptoms of peritonitis are infrequent. If the perforation is extraperitoneal, management may be expectant with placement of a ureteral catheter or double-J stent to decompress the collecting system and by withdrawing the nephrostomy tube from an intrarenal position to an intracolonic position, thus serving as a colostomy tube. The colostomy tube is left in place for a minimum of 7 days and is removed after a nephrostogram or a retrograde pyelogram showing no communication between the colon and the kidney.

31. **d. Greater than 20 mm.** Stents may be particularly advantageous with stones larger than 20 mm.

32. **c. Placement of a percutaneous nephrostomy drain.** Should a ureteral avulsion occur, the patient should undergo immediate diversion of the renal unit with the placement of a percutaneous nephrostomy drain.

33. **a. Terminate the procedure and place a ureteral stent.** When an extruded stone is noted outside the ureter, the procedure should be terminated and a ureteral stent placed.

CHAPTER REVIEW

1. EHL produces a hydraulic shockwave and cavitation bubble. It may be used in normal saline solutions.
2. Holmium laser lithotripsy causes stone vaporization by a photothermal mechanism, and when it is used, the stone should be painted.
3. Cyanide may be produced when the holmium laser is used to fragment uric acid calculi. To date, no untoward effects due to this have been reported.
4. Ultrasound breaks the stone by causing the stone to resonate at a high frequency. Considerable heat may develop at the interface.
5. Stone comminution occurs by two basic mechanisms: mechanical stresses produced by the incident shockwave and collapse of cavitation bubbles adjacent to the surface of the stone.
6. The entire ureter can be more easily accessed in the female with a rigid ureteroscope.
7. For uncomplicated ureteroscopies, a ureteral stent may be safely omitted.
8. There is a 3% to 6% incidence of ureteral stricture following ureteroscopy; therefore, follow-up imaging should be performed.
9. Struvite stones must be removed completely to minimize the risk of continued urea-splitting bacteriuria.
10. Cystine and brushite are the stones most resistant to SWL, followed by calcium oxalate monohydrate. Next, in descending order, are hydroxyapatite, struvite, calcium oxalate dihydrate, and uric acid stones.
11. When anticoagulation cannot be temporarily discontinued, the use of ureteroscopy in combination with holmium laser lithotripsy is preferred.
12. The majority of ureteral stones less than 5 mm will pass spontaneously.
13. There are three primary types of shockwave generators: electrohydraulic (Spark Gap), electromagnetic, and piezoelectric. Microexplosive generators have also been produced but have not gained mainstream acceptance.
14. Patients with existing hypertension are at increased risk for the development of perinephric hematomas as a consequence of SWL.
15. Cephalosporins are the most appropriately used antibiotics for prophylaxis of surgical procedures in noninfected stone cases, because the most common secondarily infecting organism is *S. epidermidis*.
16. Transvaginal ultrasonography may be used in the pregnant female to observe the lower ureters.
17. Fifty percent to 80% of pregnant patients will spontaneously pass the calculus.
18. Pregnancy induces a state of absorptive hypercalciuria and mild hyperuricosuria that is offset by increased excretion of urinary inhibitors such as citrate and magnesium, as well as increased urinary output. The metabolic changes in pregnancy do not influence the rate of new stone occurrence. However, paradoxically, it has been suggested that metabolic alterations in urine may contribute to accelerated encrustation of stents during pregnancy.

95

Lower Urinary Tract Calculi

Arvind P. Ganpule and Mahesh R. Desai

QUESTIONS

1. Which of the following is true about primary bladder calculi?
   a. They are described as those which form without any predisposing cause.
   b. They are more commonly found in well-developed industrialized nations.
   c. Nutritional deficiency has no role to play in the aetiopathogenesis.
   d. They occur in male children in the age group of 10 to 15 years.

2. Which of the following is not true about secondary bladder calculi?
   a. Humans with no infection, obstruction, neurological problems, and absence of foreign body rarely form stones.
   b. Homogenous nucleation is always to be blamed for crystallization in this entity.
   c. Heterogeneous nucleation occurs around the foreign body as a result of infection or due to obstruction with resulting super saturation.
   d. Among the neurogenic bladder patients, those with spinal cord injury are more prone to form bladder stones.

3. All of the following are causative factors for stone formation in neurogenic bladder patients except:
   a. completeness of neurological lesion.
   b. urinary tract infection (UTI) by *Proteus, Klebsiella*.
   c. black race.
   d. long-term catheterization.
   e. chronic inflammation.

4. Which among the following statements is false?
   a. Chemodissolution as a sole treatment would be time consuming and not completely efficient.
   b. It is not effective for preventing encrustations over catheters.
   c. This can be considered as the treatment modality as well as a prophylactic measure.
   d. Hemiacridin and Suby solutions causes acidification of urine.

5. Identify the correct statement out of the following?
   a. Extracorporeal shockwave lithotripsy (ESWL) as a modality of treatment has been considered as an option in patients with bladder calculi with artificial urinary sphincters or penile prosthesis.
   b. Transurethral surgery is completely safe even with longer OR times.
   c. Suprapubic surgery is ideal in patients who have had previous urethral or abdominal surgeries.
   d. Stones more than 2 cm should be treated with open surgery.

6. Which of the following statements is false regarding etiology of bladder calculi in patients with urinary diversions?
   a. The most commonly used segment is ileum and colon.
   b. Loss of ileum leads to enteric hyperoxaluria and can lead to formation of stones.

   c. The mucus produced also acts as a nidus for stone formation.
   d. The use of absorbable sutures reduces the incidence of bladder calculi.
   e. Clean intermittent catheterization (CIC) increases the incidence of bladder calculi in comparison with indwelling catheter.

7. The common metabolic abnormality that results in usage of ileum or colon for diversions is:
   a. hyperchloremic metabolic acidosis.
   b. hypochloremic metabolic alkalosis.
   c. hyponatremic metabolic alkalosis.
   d. hyponatremic metabolic acidosis.
   e. hyponatremic hypokalemic metabolic alkalosis.

8. All of the following are true regarding etiology of bladder calculi in patients with urinary diversions except:
   a. The most common etiological factor is persistence and recurrence of urinary tract infections.
   b. The organisms causing recurrence of infections are *Proteus, Pseudomonas, and Klebsiella*.
   c. The use of ileum causes hematuria dysuria syndrome.
   d. Mucus production leads to formation of biofilm and decreases the penetration of antibiotics.
   e. None of the above.

9. What are the treatment options available for bladder calculi in patients post urinary diversions and augmentation?
   a. Percutaneous approach
   b. Open cystolithotomy
   c. Poucholithotmy
   d. ESWL
   e. All of the above

10. The prevention strategies in case of bladder calculi in patients post urinary diversions and augmentation include all except:
    a. complete clearance of stone.
    b. eradication of infection.
    c. correction of anatomical abnormalities.
    d. use of nonabsorbable sutures.
    e. reduction of mucus formation.

11. Which of the following is false regarding treatment of bladder stone in SCI patients?
    a. ESWL is a treatment option in patients who are prone for autonomic dysreflexia.
    b. Laser and transurethral lithotripsy are ideally used for smaller calculi.
    c. Long-term use of antibiotics results in reduction of stone formation.
    d. Percutaneous or open approach are ideally used for larger calculi.
    e. None of the above.

12. The immunosuppressive drug used in transplantation that results in renal calculi is:
    a. antithymocyte globulin (ATG).
    b. mycophenolate Mofetil.
    c. calcineurin inhibitors.
    d. basiliximab.
    e. tacrolimus.

13. Regarding the epidemiology of urethral calculi, which of the following statements is true?
    a. It is more common in females with predilection for the elderly.
    b. It is more common in males with predilection for the elderly.
    c. It is more common in males with predilection for children.
    d. It is more common in females with a bimodal age distribution.
    e. It is more common in males with a bimodal age distribution.

14. Which of the following is not true about migratory urethral calculi?
    a. Migratory urethral calculi are the most common cause of urethral calculi.
    b. Structural or functional obstruction predisposes to urethral calculi.
    c. Concomitant bladder and upper tract calculi are seen in 2% and 18% of patients, respectively.
    d. Concomitant bladder and upper tract calculi are seen in 18% and 2% of patients, respectively.

15. Which of the following is true about migratory urethral calculi?
    a. Migratory urethral calculi are usually solitary and larger than primary calculi.
    b. Anterior urethral stones are more common than posterior urethral stones.
    c. The majority of patients have insidious onset of symptoms.
    d. Posterior urethral stones are palpable on digital rectal examination.

16. Which of the following is true about primary urethral calculi?
    a. Primary urethral calculi are so named because they are the primary and common cause of urethral calculi.
    b. Primary urethral calculi form primarily in the urethra irrespective of any obstruction of urethra or urinary stasis.
    c. The presence of a foreign body and urinary infection provide a conducive milieu for stone formation.
    d. The predominant composition of primary urethral calculi is calcium oxalate monohydrate.

17. Which of the following are the most commonly isolated organisms in case of infection stones?
    a. *Proteus* spp.
    b. *Escherichia coli*
    c. Enterococci
    d. All of the above

18. Which of the following is false regarding urethral calculi?
    a. Primary urethral calculi have a protracted course and insidious symptoms.
    b. Painless chronic retention occurs in 78% of patients.
    c. Patients with migratory calculi present immediately in view of sudden and drastic onset of the symptoms.
    d. Fistulous complications are more common in those who cannot report their symptoms due to decreased sensation.

19. The following statements are true about urethral calculi except:
    a. The majority of urethral stones are radiolucent and not visible on plain radiographs.
    b. Retrograde urethrogram can identify the stones as filling defect and has been the mainstay of investigation.
    c. Transrectal ultrasonography can identify the prostatic urethral calculi as a hyperechoic structure with post-acoustic shadowing.
    d. Upper tract stones may coexist and hence advocate an ultrasonography of the kidney, ureter, and bladder.

20. Which of the following is false regarding management of urethral calculi?
    a. Stones located in the posterior urethra can be pushed back into the bladder for extracorporeal shockwave lithotripsy or intracorporeal fragmentation with mechanical or electrohydraulic lithotripsy.
    b. Shockwave lithotripsy after pushback is successful, with a stone-free rate of 60%.
    c. Intracorporeal laser lithotripsy is more traumatic to the mucosa, with a success rate of 70% to 80%.
    d. For stones that do not get pushed back into the bladder, in situ fragmentation using laser or pneumatic lithotripsy should be undertaken.

21. Identify the correct statement out of the following.
    a. For stones in the anterior urethra, pushback into the bladder is hardly ever possible and is not to be attempted.
    b. A small but irregular stone can be milked out of the external meatus.
    c. Holmium laser is more traumatic than lithotripters when used for anterior urethra.
    d. A dorsal meatotomy helps in controlled removal of the stone and actually reduces urethral trauma.

22. Identify the incorrect statement out of the following.
    a. Urethral calculi amount to 0.3% to 1% of all stone disease.
    b. Normal urethra can clear stones up to a size of around 8 to 10 mm.
    c. Despite epilation, hair-bearing grafts lead to hair regrowth in 1% to 2% of patients.
    d. Nearly 22% of urethral stones having some form of lower urinary tract symptom.

ANSWERS

1. a. **They are described as those which form without any predisposing cause.** Primary bladder stones usually are described as those which form without any predisposing cause, while a secondary cause is found in most patients with certain predisposing causes. The primary bladder stones are historically known to occur associated with nutritional deficiency. These are known to be rampant in undernourished or nutritionally compromised individuals. The cause for formation of these calculi are believed to be a combination of decreased urine output, alteration in the urine pH, and other metabolic abnormalities. Vitamin deficiency and dietary compromise in the form of deficient animal proteins is responsible in the genesis of these stones. The primary bladder stones are known to form within the first 5 years of life and have a male preponderance to them.

2. b. **Homogenous nucleation is always to be blamed for crystallization in this entity.** Humans with no infection, obstruction, neurological problems, and absence of foreign body rarely form stones. Crystal formation has been implicated in formation of these stones. Homogenous nucleation rarely is to be blamed for crystallization in this entity. Heterogeneous nucleation occurs around the foreign body as a result of infection or

due to obstruction with resulting supersaturation. Among the neurogenic bladder patients, those with spinal cord injury are more prone to forming bladder stones.

3. **c. Black race** The factors implicated include complete neurological lesion, urinary tract infection caused by *Klebsiella*, and Caucasian race.

4. **b. It is not effective for preventing encrustations over catheters.** Chemodissolution as a sole treatment would be time consuming and not completely efficient. In the current era its role is limited to use in select cases as an adjunct treatment. The treatment of chemodissolution is particularly effective for encrustation over long-term catheters. This can be considered as the treatment modality as well as a prophylactic measure.

5. **a. Extracorporeal shockwave lithotripsy (ESWL) as a modality of treatment has been considered as an option in patients with bladder calculi with artificial urinary sphincters or penile prosthesis.** ESWL as a modality of treatment has been considered as an option in patients with bladder calculi with artificial urinary sphincters or penile prosthesis. Any endoscopic intervention in such a situation is fraught with jeopardizing the integrity of the prosthesis or sphincter device. It has also been considered to be a treatment option in stones in neobladders and medically high-risk patients.

6. **e. Clean intermittent catheterization (CIC) increases the incidence of bladder calculi in comparison with indwelling catheter.** CIC has been found to reduce the incidence of bladder calculi in comparison with indwelling catheter.

7. **a. Hyperchloremic metabolic acidosis** The commonly used intestinal segments at present are ileum and colon that are prone to many metabolic abnormalities, which increase the risk of stone formation. The common metabolic abnormality that results in usage of ileum or colon for diversions is hyperchloremic metabolic acidosis, which in turn may cause hypercalciuria due to decrease in absorption of calcium (Assimos, 1996).

8. **c. The use of ileum causes hematuria dysuria syndrome.** The most common etiological factor is persistence and recurrence of urinary tract infections and the organisms causing recurrence of infections are urease-splitting organisms such as *Proteus, Pseudomonas, and Klebsiella*. Mucus production leads to formation of stones by two mechanisms. It acts as a nidus for stone formation and also helps in formation of biofilm that decreases the penetration of antibiotics. The use of stomach and not the ileum results in hematuria dysuria syndrome.

9. **e. All of the above.** All the above-mentioned treatment modalities can be used in treating patients of calculi post bladder diversion and augmentation.

10. **d. Use of nonabsorbable sutures.** The prevention strategies include mainly complete removal of stone and treatment of infection, correction of anatomical abnormalities, prevention of mucus, and use of absorbable sutures.

11. **c. Long-term use of antibiotics results in reduction of stone formation.** The use of long-term antibiotics for eradication of infection can lead to reduction of gut bacteria and leads to enteric hyperoxaluria, which in turn leads to stone formation.

12. **c. Calcineurin inhibitors.** The immunosuppressive drugs causing calculi in post-transplant patients are calcineurin inhibitors and steroids.

13. **e. It is more common in males, with a bimodal age distribution.** Urethral calculi have been exceedingly more common in males, with a bimodal age distribution. The first peak occurs in early childhood and the second peak incidence occurs in the fourth or fifth decades of life. Shorter length of the female urethra and higher peak flow rates in adolescence and younger age groups may have the protective effect for the younger demographic age group.

14. **d. Concomitant bladder and upper tract calculi are seen in 18% and 2% of patients, respectively.** A vast majority of urethral calculi are migratory in nature. Any pathology, either structural or functional, affecting the urethra, such as urethral stricture, meatal stenosis, or Benign prostatic hyperplasia, can impede the normal stone passage and result in a migratory calculus, which otherwise would have been cleared. It was commonly believed that the bladder was the source of migratory

calculi, but recent evidence has suggested that the source of these migratory calculi could as well be the upper urinary tract calculi. Patients with urethral calculi had concomitant bladder and upper tract calculi in 2% and 18%, respectively.

15. **a. Migratory urethral calculi are usually solitary and larger than primary calculi.** Migratory urethral calculi are usually solitary and larger than primary calculi. Posterior urethral calculi are more common, as high as 78% in some series. Migratory urethral calculi have a drastic onset of symptoms, with only a very few presenting with lower urinary tract symptoms (LUTS). Digital rectal examination is normal except for minimal tenderness of prostate while anterior urethral calculi may be palpable.

16. **c. The presence of a foreign body and urinary infection provide a conducive milieu for stone formation.** Primary urethral calculi are named primary as they originate at the same site where they are found ultimately. In reality, they form secondary to obstruction of urethra at any level or urinary stasis in urethral diverticula. Presence of a foreign body and urinary infection provides a conducive milieu for stone formation. Most of these stones are small, round, without a core or nucleus, and the predominant composition is struvite (magnesium ammonium phosphate), although other types such as calcium phosphate and uric acid have been reported.

17. **d. All of the above.** Most of the primary calculi are small, round, without a core or nucleus, and the predominant composition is struvite (magnesium ammonium phosphate). In the presence of infection stones, the commonly isolated organisms are *E. coli, Proteus*, and enterococci.

18. **b. Painless chronic retention occurs in 78% of patients.** In a large contemporary series of urethral calculi, a vast majority of 78% had acute painful urinary retention and the remaining 22% had some form of lower urinary tract symptoms, reiterating the fact that the majority of urethral stones remain symptomatic (Kamal et al., 2004). Other authors have also observed similar findings, although the rates of urinary retention have varied from 0% to 90% in literature.

19. **a. The majority of urethral stones are radiolucent and not visible on plain radiographs.** The majority of urethral stones are radio-opaque and visible on plain radiographs. Retrograde urethrogram can identify the stones as filling defect and has been the mainstay of investigation. Transrectal ultrasonography can identify the prostatic urethral calculi as a hyperechoic structure with postacoustic shadowing. A high-frequency (10 MHz) linear transducer placed on the dorsal surface of the penis along its long axis can screen the entire urethra. Upper tract stones may coexist and hence advocate an ultrasonography of the kidney, ureter, and bladder or a cross-sectional computerized tomography, especially if there exists a strong suspicion.

20. **c. Intracorporeal laser lithotripsy is more traumatic to the mucosa, with a success rate of 70% to 80%.** Stones located in the posterior urethra can be pushed back into the bladder for extracorporeal shockwave lithotripsy or intracorporeal fragmentation with mechanical or electrohydraulic lithotripsy. Shockwave lithotripsy after pushback is successful, with a stone-free rate of roughly 60%. Intracorporeal laser lithotripsy is less traumatic to the mucosa, with a guaranteed success rate of 85% to 90%. For stones that do not get pushed back into the bladder, in situ fragmentation using laser or pneumatic lithotripsy should be undertaken.

21. **a. For stones in the anterior urethra, pushback into the bladder is hardly ever possible and is not to be attempted.** For stones in the anterior urethra, pushback into the bladder is hardly ever possible and is not to be attempted. Small stones can be milked out of the external meatus, but irregular and large stones should not be milked as they cause urethral damage. Holmium laser is least traumatic when used for anterior urethra. A ventral meatotomy helps in controlled removal of the stone and actually reduces urethral trauma.

22. **c. Despite epilation, hair-bearing grafts lead to hair regrowth in 1% to 2% of patients.** Attempts at epilation before engraftment have reduced but not eliminated the risk as the follicles persist and lead to hair growth in 3% to 6% of patients.

CHAPTER REVIEW

1. Primary bladder calculi are most common in children younger than the age of 10, with a peak incidence at 2 to 4 years. The disease is much more common in boys than in girls.

2. The most common presentation of bladder stones is hematuria with lower urinary tract symptoms.

3. Children with bladder stones often present with abdominal discomfort, dysuria, frequency, and hematuria.

4. Pulling the penis, in children, is considered pathognomic of bladder stone.

5. The options for treatment of bladder stones are medical management, extracorporeal shockwave lithotripsy, transurethral lithotripsy, suprapubic cystolithotomy, suprapubic cystolithotripsy, and open surgery.

6. The advantages of percutaneous approach in bladder stones are safety and efficacy and potentially lesser risk to the urethra.

7. Urethral calculi amount to 0.3% to 1% of all stone disease, and obstructing urethral calculus is a very rare presentation of lower urinary tract urolithiasis.

8. More commonly urethral calculi patients present with acute painful retention of urine from sudden impaction of the stone.

9. Patients with at least one symptom of prostatitis are 3.2 times more likely to harbor a significant prostatic calculus than age-matched asymptomatic group.

10. The common factors associated with prepucial calculi are severe phimosis along with poor hygiene and low socioeconomic status.

11. Plain x ray film shows calculi in 14% prepucial calculi in patients.

96   Benign Renal Tumors

William P. Parker and Matthew T. Gettman

QUESTIONS

1. A 47-year-old woman is referred for the evaluation of renal cyst disease. What features would suggest a diagnosis of autosomal dominant polycystic kidney disease?
   a. One simple (Bosniak I) renal cyst in each kidney
   b. One simple (Bosniak I) renal cyst in the right kidney and two hepatic cysts
   c. One complex (Bosniak III) renal cyst in the left kidney and one simple (Bosniak I) renal cyst in the right kidney
   d. Two simple (Bosniak I) renal cysts in each kidney
   e. Two simple (Bosniak I) renal cysts in the right kidney

2. The key finding on CT imaging that differentiates Bosniak I-IIF from Bosniak III-IV renal cysts is:
   a. enhancement on administration of intravenous contrast.
   b. high-density cystic fluid.
   c. intraseptal calcifications.
   d. septal nodularity.
   e. septal thickening.

3. A 58-year-old man undergoes a partial nephrectomy for a 4-cm renal mass. On pathologic evaluation, the mass is diffusely eosinophilic with invasion of the perirenal fat. Helpful in establishing a diagnosis of oncocytoma using immunohistochemical staining is:
   a. Cytokeratin-7.
   b. Estrogen receptor.
   c. HMB-45.
   d. Melan-A.
   e. WT1.

4. A 25-year-old man presents with a renal mass identified on axial imaging obtained during the evaluation of a pneumothorax. On examination he has multiple raised lesions around his nasal folds. What chromosome is likely altered in this patient given the likely disease?
   a. Chromosome 4
   b. Chromosome 7
   c. Chromosome 9
   d. Chromosome 16
   e. Chromosome 17

5. A 30-year-old woman with neurocognitive delay, epilepsy, and multiple cutaneous lesions presents with her family for the evaluation of bilateral fat containing renal masses. As you discuss options for management, you review the role of everolimus in the management and stabilization of renal mass growth. This medication is targeting what abnormal genetic pathway?
   a. *EHHADH* mutations resulting in decreased adenosine triphosphate (ATP) production

   b. *Hamartin* gene mutations that result in unchecked protein synthesis and cellular growth
   c. Nuclear transcription factor mutation resulting in constitutive activity
   d. *PKD1* gene mutations that impair intracellular calcium regulation
   e. *VHL* gene mutations that result in unregulated angiogenesis

6. A 44-year-old woman is referred for a suspected angiomyolipoma. All of the following radiographic findings are consistent with the diagnosis except:
   a. hyperintensity on T1 MRI sequences.
   b. hyperintensity on T2 MRI sequences.
   c. hyperintense borders on in and opposed phase MRI sequences.
   d. intralesional density of –30 Hounsfield units (HU) on non-contrast CT.
   e. hypointensity of T1 fat-suppressed MRI sequences.

7. The use of everolimus in the management of tuberous sclerosis-related angiomyolipoma is based on phase III data in which a 30% reduction in mass was observed in ____ patients.
   a. 20%
   b. 40%
   c. 60%
   d. 80%
   e. 100%

8. A 42-year-old woman presents with a hypoenhancing renal mass that is resected and determined to be a metanephric adenoma. A paraneoplastic syndrome identified in this disease is:
   a. hyperaldosteronism.
   b. hyperparathyroidism.
   c. Cushing syndrome.
   d. polycythemia.
   e. syndrome of inappropriate antidiuretic hormone secretion (SIADH).

9. A 15-year-old boy is referred to your clinic for the evaluation of a cystic renal mass. On CT, the mass has evidence of multiple septations that enhance on contrast administration. Due to concern for Wilms tumor, a radical nephrectomy is performed. The final pathology is a cystic nephroma. A finding that will aid in differentiation of Wilms tumor from cystic nephroma is:
   a. alpha-methylacyl-CoA racemase (AMACR) positivity.
   b. an absence of blastemal elements.
   c. cysts lined with hobnail epithelium in a background of spindle cell fascicles.
   d. no evidence of estrogen receptor positivity.
   e. staining for WT-1.

10. A 58-year-old man presents with renal colic and hypertensive urgency. On evaluation he is found to have a cystic mass surrounding the renal capsule and compressing the kidney. This is consistent with a diagnosis of:

    a. cystic nephroma.

    b. leiomyoma.

    c. lymphangioma.

    d. papillary adenoma.

    e. renal hemangioma.

11. A 35-year-old woman presents with hypokalemia and hypertension refractory to medical management. Evaluation reveals a small hypoechoic mass in the right kidney on ultrasound. The etiology of hypokalemia in this patient is related to:

    a. Cushing syndrome.

    b. diuretic use.

    c. hyperaldosteronism.

    d. hyperparathyroidism.

    e. SIADH.

12. A 35-year-old woman in her third trimester is brought to the emergency department unresponsive with hypotension, anemia, and is found to have a retroperitoneal hemorrhage. The most likely cause is:

    a. angiomyolipoma.

    b. clear cell renal cell carcinoma.

    c. metanephric adenoma.

    d. oncocytoma.

    e. trauma.

13. The following are common to most benign renal mass presentations EXCEPT:

    a. female gender.

    b. incidental diagnosis.

    c. older patient age.

    d. smoking history.

    e. stable size.

ANSWERS

1. **d. Two simple (Bosniak I) renal cysts in each kidney.** According to the diagnostic guidelines for autosomal dominant polycystic kidney disease, the finding of two renal cysts (unilateral or bilateral) in patients less than 30, two cysts in each kidney in patients between 30 and 59(d), and four cysts in each kidney after 60 is suggested of the disease. The other descriptors (a, b, c, e) are not sufficient for the diagnosis.

2. **a. Enhancement on administration of intravenous contrast.** The Bosniak system for classifying renal cysts defines enhancement of the solid cyst components on the administration of intravenous contrast as a concerning finding toward the risk of malignancy and is the key finding that differentiates Bosniak I-IIF from Bosniak III/IV renal cysts (a). The remainder (b, c, d, e) can be seen in Bosniak II and IIF cysts.

3. **a. Cytokeratin-7.** For differentiation of oncocytoma from eosinophilic chromophobe renal cell carcinoma (the diagnostic dilemma in this case), the ISUP (International Society of Urologic Pathology) recommends the use of cytokeratin-7, which is rarely positive in oncocytoma and is diffusely positive

in chromophobe renal cell carcinoma (a). Estrogen receptor positivity is seen in multiple other renal tumors (b), HMB-45 (c) and Melan-A (d) are positive in angiomyolipomas, and WT1 is positive in metanephric adenomas (e).

4. **e. Chromosome 17.** The likely disorder is Birt-Hogg-Dubé syndrome, which is associated with mutations in the folliculin gene on chromosome 17 (e). Chromosome 4 (a) is mutated in autosomal dominant polycystic kidney disease; chromosome 7 (b) mutations are associated with papillary adenomas; papillary renal cell carcinoma, and metanephric adenoma; chromosome 9 (c) is mutated in tuberous sclerosis; and chromosome 16 (d) in both autosomal dominant polycystic kidney disease.

5. **b. *Hamartin* gene mutations that result in unchecked protein synthesis and cellular growth.** Hamartin (b) is one of two genes mutated in tuberous sclerosis, the described disorder. In this disease, mutation results in activation of the mTOR pathway and unregulated growth. The other described mutations relate to Fanconi syndrome (a), a method for castration resistance in prostate cancer (c), polycystic kidney disease (d), and clear cell renal cell carcinoma (e).

6. **c. Hyperintense borders on in and opposed phase MRI sequences.** All of the answer choices are consistent with the diagnosis of an angiomyolipoma except for the finding of hyperintense borders on in and opposed phase imaging (c). On these sequences, angiomyolipomas will appear to have a hypointense border ("India ink artifact") due to the presence of intralesional fat.

7. **d. 80%.** The phase III randomized controlled trial of everolimus in the management of TSC-related angiomyolipomas demonstrated a 42% response of 50% or greater reduction in size, 80% response of 30% or greater reduction in size (d), and a 100% rate of stabilization or partial response. Subsequent follow-up to 4 years revealed a 92% any response rate with only 14% experiencing progression.

8. **d. Polycythemia.** Polycythemia (d) has been identified in metanephric adenoma due to tumor production of erythropoietin, IL-6, IL8, G-CSF, and GM-CSF. The remainder (a, b, c, e) of choices describe paraneoplastic syndromes not associated with metanephric adenoma.

9. **b. An absence of blastemal elements.** (b) Blastemal and embryonal elements are common to Wilms tumor and are notably absent in cystic nephroma. While answer choice (c) describes findings common to cystic nephroma, this will not definitively rule out Wilms tumor. AMACR (a) and WT1 (e) staining are used in the diagnosis of metanephric adenomas. Cystic nephromas stain positive for estrogen receptor (d).

10. **c. Lymphangioma.** Of the described choices, lymphangiomas (c) are known to present with cystic extrinsic compression of the kidney due to aberrant lymphatic development in the perirenal lymphatics. Leiomyomas (b), papillary adenomas (d), and renal hemangiomas (e) will not appear cystic and external to the kidney; while cystic nephroma (a) may appear cystic, they are most often within the renal parenchyma.

11. **e. SIADH.** This is a classic example of a juxtaglomerular tumor (JGCT). The source of hypertension in these patients is hyperproduction of renin, which results in a secondary cause of hyperaldosteronism (c). The other choices represent other paraneoplastic processes unrelated to JGCTs.

12. **a. Angiomyolipoma.** The most common cause of Wunderlich syndrome is from an angiomyolipoma (a). An additional clue to this presentation is the patient's pregnancy, where hormonal changes can result in growth of the lesion.

13. **d. Smoking history.** All of the answers suggest a benign renal mass presentation, except for smoking (d), which is a risk factor for a malignant renal mass.

CHAPTER REVIEW

1. Renal cyst disease is the most common benign renal tumor.
2. Acquired cystic kidney disease is associated with a significant increase in malignancy risk and should be followed closely.
3. Most cysts require no additional follow-up or therapy.
4. The Bosniak classification is a useful tool to estimate malignancy risk and direct therapy.
5. Renal oncocytoma is the most common benign enhancing renal mass.
6. Oncocytomas are histologically similar to chromophobe renal cell carcinoma (RCC), and immunohistochemical staining may be required to distinguish the two.
7. Oncocytoma is associated with Birt-Hogg-Dubé syndrome: characterized by pulmonary cysts, spontaneous pneumothoraces, and fibrofolliculomas.
8. When suspected, a percutaneous biopsy may provide a diagnosis when core tissue is available for additional immunohistochemical studies.
9. Active surveillance represents a reasonable treatment strategy that minimizes risk and increases certainty based on growth kinetics.
10. Angiomyolipoma is a benign tumor of dysmorphic blood vessels, smooth muscle, and adipose tissue that can be diagnosed definitively on cross-section imaging due to the presence of macroscopic fat.
11. Most patients present asymptomatically; however, angiomyolipomas (AML) is the most common cause of spontaneous retroperitoneal hemorrhage.
12. Tuberous sclerosis is associated with the development of multifocal and bilateral renal AML and is associated with activation of the mTOR pathway.
13. Treatment depends on size, presence of symptoms, and pregnancy status and should be tailored to the patient with the goal of renal function preservation.
14. The treatment of choice in patients with acute hemorrhage is selective renal angioembolization.
15. Everolimus is indicated for the management of larger, multifocal AMLs in patients with TSC and lymphangioleiomyomatosis (LAM).
16. Papillary adenomas are ≤5mm in size and are therefore not readily diagnosed on imaging.
17. Papillary adenomas share common immunohistochemical staining, genetic changes, and are found in association with papillary RCC, suggesting a commonality between these diseases.
18. Metanephric adenoma is a rare, benign enhancing renal mass. Symptoms are present in approximately 50% of patients, with a female predisposition.
19. Metanephric adenoma may exist on a continuum with Wilms tumors and papillary RCC, and can be distinguished based on histology and immunohistochemical staining.
20. Cystic nephroma and mixed epithelial and stromal tumor (MEST) are biologically related and histologically similar.
21. Frequent expression of estrogen and progesterone receptor in tumor tissue is reported with a female predisposition.
22. If feasible, a nephron-sparing approach with partial nephrectomy is the preferred management strategy.
23. Leiomyomas are described along the urinary tract, but most often from the renal capsule.
24. Radiologic examination is insufficient to confirm the diagnosis.
25. Nephron-sparing approaches are preferred when technically possible.
26. Multiple rare tumors of the kidney have been described.
27. Radiologic differentiation from renal malignancy is not possible.
28. Reninoma, a benign tumor of the renal juxtaglomerular cell apparatus, is an important but rare cause of secondary hypertension and hypokalemia.

97

Malignant Renal Tumors

Steven C. Campbell, Brian R. Lane, and Philip M. Pierorazio

QUESTIONS

1. What is the most accurate imaging study for characterizing a renal mass?
   a. Intravenous pyelography
   b. Ultrasonography
   c. Computed tomography (CT) with and without contrast enhancement
   d. CT-positron emission tomography (PET) scan
   e. Renal arteriography

2. A hyperdense renal cyst may also be termed a:
   a. probable malignancy.
   b. Bosniak II cyst.
   c. Bosniak III cyst.
   d. Bosniak IV cyst.
   e. probable angiomyolipoma.

3. The most generally accepted indication for core needle biopsy of a renal mass is a suspected clinical diagnosis of:
   a. renal cell carcinoma (RCC).
   b. renal oncocytoma.
   c. renal cyst.
   d. renal metastasis.
   e. renal angiomyolipoma.

4. According to the American Urological Association (AUA) guidelines (Fig. 97.1), recommended postoperative radiographic surveillance of the chest after radical nephrectomy for T1N0M0 RCC is:
   a. no imaging studies.
   b. chest radiograph at 1 year.
   c. chest radiograph annually for 3 years.
   d. chest CT at 1 year and then chest radiograph annually for 2 years.
   e. chest radiograph annually for 5 years.

5. The European Organization for Research and Treatment of Cancer 30904 study randomly assigned patients to radical versus partial nephrectomy. Which of the following was an inclusion criterion?
   a. Clinical T1a tumor (<4.0 cm)
   b. Tumor size <5.0 cm
   c. Estimated glomerular filtration rate (GFR) >60 mL/min/1.73 m²
   d. No hypertension
   e. Age <70 years

6. According to the AUA guidelines, following partial nephrectomy for pathologic stage T3aN0M0 RCC, it is recommended to perform surveillance abdominal CT scanning with what frequency?
   a. Never
   b. Every 6 months for at least 3 years and then annually to year 5

   c. Every year to year 5
   d. Every 2 years
   e. Every year for 2 years and then at year 5

7. Following partial nephrectomy of a solitary kidney, what is the most effective method of screening for hyperfiltration nephropathy?
   a. Urinary dipstick test for protein
   b. Albumin-to-creatinine ratio
   c. Iothalamate glomerular filtration rate (GFR) measurement
   d. Serum creatinine measurement
   e. Renal biopsy

8. The most accurate and practical assessment of renal function for routine use after nephrectomy is:
   a. serum creatinine measurement.
   b. urinary dipstick test for protein.
   c. 24-hours urinary protein measurement.
   d. iothalamate GFR measurement.
   e. serum creatinine–based estimation of GFR and analysis for proteinuria.

9. What is an important prerequisite for successful cryoablation of a renal tumor?
   a. Slow freezing
   b. Rapid thawing
   c. A single prolonged freeze-thaw cycle
   d. A double freeze-thaw cycle
   e. Freezing of tumor to a temperature of −10°C

10. Which two imaging modalities are the preferred and most accurate for demonstrating the presence and extent of an inferior vena caval tumor thrombus?
    a. Abdominal ultrasonography and CT
    b. MRI and renal artery angiography
    c. CT and MRI
    d. MRI and contrast venacavography
    e. Contrast venacavography and transesophageal ultrasonography

11. In patients undergoing complete surgical excision of RCC, the lowest 5-year survival rate is associated with which factor?
    a. Perinephric fat involvement
    b. Clear cell histology
    c. Subdiaphragmatic inferior vena caval involvement
    d. Intra-atrial tumor thrombus
    e. Lymph node involvement

12. A 45-year-old man has a 5-cm, exophytic RCC in the upper pole of a solitary left kidney and a single 2-cm left lower lung metastasis. What is the best treatment?
    a. Initial targeted therapy, then partial nephrectomy
    b. Partial nephrectomy, then targeted therapy

Renal Mass and Localized Renal Cancer[1]

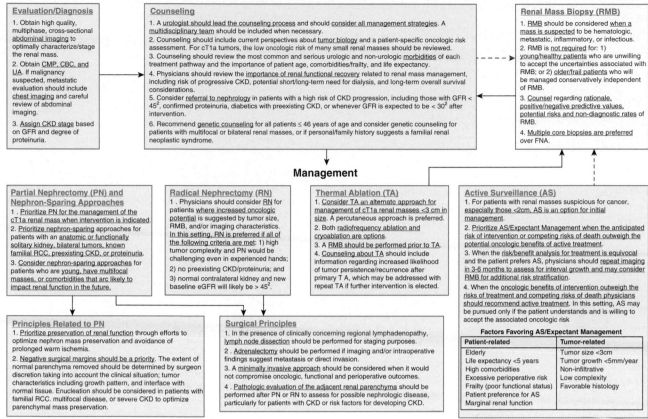

Evaluation/Diagnosis
1. Obtain high quality, multiphase, cross-sectional abdominal imaging to optimally characterize/stage the renal mass.
2. Obtain CMP, CBC, and UA. If malignancy suspected, metastatic evaluation should include chest imaging and careful review of abdominal imaging.
3. Assign CKD stage based on GFR and degree of proteinuria.

Counseling
1. A urologist should lead the counseling process and should consider all management strategies. A multidisciplinary team should be included when necessary.
2. Counseling should include current perspectives about tumor biology and a patient-specific oncologic risk assessment. For cT1a tumors, the low oncologic risk of many small renal masses should be reviewed.
3. Counseling should review the most common and serious urologic and non-urologic morbidities of each treatment pathway and the importance of patient age, comorbidities/frailty, and life expectancy.
4. Physicians should review the importance of renal functional recovery related to renal mass management, including risk of progressive CKD, potential short/long-term need for dialysis, and long-term overall survival considerations.
5. Consider referral to nephrology in patients with a high risk of CKD progression, including those with GFR < 45[2], confirmed proteinuria, diabetics with preexisting CKD, or whenever GFR is expected to be < 30[2] after intervention.
6. Recommend genetic counseling for all patients ≤ 46 years of age and consider genetic counseling for patients with multifocal or bilateral renal masses, or if personal/family history suggests a familial renal neoplastic syndrome.

Renal Mass Biopsy (RMB)
1. RMB should be considered when a mass is suspected to be hematologic, metastatic, inflammatory, or infectious.
2. RMB is not required for: 1) young/healthy patients who are unwilling to accept the uncertainties associated with RMB; or 2) older/frail patients who will be managed conservatively independent of RMB.
3. Counsel regarding rationale, positive/negative predictive values, potential risks and non-diagnostic rates of RMB.
4. Multiple core biopsies are preferred over FNA.

Management

Partial Nephrectomy (PN) and Nephron-Sparing Approaches
1. Prioritize PN for the management of the cT1a renal mass when intervention is indicated.
2. Prioritize nephron-sparing approaches for patients with an anatomic or functionally solitary kidney, bilateral tumors, known familial RCC, preexisting CKD, or proteinuria.
3. Consider nephron-sparing approaches for patients who are young, have multifocal masses, or comorbidities that are likely to impact renal function in the future.

Radical Nephrectomy (RN)
1. Physicians should consider RN for patients where increased oncologic potential is suggested by tumor size, RMB, and/or imaging characteristics. In this setting, RN is preferred if all of the following criteria are met: 1) high tumor complexity and PN would be challenging even in experienced hands; 2) no preexisting CKD/proteinuria; and 3) normal contralateral kidney and new baseline eGFR will likely be > 45[2].

Thermal Ablation (TA)
1. Consider TA an alternate approach for management of cT1a renal masses <3 cm in size. A percutaneous approach is preferred.
2. Both radiofrequency ablation and cryoablation are options.
3. A RMB should be performed prior to TA.
4. Counseling about TA should include information regarding increased likelihood of tumor persistence/recurrence after primary T A, which may be addressed with repeat TA if further intervention is elected.

Active Surveillance (AS)
1. For patients with renal masses suspicious for cancer, especially those <2cm, AS is an option for initial management.
2. Prioritize AS/Expectant Management when the anticipated risk of intervention or competing risks of death outweigh the potential oncologic benefits of active treatment.
3. When the risk/benefit analysis for treatment is equivocal and the patient prefers AS, physicians should repeat imaging in 3-6 months to assess for interval growth and may consider RMB for additional risk stratification.
4. When the oncologic benefits of intervention outweigh the risks of treatment and competing risks of death physicians should recommend active treatment. In this setting, AS may be pursued only if the patient understands and is willing to accept the associated oncologic risk

Principles Related to PN
1. Prioritize preservation of renal function through efforts to optimize nephron mass preservation and avoidance of prolonged warm ischemia.
2. Negative surgical margins should be a priority. The extent of normal parenchyma removed should be determined by surgeon discretion taking into account the clinical situation; tumor characteristics including growth pattern, and interface with normal tissue. Enucleation should be considered in patients with familial RCC, multifocal disease, or severe CKD to optimize parenchymal mass preservation.

Surgical Principles
1. In the presence of clinically concerning regional lymphadenopathy, lymph node dissection should be performed for staging purposes.
2. Adrenalectomy should be performed if imaging and/or intraoperative findings suggest metastasis or direct invasion.
3. A minimally invasive approach should be considered when it would not compromise oncologic, functional and perioperative outcomes.
4. Pathologic evaluation of the adjacent renal parenchyma should be performed after PN or RN to assess for possible nephrologic disease, particularly for patients with CKD or risk factors for developing CKD.

Factors Favoring AS/Expectant Management

Patient-related	Tumor-related
Elderly	Tumor size <3cm
Life expectancy <5 years	Tumor growth <5mm/year
High comorbidities	Non-infiltrative
Excessive perioperative risk	Low complexity
Frailty (poor functional status)	Favorable histology
Patient preference for AS	
Marginal renal function	

1. Focus is on clinically localized renal masses suspicious for RCC in adults, including solid enhanced tumors and Bosniak 3 and 4 complex cystic lesions. 2. ml/min/1.73m².

Fig. 97.1

---

c. Staged partial nephrectomy and pulmonary lobectomy

d. Simultaneous partial nephrectomy and pulmonary lobectomy

e. Simultaneous radical nephrectomy and pulmonary lobectomy

13. A healthy 75-year-old man is referred after renal biopsy of a 3.0-cm centrally located renal mass. The biopsy is definitive for renal oncocytoma. The other kidney is normal, the serum creatinine level is 1.0 mg/dL, and there is no evidence of metastatic disease. What is the best next step?

a. Open radical nephrectomy

b. Laparoscopic nephroureterectomy

c. Percutaneous thermal ablation (TA)

d. Partial nephrectomy

e. Observation with follow-up renal imaging

14. Which of the following agents demonstrated an oncologic benefit in the postoperative adjuvant setting for patients at high risk of recurrence following nephrectomy?

a. High-dose interleukin-2 (IL-2)

b. Sunitinib

c. Autologous tumor vaccine

d. Pazopanib

e. Interferon-α (IFN-α)

15. Based on the 2017 AUA Guidelines, which of the following patients would not need to be considered for genetic counseling?

a. A 45-year-old woman with a pT1a clear cell RCC.

b. A 68-year-old man with a pT1a RCC with histology suggestive of succinate dehydrogenase (SDH) deficiency

c. A 69-year-old man with 2 ipsilateral pT1a tumors, a 3.5-cm clear cell, and a 1.1-cm type 1 papillary

d. A 62-year-old woman with a pT1b chromophobe RCC and moderate-sized lung cysts

e. The 7-year-old son of a patient with von Hippel-Lindau (VHL) disease

16. Which two agents have the most similar mechanisms of action?

a. Sunitinib and temsirolimus

b. Pazopanib and axitinib

c. Pembrolizumab and ipilimumab

d. Nivolumab and cabozantinib

e. Atezolizumab and ipilimumab

17. A 48-year-old woman with a history of seizure disorder presents with recurrent gross hematuria and left flank pain. Abdominal CT shows a large left perinephric hematoma associated with a 3.0-cm left renal angiomyolipoma. There are also multiple right renal angiomyolipomas ranging in size from 1.5 to 6.5 cm. What is the best management of the left renal lesion?

a. Selective embolization

b. Radical nephrectomy

c. Observation

d. Partial nephrectomy

e. Laparoscopic exposure and renal cryoablative therapy

18. Which of the following statements is TRUE regarding cystic nephromas occurring in adults?

a. They are complex cystic lesions that are typically classified as Bosniak II to III.

b. They are malignant 2% to 5% of the time.

c. They are more common in men than in women.

d. When suspected, they should be treated by radical nephrectomy.

e. They are readily differentiated from cystic RCC on the basis of appropriate imaging studies.

19. Which environmental factor is most commonly accepted as a risk factor for RCC?

a. Radiation therapy

b. Antihypertensive medications

c. Tobacco use

d. Diuretics

e. High-fat diet

20. Which of the following manifestations is common only in certain VHL families; specifically, which is common in those with type 2 and only rarely seen in type 1 VHL?

a. RCC

b. Pancreatic cysts or tumors

c. Epididymal tumors

d. Pheochromocytoma

e. Inner ear tumors

21. Common manifestations of VHL disease include:

a. RCC, pheochromocytoma, fibrofolliculoma

b. angiomyolipoma, pheochromocytoma, fibrofolliculoma

c. RCC, pheochromocytoma, hemangioblastoma

d. angiomyolipoma, pheochromocytoma, hemangioblastoma

e. RCC, thyroid carcinoma, leiomyoma

22. What is the most common cause of death in patients with the VHL syndrome?

a. Renal failure

b. Cerebellar hemangioblastoma

c. Unrelated medical disease

d. Pheochromocytoma

e. RCC

23. The VHL syndrome tumor suppressor protein regulates the expression of which of the following mediators of biologic aggressiveness for RCC?

a. Basic fibroblast growth factor

b. Vascular endothelial cell growth factor

c. Epidermal growth factor receptor (EGFR)

d. Hepatocyte growth factor (scatter factor)

e. P-glycoprotein (multiple drug resistance efflux protein)

24. What do the hereditary papillary RCC syndrome and VHL syndrome have in common?

a. Mode of genetic transmission

b. Chromosome 3 abnormalities

c. Propensity toward tumor formation in multiple organ systems

d. Inactivation of a tumor suppressor gene

e. Nearly complete penetrance

25. Mutation of the met proto-oncogene in hereditary papillary RCC leads to:

a. increased expression of hepatocyte growth factor.

b. increased sensitivity to vascular endothelial growth factor (VEGF).

c. inactivation of a tumor suppressor gene that regulates cellular proliferation.

d. constitutive activation of the receptor for hepatocyte growth factor.

e. increased expression of VEGF.

26. P-glycoprotein is a transmembrane protein that is involved in:

a. immunotolerance.

b. resistance to high-dose IL-2 therapy.

c. resistance to cisplatin therapy.

d. resistance to radiation therapy.

e. efflux of large hydrophobic compounds, including many cytotoxic drugs.

27. Pathology demonstrates venous involvement limited to the main renal vein along with contralateral adrenal involvement with RCC. There is also a 6-cm bulky retroperitoneal lymph node replaced with cancer. What is the stage?

a. pT3aN1M0

b. pT3aN2M0

c. pT3aN1M1

d. pT3bN1M1

e. pT4N2M0

28. Which of the following is most likely to demonstrate an infiltrative growth pattern?

a. Clear cell RCC

b. Sarcomatoid variants of RCC

c. Papillary RCC

d. Chromophobe RCC

e. Oncocytoma

29. What is the most common mutation identified in sporadic clear cell RCC?

a. Activation of the met proto-oncogene

b. Activation of the VHL gene

c. Inactivation of the VHL gene

d. Inactivation of p53

e. Inactivation of genes on chromosome 9

30. Which of the following cytogenetic abnormalities is commonly associated with type 1 papillary RCC?

a. Trisomy of chromosome 7

b. Trisomy of the Y chromosome

c. Loss of chromosome 17

d. Loss of all or parts of chromosome 3

e. Loss of chromosome 7

31. What percentage of RCCs are chromophobe cell carcinomas?

a. 0% to 2%

b. 3% to 5%

c. 8% to 10%

d. 12% to 15%

e. 18% to 25%

32. Most renal medullary carcinomas are:

a. found in patients with sickle cell disease.

b. diagnosed in the fifth decade of life.

c. responsive to high-dose chemotherapy.

d. genetically and histologically similar to papillary RCC.

e. metastatic at the time of diagnosis.

33. Which paraneoplastic syndrome associated with RCC can often be managed or palliated medically?
    a. Polycythemia
    b. Stauffer syndrome
    c. Neuropathy
    d. Hypercalcemia
    e. Cachexia

34. A healthy 64-year-old man is found to have a 6.0-cm solid, heterogeneous mass in the hilum of the right kidney. CT of the abdomen and pelvis shows interaortocaval lymph nodes enlarged to 2.5 cm. A chest radiograph and a bone scan are negative, and the contralateral kidney is normal. The serum creatinine level is 1.0 mg/dL. What is the best next step?
    a. Right radical nephrectomy and regional or extended lymph node dissection
    b. Abdominal exploration, sampling of the enlarged lymph nodes, and possible radical nephrectomy pending frozen section analysis
    c. CT-guided percutaneous biopsy of the lymph nodes
    d. CT-guided percutaneous biopsy of the tumor mass
    e. Systemic therapy followed by radical nephrectomy

35. Which of the following patients would be the best candidate for percutaneous biopsy or fine-needle aspiration of a renal mass?
    a. A 42-year-old man with a 2.5-cm Bosniak III complex renal cyst
    b. An 88-year-old man with a 1.7-cm solid, enhancing renal mass
    c. A 32-year-old woman with bilateral solid, enhancing renal masses ranging in size from 1.5 to 4.0 cm
    d. A 48-year-old woman with a 3.5-cm solid, enhancing renal mass with fat density present
    e. A 38-year-old woman with a fever, a urinary tract infection, and a 3.5-cm solid/cystic, enhancing renal mass

36. A 67-year-old man undergoes radical nephrectomy and inferior vena caval thrombectomy (level 2 tumor thrombus). The primary tumor is otherwise confined to the kidney, and the lymph nodes are not involved. What is the approximate 5-year cancer-free survival rate?
    a. 0% to 15%
    b. 16% to 30%
    c. 31% to 50%
    d. 51% to 70%
    e. 71% to 90%

37. Which of the following is NOT a predictor of cancer-specific survival after nephrectomy for RCC?
    a. Pathologic stage
    b. Tumor size
    c. Nuclear grade
    d. Patient age
    e. Histologic necrosis

38. Which of the following statements about renal lymphoma is TRUE?
    a. 5% to 10% of all lymphomas involving the kidney are primary tumors.
    b. The radiographic patterns manifested by renal lymphoma are diverse and can be difficult to differentiate from RCC.
    c. Percutaneous biopsy is rarely indicated if renal lymphoma is suspected.
    d. Renal failure associated with renal lymphoma is most often due to extensive parenchymal replacement by the malignancy.
    e. The most common pattern of renal involvement is by direct extension from adjacent retroperitoneal lymph nodes.

39. Which of the following would be considered diagnostic for renal angiomyolipoma (AML)?
    a. Hyperechoic pattern on ultrasonography
    b. Enhancement of >30 Hounsfield units on CT scan
    c. Small area measuring less than −20 Hounsfield units on non-enhanced CT
    d. Aneurysmal changes on renal arteriogram
    e. Positive signal on T2 images of MRI

40. The main limitation of renal mass biopsy is:
    a. risk of needle tract seeding.
    b. difficulty differentiating the eosinophilic variants of RCC from renal oncocytoma.
    c. risk of pneumothorax.
    d. risk of hemorrhage.
    e. inability to determine subtype of RCC.

41. Which of the following tumors is most likely to be a malignant RCC?
    a. 2.5-cm hyperechoic complex cyst, with no enhancement with IV contrast
    b. 6.0-cm complex cyst with four thin septae
    c. 5.0-cm cyst with thin, curvilinear calcification
    d. 11-cm cyst with water density and homogeneous nature
    e. 3.0-cm solid lesion with fat associated with calcification

42. A common and pathogenic cytogenetic finding in children with RCC is:
    a. *VHL* mutation.
    b. *cMET* oncogene mutation.
    c. *p53* mutation.
    d. *TFE3* gene fusions.
    e. *PTEN* mutations.

43. According to the 2017 AUA Guidelines, which of the following statements about TA is TRUE?
    a. TA should be prioritized in elderly patients with comorbidities.
    b. In general, a tumor size threshold of 2.5 cm should be applied for decision making about TA.
    c. Renal mass biopsy should be performed at the time of TA whenever it might change management.
    d. Local recurrence is more common after TA than partial nephrectomy, but when repeat ablation is taken into account, similar local control rates are observed.
    e. Repeat ablation is feasible in some patients, but surgical resection is often required after failed TA.

44. What is the mechanism of action for nivolumab?
    a. Activates CTLA-4
    b. Blocks CTLA-4
    c. Activates PD-1
    d. Blocks PD-1
    e. Blocks PD-L1

45. According to the 8th edition of the AJCC TNM classification (2016), which of the following tumors would NOT be considered stage pT3a?
    a. 4.3 cm RCC with renal sinus fat invasion
    b. 12 cm RCC with involvement of the renal vein
    c. 5.6 cm RCC with invasion into the perinephric fat
    d. 4.8 cm RCC with invasion into the adrenal gland
    e. 6.4 cm RCC with collecting system involvement

46. Most tumors at various sites in the VHL syndrome share the following characteristic:
    a. Malignant behavior
    b. Hypervascularity
    c. Rapid growth rate
    d. High nuclear grade
    e. Symptomatic presentation

47. One major difference between hereditary papillary RCC syndrome and VHL syndrome is:
    a. pattern of genetic inheritance.
    b. age of onset.
    c. gender distribution.
    d. incidence of metastasis.
    e. incidence of associated tumors in nonrenal organ systems.

48. Which syndrome is most likely to exhibit aggressive behavior of RCC?
    a. VHL syndrome
    b. Hereditary papillary RCC syndrome
    c. Hereditary leiomyomatosis and RCC syndrome
    d. Birt-Hogg-Dubé (BHD) syndrome
    e. Familial oncocytosis

49. Spontaneous pneumothorax is occasionally observed in which of the following?
    a. VHL syndrome
    b. Hereditary papillary RCC syndrome
    c. Hereditary leiomyomatosis and RCC syndrome
    d. BHD syndrome
    e. Familial oncocytosis

50. Chromophobe RCC shares many characteristics with:
    a. oncocytoma.
    b. type 2 papillary RCC.
    c. clear cell RCC.
    d. mesoblastic nephroma.
    e. mixed epithelial and stromal tumor (MEST) of the kidney.

51. A finding that is diagnostic for collecting duct carcinoma is:
    a. central location and infiltrative growth pattern.
    b. aggressive clinical course.
    c. *p53* mutation.
    d. positive staining for *Ulex europaeus* lectin.
    e. sensitivity to chemotherapy.

52. Sarcomatoid differentiation is most commonly observed with which histologic subtypes of RCC?
    a. Clear cell and papillary
    b. Papillary and chromophobe
    c. Clear cell and collecting duct
    d. Clear cell and chromophobe
    e. Chromophobe and collecting duct

53. Which of the following factors has greatest utility for predicting bone metastasis from RCC?
    a. Tumor size
    b. Tumor grade
    c. Performance status (PS)
    d. Elevated alkaline phosphatase
    e. Invasion of the perinephric fat

54. The prognosis for a 3-cm tumor infiltrating the renal sinus fat is:
    a. similar to a pT1bN0 tumor.
    b. similar to a pT2aN0 tumor.
    c. similar to a pT3a tumor with invasion of the perinephric fat laterally.
    d. worse than a pT3a tumor with invasion of the perinephric fat laterally.
    e. similar to a tumor with ipsilateral adrenal involvement.

55. The single most important prognostic factor for RCC is:
    a. tumor size.
    b. tumor grade.
    c. tumor stage.
    d. histologic subtype.
    e. PS.

56. The most accurate assessment of prognosis for patients with RCC is usually provided by:
    a. tumor size.
    b. clinician judgment.
    c. tumor stage.
    d. integrated analysis of prognostic factors.
    e. PS.

57. Which of the following indicates a tumor that is NOT correctly staged according to the 2016 TNM staging system for RCC?
    a. Localized RCC, 8.5 cm: *pT2a*
    b. RCC with direct ipsilateral adrenal involvement: *pT3a*
    c. RCC with metastatic involvement of the adrenal gland: *pM1*
    d. RCC with direct invasion of the pelvicalyceal system: *pT3a*
    e. RCC with three lymph node metastases: *pN1*
    a. 2.5-cm centrally located tumor after radiofrequency ablation

58. What is the most common form of renal sarcoma?
    a. Liposarcoma
    b. Rhabdomyosarcoma
    c. Fibrosarcoma
    d. Leiomyosarcoma
    e. Angiosarcoma

59. The most useful prognostic factors for renal sarcoma are:
    a. tumor size and grade.
    b. tumor stage and grade.
    c. histologic subtype and stage.
    d. tumor stage and ploidy status.
    e. margin status and grade.

60. Which of the following renal tumors has the best prognosis?
    a. Sarcoma
    b. Carcinoid
    c. Adult Wilms
    d. Primitive neuroectodermal tumor
    e. Small cell

61. Patients with which RCC subtype are most likely to benefit from targeted therapy, such as tyrosine kinase inhibitors (TKIs)?
    a. Papillary RCC
    b. Clear cell RCC
    c. Renal medullary carcinoma
    d. Collecting duct carcinoma
    e. Chromophobe RCC

62. Agents targeting which of the following signaling pathways in clear cell RCC have significant antitumor effects in patients with metastatic disease?

    a. VEGF and EGFR

    b. *p53* and EGFR

    c. VEGF and mammalian target of rapamycin (mTOR)

    d. mTOR and transforming growth factor-α (TGF-α)

    e. All of the above

63. Of the following, which is the greatest determinant of renal function after partial nephrectomy?

    a. Surgical approach (open vs. minimally invasive)

    b. Tumor size

    c. Absence of a functioning contralateral kidney

    d. Renal function before partial nephrectomy

    e. Gender

64. Which of the following statements is TRUE regarding chronic kidney disease (CKD)?

    a. CKD due to surgery has the same impact as CKD due to medical causes.

    b. Serum creatinine below 1.4 mg/dL excludes the possibility of CKD.

    c. CKD can be diagnosed based on a single estimated GFR value less than 60 mL/min/1.73 m^2.

    d. Increasing CKD stage has been associated with an increase in morbid cardiovascular events for subjects in the general population.

    e. Choice of intervention for localized renal malignancy has little impact on development or progression of CKD.

65. Which of the following is an indication for adrenalectomy at the time of partial nephrectomy?

    a. 6-cm upper pole renal tumor

    b. 4-cm adrenal lesion measuring –20 Hounsfield units on noncontrast CT scan

    c. Bilateral adrenal hyperplasia

    d. 3-cm renal tumor adjacent to the adrenal gland on CT scan, but readily separable from the adrenal gland at surgery

    e. 1.5-cm adrenal lesion that is bright on T2-weighted MRI

66. Which of the following statements is FALSE regarding molecular imaging for renal tumors?

    a. ^{99m}Tc-sestamibi SPECT/CT is based on uptake by mitochondria, which are in abundance in oncocytomas and hybrid oncocytic/chromophobe tumors.

    b. ^{124}I-girentuximab targets carbonic anhydrase IX present on clear cell RCC.

    c. Fluorodeoxyglucose positron emission tomography (FDG-PET)-CT is useful for staging RCC.

    d. Prostate-specific membrane antigen (PSMA) imaging can identify clear cell RCC.

    e. While early studies are promising, validation studies are needed before widespread acceptance of current molecular imaging techniques.

67. Which of the following statements most accurately characterizes the role of lymphadenectomy for RCC?

    a. Offers a staging and therapeutic benefit for patients with clinically localized RCC

    b. Offers staging information but not a therapeutic benefit for all patients with RCC

    c. Offers a therapeutic benefit mostly for patients with locally advanced RCC

    d. Compliance with well-described templates is important for achieving a therapeutic benefit

    e. Demonstrated a small but statistically significant survival advantage in a randomized trial

68. According to the 2017 AUA Guidelines, which of the following patients with kidney cancer will not need to be considered for nephrology consultation?

    a. A patient with 50/50 split renal function and a preoperative GFR of 70 mL/min/1.73 m^2 who will be undergoing radical nephrectomy

    b. A patient with preoperative GFR of 42 mL/min/1.73 m^2

    c. A patient with confirmed proteinuria

    d. A diabetic with preoperative GFR <60 mL/min/1.73 m^2

    e. A patient with a solitary kidney, a preoperative GFR of 36 mL/min/1.73 m^2, and a R.E.N.A.L. 10 lesion

Pathology

1. A 49-year-old man has a biopsy of a peripheral lower pole exophytic 4-cm mass of the right kidney. The histology is depicted in Fig. 97.2 and is read as clear cell carcinoma. Metastatic workup is negative. He should be advised to:

    a. receive targeted chemotherapy.

    b. undergo radical nephrectomy.

    c. have the tumor ablated with cryotherapy.

    d. undergo partial nephrectomy.

    e. receive radiation therapy.

2. A 48-year-old woman has a right radical nephrectomy for a 6-cm mass. Preoperative metastatic workup was negative. The pathology is illustrated in Fig. 97.3 and is read as collecting duct carcinoma. She should be advised to:

    a. receive targeted chemotherapy.

    b. receive radiation therapy to the nephrectomy bed.

    c. receive platinum-based chemotherapy.

    d. follow up with her primary care physician.

    e. be followed closely because the development of metastatic disease is likely.

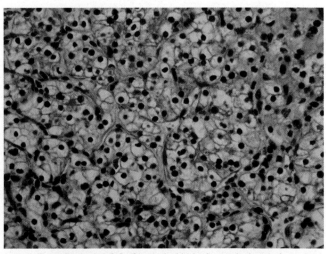

Fig. 97.2 (From Bostwick DG, Cheng L: *Urologic surgical pathology*, 2nd ed, Edinburgh, 2008, Mosby.)

Imaging

1. See Fig. 97.4. A 55-year-old man with hematuria has this contrast-enhanced CT scan for evaluation. The most appropriate therapy is:

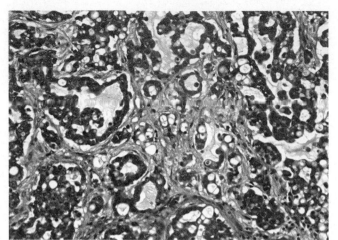

Fig. 97.3 (From Bostwick DG, Cheng L. *Urologic surgical pathology,* 2nd ed, Edinburgh, 2008, Mosby.)

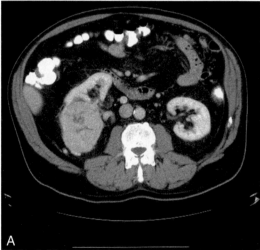

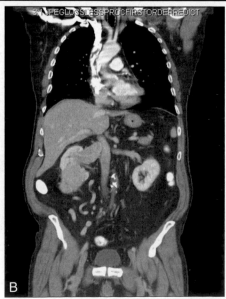

Fig. 97.4

a. laparoscopic nephron-sparing surgery.
b. radical nephrectomy.
c. open nephron-sparing surgery.
d. radiofrequency ablation.
e. cryoablation.

2. See Fig. 97.5. A 45-year-old man with no urinary symptoms has this axial contrast-enhanced CT scan. What is the most likely diagnosis?
a. Bosniak II-F lesion
b. Bosniak IV—cystic RCC
c. Bosniak II cyst
d. Bosniak III cyst
e. Bosniak I cyst

ANSWERS

1. **c. Computed tomography (CT) with and without contrast enhancement.** A dedicated triple-phase renal CT scan remains the single most important radiographic image to delineate the nature of a renal mass. In general, any renal mass that enhances with administration of intravenous contrast material on CT scanning should be considered a RCC until proved otherwise.
2. **b. Bosniak II cyst.** Category II lesions are minimally complicated cysts that are benign but have some radiologic findings that cause concern. Classic hyperdense renal cysts are small (<3 cm), round, sharply marginated, and do not enhance after administration of contrast material. Hyperdense cysts that are 3 cm or larger are classified as *Bosniak IIF* lesions.
3. **d. Renal metastasis.** The traditionally accepted indications for biopsy of a renal mass are when a renal abscess or infected cyst is suspected, or when differentiating RCC from metastatic malignancy or renal lymphoma. Core needle biopsy is now performed with increased frequency for the evaluation of renal masses in other circumstances, particularly for patients in whom a wide variety of treatment options are under consideration.
4. **c. Chest radiograph annually for 3 years.** Surveillance for recurrent malignancy after radical nephrectomy for RCC can be tailored according to the initial pathologic tumor stage. This patient is low risk (pT1N0M0), and the AUA guidelines recommend an annual chest radiograph for 3 years and only as clinically indicated beyond that time period.
5. **b. Tumor size <5.0 cm.** A solitary tumor and a normal contralateral kidney were also required, but criteria for the latter were not well defined, at least based on current perspectives about functional assessment that depend on eGFR rather than serum creatinine level.
6. **b. Every 6 months for at least 3 years and then annually to year 5.** Surveillance for recurrent malignancy after nephron-sparing surgery for RCC can be tailored according to the initial

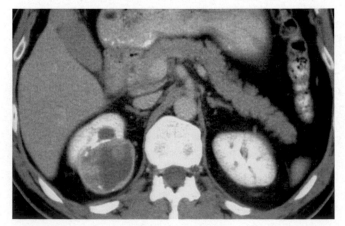

Fig. 97.5

pathologic tumor stage. This patient is intermediate to high risk, and the AUA Guidelines recommend a baseline abdominal scan (CT or MRI) within 3 to 6 months following surgery with continued imaging (ultrasonography, CT, or MRI) every 6 months for at least 3 years and annually thereafter to year 5. Imaging beyond 5 years may be performed at the discretion of the clinician.

7. **b. Albumin-to-creatinine ratio.** Patients who undergo nephron-sparing surgery for RCC may be left with a relatively small amount of renal tissue. These patients are at risk for long-term renal functional impairment from hyperfiltration renal injury. Because proteinuria is the initial manifestation of the phenomenon, an albumin-to-creatinine ratio should be obtained yearly in patients with a solitary remnant kidney to screen for hyperfiltration nephropathy. Traditionally a 24-hour urine protein was obtained on an annual basis, but this is more burdensome, and for screening purposes the albumin-to-creatinine ratio is more suitable. If positive, more rigorous testing, such as the 24-hour urine protein, can be considered to more accurately quantify the degree of proteinuria.

8. **e. Serum creatinine–based estimation of GFR and analysis for proteinuria.** Identification and classification of CKD is best performed by assessing cause, estimated GFR (eGFR), and extent of albuminuria. At present, there are several formulas in clinical use, including the MDRD and CKD-EPI formulas, each of which is an improvement over using serum creatinine alone for identification of patients with or at risk for CKD. Serum levels of creatinine are dependent on gender, muscle mass, and other factors and can therefore lead to an underestimation of kidney disease in certain populations, such as thin, elderly women. Urinary creatinine measurement is impractical and provides only marginally more valuable information than serum creatinine. Urinary protein measurement can identify patients with early signs of kidney disease (proteinuria), and there are multiple methods to assess this, including 24-hour urinary protein and spot urine studies (albumin-to-creatinine ratio, protein-to-creatinine ratio); none has been shown to be better than GFR estimation as a screening test. Direct measurement of GFR using iothalamate (or other agents) is costly and not routinely available; it is therefore impractical in most settings.

9. **d. A double freeze-thaw cycle.** Renal cryosurgery is an ablative nephron-sparing treatment option for RCC that can be performed percutaneously under radiographic guidance or laparoscopically under direct vision and ultrasound guidance. The aim of cryosurgery is to ablate the same predetermined volume of tissue that would have been removed had a conventional surgical excision been performed. Established critical prerequisites for successful cryosurgery include rapid freezing, gradual thawing, and a repetition of the freeze-thaw cycle.

10. **c. CT and MRI.** Both CT and MRI are noninvasive and accurate modalities for demonstrating both the presence and the distal extent of vena caval involvement. Although MRI has been recommended as the test of choice at most centers, many studies have demonstrated that a properly performed multiplanar CT also provides sufficient information for surgical planning, and it has become the preferred diagnostic study at many centers.

11. **e. Lymph node involvement.** In most studies, the presence of lymph node or distant metastases has carried a dismal prognosis that is much more pronounced than the other distractors.

12. **d. Simultaneous partial nephrectomy and pulmonary lobectomy.** The subset of patients with metastatic RCC and a solitary metastasis, estimated at between 1.6% and 3.2% of patients, may benefit from nephrectomy with resection of the metastatic lesion. This patient also needs partial nephrectomy to preclude the need for dialysis. Of note, both procedures could be performed with a minimally invasive approach under the same anesthesia.

13. **e. Observation with follow-up renal imaging.** Renal mass biopsy is now performed with increased frequency and should be considered in an elderly patient such as this. For those in whom nonextirpative options are being considered, biopsy can provide important information, such as a definitive nonmalignant diagnosis (as in this example). Given the benign nature of renal oncocytomas, the best answer is observation with follow-up imaging at an interval between 6 and 12 months, if clinically warranted based on the patient's overall health and life expectancy.

14. **b. Sunitinib. Sunitinib** demonstrated a significantly longer disease-free survival compared to placebo (6.8 vs. 5.6 years) in the phase 3 S-TRAC trial that randomized 615 men with pT2 (high-grade), pT3-4, or N1 clear cell RCC to sunitinib or placebo. Importantly, patients receiving therapy experienced significantly higher rates of toxic events and there was no difference in overall survival. All other therapies listed failed to demonstrate an oncologic benefit in the adjuvant setting.

15. **c. A 69-year-old man with 2 ipsilateral pT1a tumors, a 3.5-cm clear cell, and a 1.1-cm type 1 papillary.** A 69-year-old man with 2 ipsilateral pT1a tumors, a 3.5-cm clear cell and a 1.1-cm type 1 papillary probably does not need to consider genetic counseling, unless the family or personal history is otherwise suggestive of a familial syndrome. Genetic counseling is recommended for all patients with kidney cancer who are 46 years of age or younger. When histology suggests possible SDH deficiency, further testing should be pursued, and a history of chromophobe RCC and lung cysts or a prior spontaneous pneumothorax is suggestive for BHD syndrome. Relatives of patients with known familial RCC should be strongly considered for genetic counseling, and surveillance ideally will be initiated at an early age. An elderly patient with multifocal RCC may not need to be considered for genetic counseling, particularly if there is discordance in the histologies.

16. **b. Pazopanib and axitinib.** Pazopanib and axitinib both target the VEGF pathway, and specifically the VEGF receptor, and are TKI. Sunitinib and cabozantinib are also TKIs, and temsirolimus is an mTOR inhibitor. Pembrolizumab, atezolizumab, ipilimumab, and nivolumab are all checkpoint inhibitors (Fig. 97.6). Pembrolizumab and nivolumab block PD-1, while atezolizumab blocks PD-L1 and ipilimumab blocks CTLA-4.

17. **a. Selective embolization.** Most patients with acute or potentially life-threatening hemorrhage will require total nephrectomy if exploration is performed, and if the patient has TSC, bilateral disease, preexisting renal insufficiency, or other medical or urologic disease that could affect renal function in the future, selective embolization should be considered. In such circumstances, selective embolization can temporize by controlling hemorrhage and in many cases will prove to be definitive treatment. This patient almost certainly has TSC given bilateral AMLs and history of seizures.

18. **a. They are complex cystic lesions that are typically classified as Bosniak II to III.** Cystic nephromas are benign renal neoplasms that occur most commonly in middle-aged women. They appear to be genetically related to MEST but generally have a somewhat different radiographic appearance. Unlike MEST, which contain a solid stromal component and often appear as solid or Bosniak IV lesions on cross-sectional imaging, cystic nephromas are typically characterized as complex cystic lesions without a solid component.

19. **c. Tobacco use.** The most generally accepted environmental risk factor for RCC is tobacco use, although the relative associated risks have been modest, ranging from 1.4 to 2.3 when compared with controls. All forms of tobacco use have been implicated, with risk increasing with cumulative dose or pack-years. Other well-established risk factors include obesity and hypertension.

20. **d. Pheochromocytoma.** The familial form of clear cell RCC is the VHL syndrome. Major manifestations include the development of RCC, pheochromocytoma, retinal angiomas, and hemangioblastomas of the brainstem, cerebellum, or spinal cord. Penetrance for all of these traits is far from complete, and some, such as pheochromocytomas, tend to be clustered in certain families but not in others.

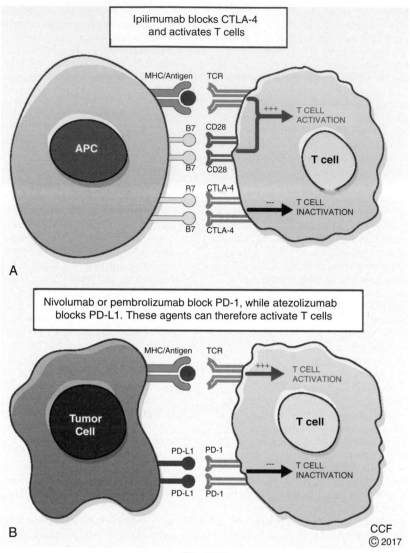

Fig. 97.6

21. **c. RCC, pheochromocytoma, hemangioblastoma.** These are the three most common tumor types occurring in VHL disease. Facial fibrofolliculomas occur in BHD syndrome, and uterine leiomyomas are commonly seen in hereditary leiomyomatosis and RCC syndrome.
22. **e. RCC.** With improved management of the central nervous system manifestations of the disease, RCC is the most common cause of mortality in patients with VHL syndrome.
23. **b. Vascular endothelial cell growth factor.** Inactivation or mutation of the VHL gene leads to dysregulated expression of hypoxia inducible factor-1, an intracellular protein that plays an important role in regulating cellular responses to hypoxia, starvation, and other stresses. This in turn leads to a several-fold upregulation of the expression of VEGF, the primary proangiogenic growth factor in RCC, contributing to the pronounced neovascularity associated with this carcinoma.
24. **a. Mode of genetic transmission.** Studies of families with hereditary papillary renal carcinoma (HPRC) have demonstrated an autosomal dominant mode of transmission, similar to VHL disease. VHL is caused by inactivation or mutation of a tumor suppressor gene, whereas HPRC is caused by activation of an oncogene.
25. **d. Constitutive activation of the receptor for hepatocyte growth factor.** Missense mutations of the *met* proto-oncogene at 7q31 were found to segregate with the disease, implicating it as the relevant genetic locus. The protein product of this gene is the receptor tyrosine kinase for the hepatocyte growth factor, which plays an important role in regulating the proliferation and differentiation of epithelial and endothelial cells in a wide

variety of organs, including the kidney. Most of the mutations in hereditary papillary RCC have been found in the tyrosine kinase domain of *met* and lead to constitutive activation.
26. **e. Efflux of large hydrophobic compounds, including many cytotoxic drugs.** P-glycoprotein is a 170-kDa transmembrane protein expressed by 80% to 90% of RCCs that acts as an energy-dependent efflux pump for a wide variety of large hydrophobic compounds, including several cytotoxic drugs.
27. **c. pT3aN1M1.** Isolated renal vein involvement is now classified as T3a, and nodal classification has been simplified such that all nodal involvement is now classified as N1. Contiguous invasion of the ipsilateral adrenal is now classified as T4, but metastatic involvement of the contralateral (or ipsilateral) adrenal gland is classified as M1, reflecting a likely hematogenous pattern of dissemination.
28. **b. Sarcomatoid variants of RCC.** Most RCCs are round to ovoid and circumscribed by a pseudocapsule of compressed parenchyma and fibrous tissue rather than a true histologic capsule. Unlike upper tract transitional cell carcinomas (TCCs), most RCCs are not grossly infiltrative, with the notable exception of some sarcomatoid variants.
29. **c. Inactivation of the VHL gene.** Chromosome 3 alterations and VHL mutations are common in conventional RCC, and mutation or inactivation of this gene has been found in over 75% of sporadic cases.
30. **a. Trisomy of chromosome 7.** The cytogenetic abnormalities associated with type 1 papillary RCC are characteristic and include trisomy of chromosomes 7 and 17.

31. **b. 3% to 5%.** Chromophobe cell carcinoma is a distinctive histologic subtype of RCC that appears to be derived from the cortical portion of the collecting duct. It represents 3% to 5% of all RCCs.

32. **e. Metastatic at the time of diagnosis.** Renal medullary carcinoma is a rare histologic subtype of RCC that occurs almost exclusively in association with sickle cell trait. It is typically diagnosed in young African Americans, often in the third decade of life. Many cases are both locally advanced and metastatic at the time of diagnosis. Most patients have not responded to therapy and have succumbed to their disease in a few to several months.

33. **d. Hypercalcemia.** Hypercalcemia has been reported in up to 13% of patients with RCC and can be due to either paraneoplastic phenomena or osteolytic metastatic involvement of the bone. The production of parathyroid hormonelike peptides is the most common paraneoplastic etiology, although tumor-derived 1,25-dihydroxyvitamin D_3 and prostaglandins may contribute in a minority of cases. Medical management includes vigorous hydration followed by diuresis with furosemide and the selective use of bisphosphonates, corticosteroids, and/or calcitonin.

34. **a. Right radical nephrectomy and regional or extended lymph node dissection.** An aggressive surgical approach is still preferred because it will likely prolong survival and represents the only realistic chance for a cure. Lymph nodes in this size range are most likely malignant, and this patient will likely need to consider adjuvant clinical trials. An extended lymph node dissection includes the interaortocaval nodes and nodes alongside and behind the ipsilateral great vessel from the crus of the diaphragm to the ipsilateral common iliac artery.

35. **e. A 38-year-old woman with a fever, urinary tract infection, and a 3.5-cm solid/cystic, enhancing renal mass.** Patients with flank pain, a febrile urinary tract infection, and a renal mass should be offered percutaneous biopsy and/or aspiration to establish a diagnosis of renal abscess rather than malignancy, and to provide drainage if abscess is confirmed.

36. **c. 31% to 50%.** Venous involvement with tumor thrombi was once thought to be a dismal sign for patients with RCC, but more recent studies suggest that many patients with tumor thrombi can be salvaged with an aggressive surgical approach. These studies document 31% to 50% 5-year survival rates for patients with IVC thrombus thrombi, as long as the tumor is otherwise confined to the kidney.

37. **d. Patient age.** Although patient age and comorbidity are important predictors of overall survival in patients with RCC and strongly affect the choice of treatment in these patients, they have no effect on the likelihood of dying of cancer-specific causes. Each of the other factors is a predictor of cancer-specific mortality from RCC and has been incorporated into one or more RCC prognostic algorithms for cancer-specific outcomes.

38. **b. The radiographic patterns manifested by renal lymphoma are diverse and can be difficult to differentiate from RCC.** Five different radiographic patterns have been described for lymphoma involving the kidney, including a solitary mass, occasionally making it difficult to differentiate from RCC.

39. **c. Small area measuring less than −20 Hounsfield units on non-enhanced CT.** The presence of even a small focus of fat, as evidenced by a density less than − 20 HU on a non-enhanced CT scan, is diagnostic for AML. The findings described in a, b, and d are all suggestive of, but not diagnostic for, renal AML.

40. **b. Difficulty differentiating the eosinophilic variants of RCC from renal oncocytoma.** The main limitation of renal mass biopsy is difficulty differentiating renal oncocytoma, the most common benign renal mass, from eosinophilic variants of conventional, papillary, and chromophobe RCC on biopsy material. While the non-diagnostic rate is between 10% and 15%, the risk of complications is low in the modern era with the use of smaller-gauge needles, and needle tract seeding with RCC appears to be a rare event.

41. **e. 3.0-cm solid lesion with fat associated with calcification.** Tumors with calcification associated with fat are uncommon but are almost always malignant RCC. In this setting the fat is thought to be a reactive process related to tumor necrosis. Calcification is virtually never seen in association with AML. The lesions described in a–c are Bosniak II renal cysts, with risk of malignancy of <10%. The lesion described in d is a simple cyst and highly likely to be benign despite its large size.

42. **d. *TFE3* gene fusions.** Mutations or translocations resulting in *TFE3* gene fusions are common in RCC occurring in the pediatric population. Although these cancers often present with advanced stage, the t(X;17) variant frequently follows an indolent course, while t(X;1) cancers can recur with late lymph node metastases.

43. **d. Local recurrence is more common after TA than partial nephrectomy, but when repeat ablation is taken into account, similar local control rates are observed.** Renal mass biopsy should always be performed prior to or concomitant with TA, as it will help guide surveillance. Most local failures of TA can be salvaged with repeat TA, and only a small minority of such patients end up requiring salvage surgery. Success rates TA, for tumors <3.0 cm have been encouraging, and this threshold is advocated in the Guidelines as a general reference point. TA can be a good choice in some elderly patients with comorbidities, but active surveillance is also a reasonable option and in reality is often a better choice for many such patients.

44. **c. Activates PD-1.** The mechanism of action of nivolumab is to block PD-1 and thus activate the immune system. Pembrolizumab also blocks PD-1, while atezolizumab blocks PD-L1 and ipilimumab blocks CTLA-4.

45. **d. 4.8 cm RCC with invasion into the adrenal gland.** Direct invasion of the adrenal gland is pT4 and metastatic involvement of the adrenal gland is pM1. All of the other characteristics are indicative of pT3a tumors, including collecting system involvement (a modification made in the 8th edition).

46. **b. Hypervascularity.** Tumors in the VHL syndrome include adrenal pheochromocytoma, retinal angiomas, cerebellar and brainstem hemangioblastoma, RCC, and others. Most are relatively slow growing and asymptomatic if patients are evaluated and screened in a proactive manner. The common feature is that almost all are hypervascular.

47. **e. Incidence of associated tumors in nonrenal organ systems.** The incidence of nonrenal tumors is low in the hereditary papillary RCC syndrome in contrast to VHL syndrome, in which patients commonly develop tumors in the eyes, spinal cord, cerebellum, adrenal glands, inner ear, epididymis, and pancreas.

48. **c. Hereditary leiomyomatosis and RCC syndrome.** Malignant behavior is particularly common in the hereditary leiomyomatosis and RCC syndrome, and proactive and aggressive surgical management is recommended.

49. **d. BHD syndrome.** Lung cysts and spontaneous pneumothoraces are well described and relatively common findings in the BHD syndrome.

50. **a. Oncocytoma.** Both chromophobe RCC and renal oncocytoma are derived from the distal tubules, and both are commonly observed in the BHD syndrome. There are also some overlapping cytogenetic changes, all suggesting a potential relationship between these renal tumors.

51. **d. Positive staining for *Ulex europaeus* lectin.** *Ulex europaeus* lectin is expressed by the normal collecting duct, and tumor staining suggests origin from this structure. Most collecting duct carcinomas are centrally located and exhibit an infiltrative growth pattern and aggressive clinical course, but this is also true for poorly differentiated TCCs of the renal pelvis or centrally located sarcomatoid RCC. Collecting duct RCC is not typically responsive to chemotherapy.

52. **d. Clear cell and chromophobe.** Sarcomatoid differentiation is most commonly found in association with clear cell and chromophobe RCC.

53. **c. Performance status (PS).** Poor PS can be used to segregate patients when deciding whether to obtain a bone scan for

metastatic RCC. Shvarts and colleagues (2004)[a] have shown that patients with good PS (ECOG PS = 0), no evidence of extraosseous metastases, and no bone pain were extremely low risk for bone metastasis and did not benefit from bone scanning. They recommended a bone scan for all other patients, and the incidence of bone metastasis in this group was >15%.

54. **d. Worse than a pT3a tumor with invasion of the perinephric fat laterally.** Invasion of the perisinus fat medially has been shown to be a poor prognostic sign. Medial invasion places the tumor in proximity to the venous system and likely increases the risk of metastatic dissemination. Ipsilateral adrenal involvement is even worse, and these are now classified as pT4 if due to direct local extension, or pM1 otherwise, consistent with a hematogenous route of dissemination.

55. **c. Tumor stage.** Although not truly a single factor because it combines tumor size with other information obtained from final pathologic analysis, tumor stage is the most powerful individual predictor of oncologic outcomes. When incorporated into a multi-predictor analysis, such as a nomogram or other multivariable analysis, the predictive ability increases further.

56. **d. Integrated analysis of prognostic factors.** Integrated analysis of a variety of factors such as tumor size, stage, and grade, PS, and histologic subtype has yielded the most accurate prognostication for RCC. Several studies have documented that nomograms and other algorithms outperform traditional staging systems, clinical opinion, individual risk factors, and chance.

57. **b. RCC with direct ipsilateral adrenal involvement: pT3a.** Several studies have demonstrated that RCC directly invading the adrenal gland is associated with poorer prognosis than RCC with perinephric or renal sinus fat invasion. Direct ipsilateral adrenal involvement is now grouped with other RCCs that extend beyond Gerota fascia as pathologic stage T4 (pT4). These patients have a high risk for disease recurrence or progression.

58. **d. Leiomyosarcoma.** Leiomyosarcoma is the most common histologic subtype of renal sarcoma, accounting for 50% to 60% of such tumors. The most common type of sarcoma in the retroperitoneum is liposarcoma.

59. **e. Margin status and grade.** Margin status and tumor grade are the primary prognostic factors for sarcoma. Patients with high-grade disease are at risk for systemic metastasis, and those with low-grade disease are at risk for local recurrence. Wide local excision with negative margins is essential for minimizing the risk of recurrence for sarcomas because these tumors are derived from the mesenchymal tissues and are typically infiltrative, and thus do not respect natural barriers.

60. **b. Carcinoid.** All of these tumor types have a relatively poor prognosis except for renal carcinoid, which tends to be associated with good outcomes in most patients.

61. **b. Clear cell RCC.** Targeted molecular therapies, such as TKI, mostly target VEGF and thus the pathways that are typically upregulated in clear cell RCC. Most objective responses have been observed in individuals with clear cell RCC. Standard of care for the treatment of metastatic non–clear cell RCC is not well defined at present.

62. **c. VEGF and mammalian target of rapamycin (mTOR).** Several clinical trials indicate that agents targeting VEGF signaling, including sunitinib, sorafenib, axitinib, pazopanib, levantanib, caboxantinib, and mTOR pathway signaling, including temsirolimus and everolimus, demonstrate substantial tumor responses or significant improvement in progression-free or overall survival.

63. **d. Renal function before partial nephrectomy.** When compared with radical nephrectomy, partial nephrectomy has been associated with better renal functional outcomes. The main determinants of renal function after partial nephrectomy are the quality of the kidney prior to surgery and the quantity of vascularized parenchymal mass that is preserved after excision of the tumor and reconstruction of the kidney. Warm ischemia time, if prolonged, can also contribute to a decline in renal function after partial nephrectomy.

64. **d. Increasing CKD stage has been associated with an increase in morbid cardiovascular events, hospitalization, and death on a longitudinal basis for subjects in the general population.** In this setting, CKD is predominantly due to medical causes. CKD due to surgical causes appears to be more stable and less deleterious than that due to medical causes.

65. **e. 1.5-cm adrenal lesion that is bright on T2-weighted MR imaging.** Several pathologic adrenal lesions can be diagnosed based on their radiographic characteristics without histologic confirmation. Lesions that are bright on T2-weighted MR imaging are suspicious for pheochromocytomas and should be surgically removed. Careful preoperative and intraoperative management are essential for safe management in this circumstance.

66. **c. Fluorodeoxyglucose positron emission tomography (FDG-PET)-CT is useful for staging RCC.** FDG-PET-CT is not useful for the staging of RCC due to high levels of visual conspicuity in the kidney and at the most common sites of metastatic disease. Sestamibi is taken up by mitochondria, which are in abundance in oncocytolmas and hybrid oncocytic/chromophobe tumors, and a strong signal is suggestive of these histologies. [124]I-girentuximab, which targets carbonic anhydrase IX primarily present on clear cell RCC, and PSMA (epithelial membrane target) remain in development for clear cell RCC.

67. **b. Offers staging information but not a therapeutic benefit for all patients with RCC.** Lymphadenectomy may be performed in patients with clinically suspicious (radiographic or intraoperative) lymphadenopathy for staging purposes and, due to lack of data indicating a reliable therapeutic benefit, need not be performed routinely in patients with localized kidney cancer and clinically negative nodes. The EORTC 30881 randomized trial of lymphadenectomy at RN failed to show a survival advantage for patients undergoing lymphadenectomy.

68. **a. A patient with 50/50 split renal function and a preoperative GFR of 70 mL/min/1.73 m² who will be undergoing radical nephrectomy.** A patient with 50/50 split renal function and a preoperative GFR of 70 mL/min/1.73m2 who will be undergoing radical nephrectomy will likely end up with a new baseline GFR of about 40-42 mL/min/1.73m2 and thus will likely not need referral to nephrology based on the 2017 AUA Guidelines for Renal Mass and Localized RCC. Per the guidelines, referral to nephrology should be considered in patients at high risk for GFR progression, including those with preoperative GFR<45 mL/min/1.73m², confirmed proteinuria, diabetics with preexisting CKD (GFR<60 mL/min/1.73m²), or whenever the GFR is expected to be <30 mL/min/1.73m² after intervention.

Pathology

1. **d. Undergo partial nephrectomy.** Notice the clear cytoplasm due to glycogen characteristic of clear cell carcinoma of the kidney. Because of the patient's young age, a nephron-sparing approach is preferred. Because the tumor is located in the lower pole, is peripheral, and is exophytic, it is ideal for this approach. These tumors are not particularly sensitive to radiation therapy, cryotherapy is not as reliable for local control, and targeted systemic therapy is not appropriate for a surgically curable lesion.

2. **e. Be followed closely because the development of metastatic disease is likely.** Collecting duct cancers have a high likelihood of being metastatic at diagnosis. None of the other therapies listed are helpful in this disease setting. Cis-platinum chemotherapy is a possibility, but in the absence of known metastasis, its role is not well defined.

Imaging

1. **b. Radical nephrectomy.** The images demonstrate a large mass in the lower pole of the right kidney, with tumor extension into the right renal vein, extending to the junction of the right renal vein with the inferior vena cava. The renal vein is enlarged, and tumor vessels are seen within the thrombus in the renal vein. These findings make radical nephrectomy the best option.

2. **b. Bosniak IV—cystic RCC.** Notice the enhancing nodules within the cyst wall with foci of dystrophic calcification making cystic RCC the most likely diagnosis.

CHAPTER REVIEW

1. A solid mass on CT scan that enhances more than 15 Hounsfield units is suggestive of RCC.
2. Twenty percent of small solid enhancing masses less than 4 cm on CT are benign, 40% of small solid enhancing masses less than 2 cm on CT are benign.
3. Hyperdense cysts (Bosniak II) contain old blood and are benign.
4. Clear cell RCCs originate from the proximal tubule; oncocytomas and chromophobe RCCs originate from the distal tubule.
5. There is ample evidence for impaired immune surveillance in RCC.
6. Bilateral involvement in RCC either synchronously or metachronously occurs in 2% to 4% of patients.
7. RCC pathologically is classified as clear cell: 70% to 80%; papillary: 10% to 15%; chromophobe: 3% to 5%; collecting duct: less than 1%; and medullary: rare.
8. Alterations in chromosome 3 are common in clear cell renal carcinoma.
9. Papillary renal cell cancer has a tendency to multifocality.
10. Paraneoplastic syndromes include hypercalcemia, hypertension, polycythemia, and hepatic dysfunction (Stauffer syndrome).
11. Stauffer syndrome is a paraneoplastic syndrome associated with RCC that results in elevated liver function tests. If hepatic function does not normalize after nephrectomy, persistent hepatic dysfunction is indicative of persistent disease.
12. Enlarged perirenal lymph nodes noted on CT may be inflammatory, particularly if they are less than 2 cm in diameter. Lymph nodes larger than 2 cm generally contain metastases.
13. Extended lymphadenectomy for renal cell carcinoma has not been shown to be beneficial for the majority of patients over conventional lymphadenectomy, which includes the renal hilar and adjacent paracaval or para-aortic lymph nodes.
14. The World Health Organization and International Society of Urologic Pathology (ISUP) grading system from 1 to 4 is used to grade the renal tumor and is based on nuclear characteristics.
15. There is an increased incidence of renal cell carcinoma in patients with acquired renal cystic disease.
16. RCC involving the vena cava that infiltrates the wall of the vena cava has an extremely poor prognosis.
17. A patient with a tumor thrombus involving the vena cava associated with metastatic regional nodal disease has a very poor prognosis.
18. A patient with a tumor thrombus involving the vena cava in which the nodes are negative and there is no invasion of the vein wall (except the ostia) has a relatively good prognosis.
19. Ipsilateral adrenalectomy as part of a radical nephrectomy is not necessary unless there is CT evidence of adrenal involvement, contiguous spread of the tumor to the adrenal, or large upper pole renal masses that are adjacent to with concern for involvement of the adrenal gland.
20. The risk for developing recurrent malignant disease is greatest in the first 3 years after surgery.
21. In a partial nephrectomy, the amount of renal parenchyma taken with the tumor does not affect oncologic outcomes provided the margin itself is negative.
22. RCCs less than 3.5 cm in general grow less than 0.5 cm per year; some may grow up to 1 cm per year.
23. Incomplete excision of a large primary tumor or debulking is rarely indicated as a sole treatment for patients with metastatic kidney cancer.
24. Sarcomas typically have a pseudocapsule that cannot be relied on for a plane of dissection because microscopic tumor will be left behind.
25. Metastatic tumors to the kidney are common, appearing in 12% of patients who die of other cancers; the most common primary lesions are those of the lung, breast, or gastrointestinal tract, melanoma, or hematologic.
26. Major poor prognostic indicators include tumors that extend beyond Gerota fascia to involve contiguous organs (pT4), have lymph node involvement (N1), or are metastatic (M1).
27. Patients with von Hippel-Lindau disease should have all tumors in a kidney treated when the largest reaches 3 cm in size.
28. Patients with a significant reduction in renal mass are at risk for developing long-term renal functional impairment from hyperfiltration renal injury. These patients should have their urinary protein excretion monitored because proteinuria is the initial manifestation of hyperfiltration injury.
29. Established critical prerequisites for successful cryosurgery include rapid freezing, gradual thawing, and a repetition of the freeze-thaw cycle.
30. Approximately 20% of angiomyolipomas are found in patients with the tuberous sclerosis (TS) syndrome, an autosomal dominant disorder characterized by mental retardation, epilepsy, and adenoma sebaceum, a distinctive skin lesion. TS, similar to VHL, is transmitted in an autosomal dominant manner.
31. Cystic nephromas are benign renal neoplasms that occur most commonly in middle-aged women.
32. The VHL syndrome's major manifestations can include the development of renal cell carcinoma, pheochromocytoma, retinal angiomas, and hemangioblastomas of the brain stem, cerebellum, or spinal cord.
33. Inactivation or mutation of the VHL gene leads to dysregulated expression of hypoxia inducible factor, an intracellular protein that plays an important role in regulating cellular responses to hypoxia, starvation, and other stresses. This in turn leads to a several-fold upregulation of the expression of vascular endothelial growth factor (VEGF).
34. Hereditary papillary renal cell carcinoma has an autosomal dominant mode of transmission.
35. Chromosome 3 alterations and VHL mutations are common in clear renal cell carcinoma, and mutation or inactivation of this gene (VHL) has been found in over 75% of sporadic cases.
36. Renal medullary carcinoma is a rare histologic subtype of RCC that occurs almost exclusively in association with sickle cell trait.
37. Most collecting duct carcinomas are centrally located and exhibit an infiltrative growth pattern mand aggressive clinical course.
38. Direct ipsilateral adrenal involvement is now grouped with other RCCs that extend beyond Gerota fascia as pathologic stage T4 (pT4).

98

Urothelial Tumors of the Upper Urinary Tract and Ureter

Panagiotis Kallidonis and Evangelos Liatsikos

QUESTIONS

1. The highest incidence of upper urinary tract carcinomas (UTUC) occurs:
   a. in Western countries
   b. in Balkan countries
   c. in Western countries and Taiwan
   d. in Balkan countries and Taiwan
   e. Similarly in all countries

2. Smoking cessation results in:
   a. similar risk for 20 years
   b. reduction of 30% to 50% with interruption for more than 10 years
   c. reduction of 60% to 70% with interruption for more than 10 years
   d. reduction of 30% to 50% with interruption for more than 20 years
   e. reduction of 60% to 70% with interruption for more than 20 years

3. UTUC related to blackfoot disease in endemic areas:
   a. is twice as common in males
   b. is twice as common in females
   c. is twice as common in males and related to younger onset of disease
   d. is twice as common in females and related to younger onset of disease
   e. both c and d

4. Inverted papillomas:
   a. are benign and only surveillance is necessary
   b. are benign but may harbor malignancy in 8% of the cases
   c. are benign but may harbor malignancy in 18% of the cases
   d. are divided into two types based on their morphology
   e. are divided into two types based on their histology

5. Micropapillary variant of urothelial carcinoma
   a. has a clinical outcome like a pure urothelial tumor
   b. is an independent predictor of progression-free survival
   c. is an independent predictor of advanced disease at diagnosis
   d. is an independent predictor of cancer-specific survival
   e. both c and d

6. Squamous cell carcinoma:
   a. is related to abuse of analgesics and chronic inflammation
   b. has an incidence 6 times higher in the renal pelvis than the ureter
   c. has an incidence 6 times higher in the ureter than the renal pelvis
   d. has an incidence 10 times higher in the renal pelvis than the ureter
   e. both a and b

7. Ureteroscopy:
   a. should be performed on all patients with urothelial cancer of the bladder
   b. does not increase the diagnostic accuracy with excretory or retrograde urography
   c. increases the diagnostic accuracy with excretory or retrograde urography
   d. both a and b
   e. both a and c

8. The performance of biopsy during ureteroscopy:
   a. has an 82% correlation with low-grade tumors
   b. has a 92% correlation with high-grade tumors
   c. successfully detects 67% of invasive tumors
   d. a and b
   e. b and c

9. In ureteroscopic biopsy:
   a. lamina propria cannot be identified
   b. the tumor grade could be correlated to the radical surgery specimen in 50% of the cases
   c. muscle layer is present in the majority of the biopsies
   d. cup biopsies have the highest yield of lamina propria layer
   e. loop biopsies have the highest yield of lamina propria layer.

10. In CT urography, a filling defect related to a radiolucent stone could be distinguished by:
   a. measuring Hounsfield units (HU) in the range of 10 to 70 HU with an average 46 HU
   b. measuring Hounsfield units (HU) in the range of 70 to 100 HU with an average 82 HU
   c. measuring Hounsfield units (HU) in the range of 80 to 250 HU with an average 100 HU
   d. measuring Hounsfield units (HU) in the range of 250 to 850 HU with an average 420 HU
   e. none of the above

11. In individual studies, recurrence in the upper tract after treatment of urothelial bladder cancer:
   a. has an incidence of 2% to 6% and a median time to recurrence >3 years
   b. has an incidence of 2% to 6% and a median time to recurrence >5 years
   c. has an incidence of up to 10% and a median time to recurrence >3 years
   d. has an incidence of up to 10% and an interval to recurrence of 17 to 170 months
   e. has an incidence of up to 10% in most of the studies, but some report higher incidence up to 25%

12. Carcinoma in situ (CIS):
   a. increases the incidence of bilateral and multifocal disease
   b. is related to a likelihood of 25% for bilateral disease
   c. has an increased probability for panurothelial disease
   d. both a and c
   e. a, b, and c

13. Important preoperative risk factors include:
    a. older age
    b. tumor location
    c. continuation of tobacco consumption
    d. both a and c
    e. a, b, and c
14. Established postoperative risk factors include:
    a. lymphovascular invasion
    b. surgical margins
    c. tumor necrosis
    d. a and b
    e. a and c

ANSWERS

1. **d. In Balkan countries and Taiwan.** The highest incidence of UTUC is observed in the Balkan countries and is related to the "Balkan nephropathy." The southeast coast of Taiwan also has a high prevalence of UTUC, which is related to the "Chinese herb nephropathy." Both nephropathies are associated with the presence of aristolochic acid in plants endemic in these countries.

2. **c. Reduction of 60% to 70% with interruption for more than 10 years.** McLaughlin et al. (1992) showed a 60% to 70% reduction in the risk for UTUC with interruption of smoking for more than 10 years.

3. **d. Is twice as common in females and related to younger onset of disease.** UTUC is twice as common in the female population in comparison to the worldwide incidence and is related to younger onset of disease in the areas endemic to blackfoot disease, such as the southwest coast of Taiwan. Blackfoot disease is related to chronic exposure to arsenic.

4. **c. Are benign but may harbor malignancy in 18% of the cases.** Inverted papillomas are considered benign. Nevertheless, studies have shown that 18% of these tumors of the ureter are malignant.

5. **b. Is an independent predictor of progression-free survival.** The micropapillary variant of the urothelial carcinoma **was** related to an independent predictor of progression-free survival (HR 3.85, $P = 0.003$) and to poorer cancer-specific survival than the nonmicropapillary UTUC ($P < .001$),

6. **e. Both a and b.** Squamous cell carcinoma has an incidence 5

times higher in the renal pelvis than in the ureter and has been associated with the abuse of analgesics and chronic inflammation.

7. **c. Increases the diagnostic accuracy with excretory or retrograde urography.** Ureteroscopy increases the diagnostic accuracy of excretory or retrograde urography alone from 75% to 85%–90%.

8. **e. b and c.** Biopsy during ureteroscopy has been reported to have a correlation with the pathohistological result of 92% for high-grade tumors and successfully detects 67% of the invasive tumors.

9. **e. Loop biopsies have the highest yield of lamina propria layer.** Loop biopsies may include the lamina propria layer in 100% of the specimens. The respective figure for cup biopsy is 62%.

10. **a. Measuring Hounsfield units (HU) in the range of 10 to 70 HU with average 46 HU.** Urothelial cancers have an average density of 46 HU and range between 10 and 70 HU.

11. **a. Has an incidence of 2% to 6% and a median time to recurrence >3 years.** Upper tract recurrence after bladder cancer treatment has an incidence of 2% to 6% and is diagnosed later with a median time to recurrence >3 years. These rates have significant fluctuation when traditional series are considered. In most of the traditional series, the recurrence rate ranges between 2% and 4% with an interval to recurrence ranging from 17 to 170 months, but there are also series with rates up to 25%.

12. **e. a, b, and c.** The presence of CIS increases the incidence of bilateral and multifocal disease. Bilateral disease has an overall incidence of 3% to 5% of UTUC cases. The presence of CIS increases this incidence to 25%. Patients with CIS have higher risk for subsequent panurothelial disease since there is a high probability for multifocal disease.

13. **e. a, b, and c.** Age is one of the most important demographic predictors of survival in UTUC. Decreased cancer-specific survival has been reported in patients of older age at the time of radical nephroureterectomy. Older age represents an independent factor for decreased survival. Being a smoker at diagnosis increases the risk for disease recurrence and mortality after radical nephroureterectomy and recurrence of the urothelial cancer in the bladder. Patients with ureteral and/or multifocal tumors seem to have a worse prognosis than those with renal pelvic tumors when the stage is adjusted.

14. **d. a and b.** Positive regional lymph nodes (LNs) is an independent factor for poor survival prognosis. Tumor stage remains the single most important factor for the oncological outcome of the UTUC patients.

CHAPTER REVIEW

1. Upper urinary tract carcinomas comprise only 5% of the urothelial cancers.
2. The highest incidence is observed in individuals age 70 to 90 years in the Balkan countries, where the UTUC represents the 40% of all renal neoplasms.
3. Multifocal presence of UTUC is diagnosed in 10% to 20% of the cases.
4. Concurrent bladder cancer is diagnosed in 17% of the cases.
5. UTUCs are twice as frequent in men as in women.
6. Familial/hereditary UTUCs are linked to hereditary nonpolyposis colorectal carcinoma syndrome (Lynch syndrome).
7. Tobacco increases the relative risk for UTUC from 2.5 to 7.
8. UTUC "amino tumors" were related to occupational exposure to carcinogenic aromatic amines.
9. Balkan nephropathy is observed as a familial not inherited condition related to the dietary exposure to aristocholic acid.
10. Patients with pelvic and ureteral tumors have been reported to have a history of analgesic abuse in 22% and 11% of the cases, respectively.

11. The excess of inorganic arsenic in drinking water from artesian wells creates a significant risk for UTUC.
12. Urothelial carcinomas represent >90% of the upper urinary tract tumors. Pure nonurothelial upper urinary tract cancers are rare conditions.
13. Variants of urothelial cancer are encountered in approximately 25% of all urothelial cancers.
14. Papillomas, inverted papillomas, and Brunn's nests are usually benign lesions.
15. UTUC develops through a gradual progression of hyperplasia to dysplasia and eventually CIS in a significant proportion of the UTUC cases.
16. CIS is difficult to diagnose with significant morphological variations.
17. The muscle invasion or invasion to the renal parenchyma or the surrounding adventitia is more likely to take place on the upper tract.
18. Localized disease: hematuria, dysuria, and flank pain.

CHAPTER REVIEW—cont'd

19. Advanced disease: flank or abdominal mass, weight loss, anorexia, bone pain.
20. Cystoscopy should always be performed.
21. Flexible ureteroscopy with biopsy is a key approach for diagnosis.
22. Computed tomography urography has the highest diagnostic accuracy.
23. Urine collection or washing of the ureter with a ureteral catheter could provide the most accurate cytologic results.
24. Ureteral tumors are in the distal ureter in 70% of cases, midureter in 25% of cases, and upper ureter in 5% of cases. Bilateral disease occurs in 3% to 5% of cases.
25. Prognosis for recurrence after radical nephroureterectomy is related to the location of the tumor and stage.
26. The recurrence rate is 2% to 4%, with an interval of 17 to 170 months.
27. Bladder recurrence occurs in 15% to 75 % of cases within 5 years.
28. CIS: higher incidence of bilateral and multifocal disease.
29. Disease spread: direct expansion of the tumor, lymphatics, and blood stream.
30. The TNM classification and staging system. The 2004/2016 WHO grading classification.
31. Age alone should not prevent a curable approach.
32. Ureteral and/or multifocal tumors have a worse prognosis than renal pelvic tumors.
33. Muscle-invasive tumors have poor prognosis.
34. Positive regional LNs have poor survival prognosis.
35. Lymphovascular invasion is a predictor of disease recurrence and survival.

99 Surgical Management of Upper Urinary Tract Urothelial Tumors

Thomas W. Jarrett, Surena F. Matin, and Armine K. Smith

QUESTIONS

1. The majority of ureteral tumors occur in the:
   a. proximal ureter.
   b. midureter.
   c. distal ureter.
   d. proximal and midureter.
   e. distal and mid ureter.

2. The most important determinant of oncologic outcome in upper tract urothelial carcinoma is:
   a. stage and grade.
   b. number of tumors.
   c. location.
   d. tumor size.
   e. tumor architecture.

3. At the time of nephroureterectomy, the ureteral stump can be safely left in place for patients with urothelial tumors of the renal pelvis.
   a. True
   b. False

4. Initial evaluation of positive cytology should include which of the following?
   a. Cystoscopy
   b. Ureteroscopy
   c. CT urography
   d. a, b, and c
   e. a and b
   f. a and c

Pathology

1. A 38-year-old woman has right flank pain and microscopic hematuria. Cytology is atypical. CT scan shows a mass in the distal right ureter with hydronephrosis. Cystoscopy is negative, and attempted ureteroscopy is unsuccessful. The distal ureter is excised, and the pathology is depicted in Fig. 99.1 and is reported as endometriosis. The patient should be advised to:
   a. have a diagnostic laparoscopy.
   b. receive ablative hormonal therapy.
   c. have periodic upper tract imaging.
   d. have cystoscopy and cytology twice yearly for the next 2 years.
   e. have a hysterectomy and bilateral salpingo-oophorectomy.

2. A 60-year-old man has a right ureteral mass excised. The pathology is low-grade noninvasive transitional cell carcinoma (TCC) (Fig. 99.2). He has no prior history of upper tract disease or bladder cancer. Management should consist of:

   a. interval cystoscopies and cytology.
   b. instillation of BCG into the right upper tract.
   c. systemic platinum chemotherapy.
   d. periodic ureteroscopies of the left system.
   e. no further follow-up.

ANSWERS

1. **e. Distal and midureter.** Ureteral tumors occur more commonly in the lower than in the upper ureter. Overall, approximately 70% of ureteral tumors occur in the distal ureter, 25% in the midureter, and 5% in the proximal ureter.

2. **a. Stage and grade.** The most well-established current predictors of survival in patients with upper tract urothelial tumors are stage and grade. The most significant decrease in survival is seen in T3 tumors, and higher-grade tumors are more likely to invade the surrounding tissues, hence presenting with higher stage. Although there have been studies showing differences in prognosis based on the tumor number, location, size, and architecture, these criteria are evolving and warrant further investigation.

3. **b. False.** Complete removal of the distal ureter and bladder cuff offers oncologic outcomes superior to those for incomplete resection. The risk of tumor recurrence in a remaining ureteral stump is 30% to 75%. In addition, adequate cystoscopic surveillance of a residual distal ureter stump after nephroureterectomy is virtually impossible, contributing to high rates of local recurrence. Therefore the entire distal ureter, including the intramural portion and the ureteral orifice, must be removed.

4. **f. a and c.** Ureteroscopy should be reserved for situations in which the diagnosis remains in question after conventional radiographic studies, and for patients in whom the treatment plan may be modified on the basis of the ureteroscopic findings. Although the risks of tumor seeding, extravasation, and dissemination are low in experienced hands, these risks are real and should preclude ureteroscopy when it is unnecessary. Because upper urinary tract tumors are often associated with bladder cancers, cystoscopy is mandatory in the evaluation to exclude coexistent bladder lesions.

Pathology

1. **c. Have periodic upper tract imaging.** With no symptoms, no further workup is indicated. The patient should be followed for possible development of a ureteral vesicle stricture at the site of the anastomosis.

2. **a. Interval cystoscopies and cytology.** Patients who have upper tract TCC have as high as a 30% incidence of bladder tumors and should be followed as for bladder cancer. Moreover, periodic upper tract imaging is necessary.

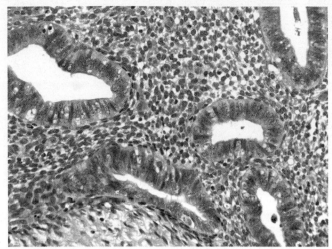

Fig. 99.1 (From Bostwick DG, Cheng L: *Urologic surgical pathology*, ed 2, Edinburgh, 2008, Mosby.)

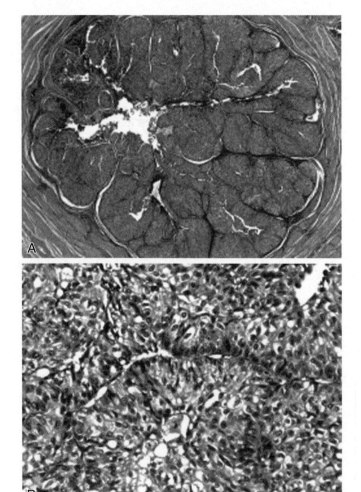

Fig. 99.2 (From Bostwick DG, Cheng L: *Urologic surgical pathology*, ed 2, Edinburgh, 2008, Mosby.)

CHAPTER REVIEW

1. Bilateral upper tract tumors occur either synchronously or metachronously in 2% to 6% of patients.
2. In renal pelvic tumors, parenchyma invasion is the most significant predictor of metastases.
3. Inverted papillomas may be associated with upper tract tumors; it is not likely that cancers arise from them.
4. Squamous cell carcinoma and adenocarcinoma, although rare in the upper tract, are usually associated with long-term obstruction, inflammation, and occasionally calculi.
5. Tumor stage and grade, lymphovascular invasion, and lymph node spread are predictors of poor prognosis. The single most important predictor of outcome is stage.
6. A significant problem with ureteroscopic biopsy is that grade may be accurate, but accurate staging can be extremely difficult.
7. There is a 30% to 50% recurrence rate in ureteral tissue left distal to an invasive ureteral cancer.
8. Patients with T3 tumors located in the renal pelvis have a better survival than those with T3 tumors located in the ureter. Of renal pelvic tumors, 50% are invasive at diagnosis.
9. An adrenalectomy is not indicated for patients undergoing a nephroureterectomy for upper tract tumors.
10. After percutaneous resection of a tumor of the renal pelvis, the nephrostomy is left indwelling to allow for revisualization several weeks later to be certain that all tumors have been removed.
11. Lymphadenectomy has prognostic and possible therapeutic value in patients with T2 to T4 disease.
12. About 70% of ureteral tumors occur in the distal ureter, 25% in the midureter, and 5% in the proximal ureter.

100 Retroperitoneal Tumors

Timothy A. Masterson, Clint Cary, and Richard S. Foster

QUESTIONS

1. Injury to the genitofemoral nerve will result in which neurologic manifestation?
   a. Loss of antegrade ejaculation
   b. Weakness with hip flexion of the lower extremity
   c. Paresthesias of the anterior thigh and lateral scrotal skin
   d. Erectile dysfunction
   e. None of the above

2. Liposarcomas of the retroperitoneum demonstrate all of the following characteristics EXCEPT:
   a. nonlipogenic components that are associated with more aggressive behavior
   b. overexpression of genes localized to chromosome 12q
   c. high frequency of local and regional recurrences
   d. excellent responsiveness to anthracycline-based chemotherapies for eradicating distant spread
   e. the need for both clinical and immunohistological characterizations to render an accurate diagnosis

3. Which of the following statements is true regarding solitary fibrous tumors?
   a. Can be associated with a paraneoplastic syndrome called Doege-Potter syndrome, which is characterized by hypoglycemia due to production of insulin-like growth factor
   b. Were previously referred to as hemangiopericytomas
   c. Are associated with uniform positivity for the *NAB2-STAT6* gene fusion product
   d. Demonstrate radiosensitivity
   e. All of the above

4. Among the spectrum of tumors classified as ganglioneuroblastomas, which of the following is true?
   a. Occur most commonly in elderly adults
   b. *N-myc* gene amplification is a negative prognostic marker
   c. Rarely, if ever, metastasize
   d. Survival rates exceed 90% at 5 years
   e. Unlike pheochromocytomas, metaiodobenzylguanidine (MIBG) scans have little value in staging disease

5. In the setting of a retroperitoneal cancer of unknown primary origin, all of the following are correct EXCEPT:
   a. PET-CT (positron emission tomography-computed tomography) offers little value in the initial workup of these patients
   b. Isochromosome i(12)p may identify patients with retroperitoneal primary germ cell tumors when assessing young, male patients
   c. Adenocarcinomas are the most common histologic subtype identified
   d. Represents up to 5% of new cancer cases worldwide
   e. Histology-specific chemotherapy is the mainstay of treatment

6. The incidence of perioperative acute respiratory distress syndrome (ARDS) in patients with prior receipt of bleomycin can be minimized by:
   a. avoidance of the Trendelenburg position
   b. keeping the FiO_2 as low as possible
   c. short operating time
   d. minimization of intra- and perioperative fluid resuscitation
   e. both b and d

7. Where is the cisterna chylae located?
   a. Immediately posterolateral to the inferior vena cava (IVC) just superior to the right renal artery
   b. Immediately posterolateral to the aorta just superior to the left renal artery
   c. Immediately posterolateral to the aorta just inferior to the left renal artery
   d. Immediately posteromedial to the aorta just superior to the right renal artery.
   e. In the retrocrural region

8. When performing a full bilateral template retroperitoneal lymph node dissection (RPLND) for a mixed germ cell tumor in the retroperitoneum, the main packets are:
   a. paracaval, suprahilar, interaortocaval, ipsilateral gonadal vein
   b. retrocrural, interaortocaval, para-aortic
   c. paracaval, interaortocaval, para-aortic, interiliac
   d. paracaval, interaortocaval, para-aortic, ipsilateral gonadal vessels
   e. retrocrural, paracaval, para-aortic, interiliac

9. How many lumbar arteries need to be identified and divided to gain total vascular control of the abdominal aorta between the renal vessels and aortic bifurcation?
   a. 2
   b. 3
   c. 6
   d. 8
   e. 9

ANSWERS

1. **c. Paresthesias of the anterior thigh and lateral scrotal skin.** The genitofemoral nerve is a sensorimotor nerve and originates from the upper L1/2 segments of the lumbar plexus. It courses from the lumbar foramina and pierces the psoas major muscles anteriorly, traveling in a caudal direction toward the internal inguinal ring. It functions to provide sensation to the anterior thigh, lateral and anterior aspects of the scrotum in males, and mons pubis in female patients. The genital branch also has motor function, providing the innervation to the cremaster muscles in males.

2. **d. Excellent responsiveness to anthracycline-based chemotherapies for eradicating distant spread.** Liposarcomas

represent soft tissue malignancies originating from adipocytes. Many tumors demonstrate aberrations of genes localized to chromosome 12q. The diagnosis of a liposarcoma can be difficult, and often requires clinical, radiographic, and histopathologic characterization to render it accurately. Surgical resection is the mainstay of treatment; however, local recurrences occur frequently in up to 40% of cases. Tumors with areas of de-differentiation are associated with more aggressive behavior, and metastatic disease responds poorly to systemic chemotherapy.

3. **e. All of the above.** All of the statements are true regarding solitary fibrous tumors. Previously referred to as hemangiopericytomas, they have been known to be associated with paraneoplastic syndromes due to endogenous insulinlike growth factor production. They are characteristically associated with the *NAB2 STAT6* gene product, which is diagnostic when present. Lastly, radiotherapy has been shown to improve surgical resection rates by decreasing positive margin rates.

4. **b. *N-myc* gene amplification is a negative prognostic marker.** Ganglioneuroblastomas are lethal tumors. While occurring most commonly in the first decade of life, they are associated with high rates of metastases. *N-myc* gene amplification has been recognized as a negative prognostic marker for disease progression. The 5-year survival rates are poor. MIBG scans and MRI have proven useful for staging of disease at time of diagnosis.

5. **a. PET-CT (positron emission tomography-computed tomography) offers little value in the initial workup of these patients.** Tumors of unknown primary origin represent a difficult challenge. Initial diagnostics of value include the use of PET-CT and histologic characterization via biopsy to provide as much information to classify these entities. In young patients, the presence of i(12)p is pathognomonic for germ cell tumors, which are treated with platinum-based chemotherapy. Overall, this entity represents 5% of all new cancer cases in the world, with adenocarcinomas comprising 50% of these tumors.

6. **e. Both b and d.** Bleomycin-induced pulmonary toxicity is a well-described side effect of the drug, seen most commonly with a greater number of cumulative doses. Minimizing risk factors associated with acute respiratory toxicity and failure remains critical to the management of postchemotherapy patients in the perioperative period. Specifically, minimizing the amount of FiO_2 received as well as reducing perioperative fluid resuscitation have both been associated with a lower risk of acute exacerbation and decompensation.

7. **d. Immediately posteromedial to the aorta just superior to the right renal artery.** The cisterna chylae is most commonly identified in the posterior and medial position relative to the aorta cephalad in location to the right renal artery.

8. **d. Paracaval, interaortocaval, para-aortic, ipsilateral gonadal vessels.** After a series of modifications made to the original template for RPLND, exclusion of the suprahilar and interiliac regions were incorporated to reduce surgical morbidity without any significant risk for relapse in select patients. As such, the current standard for a bilateral template would include the para-aortic, paracaval, and interaortocaval lymph node packets. Additionally, the ipsilateral gonadal vessels should be removed concomitantly.

9. **c. 6.** Within the retroperitoneum, the infrahilar/infrarenal aorta has paired branches that extend posterolateral off of the aorta at regular intervals. Three such paired branches exist with few exceptions, for a total number of six lumbar artery branches that require prospective identification and division to achieve total vascular control of the aorta.

CHAPTER REVIEW

1. Many tumors of the retroperitoneum (RP) grow silently over months or years, thus presenting with sizeable dimensions and adjacent organ involvement.
2. Cross-sectional imaging offers the best means of assessing size and extent of disease. Serologic testing plays an important role, specifically in germ cell tumors.
3. Fine-needle aspiration (FNA) and/or core biopsies remain an important tool in the evaluation and management of many diseases, and their diagnostic value should be considered in the initial workup of all RP masses.
4. Adjuvant and neoadjuvant therapies will continue to be expanded and incorporated as part of the multimodal approach to cancer treatment.
5. No disease process has exemplified this more than the management approach for testicular cancer patients.
6. In sarcoma, the heterogeneity across the spectrum of histologic entities and their biologic differences in response to radiation and systemic therapies restrict one's ability to make sweeping recommendations as to the timing and sequencing of different therapies.
7. Accordingly, using a multidisciplinary team to explore all available options to ensure optimal management of the RP mass offers patients the greatest chance of a successful outcome.

101 Open Surgery of the Kidney

Aria F. Olumi and Michael L. Blute

QUESTIONS

1. A healthy 45-year-old man with no family history of cancer is found to have a 6-cm enhancing mass in the upper pole of his right kidney. A 2-cm solitary nodule is noted on preoperative chest radiography. Computed tomography (CT) confirms a solitary nodule in the lower lobe of the right lung. What is the most appropriate treatment course?

   a. Systemic chemotherapy alone

   b. Radical right nephrectomy and postoperative chemotherapy

   c. Biopsy of pulmonary nodule

   d. Radical nephrectomy and simultaneous pulmonary metastasectomy

   e. Radical nephrectomy with staged resection of pulmonary nodule 6 weeks postoperatively

2. What is the preferred technique for radical nephrectomy and removal of tumor thrombus above the level of the diaphragm in the absence of significant metastatic disease?

   a. Flank incision with extensive liver mobilization and removal of tumor through an incision in the diaphragm

   b. Flank incision with cardiopulmonary bypass and deep hypothermic circulatory arrest (CPB-DHCA)

   c. Chevron incision with CPB-DHCA

   d. Chevron incision with Pringle maneuver

   e. Midline incision with CPB-DHCA

3. Deep hypothermic circulatory arrest (DHCA) can have irreversible neurologic effects after what period of time?

   a. 10 minutes

   b. 20 minutes

   c. 40 minutes

   d. 60 minutes

   e. 90 minutes

4. In a 45-year-old man with a normal contralateral kidney and no family history of kidney cancer, in which of the following clinical scenarios would partial nephrectomy be indicated?

   a. Two tumors less than 3 cm each in the upper and lower pole

   b. Single 8-cm tumor in the upper pole

   c. Single 2-cm tumor in a hilar location with small renal vein tumor thrombus

   d. Single 4-cm tumor in any location

   e. All of the above

5. What is the strongest modifiable risk factor for renal insufficiency after partial nephrectomy?

   a. Duration of renal ischemia

   b. Surgical approach

   c. Administration of nephrotoxins

   d. Resection margin

   e. Administration of heparin

6. During a posterior right lumbotomy approach, what is the order of appearance of the renal artery, renal vein, and renal pelvis?

   a. Artery, renal pelvis, vein

   b. Artery, vein, renal pelvis

   c. Renal pelvis, artery, vein

   d. Vein, renal pelvis, artery

   e. Renal pelvis, vein, artery

7. Match the following T stage with the tumor characteristics.

   1. T3c

   2. T1a

   3. T3a

   4. T4

   5. T2b

   a. Greater than 10 cm confined to capsule

   b. Less than 4 cm confined to capsule

   c. 6 cm invading adrenal gland

   d. 5 cm with renal sinus fat invasion

   e. 13 cm with renal vein thrombus invading the wall of the inferior vena cava

8. Five days after left partial nephrectomy for a hilar tumor, there is persistent drainage from the Penrose drain site. Laboratory analysis of the drain fluid demonstrates elevated amylase levels. Imaging studies demonstrate small bowel dilation consistent with ileus and fluid around the tail of pancreas. What is the ideal management?

   a. Antibiotics

   b. Immediate surgical exploration

   c. Percutaneous drain placement

   d. Nasogastric tube placement, parenteral nutrition, and conservative management

   e. Nasogastric tube placement, low-fat diet, and conservative management

9. Which segmental branch of the renal artery is most consistent and supplies 25% of the arterial supply to the renal unit?

   a. Apical (superior) segmental artery

   b. Anterior superior segmental artery

   c. Posterior segmental artery

   d. Anterior inferior segmental artery

   e. The basilar (inferior) segmental artery

10. What maneuver refers to the reflection of the second and third portions of the duodenum in a medial direction to expose the right renal vessels and ventral inferior vena cava?

    a. Cattell maneuver

    b. Langenbeck maneuver

    c. Sorcini maneuver

    d. Kocher maneuver

    e. Pringle maneuver

11. What partial nephrectomy technique should be used as a last resort in a solitary kidney?
    a. Enucleation
    b. Wedge resection
    c. Cryotherapy
    d. Polar resection
    e. Extracorporeal repair and autotransplantation

12. The subcostal nerve may be inadvertently transected during an anterior subcostal incision for a radical nephrectomy. Between what two layers does this nerve run?
    a. Posterior peritoneum and transversalis fascia
    b. Scarpa fascia and external oblique muscle
    c. External oblique and internal oblique
    d. Internal oblique and transversalis
    e. Skin and Scarpa fascia

13. What is the motor deficit resulting from transaction of the subcostal nerve?
    a. Winged scapula
    b. Hemidiaphragmatic paralysis
    c. Paresis of the flank musculature and flank bulge
    d. Inability to flex ipsilateral adductor muscle
    e. Weakness of contralateral rectus abdominis muscle

14. What percentage of patients have multiple renal arteries?
    a. 0% to 2%
    b. 2% to 10%
    c. 10% to 20%
    d. 20% to 30%
    e. More than 30%

15. Which of the following is NOT an indication for simple nephrectomy?
    a. Nonfunctional chronically infected kidney
    b. Nonfunctional persistently hydronephrotic kidney causing pain
    c. Renovascular hypertension refractory to medical and nephron-sparing surgical intervention
    d. Polycystic kidney with minimal function and recurrent infections
    e. Kidney with 8-cm enhancing upper pole hilar mass

16. Two days after cardiopulmonary bypass and circulatory arrest (20 minutes) for an extensive right-sided renal mass with thrombus extending into the atrium, using traditional median sternotomy, a relatively healthy 36-year-old patient is unable to be extubated and has no purposeful right-sided movement. Imaging reveals a large left-sided cerebrovascular infarct. What clinical scenario can explain this event?
    a. Pulmonary air embolism
    b. Cerebral ischemia from bypass and circulatory arrest
    c. Tension pneumothorax
    d. Right main stem bronchial intubation
    e. Unrecognized paradoxical embolism

17. Which form of therapy has been considered the gold standard for localized renal cell carcinoma?
    a. Chemotherapy
    b. Immunotherapy
    c. Radiation
    d. Hormonal therapy
    e. Surgical resection

18. On postoperative day 2 after radical nephrectomy for a 14-cm complex left renal tumor using an anterior midline incision, there are overt signs of peritonitis. The patient is 72 years old with significant atherosclerotic disease. At exploration, the entire small bowel is necrotic and nonviable. What artery was inadvertently ligated?
    a. Celiac
    b. Left gastric
    c. Inferior mesenteric
    d. Superior mesenteric
    e. Right gastroepiploic

19. During resection of a large right renal mass, the main renal artery is identified, ligated, and divided, but the renal vein fails to decompress. What is the most likely explanation for this?
    a. Renal vein tumor thrombus
    b. Subclinical renal arteriovenous malformation
    c. Bleeding disorder
    d. Arterial collateral branch vessels
    e. Extensive venous collateral obstruction

20. What is most appropriate setting for a thoracoabdominal incision?
    a. Large right upper pole renal mass with tumor thrombus in the renal vein
    b. 5-cm right renal tumor in a hilar location
    c. Large left lower pole tumor with extensive lymphadenopathy
    d. Large right renal mass with tumor thrombus to the retrohepatic level
    e. A 10-cm right lower pole tumor with arteriovenous malformation

21. What is the most common complication associated with performing CPB-DHCA for the removal of large renal cell tumor thrombus?
    a. Pulmonary air emboli
    b. Intestinal ischemia
    c. Bleeding and coagulopathy
    d. Lower extremity tumor emboli
    e. Tumor emboli

22. Which of the following is NOT a proposed benefit of renal artery embolization (RAE)?
    a. Shrinkage of an arterialized tumor thrombus to ease surgical removal
    b. Reduced blood loss
    c. Facilitation of dissection due to tissue plane edema
    d. Ability to ligate the renal vein before the renal artery at time of nephrectomy
    e. Modulation of the immune response
    f. None of the above

23. What is the most common complication after RAE?
    a. Groin hematoma from puncture site
    b. Paraplegia from spinal artery occlusion
    c. Coil migration
    d. Postinfarction syndrome (pain, nausea, and fever)
    e. Adrenal insufficiency

24. What is the most common complication after partial nephrectomy for nonexophytic renal masses?
    a. Hemorrhage
    b. Renal failure
    c. Rhabdomyolysis
    d. Hydronephrosis
    e. Urinary leak

25. Ten days after a left partial nephrectomy for a 4.5-cm hilar tumor, there is persistent fluid output from the surgical drain. No ureteral stent was placed at the time of surgery, and a small opening in the collecting system was oversewn. The creatinine concentration of the drain fluid is 34.5 mg/dL, consistent with urine. Despite conservative management, the volume fails to decline. A retrograde pyelogram demonstrates a moderate amount of contrast extravasation, confirming the urinary fistula. What is the most appropriate management at this time?
    a. Immediate reexploration and repair
    b. Percutaneous nephrostomy tube placement
    c. Removal of surgical drain
    d. Internalized ureteral stent placement
    e. Internalized ureteral stent placement, continued surgical drain monitoring, and placement of Foley catheter

ANSWERS

1. **d. Radical nephrectomy and simultaneous pulmonary metastasectomy.** This patient would be best managed with a radical nephrectomy and simultaneous removal of the pulmonary nodule. Systemic therapy is not a primary treatment unless there is extensive metastatic disease at presentation. Given his age and lack of medical problems, there is no reason to delay the removal of his kidney and the pulmonary nodule. The tumor location and pulmonary nodule both can be accessed through one incision (i.e., thoracoabdominal).

2. **c. Chevron incision with CPB-DHCA.** CPB-DHCA has been established as the most prudent course for the removal of these tumor thrombi. The chevron incision provides the best exposure. Alternatives to CPB, including extensive liver mobilization and intrapericardial resection, carry an increased risk of bleeding.

3. **c. 40 minutes.** The duration of DHCA can vary depending on the degree of tumor thrombus. Vena cava resection and substitution can add additional time if there is significant tumor invasion into the wall of the vena cava. Studies have suggested that irreversible neurologic effects may be observed after 40 minutes of DHCA.

4. **d. Single 4-cm tumor in any location.** In patients with a normal contralateral kidney, the current literature supports elective partial nephrectomy for single T1 tumors.

5. **a. Duration of renal ischemia.** Duration of renal ischemia is the strongest modifiable risk factor for renal insufficiency after partial nephrectomy.

6. **c. Renal pelvis, artery, vein.** The renal pelvis is the first structure one encounters with the posterior right lumbotomy incision, followed by the artery and vein. This approach can be used to repair ureteropelvic junction obstruction, especially in children or patients with multiple prior abdominal and/or flank surgeries.

7. a: T2b; b: T1a; c: T4; d: T3a; e: T3c.

8. **d. Nasogastric tube placement, parenteral nutrition, and conservative management.** Conservative management of a pancreatic fistula should be the first approach in this patient. Initial nasogastric tube placement can help resolve the ileus. Parenteral nutrition will limit any pancreatic secretions from oral intake.

9. **c. Posterior segmental artery.** The posterior division is the first and most consistent branch point of the renal artery and supplies approximately one-fourth of the blood supply.

10. **d. Kocher maneuver.** Mobilization of the second and third portions of the duodenum is referred to as a *Kocher maneuver.* The Pringle maneuver is the temporary occlusion of the porta hepatis. The Langenbeck maneuver is the division of the coronary and right triangular ligaments, providing medial rotation of the right lobe of the liver and exposure of the suprarenal inferior vena cava.

11. **e. Extracorporeal repair and autotransplantation.** All patients with solitary kidneys are high-risk candidates for partial nephrectomy and may have transient renal impairment postoperatively. The degree and duration of renal impairment may be increased owing to risks associated with renal autotransplantation (hemorrhage, thrombosis, lymphocele, stenosis).

12. **d. Internal oblique and transversalis.** The subcostal nerve runs between these two layers. Caution must be taken not to sever this nerve during flank incisions.

13. **c. Paresis of the flank musculature and flank bulge.** Damage to the subcostal nerve results in denervation and paresis of the flank musculature, leading to chronic postoperative pain or flank bulge.

14. **d. 20% to 30%.** Multiple postmortem and radiographic studies estimate that 25% of the general population have supernumerary renal arteries.

15. **e. Kidney with 8-cm enhancing upper pole hilar mass.** There should be little reservation about performing a radical nephrectomy for an enhancing mass, especially in the upper pole. Almost all nonmalignant disease affecting the kidney can be treated via a simple approach.

16. **e. Unrecognized paradoxical embolism.** This rare but devastating clinical situation occurs in patients with a patent foramen ovale. An embolism may originate from tumor thrombus manipulation or from deep venous thromboembolism.

17. **e. Surgical resection.** There have been numerous studies to suggest that surgical resection is the mainstay of therapy for kidney cancer.

18. **d. Superior mesenteric.** Ligation of the superior mesenteric artery produces ischemia in the bowel distribution above. The superior mesenteric artery can be mistaken for the left renal artery from the anterior approach. Visualizing the artery from a posterior position as it enters the hilum will help to minimize this complication.

19. **d. Arterial collateral branch vessels.** Failure of the renal vein to decompress after ligation of the main renal artery indicates additional arterial inflow, which may be secondary to a missed lower or upper pole artery or extensive collateral arteries.

20. **a. Large right upper pole renal mass with tumor thrombus in the renal vein.** The thoracoabdominal incision is ideal for larger tumors involving the upper pole. The incision is also ideal for managing tumor thrombus extending into the renal vein. The inferior vena cava can be nicely exposed via this approach.

21. **c. Bleeding and coagulopathy.** Intraoperatively, the administration of heparin in addition to hypothermia leads to significant coagulopathy. The bleeding from heparin is typically limited to an "ooze" intraoperatively and should not consume time and energy during the operation. After tumor removal, the rewarming process helps to promote coagulation.

22. **f. None of the above.** Proposed benefits of preoperative RAE include shrinkage of an arterialized tumor thrombus to ease surgical removal, reduced blood loss, facilitation of dissection due to tissue plane edema, ability to ligate the renal vein before the renal artery at time of nephrectomy, and modulation of the immune response.

23. **d. Postinfarction syndrome (pain, nausea, and fever).** The triad of fever, flank pain, and nausea occurs in up to 75% of patients after angioembolization. Fevers can often exceed 39.4°C (103°F) and are best managed with antipyretics.

24. **e. Urinary leak.** Partial nephrectomy for nonexophytic masses has an increased risk of entering the collecting system. Even when the collecting system is closed under direct vision, there may still be extravasation of urine that collects in the perirenal space. The use of postoperative surgical drains is imperative in the management of these collections to reduce the risk of infections. In addition, the drain output volume can be observed to determine if collections are resolving. Renal failure is rare unless operating on a solitary kidney or on a patient with marginal renal function. Rhabdomyolysis can be encountered secondary to patient positioning and increased body mass index.

25. **e. Internalized ureteral stent placement, continued surgical drain monitoring, and placement of Foley catheter.** Placement of a ureteral stent can promote urine drainage into the bladder. Keeping a Foley catheter in place reduces urine reflux.

CHAPTER REVIEW

1. The right renal artery is posterior to the inferior vena cava.
2. Renal arteries are end arteries; ligation results in infarction of the segment that they supply.
3. The renal venous network intercommunicates.
4. Lumbar veins often enter the left renal vein and, not infrequently, the right renal vein. They enter posteriorly. Care must be taken when encircling the renal vein not to tear one of these lumbar veins.
5. There is no conclusive evidence that renal artery embolization has any immunologic therapeutic benefit.
6. The renal artery is always ligated before the renal vein when performing a nephrectomy; each vessel is ligated individually.
7. Patients with a glomerular filtration rate of less than 60 mL/min or those with significant proteinuria are at risk for postoperative renal failure following renal surgery—particularly when a nephrectomy is performed.
8. Adrenalectomy is not recommended as part of a radical nephrectomy unless imaging shows adrenal involvement with tumor or an upper pole tumor is contiguous with the adrenal.
9. Transesophageal echocardiography is an excellent modality to determine the level of the vena cava tumor thrombus immediately before the surgical event.
10. In patients with vena cava tumor thrombi cephalad to the hepatic venous outflow who require CPB, either mild hypothermia and no circulatory arrest or significant hypothermia with circulatory arrest may be performed. Each technique has its advantages and disadvantages. The method used is at the discretion of the surgeon.
11. The addition of a lymphadenectomy to a radical nephrectomy for renal cell carcinoma has a questionable impact on progression-free and overall survival. It may be considered in patients who have enlarged lymph nodes on preoperative imaging, those in whom cytoreductive surgery is being performed, and those with ominous pathologic findings of the primary renal tumor.
12. Ligation of the right renal vein will result in failure of the right renal unit due to lack of venous collateral vessels.
13. Ligation of the left renal vein is possible because collateral venous drainage may occur through lumbar and gonadal vessels.
14. The renal vein ostium of the vena cava should be excised in patients with vena cava tumor thrombi, because invasion of the vena cava vein wall at this site is not uncommonly found.
15. Twenty-five percent of the general population have supernumerary renal arteries.
16. The superior mesenteric artery can be mistaken for the left renal artery from the anterior approach. Rarely, the hepatic artery can be mistaken for the right renal artery. Visualizing the artery from a posterior position relative to the renal vein as it enters the hilum will help identify the renal artery.
17. Proposed benefits of preoperative renal artery embolization include shrinkage of an arterialized vena cava tumor thrombus to ease surgical removal, reduced blood loss, facilitation of dissection due to tissue plane edema, and the ability to ligate the renal vein before the renal artery at time of nephrectomy. These patients may develop the postinfarction syndrome (pain, nausea, and fever). The triad of fever, flank pain, and nausea occurs in up to 75% of patients after angioembolization.

102 Laparoscopic and Robotic Surgery of the Kidney

Daniel M. Moreira and Louis R. Kavoussi

QUESTIONS

1. The following statements are true regarding laparoscopic and robotic renal surgery in obese patients, EXCEPT:
   a. Obesity is associated with distorted anatomy and limited range of instrument motion.
   b. Morbid obesity (body mass index [BMI] >40) is a contraindication to laparoscopic or robotic surgery.
   c. Complication rates are higher among obese patients.
   d. Conversion to open surgery is more common in obese patients.
   e. Longer surgical instruments are sometimes required to complete the procedure.

2. The following statements are true regarding laparoscopic and robotic surgical approaches to renal surgery, EXCEPT:
   a. Transperitoneal is the most widely used approach.
   b. Retroperitoneal partial nephrectomy is best suited for anterior renal tumors.
   c. Disadvantages of retroperitoneal approach include the limited working space and decreased instrument triangulation.
   d. The advantages of robotic approach include greater degree of instrument motion, elimination of tremor, and the ability to scale motions.
   e. Advantages of transperitoneal approach include familiar anatomic landmarks and more flexibility of trocar placement.

3. The following statements are true regarding laparoendoscopic single site (LESS) and natural orifice transluminal endoscopic surgery (NOTES) compared to conventional laparoscopic renal surgery, EXCEPT:
   a. For both LESS and NOTES, conventional laparoscopic instrumentation cannot be used, and flexible or articulated instruments are required.
   b. LESS consolidates all laparoscopic ports in a single skin incision.
   c. LESS and NOTES are associated with improving cosmesis and reduced postoperative pain.
   d. LESS has limited triangulation due to the clustering of instruments entering the intracorporal working space.
   e. NOTES uses one or more patent natural orifices of the body for access.

4. The following are indications for renal cysts disease treatment, EXCEPT:
   a. cyst-associated pain.
   b. ureteral obstruction.
   c. suspicion for malignancy.
   d. infection.
   e. autosomal dominant polycystic kidney disease.

5. The following statements are true regarding laparoscopic and robotic renal surgery for renal cystic disease, EXCEPT:
   a. Symptomatic benign cysts can be initially managed with percutaneous needle aspiration.
   b. Multiple or bilateral cysts should not be treated in the same operation.
   c. Laparoscopic management of symptomatic renal cysts is associated with greater than 90% symptom improvement.
   d. If a sclerosing agent is used, it should not be injected into the collecting system.
   e. Most renal cysts do not require surgical intervention.

6. The following statements are true regarding laparoscopic renal biopsy, EXCEPT:
   a. It is indicated in cases of hematuria and proteinuria of glomerular origin and/or unexplained renal failure.
   b. The most common complication is bleeding.
   c. Ultrasound guidance can facilitate the localization of the kidney in cases of abundant retroperitoneal and perinephric adipose tissue.
   d. A 5-mm biopsy forceps or an 18-gauge Tru-Cut needle can be used for tissue sampling.
   e. It is contraindicated in cases of multiple renal cysts or solitary kidney.

7. The following statements are true regarding nephropexy and nephrolysis, EXCEPT:
   a. Nephrolysis consists of the renal mobilization with skeletonization of the hilar vessels and upper ureter.
   b. Nephrolysis is an effective treatment for severe refractory chyluria.
   c. Nephropexy is indicated in cases of nephroptosis associated with pain or vascular or urinary obstruction.
   d. Nephropexy can be accomplished with either suture fixation or the use of foreign material, such as mesh or tissue adhesive.
   e. Laparoscopic nephropexy is associated with greater than 80% resolution of nephroptosis but almost no pain improvement.

8. The following statements are true regarding calyceal diverticulectomy, EXCEPT:
   a. Most cases of calyceal diverticulectomy require hilar clamping.
   b. Indications for surgical intervention include chronic pain, recurrent urinary tract infection, gross hematuria, and decline in renal function.
   c. Calyceal diverticulectomy involves widening of the infundibular drainage to prevent urinary stasis or complete ablation of the diverticula cavity.
   d. Injection of dye via a preoperatively placed externalized ureteral catheter is helpful in localizing the diverticulum.
   e. Laparoscopic, robotic, or LESS transperitoneal or retroperitoneal approaches can be used.

9. The following are advantages of laparoscopic over open radical nephrectomy, EXCEPT:
   a. improved cosmesis.
   b. shorter hospital stay.
   c. improved cancer-specific survival.

d. less analgesic use.

e. shorter convalescence time.

10. Which of the following is an absolute contraindication to laparoscopic radical nephrectomy?

a. Tumor size greater than 14 cm

b. Age older than 80 years

c. Uncorrected coagulopathy

d. Renal vein thrombus

e. Multiple prior abdominal surgeries

11. Regarding laparoscopic radical nephrectomy, the following statement is CORRECT:

a. En bloc hilar vessel stapling is unsafe and should not be attempted.

b. The use of a retrieval bag is not needed in cases of tumor extraction after morcellation.

c. Metastatic renal cell carcinoma is an absolute contraindication.

d. Clips alone are contraindicated for the ligation of the renal artery.

e. Adrenal gland should be bluntly hand-dissected away from the upper pole during hand-assisted nephrectomy.

12. Compared to traditional laparoscopic nephrectomy, hand-assisted nephrectomy is associated with higher:

a. local recurrence.

b. wound-related complications.

c. pain scores.

d. conversion to open surgery.

e. costs.

13. Regarding minimally invasive partial nephrectomy, the following statement is CORRECT:

a. Central and hilar tumors are a contraindication to laparoscopic partial nephrectomy.

b. Compared to open partial nephrectomy, robot-assisted partial nephrectomy in solitary kidney is associated with higher conversion to radical nephrectomy.

c. The placement of a drain is generally considered unnecessary when the incision in the pelvicalyceal system is repaired with running suture.

d. Suture renorrhaphy is the most reliable technique to achieve hemostasis of the partial nephrectomy bed.

e. Multiple ipsilateral renal tumors should not be removed in the same setting.

14. Regarding warm renal ischemia and hilar control, the following statement is INCORRECT:

a. Hilar control can be accomplished by using bulldog clamps or a laparoscopic Satinsky clamp.

b. Renal artery–only clamping is a safe alternative to artery and vein clamping.

c. Parenchymal compression is best suited for peripheral tumors.

d. Off-clamp partial nephrectomy is a suitable option for the resection of small, exophytic, and noninfiltrating tumors.

e. Hilar unclamping before the completion of the renorrhaphy is contraindicated.

15. Regarding laparoscopic thermal ablation, the following statement is INCORRECT:

a. Compared to partial nephrectomy, the advantages of thermal ablation include less blood loss, short operative time, and fewer complications.

b. The advantages of the laparoscopic approach over percutaneous ablation include direct tumor visualization, mobilization of the kidney, and dissection and retraction of surrounding structures.

c. Contact of the iceball with the renal collecting system, ureter, renal vasculature, or adjacent organs should be avoided.

d. Intraoperative monitoring of radiofrequency ablation is based on direct temperature measurement or measurement of electrical impedance.

e. Temperatures greater than 105°C throughout the tumor are recommended for an adequate thermal damage.

16. Regarding complications of minimally invasive renal surgery, the following statement is INCORRECT:

a. Advanced age is a major risk factor for complications.

b. Partial nephrectomy is associated with higher complication rates compared to radical nephrectomy and simple nephrectomy.

c. Large tumors, obesity, and prior abdominal surgery are associated with a higher complication rate.

d. Chronic pyelonephritis, such as xanthogranulomatous pyelonephritis, is associated with greater rate of conversion to open surgery.

e. The most common postoperative complications are bleeding, wound infection, pneumonia, and prolonged ileus.

17. Regarding complications of minimally invasive renal surgery, the following statement is INCORRECT:

a. Most of the life-threatening intraoperative complications occur during the access phase and dissection of the renal hilum.

b. Most cases of urinary leak require ureteral stenting or percutaneous nephrostomy placement.

c. Mild to moderate venous bleeding can be controlled by applying direct pressure.

d. Factors associated with urinary leak include large tumor size, hilar location, pelvicalyceal repair, and prolonged warm ischemia time.

e. Stapler malfunction is associated with a 20% conversion rate to open surgery and 2% mortality rate.

18. Regarding complications of minimally invasive renal surgery, the following statement is INCORRECT:

a. Persistent and increased trocar site pain without significant erythema or purulent drainage is a common sign of visceral injury.

b. Splenic injuries are most commonly caused by vigorous traction on splenic ligaments.

c. Gallbladder injuries are best managed by primary surgical repair.

d. Capsular pancreatic injuries can be managed by closing the defect with nonabsorbable suture and/or drain placement.

e. Most liver injuries can be managed with topical hemostatic therapy and argon beam coagulation.

19. A 55-year-old woman presents to the emergency department on postoperative day 5 after laparoscopic left radical nephrectomy complaining of vomiting, fever, and diffuse abdominal pain. Computed tomography (CT) scan with oral contrast shows leakage of contrast from the ascending colon. The most likely cause of this injury is:

a. bowel ischemia.

b. trocar placement.

c. blunt dissection.

d. electrocautery.

e. abdominal wall closure.

20. A 71-year-old woman presents to emergency department with new-onset gross hematuria on postoperative day 6 after an uncomplicated laparoscopic right partial nephrectomy. Her blood pressure is 90/56 mm Hg and heart rate is 112 beats/min. Hematocrit is 21%. After fluid resuscitation, her vital signs normalized, but the hematuria worsens and requires continuous bladder irrigation. The best next step is:

    a. cystoscopy and retrograde pyelogram.

    b. radical nephrectomy.

    c. renal angiography and embolization.

    d. admission to intensive care unit and blood transfusion.

    e. CT scan with intravenous contrast.

ANSWERS

1. **b. Obesity is associated with distorted anatomy and limited range of instrument motion.** Although morbid obesity is associated with distorted anatomy, limited range of instrument motion, and higher complication and conversion rates, it is not a contraindication to laparoscopic or robotic renal surgery. In general, obese patients benefits from minimally invasive surgery given it provides less incisional pain and shorter convalescence.

2. **b. Retroperitoneal partial nephrectomy is best suited for anterior renal tumors.** Although anterior renal tumors can be resected with retroperitoneal partial nephrectomy, this technique is best suited for posterior tumors. A study comparing 100 transperitoneal and 63 retroperitoneal laparoscopic partial nephrectomies found that 77% of the posterior tumors were managed via retroperitoneal approach and 97% of the anterior tumors were managed with transperitoneal surgery.

3. **a. For both LESS and NOTES, conventional laparoscopic instrumentation cannot be used, and flexible or articulated instruments are required.** Although LESS has limited triangulation due to the clustering of instruments entering the intracorporeal working space, conventional laparoscopic instrumentation can be used. Flexible or articulated instruments are helpful but not required in cases of LESS or NOTES.

4. **e. Autosomal dominant polycystic kidney disease.** Cyst-associated pain, urinary obstruction, suspicion for malignancy, and infection are traditional indications for operative management of renal cysts. Autosomal dominant polycystic kidney disease alone is not an indication for surgical intervention unless it is accompanied by complications, pain, suspicion for malignancy, etc.

5. **b. Multiple or bilateral cysts should not be treated in the same operation.** Although most renal cysts do not require surgical intervention, multiple or bilateral cysts can and frequently are treated in the same operation, with greater than 90% symptom improvement and radiologic resolution.

6. **e. It is contraindicated in cases of multiple renal cysts or solitary kidney.** Although renal biopsy is typically done percutaneously under CT or ultrasound guidance, there are circumstances where a laparoscopic biopsy may be preferred, including failed previous attempts at percutaneous biopsy, renal anatomic abnormalities, bleeding diathesis, morbid obesity, multiple renal cysts, or a solitary kidney.

7. **e. Laparoscopic nephropexy is associated with greater than 80% resolution of nephroptosis but almost no pain improvement.** Laparoscopic nephropexy is associated with a 90% to 100% pain improvement, 80% to 95% resolution of the 5-cm renal descent, and 90% improvement in renal function measured by nuclear medicine scan. Nephrolysis consists of the renal mobilization with skeletonization of the hilar vessels and upper ureter and is an effective treatment for severe refractory chyluria.

8. **a. Most cases of calyceal diverticulectomy require hilar clamping.** Given most cases of calyceal diverticulectomy have low bleeding risk, hilar control is usually not required.

9. **c. Improved cancer-specific survival.** Advantages of laparoscopic radical nephrectomy include improved cosmesis, shorter hospital stay, less analgesic requirement, and shorter convalescence time. Oncologic outcomes including recurrence, progression to metastatic disease, and cancer-specific survival are comparable with open radical nephrectomy.

10. **c. Uncorrected coagulopathy.** Uncorrected coagulopathy is an absolute contraindication to laparoscopic renal surgery, as are untreated infection and hypovolemic shock. Laparoscopic partial nephrectomy has been reported as a feasible and safe approach in the management of select large renal masses, elderly patients, renal vein thrombosis, and multiple prior abdominal surgeries.

11. **d. Clips alone are contraindicated for the ligation of the renal artery.** Although previously there have been concerns of arteriovenous fistula formation in cases of en bloc hilar vessel stapling, this approach has been shown to be a safe alternative. The use of a retrieval bag is mandatory in cases of tumor extraction after morcellation to prevent tumor spillage. Cytoreductive laparoscopic nephrectomy is safe and effective in patients with metastatic renal cell carcinoma. The hand should not be used to bluntly dissect the adrenal gland free from the upper pole because this will typically result in bleeding. Clips alone are contraindicated for the ligation of the renal artery due to reports of fatal cases of clip failure.

12. **b. Wound-related complications.** Hand-assisted laparoscopic nephrectomy offers recovery, morbidity and cost that are comparable with those of pure laparoscopy surgery. Recurrence-free, cancer-specific, and overall survivals are similar between surgical techniques. The rate of wound-related complications such as wound infection and incisional hernia are slightly higher in hand-assisted approach compared to pure laparoscopy.

13. **d. Suture renorrhaphy is the most reliable technique to achieve hemostasis of the partial nephrectomy bed.** Minimally invasive partial nephrectomy for central and hilar tumors can be performed safely by an experienced surgeon with perioperative outcomes comparable with those of peripheral tumors. Minimally invasive partial nephrectomy for tumors in a solitary kidney is safe and offers comparable outcomes to open surgery. Repeat renal surgery can pose a technical challenge and is associated with higher blood loss and complication rates compared to first-time renal surgery. Although the laparoscopic resection of multiple tumors is associated with long operative time and hospitalization, in experience hands it is associated with comparable blood loss, complication rates, and renal functional outcomes as resection of a solitary tumor. The placement of a drain is usually recommended in most cases of pelvicalyceal system, even cases that are repaired with running sutures, to reduce the risk of perinephric urinoma. Although there are other means of achieving hemostasis of the partial nephrectomy bed such as the use of clips and tissue sealants, suture renorrhaphy is considered the most reliable technique to achieve hemostasis.

14. **e. Hilar unclamping before the completion of the renorrhaphy is contraindicated.** During radiofrequency ablation, thermal damage occurs through frictional heating due to ionic oscillation by a monopolar or bipolar high-frequency alternating current which can induce temperatures between 60°C and 100°C throughout the tumor. Temperatures greater than 105°C should be avoided to prevent tissue vaporization.

15. **e. Temperatures greater than 105°C throughout the tumor are recommended for an adequate thermal damage.** Hilar control can be accomplished by using bulldog clamps on the renal artery with or without venous clamping, or a laparoscopic Satinsky clamp for en bloc hilar clamping. Studies evaluating early unclamping (before the completion of the renorrhaphy) found this technique to be associated with shorter warm ischemia time and comparable estimated blood loss and complication rates.

16. **a. Advanced age is a major risk factor for complications.** Advanced age alone is not a major risk factor for complications. Obesity, comorbidities, prior abdominal surgery, and larger and more anatomically complex tumors have all been associated with higher complication rates.

17. **b. Most cases of urinary leak require ureteral stenting or percutaneous nephrostomy placement.** Factor associated with urinary leak include large tumor size, hilar location, pelvicalyceal repair, and prolonged operative and warm ischemia time. Most cases of urinary leak require no intervention other than percutaneous drainage. When conservative management fails or there is evidence of distal obstruction, additional intervention may be required, such as ureteral stenting and bladder decompression.

18. **c. Gallbladder injuries are best managed by primary surgical repair.** Gallbladder injuries are best managed by cholecystectomy.

19. **d. Electrocautery.** Although bowel injury can occur at any point during the procedure, the most common case of unrecognized injury is the use of thermal energy adjacent to the bowel, responsible for nearly 50% of the cases. Thermal injuries usually present later than nonthermal bowel injuries.

20. **c. Renal angiography and embolization.** Significant gross hematuria after partial nephrectomy suggests postoperative bleeding from an arteriovenous fistula or pseudoaneurysm. Although a CT scan with intravenous contrast may help to diagnose and localize a postoperative bleed, this will ultimately delay treatment. Immediate renal angiogram with selective arterial embolization allows for diagnosis, localization, and definitive treatment in the same setting.

CHAPTER REVIEW

1. Minimally invasive renal surgery provides less incisional pain, shorter convalescence, and better cosmesis compared to open surgery, with comparable efficacy and long-term outcomes.
2. The indications for minimally invasive renal surgery are generally similar to those for open renal surgery.
3. The basic principles of oncologic surgery, including complete tumor excision with negative margins associated with maximization of renal parenchyma preservation when feasible, should be followed when using minimally invasive approaches to treat renal tumors.
4. Familiarity with the anatomic landmarks, surgical techniques, and instrumentation and knowledge of each procedure and its potential pitfalls are key for successful minimally invasive surgery.

103 Nonsurgical Focal Therapy for Renal Tumors

Chad R. Tracy and Jeffrey A. Cadeddu

QUESTIONS

1. Nephron-sparing surgery (partial nephrectomy):
   a. is the predominant treatment modality used in the United States for the management of small renal masses.
   b. offers equivalent cancer-specific and overall survival compared with radical nephrectomy.
   c. when performed laparoscopically, it is associated with fewer complications than radiofrequency ablation (RFA) or cryoablation.
   d. offers metastatic recurrence-free survival and cancer-specific survival similar to that of radiofrequency ablation and cryoablation.
   e. was not impacted by the advent of hand-assisted laparoscopic radical nephrectomy.

2. With regard to deciding on a particular ablation modality, which of the following should be considered?
   a. RFA is associated with less postoperative hemorrhage than cryoablation.
   b. Both RFA and cryoablation are subject to "heat sink."
   c. The American Urological Association (AUA) guidelines currently recommend consideration of ablation for primary treatment of T1a renal tumors, even for younger, healthier patients, with the understanding that recurrence rates may be higher and salvage procedure more difficult.
   d. All of the above.
   e. Both a and b are true.

3. The critical treatment temperature threshold during cryoablation at which irreparable cell damage is achieved is:
   a. $0°C$.
   b. $-60°C$.
   c. $-20°C$.
   d. $-40°C$.
   e. $-19.4°C$.

4. Critical parameters for successful renal cryosurgery include:
   a. a double freeze-thaw cycle.
   b. achieving a critical target temperature.
   c. treatment under real-time image guidance.
   d. treatment to beyond 1 cm of the targeted lesion.
   e. all of the above.

5. Compared with renal cryoablation, the primary disadvantage of RFA is:
   a. higher risk of hemorrhage following RFA.
   b. inability to use RFA laparoscopically.
   c. inability to monitor treatment under image guidance.
   d. inferior cancer-specific survival.
   e. none of the above.

6. Recent meta-analyses have demonstrated:
   a. higher local recurrence rates with ablative technologies when compared with partial or radical nephrectomy.
   b. no evidence for the superiority of one ablation technology versus the other with regard to oncologic outcomes or complications.
   c. a lack of uniformity regarding evaluation, patient selection, treatment, and follow-up of patients undergoing renal tumor ablation.
   d. fewer complications with renal tumor ablation compared with extirpative treatments.
   e. all of the above.

7. The most important technique to increase the size of RF lesions is:
   a. using higher RF currents.
   b. applying RF currents faster to achieve better heating.
   c. clamping hilar vessels.
   d. reducing impedance by improving current conductivity.
      using "dry" RFA.

8. Compared to radiofrequency ablation and cryoablation, newer technologies may have which of the following advantages?
   a. High-intensity focused ultrasound (HIFU) requires no percutaneous needle placement, yet results in equivalent oncologic outcomes.
   b. Irreversible electroporation (IRE) has a potential advantage for treating central tumors due to its nonthermal mechanism that preserves tissue scaffolding, large blood vessels, and urothelium.
   c. Microwave ablation works through a similar mechanism to RFA and is therefore similarly limited by tissue charring and heat sink.
   d. Stereotactic body radiation therapy (SBRT) is highly effective at treating renal cell carcinoma but is limited due to mobility of the kidney with respiration.
   e. Routine use of selective embolization has consistently demonstrated improved outcomes for ablation of all renal mass, regardless of location.

9. Following tumor ablation, the most reliable method of documenting treatment success is:
   a. biopsy of the treatment area with hematoxylin and eosin (H&E) staining.
   b. biopsy of the treatment area with reduced nicotinamide adenine dinucleotide (NADH) diaphorase staining.
   c. follow-up computed tomography (CT) or magnetic resonance imaging (MRI) with contrast that demonstrates complete loss of contrast enhancement and stable or decreased size of the treated area.
   d. follow-up CT or MRI without contrast that demonstrates a decrease in size of the treated area.
   e. all of the above.

ANSWERS

1. **d. Offers metastatic recurrence-free survival and cancer-specific survival similar to that of radiofrequency ablation and cryoablation.** Nephron-sparing surgery is considered the gold-standard treatment for small renal masses but is underused in the United States. Partial nephrectomy offers equivalent oncologic outcomes when compared with radical nephrectomy and demonstrates superior renal functional preservation. Laparoscopic partial nephrectomy offers excellent cancer-specific end points but is technically challenging and is associated with significant complications. Cryoablation and radiofrequency ablation are associated with significantly fewer complications than laparoscopic partial nephrectomy. There is no significant difference in metastatic recurrence free survival between extirpative and ablative treatments. Cancer-specific survival (CSS) following RFA is comparable to laparoscopic partial nephrectomy. CSS is comparable between open partial nephrectomy and both RFA and cryoablation. Preliminary studies suggest that the technical ease and minimal morbidity of hand-assisted laparoscopic nephrectomy may ultimately lead to fewer nephron-sparing procedures.

2. **e. Both a and b are true.**

3. **d. –40°C.** Experimental evidence suggests that irreversible cellular damage is achieved in normal renal parenchyma at –19.4°C. However, tumor cells require lower treatment temperatures to achieve uniform cellular necrosis. The recommended treatment temperature during renal cryosurgery is –40°C.

4. **e. All of the above.** Animal studies have demonstrated that a single freeze-thaw cycle is inferior to a double freeze-thaw cycle with respect to adequacy of tissue ablation and local tumor control. As mentioned, complete cellular necrosis is consistently achieved at a targeted temperature of –40°C. Campbell and colleagues (1998)[a] demonstrated that the aforementioned threshold temperature of –40°C was achieved 3.1 mm inside the edge of the evolving ice ball. To guarantee that the tumor is completely ablated with a margin of normal tissue, the ice ball is generally carried 5 to 10 mm beyond the edge of the tumor when viewed under real-time imaging.

5. **c. Inability to monitor treatment under image guidance.** The primary disadvantage when employing RFA for the treatment of renal lesions is difficulty in monitoring treatment under real-time image guidance. The risk of hemorrhage is higher with cryoablation. RFA may be employed laparoscopically, percutaneously, or openly. Cancer-specific survival is equivalent between RFA and cryoablation.

6. **e. All of the above.** Three recent meta-analyses evaluated outcomes following partial nephrectomy, radical nephrectomy, cryoablation, and RFA for the treatment of small renal masses. Both RFA and cryoablation demonstrated higher local recurrence rates when compared with partial or radical nephrectomy. However, the majority of published studies on cryoablation and RFA have enrolled small numbers of patients and used disparate operative and follow-up protocols. The pathology is either not obtained or is difficult to interpret, and the reliability of radiographic imaging remains unknown. Although the aggregate duration of follow-up is too short to derive irrefutable conclusions, treatment outcomes with cryoablation and RFA appear comparable. In general, complications occur with equal or less frequency with tumor ablation when compared with partial or radical nephrectomy.

7. **d. Reducing impedance by improving current conductivity.** The electrically conductive agent facilitates the delivery of energy from the electrode to surrounding tissue, rendering it a much larger, "virtual" electrode. Impedance remains lower, and larger volumes are ablated. One technique to accomplish this is to employ saline-cooled electrodes, which reduce charring at the tip of the electrode and thereby reduce impedance.

8. **b. Irreversible electroporation (IRE) has a potential advantage for treating central tumors due to its nonthermal mechanism that preserves tissue scaffolding, large blood vessels, and urothelium.** IRE is produced through a series of electrical pulses delivered by a single (bipolar) or multiple (monopolar) electrodes. With appropriate modulation it is able to ablate a substantial and reproducible amount of tissue by increasing cell membrane permeability that ultimately leads to cell death. Because it is nonthermal, studies have confirmed its ability to spare the urothelium and larger blood vessels.

9. **c. Follow-up computed tomography (CT) or magnetic resonance imaging (MRI) with contrast that demonstrates complete loss of contrast enhancement and stable or decreased size of the treated area.** Complete loss of contrast enhancement on follow-up CT or MRI has been considered a sign of complete tissue destruction. Following cryoablation, the treated area demonstrates a decrease in size of approximately 50% in the year following treatment. Following RFA, the treated area may not demonstrate a decrease in size. Any increase in size following treatment should be viewed as an ominous sign, and intervention should be directed accordingly. Postablative biopsy, although helpful, yields ambiguous results following RFA. Its use and interpretation remain controversial.

CHAPTER REVIEW

1. Currently, a double freeze-thaw cycle is suggested for cryotherapy with a period of time during each cycle in which the temperature is maintained at –40°C.
2. Radiofrequency waves generate heat by causing ionic agitation in the tissue through which they pass; charring at the probe tip prevents adequate conduction of the wave from the probe into tissue; to prevent heat at the probe becoming excessive with resultant charring, the probes are cooled.
3. CT or MRI is used to follow patients after ablative therapy. There should be a complete lack of contrast enhancement at the tumor site. Successful cryoablation on follow-up imaging often reveals up to a 50% reduction in size of the lesion. RF ablation followed over the long term often shows a slight reduction in size and cavitation.
4. The tumor should be biopsied to confirm its malignant nature before ablative therapy is performed.
5. The most common complication following cryoablation is hemorrhage; a serious complication following radiofrequency ablation is ureteral/collecting system injury. Bleeding is less common following radiofrequency ablation.
6. High-intensity focused ultrasonography generates heat by focusing the ultrasound waves at a point; unfortunately, skin burns are a common complication of this technology.
7. There is no significant difference in metastatic recurrence-free survival between extirpative and ablative treatments. Cancer-specific survival (CSS) following RFA is comparable to laparoscopic partial nephrectomy. CSS is comparable between open partial nephrectomy and both RFA and cryoablation.

104 Treatment of Advanced Renal Cell Carcinoma

Ramaprasad Srinivasan and W. Marston Linehan

QUESTIONS

1. What is the approximate overall objective response rate to interleukin-2 (IL-2) monotherapy in patients with metastatic renal cell carcinoma (RCC)?
   a. 5%
   b. 10%
   c. 15%
   d. 25%
   e. 35%

2. Which of the following regarding IL-2 therapy for metastatic RCC is TRUE?
   a. IL-2 has demonstrable efficacy in clear cell as well as papillary RCC.
   b. Randomized studies have demonstrated a survival benefit associated with high-dose IL-2.
   c. Low-dose subcutaneous and high-dose intravenous IL-2 have comparable efficacy.
   d. Durable complete responses are seen in a small proportion of patients receiving high-dose IL-2.
   e. Newer formulations have led to better tolerability of high-dose IL-2.

3. In the Memorial Sloan-Kettering Cancer Center (MSKCC) prognostic scheme for patients with metastatic RCC undergoing therapy with cytokine or chemotherapy, which of the following is NOT a predictor of poor outcome?
   a. Karnofsky performance status greater than 80%
   b. Elevated lactate dehydrogenase
   c. Elevated calcium
   d. Decreased hemoglobin
   e. Interval from diagnosis to systemic therapy initiation of <1 year

4. A 50-year-old man with a 12-cm left renal renal mass, identified on a CT scan to evaluate abdominal pain, is referred for further management. He is otherwise healthy except for mild fatigue that has developed over the past 3 months; laboratory evaluation reveals a hemoglobin of 9.8 mg/dL and an elevated corrected calcium (10.8 mg/dL) but an otherwise normal chemistry panel and complete blood count. A CT scan of the chest reveals multiple pulmonary nodules consistent with metastatic disease. A biopsy of the renal mass reveals clear cell RCC, Fuhrman grade 3. Which of the following is true with regard to surgical management of this patient?
   a. Cytoreductive nephrectomy should be performed since this patient appears to be otherwise healthy with a good performance status.
   b. Systemic therapy should be offered to this patient since he is unlikely to benefit from cytoreductive nephrectomy.
   c. Sytemic therapy should be commenced, with cytoreductive nephrectomy after six cycles of sunitinib.
   d. The patient has high-risk disease and should commence therapy with everolimus.

5. Which of the following statements about cytokine therapy for metastatic renal cell carcinoma is TRUE?
   a. Lymphokine-activated killer (LAK) cells augment the efficacy of both interferon-α (IFN-α) and IL-2.
   b. Randomized trials have demonstrated a significant survival advantage for combined IL-2 and interferon versus either agent given as monotherapy.
   c. The combination of IL-2 and interferon leads to higher overall response rates than either agent alone.
   d. The complete response rate with interferon-α monotherapy is 10%.

6. Which of the following metastatic RCC tumors is most likely to benefit from cytokine therapy?
   a. Papillary carcinoma
   b. Clear cell carcinoma
   c. Medullary carcinoma
   d. Collecting duct carcinoma
   e. Chromophobe carcinoma

7. A 58-year-old woman had a nephrectomy 6 years previously for a grade 2 clear cell carcinoma. She was incidentally found to have three left-sided pulmonary nodules (two <1.0 cm, other 2.5 cm). A physical examination is normal, as are all blood chemistries. Computed tomography (CT) of the brain, lungs, abdomen, and pelvis show three pulmonary nodules with no associated hilar or mediastinal adenopathy, and a bone scan is normal. Which of the following is the most appropriate next step in her management?
   a. Therapy with high-dose IL-2
   b. Biopsy of a pulmonary nodule
   c. Mediastinoscopy followed by resection of the pulmonary nodules
   d. Observation
   e. IFN-α therapy

8. The sirolimus analogs temsirolimus and everolimus act primarily on which of the following pathways?
   a. Vascular endothelial growth factor (VEGF)
   b. Platelet-derived growth factor (PDGF)
   c. Raf-1
   d. Mechanistic target of rapamycin (mTOR)
   e. C-met

9. The overall response rate in metastatic clear cell RCC patients receiving front-line therapy nivolumab in combination with ipilimumab is:
   a. 15% to 20%.
   b. 30% to 40%.
   c. 60% to 70%.
   d. less than 10%.
   e. greater than 70%.

10. A newly diagnosed patient with metastatic clear cell RCC is referred for discussion of systemic therapy options. You

determine that he has intermediate risk disease based on standard prognostic criteria and that systemic therapy should be commenced. Which of the following decisions would be supported by data from randomized phase 3 studies?

a. Sunitinib is the most appropriate choice for initial treatment of this patient

b. Initiate therapy with a combination of nivolumab and ipilimumab since it is associated with better response rates and overall survival compared with sunitinib

c. Initiate therapy with a combination of pazopanib and nivolumab

d. Initiate therapy with a combination of lenvatinib and everolimus

11. Which of the following agents has been shown to prolong progression-free survival in patients with metastatic clear cell RCC who have progressed on first-line therapy with VEGFR antagonists?

a. Axitinib

b. Bevacizumab + IFN-α

c. High-dose IL-2

d. Bevacizumab

e. Low-dose subcutaneous IL-2

12. Randomized trials in patients with previously untreated metastatic clear cell RCC have demonstrated that:

a. the combination of pembrolizumab and axitinib is associated with better overall survival compared to sunitinib.

b. the combination of avelumab in combination with axitinib is associated with better progression free survival compared to sunitinib.

c. cabozantinib is associated with a better response rate and progression free survival compared to sunitinib.

d. all of the above.

e. none of the above.

13. Which of the following agents has been shown in randomized phase 3 trials to prolong survival in "poor-risk" metastatic RCC patients?

a. IL-2

b. Sunitinib

c. Sorafenib

d. Temsirolimus

e. IFN-α

14. Which of the following molecules is not known to be up-regulated as a consequence of VHL inactivation in clear cell RCC?

a. VEGF

b. PDGF

c. TGF-α

d. Glut-1

e. Raf-1

15. In what proportion of sporadic clear cell tumors are mutations or promoter hypermethylation of the *VHL* gene seen?

a. 70% to 90%

b. 10% to 20%

c. 100%

d. Less than 10%

16. A 47-year-old man presents with multiple metastatic lesions to the lungs and liver 8 months following a radical nephrectomy

for a 9-cm papillary type I renal tumor. Which of the following statements about his systemic treatment options is TRUE?

a. Sunitinib is associated with a 30% to 40% overall RECIST response rate in this subtype of RCC.

b. Sorafenib is associated with better long-term outcomes than sunitinib in papillary type I RCC.

c. mTOR inhibitors improve survival in patients with metastatic papillary RCC.

d. Enrollment in a phase 2 trial evaluating a novel inhibitor of MET activity is a reasonable consideration in this patient.

ANSWERS

1. **c. 15%.** Although response rates of 30% or more were reported in early phase 2 studies with IL-2, the overall response rate with this agent was determined to be approximately 15% in larger studies and meta-analysis.

2. **d. Durable complete responses are seen in a small proportion of patients receiving high-dose IL-2.** Complete responses are seen in 7% to 9% of metastatic clear cell RCC patients receiving high-dose IL-2, with the majority of these remaining disease-free for more than 15 years. The efficacy of IL-2 has not been adequately evaluated in patients with non–clear cell histologies, and the use of this agent is largely restricted to clear cell RCC patients. There are no randomized phase 3 studies demonstrating survival benefit with IL-2. While IL-2 use is limited in current clinical practice, it may be considered in well-selected patients because of its ability to provide durable responses in some patients.

3. **a. Karnofsky performance status greater than 80%.** A Karnofsky performance score below 80% was determined to be an adverse prognostic feature and is one of the factors used to predict outcome in the MSKCC prognostic system for patients with metastatic RCC. All other factors listed have been associated with poor outcome.

4. **b. Systemic therapy should be offered to this patient since he is unlikely to benefit from cytoreductive nephrectomy.** This patient has multiple poor prognostic indicators and is not likely to benefit from cytoreductive nephrectomy. While data from a randomized phase 3 study conducted in the era of cytokine therapy, as well as retrospective data in patients receiving therapy with VEGFR-targeted agents, suggest a benefit for cytoreductive nephrectomy in well-selected patients, a recent phase 3 study that randomized newly diagnosed intermediate and poor-risk patients with metastatic clear cell RCC to receive either cytoreductive nephrectomy followed by sunitinib or sunitinib alone (CARMENA) demonstrated no benefit for surgery preceding systemic therapy. There are insufficient data to support routine cytoreductive nephrectomy following suntinib; a study evaluating this approach (SURTIME) was closed early because of slow accrual. Everolimus is not appropriate in the front-line setting.

5. **c. The combination of IL-2 and interferon leads to higher overall response rates than either agent alone.** In a randomized phase 3 study, the combination of IL-2 and interferon was associated with a higher response rate than either agent given alone, although this did not translate to an improved long-term outcome (overall survival) in the combination arm. The addition of LAK cells to cytokine therapy does not appear to improve outcome.

6. **b. Clear cell carcinoma.** Clear cell RCC is the histology most likely to respond to cytokine therapy. Although there are inadequate data to make definitive determinations about the activity of cytokines such as IL-2 or interferons in other histologic subtypes, these agents do not appear particularly effective in non–clear cell RCC variants.

7. **c. Mediastinoscopy followed by resection of the pulmonary nodules.** Patients with metachronous pulmonary nodules related to remote renal tumors may have prolonged survival following resection of the nodule(s) as demonstrated by several retrospective studies.
8. **d. Mechanistic target of rapamycin (mTOR).** mTOR (mammalian target of rapamycin) is the primary target of sirolimus (rapamycin) and its analogs.
9. **b. 30% to 40%.** Objective overall response rates in metastatic clear cell RCC patients treated with nivolumab in combination with ipilimumab was 42% in a randomized phase 3 study comparing this combination with sunitinib.
10. **b. Initiate therapy with a combination of nivolumab and ipilimumab since it is associated with better response rates and overall survival compared with sunitinib.** Nivolumab, in combination with ipilimumab, was superior to sunitinib in patients with previously untreated metastatic clear cell RCC. Sunitinib is no longer considered the standard of care in these patients. Lenvatinib plus everolimus has not been evaluated in this setting, and the combination of pazopanib and a PD1 inhibitor is deemed to have an unacceptable side effect profile.
11. **a. Axitinib.** In a randomized phase 3 trial, axitinib has been shown to prolong progression free survival compared with sorafenib in patients with metastatic clear cell RCC who have progressed on front-line therapy with either a VEGFR inhibitor or cytokine therapy.
12. **d. All of the above.** In separate randomized phase 3 studies, axitinib, in combination with either pembrolizumab or avelumab, was shown to be superior to sunitinib in previously untreated patients with metastatic clear cell RCC. Cabozantinib was associated with a higher response rate and PFS compared with sunitinib in patients with intermediate or poor-risk prognostic features in a randomized phase 2 study.
13. **d. Temsirolimus.** In a randomized phase 3 study, temsirolimus was associated with better overall survival than IFN-α (median 10.9 vs. 7.3 months) in metastatic RCC patients presenting with three or more predefined factors predictive of poor prognosis.
14. **e. Raf-1.** Raf-1 is a mediator of growth factor signaling pathways but has not been shown to be upregulated in RCC as a consequence of VHL inactivation/HIF upregulation.
15. **a. 70% to 90%.** Based on numerous recent studies, it is estimated that VHL inactivation by mutation or promoter hypermethylation occurs in 70% to 90% of clear cell renal tumors.
16. **d. Enrollment in a phase 2 trial evaluating a novel inhibitor of MET activity is a reasonable consideration in this patient.** There is no conclusive evidence suggesting that standard agents with activity in clear cell RCC (including VEGF pathway inhibitors and mTOR inhibitors) have a favorable impact on outcome in patients with metastatic papillary RCC, and patients with these tumors are appropriate candidates for rational targeted therapy approaches. The presence of activating c-met mutations in some papillary tumors has kindled interest in the evaluation of *Met* pathway antagonists in this patient population.

CHAPTER REVIEW

1. Two randomized studies have demonstrated improved survival in carefully selected metastatic RCC patients undergoing cytoreductive nephrectomy followed by cytokine therapy (IFN-α) compared with those receiving cytokine therapy alone.
2. Several patient and/or disease characteristics appear to influence outcome; patients with poor performance status, comorbid medical conditions, rapidly progressive disease, presence of brain metastases, and so on, are unlikely to benefit from this approach.
3. Although several retrospective studies suggested that cytoreductive nephrectomy may be of benefit in the era of VEGFR-targeted therapy, a randomized study failed to demonstrate an advantage in intermediate and poor prognosis patients. These data, however, do not specifically address the utility of nephrectomy in patients with relatively low metastatic burden and other favorable features, who may benefit from this approach.
4. It is our current practice to offer cytoreductive nephrectomy to well-selected patients with metastatic clear cell RCC
5. Resection of isolated metastatic lesions is appropriate in selected patients.
6. Several retrospective studies have suggested that patients undergoing complete resection of isolated metastatic foci may experience long disease-free intervals, with median overall survival rates of 35% to 50% in some reports.
7. Several factors are associated with an improved outcome after metastasectomy, including complete resection, presence of solitary metastatic lesions, age younger than 60 years, smaller tumor size, presence of pulmonary metastases, and development of metachronous metastatic disease.
8. There are no prospective, randomized studies demonstrating a favorable outcome with metastasectomy. It is therefore possible that the favorable outcome after resection of limited metastatic disease may be a reflection of patient selection bias, differences in tumor biology and natural history, or other confounding factors not related to resection.
9. In some patients with advanced RCC, cytoreductive nephrectomy may help alleviate symptoms related to the primary tumor (e.g., intractable pain, hematuria) or paraneoplastic manifestations.
10. However, nonsurgical options are often effective in palliating symptoms associated with RCC; cytoreductive nephrectomy is hence infrequently performed with purely palliative intent.
11. Resection of metastatic lesions (often in combination with radiation or systemic therapy) is sometimes performed for relief of symptoms or to prevent life-threatening or disabling sequelae.

105   Surgical and Radiographic Anatomy of the Adrenals

Ravi Munver and John Stites

QUESTIONS

1. Which of the following statements is (are) TRUE?
   a. The weight of each of the glands is approximately 10 g.
   b. The adrenal glands are in close proximity to the crus of the diaphragm.
   c. The right gland is crescentic in shape.
   d. The left adrenal gland lies adjacent to the splenic vessels.
   e. Both b and d.

2. Which of the following statements is (are) TRUE?
   a. The right renal vein is longer than the left renal vein.
   b. The right adrenal vein is longer than the left adrenal vein.
   c. The right kidney is typically located lower in the retroperitoneum than the left kidney.
   d. The right adrenal gland is typically located higher in the retroperitoneum than the left adrenal gland.
   e. Both c and d.

3. The adrenal arteries are branches from:
   a. the aorta.
   b. the inferior phrenic arteries.
   c. the renal arteries.
   d. the celiac arterial trunk.
   e. a, b, and c.

4. In cases of renal ectopia, the ipsilateral adrenal gland is typically:
   a. absent.
   b. found in its normal anatomic position in the upper retroperitoneum.
   c. found in association with the contralateral adrenal gland.
   d. found closely applied to the superior pole of the ectopic kidney.
   e. found closely associated with the ipsilateral renal artery.

5. In cases of unilateral renal agenesis, the ipsilateral adrenal gland is commonly:
   a. absent.
   b. found in its normal anatomic position in the upper retroperitoneum.
   c. found in association with the contralateral adrenal gland.
   d. found just inside the ipsilateral internal inguinal ring.
   e. found in an ectopic, intrathoracic location.

6. As one proceeds outward from the adrenal medulla, the three separate functional layers of the adrenal cortex, in correct order, are:
   a. zona reticularis, zona fasciculata, and zona glomerulosa.
   b. zona fasciculata, zona reticularis, and zona glomerulosa.
   c. zona glomerulosa, zona fasciculata, and zona reticularis.
   d. zona glomerulosa, zona reticularis, and zona fasciculata.
   e. zona reticularis, zona glomerulosa, and zona fasciculata.

7. Which of the following statements is (are) FALSE?
   a. The adrenal medulla produces catecholamines in response to stimulation from the sympathetic nervous system.
   b. The zona glomerulosa produces aldosterone in response to angiotensin II.
   c. The zona fasciculata of the adrenal cortex produces glucocorticoids in response to adrenocorticotropic hormone (ACTH).
   d. The zona reticularis of the adrenal cortex produces androgens in response to luteinizing hormone (LH).
   e. Both b and c.

8. Which of the following statements is TRUE?
   a. Ultrasound imaging cannot differentiate between solid and cystic masses of the adrenal gland.
   b. Contrast resolution of magnetic resonance imaging (MRI) is inferior to that of computed tomography (CT) in enabling differentiation of adrenal masses.
   c. CT is the most widely used modality for imaging the adrenal glands.
   d. Normal adrenal tissue has a density of greater than 10 Hounsfield units on noncontrast CT imaging.
   e. MRI, via T1-weighted and T2-weighted images, can provide functional data about adrenal masses.

ANSWERS

1. **e. Both b and d.** Both adrenal glands are in close proximity to the crus of the diaphragm. The left adrenal gland is in contact with the medial aspect of the upper pole of the left kidney. The adjacent structures include the splenic vessels and body of the pancreas anteriorly, the aorta medially, and the psoas muscle posteriorly.

2. **e. Both c and d.** The right kidney is typically located lower in the retroperitoneum than the left kidney. The right adrenal gland lies more superiorly in the retroperitoneum than the left adrenal gland.

3. **e. a, b, and c.** The three main adrenal arteries each branch into cascades of 10 to 50 smaller arteries, which then supply each adrenal gland. The three major arterial sources for each gland are: (1) superior branches from the inferior phrenic artery, (2) middle branches directly from the aorta, and (3) inferior branches from the ipsilateral renal artery.

4. **b. Found in its normal anatomic position in the upper retroperitoneum.** In cases of renal ectopia, the adrenal gland is usually found in approximately its normal anatomic position.

5. **b. Found in its normal anatomic position in the upper retroperitoneum.** In cases of renal agenesis, the adrenal gland on the involved side is typically present.

6. **a. Zona reticularis, zona fasciculata, and zona glomerulosa.** The adult adrenal gland consists of an outer cortex, which makes up approximately 90% of the adrenal mass, and an inner medulla. The adrenal cortex consists of three concentric zones: the outer zona glomerulosa comprising approximately 15% of the cortex, the middle zona fasciculata 80% of the cortex, and the inner zona reticularis 5% to 7% of the cortex. The zona glomerulosa produces aldosterone, zona fasciculata produces glucocorticoids, and zona reticularis produces sex steroids.

7. **d. The zona reticularis of the adrenal cortex produces androgens in response to luteinizing hormone (LH).** The production of androgen by the zona reticularis is regulated by pituitary release of ACTH.

8. **c. CT is the most widely used modality for imaging the adrenal glands.** Ultrasound imaging can be used to differentiate between solid and cystic adrenal masses. Normal adrenal tissue has a density of less than or equal to 10 Hounsfield units (HU) on noncontrast CT imaging. MRI, via T1-weighted and T2-weighted images, is superior to CT and enables differentiation of adrenal masses. Although CT and MRI provide excellent morphologic information, these studies cannot provide functional data.

CHAPTER REVIEW

1. The adrenals are enclosed within the Gerota fascia.
2. The right adrenal vein is short and enters the vena cava posterolaterally.
3. Adrenal rests are found in proximity to the celiac axis and along the path of gonadal descent. In patients with congenital adrenal hyperplasia, adrenal rests along the spermatic cord may become quite large.
4. The right kidney is typically located lower in the retroperitoneum than the left kidney. The right adrenal gland lies more superiorly in the retroperitoneum than the left adrenal gland. Both adrenal glands are in close proximity to the crus of the diaphragm.
5. In cases of renal ectopia, the adrenal gland is usually found in approximately its normal anatomic position.
6. The zona glomerulosa produces aldosterone, the zona fasciculata produces glucocorticoids, and the zona reticularis produces sex steroids.
7. The production of androgen by the zona reticularis is regulated by pituitary release of adrenocorticotropic hormone (ACTH).
8. Normal adrenal tissue has a density of less than or equal to 10 Hounsfield units (HU) on noncontrast CT imaging.

106 Pathophysiology, Evaluation, and Medical Management of Adrenal Disorders

Alexander Kutikov, Paul L. Crispen, and Robert G. Uzzo

QUESTIONS

1. At birth the adrenal cortex:
   a. is completely developed.
   b. weighs half as much as the adrenal cortex in adults.
   c. is composed of fetal and adult components.
   d. will continue to enlarge until 12 months of age.
   e. is composed of a single histologic zone.

2. Adrenal rest tissue within the testis can mimic testicular cancer in patients with:
   a. neuroblastoma.
   b. pheochromocytoma.
   c. primary aldosteronism.
   d. congenital adrenal hyperplasia.
   e. cryptorchidism.

3. In cases of renal agenesis, the ipsilateral adrenal gland is typically:
   a. absent.
   b. in the normal location.
   c. located at the level of the eighth thoracic vertebral body.
   d. located at the level of the first lumbar vertebral body.
   e. at a location dependent on the cause of renal agenesis.

4. The most abundant product of the adrenal cortex is:
   a. mineralocorticoids.
   b. glucocorticoids.
   c. adrenal androgens.
   d. catecholamines.
   e. adrenocorticotropic hormone (ACTH).

5. Aldosterone synthase (CYP11B2) is unique to:
   a. the zona glomerulosa.
   b. the zona fasciculata.
   c. the zona reticularis.
   d. the adrenal medulla.
   e. the distal renal tubule.

6. The only zone of the adrenal cortex that does not atrophy upon pituitary failure is:
   a. the zona glomerulosa.
   b. the zona fasciculata.
   c. the zona reticularis.
   d. the adrenal medulla.
   e. none of the above.

7. Presence of the phenylethanolamine-*N*-methyltransferase (PNMT) enzyme in the adrenal medulla is significant because:
   a. the enzyme catalyzes degradation of catecholamines to metanephrines.
   b. the enzyme catalyzes conversion of catecholamines to vanillylmandelic acid (VMA).
   c. the enzyme converts tyrosine to dopamine.
   d. the enzyme catalyzes the conversion of norepinephrine to epinephrine.
   e. all of the above.

8. Metanephrines:
   a. refers to the term used for catecholamines and their byproducts.
   b. refers to the combined term for methylated metabolites of norepinephrine (normetanephrine) and epinephrine (metanephrine).
   c. refers to precursors to normetanephrines.
   d. are rarely helpful in establishing a diagnosis of pheochromocytoma.
   e. refers to the term used to describe epinephrine and norepinephrine in the context of pheochromocytoma symptomatology.

9. The term *free metanephrines*:
   a. is interchangeable with the term *total metanephrines*.
   b. is interchangeable with the term *fractionated metanephrines*.
   c. refers to normetanephrine and metanephrine that are not conjugated by a sulfate moiety.
   d. refers to normetanephrine and metanephrine that are not bound to albumin.
   e. refers to all of the above.

10. The most common cause of Cushing syndrome (exclusive of exogenous steroid intake) is:
    a. Cushing disease.
    b. a cortisol-producing adrenal adenoma.
    c. ectopic ACTH production by a lung malignancy.
    d. an adrenal carcinoma.
    e. a pheochromocytoma.

11. What common urologic ailment can be found in up to 50% of patients with Cushing syndrome?
    a. Testicular cancer
    b. Torsion of the appendix testis
    c. Urolithiasis
    d. Fournier gangrene
    e. Stress urinary incontinence

12. How does one perform a low-dose dexamethasone suppression test (LDDST)?
    a. Admit the patient and measure serum cortisol levels every 6 hours while the patient is on a dexamethasone drip
    b. Measure the patient's saliva cortisol level at midnight
    c. Obtain a 24-hour urine cortisol measurement after the patient receives 1 mg of dexamethasone with the first void
    d. Have the patient take 10 mg of dexamethasone at 11 PM and measure urinary cortisol the next morning
    e. Have the patient take 1 mg of dexamethasone at 11 PM and measure serum cortisol the next morning

13. The adrenal surgeon plays no role in the management of Cushing disease.
    a. True
    b. False

14. What percentage of patients presenting with primary aldosteronism are hypokalemic?
    a. 5% to 12%
    b. 9% to 37%
    c. 33% to 50%
    d. 55% to 75%
    e. 63% to 91%

15. Elevated aldosterone in patients with familial hyperaldosteronism type I is mediated by:
    a. renin.
    b. sodium.
    c. angiotensin II.
    d. cortisol.
    e. ACTH.

16. What percentage of patients with a positive screening test will be diagnosed with primary aldosteronism after confirmatory testing?
    a. 2% to 10%
    b. 20% to 40%
    c. 30% to 50%
    d. 50% to 70%
    e. 75% to 90%

17. What is the most common subtype of primary aldosteronism?
    a. Idiopathic hyperplasia
    b. Aldosterone-producing adenoma
    c. Unilateral adrenal hyperplasia
    d. Familial hyperaldosteronism type I
    e. Adrenocortical carcinoma

18. The primary determinant of potentially surgically correctable primary aldosteronism is:
    a. blood pressure.
    b. patient age.
    c. demonstration of lateralized aldosterone secretion.
    d. response to medical therapy.
    e. plasma aldosterone levels.

19. Which class of antihypertensives is contraindicated during the evaluation of primary aldosteronism?
    a. Calcium channel blockers
    b. Alpha blockers
    c. Beta blockers
    d. Aldosterone-receptor blockers
    e. Angiotensin-converting enzyme inhibitors

20. What percentage of patients with incidental adrenal masses prove to have pheochromocytoma?
    a. 1%
    b. 5%
    c. 10%
    d. 25%
    e. 35%

21. What subtype is assigned to patients with a von Hippel-Lindau (VHL) mutation and a history of pheochromocytoma but no other stigmata of the VHL syndrome?

    a. Type 1
    b. Type 2A
    c. Type 2B
    d. Type 2C
    e. None of the above

22. What genetic abnormality is strongly linked with malignant pheochromocytoma?
    a. *RET* mutation
    b. *VHL* mutation
    c. *SDHB* mutation
    d. *SDHD* mutation
    e. All of the above

23. What test is considered the cornerstone for modern pheochromocytoma biochemical testing?
    a. Plasma catecholamines
    b. Plasma-free metanephrines or fractionated urinary metanephrines
    c. VMA testing
    d. Fasting morning urinary norepinephrine
    e. Adrenal vein sampling for catecholamines

24. With regard to preoperative pheochromocytoma blockade, β-blockers should be started:
    a. 2 weeks prior to adrenalectomy.
    b. at least several days prior to α-blockers.
    c. to control tachycardia and arrhythmias that can result upon initiation of α blockade.
    d. in conjunction with metyrosine.
    e. never, because β-blockers can be lethal in patients with pheochromocytomas.

25. Patients with adrenal crisis can exhibit all of the following symptoms EXCEPT:
    a. hypotension unresponsive to fluid resuscitation.
    b. abdominal pain.
    c. nausea.
    d. fever.
    e. priapism.

26. All of the following lesions can be extra-adrenal EXCEPT:
    a. myelolipoma.
    b. ganglioneuroma.
    c. aldosteronoma.
    d. pheochromocytoma.
    e. oncocytoma.

27. A 25-year-old woman is diagnosed with a left adrenal mass, with abundant stippled calcifications, that exhibits imaging features inconsistent with adrenal adenoma. The patient complains of a severe bout of diarrhea that started approximately 8 months ago. Adrenalectomy reveals a ganglioneuroma. At her postoperative visit she is grateful, because her gastrointestinal (GI) complaints vanished following surgery. The substance responsible for diarrhea in this patient is most likely:
    a. metanephrine.
    b. epinephrine.
    c. norepinephrine.
    d. VMA.
    e. vasoactive intestinal polypeptide (VIP).

28. What percentage of adrenal cysts is associated with malignancy in surgical series?

a. 1%

b. 3%

c. 7%

d. 12%

e. 15%

29. Adrenocortical carcinoma in children:

a. has a more favorable 5-year survival rate compared with adults.

b. uses the same pathologic staging system as adults.

c. is rarely associated with virilization.

d. has equal female and male incidence in children older than 10 years.

e. is frequently metastatic to the central nervous system.

30. The most common hormone secreted by adrenocortical carcinoma is:

a. aldosterone.

b. testosterone.

c. dehydroepiandrosterone (DHEA).

d. cortisol.

e. androstenedione.

31. The Weiss criteria for identifying malignant adrenal tumors should be applied with caution in tumors with:

a. necrosis.

b. high mitotic index.

c. inferior vena cava (IVC) invasion.

d. liver metastasis.

e. oncocytic features.

32. In patients presenting with metastatic adrenocortical carcinoma, the systemic agent of choice is:

a. valrubicin.

b. mitotane alone or in combination with additional cytotoxic agents.

c. gemcitabine and cisplatin.

d. docetaxel (Taxotere).

e. bleomycin, etoposide, and cisplatin.

33. In the treatment of pathologically localized adrenocortical carcinoma:

a. adjuvant radiation therapy decreases systemic progression.

b. complete surgical resection offers the best chance of cure.

c. increased Ki-67 expression has been associated with improved survival.

d. the tumor's functional status is an independent predictor of survival.

e. adjuvant therapy with mitotane has no proven benefit.

34. A 50% false-positive rate can be seen during low-dose dexamethasone suppression testing in:

a. men with testicular cancer.

b. women taking oral contraceptives.

c. men with history of orchiopexy.

d. patients with brain malignancy.

e. patients with pheochromocytoma.

35. The adrenal gland should be resected whenever one performs a radical nephrectomy.

a. True

b. False

36. A 55-year-old woman presents for the evaluation of an adrenal mass. Past medical history is significant for severe hypertension requiring four oral medications for adequate blood pressure control. A noncontrast computed tomography (CT) scan of the abdomen reveals a 3-cm left adrenal mass, with an average attenuation of 7 Hounsfield units (HU). Appropriate initial screening should include:

a. free-fractionated plasma metanephrines, plasma aldosterone concentration, and plasma renin activity.

b. LDDST and serum catecholamines.

c. late-night salivary cortisol test, plasma aldosterone concentration, plasma renin activity, and plasma free metanephrines.

d. plasma aldosterone concentration and plasma renin activity.

e. 24-hour urinary-fractionated metanephrines and serum cortisol concentration.

37. A 62-year-old man presents for postoperative surveillance of renal cell carcinoma. Three years prior, a right nephrectomy was performed for T2N0M0 grade III clear cell renal cell carcinoma. A current abdominal CT scan reveals a 3.5-cm right adrenal mass with an average attenuation of 32 HU prior to contrast administration. A CT washout study is performed, and absolute percent washout is calculated to be 52%. No other suspicious lesions are noted within the chest, abdomen, or pelvis. The next step in management should be:

a. observation.

b. adrenalectomy.

c. percutaneous biopsy.

d. initiation of an oral tyrosine kinase inhibitor.

e. assessment of the adrenal tumor's functional status.

38. A 58-year-old woman has been diagnosed with primary aldosteronism based on appropriate screening and confirmatory testing. A CT scan of the abdomen reveals a 1.0-cm left adrenal mass. Adrenal vein sampling is performed with the results outlined below. Results of adrenal vein sampling:

Right cortisol gradient 2.7:1

Left cortisol gradient 3.4:1

Aldosterone ratio (left:right) 2.5:1

The next step in management would be:

a. repeat adrenal vein sampling with ACTH stimulation.

b. counseling for left adrenalectomy.

c. counseling for right adrenalectomy.

d. initiation of medical management based on diagnosis of bilateral adrenal hyperplasia.

e. ^{131}I-iodomethyl-norcholesterol (NP-59) scintigraphy to confirm lateralization.

39. A 43-year-old woman undergoes an uneventful right laparoscopic adrenalectomy for a 4.5-cm pheochromocytoma. The pathology report states that the lesion is benign and that the margins are negative. On postoperative day 1, she is ready for discharge and wants to know if any additional follow-up is necessary. You inform her that the following is required:

a. Consideration of genetic screening

b. Repeat metabolic testing in 2 weeks

c. Cross-sectional imaging in 6 months

d. Biochemical testing in 6 months and then lifelong biochemical testing

e. All of the above

PATHOLOGY

1. A 60-year-old woman is noted to have a 4-cm left adrenal mass on an abdominal CT scan. The endocrine workup is negative, and the

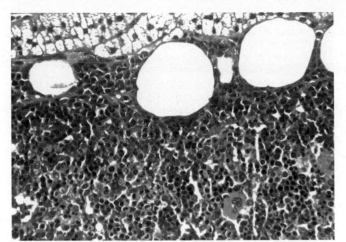

Fig. 106.1 (From Bostwick DG, Cheng L: *Urologic surgical pathology*, ed 2, Edinburgh, 2008, Mosby.)

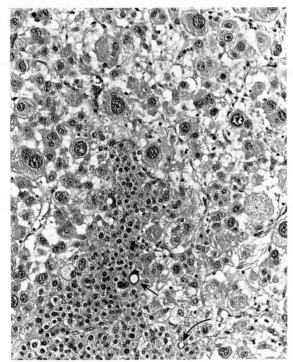

Fig. 106.2 (From Bostwick DG, Cheng L: *Urologic surgical pathology*, ed 2, Edinburgh, 2008, Mosby.)

mass is excised laparoscopically. The pathology, depicted in Fig. 106.1, is reported as a myolipoma. The next step in management is:

a. no additional therapy is indicated because this is a benign tumor.

b. ask the pathologist to grade the tumor.

c. the patient should receive mitotane.

d. the patient should be followed carefully for development of hypertension.

e. a metaiodobenzylguanidine (MIBG) scan should be obtained.

2. A 45-year-old man has an incidentally discovered 6-cm adrenal mass. Hormonal workup is negative. The mass is laparoscopically removed. The pathology is depicted in Fig. 106.2 and is read as adrenal corticocarcinoma. On separate stains the lesion stains positive for Ki-67. The next step in management is:

a. request a pathologic grade.

b. stain for catecholamines.

c. inquire as to whether any fat was observed in the specimen.

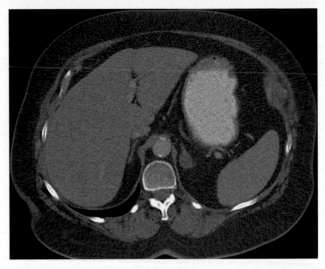

Fig. 106.3

d. short-term follow-up with imaging.

e. adjuvant mitotane.

IMAGING

1. See Fig. 106.3. A 42-year-old man with lung cancer has this CT scan. The right adrenal nodule has attenuation measurements of 7 HU. The most likely diagnosis is:

a. adrenal adenoma.

b. adrenal metastasis.

c. indeterminate adrenal nodule.

d. pheochromocytoma.

e. adrenal myelolipoma.

ANSWERS

1. **c. Is composed of fetal and adult components.** The adrenal gland weighs twice as much as the adult gland and begins to atrophy at birth. Development of the gland continues during the first 3 years of life, with the zona reticularis developing last.

2. **d. Congenital adrenal hyperplasia.** Testicular adrenal rests must be remembered when evaluating patients with congenital adrenal hyperplasia and testicular masses to avoid an unnecessary orchiectomy.

3. **b. In the normal location.** Reports of adrenal agenesis are extremely rare.

4. **c. Adrenal androgens.** Although adrenal androgens are arguably the least physiologically significant compounds produced by the adrenals, the glands produce more than 20 mg of these compounds per day. Meanwhile, only 100 to 150 mcg/d of aldosterone and approximately 10 to 20 mg/d of cortisol are produced by the glands.

5. **a. The zona glomerulosa.** The zona glomerulosa cells are the sole source of aldosterone in humans.

6. **a. The zona glomerulosa.** Production of aldosterone in the zona glomerulosa is primarily regulated by angiotensin II through the renin-angiotensin-aldosterone system and potassium levels. Elevation of ACTH can also increase aldosterone secretion, but this is a much less potent stimulus. Therefore, in pituitary failure, when ACTH levels fall, the zona glomerulosa fails to atrophy.

7. **d. The enzyme catalyzes the conversion of norepinephrine to epinephrine.** PNMT is virtually unique to the adrenal medulla (the brain and organ of Zuckerkandl also express the protein). Therefore the presence of PNMT results in epi-

nephrine being virtually a unique product of the adrenal gland.

8. **b. Refers to the combined term for methylated metabolites of norepinephrine (normetanephrine) and epinephrine (metanephrine).** The enzyme catechol-O-methyltransferase catalyzes the methylation of norepinephrine to normetanephrine and epinephrine to metanephrine. The term *normetanephrines* is not used.

9. **c. Refers to normetanephrine and metanephrine that are not conjugated by a sulfate moiety.** Free metanephrines are unsulfonated normetanephrine and metanephrine, whereas total metanephrines refers to both conjugated and free compounds. The term *fractionated metanephrines* refers to laboratory reports that differentiate between metanephrine and normetanephrine concentrations (i.e., instead of only reporting metanephrine concentration, state the concentration of metanephrine and normetanephrine separately).

10. **a. Cushing disease.** Cushing disease, which describes overproduction of ACTH by the pituitary, accounts for some 70% of endogenous Cushing syndrome.

11. **c. Urolithiasis.** Urolithiasis is seen in up to 50% of patients with Cushing syndrome; therefore stone formers with cushingoid features deserve a hypercortisolemia workup. The astute urologist should also remember that Cushing patients can also exhibit hypogonadal hypogonadism and should have a low threshold for a hypercortisolism workup in men with low testosterone and low gonadotropin levels.

12. **e. Have the patient take 1 mg of dexamethasone at 11 PM and measure serum cortisol the next morning.** Despite its intimidating name and rather complex physiologic underpinnings, the test is remarkably simple to administer. Write the patient a prescription for 1 mg of dexamethasone and ask that it be taken by mouth at 11 PM. The next morning, determine the patient's serum cortisol level. If the cortisol level is 5 mcg/dL or higher (i.e., not suppressed), then the patient likely has hypercortisolemia. Be aware that women on birth control will have false-positive results.

13. **b. False.** ACTH-secreting pituitary adenomas are treated with transsphenoidal surgical resection. However, a cure is seen in only 60% to 80% of patients. Among those who are cured, there is approximately 25% relapse. One option for patients who are refractory to neurosurgical treatment is a bilateral adrenalectomy. However, this treatment should not be performed hastily. It is crucial that a thoughtful multidisciplinary decision be made. Up to 30% of patients with Cushing disease who undergo bilateral adrenalectomy may develop Nelson syndrome—progressive growth of the pituitary adenoma causing increased intracranial pressure and compression of the ocular chiasm.

14. **b. 9% to 37%.** Although hypokalemia has been classically described as a common finding in primary aldosteronism, only 9% to 37% of newly diagnosed patients are hypokalemic.

15. **e. ACTH.** Because of the chimeric fusion of the promoter region of 11β-hydroxylase and the coding region of aldosterone synthase, aldosterone production is mediated by ACTH in familial hyperaldosteronism type I.

16. **d. 50% to 70%.** Fifty percent to 70% of patients with a positive screening test will be diagnosed with primary aldosteronism following confirmatory testing.

17. **a. Idiopathic hyperplasia.** This subtype of primary aldosteronism accounts for approximately 60% of cases.

18. **c. Demonstration of lateralized aldosterone secretion.** Lateralization of aldosterone secretion is the primary determinant of successful surgical treatment of primary aldosteronism.

19. **d. Aldosterone-receptor blockers.** Aldosterone-receptor blockers (spironolactone and eplerenone) are contraindicated during the evaluation of primary aldosteronism. Patients requiring these agents for blood pressure control should be transitioned to other medications during testing for at least 6 weeks.

20. **b. 5%.** Incidentally discovered lesions account for 10% to 25% of all pheochromocytomas.

21. **d. Type 2C.** Type 1 = VHL patient with no evidence or family history of pheochromocytoma. Type 2 patients are those with evidence or family history of pheochromocytoma. Type 2 is further subdivided. Type 2A = patients with concomitant RCC; type 2B = no evidence of renal malignancy; type 2C = patients with pheochromocytoma and evidence of a *VHL* gene mutation but no other stigmata of VHL.

22. **c. *SDHB* mutation.** Patients with multiple endocrine neoplasia (types 2A and 2B) possess a mutation in the *RET* proto-oncogene. Approximately half of these patients develop pheochromocytoma, but only about 3% of those with pheochromocytoma exhibit malignant potential. Ten percent to 20% of patients with VHL develop pheochromocytomas, but only 5% of those with pheochromocytoma have malignant disease. Pheochromocytoma among patients with neurofibromatosis type 1 is rare (1%), but malignant disease can be seen in more than 10%. Familial paraganglioma syndrome type 4 (*SDHB* mutation) carries the highest risk of malignancy (30% to 50%) among patients with the condition who develop pheochromocytoma (≈20%). Its pathologic cousin, familial paraganglioma syndrome type 1 (*SDHD* mutation), carries a negligible risk (<3%) of malignancy among patients who develop pheochromocytomas (≈20%).

23. **b. Plasma-free metanephrines or fractionated urinary metanephrines.** Methylated metabolites of catecholamines are known as *metanephrines*. Therefore normetanephrine (from norepinephrine) and metanephrine (from epinephrine) are collectively known as *metanephrines*. The vast majority of methylation occurs within the adrenal medulla or pheochromocytoma, when present. Because this conversion of catecholamines to metanephrines is an uninterrupted process within pheochromocytomas, testing for these compounds is a much more sensitive means of tumor detection than the measurement of catecholamine levels, which may be paroxysmal. Furthermore, measurement of levels of metanephrines is rather specific. Controversy exists regarding whether measurement of plasma-free metanephrines versus fractionated urinary metanephrine should be used as the initial test. The term "free" indicates that the metanephrines being measured are not conjugated by a sulfate moiety, whereas the term "fractionated" simply indicates that normetanephrine and metanephrine levels are reported as separate values.

24. **c. To control tachycardia and arrhythmias that can result upon initiation of α blockade.** Beta-blockade should never be started prior to appropriate α blockade. In the absence of α blockade, β antagonists cause a potentiation of the action of epinephrine on the $α_1$ receptor, due to blockade of the arteriolar dilation at the $β_2$ receptor. Nevertheless, β blockade is at times necessary to control reflex tachycardia and arrhythmias that can result from α blockade.

25. **e. Priapism.** Patients with adrenal crisis are easily misdiagnosed with an acute abdomen. Children can exhibit hypoglycemic seizures. Persistent painful erections are generally not associated with adrenal insufficiency.

26. **c. Aldosteronoma.** All listed lesions, other than an aldosterone-producing adenoma, can develop outside of the adrenal gland.

27. **e. Vasoactive intestinal polypeptide (VIP).** Ganglioneuromas are rare lesions that can arise in the adrenal glands and can secrete VIP, causing profound diarrhea in some patients. Nevertheless, most ganglioneuromas are asymptomatic.

28. **c. 7%.** In a meta-analysis accounting for 515 adrenal cysts, the incidence of associated adrenal malignancy was 7%.

29. **a. Has a more favorable 5-year survival rate compared with adults.** The 5-year survival rate in children with adrenal cortical carcinoma is 54% compared with only 20% to 47% in adults.

30. **d. Cortisol.** Up to 74% of functional adrenocortical tumors produce excess cortisol.

31. **e. Oncocytic features.** The Weiss criteria should be applied with caution in pediatric cases and in those with oncocytic features.

32. **b. Mitotane alone or in combination with additional cytotoxic agents.** Mitotane has adrenolytic activity and is the first-line agent of choice in patients with metastatic adrenocortical

carcinoma. The addition of streptozotocin or etoposide, doxorubicin, and cisplatin to mitotane has been shown to improve progression free survival compared to the use of mitotane alone.

33. **b. Complete surgical resection offers the best chance of cure.** Adjuvant radiation therapy has demonstrated a decreased rate of local recurrence but has not been shown to improve overall survival. Adjuvant mitotane therapy has been shown to significantly improve recurrence-free and overall survival. A tumor's functional status has not been consistently demonstrated to impact survival.

34. **b. Women taking oral contraceptives.** The urologist must be aware that the LDDST can yield as high as a 50% false-positive rate in women using oral contraceptives, because the contraceptives increase total (but not bioavailable) cortisol levels by raising the patient's cortisol-binding globulin concentrations.

35. **b. False.** The classic description by Robson in the 1950s suggested that radical nephrectomy should include adrenalectomy. Today, however, adrenalectomy is believed to be necessary only for large (T2) upper pole tumors, in cases in which an abnormality in the gland can be seen on preoperative imaging and in cases in which a vein thrombus is present to the level of the adrenal gland.

36. **c. Late-night salivary cortisol test, plasma aldosterone concentration, plasma renin activity, and plasma-free metanephrines.** All patients presenting with an adrenal mass should be evaluated for cortisol and catecholamine hypersecretion. Given the patient's history of hypertension, evaluation of primary aldosteronism should also be undertaken. Choice c is the best answer.

37. **e. Assessment of the adrenal tumor's functional status.** Although there is a high probability that the adrenal lesion, in this case, represents a recurrence of the patient's renal cell carcinoma, the functional status of the adrenal mass should be assessed. A pheochromocytoma may always be lurking.

38. **b. Counseling for left adrenalectomy.** Both the right and left cortisol gradients suggest proper catheter placement for adrenal vein sampling. The aldosterone ratio of 2.5:1 demonstrates left lateralization of autonomous aldosterone secretion, and counseling for left adrenalectomy is appropriate.

39. **e. All of the above.** The patient is less than 50 years old; therefore genetic screening is recommended. Up to 25% of patients who appear to have sporadic pheochromocytoma on presentation turn out to have germline mutations upon genetic testing. Repeat metabolic testing at 2 weeks after resection is prudent. Most experts recommend additional biochemical testing at 6 months, followed by annual lifelong screening. More than 15% of patients will demonstrate recurrence of pheochromocytoma in the first 10 years after a successful resection. Recurrent disease has been reported more than 15 years following adrenalectomy; therefore lifelong annual biochemical screening is advised. Although cross-sectional imaging is not absolutely required in the face of a negative biochemical workup, most surgeons obtain at least one study at some point during the postoperative follow-up.

PATHOLOGY

1. **a. No additional therapy is indicated because this is a benign tumor.** This is a benign myolipoma. Notice that it consists of fat mixed with hematopoietic elements.

2. **d. Short-term follow-up with imaging.** The marked nuclear variability, increased mitotic figures, and positive staining for Ki-67 all strongly suggest adrenal corticocarcinoma. No further pathologic information is necessary. These patients have a high risk of developing metastatic disease, at which time mitotane would be considered.

IMAGING

1. **a. Adrenal adenoma.** Adrenal nodules that are less than 10 HU in density are almost always benign nodules, most often adrenal adenomas.

CHAPTER REVIEW

1. The right adrenal gland is triangular in shape; the left is crescent shaped.
2. The zona glomerulosa secretes mineralocorticoids, the zona fasciculata secretes glucocorticoids, and the zona reticularis secretes sex steroids.
3. The production of cortisol is circadian, with the peak occurring in the early morning and the nadir at 11:00 PM.
4. Adrenal androgens are under the control of ACTH.
5. Ectopic ACTH production almost always originates from malignant tissue.
6. Renin release is stimulated by low renal perfusion pressure, increased renal sympathetic nervous activity, and low sodium.
7. Mineralocorticoid production results in sodium retention and volume expansion initially; however, with continued production, the kidney escapes from the sodium-retentive action of the hormone.
8. Sodium loading reduces endogenous aldosterone and renin production in those patients who do not have autonomous aldosterone secretion from aldosterone producing tumors.
9. The predictors of persistent hypertension following adrenalectomy for primary aldosteronism include (1) age older than 50 years, (2) the requirement for more than two antihypertensive agents preoperatively, (3) a first-degree relative with hypertension, (4) prolonged duration of hypertension prior to adrenalectomy, and (5) renal insufficiency.
10. Ki-67 staining of adrenal tissue is perhaps the best indicator of malignancy.
11. Chromogranin A elevation in the serum has been used as a confirmatory test in patients with pheochromocytoma.
12. Restoration of intravascular volume is the most important component of preoperative preparation in patients with pheochromocytoma.
13. The most frequent cause of adrenal insufficiency in the United States is autoimmune adrenalitis; in developing countries, it is tuberculosis.
14. Patients with congenital adrenal hyperplasia have a high risk for developing benign adrenal corticoadenomas.
15. The Weiss criteria distinguish benign from malignant adrenal tumors. The presence of three or more of the Weiss criteria is associated with malignancy. When oncocytic features are present, the criteria should be used with caution.
16. An attenuation of less than 10 Hounsfield units on unenhanced computed tomography scan is strongly suggestive of an adrenal adenoma.
17. There are four histologic types of adrenal cysts: (1) pseudocyst, (2) endothelial, (3) epithelial, and (4) parasitic.
18. Positron emission tomography (PET) scan is the preferred imaging modality for pheochromocytoma.
19. Pheochromocytomas recur in up to 16% of patients who have had a complete surgical resection; 50% of the recurrences are malignant.
20. Metastases to the adrenal are common.
21. Production of aldosterone in the zona glomerulosa is primarily regulated by angiotensin II through the renin-angiotensin-aldosterone system and potassium levels.
22. Epinephrine is virtually a unique product of the adrenal gland, and when it is the dominant catechol produced by a tumor, an adrenal origin is suggested.

23. Cushing disease is a result of an overproduction of ACTH by the pituitary. It accounts for some 70% of endogenous Cushing syndrome.

24. Urolithiasis is seen in up to 50% of patients with Cushing syndrome.

25. Up to 30% of patients with Cushing disease who undergo bilateral adrenalectomy may develop Nelson syndrome—progressive growth of the pituitary adenoma causing increased intracranial pressure and compression of the ocular chiasm.

26. Although hypokalemia has been classically described as a common finding in primary aldosteronism, only 9%–37% of newly diagnosed patients are hypokalemic

27. Conversion of catecholamines to metanephrines is an uninterrupted process within pheochromocytomas; testing for these compounds is a much more sensitive means for tumor detection than the measurement of catecholamine levels, which may be paroxysmal.

28. Ganglioneuromas are rare lesions that can arise in the adrenal glands and can secrete the vasoactive intestinal polypeptide, causing profound diarrhea in some patients.

29. All patients presenting with an adrenal mass should be evaluated for cortisol and catecholamine hypersecretion.

107 Surgery of the Adrenal Glands

Sey Kiat Lim and Koon Ho Rha

QUESTIONS

1. Which of the following statements regarding the anatomy of the right adrenal gland is TRUE?
   a. Its vein drains into the right renal vein.
   b. It is usually located on the upper pole and lateral border of the right kidney.
   c. The medulla is innervated by preganglionic sympathetic nerve fibers.
   d. It is usually located more caudal than the left adrenal gland and is closely related to the diaphragm.
   e. The right adrenal gland only receives arterial supply from the right renal artery.

2. What is the risk of malignancy in an incidentaloma of more than 6 cm?
   a. 2%
   b. 6%
   c. 10%
   d. 25%
   e. 50%

3. Absolute contraindications to laparoscopic adrenalectomy include:
   a. significant abdominal adhesions.
   b. adrenal mass greater than 12 cm in size.
   c. invasive adrenal cortical carcinoma with thrombus in the inferior vena cava.
   d. malignant pheochromocytoma.
   e. all of the above.

4. Which of the following statements regarding the perioperative management of pheochromocytoma is FALSE?
   a. Preoperative sympatholytic therapy with α-adrenergic blockers should be started for at least 2 weeks before surgery.
   b. Phenoxybenzamine may lead to tachycardia, and β-adrenergic blockade should be started before phenoxybenzamine administration.
   c. Vasopressins and aggressive fluid infusion are often necessary after ligation of the adrenal vein or excision of a pheochromocytoma.
   d. The adrenal vein should be ligated early during surgical excision of a pheochromocytoma.
   e. Intravenous drugs with short half-lives are preferred versus longer-acting drugs for controlling blood pressure fluctuations during surgical excision of a pheochromocytoma.

5. The lumbodorsal posterior approach to open adrenalectomy is not ideal in any of the following circumstances EXCEPT:
   a. large adrenal tumors.
   b. bilateral adrenal hyperplasia.
   c. bilateral small adrenocortical carcinoma.
   d. patients with ventilatory difficulties.
   e. b and c.

6. In bilateral adrenalectomy, steroids replacement should be started:
   a. on induction of general anesthesia.
   b. after ligation of the right adrenal vein.
   c. after excision of both adrenal glands.
   d. during closing of the abdominal incision.
   e. in the recovery room after surgery.

7. A 57-year-old male with no significant medical problems presented with a right-sided abdominal mass. Computed tomographic (CT) imaging showed an 18-cm right adrenal tumor with invasion of the upper pole of the right kidney and tumor thrombus extending into the retrohepatic inferior vena cava. Which is the best surgical approach for this patient?
   a. Open lumbodorsal posterior approach
   b. Open anterior transabdominal approach
   c. Open thoracoabdominal approach
   d. Laparoscopic transperitoneal approach
   e. Robot-assisted laparoscopic transperitoneal approach

8. Which of the following is NOT a possible approach to the left adrenal gland in the anterior transabdominal approach?
   a. Through the gastrocolic ligament
   b. Through the lienorenal ligament
   c. Through the transverse mesocolon
   d. Through the lesser omentum
   e. All the above are possible approaches

9. Which of the following statements on partial adrenalectomy is FALSE?
   a. The adrenal gland is usually exposed but not mobilized.
   b. The arterial supply of the adrenal gland can be ligated without devascularizing the gland.
   c. It is generally safe to ligate the main adrenal vein if the adrenal gland is not mobilized.
   d. A repeat partial adrenalectomy is indicated in a small local recurrence of an adrenal mass previously treated with partial adrenalectomy.
   e. Partial adrenalectomy may be indicated in multiple endocrine neoplasia type IIA.

10. During a right adrenalectomy, severe bleeding is encountered. The possible causes include all of the following EXCEPT:
    a. right adrenal vein avulsion at the origin on the inferior vena cava.
    b. avulsion of the right hepatic vein branch.
    c. disruption of the adrenal capsule.
    d. inadvertent ligation of the upper pole renal artery.
    e. all of the above.

11. Which of the following is not an advantage of retroperitoneal adrenalectomy when compared to transperitoneal approach?
    a. Reducing the risk of injury to bowels and abdominal organs
    b. Larger working space and clearer anatomical landmarks

c. Lower incidence of hemodynamic and respiratory morbidities

d. Usually the approach of choice in patients with multiple previous abdominal surgeries

e. All of the above are advantages of the retroperitoneal approach over the transperitoneal approach

12. With regard to intraoperative complications during adrenalectomy, which of the following is NOT the appropriate management?

a. In an event when splenectomy is performed for uncontrollable splenic hemorrhage, pneumococcus, *Haemophilus influenzae* type B (Hib), and meningococcus vaccinations should be given intraoperatively or immediately postoperatively.

b. Postoperative drainage high in triglycerides and amylase is indicative of pancreas injury. Management consists of bowel rest with parenteral nutrition.

c. Small diaphragmatic injuries if recognized intraoperatively should be repaired and a chest drain inserted.

d. Inadvertent ligation of the superior mesenteric vein should be managed with revascularization and bowel resection.

e. All of the above are appropriate management.

ANSWERS

1. **c. The medulla is innervated by preganglionic sympathetic nerve fibers.** The right adrenal vein drains directly into the inferior vena cava and derives its arterial supply through the superior, middle, and inferior adrenal arteries from the inferior phrenic artery, the abdominal aorta, and the renal artery, respectively. It is usually more cephalad than the left adrenal gland and is located at the upper pole and medial border of the right kidney. It is closely related to the diaphragm posteriorly, and thus extra care should be taken during surgical dissection, especially of large tumors.

2. **d. 25%.** Of adrenal lesions larger than 6 cm, 25% are adrenal cortical carcinomas, and these larger lesions should be resected. Risk of malignancy in lesions smaller than 4 cm is 2%. Approximately 6% of adrenal lesions between 4 and 6 cm are malignant, and surgical resection can be considered in appropriate individuals.

3. **c. Invasive adrenal cortical carcinoma with thrombus in the inferior vena cava.** Previous abdominal surgeries may result in dense intra-abdominal adhesions that may make surgery difficult. With improved laparoscopic techniques and equipment, large adrenal tumors are no longer considered absolute contraindication to the laparoscopic approach. Literature had described the feasibility of resecting large adrenal tumors laparoscopically. However, the risk of open conversion is greater in such large tumors. Invasion of adrenal cortical carcinoma into surrounding structures will make laparoscopic resection very difficult, and extension of tumor into the inferior vena cava should be considered an absolute contraindication to the laparoscopic approach.

4. **b. Phenoxybenzamine may lead to tachycardia, and β-adrenergic blockade should be started before phenoxybenzamine administration.** Preoperative sympatholytic therapy with α-adrenergic blockers for at least 2 weeks before surgery helps in both hemodynamic and glucose control and should be continued until the day of surgery. Phenoxybenzamine, being nonselective, may lead to tachycardia, and β-adrenergic blockade may be necessary. Because phenoxybenzamine is an irreversible noncompetitive α-adrenergic blocker, prolonged hypotension in the immediate postoperative period and central nervous system effects such as somnolence may be expected. β-Adrenergic blockade, if needed, must be given with caution in patients with myocardial depression and started

only after phenoxybenzamine therapy. Aggressive fluid management with volume repletion is necessary after removal of pheochromocytoma or ligation of the adrenal vein, because hypotension can occur as a result of sudden loss of tonic vasoconstriction. The adrenal vein should be ligated early during the resection of pheochromocytoma to avoid the systemic release of catecholamines during manipulation of the adrenal gland. Lastly, drugs with rapid onset and short half-lives, such as nitroprusside, phentolamine, nitroglycerin, or nicardipine, are generally preferred in intraoperative hypertensive episodes, because hypotension can occur after ligation of the adrenal vein or excision of the pheochromocytoma.

5. **b. Bilateral adrenal hyperplasia.** Although the posterior approach is the most direct route to the adrenal glands and no major muscles are divided, surgical exposure is limited. In addition, access to the adrenal vein and great vessels is more difficult, which may be problematic in event of excessive intraoperative bleeding. Thus this approach is not ideal in large adrenal tumors or adrenocortical carcinoma. The prone position will also make ventilating the patient difficult. However, this approach provides ready access to both adrenal glands through two separate incisions and is ideal for bilateral adrenal hyperplasia or small benign adrenal tumors.

6. **c. After excision of both adrenal glands.** It is generally recommended that steroid replacement be started as soon as both adrenal glands are excised to minimize acute adrenal insufficiency. Patients can present with back/abdominal pain, nausea, vomiting, diarrhea, hypotension, fever, hypoglycemia, and hyperkalemia.

7. **c. Open thoracoabdominal approach.** Surgical exposure is limited with the lumbodorsal posterior approach, and this approach should not be used for large tumors or adrenocortical carcinoma. Although the open anterior transabdominal approach using the subcostal or chevron incision gives a fairly good and adequate exposure for most cases, this approach might not be adequate in this case in view of the involvement of the retrohepatic inferior vena cava. The open thoracoabdominal approach is generally reserved for large and invasive tumors with extensive involvement of surrounding structures or vena cava that cannot be safely removed via the anterior transabdominal approach. The thoracoabdominal approach is particularly useful in right-sided tumors, because the liver and inferior vena cava can limit exposure, whereas on the left side, the spleen and pancreas can generally be elevated to provide adequate exposure. Minimally invasive approaches such as conventional laparoscopic or robot-assisted laparoscopic approach are usually contraindicated in such large tumors with extensive involvement of the great vessels.

8. **e. All the above are possible approaches.**

9. **d. A repeat partial adrenalectomy is indicated in a small local recurrence of an adrenal mass previously treated with partial adrenalectomy.** The arterial supply of the adrenal gland forms a plexus circumferentially around the gland and can usually be taken without fear of devascularizing the adrenal cortex, and the gland will remain viable as long it remains attached to the kidney or to an area of unmobilized connective tissue. The venous system drains into a central adrenal vein, and the main adrenal vein can be taken as long as the remnant adrenal gland remains in situ without mobilization. However, it would be prudent to preserve the main adrenal vein as long as it is safe and adequate margins can be obtained. A local recurrence after a previous partial adrenalectomy, regardless of size of recurrence, is an absolute contraindication to a repeat partial adrenalectomy. Multiple endocrine neoplasia type IIA is associated with adrenal tumors, and therefore partial adrenalectomy may be indicated in these patients.

10. **d. Inadvertent ligation of the upper pole renal artery.** All of the vascular injuries noted cause bleeding except ligation of an upper pole renal artery. Ligation of this artery would result in upper pole devascularization, not hemorrhage.

11. **b. Larger working space and clearer anatomical landmarks.** The main advantage of the retroperitoneal approach is that entry into the peritoneum is avoided, and thus complications such as visceral and bowel injuries are minimized. In the absence of pneumoperitoneum, hemodynamic and respiratory morbidities are also reduced. In addition, dense intraperitoneal adhesions arising from previous surgery or inflammation are averted by operating in the retroperitoneum. The main disadvantage of the retroperitoneal approach is the limited working space that makes dissection of large tumors difficult. Finally, the lack of anatomic landmarks and the abundant retroperitoneal adipose tissues may pose a significant challenge to surgeons inexperienced with the retroperitoneum. The main advantage of the lateral approach over the posterior approach is the ease of conversion into the transperitoneal approach should difficulties be encountered. In contrast, the prone retroperitoneal approach allows for bilateral adrenalectomy without patient repositioning.

12. **a. In an event when splenectomy is performed for uncontrollable splenic hemorrhage, pneumococcus, *Haemophilus influenzae* type B (Hib), and meningococcus vaccinations should be given intraoperatively or immediately postoperatively.** Vaccinations should be given only after patients have recovered adequately from their surgeries (usually just before discharge from hospital) and not intraoperatively or immediately postoperatively. Diaphragmatic injuries, even if small, should be repaired due to the risk of abdominal content herniation and bowel strangulations. Ligation of the superior mesenteric vein is potentially fatal due to large segments of bowel congestion. Management must include revascularization and resection of unhealthy segment of bowels if necessary.

CHAPTER REVIEW

1. The right adrenal vein enters the inferior vena cava in a posterior lateral position. When torn, the vena cava must be rotated to gain access to suture the defect.

2. Local regional recurrence in the adrenal cortical carcinoma occurs in 60% of cases.

3. It is important to note that the tail of the pancreas can lie adjacent to the upper pole of the left kidney and adrenal. Care must be taken not to injure this organ.

4. In a thoracoabdominal incision, the diaphragm should not be incised radially but, rather, circumferentially because the former results in a phrenic nerve injury with an atonic diaphragm lateral to the incision.

5. An Addisonian crisis is most commonly seen after excision of an adrenal tumor that secretes cortisol as the contralateral adrenal is suppressed.

6. In removing large adrenal masses, it is important to be careful not to ligate an upper pole renal artery branch because this will result in an infarction of the renal segment that is served by this artery.

7. The most common sites from which metastases occur to the adrenal are lung, breast, kidney, and melanoma.

8. Before resecting aldosterone-secreting tumors, consideration should be given to preoperative administration of spironolactone and correction of hypokalemia and hypomagnesemia if they exist.

9. Twenty-five percent of adrenal lesions greater than 6 cm are adrenal cortical carcinomas, and these larger lesions should be resected. The risk of malignancy in lesions less than 4 cm is 2%.

10. Preoperative sympatholytic therapy with α-adrenergic blockers for at least 2 weeks before surgery in patients with a pheochromocytoma is necessary because it restores vascular volume and helps in both hemodynamic and glucose control. If a β blocker is necessary to control cardiac arrhythmias, it should be begun after full alpha blockade has been achieved.

108   Surgical, Radiographic, and Endoscopic Anatomy of the Female Pelvis

Priya Padmanabhan

QUESTIONS

1. The uterine vessels are found _____ to the ureter.
   a. laterally
   b. posteriorly
   c. anteriorly
   d. medially
   e. running together in a common sheath

2. All of the following are TRUE EXCEPT:
   a. The angle between the inferior pubic rami is obtuse in women.
   b. The female pelvis is larger and broader than the male pelvis.
   c. The female inlet is heart shaped (as compared with the oval-shaped male inlet).
   d. The female pelvis is shorter and wider, with a less pronounced sacral promontory.
   e. Female pelvic inlet faces anteriorly, allowing pressure of the intra-abdominal and intrapelvic contents to be directed to the bony pelvis.

3. In contrast to that of the male, the female bladder neck:
   a. has extensive adrenergic innervation.
   b. has a thickened middle smooth muscle layer.
   c. is largely responsible for urinary continence.
   d. is surrounded by type I (slow-twitch) fibers.
   e. has longitudinal smooth muscle fibers that extend to the external meatus.

4. Relative to the anterior portion of the uterosacral ligament, the ureter:
   a. lies inferior.
   b. lies posterior.
   c. lies superior.
   d. lies lateral.
   e. runs along with it.

5. To avoid denervation of the striated urethral sphincter, incisions through the vaginal wall to enter the retropubic space should be made:
   a. perpendicular to the urethra.
   b. over the urethra.
   c. close to the lateral margins of the urethra.
   d. cephalad to the bladder neck.
   e. far lateral in the vaginal wall, parallel to the urethra.

6. The levator ani muscles make up the largest portion of the pelvic cavity floor. This consists of the:
   a. iliopsoas, puborectalis, and obturator internus.
   b. obturator externus, psoas major, and psoas minor.
   c. coccygeus, pubococcygeus, and iliopsoas.
   d. iliococcygeus, puborectalis, and pubococcygeus.
   e. obturator internus, pubococcygeus, and psoas minor.

7. A Maritus (labial fat pad) rotational flap used in the repair of vesicovaginal fistula receives blood supply from the:
   a. terminal branches of the internal pudendal artery and vein.
   b. superficial inferior epigastric vessels.
   c. inferior epigastric vessels.
   d. accessory pudendal vessels.
   e. external pudendal vessels.

8. Translabial ultrasound is valuable because it does not distort or compress the tissue. It is commonly used to visualize:
   a. transvaginal mesh.
   b. urethral bulking agents.
   c. urethral implants.
   d. bladder wall thickness.
   e. all of the above.

9. The round ligament:
   a. terminates in the uterus.
   b. is the main source of blood supply to the ovaries.
   c. terminates in the labia.
   d. is the male homolog of the spermatic cord.
   e. is NOT part of the broad ligament.

10. All of the following are true regarding the perineal body EXCEPT:
    a. Damage to the perineal body during labor can cause damage to fibers of the internal anal sphincter.
    b. It is the convergence of the bulbospongiosus, external anal sphincter and superficial and deep transverse perineal muscles.
    c. Perineal body attaches to the posterior border of the perineal membrane.
    d. Perineal body is made up of muscle and collagenous and elastic fibers and lies at the central point of the perineum.
    e. Episiotomy is angled laterally to avoid damage to fibers of the external anal sphincter.

11. The transversalis fascia is:
    a. part of the inner stratum.
    b. part of the outer stratum.
    c. part of the intermediate stratum.
    d. continuous with the endopelvic fascia.
    e. b and d.

12. After a sacrospinous ligament fixation, the patient wakes up with pain in the posterior and lower leg. The nerve that was likely compromised is the:
    a. femoral nerve.
    b. pudendal nerve.
    c. sacral plexus.
    d. obturator nerve.
    e. a and b.

13. The arcus tendineus fascia pelvis:
    a. is present in females.
    b. attaches from the ischial spine to the sacrum.
    c. is also known as the tendinous arc.
    d. is present only in males.
    e. all of the above.

14. Please identify the correct pair(s) of arterial supply and lymphatic drainage of the vagina.
    a. Uterine arteries: superficial inguinal nodes
    b. Internal pudendal artery: sacral common iliac and superficial inguinal nodes
    c. Vaginal arteries: external iliac nodes
    d. Uterine arteries: sacral common iliac nodes
    e. Internal pudendal artery: external iliac nodes

15. Squamous metaplasia of the bladder:
    a. is a premalignant lesion.
    b. is a sign of an underlying serious infection.
    c. should always be treated with surgical resection.
    d. is a normal finding in premenopausal females.
    e. is none of the above.

16. The levator ani attaches to all of the following EXCEPT:
    a. perineal body.
    b. pubis.
    c. coccyx.
    d. vagina.
    e. arcus tendineus fascia pelvis.

17. The ureter can be injured during a hysterectomy:
    a. at the time of the division of the ovarian artery.
    b. at the time of the division of the uterine artery.
    c. at the time of the division of the cardinal artery.
    d. while dissecting out the cervix.
    e. all of the above.

18. During a sacrospinous ligament vault suspension, significant bleeding is encountered. The bleeding vessels most likely originate from the:
    a. anterior division of the internal iliac artery.
    b. posterior division of the internal iliac artery.
    c. perineal artery.
    d. mesenteric artery.
    e. epigastric artery.

19. The peritoneum may be accessed transvaginally through the:
    a. posterior fornix.
    b. anterior fornix.
    c. rectovaginal septum.
    d. lateral fornices.
    e. vesicovaginal space.

20. The cavernous nerve, responsible for clitoral engorgement during sexual activity, is derived from:
    a. the pudendal nerve.
    b. the dorsal nerve of the clitoris.
    c. the superior hypogastric plexus.
    d. the inferior hypogastric plexus.
    e. the obturator nerve

ANSWERS

1. **c. Anteriorly.** In women, the ureter first runs posterior to the ovary, then turns medially to run deep to the base of the broad ligament before entering a loose connective tissue tunnel through the substance of the cardinal ligament.
2. **c. The female inlet is heart shaped (as compared with the oval-shaped male inlet).** The female inlet is oval in shape (as compared with the heart-shaped male inlet) and wider, which contributes to the weakness of the pelvic floor.
3. **e. Has longitudinal smooth muscle fibers that extend to the external meatus.** At the female bladder neck, the inner longitudinal fibers converge radially to pass downward as the inner longitudinal layer of the urethra. The middle circular layer does not appear to be as robust as that of the male. The female bladder neck differs strikingly from the male in possessing little adrenergic innervation.
4. **d. Lies lateral.** The uterosacral originates from the greater sciatic foramen and inserts into the lateral aspect of the fascia surrounding the cervix, isthmus of the uterus, and vaginal wall. The ureter lies lateral to the anterior portion of the uterosacral ligament (closest to the cervix).
5. **e. Far lateral in the vaginal wall, parallel to the urethra.** Somatic and autonomic nerves to the urethra travel on the lateral walls of the vagina near the urethra. During transvaginal incontinence surgery, the anterior vaginal wall should be incised laterally to avoid these nerves and prevent type III urinary incontinence.
6. **d. Iliococcygeus, puborectalis, and pubococcygeus.** This is innervated by the fourth sacral nerve. The name of each component is derived from their attachments.
7. **e. External pudendal vessels.** The labial fat pads received blood supply from the external pudendal branches of the femoral vessels.
8. **e. All of the above.**
9. **c. Terminates in the labia.** The round ligament exits at the internal inguinal ring and crosses over the external iliac artery, terminating in the mons pubis of the labia. The male homolog of the round ligament is the gubernaculum.
10. **a.** Damage to the perineal body during labor can cause damage to fibers of the internal anal sphincter.
11. **e. b and c.** The transversalis fascia is part of the outer stratum and is continuous with the endopelvic and lateral pelvic fascia. Both the transversalis and endopelvic fascia play important roles at the exit points of the pelvic organs. The endopelvic fascia extends from the uterine artery down to where the vagina and levator ani fuse.
12. **c. Sacral plexus.** During an sacrospinous ligament fixation, the sacral plexus is in jeopardy of being injured because it lies immediately posterior to the sacrospinous ligament as it leaves through the greater sciatic foramen. The pudendal nerve may also be injured during this repair.
13. **c. Is also known as the tendinous arc.** The arcus tendineus fascia pelvis, or tendinous arc, is a thickened band of the pelvic

fascia that runs from the ischial spine to the pubic bone. It originates from the pubic bone laterally and is connected to the pubovesical ligament medially and the tendinous arch of the levator ani.

14. **b. Internal pudendal artery: sacral, common iliac, and superficial inguinal nodes.** The superior part: blood supply—uterine arteries/drainage—internal and external iliac nodes middle and inferior: blood supply—vaginal arteries/drainage—internal and external iliac nodes Inferior vagina: blood supply—internal pudendal artery/drainage—sacral, common iliac, and superficial inguinal nodes.

15. **d. Is a normal finding in premenopausal females.** Premenopausal women can have normal signs of squamous metaplasia at the trigone and base of the bladder. This is a nonkeratinizing metaplasia or vaginal metaplasia that is hormonally responsive and is a normal variant.

16. **e. Arcus tendineus fascia pelvis.** The tendinous arc of the levator ani serves as the origin of the muscles of the pelvis diaphragm: pubococcygeus and iliococcygeus. The muscle

bordering this hiatus has been referred to as "puboviscceral" because it provides a sling for (pubourethralis, puborectalis), inserts directly into (pubovaginalis, puboanalis, levator prostate), or inserts into a structure intimately associated with the pelvic viscera. The coccygeus muscle extends from the sacrospinous ligament to the lateral border of the sacrum and coccyx to complete the pelvic diaphragm.

17. **e. All of the above.** The ureter is vulnerable to injury because it comes in close proximity to many of the structures that are dissected and divided during a radical hysterectomy. It crosses the infundibulopelvic ligament under the ovarian artery and is just medial to the uterine artery. It also passes through the cardinal ligament and lies in close proximity to the cervix.

18. **b. Posterior division of the internal iliac artery.**

19. **a. Posterior fornix.** Because the apex of the vagina is covered with the peritoneum of the rectouterine pouch, the peritoneal cavity may be accessed through the posterior fornix.

20. **d. The inferior hypogastric plexus.**

CHAPTER REVIEW

1. The pelvic inlet faces anteriorly, allowing pressure of the intra-abdominal and intrapelvic contents to be directed to the bony pelvis, rather than the muscles and the fascia. The bony pelvis should be visualized in the supine position.

2. The arcus tendinous fascia pelvis (ATFP) and arcus tendinous levator ani (ATLA) are two distinct structures, serving as key players in fascial attachment. ATFP is the main point for fascial attachment. The levator ani muscles attach to the ATFP and cover the obturator internus.

3. The ischial spine and sacrospinous ligament are important landmarks during vault suspension to avoid injury to the sacral plexus and pudendal nerve.

4. The sustained resting tone of the pelvic floor muscles (pubococcygeus, puborectalis, and iliococcygeus) support pelvic viscera, resists increases in intra-abdominal pressure, and is crucial in passive control of urinary and fecal continence.

5. Translabial ultrasound is useful for visualization of transvaginal mesh, urethral bulking agents, and urethral implants.

6. Magnetic resonance imaging (MRI) is the most comprehensive and conclusive imaging modality available to image the female pelvis without the use of radiation.

7. T2-weighted MRI is the best imaging technique to visualize and localize urethral diverticula and to differentiate them from other benign vaginal masses.

109

Surgical, Radiographic, and Endoscopic Anatomy of the Male Pelvis

Jen-Jane Liu, Bryan R. Foster, and Christopher L. Amling

QUESTIONS

1. The greater and lesser sciatic foramina are separated by the:
   a. sacrotuberous ligament.
   b. Cooper (pectineal) ligament.
   c. arcuate line.
   d. sacrospinous ligament.
   e. piriformis muscle.

2. During inguinal incisions, the vessels invariably encountered in Camper fascia are the:
   a. superficial inferior epigastric artery and vein.
   b. superficial circumflex iliac artery and vein.
   c. external pudendal artery and vein.
   d. gonadal artery and veins.
   e. accessory obturator vein.

3. Rupture of the penile urethra at the junction of the penis and scrotum can result in urinary extravasation into all of the following structures EXCEPT the:
   a. anterior abdominal wall up to the clavicles.
   b. scrotum.
   c. penis, deep to the dartos fascia.
   d. perineum in a "butterfly" pattern.
   e. buttock.

4. Accessory obturator veins (from the external iliac artery) and accessory obturator arteries (from the inferior epigastric artery) are encountered in:
   a. 50% and 25% of patients, respectively.
   b. 5% and 50% of patients, respectively.
   c. 50% and 75% of patients, respectively.
   d. 25% and 50% of patients, respectively.
   e. 25% and 5% of patients, respectively.

5. A retractor blade has rested on the psoas muscle during a prolonged procedure, resulting in a femoral nerve palsy. Postoperatively, the patient will experience:
   a. inability to flex the hip and numbness over the anterior thigh.
   b. inability to flex the knee and numbness over the thigh.
   c. numbness over the anterior thigh only.
   d. inability to extend the knee and numbness over the anterior thigh.
   e. inability to flex the knee only.

6. Autonomic nerves contributing to the pelvic plexus include the:
   a. superior hypogastric nerves from the para-aortic plexuses.
   b. pelvic sympathetic trunks.
   c. pelvic parasympathetic neurons from the sacral spinal cord.
   d. a and c only.
   e. a, b, and c.

7. To preserve the vascular supply to the ureter, incisions in the peritoneum should be made:
   a. medially in the abdomen and laterally in the pelvis.
   b. laterally in the abdomen and medially in the pelvis.
   c. always medial to the ureter.
   d. always lateral to the ureter.
   e. directly over the ureter.

8. All of the following features of the ureterovesical junction cooperate to prevent vesicoureteral reflux EXCEPT:
   a. fixation of the ureter to the superficial trigone.
   b. sphincteric closure of the ureteral orifice.
   c. detrusor backing.
   d. telescoping of the bladder outward over the ureter.
   e. passive closure of the intramural ureter caused by bladder filling.

9. Which of the following statements about the trigone is TRUE?
   a. Epithelium is thicker than the rest of the bladder and densely adherent.
   b. Superficial smooth muscle is a continuation of Waldeyer sheath.
   c. Smooth muscle enlarges to form thick fascicles.
   d. Smooth muscle of the ureter forms the interureteric ridge (Mercier bar).
   e. When the bladder empties, the trigone is thrown into thick folds.

10. Arterial supply to the bladder includes:
    a. the superior vesical artery.
    b. the inferior vesical artery.
    c. the obturator artery.
    d. the inferior hemorrhoidal artery.
    e. all of the above.

11. Which of the following statements concerning the male striated urethral sphincter is TRUE?
    a. It is composed of type I (slow-twitch) and type II (fast-twitch) fibers.
    b. It is bounded above by the superior fascia.
    c. It receives motor blanches from the dorsal nerve of the penis.
    d. It is shaped like a signet ring and is 2 to 2.5 cm in length.
    e. It is densely supplied with proprioceptive muscle spindles.

12. The first branch of the pudendal nerve in the perineum is the:
    a. dorsal nerve of the penis.
    b. inferior rectal nerve(s).
    c. perineal nerve.
    d. posterior femoral cutaneous branches.
    e. posterior scrotal branches.

13. Lymphatic drainage from the scrotum travels:
    a. through perianal nodes to reach the pelvis.
    b. directly to the deep pelvic lymph nodes.
    c. through the superficial and deep inguinal lymph nodes.
    d. to prepubic nodes.
    e. to para-aortic lymph nodes along with testicular drainage.

14. Which layers of the scrotum and testicular tunics usually need to be debrided in patients with Fournier gangrene?
    a. The scrotal skin only
    b. The scrotal skin and dartos layer
    c. The scrotal skin, dartos layer, and external spermatic fascia
    d. The scrotal skin, dartos layer, and external cremasteric and internal spermatic fasciae, leaving the tunica vaginalis intact
    e. All tissues, including the tunica vaginalis

15. Lymphatic drainage from the bladder passes through the:
    a. external iliac lymph nodes.
    b. obturator and internal iliac lymph nodes.
    c. internal and common iliac lymph nodes.
    d. common iliac, periureteral, and para-aortic lymph nodes.
    e. a, b, and c.

16. To preserve potency during a radical cystectomy, ligation of the lateral and posterior vascular pedicles is best carried out:
    a. close to their origin from the internal iliac vessels.
    b. near the bladder.
    c. from beneath the bladder after rotating the prostate cephalad.
    d. as they cross the ureter.
    e. lateral to the rectum.

17. Which imaging modality/procedure would be optimal to assess degree of invasion of a bulbar urethral tumor?
    a. CT scan with contrast
    b. Retrograde urethrogram with fluoroscopy
    c. MRI of the pelvis with contrast with T1- and T2-weighted images
    d. Endoscopy with direct visualization
    e. Ultrasound of the perineum

18. During transurethral resection of the prostate, what maneuver is most likely to result in urinary incontinence?
    a. Undermining of the floor of the bladder neck
    b. Deep resection distal to the verumontanum
    c. Superficial resection of the ejaculatory ducts
    d. Deep resection of intravesical protrusion of the prostate
    e. Deep resection of the lateral lobes of the prostate proximal to the verumontanum

ANSWERS

1. **d. Sacrospinous ligament.** The sacrospinous ligament separates the greater and lesser sciatic foramina.
2. **a. Superficial inferior epigastric artery and vein.** The superficial inferior epigastric vessels are encountered during inguinal incisions and can cause troublesome bleeding during placement of pelvic laparoscopic ports or in an inguinal incision.
3. **e. Buttock.** Blood and urine can accumulate in the scrotum and penis deep to the dartos fascia after an anterior urethral injury. In the perineum, their spread is limited by the fusions of Colles fascia to the ischiopubic rami laterally and to the posterior edge of the perineal membrane; the resulting hematoma is therefore butterfly shaped. These processes will not

extend down the leg or into the buttock, but they can freely travel up the anterior abdominal wall deep to Scarpa fascia to the clavicles and around the flank to the back.

4. **a. 50% and 25% of patients, respectively.** In half of patients, one or more accessory obturator veins drain into the underside of the external iliac vein and can easily be torn during lymphadenectomy. In 25% of people, an accessory obturator artery arises from the inferior epigastric artery and runs medial to the femoral vein to reach the obturator canal.
5. **d. Inability to extend the knee and numbness over the anterior thigh.** The femoral nerve (L2, L3, and L4) supplies sensation to the anterior thigh and motor innervation to the extensors of the knee.
6. **e. a, b, and c.** The presynaptic sympathetic cell bodies reach the pelvic plexus by two pathways: (1) the superior hypogastric plexus and (2) the pelvic continuation of the sympathetic trunks. Presynaptic parasympathetic innervation arises from the intermediolateral cell column of the sacral cord.
7. **b. Laterally in the abdomen and medially in the pelvis.** Blood supply to the pelvic ureter enters laterally; thus the pelvic peritoneum should be incised only medial to the ureter.
8. **b. Sphincteric closure of the ureteral orifice.** The intravesical portion of the ureter lies immediately beneath the bladder urothelium and is therefore quite pliant; it is backed by a strong plate of detrusor muscle. With bladder filling, this arrangement is thought to result in passive occlusion of the ureter, like a flap valve.
9. **d. Smooth muscle of the ureter forms the interureteric ridge (Mercier bar).** Fibers from each ureter meet to form a triangular sheet of muscle that extends from the two ureteral orifices to the internal urethra meatus. The edges of this muscular sheet are thickened between the ureteral orifices (the interureteric crest, or Mercier bar) and between the ureters and the internal urethral meatus (Bell muscle).
10. **e. All of the above.** In addition to the vesical branches, the bladder may be supplied by any adjacent artery arising from the internal iliac artery.
11. **d. It is shaped like a signet ring and is 2 to 2.5 cm in length.** The membranous urethra spans on average 2 to 2.5 cm (range: 1.2 to 5 cm). In the male it is surrounded by the striated (external) urethral sphincter, which is often incorrectly depicted as a flat sheet of muscle sandwiched between two layers of fasciae. The striated sphincter is actually shaped like a signet ring, broad at its base and narrowing as it passes through the urogenital hiatus of the levator ani to meet the apex of the prostate.
12. **a. Dorsal nerve of the penis.** The pudendal nerve follows the vessels in their course through the perineum. Its first branch, the dorsal nerve of the penis, travels ventral to the main pudendal trunk in the Alcock canal.
13. **c. Through the superficial and deep inguinal lymph nodes.** The penis, scrotum, and perineum drain into the inguinal lymph nodes. These nodes can be divided into superficial groups and deep groups.
14. **b. The scrotal skin and dartos layer.** The external, cremasteric, and internal spermatic fasciae are embryologically distinct from the scrotal and dartos layers and have their own blood and nerve supplies. It is uncommon for them to be involved in the necrotic process in Fournier gangrene; therefore they can be spared. (In practice, in patients with Fournier gangrene, all scrotal tissue is debrided to the tunica vaginalis.)
15. **e. a, b, and c.** In the bladder, the bulk of the lymphatic drainage passes to the external iliac lymph nodes. Some anterior and lateral drainage may go through the obturator and internal iliac nodes, and portions of the bladder base and trigone may drain into the internal and common iliac groups. Complete lymph node dissection during radical cystectomy should encompass all of these lymph node groups.
16. **b. Near the bladder.** The bladder vasculature pierces the pelvic autonomic plexuses near the origin of the arteries from the internal iliac arteries. Ligation of these vessels proximally will

injure the pelvic autonomic nervous plexuses. Ligation is best carried out near the bladder to avoid nerve damage.

17. **c. MRI of the pelvis with contrast with T1 and T2-weighted images.** MRI has superior soft tissue spatial resolution that is well suited to imaging of the pelvic floor and external genitalia structures. Tumors typically enhance on T1 imaging when gadolinium contrast is administered, and T2 images show organ anatomy and detail well, enabling invasion to be determined.

18. **b. Deep resection distal to the verumontanum.** The striated urethral sphincter is located just distal to the verumontanum, and its coaptation can be noted visually during cystourethroscopy. Deep resection in this area may damage the striated urethral sphincter and result in urinary incontinence.

CHAPTER REVIEW

1. Scarpa fascia on the abdomen forms a distinct layer and is continuous with Colles fascia in the perineum medially. It fuses with the deep fascia of the thigh laterally. Colles fascia is continuous with the dartos fascia of the penis. Thus, urinary extravasation and infections confined by these fascia attachments do not extend down the legs or into the buttocks but may travel cephalad to the clavicles.

2. The internal oblique and the transversalis fascia fuse to form the conjoin tendon, which reinforces the posterior wall of the inguinal canal.

3. A direct hernia of the inguinal canal occurs medial to the inferior epigastric vessels; an indirect hernia occurs lateral to these vessels.

4. The superior vesicle artery arises from the proximal portion of the obliterated umbilical artery. The obliterated umbilical artery may be used to find the superior vesicle artery.

5. In 25% of people there is an accessory obturator artery that arises from the inferior epigastric artery and courses medial to the femoral vein.

6. The genitofemoral nerve courses along the ventral surface of the psoas muscle; the femoral nerve runs in the substance of the psoas muscle. Retractors compressing the muscle may result in nerve palsy. Sutures placed perpendicular to the muscle fibers may entrap the nerves.

7. The obturator nerve supplies the adductors of the thigh.

8. The male bladder neck receives abundant sympathetic innervation. The female bladder neck receives little sympathetic innervation.

9. The blood supply to the prostate enters at the 4 and 8 o'clock positions. It is important to understand this in prostatectomy when securing hemostasis.

10. Although lymphatic supply from the prostate is primarily to the obturator and internal iliac nodes, it may drain directly to the presacral and external iliac nodes.

11. Denonvilliers fascia separates the prostate from the rectum.

12. Scrotal lymphatics do not cross the median raphe; drainage is to the ipsilateral inguinal nodes. Lymphatics from the penis cross over extensively and may drain to either or both groin nodes irrespective of the side of the penis involved.

13. The cavernosal nerves pass by the tips of the seminal vesicles and lie within the leaves of the lateral endopelvic fascia and course very close to the apex of the prostate, where they are most vulnerable to injury.

14. The ureter is anterior (ventral) to the common iliac artery.

15. The blood supply to the pelvic ureter enters laterally.

16. The bladder is an intra-abdominal organ in the infant and may project above the umbilicus.

17. The muscle of the trigone has three layers: (1) the superficial layer, derived from the longitudinal muscle of the ureter; (2) the deep layer, which arises from Waldeyer sheath on the ureter and inserts at the bladder neck; and (3) the detrusor layer.

18. The bladder has a lateral pedicle that is lateral to the ureter and a posterior pedicle that is posteromedial to the ureter.

110 Physiology and Pharmacology of the Bladder and Urethra

Toby C. Chai and Lori A. Birder

QUESTIONS

1. The lower urinary tract is innervated by three sets of peripheral nerves. Which of the following is correct?
   a. Pelvic parasympathetic nerves arise at the sacral spinal cord level and excite the bladder and urethra.
   b. Sympathetic nerves inhibit the bladder body and excite the bladder neck and urethra.
   c. Pudendal (somatic) nerves excite the bladder body and the external urethral sphincter.
   d. All of the above are true.
   e. None of the above are true.

2. "Sensing" bladder volume is relevant during bladder storage. Which of the following is correct?
   a. It has been speculated the sense of imminent micturition arises in the urethra.
   b. Bladder filling has been shown to correlate with episodic bursts of sensation and afferent discharge.
   c. Nathan first described sensations of awareness during bladder filling.
   d. Sensations of awareness during bladder distension can be mapped to the urinary bladder.
   e. All are correct.

3. Bladder afferents can be:
   a. characterized by responses to receptive field stimulation.
   b. classified according to ability to respond to a diverse range of chemical mediators.
   c. silent initially but sensitized during inflammatory processes.
   d. variable in both morphology and function depending upon species.
   e. all of the above.

4. Sensitization of afferents in bladder pathology can:
   a. open ion channels in the nerve terminals.
   b. release a number of inflammatory mediators.
   c. develop rapidly and be relatively short lived.
   d. be resolved easily.
   e. a, b, and c only.

5. Patients with irritable bowel syndrome (IBS) often report changes in bladder function. Which of the following statements is correct?
   a. This is an example of cross-organ sensitization.
   b. In animal models, colonic inflammation rarely leads to bladder dysfunction.
   c. Cross-organ sensitization only occurs between the gastrointestinal tract and the urinary bladder.
   d. The mediators, which are responsible for these conditions, have been well described.
   e. None are true.

6. In terms of nerves innervating the detrusor:
   a. the majority express acetylcholinesterase enzyme.
   b. acetylcholine and adenosine triphosphate (ATP) appear to provide the majority of the excitatory input.
   c. release of both acetylcholine and ATP result in smooth muscle contraction.
   d. additional substances released from efferent nerves include nitric oxide (NO) and vasoactive intestinal polypeptide.
   e. all are correct.

7. In terms of adrenergic influences:
   a. reflex bladder activity can be modulated by α-1 adrenergic mechanisms.
   b. α-1 adrenergic mechanisms control blood pressure and tissue blood flow.
   c. the β-3 adrenergic receptors are present at a number of sites (both peripherally and centrally).
   d. β-3 receptor agonists, via effects on a number of sites, are a promising treatment for overactive bladder.
   e. all are correct.

8. Which of the following is TRUE about ATP?
   a. It is the main excitatory neurotransmitter for bladder contraction in humans.
   b. It can activate two main families of purinergic receptors: P2X and P2Y.
   c. Purinergic neurotransmission plays an important role in bladder overactivity and bladder pain.
   d. b and c are true.
   e. All are correct.

9. During bladder storage:
   a. bladder accommodation is dependent upon activation of sympathetic pathways.
   b. bladder accommodation is dependent upon quiescence of parasympathetic efferent pathways.
   c. intravesical pressure measurements are low when below the voiding threshold.
   d. the sympathetic reflex provides negative feedback.
   e. all are true.

10. During storage phase of the bladder:
    a. the urothelium plays an important role in accommodating urine storage.
    b. the urothelium is only a barrier and exhibits no other functions.
    c. increase of urothelial mediators during bladder filling can influence smooth muscle tone.
    d. the urothelial surface cells change shape during bladder filling.
    e. a, c, and d are correct.

11. The guarding reflex is a mechanism for maintaining continence and is characterized by:
    a. activation of pudendal motoneurons.
    b. increased outlet resistance.
    c. activation of external urethral sphincter motoneurons.
    d. activation of afferent input from the urethra or pelvic floor that leads to closure of the urethral outlet.
    e. all of the above.

12. Electrical stimulation of the sacral nerve roots is known to be:
    a. an effective treatment for refractory overactive bladder.
    b. an effective treatment for non-obstructive urinary retention.
    c. effective by modulation of central nervous system pathways.
    d. a better treatment compared with posterior tibial nerve stimulation.
    e. a, b, and c are correct.

13. In terms of bladder emptying:
    a. switching between bladder storage and emptying can occur involuntarily (reflex emptying) or voluntarily.
    b. reflex voiding only occurs in the normal adult.
    c. initial expulsion of urine consists of initial contraction of the urethral sphincter.
    d. relaxation of the urethral smooth muscle during micturition is achieved by release of acetylcholine.
    e. none are true.

14. The facilitatory urethra to bladder reflex was characterized by:
    a. Barrington.
    b. Delancey.
    c. de Groat.
    d. increased urethral afferent activation promoting bladder emptying.
    e. a and d are correct.

15. An essential control center for micturition in healthy individuals is:
    a. the dorsal pontine tegmentum.
    b. Barrington nucleus.
    c. the pontine micturition center (PMC).
    d. the M region.
    e. all of the above.

16. In terms of cerebral control of voiding in humans:
    a. coordinated relaxation and contraction of urethra and bladder is driven by a long-loop spinobulbospinal reflex.
    b. afferents activated during bladder filling synapse in the central periaqueductal gray (PAG) and PMC regions.
    c. spinobulbospinal voiding-reflex pathway functions as a "switch."
    d. absence of the "switch" would lead to incontinence.
    e. all of the above.

17. In terms of continence and brain–bladder control:
    a. it involves limbic areas associated with basic emotion and safety.
    b. it involves cortical circuits concerned with social propriety.
    c. the PAG and PMC form the main brainstem "switch."
    d. all of the above.

18. The contraction of detrusor by cholinergic muscarinic receptor agonists is characterized by:
    a. inositol triphosphate (ISP) hydrolysis and release of intracellular calcium.

    b. decreased calcium flux through nifedipine-sensitive calcium channels.
    c. involvement of the muscarinic M1 subtype only.
    d. stimulation of the Rho-kinase pathway.
    e. none of the above.

19. Stimulation of β-adrenergic receptors in human detrusor is characterized by:
    a. relaxation of detrusor smooth muscle.
    b. involvement of β-2 and β-3 subtype receptors.
    c. accumulation of cyclic adenosine monophosphate (cAMP).
    d. all of the above.

20. Urethral tone and intraurethral pressure are influenced by:
    a. α adrenergic receptors.
    b. sympathetic innervation.
    c. number of intramural ganglia.
    d. parasympathetic innervation.
    e. a and b are correct.

21. Which transgenic animal models has (have) been published showing detrusor overactivity?
    a. Increased M3
    b. Decreased P2X3/P2X2
    c. Decreased BK
    d. Decreased β1-integrin
    e. c and d are correct

22. The lamina propria (LP) of the bladder is thought to be the critical compartment because of which cell(s) that can mediate interaction between urothelium and nerves within the LP?
    a. Fibroblasts
    b. Ganglion cells
    c. Myofibroblasts
    d. Interstitial cells
    e. c and d are correct

23. The primary mechanism of action of onabotulinumtoxinA is:
    a. blockade of intracellular vesicle fusion in presynaptic nerves.
    b. suppression of afferent nerves in the LP.
    c. blockade of M3 receptor on detrusor myocyte.
    d. opening of BK channel on detrusor myocyte.
    e. blockade of voltage-dependent calcium channels on detrusor myocyte.

24. What distinguishing feature(s) in the bladder urothelium distinguish(es) it from the LP, detrusor, and serosal compartments?
    a. Presence of connexin-43 (Cx43)
    b. Presence of purinergic receptors
    c. Presence of tight junction proteins
    d. Presence of uroplakins
    e. c and d are correct

25. During acute bacterial cystitis, uropathogenic bacteria induce a host immune response due to their interaction with which of the following receptors on the urothelial cell?
    a. TRPV1
    b. M2
    c. NK-A
    d. TLR4
    e. P2X3

26. Maintenance of normal bladder compliance during urinary storage is (are) due to:
    a. passive viscoelastic properties.
    b. active neural signaling.
    c. modulation of filling rate.
    d. all of the above.
    e. a and b are correct.

27. Cx43 is important in regulating detrusor contractility because:
    a. it regulates acetylcholine release by efferent nerves.
    b. it breaks down acetylcholine in the neuromuscular junction.
    c. it allows for passage of ions between adjoining detrusor myocytes.
    d. it has a circadian rhythm of expression.
    e. c and d are correct.

28. Which urethral mechanisms are involved in maintenance of continence in the female?
    a. Network of submucosal vascularity
    b. Guarding reflex
    c. Hammock hypothesis
    d. Sympathetic tone
    e. All are correct

29. G-coupled proteins:
    a. mediate many different receptor functions.
    b. enzymatically cleave ATP to adenosine diphosphate (ADP).
    c. regulate protein folding in the endoplasmic reticulum (ER).
    d. help to regulate intracellular calcium concentrations.
    e. a and d are correct.

30. Urothelial barrier function is maintained by which of the following?
    a. Gap junctions
    b. Uroplakins
    c. TLR4 receptor
    d. Aquaporin channels
    e. Mucinous layer

31. In supraspinal spinal cord injury (SCI), mechanisms associated with neurogenic detrusor overactivity include:
    a. activity of C-fiber afferent fibers.
    b. nerve growth factor (NGF).
    c. activation of G-coupled protein receptors on detrusor muscle.
    d. contractions of the external sphincter.
    e. all are correct.

32. Membrane potential of a cell:
    a. requires energy to maintain, even at rest.
    b. at rest, is maintained by low intracellular potassium and high extracellular potassium.
    c. at rest, is maintained by low intracellular sodium and high intracellular chloride.
    d. becomes electrically more negative during an action potential in a neuron.
    e. changes during an action potential due to influx of anions into the detrusor myocyte.

33. Which of the following mechanisms is unique to M2 muscarinic receptor activation when compared to M3 muscarinic receptor activation?
    a. Mediates rise in intracellular calcium when activated
    b. Uses G-coupled proteins
    c. Involves cAMP downstream
    d. Causes detrusor contraction
    e. Causes detrusor relaxation

34. Isolated nocturia complaints are due to:
    a. nocturnal polyuria.
    b. sleep apnea.
    c. detrusor overactivity.
    d. peripheral edema.
    e. a, b, and d are correct.

35. Which of the following declines with aging?
    a. Bladder sensation
    b. ATP content of bladder
    c. Detrusor contractile responses to α adrenergic stimulation
    d. Detrusor contractile responses to cholinergic or electrical stimulation
    e. Bladder capacity

36. Urine from bladder pain syndrome/interstitial cystitis (BPS/IC) patients has been found to contain:
    a. a protein that inhibits urothelial cell growth in culture.
    b. a virus that induces T cell–mediated inflammation.
    c. a protozoan that invades the urothelial cell.
    d. an increased level of ATP.
    e. a and d are correct.

37. The "motor-sensory" hypothesis is used to explain mechanism of action in treating:
    a. bladder underactivity with a muscarinic agonist.
    b. neurogenic detrusor overactivity with TRPV1 blocker.
    c. idiopathic detrusor overactivity with onabotulinumtoxinA.
    d. urinary urgency with antimuscarinics.
    e. urinary frequency with α-blockers.

38. The reason that some women void without measurable increase in Pdet is because:
    a. the detrusor does not need to contract during voiding in women.
    b. the urethra contains smooth, in addition to striated, muscle fibers.
    c. there is a reduced parasympathetic innervation to the female bladder.
    d. Pdet is not the only measure of the bladder's mechanical work ability.
    e. the female bladder has increased viscoelastic properties.

39. Differences between smooth and striated muscles include:
    a. actinomyosin cross-bridge cycling in smooth muscle only.
    b. visible striations in striated muscle only.
    c. release of acetylcholine by prejunctional motor neurons in smooth muscle only.
    d. lack of intermediate filaments in skeletal muscles only.
    e. b and d are correct.

40. Bladder outlet obstruction results in:
  a. change in collagen subtype proportions.
  b. afferent and efferent neuronal hypertrophy.
  c. urothelial hyperplasia.
  d. C-fiber–mediated micturition reflex.
  e. a, b, and d are correct.

41. The principle behind neuromodulation in treating overactive bladder is:
  a. inhibition of detrusor interstitial cell activity.
  b. block of release of postganglionic neuronal acetylcholine.
  c. activation of C-fiber afferents.
  d. inhibition of somatic afferent processing in spinal cord.
  e. excitation of sacral sympathetic nerve fibers.

42. Which of the following animal models best mimics human BPS/IC?
  a. Social stress model
  b. Water avoidance stress model
  c. Acetic acid infusion into bladder
  d. Cyclophosphamide intraperitoneal injection
  e. Bowel radiation model

43. Etiologic causes for stress urinary incontinence may include:
  a. decreased urethral support.
  b. loss of urothelial seal.
  c. decreased serotonin in sacral spinal cord.
  d. shortened urethra.
  e. a, b, and c are correct.

44. The neurotransmitter released by sympathetic preganglionic neurons at the ganglia is:
  a. acetylcholine.
  b. norepinephrine.
  c. ATP.
  d. epinephrine.
  e. NO.

45. The action potential in either an afferent or efferent neuron is due to:
  a. influx of Na.
  b. influx of K.
  c. influx of Cl.
  d. influx of Ca.
  e. efflux of Ca.

ANSWERS

1. b. Sympathetic nerves inhibit the bladder body and excite the bladder neck and urethra.
2. e. All are correct.
3. e. All of the above.
4. e. a, b, and c only.
5. a. This is an example of cross-organ sensitization.
6. e. All are correct.
7. e. All are correct.
8. d. b and c are true.
9. e. All are true.
10. e. a, c, and d are correct.
11. e. All of the above.
12. e. a, b, and c are correct.
13. a. Switching between bladder storage and emptying can occur involuntarily (reflex emptying) or voluntarily.
14. e. a and d are correct.
15. e. All of the above.
16. e. All of the above.
17. d. All of the above.
18. a. inositol triphosphate (ISP) hydrolysis and release of intracellular calcium.
19. d. All of the above.
20. e. a and b are correct.
21. e. c and d are correct.
22. e. c and d are correct.
23. a. Blockade of intracellular vesicle fusion in presynaptic nerves.
24. e. c and d are correct.
25. d. TLR4
26. e. a and b are correct.
27. e. c and d are correct.
28. e. All are correct.
29. e. a and d are correct.
30. b. Uroplakins.
31. e. All are correct.
32. a. Requires energy to maintain, even at rest.
33. c. Involves cAMP downstream.
34. e. a, b, and d are correct.
35. a. Bladder sensation.
36. e. a and d are correct.
37. d. Urinary urgency with antimuscarinics.
38. d. Pdet is not the only measure of bladder's mechanical work ability.
39. e. b and d are correct.
40. e. a, b, and d are correct.
41. d. Inhibition of somatic afferent processing in spinal cord.
42. b. Water avoidance stress model.
43. e. a, b, and c are correct.
44. a. Acetylcholine.
45. a. Influx of Na.

CHAPTER REVIEW

1. The bladder has two parts: the body, which lies above the ureteral orifices, and the base, consisting of the trigone and bladder neck.
2. Smooth muscle is able to adjust its length over a much wider range than skeletal muscle. Thus an empty bladder has a small intravesical space despite the amount of smooth muscle it contains.
3. There is a complete, competent ring of smooth muscle around the bladder neck in the male. This does not occur in the female.
4. In women the density of adrenergic innervation in the bladder neck is less than in men.
5. Myofibroblasts in the LP modulate physiologic interactions between the urothelium and detrusor.
6. Bladder wall blood flow is reduced by distention; in patients with decreased compliance, this effect is pronounced.
7. In the female, the external urethral sphincter covers the ventral surface of the urethra in a horseshoe configuration.
8. The levator ani pelvic floor muscle does not surround the ventral aspect of the urethra in either the male or the female.
9. The external urethral sphincter is composed of (1) periurethral striated muscle of the pelvic floor and (2) striated muscle within the urethra.
10. The bladder urothelium serves a barrier function but is permeable to water to a limited degree and can actively transport sodium.
11. There is no definite evidence that the glycosaminoglycan (GAG) layer acts as a primary epithelial barrier.

12. Urothelial cells release chemical mediators such as NO, ATP, acetylcholine, and substance P that have excitatory and inhibitory actions on afferent nerves in the bladder wall.
13. Prostaglandins are released from the urothelium.
14. Uroplakin and tight junction proteins are important in maintaining the urothelial barrier function.
15. The normal bladder at rest may be spontaneously active.
16. A low voiding pressure in women does not equate with impaired detrusor contractility.
17. The parasympathetic nerves from S2 to S4 excite the bladder and relax the urethra. They have afferent fibers. The lumbar sympathetic nerves inhibit the bladder body and excite the bladder base and urethra. They also have afferent fibers. The pudendal nerves (S2 to S4) excite the external urethral sphincter. Afferent nerve fibers travel with the pudendal nerve as well.
18. There may be parasympathetic afferent and efferent nerve interconnections at the level of the intramural ganglia.
19. Pelvic nerve afferents monitor bladder volume and amplitude of the bladder contraction.
20. The bladder neck and proximal urethra contain the largest density of bladder nerves.
21. Decreased afferent sensitivity or excitability in certain pathologic conditions, as well as aging, may be an important cause of impaired voiding.
22. Activation of the parasympathetic pathway during voiding triggers the release of NO, which is a major inhibitor of urethral smooth muscle.
23. Cross organization may occur between bladder and bowel, uterus, pelvic urethra, vagina, and prostate. This may contribute to the chronic pelvic pain syndrome.
24. A substantial proportion of the C-fiber afferent population is silent; pathologic conditions may recruit mechanosensitive C-fibers to form a new functional afferent pathway.
25. Activation of the central serotonergic system can suppress voiding by inhibiting the parasympathetic excitatory input to the urinary bladder.
26. The bladder sympathetic reflex promotes closure of the urethral outlet and inhibits neurally mediated contractions of the bladder.
27. While the bladder fills, the external sphincter activity increases (guarding reflex)—i.e., pudendal motor neurons are activated by bladder afferent input.
28. The dorsal pontine tegmentum is the control center for micturition.
29. Stimulation of β-2 and β-3 receptors relaxes the detrusor.
30. Sex steroids modulate receptors and influence growth of bladder tissues.
31. After SCI, a C-fiber–mediated spinal reflex develops and may play a role in the development of detrusor overactivity.
32. Alterations of neural networks occur in the central nervous system following obstruction of the lower urinary tract.
33. Obstruction-induced detrusor overactivity may be due to denervation supersensitivity.
34. With aging detrusor contractility, bladder sensation and urethral pressure decline.
35. Sacral neuromodulation is thought to have its beneficial effect by somatic inhibition of sensory processing in the spinal cord.
36. The hammock hypothesis of urinary continence suggests that the urethra has a fixed dorsal surface due to its attachments to the pubis, pelvic muscles, and fascia, which allow ventral wall compression of the urethra against the fixed dorsal wall.

111 Pathophysiology and Classification of Lower Urinary Tract Dysfunction: Overview

Elizabeth Timbrook Brown, Alan J. Wein, and Roger R. Dmochowski

QUESTIONS

1. Which of the following best describes normal bladder behavior during the filling-storage phase of the micturition cycle?
   a. Low compliance due to elastic properties
   b. High compliance due to elastic properties
   c. Low compliance due to elastic and viscoelastic properties
   d. High compliance due to elastic and viscoelastic properties
   e. High compliance due to a low relaxation coefficient of the lamina propria

2. A patient who has significantly and urodynamically dangerous decreased compliance because of a replacement by collagen of other components of the stroma is generally best managed by:
   a. pharmacologic regimen.
   b. hydraulic distention.
   c. nerve section.
   d. augmentation cystoplasty.
   e. neuromodulation.

3. The "guarding reflex" refers to the:
   a. abrupt increase in striated sphincter activity seen with a cough during normal bladder filling/storage.
   b. spinal sympathetic inhibition of parasympathetic ganglion activity.
   c. gradual increase in striated sphincter activity seen during normal bladder filling/storage.
   d. gradual inhibition of the pontine-mesencephalic micturition center by the cerebral cortex during normal bladder filling/storage.
   e. gradual inhibition of the sacral spinal cord ventral nuclei by the pontine-mesencephalic brainstem during normal bladder filling/storage.

4. The primary effect of the spinal sympathetic reflexes that are evoked in animals during bladder filling and that facilitate bladder filling/storage is:
   a. neurally mediated stimulation of the α-adrenergic receptors in the area of the smooth sphincter.
   b. neurally mediated stimulation of the β-adrenergic receptors in the bladder body smooth musculature.
   c. direct inhibition of detrusor motor neurons in the sacral spinal cord.
   d. neurally mediated inhibition of cholinergic receptors in the area of the bladder body.
   e. neurally mediated sympathetic modulation of cholinergic ganglionic transmission.

5. The organizational center for the micturition reflex in an intact neural axis is the:
   a. pontine mesencephalic formation in the brainstem.
   b. frontal area of the cerebral cortex.
   c. parietal area of the cerebral cortex.
   d. cerebellum.
   e. sacral spinal cord.

6. IVCs are most commonly seen in association with:
   a. sacral spinal cord neurologic disease or injury.
   b. infrasacral neurologic disease or injury.
   c. suprasacral neurologic disease or injury.
   d. peripheral nerve neurologic disease or injury.
   e. interstitial cystitis.

7. Using the functional classification system, the usual lower urinary tract dysfunction seen after a stroke would be categorized as:
   a. failure to store because of the bladder (overactivity).
   b. combined deficit (failure to store because of the bladder, failure to empty because of striated sphincter dyssynergy).
   c. combined deficit (failure to store because of the bladder, failure to empty because of a nonrelaxing outlet).
   d. failure to store because of the bladder (hypersensitivity).
   e. failure to store because of the outlet.

8. In the International Continence Society (ICS) classification system, the disorder described in question 7 would be characterized as:
   a. during storage, overactive neurogenic detrusor activity, increased sensation, low bladder capacity, and incompetent urethral closure mechanism; and during voiding, normal detrusor activity and abnormal urethral function (dysfunctional voiding).
   b. during storage, normal detrusor function, increased sensation, low bladder capacity, and normal urethral closure mechanism; and during voiding, normal detrusor activity and abnormal urethral function (dysfunctional voiding).
   c. during storage, overactive neurogenic detrusor activity, normal sensation, normal bladder capacity, and incompetent urethral closure mechanism; and during voiding, normal detrusor activity and normal urethral function.
   d. during storage, stable detrusor activity, reduced sensation, low bladder capacity, and normal urethral closure mechanism; and during emptying, normal detrusor activity and abnormal urethral function (dysfunctional voiding).
   e. during storage, overactive neurogenic detrusor activity, normal sensation, low capacity, normal compliance, and normal urethral closure function; and during emptying, normal detrusor activity and normal urethral function.

9. In the current ICS terminology, "detrusor hyperreflexia" has been replaced by:
   a. detrusor instability.
   b. idiopathic detrusor overactivity.
   c. hyperactive bladder.
   d. neurogenic detrusor overactivity.
   e. neurogenic detrusor instability.

10. In the Krane-Siroky urodynamic classification system, a patient with post–cerebrovascular accident voiding dysfunction characterized by urgency, frequency, and urge incontinence would most commonly be characterized as having:

    a. detrusor areflexia, striated sphincter dyssynergia, and smooth sphincter dyssynergia.

    b. detrusor overactivty, striated sphincter synergia, and smooth sphincter dyssynergia.

    c. detrusor overactivty, striated sphincter dyssynergia, and smooth sphincter synergia.

    d. detrusor areflexia, striated sphincter synergia, and smooth sphincter dyssynergia.

    e. detrusor overactivty, striated sphincter synergia, and smooth sphincter dyssynergia.

11. In the Lapides classification system, a patient with post–cerebrovascular accident voiding dysfunction characterized by urgency, frequency, and urge incontinence would most commonly be characterized as having:

    a. sensory neurogenic bladder.

    b. motor paralytic bladder.

    c. uninhibited neurogenic bladder.

    d. reflex neurogenic bladder.

    e. autonomous neurogenic bladder.

12. A reflex neurogenic bladder, as described in the Lapides system classification, is characteristically seen in which of the following?

    a. Traumatic spinal cord injury between the sacral spinal cord and the brainstem

    b. Traumatic spinal cord injury between the sacral spinal cord and conus medullaris

    c. Cerebrovascular accident and insulin-dependent diabetes mellitus

    d. Non-insulin-dependent diabetes mellitus

    e. Multiple sclerosis

13. In the Bors-Comarr system of classification, the term *unbalanced*, when applied to a patient with an upper motor neuron (UMN) lesion, implies:

    a. cerebellar lesion.

    b. involuntary bladder contractions during filling.

    c. areflexic bladder.

    d. decreased bladder compliance during filling.

    e. sphincter dyssynergia.

14 In the Bors-Comarr system, a patient with post–cerebrovascular accident voiding dysfunction characterized by urgency, frequency, and urge incontinence would most commonly be characterized as having:

    a. a UMN lesion, complete, and balanced.

    b. a UMN lesion, complete, and imbalanced.

    c. a lower motor neuron (LMN) lesion, complete, and imbalanced.

    d. an LMN lesion, incomplete, and balanced.

    e. a UMN lesion/LMN lesion, complete, and balanced.

15. Which of the following is an absolute requirement for a patient to be included in the symptom syndrome of overactive bladder?

    a. Nocturia

    b. Urinary frequency

    c. Urgency

    d. Urgency incontinence

    e. Detrusor overactivity

16. Which of the following pathophysiologic factors is shared by men and women with urinary incontinence (failure to store) due to outlet underactivity?

    a. Bladder neck hypermobility

    b. Intrinsic sphincter dysfunction

    c. Proximal urethral hypermobility

    d. Nonrelaxing striated sphincter

    e. Bladder neck dysfunction

ANSWERS

1. **d. High compliance due to elastic and viscoelastic properties.** The normal adult bladder response to filling at a physiologic rate is an almost imperceptible change in intravesical pressure. During at least the initial stages of bladder filling, after unfolding of the bladder wall from its collapsed state, this high compliance ($\Delta V/\Delta P$) of the bladder is due primarily to its elastic and viscoelastic properties. Elasticity allows the constituents of the bladder wall to stretch to a certain degree without any increase in tension. Viscoelasticity allows stretch to induce a rise in tension followed by a decay (stress relaxation) when the filling (stretch stimulus) slows or stops.

2. **d. Augmentation cystoplasty.** The viscoelastic properties of the stroma (bladder wall less smooth muscle and epithelium) and the urodynamically relaxed detrusor muscle account for the passive mechanical properties and normal bladder compliance seen during filling. The main components of stroma are collagen and elastin. When the collagen component increases, compliance decreases. This can occur with various types of injury, chronic inflammation, bladder outlet obstruction, and neurologic decentralization. Once decreased compliance occurs because of a replacement by collagen of other components of the stroma, it is generally unresponsive to pharmacologic manipulation, hydraulic distention, or nerve section. Most often, under those circumstances, augmentation cystoplasty is required to achieve satisfactory reservoir function.

3. **c. Gradual increase in striated sphincter activity seen during normal bladder filling/storage.** There is a gradual increase in urethral pressure during bladder filling, contributed to by at least the striated sphincter element and perhaps by the smooth sphincteric element as well. The rise in urethral pressure seen during the filling/storage phase of micturition can be correlated with an increase in efferent pudendal nerve impulse frequency and in electromyographic activity of the periurethral striated musculature. This constitutes the efferent limb of a spinal somatic reflex, the so-called *guarding reflex*, which results in a gradual increase in striated sphincter activity during normal bladder filling and storage.

4. **e. Neurally mediated sympathetic modulation of cholinergic ganglionic transmission.** Does the nervous system affect the normal bladder response to filling? At a certain level of bladder filling, spinal sympathetic reflexes facilitatory to bladder filling/storage are clearly evoked in animals, a concept developed over the years by deGroat and colleagues, who have also cited indirect evidence to support such a role in humans. This inhibitory effect is thought to be mediated primarily by sympathetic modulation of cholinergic ganglionic transmission. Through this reflex mechanism, two other possibilities exist for promoting filling/storage. One is neurally mediated stimulation of the predominantly α-adrenergic receptors in the area of the smooth sphincter, the net result of which would be to cause an increase in resistance in that area. The second is neurally mediated stimulation of the predominantly β-adrenergic receptors (inhibitory) in the bladder body smooth musculature, which would cause a decrease in bladder wall tension. McGuire has also cited evidence for direct inhibition of detrusor motor neurons in the sacral spinal cord during bladder filling that is due to increased afferent pudendal nerve activity generated by receptors in the

striated sphincter. Good evidence also seems to exist to support a tonic inhibitory effect of other neurotransmitters on the micturition reflex at various levels of the neural axis. Bladder filling and consequent wall distention may also release autocrine-like factors that influence contractility (e.g., nitric oxide, prostaglandins, peptides).

5. **a. Pontine mesencephalic formation in the brainstem.** Although the origin of the parasympathetic neural outflow to the bladder, the pelvic nerve, is in the sacral spinal cord, the actual organizational center for the micturition reflex in an intact neural axis is in the brainstem, and the complete neural circuit for normal micturition includes the ascending and descending spinal cord pathways to and from this area and the facilitatory and inhibitory influences from other parts of the brain.

6. **c. Suprasacral neurologic disease or injury.** Involuntary contractions (IVCs) are most commonly seen associated with suprasacral neurologic disease or after suprasacral neurologic injury; however, they may also be associated with aging, inflammation or irritation of the bladder wall, bladder outlet obstruction, or stress urinary incontinence, or they may be idiopathic.

7. **a. Failure to store because of the bladder (overactivity).** The classic symptoms of post-stroke lower urinary tract dysfunction are urgency, frequency, and possible urgency incontinence. The urodynamic findings are generally detrusor overactivity (DO) during filling/storage with normal sensation and synergic sphincter activity during voluntary or involuntary emptying, unless the patient attempts to inhibit the DO with striated sphincter contraction. This translates simply in the functional system to a failure to store because of the bladder.

8. **e. During storage, overactive neurogenic detrusor activity, normal sensation, low capacity, normal compliance, and normal urethral closure function; and during emptying, normal detrusor activity and normal urethral function.** The micturition dysfunction of a stroke patient with urgency incontinence would most likely be classified during storage as overactive neurogenic detrusor function, normal sensation, low capacity, normal compliance, and normal urethral closure function. During voiding, the dysfunction would be classified as normal detrusor activity and normal urethral function, assuming that no anatomic obstruction existed.

9. **d. Neurogenic detrusor overactivity.** The Standardization Subcommittee of the ICS made some changes in definitions of terms (published as a committee report in 2002). One change was to eliminate the terms *detrusor hyperreflexia* and *instability* and replace them with the terms *neurogenic detrusor overactivity* and *idiopathic detrusor overactivity* (Abrams P et al., 2003).[a]

10. **b. Detrusor overactivty striated sphincter synergia, and smooth sphincter dyssynergia.** When exact urodynamic classification is possible, this system provides a truly precise description of the voiding dysfunction that occurs. If a normal or hyperreflexic detrusor exists with coordinated smooth and striated sphincter function and without anatomic obstruction, normal bladder emptying should occur. *Detrusor overactivty* is most commonly associated with neurologic lesions above the sacral spinal cord. Striated sphincter dyssynergia is most common after complete suprasacral spinal cord injury, following the period of spinal shock. Smooth sphincter dyssynergia is seen most classically in autonomic overactivty, when it is characteristically associated with detrusor overactivty and striated sphincter dyssynergia. *Detrusor areflexia* may be secondary to bladder muscle decompensation or to various other conditions that produce inhibition at the level of the brainstem micturition center, sacral spinal cord, bladder ganglia, or bladder smooth muscle. Patients with a voiding dysfunction secondary to detrusor areflexia generally attempt bladder emptying by abdominal straining, and their continence status and the ef-

ficiency of their emptying efforts are determined by the status of their smooth and striated sphincter mechanisms.

11. **c. Uninhibited neurogenic bladder.** Lapides contributed significantly to the classification and care of the patient with neuropathic voiding dysfunction by slightly modifying and popularizing a system originally proposed by McLellan in 1939. Lapides' classification differs from that of McLellan in only one respect, and that is the division of the group "atonic neurogenic bladder" into sensory neurogenic bladder and motor neurogenic bladder. This remains one of the most familiar systems to urologists and nonurologists because it describes in recognizable shorthand the clinical and cystometric conditions of many types of neurogenic voiding dysfunction. An uninhibited neurogenic bladder was described originally as resulting from injury or disease to the "corticoregulatory tract." The sacral spinal cord was presumed to be the micturition reflex center, and this corticoregulatory tract was believed to normally exert an inhibitory influence on the sacral micturition reflex center. A destructive lesion in this tract would then result in overfacilitation of the micturition reflex. Cerebrovascular accident, brain or spinal cord tumor, Parkinson disease, and demyelinating disease were listed as the most common causes in this category. The voiding dysfunction is most often characterized symptomatically by frequency, urgency, and urge incontinence, as well as urodynamically by normal sensation with DO at low filling volumes. Residual urine is characteristically low unless anatomic outlet obstruction or true smooth or striated sphincter dyssynergia occurs. The patient can generally initiate a bladder contraction voluntarily but is often unable to do so during cystometry because sufficient urine storage cannot occur before the DO is stimulated.

12. **a. Traumatic spinal cord injury between the sacral spinal cord and the brainstem.** Reflex neurogenic bladder describes the post-spinal shock condition that exists after complete interruption of the sensory and motor pathways between the sacral spinal cord and the brainstem. Most commonly, this occurs in traumatic spinal cord injury and transverse myelitis, but it may occur with extensive demyelinating disease or any process that produces significant spinal cord destruction as well. Typically, there is no bladder sensation and there is inability to initiate voluntary micturition. Incontinence without sensation generally results because of low-volume DO. Striated sphincter dyssynergia is the rule. This type of lesion is essentially equivalent to a complete UMN lesion in the Bors-Comarr system.

13. **e. Sphincter dyssynergia.** This system applies only to patients with neurologic dysfunction and considers three factors: (1) the anatomic localization of the lesion; (2) the neurologic completeness or incompleteness of the lesion; and (3) a designation as to whether lower urinary tract function is balanced or unbalanced. The latter terms are based solely on the percentage of residual urine relative to bladder capacity. Unbalanced signifies the presence of greater than 20% residual urine in a patient with a UMN lesion or 10% in a patient with an LMN lesion. This relative residual urine volume was ideally meant to imply coordination (synergy) or dyssynergia between the smooth and striated sphincters of the outlet and the bladder, during bladder contraction or during attempted micturition by abdominal straining or the Credé method.

14. **a. A UMN lesion, complete, and balanced.** In this system, UMN bladder refers to the pattern of micturition that results from an injury to the suprasacral spinal cord after the period of spinal shock has passed, assuming that the sacral spinal cord and the sacral nerve roots are intact and that the pelvic and pudendal nerve reflexes are intact. LMN bladder refers to the pattern resulting if the sacral spinal cord or sacral roots are damaged and the reflex pattern through the autonomic and somatic nerves that emanate from these segments is absent. This system implies that if skeletal muscle spasticity exists be-

---

[a] Sources referenced can be found in *Campbell-Walsh-Wein Urology, 12th Edition*, on the Expert Consult website.

low the level of the lesion, the lesion is above the sacral spinal cord and is by definition a UMN lesion. This type of lesion is characterized by DO during filling. If flaccidity of the skeletal musculature below the level of a lesion exists, an LMN lesion is assumed to exist, implying detrusor areflexia. Exceptions occur and are classified in a mixed lesion group characterized either by DO with a flaccid paralysis below the level of the lesion or by detrusor areflexia with spasticity or normal skeletal muscle tone neurologically below the lesion level. UMN lesion, complete, and imbalanced implies a neurologically complete lesion above the level of the sacral spinal cord that results in skeletal muscle spasticity below the level of the injury. DO occurs during filling, but a residual urine volume of greater than 20% of the bladder capacity is left after bladder contraction, implying obstruction in the area of the bladder outlet during the involuntary detrusor contraction. This obstruction is generally due to striated sphincter dyssynergia, typically occurring in patients who are paraplegic and quadriplegic with lesions between the cervical and the sacral spinal cord. Smooth sphincter dyssynergia may be seen as well in patients with lesions above the level of T6, usually in association with autonomic DO. LMN lesion, complete, and imbalanced implies a neurologically complete lesion at the level of the sacral spinal cord or of the sacral roots, resulting in skeletal muscle flaccidity below

that level. Detrusor areflexia results, and whatever measures the patient may use to increase intravesical pressure during attempted voiding are not sufficient to decrease residual urine to less than 10% of bladder capacity.

15. **c. Urgency.** Overactive bladder is defined (ICS) as urgency, with or without urinary urgency incontinence, usually with frequency and nocturia. One-third of the patients have incontinence, but two-thirds do not. Frequency and nocturia are usually but not always present. Detrusor overactivity is a urodynamic term indicating an involuntary bladder contraction. Urgency may or may not be associated with detrusor overactivity on a urodynamic study.

16. **b. Intrinsic sphincter dysfunction.** Failure to store because of outlet underactivity in the female is due to a combination of a failure of support, generally accompanied by hypermobility of the bladder outlet and intrinsic sphincter dysfunction (ISD). It is impossible to have effort-related incontinence in the woman without some element of ISD. Outlet-related incontinence in the male is most commonly seen after prostatectomy, and there is no pathophysiologic factor of hypermobility involved. The condition is essentially ISD. A nonrelaxing striated sphincter would not produce urinary incontinence, nor would bladder neck dysfunction.

CHAPTER REVIEW

1. The spinal sympathetic reflexes are facilitatory to bladder filling/storage.
2. The micturition cycle is divided into two phases: (1) bladder filling/urine storage and (2) bladder empting/voiding.
3. There are two urethral sphincters: (1) the smooth urethral sphincter is the smooth musculature of the bladder neck and proximal urethra; the smooth sphincter is not under voluntary control; and (2) the striated sphincter, which has two parts—the striated intramural sphincter, called the rhabdosphincter, and the external striated sphincter, which is part of the levator musculature. This sphincter is under voluntary control.
4. While collagen content of the bladder wall increases, compliance decreases.
5. There is increased afferent input when inflammation or irritation occurs, causing hypersensitivity to pain.
6. The hammock hypothesis of continence proposes that there is a fixed dorsal portion of the urethra due to fascial attachments against which the ventral aspect of the urethra is compressed.
7. Increases in intra-abdominal pressure are transmitted to the proximal urethra (as well as the mid-urethra in females).
8. The bladder response to filling at a physiologic rate is an almost imperceptible change in intravesical pressure.
9. Elasticity allows the constituents of the bladder wall to stretch to a certain degree without any increase in tension. Viscoelasticity allows stretch to induce a rise in tension followed by a decay (stress relaxation) when the filling (stretch stimulus) slows or stops.
10. IVCs are most commonly seen associated with suprasacral neurologic disease or after suprasacral neurologic injury; however, they may also be associated with aging, inflammation, or irritation of the bladder wall, bladder outlet obstruction, or stress urinary incontinence, or they may be idiopathic.
11. Overactive bladder is defined (ICS) as urgency, with or without urinary urgency incontinence, usually with frequency and nocturia.
12. It is impossible to have effort-related incontinence in the woman without some element of ISD.

112 Evaluation and Management of Women With Urinary Incontinence and Pelvic Prolapse

Alvaro Lucioni and Kathleen C. Kobashi

QUESTIONS

1. Which of the following is *not* a risk factor for urinary incontinence?
   a. Increased BMI
   b. Male gender
   c. Fecal incontinence
   d. Smoking
   e. Increased age

2. A 57-year-old woman is advised to start on estrogen replacement therapy. She should be told that:
   a. past history of birth control pill or systemic hormone use can increase the risk of stress incontinence.
   b. active systemic exogenous estrogen can decrease stress incontinence.
   c. low endogenous estrogen level is a risk for the development of stress incontinence.
   d. hormone replacement has no established effect on continence.
   e. systemic estrogen therapy is preferential to vaginal therapy for incontinence.

3. Patients with vaginal vault prolapse and no symptoms of stress urinary incontinence should undergo a sacrocolpopexy only (i.e., no sling):
   a. regardless of preoperative testing.
   b. if stress urinary incontinence was only demonstrated on physical examination.
   c. if no stress urinary incontinence was demonstrated on either physical examination or urodynamic testing.
   d. if stress urinary incontinence was demonstrated only during urodynamic evaluation.
   e. if they had a previous history of a bulking agent.

4. A 49-year-old woman has prolapse that is recorded as Aa-3, Ba-3, Ap-3, Bp-3. She has:
   a. no prolapse.
   b. stage 1 prolapse.
   c. stage 2 prolapse.
   d. stage 3 prolapse.
   e. stage 4 prolapse.

5. A patient is suspected of having a urinary tract–vaginal fistula. Which is the best dye test method to facilitate diagnosis of an isolated ureterovaginal fistula?
   a. Oral pyridium.
   b. Intravesical indigo carmine.
   c. Intravenous indigo carmine.
   d. Simultaneous oral pyridium and intravenous indigo carmine.
   e. Simultaneous oral pyridium and intravesical indigo carmine.

6. A healthy 65-year-old woman has bothersome prolapse and stress urinary incontinence (SUI). Exam shows stage 3 anterior prolapse and no apical or posterior prolapse or stress incontinence. On urodynamics she has a stable bladder and no SUI. The next step is repeat stress testing with:
   a. the urethral catheter removed.
   b. the prolapse reduced.
   c. the prolapse reduced and the urethral catheter removed.
   d. both the rectal and urethral catheters removed.
   e. a smaller-caliber urethral catheter.

7. The Pelvic Organ Prolapse Quantification (POP-Q) system:
   a. is a simple six-point quantification system for pelvic prolapse.
   b. was created in an effort to quantify pelvic organ prolapse and urinary incontinence.
   c. includes six specific points of position measurement in relation to the introitus.
   d. includes a simplified five-level staging system that does not require listing each of the points specifically.
   e. includes measurement of the total vaginal length performed *without* reduction of the prolapse.

8. A 34-year-old female is undergoing urodynamics for symptoms of urinary hesitancy. She is noted to have an absence of electromyography (EMG) recruitment with a squeezing of the clitoris. This represents a:
   a. disruption at the level of sacral nerve roots 2 to 4.
   b. dysfunction in the cauda equina.
   c. positive bulbocavernosus reflex (BCR).
   d. normal finding in 30% of normal females.
   e. problem with technique in assessing for the BCR.

9. The Food and Drug Administration (FDA) issued a mandate ordering the manufacturers to stop the sale and distribution of all remaining surgical mesh indicated for:
   a. slings.
   b. transvaginal prolapse repairs.
   c. transabdominal prolapse repairs.
   d. all prolapse repairs.
   e. all slings and pelvic prolapse repairs.

10. A 62-year-old man has bothersome urinary frequency and urgency associated with rare leakage. He has no obstructive symptoms, and postvoid residual (PVR) is 20 mL. Urine analysis (UA) is negative. The only therapy he has tried is a 2-week course of oxybutynin, but he is currently on no medications. The next step is:
    a. behavioral therapy, including dietary modification, fluid management, and bladder training.
    b. alpha-blocker therapy.
    c. repeat a trial of antimuscarinic therapy.
    d. beta-3 agonist therapy.
    e. combination antimuscarinic and beta-3 agonist therapy.

11. "Eyeball urodynamics" can provide information regarding:
    a. detrusor compliance.

b. bladder outlet obstruction.

c. abdominal leak point pressure.

d. detrusor leak point pressure.

e. detrusor-sphincter coordination.

12. Multichannel urodynamics:

a. is the most accurate diagnostic tool available for the evaluation of incontinence.

b. should be used in all patients with incontinence.

c. includes three directly measured values: detrusor pressure (Pdet), vesical pressure (Pves), and abdominal pressure (Pabd).

d. is not helpful in determining if a patient is at risk of developing upper tract deterioration.

e. all of the above.

13. Urodynamics should be considered:

a. when conservative measures have failed.

b. when the clinical picture is unclear.

c. when the symptoms cannot be confirmed by the clinician.

d. in patients who have undergone previous pelvic floor reconstruction.

e. all of the above.

14. Electromyelogram should:

a. be performed on all patients undergoing urodynamics.

b. demonstrate recruitment during the filling phase.

c. be active during coughing.

d. be silent with bulbocavernosus reflex (BCR).

e. be active during the voiding phase.

15. A 50-year-old lady presents with pure stress urinary incontinence. She has no other lower urinary tract symptoms (LUTS) and no previous pelvic surgeries. According to the American Urological Association/Society of Urodynamics, Female Pelvic Medicine & Urogenital Reconstruction (AUA/SUFU) SUI guideline, the initial evaluation of this patient should include a thorough history with assessment of symptoms and the following:

a. Physical and pelvic exam with demonstration of SUI, urinalysis, postvoid residual, cystoscopy.

b. Physical and pelvic exam with demonstration of SUI, urinalysis, postvoid residual, cystoscopy, urodynamics.

c. Physical and pelvic exam with demonstration of SUI, urinalysis, cystoscopy, urodynamics.

d. Physical and pelvic exam with demonstration of SUI, urinalysis, postvoid residual.

e. Physical and pelvic exam with demonstration of SUI, urinalysis, postvoid residual, urodynamics.

ANSWERS

1. **b. Male gender.** Obesity, advanced age, female gender, smoking, and associated pelvic floor disorders are risk factors for the development of urinary incontinence.

2. **a. Past history of birth control pill or systemic hormone use can increase the risk of stress incontinence.** Evidence shows that the use of exogenous hormones, currently or in the past, can increase the risk of development or exacerbation of existing stress incontinence such that local hormone replacement therapy is no longer considered part of the routine treatment for stress incontinence. However, local hormone replacement therapy can be helpful in the treatment of urgency incontinence. Vaginal hormone replacement is preferred to systemic therapy for treatment of lower urinary tract symptoms. Low endogenous hormone levels do not increase the risk of stress incontinence.

3. **c. If no stress urinary incontinence was demonstrated on either physical examination or urodynamic testing.** According to the AUA guidelines on surgical treatment of female stress urinary incontinence, a physician should demonstrate objective evidence of stress urinary incontinence prior to considering surgical management. Stress urinary incontinence could be demonstrated on physical exam or urodynamic testing. Based on the CARE and OPUS trials, patients with objective evidence of stress urinary incontinence should be counseled to consider concomitant surgical management of stress urinary incontinence. Patients with previous history of anti-incontinence procedure and objective evidence of stress urinary incontinence should still be counseled on surgical management of incontinence. If there is no objective evidence of stress urinary incontinence, one may consider not proceeding with surgical management of incontinence at time of prolapse repair.

4. **a. No prolapse.** The Pelvic Organ Prolapse-Quantification ("POP-Q") system is a 9-measure system that was created in an effort to provide objectivity to POP quantification. Six vaginal points labeled Aa, Ba, C, D, Ap, and Bp are measured in relation to the hymenal ring during a Valsalva maneuver. Aa and Ba represent points along the anterior vaginal wall, while Ap and Bp represent the posterior wall. Point C is the most distal point of the vaginal cuff or cervix, and D is the distance to the posterior fornix and is measured only if the cervix is still present. Points above the hymen are considered negative and points below the hymen are positive with a maximal established range of –3 to +3. The remaining three points are the genital hiatus (gh), which represents the size of the vaginal opening; the perineal body (pb), which represents the distance between the vagina and the anus; and the total vaginal length (tvl), which is measured by reducing the prolapse and measuring the depth of the vagina. A staging system based upon the above measurements ranges from stage 0 (no prolapse), in which all A and B points are –3, to stage 4, in which the leading edge is an absolute number that is no less than tvl –<2 cm (and is preceded by a "+" since it is below the hymen).

5. **a. Oral pyridium.** Oral pyridium will be excreted in the urine, so it will discolor a vaginal tampon whether the fistula is vesicovaginal or ureterovaginal or both. Intravenous indigo carmine would also demonstrate tampon staining in a similar pattern, but this is not practical as it involves the need for intravenous access. Presumably, staining higher on the tampon would indicate a ureterovaginal fistula, while lower staining would suggest a vesicovaginal fistula, but it can be difficult to differentiate with certainty as the dye can diffuse and 12% of patients with a vesicovaginal fistula have a concomitant ureteral fistula. Direct placement of dye (i.e., indigo carmine or methylene blue) into the bladder would only discolor the tampon if there is involvement of the bladder, but an isolated ureterovaginal fistula would be missed with this method. The best dye administration to evaluate for an isolated ureterovaginal fistula would be simultaneous intravesical blue dye and oral pyridium that would reveal orange staining only.

6. **b. The prolapse reduced.** When a patient who has subjective SUI and high-grade prolapse does not elicit SUI on urodynamics (UDS) studies, the AUA/SUFU urodynamics guidelines recommend reduction of the prolapse and repeat stress testing. In patients who have SUI with no prolapse, the next step is to repeat stress testing with the urethral catheter removed. In this situation, one would first repeat stress testing with the prolapse adequately reduced followed by removal of the urethral catheter. While downsizing the catheter or removing all catheters might result in demonstration of the leakage, this is not necessary or recommended by guidelines.

7. **d. Includes a simplified five-level staging system that does not require listing each of the points specifically.** POP-Q is a nine-point system that was created to objectify the assessment of pelvic organ prolapse. It measures six specific points in the vagina in relation to the hymen. The remaining three points include the total vaginal length, measured with the vagina completely reduced, the perineal body, and the genital hiatus. It has been simplified into to a five-stage system that does not require specific listing of each of the nine points.

8. **d. Normal finding in 30% of normal females.** BCR represents S2-4 and is present in all normal males and 70% of normal females. It is elicited by squeezing the glans penis or clitoris. During urodynamics, a positive is represented by increased EMG activity.

9. **b. Transvaginal prolapse repairs.** In 2019, the FDA released a mandate ordering the manufacturers to halt the sale and distribution of mesh placed transvaginally specifically for the repair of pelvic prolapse (https://www.fda.gov/news-events/press-announcements/fda-takes-action-protect-womens-health-orders-manufacturers-surgical-mesh-intended-transvaginal). Although the mandate excluded slings and transabdominally placed mesh for prolapse repair, unfortunately, subsequent media communication regarding mesh litigation created patient confusion and concern about the use of mesh in the pelvic floor in general. This prompted a response from the Society of Urodynamics, Female Pelvic Medicine and Urogenital Reconstruction (SUFU) (https://sufuorg.com/about/news/message-about-fda-statement-on-mus.aspx).

10. **a. Behavioral therapy, including dietary modification, fluid management, and bladder training.** Technically, this patient has not yet tried the first line of therapy according to the OAB guidelines. The best response is behavioral therapy that entails bladder exercises to train the bladder to overcome the sense of urgency when it occurs, pelvic floor exercises, fluid management, and avoidance of bladder irritants. Responses c, d, and e are all reasonable options to try in conjunction with behavioral therapy. Alpha-blockade would not be helpful in this situation in which the patient has no obstructive symptoms.

11. **a. Detrusor compliance.** "Eyeball UDS" is a simple alternative to full multichannel UDS that can provide ample information in selected patients. The study can determine bladder sensation, compliance, stability, and capacity as well as outlet competence and PVR. A 60-mL catheter tip syringe with the barrel removed is placed into the end of the catheter through which the bladder is filled by gravity. The height of the meniscus above the bladder represents the intravesical pressure. During the filling phase, a rise and fall in the meniscus may represent bladder overactivity, whereas a consistent gradual rise suggests compromised detrusor compliance. Because of the absence of the abdominal pressure (Pabd) channel, no information about the contribution of abdominal pressure is gleaned, and it is therefore not possible to definitively establish the presence or absence of significant outlet obstruction. Similarly, there is no information about urethral function or EMG afforded by this method, thereby making c, d, and e incorrect responses.

12. **a. Is the most accurate diagnostic tool available for the evaluation of incontinence.** Multichannel urodynamics is currently the most accurate diagnostic tool available for the evaluation of urinary incontinence. Whether it is necessary in the assessment of all patients with urinary incontinence remains controversial. Findings on urodynamics, which include direct measurements of vesical and abdominal pressures (Pves and Pabd, respectively) and a calculated measure of detrusor pressure (Pdet), can provide helpful information including findings such as elevated Pdet that may suggest a patient is at increased risk of developing upper deterioration.

13. **e. All of the above.** While a clinician may reasonably forego performing UDS on the index patient with SUI and no urinary urgency, the guidelines state that UDS may be considered in patients who are considering undergoing invasive, potentially morbid, or irreversible treatments. This is left to the clinician, and the philosophy is that if the study may answer an unanswered question or somehow change the course of care, it may be considered. However, any patient with a picture complicated by issues such as previous pelvic or anti-incontinence surgery, radiation therapy, neurologic disease, or difficult or unclear diagnosis should be considered for urodynamics.

14. **c. Be active during coughing.** EMG should be used in selected patients. Recruitment should occur with BCR in all men and 70% of women and in the face of increased intra-abdominal pressure, such as with coughing. It should be silent during voiding to allow passage of urine without outlet resistance.

15. **d. Physical and pelvic exam with demonstration of SUI, urinalysis, postvoid residual.** According to AUA/SUFU guidelines, the initial evaluation of patients with SUI desiring to undergo surgical intervention should include the following: history with assessment of symptoms, physical examination (including pelvic exam), objective demonstration of SUI, assessment of postvoid residual, and urinalysis. Additional evaluations such as cystoscopy and urodynamics should be limited to patients who cannot be undiagnosed based on initial evaluation or who demonstrate SUI, neurogenic bladder, abnormal urinalysis, urgency-predominant mixed urinary incontinence, elevated PVR, high-grade prolapse, and evidence of significant voiding dysfunction.

CHAPTER REVIEW

1. Pelvic floor disorders (PFDs) are a prevalent worldwide health concern.
2. Careful history and physical with objective demonstration of incontinence are integral in the proper evaluation of patients with PFDs.
3. Supplementary evaluation including urinalysis, postvoid residual, urodynamics, endoscopy, and radiologic imaging can be helpful in facilitating a complete and accurate diagnosis.
4. A variety of surgical and nonsurgical treatment options are available for treatment of urinary incontinence and pelvic organ prolapse.
5. The severity of PFD symptoms should be taken into account when considering treatment.
6. A thorough history is essential in the diagnostic evaluation of patients with PFDs.
7. Queries specific to the character, severity, duration, and quantity of incontinence and other symptoms related to pelvic floor function should be performed.
8. Attention should be paid to the impact of PFD symptoms on quality of life (QoL).
9. When appropriate, the clinician should present questions specific to the female with potential pelvic organ prolapse and the male with potential prostate issues.
10. Queries regarding past medical and surgical history, obstetric and gynecologic history, radiation therapy, trauma, and medications may provide important information.
11. A properly performed physical examination is imperative in the evaluation of patients with PFDs.
12. The Centers for Medicare/Medicaid require specific elements of both male and female genitourinary examination in order to meet coding guidelines (see Table 112.4).
13. Assessment of pelvic organ prolapse (POP) should ideally be performed in both the supine and standing positions.
14. Several classification and quantification systems are available for assessment of POP, the most widely used of which (Baden-Walker and POP-Q) are illustrated in Figs. 112.1 and 112.2.
15. A neurological examination and rectal examination should be performed in appropriate patients in order to obtain complete clinical information important in the assessment of lower urinary tract and pelvic floor function.
16. It has been demonstrated that patient subjective history alone often does not reflect an accurate or complete picture of their symptomatology complex.
17. Several instruments designed to facilitate symptom quantification have been developed and include tools such as voiding diaries, symptom and QoL questionnaires, and pad tests.
18. Voiding diaries can be both diagnostic and therapeutic, as they can provide patients with insights into behaviors that may be contributing to their voiding symptoms.
19. Pad tests may be helpful, particularly in the academic setting, to quantify incontinence symptoms. Loss of up to 8 g of urine in 24 hours may be considered normal, although the International Consultation on Incontinence (ICI) considers loss of greater than 1.3 g to be a positive 24-hour test.
20. Validated questionnaires are available to assess symptoms and quality of life in patients with PFDs.
21. Urodynamics (UDS) is the most accurate tool available for the assessment of LUT function and provides information regarding urine storage and emptying as they are affected by the bladder and the bladder outlet.
22. Although the use of routine UDS for straightforward incontinence is a topic of discussion, UDS should be strongly considered prior to intervention in patients who have a complex clinical picture due to failed previous treatment or surgery, mixed incontinence, obstructive symptoms, significantly elevated PVR, neurologic disease, or other medical conditions that may contribute to the LUT function, such as diabetes mellitus, pelvic prolapse, or history of radiation therapy.
23. "Eyeball UDS" may provide an approximate picture of the bladder capacity, sensation, stability, compliance, and outlet resistance when formal UDS is not available.

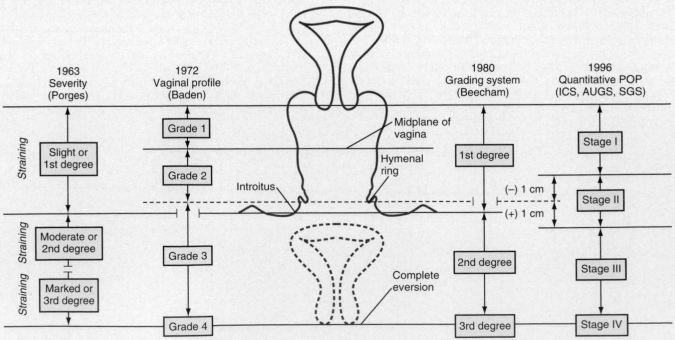

Fig. 112.1 Visual comparison of systems used to quantify pelvic organ prolapse (POP). *AUGS*, American Urogynecologic Society; *ICS*, International Continence Society; *SGS*, Society of Gynecologic Surgeons. (From Theofrastous JP, Swift SE: The clinical evaluation of pelvic floor dysfunction. *Obstet Gynecol Clin North Am* 25:783–804, 1998.)

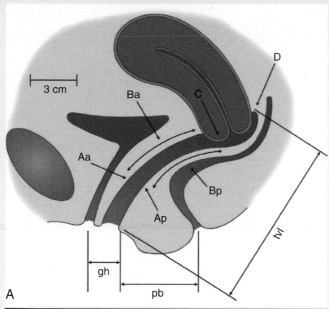

24. Multichannel UDS offers extensive evaluation of LUT function. It involves direct measurement of bladder and intra-abdominal pressure (Pves and Pabd, respectively) and a calculated assessment of detrusor pressure that is independent of abdominal pressure (Pdet). Pves-Pabd=Pdet.
25. Fluoroscopic imaging provides useful adjunctive information, such as the position and status of the bladder base and bladder neck, the presence of vesicoureteral reflux, and direct visualization of urinary leakage under real-time circumstances. Video imaging should be considered when the diagnosis cannot be made with certainty without simultaneous understanding of the anatomy in conjunction with the functional findings.

Point	Description	Range of values
Aa	Anterior vaginal wall 3 cm proximal to the hymen	−3 cm to +3 cm
Ba	Most distal position of remaining upper anterior vaginal wall	−3 cm to +tvl
C	Most distal edge of cervix or vaginal cuff scar	−
D	Posterior fornix (N/A if posthysterectomy)	−
Ap	Posterior vaginal wall 3 cm proximal to the hymen	−3 cm to +3 cm
Bp	Most distal position of remaining upper posterior vaginal wall	−3 cm to +tvl
gh (genital hiatus)	Measured from middle of external urethral meatus to posterior midline hymen	−
pb (perineal body)	Measured from posterior margin of gh to middle of anal opening	−
tvl (total vaginal length)	Depth of vagina when point D or C is reduced to normal position	−

Fig. 112.2 (A) Landmarks for the POP-Q system. (B) POP-Q points of reference. A, From Bump RC, Mattiasson A, Bo K, et al: The standardization of terminology of female pelvic organ prolapse and pelvic floor dysfunction. *Am J Obstet Gynecol* 175:10–17, 1996.

113 Evaluation and Management of Men With Urinary Incontinence

Riyad Tasher Al Mousa and Hashim Hashim

QUESTIONS

1. Which of the following is the definition of stress urinary incontinence (UI)?
   a. Leakage of urine with urgency
   b. Leakage of urine with an increase in intra-abdominal pressure
   c. Leakage of urine while asleep
   d. Leakage of urine with urgency and effort
   e. Leakage of urine without being aware of it

2. Which of the following symptoms is not considered a bladder storage symptom?
   a. Frequency
   b. Urgency
   c. Hesitancy
   d. Nocturia
   e. UI

3. Which of the following is not a potential risk factor for UI in men?
   a. Age
   b. Race
   c. Urological infection
   d. Cognitive impairment
   e. Prostatectomy

4. Initial assessment of men with UI includes all of the following EXCEPT:
   a. flow test.
   b. invasive urodynamics.
   c. frequency/volume chart.
   d. urinalysis.
   e. quality-of-life questionnaire.

5. Which of the following is not a treatment for urgency urinary incontinence (UUI)?
   a. Bladder training
   b. Pelvic floor muscle training
   c. Antimuscarinics
   d. Duloxetine
   e. Botox

6. Which of the following is not a treatment for stress urinary incontinence (SUI) in men?
   a. Pelvic floor muscle training
   b. Penile clamp
   c. Antimuscarinics
   d. Male sling
   e. Artificial urinary sphincter

7. Which of the following is not measured by the International Prostate Symptom Score (AUA-SI)?
   a. Urgency
   b. Frequency
   c. Nocturia
   d. Incontinence
   e. Straining

ANSWERS

1. **b. Leakage of urine with an increase in intra-abdominal presssure.** Leakage of urine with urgency is known as UUI. Leakage of urine while asleep is nocturnal enuresis. Leakage of urine on urgency and effort is mixed UI, and leakage of urine without being aware of it is insensible UI.
2. **c. Hesitancy.** Frequency, urgency, nocturia, and urinary incontinence are all bladder storage symptoms, while hesitancy is a voiding symptom.
3. **b. Race.** Potential risk factors for UI in men include increased age, urological infection, neurological and cognitive impairment, prostatectomy, and drugs. Ethnicity and race were not shown to have any statistical significance as a potential risk factor for UI in men.
4. **b. Invasive urodynamics.** Men with UI should be assessed with noninvasive baseline investigations including a flow test, frequency/volume chart or bladder diary, urinalysis to exclude infection and blood in the urine, and a quality-of-life questionnaire to assess the impact of the incontinence on quality of life. Invasive urodynamics, including filling cystometry and pressure flow studies, is reserved for use following failure of conservative and medical therapies and when it will alter the management of the patient.
5. **d. Duloxetine** Bladder training, pelvic floor muscle training, and antimuscarinics are first-line treatments of patients with UUI. If these fail, then patients can be treated with cystoscopic intradetrusor botulinum toxin-A injections. Duloxetine is a serotonin, norepinephrine reuptake inhibitor that has been licensed for the treatment of SUI in women but not for the treatment of UUI.
6. **c. Antimuscarinics.** Antimuscarinics are licensed for the treatment of overactive bladder syndrome and not SUI.
7. **d. Incontinence.** The IPSS or AUA-SI assesses three storage symptoms (urgency, frequency, nocturia), three voiding symptoms (intermittency, weak stream, straining), and one post-micturition symptom (incomplete emptying). It does not assess for UI (see Fig. 113.1AB).

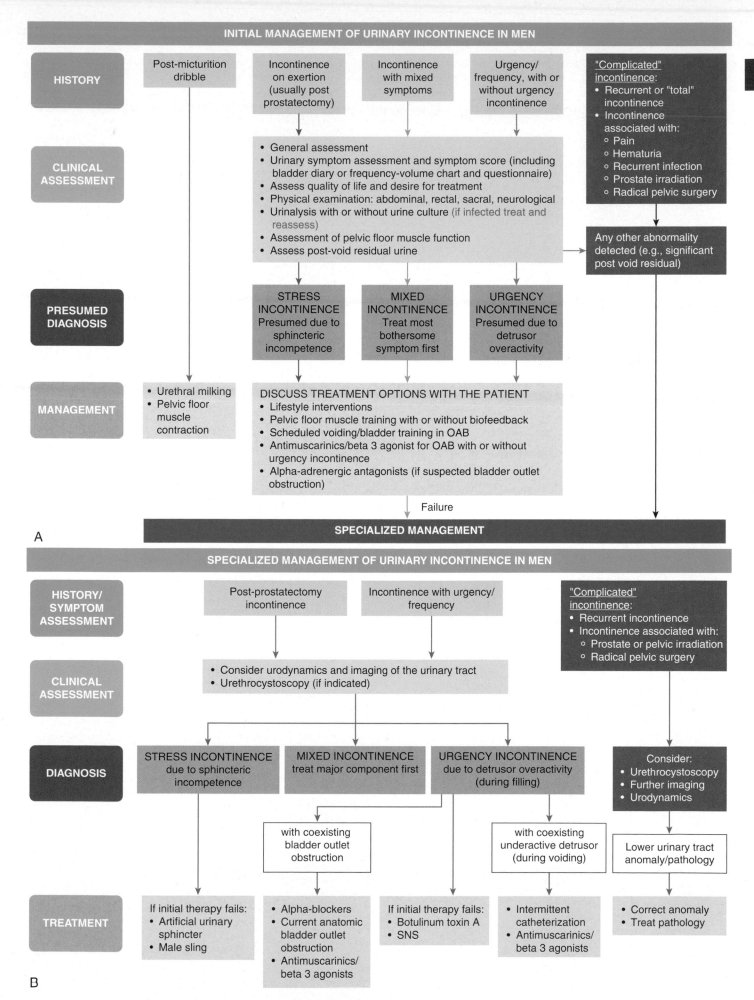

Fig. 113.1

CHAPTER REVIEW

1. UI is defined by the International Continence Society as the complaint of any involuntary loss of urine. It is part of the storage lower urinary tract symptoms (LUTS).

2. UI can result from a variety of causes and can become a social and hygienic problem that affects quality of life (QoL).

3. Potential risk factors for UI include increased age, infection, functional and cognitive impairment, neurological disorders, diabetes, prostatectomy, drugs, and alcohol.

4. UI in men is prevalent but less so than in women, and it can reach up to 39% of all men.

5. There are different types of UI in men, including SUI, UUI, a mixture of the two, and several other types. It is important to know the differences among them, as this affects management.

6. It is important to assess these patients appropriately to formulate a management plan that will help improve the patient's QoL. Depending on the etiology, initial treatment is usually conservative and medical, with surgical therapies reserved for those who fail initial treatment and in whom the UI is affecting their QoL.

114 Urodynamic and Video-Urodynamic Evaluation of the Lower Urinary Tract

Benjamin M. Brucker and Victor W. Nitti

QUESTIONS

1. Indications for urodynamic studies:
   a. are supported by high-quality, level 1 evidence for most conditions.
   b. are better defined for men than for women.
   c. are best defined by the clinician who has clear-cut reasons for performing the study and will use the information obtained to guide treatment.
   d. are of little value in assessing a patient with neurogenic lower urinary tract dysfunction.
   e. are only useful in women when incontinence is seen clinically.

2. The American Urological Association/Society for Urodynamics and Female Urology Urodynamics (AUA/SUFU) guidelines and recommendations:
   a. are all supported by level 1 or 2 evidence.
   b. do not apply to patients with neurogenic lower urinary tract dysfunction.
   c. are intended to assist the clinician in the appropriate selection of urodynamic tests, following evaluation and symptom characterization.
   d. include recommendations on standardization of urodynamic equipment.
   e. do not consider expert opinion.

3. Which of the following tests assesses bladder compliance?
   a. Cystometrogram (CMG)
   b. Micturitional urethral pressure profile
   c. Postvoid residual volume
   d. Voiding pressure flow study
   e. Electromyogram

4. Detrusor pressure:
   a. can be measured directly via a transurethral catheter.
   b. should remain low (near zero) during bladder filling.
   c. rises abruptly and does not return to baseline with detrusor overactivity.
   d. rises before the external sphincter relaxes in normal voluntary micturition.
   e. is obtained by adding the abdominal pressure to the vesicle pressure.

5. Detrusor overactivity (DO):
   a. is synonymous with overactive bladder.
   b. is necessary to make a diagnosis of urodynamic bladder outlet obstruction.
   c. can be seen on urodynamics of asymptomatic men and women.
   d. is commonly associated with renal deterioration.
   e. is a diagnosis made based on history alone.

6. The hallmark of bladder outlet obstruction is:
   a. incomplete bladder emptying.
   b. low pressure–low flow voiding dynamics.
   c. high pressure–low flow voiding dynamics.
   d. impaired detrusor contractility.
   e. elevated postvoid residual.

7. The external urethral sphincter should normally:
   a. relax with an involuntary bladder contraction in a neurologically normal person.
   b. relax prior to a voluntary detrusor contraction in a neurologically normal person.
   c. progressively relax while the bladder fills.
   d. always contract when the detrusor contracts.
   e. contract during urination in a neurologically normal person.

8. Video-urodynamics (VUDS):
   a. is the most precise measure of lower urinary tract function and should be used in all cases in which urodynamics are to be performed.
   b. is required to assess obstruction in a man.
   c. is the procedure of choice for documenting bladder neck dysfunction in men and women.
   d. is impractical to perform in spinal cord–injured patients.
   e. is needed to confirm detrusor overactivity.

9. Urethral function tests such as abdominal leak point pressure (ALPP) and maximum urethral closure pressure (MUCP):
   a. can precisely define intrinsic sphincter deficiency (ISD).
   b. should be done routinely before all surgery for stress incontinence.
   c. are the most important part of the urodynamic assessment of women with stress urinary incontinence (SUI).
   d. should not be used as a single factor to grade the severity of incontinence.
   e. can only be performed during ambulatory urodynamics.

10. Which of the following conditions/factors may result in inaccurate measurement of bladder compliance?
    a. Prior radiation to the pelvis
    b. Use of fluid-filled urodynamic catheters
    c. Presence of vesicoureteral reflux
    d. Bladder outlet obstruction
    e. History of genitourinary (GU) tuberculosis (TB)

11. According to the Functional Classification System, the symptom of stress incontinence can be classified as:
    a. failure to store secondary to an overactive bladder outlet.
    b. failure to store secondary to an overactive bladder.
    c. failure to store secondary to an underactive bladder outlet.
    d. failure to empty secondary to an underactive bladder outlet.
    e. failure to empty secondary to an overactive bladder outlet.

12. During multichannel urodynamics, what is the best measure that allows the clinician to look for abdominal straining occurring during micturition?

    a. Rectal or vaginal catheter pressure

    b. Bladder catheter pressure

    c. Uroflow pattern

    d. Electromyogram activity and uroflow velocity

    e. Postvoid residual

13. For women with stress incontinence, urodynamics have the most useful role in which of the following scenarios?

    a. In women who are considering surgical correction who also have urgency incontinence symptoms or difficulty emptying the bladder

    b. In predicting outcomes of surgery for women with pure stress incontinence

    c. In predicting the likelihood of voiding dysfunction in women with pure stress incontinence

    d. In predicting outcomes of conservative, nonsurgical treatments for women with mixed incontinence

    e. Prior to starting conservative, nonsurgical treatments for women with pure incontinence

ANSWERS

1. **c. Are best defined by the clinician who has clear-cut reasons for performing the study and will use the information obtained to guide treatment.** Urodynamics studies have been used for decades, yet clear-cut, level-1 evidenced-based "indications" for its use are surprisingly lacking. There are a number of reasons for this. It is difficult to conduct proper randomized controlled trials on urodynamics for conditions in which lesser levels of evidence and expert opinion strongly suggest clinical utility and in which "empiric treatment" is potentially harmful or even life-threatening (e.g., neurogenic voiding dysfunction). In addition, symptoms can be caused by a number of different conditions, and it is difficult to study pure or homogeneous patient populations. Given the current state of evidence for urodynamic studies, what is most important is that the clinician has clear-cut reasons for performing the study and that the information obtained will be used to guide treatment of the patient. Despite having established nomograms for bladder outlet obstruction in men, the indications for urodynamics in men are no more clear-cut than they are in women. Urodynamics probably have the most important role in the diagnosis and management of patients with neuropathic voiding dysfunction. In straightforward cases of pure SUI where incontinence is seen clinically, urodynamics may not be needed.

2. **c. Are intended to assist the clinician in the appropriate selection of urodynamic tests, following evaluation and symptom characterization.** The intent of the guideline was to assist clinicians in the appropriate selection of tests rather than to provide absolute indications for urodynamics. The review of literature produced few articles offering a high level of evidence, and most of the recommendations are based on lower levels of evidence, expert opinion, and clinical principles.

3. **a. Cystometrogram (CMG).** Compliance is the change in bladder volume/change in bladder pressure. Bladder pressure during filling is assessed by CMG.

4. **b. Should remain low (near zero) during bladder filling.** Detrusor pressure normally remains low during filling, as the bladder is highly compliant. It cannot be measured directly with a transurethral catheter, but must be obtained via subtraction of abdominal pressure from vesicle pressure. With detrusor overactivity, pressure usually returns to baseline after the involuntary contraction abates.

5. **c. Can be seen on urodynamics of asymptomatic men and women.** DO is defined as involuntary bladder contractions

on CMG. Overactive bladder is a symptom complex with the hallmark symptom of urinary urgency and is not diagnosed on urodynamics. DO has been reported to occur in studies on asymptomatic men and women. Impaired compliance, not DO, is associated with renal deterioration. DO is an observation made during urodynamics.

6. **c. High pressure–low flow voiding dynamics.** Obstruction is defined by high pressure low flow voiding. It may or may not be accompanied by incomplete bladder emptying. Impaired detrusor contractility may sometimes, but not always, be a long-term consequence of obstruction.

7. **b. Relax prior to a voluntary detrusor contraction in a neurologically normal person.** In a neurologically normal person, the external sphincter progressively contracts with bladder filling and will also contract during an involuntary bladder contraction (guarding reflex). External sphincter relaxation is the first step in the micturition cycle and precedes the detrusor contraction. In detrusor external sphincter dyssynergia, an abnormal neurologic condition, the external sphincter contracts when the detrusor does. Intermittent or fluctuating flow rate of urine due to intermittent contractions of the external sphincter in a neurologically normal person is considered dysfunctional voiding.

8. **c. Is the procedure of choice for documenting bladder neck dysfunction in men and women.** Although VUDS provides the most precise evaluation of voiding function and dysfunction and is particularly useful when anatomic structure and function are important, it is not practical or necessary for all centers to have VUDS capabilities. VUDS is useful for a number of conditions when an accurate diagnosis cannot otherwise be obtained (e.g., by conventional urodynamics), including complicated voiding dysfunction or known or suspected neuropathic voiding dysfunction (adults and children), unexplained urinary retention in women, prior radical pelvic surgery, urinary diversion, preceding or following renal transplant, or prior pelvic radiation. VUDS is the procedure of choice for documenting bladder neck dysfunction in men and women. VUDS is not specifically needed to diagnose DO.

9. **d. Should not be used as a single factor to grade the severity of incontinence.** Urethral function tests such as ALPP and MUCP have not been shown to be consistently useful in defining ISD or outcomes of treatments for SUI. They may be useful for some clinicians, but are by no means mandatory. According to the International Continence Society, "Urethral function measurements of leak point pressures and urethral closure pressures are not used as a single factor to grade the severity of incontinence." Urodynamics are not necessary before surgical treatment of SUI for all women, but if it is done, the AUA/SUFU Guideline states that ALPP or MUCP should be preformed. ALPP can be reported as part of ambulatory urodynamics; however, it is not a measure that is unique to this method.

10. **c. Presence of vesicoureteral reflux.** Bladder outlet obstruction and radiation can cause a decrease in compliance, but should not affect its accurate measurement. GU TB also can cause significant bladder fibrosis and impaired compliance. Reflux can make compliance look worse than it actually is secondary to the "pop-off" it creates. Fluoroscopy or VUDS is necessary in some cases (e.g., neurogenic bladder) to assess for reflux during filling. In addition, filling rate and involuntary detrusor contractions can also make compliance look worse than it actually is. There are no data to support the proposition that fluid-filled catheters or air charge catheters will result in inaccurate measures of compliance, which is a measure of change volume over pressure.

11. **c. Failure to store secondary to an underactive bladder outlet.** Stress incontinence is a symptom caused by failure to store urine during increases in abdominal pressure. It can be caused by a loss of outlet resistance or an underactive bladder outlet.

12. **a. Rectal or vaginal catheter pressure.** Rectal and or vaginal pressure are used to measure abdominal pressure throughout urodynamics. Patients who are straining to void will exhibit

increases in abdominal pressure measurements. Flow patterns can be suggestive of abdominal straining, but are not as accurate as measuring abdominal pressure. Postvoid residual may allow clinicians to understand how well the patient is emptying his or her bladder but does not give information about how voiding is accomplished. Similarly, EMG may be increased from abdominal straining, but there are many other causes of increased EMG activity during voiding. Bladder catheter pressure will increase with abdominal straining. The difference between the bladder catheter and the rectal or vaginal catheter allows for calculation of the detrusor pressure.

13. **a. In women who are considering surgical correction who also have urgency incontinence symptoms or difficulty emptying the bladder.** UDS in women with pure stress or stress-predominant mixed incontinence and normal emptying has not been shown in randomized controlled trials to be more beneficial than office evaluation alone and has not been shown to predict outcomes of surgery in the same population. Women with significant mixed incontinence and emptying problems have not been studied in randomized controlled trials, and it is felt that UDS is beneficial in these women.

CHAPTER REVIEW

1. Urodynamics are performed in an unnatural setting and therefore does not always predict the findings with normal activity.
2. Normal uroflow is a bell-shaped curve.
3. EMG patch electrodes measure perineal muscle function with the assumption that it is reflective of urethral external sphincter function.
4. To specifically measure external sphincter function, needle electrodes must be used.
5. Mean values for compliance are 40–120 mL/cm H_2O.
6. Measurement of compliance is difficult to interpret; therefore, pressures during filling are more often used to predict outcome.
7. There are two types of leak-point pressures: (a) abdominal leak-point pressure, which is defined as the intravesical pressure at which urine leakage occurs due to increased abdominal pressure; and (b) detrusor leak-point pressure, which is a measure of detrusor pressure at which urine leakage occurs in the absence of a detrusor contraction or increased abdominal pressure. This measure is generally used in patients with decreased compliance or lower motor neuron disease.
8. Detrusor pressures that are sustained above 40 cm H_2O lead to deterioration of the upper tracts.
9. Maximum urethra closure pressure is defined as the difference between peak urethral pressure and intravesical pressure and is normally between 40 and 60 cm H_2O.
10. Bladder outlet obstruction index is defined by the equation: BOOI = Pdet Qmax − 2(Qmax). In men, a value greater than 40 is considered obstructed; a value less than 20 is considered unobstructed.
11. A uroflow less than 12 mL/sec and Pdet greater than 25 cm H_2O predict outlet obstruction in women.
12. Detrusor external sphincter dyssynergia can be due to a neurologic lesion (above the sacral micturition center) or a learned disorder. The latter is considered dysfunctional voiding.
13. Internal sphincter dyssynergia must be diagnosed by VUDS.
14. Stress incontinence, which is observed only when a coexisting prolapse is reduced, is referred to as occult or latent stress incontinence.
15. For internal sphincter dyssynergia to occur, the spinal cord lesion must be above the sympathetic outflow (T-10-L-1).
16. VUDS is the procedure of choice for documenting bladder neck dysfunction in men and women.
17. In a neurologically normal person, the external sphincter progressively contracts with bladder filling and will also contract during an involuntary bladder contraction (guarding reflex). External sphincter relaxation is the first step in the micturition cycle and precedes the detrusor contraction.

115 Urinary Incontinence and Pelvic Prolapse: Epidemiology and Pathophysiology

Gary E. Lemack and Maude Carmel

QUESTIONS

1. An example of a lower urinary tract (LUT) symptom is:
   a. urine loss while playing tennis.
   b. urodynamic stress incontinence with Valsalva leak point pressure (VLPP) of 60 cm H_2O.
   c. a symptom score of 19 on the AUA Symptom Index.
   d. the finding of urinary incontinence on a supine stress test.
   e. the presence of stage 2 anterior pelvic organ prolapse on a cystogram.

2. Which of the following is consistent with the diagnosis of urgency urinary incontinence?
   a. Leakage of urine with coughing and a VLPP of 60 cm H_2O
   b. Leakage of urine with detrusor overactivity
   c. Leakage of urine while coughing and detrusor leak point pressure of 50 cm H_2O
   d. Leakage of urine while coughing and leakage of urine with urgency
   e. Leakage of urine and feces while straining

3. The most common form of urinary incontinence (UI) in a woman aged 40 years is:
   a. stress incontinence.
   b. urgency incontinence.
   c. mixed incontinence.
   d. detrusor overactivity incontinence.
   e. continuous incontinence.

4. What factor has been associated with LUTS but not urinary incontinence in women?
   a. Advancing age.
   b. Caucasian race.
   c. Number of prior vaginal delivereries.
   d. Caffeine intake.
   e. Large birth weight.

5. Later in life, when compared with a woman who had her first child at the age of 36, a woman delivering her first child at 23 years of age would be:
   a. more likely to experience SUI.
   b. equally likely to experience SUI.
   c. more likely to experience UUI.
   d. equally likely to experience UUI.
   e. less likely to experience MUI.

6. The symptom most closely associated with the presence of advanced pelvic organ prolapse is the sensation of:
   a. pelvic pressure.
   b. pelvic pain.
   c. constipation.
   d. voiding difficulty.
   e. vaginal bulge.

7. Which of the following Pelvic Organ Prolapse Quantification System (POP-Q) scores is implausible?
   a. Aa of −2
   b. Ap of +4
   c. Ba of +5
   d. Bp of 0
   e. C of −8

8. A woman with POP-Q scores of Aa −2, Ba 0, C −5, Ap +1, Bp +1 would be considered to have what stage prolapse?
   a. Stage 0
   b. Stage 1
   c. Stage 2
   d. Stage 3
   e. Stage 4

9. A patient with a POP-Q score of Aa −2 , Ba −2, Ap +2, Bp +2, and C 0 should be counseled to undergo:
   a. anterior colporrhaphy.
   b. posterior colporrhaphy.
   c. anterior and posterior colporrhaphy.
   d. posterior colporrhaphy and sacrospinous fixation.
   e. sacrospinous fixation.

10. During bladder contraction, which is most active?
    a. Pelvic nerve
    b. Hypogastric nerve
    c. Pudendal nerve
    d. A-delta nerves
    e. Onuf nucleus

ANSWERS

1. **a. Urine loss while playing tennis.** A LUT symptom is one that is recognizable by the patient. A sign is one that is observable by a clinician (i.e., urine loss during a supine stress test). A VLPP result is a urodynamic observation, whereas a cystogram report of a cystocele is a radiologic observation.

2. **b. Leakage of urine with detrusor overactivity.** Urgency urinary incontinence may be associated with detrusor overactivity (DO), though DO need not be present for the diagnosis, merely sense of urgency with loss of urine. Mixed incontinence is the symptomatic complaint of both stress urinary incontinence and urgency incontinence.

3. **a. Stress incontinence.** Stress urinary incontinence (SUI) is the most common form of UI in young women. In contrast, urge UI and mixed UI appear to become more prevalent forms of UI with aging. Continuous incontinence is uncommon—often associated with iatrogenic injuries to the lower urinary tract resulting in fistulae.

4. **d. Caffeine intake.** Caffeine consumption has been associated with urinary urgency, but most studies have not necessarily noted an association with urinary incontinence. All other factors mentioned have been associated with a form of UI.

5. **a. More likely to experience SUI.** Younger age at time of first pregnancy has been associated with a greater likelihood of developing SUI later in life.

6. **e. Vaginal bulge.** Although all of the symptoms described can be associated with POP, only the specific complaint of a vaginal bulge has been consistently demonstrated to be associated with the presence of POP. All others can be associated with other conditions distinct from the presence of POP. For example, pelvic pressure can be related to pelvic floor dysfunction or a variety of other conditions, and pelvic pain can be associated with various forms of pelvic pathology including adnexal pathology.

7. **b. Ap of + 4.** POP-Q points are measured by their distance from the hymenal ring (in centimeters). By definition, Aa and Ap are the points 3 cm from the hymen on the anterior and posterior vaginal walls, respectively. It would be impossible for this point to be greater than 3 cm proximal (or distal) to the hymen. In advanced prolapse, this point could be up to 3 cm distal to the hymen. C point represents the distance from the hymen to the cervix or vaginal cuff (post hysterectomy). Ba and Bp point represent the leading edge of the most advanced aspect of the prolapse on the anterior and posterior vaginal walls, respectively. As such, they can be well beyond + 3 in advanced prolapse.

8. **c. Stage 2.** Staging in POP-Q is based on the leading edge of prolapse. This equates to the highest (positive) number associated with the points listed (Aa, Ba, Ap, Bp, C). The leading edge of the most advanced POP is greater than 1 cm proximal to the hymen in patients with stage 1 prolapse. Stage 2 patients will have their leading edge between 1 cm proximal to and distal to the hymen. Stage 3 indicates a leading edge greater than 1 cm beyond the hymen but not completely everted (stage 4).

9. **d. Posterior colporrhaphy and sacrospinous fixation.** This patient has both posterior compartment prolapse (based on Ap and Bp points beyond the hymen) and apical prolapse (C point at the hymen) based on the POP-Q score. Therefore the patient should be counseled to have both posterior repair of some type (posterior colporrhaphy in this example) and apical repair (sacrospinous fixation in this example).

10. **a. Pelvic nerve.** During bladder contraction, parasympathetic transmission (via the pelvic nerve) is active and sympathetic transmission (via the hypogastric nerve) is suppressed. Pudendal innervation to the external sphincter is suppressed. Pudendal innervation is derived from Onuf nucleus in the sacral cord. A-delta nerves (afferent) are active during storage and are involved in the spinal reflex mechanism that promotes closure of the bladder neck.

CHAPTER REVIEW

1. Pelvic organ prolapse may mask incontinence.
2. The prevalence of urinary incontinence in women is between 25% and 40%. Ten percent of women experience weekly incontinence episodes. Fecal incontinence occurs in 17% of women with pelvic organ prolapse.
3. The female bladder neck is weaker than the male bladder neck and is often incompetent.
4. In women, the majority of the urethra should be considered an active area of sphincter control; however, in the female the most important portion of continence is the mid-urethra.
5. A Valsalva leak point pressure of less than 60 cm H_2O indicates but does not confirm intrinsic sphincter dysfunction.
6. Twelve percent of men report terminal dribbling.
7. Rates of overactive bladder increase with age.
8. Oral estrogen treatment is associated with the development of incontinence. Topical estrogen therapy is not linked to stress incontinence.
9. Intrinsic properties of the urethra mucosa and urethra wall are important in maintaining continence in women.
10. The anterior vaginal wall provides posterior support of the urethra allowing for compression of the mid-urethra. The urethra is attached laterally to the arcus tendineus by the urethra pelvic ligaments.
11. Urge UI and mixed UI appear to become more prevalent forms of UI with aging.
12. Age is strongly correlated with the development of UI of all types. White women appear to be at greater risk for UI when compared with African American and Asian women in particular.
13. POP-Q points are measured by their distance from the hymenal ring (in centimeters). By definition, Aa and Ap are the points 3 cm from the hymen on the anterior and posterior vaginal walls, respectively. Ba and Bp point represent the leading edge of the most advanced aspect of the prolapse on the anterior and posterior vaginal walls, respectively. Thus they can be well beyond + 3 in advanced prolapse. C point represents the distance from the hymen to the cervix or vaginal cuff (post hysterectomy).
14. The leading edge of the most advanced POP is greater than 1 cm proximal to the hymen in patients with stage 1 prolapse. Stage 2 patients will have their leading edge between 1 cm proximal to and distal to the hymen. Stage 3 indicates a leading edge greater than 1 cm beyond the hymen but not completely everted.

116 Neuromuscular Dysfunction of the Lower Urinary Tract

Casey Kowalik, Alan J. Wein, and Roger R. Dmochowski

QUESTIONS

1. What is the general pattern of voiding dysfunction secondary to neurologic lesions above the level of the brainstem?
   a. Involuntary bladder contractions, smooth sphincter dyssynergia, striated sphincter synergy
   b. Involuntary bladder contractions, smooth sphincter synergy, striated sphincter synergy
   c. Involuntary bladder contractions, smooth sphincter synergy, striated sphincter dyssynergia
   d. Detrusor hypocontractility, smooth sphincter synergy, striated sphincter synergy
   e. Detrusor areflexia, smooth sphincter synergy, striated sphincter synergy

2. What is the general pattern of voiding dysfunction that results from complete lesions of the spinal cord above the level of S2 after recovery from spinal shock?
   a. Involuntary bladder contractions, smooth sphincter dyssynergia, striated sphincter synergy
   b. Involuntary bladder contractions, smooth sphincter synergy, striated sphincter synergy
   c. Involuntary bladder contractions, smooth sphincter synergy, striated sphincter dyssynergia
   d. Detrusor hypocontractility, smooth sphincter synergy, striated sphincter synergy
   e. Detrusor areflexia, smooth sphincter synergy, striated sphincter synergy

3. Which of the following is the most common long-term expression of lower urinary tract dysfunction after a cerebrovascular accident (CVA)?
   a. Detrusor areflexia
   b. Lack of sensation of filling
   c. Impaired bladder contractility
   d. Striated sphincter dyssynergia
   e. Detrusor overactivity

4. A 65-year-old man who has sustained a stroke but is otherwise in good health has symptoms of hesitancy, straining to void, urgency, and frequency. The optimal next step in management is:
   a. anticholinergic therapy.
   b. transurethral resection of the prostate (TURP).
   c. transurethral incision of the bladder neck and prostate.
   d. clean intermittent catheterization.
   e. full urodynamic evaluation.

5. The most common pattern of micturition in children and adults who have cerebral palsy (CP) and no other complicating neurologic condition is:
   a. abnormal filling/storage because of detrusor overactivity; normal emptying.
   b. normal filling/storage; normal emptying.

   c. normal filling/storage; abnormal emptying because of smooth sphincter dyssynergia.
   d. normal filling/storage; abnormal emptying because of striated sphincter dyssynergia.
   e. abnormal filling/storage because of detrusor overactivity; abnormal emptying because of striated sphincter dyssynergia.

6. The most common urodynamic findings in individuals with CP who do exhibit lower urinary tract dysfunction are:
   a. detrusor areflexia, coordinated sphincters.
   b. detrusor overactivity, smooth sphincter dyssynergia, striated sphincter dyssynergia.
   c. detrusor overactivity, smooth sphincter synergy, striated sphincter dyssynergia.
   d. decreased detrusor compliance, coordinated sphincters.
   e. detrusor overactivity, coordinated sphincters.

7. The most common urodynamic abnormality found in patients with voiding dysfunction secondary to Parkinson disease (PD) is:
   a. impaired sensation during filling.
   b. striated sphincter dyssynergia.
   c. striated sphincter bradykinesia.
   d. detrusor overactivity.
   e. impaired detrusor contractility.

8. Urodynamic findings that may distinguish multiple system atrophy (MSA) from PD include:
   a. sphincteric insufficiency
   b. detrusor overactivity
   c. detrusor areflexia
   d. lack of sensation during filling
   e. decreased bladder capacity

9. The most common urodynamic findings in individuals with multiple sclerosis (MS) who have lower urinary tract dysfunction are:
   a. detrusor overactivity, smooth sphincter dyssynergia
   b. detrusor overactivity, smooth sphincter synergia
   c. detrusor areflexia, impaired filling sensation
   d. detrusor areflexia, striated sphincter dyssynergia
   e. normal filling and storage

10. The incidence of upper urinary tract deterioration is greatest in which of the following?
    a. MS
    b. MSA
    c. PD
    d. Spinal cord injury (SCI)
    e. Diabetes

11. All of the following are risk factors for upper urinary tract deterioration in a patient with a suprasacral SCI except:
    a. high-pressure storage.
    b. high detrusor leak-point pressure.
    c. chronic bladder overdistention.
    d. high abdominal leak-point pressure.
    e. vesicoureteral reflux with infection.

12. In spinal shock, findings generally include all of the following EXCEPT:
    a. acontractile bladder.
    b. areflexic bladder.
    c. open bladder neck.
    d. absent guarding reflex.
    e. maximal urethral closure pressure above normal.

13. The presence of true striated sphincter dyssynergia implies a neurologic lesion between the:
    a. pons and the sacral spinal cord.
    b. cerebral cortex and the pons.
    c. cervical and the sacral spinal cord.
    d. sacral spinal cord and the striated sphincter.
    e. cauda equina and the striated sphincter.

14. Which of the following is least characteristic as a finding in autonomic hyperreflexia?
    a. Headache before bladder contraction
    b. Hypertension
    c. Flushing above the level of the lesion
    d. Tachycardia
    e. Sweating above the level of the lesion

15. A patient with a history of cervical SCI is undergoing urodynamic evaluation and currently has 350 cc infused volume. He begins to complain of headache and develops hypertension and bradycardia. What is the next step?
    a. Continue filling and reassure him
    b. Administer an antibiotic
    c. Give terazosin 5 mg immediately
    d. Empty his bladder
    e. Apply 2% nitroglycerin paste

16. The sacral spinal cord terminates in the cauda equina at approximately the spinal column level of:
    a. T10.
    b. L1.
    c. L2.
    d. L3.
    e. S1.

17. Patients who have voiding dysfunction secondary to lumbar disk disease most commonly present with which of the following symptoms and urodynamic findings?
    a. Retention; involuntary bladder contractions
    b. Incontinence; involuntary bladder contractions
    c. Retention; decreased bladder compliance
    d. Difficulty voiding; normal bladder compliance
    e. Incontinence; normal bladder compliance

18. The clinical picture of cauda equina syndrome (CES) varies widely. Which of the following is typically not seen with CES?
    a. Urinary incontinence
    b. Loss of bowel control
    c. Perineal sensory loss
    d. Sexual dysfunction
    e. Limb spasticity

19. The combination that best describes the type of permanent voiding dysfunction that can occur after radical pelvic surgery is:
    a. stress incontinence; detrusor areflexia.
    b. urgency incontinence; detrusor overactivity.
    c. reflex incontinence; detrusor areflexia.
    d. urgency incontinence; detrusor overactivity.
    e. stress incontinence; detrusor overactivity.

20. What is optimal management for a 65-year-old man who has had a first occurrence of urinary retention after radical pelvic surgery?
    a. Anticholinergic therapy
    b. Clean intermittent catheterization
    c. TURP
    d. External sphincterotomy
    e. Bethanechol chloride

21. The urodynamic parameter most likely to distinguish urinary retention due to prostatic obstruction from urinary retention due to "classic diabetic cystopathy" is:
    a. uroflow.
    b. residual urine volume.
    c. bladder compliance.
    d. vesical pressure.
    e. detrusor pressure.

22. Detrusor-striated sphincter dyssynergia is least expected to occur with which of the following conditions?
    a. MS
    b. SCI
    c. Stroke
    d. Autonomic hyperreflexia
    e. Transverse myelitis

23. Treatment options for DSD can include all of the following except:
    a. intermittent catheterization
    b. injection of onabotulinum toxin into the sphincter
    c. sacral neuromodulation
    d. sphincterotomy
    e. urinary diversion

24. Differentiation of bladder neck obstruction from dysfunctional voiding is most easily and accurately made by:
    a. filling cystometry.
    b. voiding cystometry.
    c. cystourethroscopy.
    d. flowmetry and residual urine determination.
    e. video-urodynamics study.

25. According to the AUA consensus statement on non-neurogenic urinary retention,
    a. non-neurogenic urinary retention is defined as a postvoid residual > 300 mL on a single occasion.
    b. low-risk and high-risk patients should be distinguished and patients with high-risk features should be treated.
    c. low-risk patients include those with hydronephrosis, recurrent UTIs, and chronic kidney disease.

d. if long-term catheterization is needed, then an indwelling urethral catheter is preferred.

e. patients with low-risk urinary retention do not need to be followed long term.

26. Which of the following is not a typical finding in a patient with Fowler syndrome?

a. Female younger than 30 years

b. Unable to void for a day or more with no urgency

c. Bladder capacity of less than 1 L

d. Increasing lower abdominal discomfort

e. Electromyographic (EMG) abnormalities

27. Which of the following with the typical history is the most specific study to make the diagnosis of Fowler syndrome?

a. Striated sphincter needle EMG recording

b. Striated sphincter patch EMG recording

c. Neurologic examination

d. Spinal magnetic resonance imaging (MRI) examination

e. Detrusor pressure/urinary flow recording

28. Which of the following has proved to be successful in treating the urologic manifestations of Fowler syndrome?

a. Estrogen therapy

b. Progesterone therapy

c. Baclofen therapy

d. Botulinum toxin injection therapy

e. Neuromodulation

29. A 65-year-old female presents with a history of pelvic radiation for treatment of cervical cancer 30 years ago. What urodynamic findings would you expect?

a. Reduced bladder capacity

b. Increased postvoid residual

c. Normal compliance

d. Decreased flow rate

e. Bladder outlet obstruction

30. In the medical management of neurogenic detrusor overactivity (NDO), which of the following is least likely to worsen constipation?

a. Oxybutynin

b. Mirabegron

c. Tolterodine

d. Tamsulosin

e. Trospium

31. Increasing numbers of individuals with myelomeningocele are surviving into adulthood and older age. Critical for stability of function is recognition that the spinal cord may be tethered. Regarding the tethered spinal cord,

a. the level of tethering as demonstrated by MRI is predictive of findings on urodynamics.

b. urodynamics often shows improvement after detethering.

c. tethered cord syndrome is not usually associated with bowel or leg dysfunction.

d. there are no predictors for social continence after detethering.

e. the symptomatic tethered cord, associated with worsening ambulation, can be managed non-operatively.

32. Guillain-Barré syndrome is a demyelinating disorder. It is:

a. not usually identified as a clinical entity having sporadic clinical manifestation.

b. not caused by an acute inflammatory disorder.

c. not usually associated with an antecedent acute infectious illness.

d. associated with lower urinary tract function, usually in less than 5% of cases.

e. associated with voiding dysfunction, which is usually reversible

33. In a patient with voiding dysfunction secondary to myelomeningocele who has slightly decreased compliance, detrusor areflexia, and low-pressure moderate to severe vesicoureteral reflux, which of the following urodynamic changes would be most likely after ureteral reimplantation alone?

a. Compliance increased

b. Voiding pressure decreased

c. Valsalva leak-point pressure decreased

d. Maximum urethral closure pressure decreased

e. Maximum bladder capacity decreased

34. Which of the following is true about patients with myelomeningocele?

a. Myelomeningoceles most commonly occur at the cervical level.

b. The level of the lesion correlates poorly with urodynamic findings.

c. Neurologic examination of patients with myelomeningocele accurately predicts urodynamic findings.

d. Patients rarely have lower urinary tract dysfunction.

e. Life-long follow-up is not necessary.

35. Findings consistent with herpes virus infection may include all of the following except:

a. vesicles in the bladder on cystoscopy

b. urinary retention

c. detrusor overactivity

d. rash on the palms and soles of feet

e. fever, malaise

ANSWERS

1. **b. Involuntary bladder contractions, smooth sphincter synergy, striated sphincter synergy.** Neurologic lesions above the level of the brainstem that affect micturition generally result in involuntary bladder contractions with smooth and striated sphincter synergy. Sensation and voluntary striated sphincter function are generally preserved. Areflexia may occur either initially or as a permanent dysfunction.

2. **c. Involuntary bladder contractions, smooth sphincter synergy, striated sphincter dyssynergia.** Patients with complete lesions of the spinal cord between spinal cord levels T6 and S2, after they recover from spinal shock, generally exhibit involuntary bladder contractions without sensation of the contraction, smooth sphincter synergy, but striated sphincter dyssynergia. Those with lesions above T6 may experience, in addition, smooth sphincter dyssynergia and autonomic hyperreflexia.

3. **e. Detrusor overactivity.** The most common long-term expression of lower urinary tract dysfunction after a CVA is detrusor overactivity. Sensation is variable but is classically described as generally intact, and thus the patient has urgency and frequency with detrusor overactivity.

4. **e. Full urodynamic evaluation.** Poor flow rates and high residual urine volumes in a male with pre-CVA symptoms of prostatism generally indicate prostatic obstruction, but a full urodynamic evaluation is advisable before committing a patient to mechanical outlet reduction primarily to exclude detrusor hyperactivity with impaired contractility as a cause of symptoms.

5. **b. Normal filling/storage; normal emptying.** Most children and adults with only CP have urinary control and what seems to be normal filling/storage and normal emptying. The actual incidence of voiding dysfunction is somewhat vague because the few available series report findings predominantly in those who present with voiding symptoms. One study estimated that a third or more of children with CP are so affected. When an adult with CP presents with an acute or subacute change in voiding status, however, it is most likely unrelated to CP.

6. **e. Detrusor overactivity, coordinated sphincters.** In those individuals with CP who exhibit significant dysfunction, the type of damage that one would suspect from the most common urodynamic abnormalities seems to be localized above the brainstem. This is commonly reflected by detrusor overactivity and coordinated sphincters. Spinal cord damage can occur, however, and probably accounts for those individuals with CP who seem to have evidence of striated sphincter dyssynergia.

7. **d. Detrusor overactivity.** The most common urodynamic finding is detrusor overactivity. The pathophysiology of detrusor overactivity most widely proposed is that the basal ganglia normally have an inhibitory effect on the micturition reflex, which is abolished by the cell loss in the substantia nigra.

8. **a. Sphincteric insufficiency.** Patients with MSA usually have sphincteric insufficiency, while patients with PD rarely have external sphincter acontractility. For this reason, a bladder outlet treatment is rarely indicated in MSA patients. Decreased compliance may also occur in MSA.

9. **b. Detrusor overactivity and smooth sphincter synergia.** In terms of urodynamic findings, detrusor overactivity is the most common abnormality detected and, in general, the smooth sphincter is synergic and sensation is intact. There can also be coexisting striated sphincter dyssynergia and/or impaired detrusor contractility.

10. **d. Spinal cord injury (SCI).** Progressive neurologic diseases cause upper tract damage much less commonly than SCI, even when associated with severe disability and spasticity.

11. **d. High abdominal leak-point pressure.** As with all patients with neurologic impairment, a careful initial evaluation and periodic follow-up evaluation must be performed to identify and correct the following risk factors and potential complications: bladder overdistention, high-pressure storage, high detrusor leak-point pressure, vesicoureteral reflux, stone formation (lower and upper tracts), and complicating infection, especially in association with reflux.

12. **c. Open bladder neck.** Spinal shock includes a suppression of autonomic activity and somatic activity, and the bladder is acontractile and areflexic. Radiologically, the bladder has a smooth contour with no evidence of trabeculation. The bladder neck is generally closed and competent unless there has been prior surgery or, in some cases, thoracolumbar and presumably sympathetic injury. The smooth sphincter mechanism seems to be functional. Some EMG activity may be recorded from the striated sphincter, and the maximum urethral closure pressure is lower than normal but still maintained at the level of the external sphincter zone; however, the normal guarding reflex is absent and there is no voluntary control.

13. **a. Pons and the sacral spinal cord.** A diagnosis of striated sphincter dyssynergia implies a neurologic lesion that interrupts the neural axis between the pontine-mesencephalic reticular formation and the sacral spinal cord.

14. **d. Tachycardia.** Symptomatically, autonomic hyperreflexia is a syndrome of exaggerated sympathetic activity in response to stimuli below the level of the lesion. The symptoms are pounding headache, hypertension, and flushing of the face and body above the level of the lesion with sweating. Bradycardia is a usual accompaniment, and an arrhythmia may be present.

15. **d. Empty his bladder.** Immediate treatment of autonomic dysreflexia is to remove the cause, which in this case is bladder distension. The current recommendation for the acute pharmacologic treatment of autonomic dysreflexia is placement of 2% nitroglycerin paste above the level of the lesion for rapid blood pressure reduction secondary to vasodilation after removal of the stimulus.

16. **c. L2.** Spinal column (bone) segments are numbered by the vertebral level, and these have a different relationship to the spinal cord segmental level at different locations. The sacral spinal cord begins at approximately spinal column level T12-L1. The spinal cord terminates in the cauda equina at approximately the spinal column level of L2.

17. **d. Difficulty voiding; normal bladder compliance.** A study reported on findings in 114 patients with lumbar disk protrusion who were prospectively studied. The authors found detrusor areflexia in 31 (27.2%) and normal detrusor activity in the remaining 83. All 31 patients with detrusor areflexia reported difficulty voiding with straining. Patients with voiding dysfunction generally present with these symptoms or in urinary retention. The most consistent urodynamic finding is that of a normally compliant areflexic bladder associated with normal innervation or findings of incomplete denervation of the perineal floor musculature.

18. **e. Limb spasticity.** CES is characterized by perineal sensory loss with loss of voluntary control of both anal and urethral sphincter and of sexual dysfunction. CES is a lower motor neuron disease, so would not expect limb spasticity which is a characteristic of upper motor neuron disease.

19. **a. Stress incontinence; detrusor areflexia.** When permanent voiding dysfunction occurs after radical pelvic surgery, the pattern is generally one of a failure of voluntary bladder contraction, or impaired bladder contractility, with obstruction by what seems urodynamically to be residual fixed striated sphincter tone, which is not subject to voluntarily induced relaxation. Often, the smooth sphincter area is open and nonfunctional. Decreased compliance is common in these patients, and this, with the "obstruction" caused by fixed residual striated sphincter tone, results in both storage and emptying failure. These patients often experience leaking across the distal sphincter area and, in addition, are unable to empty the bladder because although intravesical pressure may be increased, there is nothing that approximates a true bladder contraction. The patient often presents with urinary incontinence that is characteristically most manifest with increases in intra-abdominal pressure. This is usually most obvious in females because the prostatic bulk in males often masks an equivalent deficit in urethral closure function. Alternatively, patients may present with variable degrees of urinary retention.

20. **b. Clean intermittent catheterization.** The temptation to perform a prostatectomy should be avoided unless a clear demonstration of outlet obstruction at this level is possible. Otherwise, prostatectomy simply decreases urethral sphincter function and thereby may result in the occurrence or worsening of sphincteric urinary incontinence. Most of these dysfunctions will be transient, and the temptation to "do something" other than perform clean intermittent catheterization initially after surgery in these patients, especially in those with little or no preexisting history of voiding dysfunction, cannot be too strongly discouraged.

21. **e. Detrusor pressure.** Detrusor contractility is classically described as being decreased in the end-stage diabetic bladder. Current evidence points to both sensory and motor neuropathy as being involved in the pathogenesis, the motor aspect per se contributing to the impaired detrusor contractility. The typically described classic urodynamic findings include impaired bladder sensation, increased cystometric capacity, decreased bladder contractility, impaired uroflow, and, later, increased residual urine volume. The main differential diagnosis, at least in men, is generally bladder outlet obstruction because both conditions commonly produce a low flow rate. Pressure/flow urodynamic studies easily differentiate the two.

22. **c. Stroke.** True detrusor sphincter dyssynergia should exist only in patients who have an abnormality in pathways between the sacral spinal cord and the brainstem pontine micturition center, generally due to neurologic injury or disease.

23. **c. Sacral neuromodulation.** Therapy for DSD is designed to either eliminate or significantly minimize the abnormal sphincter activity or to bypass the sphincter itself.

24. **e. Video-urodynamics study.** Objective evidence of outlet obstruction in these patients is easily obtainable by urodynamic study. Once obstruction is diagnosed, it can be localized at the level of the bladder neck by video-urodynamics study, cystourethrography during a bladder contraction, or micturitional urethral profilometry.

25. **b. Low-risk and high-risk patients should be distinguished and patients with high-risk features should be treated.** Following a thorough history and physical examination, if a high-risk variable is present, such as hydronephrosis, hydroureter, chronic kidney disease, recurrent UTI, or urinary incontinence with skin sequalae, then treatment is recommended.

26. **c. Bladder capacity of less than 1 L.** The criteria for Fowler syndrome include a bladder capacity of more than 1 L with no sensation of urgency.

27. **a. Striated sphincter needle EMG recording.** *Fowler syndrome* refers particularly to a syndrome of urinary retention in young women in the absence of overt neurologic disease. The typical history is that of a woman younger than 30 years, who has found herself unable to void during the preceding day but with no sensation of urgency. MRI studies of the brain and the entire spinal cord are normal. On concentric needle electrode examination of the striated muscle of the urethral sphincter, however, Fowler and colleagues described a unique EMG abnormality. This abnormal activity, localized to the urethral sphincter, consists of a type of activity that would be expected to cause inappropriate contraction of the muscle. Sphincter activity consists of two components: complex repetitive discharges and decelerating bursts. This abnormal activity impairs sphincter relaxation.

28. **e. Neuromodulation.** Fowler reports that efforts to treat this condition by hormonal manipulation, pharmacologic therapy, or injections of botulinum toxin have been unsuccessful. This condition is highly responsive to neuromodulation, even in women who have had retention for many months or years.

29. **a. Reduced bladder capacity.** Radiation effects on the bladder evolve over time and may be progressive. Most commonly urodynamics will demonstrate reduced bladder capacity. Patients may also have reduced compliance and detrusor overactivity.

30. **b. Mirabegron.** Mirabegron is a β3 agonist that has shown efficacy in the treatment of NDO. Mirabegron avoids the anticholinergic effects of constipation and dry mouth, but can have cardiovascular side effects including mild elevations in blood pressure and small, dose-dependent increases in heart rate.

31. **b. Urodynamics often show improvement after detethering.** Despite efforts at improved radiographic visualization of the spinal cord, imaging does not correlate with physical findings or connote overall responsiveness to surgical intervention because detethering remains a critical aspect of management and control of tethered cord. Cord tethering affects both bowel and leg function, as well as bladder function. Urodynamics is improved by detethering, and this parallels functional improvement in those individuals who have undergone the surgical procedure. The successful management of the tethered cord remains a critical aspect of long-term care in the myelomeningocele population.

32. **e. Associated with voiding dysfunction, which is usually reversible.** Guillain-Barré syndrome is an acute inflammatory disorder thought to be due to some inflammatory process because most patients do have evidence of acute inflammatory conditions before development of the syndrome. The syndrome is characterized by a distinct presenting scenario (ascending paralysis). Lower urinary tract dysfunction has been reported in as few as 25% to as many as 80% of cases and is usually reversible with resolution of the disorder.

33. **e. Maximum bladder capacity decreased.** One must remember the potential artifact that significant reflux can introduce into urodynamic studies. Measured bladder capacity may be more, and measured pressures at given inflow volumes may be less, than those after reflux correction. The apparent significance of detrusor overactivity may thus be underestimated.

34. **b. The level of the lesion correlates poorly with urodynamic findings.** Myelomeningocele lesions most commonly occur in the lumbosacral region. The incidence of lower urinary tract dysfunction is estimated to be about 90%, and patients with lower urinary tract dysfunction require life-long follow-up with a urologist.

35. **d. Rash on the palms and soles of feet.** Invasion of the sacral dorsal root ganglia and posterior nerve roots with herpes zoster virus may produce urinary retention, detrusor areflexia, or detrusor overactivity. A rash on the palms and soles is associated with syphilis.

CHAPTER REVIEW

1. In general, complete spinal cord injury above the sacral spinal cord, but below the area of the sympathetic outflow, results in detrusor overactivity, absent sensation below the level of the lesion, smooth sphincter synergia, and striated sphincter dyssynergia.
2. Lesions at or above the spinal cord level of T7 or T8 (the spinal column level of T6) may result in smooth sphincter dyssynergia as well.
3. Neurologic examination is no substitute for urodynamic evaluation in these patients when one is determining risk factors and treatment.
4. A careful initial evaluation and periodic, routine follow-up evaluation must be performed to identify and correct risk factors and potential complications: high-pressure storage, high detrusor leak point pressure, vesicoureteral reflux (VUR), stone formation (lower and upper tracts), and complicating infection, especially in association with reflux.
5. Avoid use of long-term antibiotics to prevent infection in patient performing clean intermittent catheterization (CIC).
6. Ongoing investigations with ventral nerve surgery and use of stem cells may completely change the paradigm of suprasacral cord injury management in the future.
7. Potential risk factors and complications are those previously described, with particular emphasis on storage pressure, which can result in silent upper tract decompensation and deterioration in the absence of VUR.
8. Treatment is usually directed toward producing or maintaining low-pressure storage while circumventing emptying failure with CIC when possible. Pharmacologic and electrical stimulation may be useful in promoting emptying in certain circumstances.

117 Overactive Bladder

W. Stuart Reynolds and Joshua A. Cohn

QUESTIONS

1. Which definition or definitions appear in the current International Continence Society (ICS) terminology (2002)?
   a. Detrusor hyperreflexia
   b. Overactive bladder
   c. Idiopathic detrusor overactivity
   d. Detrusor instability
   e. b and c

2. Which symptoms are included in overactive bladder syndrome (OAB)?
   a. Dysuria
   b. Straining
   c. Urgency incontinence
   d. Bladder pain
   e. Stress incontinence

3. In the community, what percentage of adults have overactive bladder symptoms?
   a. Less than 5%
   b. 5% to 10%
   c. 10% to 20%
   d. 20% to 50%
   e. More than 50%

4. Mixed incontinence includes:
   a. stress urinary incontinence.
   b. continuous incontinence.
   c. postmicturition leakage.
   d. incontinence during sexual intercourse.
   e. giggle incontinence.

5. Which features are characteristics of urgency?
   a. A normal sensation.
   b. It builds up slowly.
   c. It is usually felt suprapubically.
   d. It develops quickly and may lead to incontinence.
   e. a and b.

6. Which statements are TRUE for detrusor overactivity (DO)?
   a. It is characterized by phasic involuntary detrusor contractions during bladder filling.
   b. It is always accompanied by a feeling of urgency.
   c. It is a urodynamic diagnosis.
   d. It is a feature of the voiding phase of micturition.
   e. a and c.

7. Detrusor overactivity can be diagnosed:
   a. only if involuntary filling phase contractions are greater than 15 cm H_2O in amplitude.
   b. if an involuntary contraction is seen during bladder filling, irrespective of size.
   c. if there is urgency incontinence but no contraction.
   d. if leakage occurs during exercise.
   e. before urodynamics if the patient has overactive bladder syndrome.

8. Which statement is FALSE with respect to the hypotheses of detrusor pathophysiology?
   a. Afferent sensitization signifies an increased afferent firing rate in response to a standardized stimulus.
   b. The myogenic and integrative hypotheses require abnormal propagation of excitation in the bladder wall.
   c. Synaptic reorganization in the spinal cord may contribute to neurogenic detrusor overactivity.
   d. Detrusor overactivity requires volitional control.
   e. Synergic coordination of bladder and outlet are determined at the brainstem/midbrain level.

9. Which of the following statements is correct regarding symptom assessment tools?
   a. OAB can be diagnosed from the frequency volume chart.
   b. A validated questionnaire is mandatory for diagnosis of OAB.
   c. Modular components of the International Consultation on Incontinence Questionnaire system (ICIQ) have undergone formal validation.
   d. A high urgency score is diagnostic of detrusor overactivity.
   e. a and b.

ANSWERS

1. **e. b and c.** Detrusor hyperreflexia has been replaced by neurogenic detrusor overactivity. The concept of tone is poorly understood; hence, the term *detrusor instability* is not recommended.

2. **c. Urgency incontinence.** Urgency incontinence is experienced by a large proportion of patients with OAB.

3. **c. 10% to 20%.** Two large prevalence surveys in North America and Europe have shown the prevalence at 16%, whereas the EPIC study put the figure at nearly 12%. Prevalence of at least one lower urinary tract symptom is greater than 50% according to the EPIC study.

4. **a. Stress urinary incontinence.** This is one of the two constituents of mixed incontinence, along with urgency urinary incontinence.

5. **d. It develops quickly and may lead to incontinence.** Urgency is thought to be a symptom of rapid onset. Urgency leads to urgency incontinence in the susceptible patient, but not invariably.

6. **e. a and c.** Involuntary contractions seen on urodynamic assessment are characteristic of detrusor overactivity.

7. **b. If an involuntary contraction is seen during bladder filling, irrespective of size.**

8. **d. Detrusor overactivity requires volitional control.** Patients are unable to inhibit overactive contractions voluntarily.

9. **c. Modular components of the International Consultation on Incontinence Questionnaire system (ICIQ) have undergone formal validation.** The ICIQ generates new tools and adopts established tools for a system that allows selection of appropriate symptom assessment for specific clinical contexts.

CHAPTER REVIEW

1. DO is a urodynamic diagnosis. OAB is a symptom-based diagnosis, defined as urgency with or without urgency incontinence, usually with frequency and nocturia with no proven infection or other obvious pathology.
2. The pattern of voided volumes in patients with OAB is erratic.
3. Urgency with at least one other symptom is essential to the diagnosis of OAB.
4. The etiology of DO has been hypothesized to be due to neurogenic or myogenic disorders. Neurogenic disorders may involve (1) reduced suprapontine inhibition, (2) overexpression of primitive spinal bladder reflexes, (3) synaptic plasticity in which new reflexes develop as a response to C-fiber afferent neurons, and (4) sensitization of peripheral afferent terminals. Myogenic disorders involve spontaneous excitation, which may be a result of upregulation of surface membrane receptors.
5. A frequency voiding chart or voiding diary is essential for assessing OAB.
6. The two main urodynamic findings with overactive bladder are DO and increasing filling sensation.
7. Treatment of OAB should begin with conservative management, including lifestyle changes, followed by pharmacotherapy and, finally, for intractable cases, surgical therapy that involves either nerve stimulation or surgical procedures on the bladder itself.
8. Aging, neurologic disease, female gender, bladder outlet obstruction, and the metabolic syndrome are potential contributors to OAB.

118 The Underactive Detrusor

Christopher R. Chapple and Nadir I. Osman

QUESTIONS

1. Which of the following is NOT part of the International Continence Society's (ICS's) definition of detrusor underactivity (DUA)?
   a. A contraction of reduced duration
   b. Prolonged bladder emptying
   c. Incomplete bladder emptying
   d. A contraction of reduced strength
   e. A contraction of reduced speed

2. A symptom syndrome of "underactive bladder" (UAB) is defined as:
   a. reduced desire to void, usually accompanied by urinary frequency or nocturia, with or without incontinence that predominates at night.
   b. reduced desire to void, associated with incomplete bladder emptying.
   c. symptoms of impaired bladder emptying in the absence of bladder outlet obstruction.
   d. infrequent voiding, associated with voiding symptoms and increased postvoid residual.
   e. There is currently no recognized definition for UAB.

3. What is the ultrastructural pattern associated with DUA, according to the classification of Elbadawi?
   a. Dense band pattern
   b. Degeneration pattern
   c. Dysfunction pattern
   d. Disjunction pattern
   e. Myelohypertrophy pattern

4. Most current diagnostic criteria estimate which aspect of detrusor contraction?
   a. Efficiency
   b. Sustainability
   c. Speed
   d. Strength
   e. Duration

5. Which of the following criteria is not thought to be affected by the presence of bladder outlet obstruction?
   a. Detrusor contraction duration
   b. Bladder contractility index
   c. Detrusor contraction coefficient
   d. Projected isovolumetric pressure
   e. Watt factor

6. Which of the following statements regarding parasympathomimetic agents in DUA is TRUE?
   a. Muscarinic agonists show good efficacy in restoring contractility.
   b. Muscarinic agonists are more likely to be effective in patients with complete bladder denervation.

   c. Muscarinic agonists can cause severe cardiac depression.
   d. Anticholinesterases can cause uterine contraction.
   e. None of the above.

7. What is the proposed mechanism of action of intravesical electrotherapy (IVE)?
   a. Direct stimulation of detrusor myocytes
   b. Stimulation of mechanoreceptive afferent nerves
   c. Direct stimulation of efferent nerves
   d. Inhibition of pathologic urethral afferent signaling
   e. None of the above

8. Which of the following features appears to be associated with more positive outcomes in the treatment of DUA?
   a. Neurogenic etiology
   b. Older age
   c. Intact bladder sensation
   d. Myogenic etiology
   e. Acontractile bladder

9. Which of these neurologic disorders is most frequently associated with DUA on urodynamics?
   a. Parkinson disease
   b. Multiple sclerosis
   c. Multisystem atrophy
   d. Cerebrovascular accident—postacute phase
   e. Brain tumor

10. What is the natural history of DUA in men without known neurogenic bladder dysfunction?
    a. Deterioration in symptoms but not urodynamic parameters
    b. No significant change in urodynamic parameters for at least 10 years
    c. Improvement in contractility in at least 50% of individuals
    d. Most will require bladder outlet surgery by 10 years
    e. No studies are available

ANSWERS

1. **e. A contraction of reduced speed.** The 2002 standardization report of the ICS defines DUA as "a contraction of reduced strength and/or duration, resulting in prolonged bladder emptying and/or failure to achieve complete bladder emptying within a normal time span." An acontractile detrusor is separately defined as "one that cannot be demonstrated to contract during urodynamic studies."

2. **e. There is currently no recognized definition for UAB.** A symptom syndrome of "underactive bladder" is difficult to rationally define because of the absence of studies correlating individual symptoms to the underlying detrusor abnormality. Even then, empirical evidence would suggest that symptoms of DUA are very diverse and overlap significantly with those of overactive bladder (OAB).

3. **b. Degeneration pattern.** The "degeneration" pattern is associated with DUA and consists of widespread disrupted detrusor myocytes and axonal degeneration. Elbadawi proposed that distinct ultrastructural patterns observed by electron microscopy characterized the normally contractile aging detrusor and different bladder dysfunctions. Although the applicability of this classification system is disputed, other groups have noted similar findings.

4. **d. Strength.** Most criteria focus on contraction strength as derived from detrusor pressure at maximal flow.

5. **e. Watt factor.** The watt factor is a mathematical calculation and provides a measure of bladder power. Its major advantages are that it minimally depends on volume and is not affected by increased outlet resistance. However, it is a complex calculation with no validated cutoffs.

6. **c. Muscarinic agonists can cause severe cardiac depression.** Muscarinic agonists have been associated with reports of severe myocardial depression leading to cardiac arrest. This, and their lack of efficacy, has led to their nonuse in clinical practice.

7. **b. Stimulation of mechanoreceptive afferent nerves.** IVE activates mechanosensitive bladder afferents (myelinated Aδ fibers) and restores bladder sensation. It is postulated that repeat activation of this pathway upregulates its performance during volitional voiding.

8. **c. Intact bladder sensation.** Intact bladder sensation is necessary to normally trigger the micturition reflex. Its presence suggests some residual bladder innervation and was found to be associated with better responses to some treatments of DUA (e.g., urethral sphincter botulinum neurotoxin A and muscarinic agonists)

9. **c. Multisystem atrophy.** Multisystem atrophy is a neurodegenerative disease that may be confused with Parkinson disease. It is associated with autonomic dysfunction and DUA in at least half of patients because of atrophy of parasympathetic nerves.

10. **b. No significant change in urodynamic parameters for at least 10 years.** There are very few data on the natural history of DUA. A longitudinal follow-up study (10 years) by Thomas et al. showed no significant symptomatic or urodynamic deterioration in men with DUA managed conservatively at 10 years.

CHAPTER REVIEW

1. Detrusor underactivity (DUA) is a contraction of reduced strength and/or duration, resulting in prolonged bladder emptying and/or failure to achieve complete bladder emptying within a normal time span.

2. DUA often coexists with other lower urinary tract dysfunctions in the elderly.

3. Normal aging results in a reduction in autonomic innervation and a decline in sensory function in the lower urinary tract.

4. Diabetes mellitus impairs detrusor function through both myogenic and autonomic dysfunction.

5. Lumbosacral spinal cord trauma or disk disease and pelvic surgery can lead to injury of the pelvic plexus.

6. Afferent nerves play a central role in the initiation and maintenance of a detrusor contraction.

7. Treatment strategies to address DUA include timed voiding, double voiding, pelvic floor physiotherapy, and intermittent self-catheterization.

8. Intravesical electrotherapy activates mechanosensitive bladder afferents (myelinated Aδ fibers) and restores bladder sensation. It is postulated that repeat activation of this pathway upregulates its performance during volitional voiding.

119 Nocturia

Stephen D. Marshall and Jeffrey P. Weiss

QUESTIONS

1. Nocturnal polyuria is defined as:
   a. nocturnal polyuria index (NPi) greater than 0.33.
   b. nocturnal urine volume (NUV) greater than 6.4 mL/kg.
   c. NUV greater than 54 mL/h.
   d. a and b.
   e. a, b, and c.

2. All of the following statements are true about nocturia EXCEPT:
   a. nocturia is voiding that is preceded and followed by sleep.
   b. the prevalence of nocturia increases with age.
   c. nocturia impairs sleep efficiency, sleep latency, and slow-wave sleep and is associated with increased mortality.
   d. one or more voids per night appear to be clinically significant.
   e. nocturia is associated with falls.

3. When instructing a patient how to complete a frequency-volume chart, it is essential to:
   a. tell the patient to record what time he or she goes to sleep.
   b. tell the patient to record what time he or she awakens.
   c. tell the patient to record how much he or she drinks during the day.
   d. a and b.
   e. a, b, and c.

4. Factors that inhibit antidiuretic hormone (ADH) secretion include all of the following EXCEPT:
   a. hyperkalemia.
   b. atrial natriuretic peptide (ANP).
   c. hypercalcemia.
   d. prostaglandin E2 (PGE2).
   e. lithium.

5. A 75-year-old obese man (100 kg) with a short neck reports frequent urination during the nighttime and completes a voiding diary. His 24-hour voided volume is 2000 mL, and his NUV is 1000 mL. Based on these diary findings, this man has:
   a. global polyuria.
   b. nocturnal polyuria.
   c. diminished nocturnal bladder capacity.
   d. diminished global bladder capacity.
   e. none of the above.

6. According to a recent study, which of the following showed the greatest decline in nocturia severity and greatest improvement of health-related quality of life (HRQL) in men with benign prostatic hyperplasia (BPH) and nocturia?
   a. Watchful waiting.
   b. α-Blockers.

   c. Transurethral resection of the prostate (TURP).
   d. Transurethral microwave treatment (TUMT).
   e. There was no difference among these treatments.

7. When bound to V2 receptors in the renal collecting tubules, desmopressin:
   a. increases water permeability.
   b. enhances water reabsorption.
   c. dilutes extracellular fluid.
   d. concentrates urine.
   e. all of the above.

8. Current thinking is that desmopressin is most appropriate to treat:
   a. nocturnal polyuria.
   b. global polyuria.
   c. decreased global bladder capacity.
   d. decreased nocturnal bladder capacity.
   e. all of the above.

9. Which of the following have caused statistically but minimally clinically significant reductions in nocturia episodes?
   a. α-Blockers
   b. 5α-Reductase inhibitors
   c. Antimuscarinics
   d. α-Blockers and antimuscarinics
   e. All of the above

10. Regarding the frequency volume chart (voiding diary), which of the following statements is FALSE?
    a. NUV is defined as the total volume of all voids preceded and followed by sleep.
    b. The first morning void counts toward total number of daily voiding episodes.
    c. Nighttime may be during daylight hours.
    d. Maximum voided volume is the single greatest urine volume measured during a 24-hour period.
    e. Nocturia or enuresis occurs when the nocturia index (Ni) is greater than 1.

11. When prescribing desmopressin to an elderly patient (>65 years), it is advisable to:
    a. check a baseline serum sodium level
    b. check a serum sodium level within 7 days and then 28 days after initial or incremental dosing
    c. check a serum sodium level every 6 months or as often as indicated
    d. avoid prescribing in those with baseline serum sodium below 130 mmol/L
    e. all of the above

ANSWERS

1. **e. a, b, and c.** Nocturnal polyuria is defined as NPi greater than 0.20 in young adults and greater than 0.33 in adults older than 65 years when 24-hour urine production is within normal limits. Other definitions include NUV greater than 0.9 mL/min (54 mL/h) and NUV greater than 1.5 mL/min (90 mL/h). A universally accepted definition of nocturnal polyuria has yet to be identified.

2. **c. One or more voids per night appear to be clinically significant.** Several studies have shown that two or more voids per night generate bother and impair quality of life.

3. **d. a and b.** Although having the patient record how much he drinks during the day may be helpful, it is essential that the patient record the time he goes to sleep and the time he awakens to know the number of nocturnal voids and NUV.

4. **a. Hyperkalemia.** Factors that inhibit antidiuretic hormone (ADH) and cause diuresis (inhibit water reabsorption) include PGE2, ANP, hypercalcemia, hypokalemia, lithium, and tetracyclines. Reversal of water diuresis, accordingly, may occur through stimulation of V2 receptors, either by endogenous arginine vasopressin or a congener thereof, such as desmopressin.

5. **b. Nocturnal polyuria.** This patient suffers from nocturnal polyuria as defined by his NPi. His NPi can be calculated by dividing his NUV by his 24-hour voided volume:

$$NPi = NUV / 24 - hour\ voided\ volume$$

$$= 1000\ mL / 2000\ mL = 0.5$$

He has nocturnal polyuria because his NPi is greater than 0.33. Global polyuria is defined as 24-hour urine volume greater than 40 mL/kg. Diminished nocturnal bladder capacity and global bladder capacity cannot be determined by the information provided in this scenario.

6. **c. Transurethral resection of the prostate (TURP).** After 6 to 12 months, watchful waiting, α-blockers, TURP, and TUMT yielded reduction in nocturia episodes by 7%, 17%, 75%, and 32%, respectively. Improvements in HRQL were most strongly associated with treatment-associated declines in nocturia severity.

7. **e. All of the above.** When bound to V2 receptors in the renal collecting tubules, desmopressin increases water permeability, enhances water reabsorption, dilutes extracellular fluid, and concentrates urine.

8. **a. Nocturnal polyuria.** Current thinking is that desmopressin would be the most appropriate therapy for patients with nocturia related to nocturnal polyuria.

9. **e. All of the above.** α-blockers, 5α-reductase inhibitors, antimuscarinics, and antimuscarinics + α-blockers have been found to produce a statistically significant reduction in nocturia episodes, yielding minimal clinical significance.

10. **a. NUV is defined as the total volume of all voids preceded and followed by sleep.** This is incorrect. NUV is the total volume of urine passed during the night and the first morning void.

11. **e. All of the above.** When prescribing desmopressin to a patient older than 65 years of age, it is advisable to closely monitor serum sodium AND to avoid prescribing it to elderly patients with baseline hyponatremia.

CHAPTER REVIEW

1. There is a clear impact of aging on the prevalence of nocturia. Younger people are more likely to manifest decreased nocturnal bladder capacity, whereas older people manifest overproduction of urine.

2. Accumulation of fluid in the dependent parts of the body (third spacing) and return of fluid to the circulating volume when the patient is recumbent may be an underlying cause of nocturia.

3. The pathophysiology of nocturia may be related to increased mean arterial blood pressure when supine and an alteration of circadian rhythm of ADH (ordinarily there is an increased production of ADH at night during the hours of sleep).

4. Twenty percent of people aged 20–40 years awake to void two or more times compared with 60% of those 70 years or older.

5. Two or more voids a night are clinically significant.

6. Obstructive sleep apnea is a common cause of nocturia.

7. Desmopressin may result in hyponatremia; women are more sensitive to the drug than are men.

120 Pharmacologic Management of Lower Urinary Tract Storage and Emptying Failure

Karl-Erik Andersson and Alan J. Wein

QUESTIONS

(Multiple answers are possible throughout.)

1. The effects of administration of an antimuscarinic agent to an individual with an overactive bladder (OAB) include all of the following EXCEPT:
   a. increased total bladder capacity.
   b. depressed amplitude of involuntary bladder contractions.
   c. increased outlet resistance.
   d. increased volume to the first involuntary bladder contraction.
   e. increased mean volume voided.

2. Which of the following muscarinic receptor subtypes is the most common in human detrusor smooth muscle?
   a. M_1
   b. M_2
   c. M_3
   d. M_4
   e. M_5

3. Which of the following muscarinic receptor subtypes is predominantly responsible for the mediation of bladder contraction in human detrusor smooth muscle?
   a. M_1
   b. M_2
   c. M_3
   d. M_4
   e. M_5

4. The use of antimuscarinic agents to treat OAB is limited by their lack of uroselectivity. Which of the following is NOT a recognized side effect of antimuscarinic agents?
   a. Dry mouth
   b. Constipation
   c. Cognitive dysfunction
   d. Bradycardia
   e. Blurred vision

5. Which of the following characteristics increases the possibility for an antimuscarinic agent to pass the blood-brain barrier?
   a. High lipophilicity
   b. Large molecular size
   c. Low electrical charge
   d. Quaternary ammonium structure
   e. Small molecular size

6. Anticholinergics exert their favorable effects on OAB by affecting:
   a. peripheral afferent (sensory) transmission.
   b. ganglionic transmission.
   c. central neural afferent transmission.
   d. muscarinic receptors on the detrusor smooth muscle.
   e. nicotinic receptors on the detrusor smooth muscle.

7. The Committee on Pharmacologic Treatment of the Fifth (2013) International Consultation on Incontinence assessed agents according to the Oxford Guideline, according to level of evidence and grade of recommendation with respect to treatment of detrusor overactivity (DO). Which of the following (multiple answers are possible) did NOT receive a level of evidence rating of 1 and a grade of recommendation of A?
   a. Fesoterodine
   b. Flavoxate
   c. Trospium
   d. Solifenacin
   e. Oxybutynin

8. Which of the following is NOT a class effect of antimuscarinics?
   a. Accommodation paralysis
   b. Constipation
   c. Increased heart rate
   d. Prolongation of the QT interval
   e. Dry mouth

9. Of the following choices, which are correct? The bladder contains how many β-receptor subtypes (answer 1) _____ with the (answer 2) _____ having the most important functional role.
   a. one; β_2
   b. two; β_2
   c. three; β_3
   d. four; β_2
   e. five; β_5

10. Which of the following pharmacologic actions is most likely responsible for the effects of oxybutynin when given systemically?
    a. Antimuscarinic, direct muscle relaxant, and local anesthetic actions, equally
    b. Direct muscle relaxant effect alone
    c. Direct muscle relaxant effect and local anesthetic action
    d. Antimuscarinic and direct muscle relaxant effects
    e. Antimuscarinic effect

11. Which of the following muscarinic receptor subtypes are NOT known to be involved in the potential antimuscarinic side effects of dry mouth, constipation, tachycardia, drowsiness, and blurred vision?
    a. M_1
    b. M_2
    c. M_3
    d. M_4
    e. M_5

12. The primary adverse event reported with the use of oxybu-tynin-transdermal has been:
    a. tachycardia.
    b. dry mouth.
    c. constipation.
    d. application site reactions.
    e. blurred vision.

13. Which of the following agents is relatively selective for M_3 receptor blockade?
    a. Darifenacin
    b. Oxybutynin
    c. Solifenacin
    d. Tolterodine
    e. Trospium

14. Mirabegron probably exerts its favorable effect on OAB by:
    a. activating the β_3 adrenergic receptor.
    b. competitive blockade of the β_3 receptor.
    c. inhibiting filling-induced activity in bladder afferent nerves.
    d. activating the α-adrenergic receptor.
    e. inhibiting the α-adrenergic receptor.

15. Of the following agents, which is actively excreted by the kidney in the proximal convoluted tubules?
    a. Darifenacin
    b. Oxybutynin
    c. Solifenacin
    d. Tolterodine
    e. Trospium

16. Which is (are) TRUE about tadalafil?
    a. It improves International Index of Erectile Function (IIEF) scores.
    b. It improves International Prostate Symptom Score (IPSS) scores.
    c. It improves peak flow rates.
    d. It is approved for the treatment of lower urinary tract symptoms (LUTS) due to benign prostatic obstruction (BPO).
    e. It decreases detrusor pressure at peak flow.

17. Which of the following is NOT listed as a common side effect of imipramine?
    a. Systemic antimuscarinic effects
    b. Weakness, fatigue
    c. Priapism
    d. Cardiac arrhythmia
    e. Hepatic dysfunction

18. In men with BPO and OAB, adding an antimuscarinic to an α-adrenergic blocking agent will:
    a. significantly increase residual urine volume.
    b. significantly decrease detrusor pressure at peak flow.
    c. significantly decrease peak and mean flow rate.
    d. cause a, b, and c.
    e. none of the above.

19. Intravesical botulinum toxin subtype A:
    a. activates synaptosomal-associated protein (SNAP) 25 and the soluble N-ethylmaleimide-sensitive factor attachment *protein* (SNARE) complex.
    b. acts only on smooth muscle.

    c. inhibits the peripheral release of acetylcholine.
    d. is effective only in patients with both OAB and DO.
    e. reduces firing from bladder afferents.

20. Vaginal estrogen is effective in the treatment of:
    a. urogenital atrophy.
    b. stress urinary incontinence (SUI).
    c. urgency urinary incontinence.
    d. mixed urinary incontinence.
    e. anterior vaginal prolapse.

21. The side effects of the alpha-adrenergic agonists include all of the following EXCEPT:
    a. tremor.
    b. palpitations.
    c. hypertension.
    d. somnolence.
    e. respiratory difficulties.

22. Which of the following has been reported to increase stroke risk in women younger than 50 years?
    a. Phenylpropanolamine
    b. Ephedrine
    c. Pseudoephedrine
    d. Midodrine
    e. Clenbuterol

23. In theory, which of the following agents, from the standpoint of potential efficacy and safety, would be preferred for the treatment of SUI in a hypertensive individual?
    a. Ephedrine
    b. Propranolol
    c. Phenylpropanolamine
    d. Pseudoephedrine
    e. Clenbuterol

24. Which of the following statements is NOT true with respect to duloxetine hydrochloride?
    a. It significantly increases sphincteric muscle activity during filling/storage in an animal model.
    b. It is a serotonin-norepinephrine reuptake inhibitor.
    c. It is lipophilic and well absorbed.
    d. It is effective in decreasing SUI episodes in women.
    e. It is not metabolized by the liver.

25. Oral estrogen with or without progesterones in postmenopausal women:
    a. improves mixed urinary incontinence.
    b. worsens the risk of incontinence.
    c. worsens urinary incontinence in women with incontinence.
    d. improves SUI.
    e. improves urgency incontinence.

26. A 75-year-old man placed on desmopressin therapy 3 days previously presents with a change of mental status and mental confusion. The most likely cause is:
    a. cognitive dysfunction due to antimuscarinic effect.
    b. hyponatremia.
    c. hypernatremia.
    d. hypokalemia.
    e. hyperkalemia.

27. With regard to bethanechol chloride, the least objective evidence exists to support which of the following statements?

    a. It has relatively selective in vitro action on urinary bladder and bowel.

    b. It has little or no nicotinic action.

    c. It is cholinesterase resistant.

    d. It causes in vitro contraction of bladder and smooth muscle.

    e. It facilitates bladder emptying.

28. What oral dose of bethanechol chloride is required to produce the same urodynamic effects, at least in a denervated bladder, at the subcutaneous dose of 5 mg?

    a. 200 mg

    b. 100 mg

    c. 50 mg

    d. 25 mg

    e. 10 mg

29. Prostaglandins have been hypothesized to affect bladder activity through all of the following actions EXCEPT:

    a. neuromodulation of efferent and afferent neurotransmission.

    b. sensitization to sensory stimuli (activation occurs with a lower degree of filling).

    c. activation of certain sensory nerves.

    d. potentiation of acetylcholine release from cholinergic nerve terminals.

    e. potentiation of adenosine triphosphate release from bladder mucosa.

30. With respect to α- and β-adrenergic receptors in the lower urinary tract and prostate, all the following are true EXCEPT:

    a. α receptors outnumber β receptors in the smooth muscle of the bladder base and proximal urethra.

    b. β receptors outnumber α receptors in the bladder body.

    c. α_1 receptors are more common than α_2.

    d. Lower urinary tract and prostate adrenergically induced smooth muscle contraction is mediated largely by α_1 receptors.

    e. Proximal urethral smooth muscle contraction is mediated primarily by α_1 receptors.

31. Which of the following α-adrenergic blocking agents has significant antagonistic properties at both α_1 and α_2 receptor sites?

    a. Prazosin

    b. Terazosin

    c. Phenoxybenzamine

    d. Doxazosin

    e. Tamsulosin

32. Available data suggest that which of the following side effects is more common with tamsulosin than with either terazosin or doxazosin?

    a. Dizziness

    b. Asthenia

    c. Postural hypotension

    d. Palpitations

    e. Retrograde ejaculation

33. Which of the following agents or classes of agents, when administered systemically, will selectively relax the striated musculature of the pelvic floor?

    a. Benzodiazepines

    b. Dantrolene

    c. Baclofen

    d. Botulinum toxin

    e. None of the above

34. Which of the following is the most widely distributed inhibitory neurotransmitter in the mammalian central nervous system?

    a. γ-Aminobutyric acid (GABA)

    b. Glycine

    c. Glutamate

    d. Dopamine

    e. Norepinephrine

35. Baclofen (Lioresal) acts to decrease striated sphincter activity by which of the following mechanisms?

    a. Facilitating neuronal hyperpolarization through the $GABA_A$ receptor

    b. Activating the $GABA_B$ receptor and depressing monosynaptic and polysynaptic excitation of motor neurons and interneurons in the spinal cord

    c. Inhibiting excitation-contraction coupling in skeletal muscle by decreasing calcium release from the sarcoplasmic reticulum

    d. Inhibiting excitation-contraction coupling by preventing calcium entry into the cell

    e. Inhibiting acetylcholine release at the neuromuscular junction

36. All of the following statements are true with regard to botulinum toxin EXCEPT:

    a. It has been reported to be useful in the treatment of striated sphincter dyssynergia via direct sphincteric injection.

    b. It has been reported to be useful in the treatment of DO by direct intradetrusor injection.

    c. It inhibits the release of acetylcholine and other transmitters at the neuromuscular junction of somatic nerve and striated muscle and the autonomic nerves in smooth muscle.

    d. It has been reported to be of use, via periurethral striated muscle injections, in the treatment of SUI.

    e. The immunologic subtype utilized for urologic use has primarily been type A.

37. All of the following statements are true regarding the action of atropine and atropine-like agents (antimuscarinic agents) in patients with OAB and DO EXCEPT:

    a. Volume to first involuntary contraction increases.

    b. Total bladder capacity increases.

    c. Heart rate decreases.

    d. Urgency episodes decrease.

    e. Amplitude of the DO contractions decreases.

38. Which of the following statements is FALSE with respect to atropine resistance?

    a. It is secondary to release of norepinephrine from pelvic nerve in addition to acetylcholine.

    b. It is of little importance in normal human detrusor function.

    c. Its importance in treatment of DO in humans remains to be established.

    d. It applies to the response of the whole bladder to pelvic nerve stimulation, but not to the response of the detrusor to exogenous cholinergic stimulation.

    e. It is commonly invoked as a cause for only partial clinical improvement in the treatment of OAB with antimuscarinic agents.

39. Which statement is FALSE regarding M_3 receptors?
    a. They are less common than M_2 receptors in detrusor smooth muscle.
    b. They are more common than M_2 receptors in urothelium.
    c. They are the most important muscarinic receptor for detrusor contraction.
    d. They are blocked by atropine.
    e. When activated, they lead to an increase in intracellular calcium in detrusor smooth muscle cells.

40. All of the following are well-known potential adverse events of antimuscarinic therapy EXCEPT:
    a. constipation.
    b. cognitive dysfunction.
    c. increased heart rate.
    d. blurred vision.
    e. hyperhidrosis.

41. Match the side effects with the predominate muscarinic receptor subtype.
    1. M1
    2. M2
    3. M3
    4. M4
    5 M5
    6. none
    a. constipation
    b. dry mouth
    c. cognitive dysfunction
    d. increased heart rate
    e. increased QT interval

42. When used in the usual dosages for the treatment of OAB in a patient who is not on clean intermittent catheterization, antimuscarinic agents act primarily by (more than one response may be correct):
    a. reducing detrusor voiding contraction.
    b. decreasing activity in C fibers.
    c. decreasing activity in Aδ fibers.
    d. reducing the micromotions caused by the release of small packets of acetylcholine.
    e. reducing excitation of afferent nerves from the urothelium and detrusor.

43. An 80-year-old man has OAB-wet and cognitive dysfunction. Theoretically, the antimuscarinic drug that would be expected to be the safest with respect to worsening his cognition is:
    a. solifenacin.
    b. oxybutynin ER.
    c. fesoterodine.
    d. trospium.
    e. tolterodine.

44. Activation of detrusor smooth muscle by both acetylcholine and adenosine triphosphate requires:
    a. increase in intracellular potassium concentration.
    b. decrease in intracellular potassium concentration.
    c. increase in intracellular calcium concentration.
    d. increase in intracellular cyclic guanosine monophosphate (GMP).
    e. increase in intracellular cyclic adenosine monophosphate (AMP).

45. Which of the following have 1A or 1B ratings (modified Oxford system) for treatment of DO?
    a. Flavoxate
    b. Dicyclomine
    c. Estrogen
    d. Tamsulosin
    e. Tolterodine
    f. Fesoterodine
    g. Darifenacin
    h. Solifenacin
    i. Propiverine
    j. Oxybutynin
    k. Trospium

46. Which of the following drugs can produce or aggravate SUI in a woman?
    a. Alfuzosin
    b. Nifedipine
    c. Tamsulosin
    d. Oxybutynin
    e. Propantheline
    f. Flavoxate
    g. Fesoterodine
    h. Duloxetine

47. Intravesical DMSO is:
    a. generally used in a 70% solution.
    b. generally used in a 50% solution.
    c. useful for the treatment of neurogenic DO.
    d. useful for the treatment of bladder pain syndrome (interstitial cystitis).
    e. useful for the treatment of idiopathic DO.

48. Regarding the vanilloids, which of the following is/are TRUE?
    a. They act primarily to render C fibers insensitive.
    b. They act primarily to render Aδ fibers insensitive.
    c. When delivered intravesically, they cause a biphasic (excitation then blockade) effect.
    d. Resiniferatoxin is much more potent than capsaicin for desensitization but proportionately less so for excitation.
    e. Capsaicin is more potent than resiniferatoxin for desensitization.

49. A 30-year-old paraplegic man is wet between intermittent catheterizations (catheterizes five times per day). He is on solifenacin, 10 mg daily, and reports moderate dry mouth and increased difficulty in his bowel regimen. A reasonable next step in treatment is to:
    a. increase dose of solifenacin.
    b. add oxybutynin ER, 10 mg daily.
    c. add darifenacin, 7.5 mg daily.
    d. add darifenacin, 15 mg daily.
    e. use intradetrusor botulinum toxin.

50. Generally, treatment with intradetrusor botulinum toxin:
    a. must be repeated every 3 to 12 months.
    b. improves quality of life in patients incontinent due to neurogenic DO.
    c. loses efficacy with repeat treatments.
    d. can cause urinary retention.
    e. requires general anesthesia.

51. The Heart and Estrogen/Progestin Replacement Study (HERS), Women's Health Initiative (WHI), and Nurses' Health Study compositely showed that:
    a. oral estrogen plus progesterone worsened urinary incontinence in older postmenopausal women with incontinence.
    b. oral estrogen plus progesterone increased the incidence of SUI and urgency urinary incontinence in those continent at baseline.
    c. oral estrogen and progesterone worsened the frequency of incontinence in those incontinent at baseline.
    d. transvaginal estrogen improves SUI in postmenopausal women.
    e. the risk of developing incontinence was increased in postmenopausal women taking estrogen alone or estrogen with progestin.

52. Adrenergically induced smooth muscle contraction in the human lower urinary tract is mediated primarily by which receptor?
    a. α_{1D}
    b. β_3
    c. β_2
    d. α_{1A}
    e. α_2

ANSWERS

1. **c. Increased outlet resistance.** Atropine and atropine-like agents will depress normal bladder contractions and involuntary bladder contractions of any cause. In such patients, the volume to the first involuntary bladder contraction will generally be increased, the amplitude of the involuntary bladder contraction decreased, and the total bladder capacity increased. Outlet resistance, at least as reflected by urethral pressure measurements, does not seem to be clinically affected.

2. **b. M_2.** On the basis of existing knowledge, it is now recommended that the designations M_1 to M_5 be used to describe both the pharmacologic subtypes and the molecular subtypes of muscarinic acetylcholine receptors. The human urinary bladder smooth muscle contains a mixed population of M_2 and M_3 subtypes, with M_2 receptors predominant (M_2 receptors predominate at least 3:1 versus M_3 receptors not only on detrusor cells but also on other bladder structures, which may be of importance for detrusor activation).

3. **c. M_3.** The minor population of M_3 receptors is generally accepted at this time as primarily responsible for the mediation of bladder contraction.

4. **d. Bradycardia.** In general, drug therapy for lower urinary tract dysfunction is hindered by a concept that can be expressed in one word: uroselectivity. The clinical utility of available antimuscarinic agents is limited by their lack of selectivity, responsible for the classic peripheral antimuscarinic side effects of dry mouth, constipation, blurred vision, tachycardia, and effects on cognitive function.

5. **a, c, and e.** High lipophilicity, small molecular size, and low electrical charge increase the possibilities for an antimuscarinic agent to pass the blood-brain barrier. Quaternary ammonium compounds pass into the central nervous system to a limited extent. Tertiary amines pass the blood-brain barrier to a greater extent.

6. **a and d.** The traditional view was that in OAB/DO, antimuscarinics act by blocking the muscarinic receptors on the detrusor muscle that are stimulated by acetylcholine released from the activated cholinergic (parasympathetic) nerves. However, antimuscarinic drugs act mainly during the storage phase of micturition, decreasing urgency and increasing bladder capacity, and during this phase there is normally no parasympathetic input to the lower urinary tract. There is good experimental evidence that antimuscarinics decrease the activity in both C and Aδ afferent fibers during the filling/storage phase of micturition.

7. **b. Flavoxate.** A level of 1 implies the presence of systematic reviews, meta-analysis, and good-quality randomized controlled clinical trials. A grade of recommendation of A means that the agent is highly recommended based on level 1 evidence. Flavoxate received a level of evidence of 2, meaning that either randomized control trials and/or good-quality prospective cohort studies existed regarding its use, but a grade of recommendation of D, meaning that no recommendation for use is possible because of inconsistent/inconclusive evidence.

8. **d. Prolongation of the QT interval.** Well-known peripheral antimuscarinic side effects include blurred vision due to accommodation paralysis, constipation due to impaired bowel motility, increase in heart rate due to some blockade of M_2 cardiac receptors, and dry mouth due primarily to blockade of M_3 receptors in the salivary glands. QT prolongation is not related to muscarinic blockade but rather linked to inhibition of the hERG potassium channel in the heart. Some antimuscarinic drugs may in fact cause this, but this is not a class effect.

9. **c. Three; β_3.** Three cloned subtypes of β-adrenergic receptors, β_1, β_2, β_3, have been identified in the detrusor of most species, including humans. Studies have revealed a predominant expression of the β_3 receptor, and there is functional evidence for an important role in both normal and neurogenic bladders. The β_3 agonist mirabegron represents the first drug in this class to be developed for treatment of OAB.

10. **e. Antimuscarinic effect.** Oxybutynin has several pharmacologic effects, some of which seem difficult to relate to its effectiveness in the treatment of DO. It has antimuscarinic, direct muscle relaxant, and local anesthetic actions. The local anesthetic action and direct muscle relaxant effect may be of importance when the drug is administered intravesically but probably play no role when it is given orally. In vitro, oxybutynin was shown to be 500 times weaker as a smooth muscle relaxant than as an antimuscarinic agent. Most probably, when given systematically, oxybutynin acts mainly as an antimuscarinic drug.

11. **d and e.** The M_3 receptor has a primary role in salivation, bowel motility, and visual accommodation. The M_1 receptor is thought to be involved in cognition. The M_2 receptor is the primary cholinergic receptor in the heart, causing bradycardia when activated and, potentially, tachycardia, when blocked. The M_4 and M_5 receptors do not at this time seem to have a primary role in any of these organ systems.

12. **d. Application site reactions.** The transdermal delivery of oxybutynin alters oxybutynin metabolism, reducing production of the primary metabolite, responsible for most of the side effects, to an even greater extent than extended-release oxybutynin. The primary adverse event for this preparation has been application-site reaction: pruritus in 14% and erythema in 8.3%.

13. **a. Darifenacin.** Darifenacin is relatively selective for M_3 receptor blockade, meaning that, in vitro, the affinity for M_3 receptors is greater than for the other muscarinic receptors. This is only a relative selectivity, however, and whether this translates into either greater efficacy or greater tolerability has yet to be established.

14. **a and c.** Mirabegron is a β_3 agonist, the first commercially available and approved drug of its type, approved for the treatment of OAB. It acts not only by stimulating the B$_3$ receptors in the bladder (causing detrusor relaxation) but also by inhibiting filling-induced activity in both mechanosensitive Aδ and C-fiber primary bladder afferents, at least in an animal model.

15. **e. Trospium.** Darifenacin, oxybutynin, solifenacin, and tolterodine are all actively metabolized in the liver by the cytochrome P450 enzyme system. Trospium chloride is not metabolized to any significant degree in the liver. It is actively excreted by the proximal convoluted tubules in the kidney.

16. **a, b, and d.** Tadalafil is a phosphodiesterase (PDE)-5 inhibitor. Phosphodiesterase inhibitors enhance the presumed cyclic AMP and cyclic GMP relaxation of lower urinary tract smooth muscles as well as blood vessels in the penis. It was originally developed for the treatment of erectile dysfunction and improved IIEF scores. The observation that patients treated for erectile dysfunction with PDE-5 inhibitors had an improvement of their lower urinary tract symptoms led to interest in use of these drugs to treat LUTS and OAB. **PDE-5 inhibitors significantly improve IPSS scores but do not improve peak flow rates compared with placebo.** Similarly, they do not change detrusor pressure at peak flow. The mechanism behind the beneficial effect of these substances on LUTS/OAB and their site(s) of action largely remains to be elucidated. They are effective, however, and in fact tadalafil, at the time of this writing, has been approved for the treatment of LUTS due to benign prostatic obstruction.

17. **c. Priapism.** The most frequent side effects of the tricyclic antidepressants are those attributable to their systemic antimuscarinic activity. Allergic phenomena (including rash), hepatic dysfunction, obstructive jaundice, and agranulocytosis may also occur, but rarely. Central nervous system side effects may include weakness, fatigue, parkinsonian effect, fine tremor noted most in the upper extremities, manic or schizophrenic picture, and sedation, probably from an antihistaminic effect. Postural hypotension may also be seen, presumably on the basis of selective blockade (a paradoxic effect) of α_1-adrenergic receptors in some vascular smooth muscle. Tricyclic antidepressants can also cause excess sweating of obscure cause and a delay of orgasm or orgasmic impotence, the cause of which is likewise unclear. They can also produce arrhythmias and interact in deleterious ways with other drugs, and so caution must be observed in their use in patients with cardiac disease. They have not been reported to cause priapism.

18. **e. None of the above.** Several randomized control trials have demonstrated that the combination treatment of antimuscarinic drugs and α_1-adrenergic receptor antagonist is more effective at reducing male lower urinary tract symptoms than α-blockers alone in men with BPO and OAB. Used in the recommended doses, and in men whose voiding was not significantly compromised previously, none of the parameters related to emptying changed appreciably (detrusor pressures, flow rates, residual voided volume).

19. **c and e.** Botulinum toxin-A cleaves SNAP 25 and renders the SNARE complex inactive as its primary mechanism of action. It acts on both striated muscle and smooth muscle and in fact was first studied in striated muscle. It blocks acetylcholine release and reduces firing from bladder afferents. It is effective in both neurogenic and idiopathic DO and also in patients with OAB. Successful OAB treatment does not appear to be related to the existence of DO.

20. **a. Urogenital atrophy.** The evidence supporting the use of estrogens in lower urinary tract dysfunction remains controversial, but considerable data support the use of vaginal estrogen in urogenital atrophy. The vaginal route improves dryness, pruritus, and dyspareunia and provides a greater improvement in physical findings than oral administration.

21. **d. Somnolence.** Potential side effects of all of these agents include blood pressure elevation, anxiety, and insomnia due to stimulation of the central nervous system; headache; tremor; weakness; palpations; cardiac arrhythmias; and respiratory difficulties. They should be used with caution in patients with hypertension, cardiovascular disease, or hyperthyroidism.

22. **a. Phenylpropanolamine.** The risk of hemorrhagic stroke in women younger than 50 years has been reported to be 16 times higher in those who have been taking phenylpropanolamine, an α-adrenergic agonist, as an appetite suppressant, and 3 times higher in women who have been taking the drug for less than 24 hours as a cold remedy, although the latter was not statistically significant (the former was). Phenylpropanolamine has been removed from the market in the United States.

23. **b. Propranolol.** Theoretically, β-adrenergic blocking agents, such as propranolol, might be expected to "unmask" or potentiate an α-adrenergic effect, thereby increasing urethral resistance. Such treatment has been suggested as an alternative treatment to α-adrenergic agonists in patients with sphincteric incontinence and hypertension. Some studies support such usage, but they are not randomized or controlled. The other compounds listed are α-adrenergic agonists and are a risk factor for increased blood pressure.

24. **e. It is not metabolized by the liver.** Duloxetine hydrochloride is a serotonin-norepinephrine reuptake inhibitor that has been shown, in an animal model, to significantly increase urethral sphincteric muscle activity during the filling/storage phase of micturition. It is lipophilic, well absorbed, and extensively metabolized by the liver. It is still approved as a treatment for SUI in some countries. It was withdrawn from the FDA approval process in the United States but is licensed in the European Union for the treatment of SUI in women with moderate to severe incontinence, defined as 15 or more episodes per week.

25. **b and c.** The results of the HERS study, the WHI study, and the Nurses' Health Study all suggest that there is no evidence that estrogens with or without progesterone should be used in the treatment of urinary incontinence. In fact, estrogen with or without progesterone increases the risk of urinary incontinence among continent postmenopausal women and worsens urinary incontinence in those already with incontinence.

26. **b. Hyponatremia.** Side effects are relatively uncommon during desmopressin treatment, but there is a risk of water retention and hyponatremia. It is recommended that serum sodium concentration be measured in elderly patients before and after a few days of treatment.

27. **e. It facilitates bladder emptying.** Many acetylcholine-like drugs exist, but only bethanechol chloride (Urecholine, Duvoid, others) exhibits a relatively selective in vitro action on the urinary bladder and gut with little or no nicotinic action. Bethanechol chloride is cholinesterase resistant and causes an in vitro contraction of smooth muscle from all areas of the bladder. Although it has been reported to increase gastrointestinal motility and has been used in the treatment of gastroesophageal reflux, and although anecdotal success in specific patients with voiding dysfunction seems to occur, there is no evidence to support its success in facilitating bladder emptying in a series of patients when the drug was the only variable.

28. **a. 200 mg.** It is generally agreed that, at least in a "denervated" bladder, an oral dose of 200 mg is required to produce the same urodynamic effects as a subcutaneous dose of 5 mg.

29. **e. Potentiation of adenosine triphosphate release from bladder mucosa.** Prostanoids are synthesized both locally in bladder muscle and mucosa, with synthesis initiated by various physiologic stimuli such as detrusor muscle stretch, mucosal injury, and neural stimulation; directly by adenosine triphosphate; and by mediators of inflammation. Prostanoids have been variably reported to be useful in facilitating bladder emptying with intravesical administration. Possible roles include (1) neuromodulators of efferent and afferent transmission; (2) sensitization; (3) activation of certain sensory nerves; and (4) potentiation of acetylcholine (but not ATP) release from cholinergic nerve terminals through prejunctional prostanoid receptors.

30. **c. α_1 Receptors are more common than α_2.** The human lower urinary tract contains more α_2 than α_1 receptors, but adrenergically induced human lower urinary tract smooth muscle contraction and prostate smooth muscle contraction are mediated largely, if not exclusively, by α_1 adrenergic receptors. The remainder of the statements are true.

31. **c. Phenoxybenzamine.** Phenoxybenzamine (Dibenzyline) was the α-adrenolytic agent originally used for the treatment of voiding dysfunction. It and phentolamine have blocking properties at both α-adrenergic receptor sites. Prazosin hydrochloride (Minipress) was the first potent selective α-adrenergic antagonist used to lower outlet resistance. Terazosin (Hytrin) and doxazosin (Cardura) are two highly selective postsynaptic α_1-adrenergic blockers. Most recently, alfuzosin and tamsulosin (Flomax), both highly selective α_1-adrenergic blockers, have appeared and are marketed solely for the treatment of benign prostatic hyperplasia because of some reports suggesting preferential action on prostatic rather than vascular smooth muscle.

32. **e. Retrograde ejaculation.** Available data suggest that retrograde ejaculation and rhinitis are more common with tamsulosin, whereas dizziness and asthenia are more common with terazosin and doxazosin.

33. **e. None of the above.** There is no class of pharmacologic agents that will selectively relax the striated musculature of the pelvic floor. Botulinum toxin-A when injected directly into the striated sphincter will relax it, but this "relative selectivity" is because of where it is locally injected.

34. **a. γ-Aminobutyric acid (GABA).** GABA and glycine have been identified as major inhibitory transmitters in the central nervous system. GABA is the most widely distributed inhibitory neurotransmitter in the mammalian central nervous system. It appears to mediate the inhibitory actions of local interneurons in the brain and presynaptic inhibition within the spinal cord.

35. **b. Activating the GABA$_B$ receptor and depressing monosynaptic and polysynaptic excitation of motor neurons and interneurons in the spinal cord.** Benzodiazepines potentiate the action of GABA by facilitating neuronal hyperpolarization through the GABA$_A$ receptor. Baclofen (Lioresal) depresses monosynaptic and polysynaptic excitation of motor neurons and interneurons in the spinal cord by activating GABA$_B$ receptors. Dantrolene (Dantrium) exerts its effects by a direct peripheral action on skeletal muscle. It is thought to inhibit the excitation-induced release of calcium ions from the sarcoplasmic reticulum of striated muscle fibers, thereby inhibiting excitation-contraction coupling and diminishing the mechanical force of contraction. Botulinum A toxin (Botox) is an inhibitor of acetylcholine release at the neuromuscular junction of somatic nerves on striated muscle.

36. **d. It has been reported to be of use, via periurethral striated muscle injections, in the treatment of SUI.** Intrasphincteric injection of botulinum toxin A was first reported useful in the treatment of striated sphincteric dyssynergia in 1990. The toxin blocks the release of acetylcholine and other transmitters from presynaptic nerve endings by interacting with the protein complex necessary for docking vesicles. This results in decreased muscle contractility and muscle atrophy at the injection site. The drug has been reported to be of use as well in the treatment of neurogenic DO and cases of non-neurogenic DO. There are seven immunologically distinct antigenic subtypes. Types A and B are in clinical use in urology, but most studies and treatments have been carried out with botulinum toxin type A (Botox). Intrasphincteric injections of botulinum toxin are not useful for SUI. In fact, they can cause SUI in females.

37. **c. Heart rate decreases.** Those with an M$_2$ receptor blockade profile can increase heart rate, but the clinical significance of this is unknown.

38. **a. It is secondary to release of norepinephrine from pelvic nerve in addition to acetylcholine.** The most common neurotransmitter mentioned as the prime alternate in atropine resistance is adenosine triphosphate. Norepinephrine is released by postganglionic sympathetic nerves (e.g., hypogastric), not by parasympathetic ones (e.g., pelvic).

39. **b. They are more common than M$_2$ receptors in urothelium.** M$_2$ receptors outnumber M$_3$ in urothelium as well as detrusor smooth muscle. All other statements are true.

40. **e. Hyperhidrosis.** If anything, antimuscarinic agents can cause decreased sweating. All the others are antimuscarinic side effects.

41. **a: 3; b: 3; c: 1; d: 2; e: 6.** Increased QT interval, caused by some antimuscarinic compounds, is not an antimuscarinic property. All the others are antimuscarinic and are caused primarily by blockade of the indicated receptor subtype.

42. **b, c, d, and e.** At the dose employed for OAB treatment, antimuscarinic agents do not cause significant reduction in the voiding contraction of voluntary micturition. They have been implicated in all the others. C and Aδ fibers refer to afferent nerves carrying noxious and "normal" stimuli, respectively.

43. **d. Trospium.** Trospium, as a quaternary amine, is lipophobic and does not penetrate well through the blood-brain barrier. The others, all tertiary amines, do pass the blood-brain barrier to a greater extent.

44. **c. Increase in intracellular calcium concentration.** This occurs through both extracellular influx and mobilization of intracellular calcium.

45. **e, f, g, h, i, j, and k.** Propiverine is a drug with "mixed action" and currently is not available in the United States, but is in Europe.

46. **a and c.** The α-adrenergic antagonists can decrease outlet resistance and thereby irritate or worsen SUI. Nifedipine is a calcium antagonist; fesoterodine and propantheline are anticholinergic agents; duloxetine is a serotonin-norepinephrine reuptake inhibitor; oxybutynin is primarily an antimuscarinic agent with some direct smooth muscle relaxant effects on the bladder; and flavoxate has mixed actions and questionable effects.

47. **b and d.** DMSO is a naturally occurring compound with multiple pharmacologic actions used in a 50% solution for the treatment of bladder pain syndrome (including interstitial cystitis). It is not useful for the treatment of DO.

48. **a, c, and d.** It is possible that vanilloids have some effects on Aδ fibers as well. They cause an initial excitation followed by a long-lasting blockade. Resiniferatoxin is 1000 times more potent than capsaicin for desensitization and a few hundred times more potent for excitation.

49. **e. Use intradetrusor botulinum toxin.** Adding or increasing antimuscarinic medication will simply increase the severity of the adverse events already experienced. Intradetrusor botulinum toxin has been shown to be very effective in neurogenic DO and should be considered if following failure of, or intolerance to, antimuscarinic therapy.

50. **a, b, and d.** Repeat injections (two to nine) have not lost efficacy over time. The injections can be done without general anesthesia (local). Intravesical botulinum toxin A is effective in reducing neurogenic DO and does improve quality of life in such patients.

51. **a, b, c, and e. a** is from the HERS, **b** and **c** from the WHI, and **e** from the Nurses' Health Study. Although many clinicians prescribe transvaginal estrogen or estrogen plus progestin cream for symptoms of OAB or/and SUI, there is no real evidence that estrogen, with or without progesterone, is useful in the treatment of urinary incontinence.

52. **d.** α_{1A}. More α_2 than α_1 receptors are present, but adrenergically induced contraction is mediated largely by the α_{1A} (and in the detrusor, α_{1D}). β receptors cause smooth muscle relaxation. The β_3 subtype is the predominant β receptor in the human detrusor.

CHAPTER REVIEW

1. The major neurohumoral stimulus for physiologic bladder contraction is acetylcholine-induced stimulation of post-ganglionic parasympathetic muscarinic cholinergic receptor sites in the bladder.
2. The muscarinic receptor functions may be changed in different urologic disorders without an overt neurogenic cause.
3. Behavioral therapy should always be used in conjunction with drug therapy for overactive bladder (OAB).
4. Calcium channel antagonists are not effective in treating OAB.
5. Potassium channel openers available today are not effective in treating OAB.
6. The use of estrogens to treat stress urinary incontinence (SUI) has resulted in worsening of preexisting urinary incontinence in patients with SUI and urgency urinary incontinence and new-onset incontinence in patients who have not had it. The use of vaginal estrogen in the treatment of urogenital atrophy improves dryness, pruritus, dyspareunia, and physical findings. The vaginal route is more effective than oral administration.
7. Intravesical oxybutynin has shown some efficacy in treating OAB as well as in treating intestinal augmented OABs.
8. Antimuscarinics may have effects on cognitive function, particularly in the elderly.
9. Antimuscarinics may be divided into tertiary and quaternary amines. The latter are not well absorbed and have limited ability to enter the central nervous system, unlike the tertiary amines.
10. Antimuscarinics may have adverse cardiac effects.
11. α_1-adrenergic blockers are not effective in women.
12. The human urinary bladder smooth muscle contains a mixed population of M_2 and M_3 subtypes, with M_2 receptors predominant (M_2 receptors predominant at least 3:1 versus M_3). M_3 receptors are primarily responsible for the mediation of bladder contraction.
13. Mirabegron is a β_3 agonist, the first commercially available drug of its type approved for the treatment of overactive bladder.
14. PDE-5 inhibitors significantly improve International Prostate Symptom Score scores but do not improve peak flow rates when compared with placebo.
15. Urinary tract smooth muscle contraction and prostate smooth muscle contraction are mediated largely, if not exclusively, by α_1-adrenergic receptors.

121 Conservative Management of Urinary Incontinence: Behavioral and Pelvic Floor Therapy, Urethral and Pelvic Devices

Diane K. Newman and Kathryn L. Burgio

QUESTIONS

1. A person with cognitive impairment may not be a candidate for which behavioral interventions:
   a. prompted voiding
   b. timed voiding
   c. bladder training
   d. habit training

2. A bladder diary is integral to behavioral therapy because it can:
   a. help determine functional bladder capacity
   b. provide information about symptom improvement
   c. determine adherence to pelvic floor muscle training
   d. improve understanding of patient's voiding pattern
   e. all of the above
   f. b and d

3. Which of the following are true about pelvic floor muscle training?
   a. Pelvic floor muscle training is effective for treating stress, urge, or mixed incontinence in men and women of any age.
   b. Pelvic floor muscle training is appropriate for stress or mixed incontinence, but not for urgency incontinence.
   c. Pelvic floor muscle training works for women, but not for men.
   d. Pelvic floor muscle training is not effective for older people.
   e. Pelvic floor muscle training is useful for mild-moderate incontinence, but not severe incontinence.

4. When teaching the urge suppression technique, patients are encouraged to:
   a. Stay near a bathroom as much as possible, so they won't have far to go when they feel an urge to void.
   b. Stay away from the bathroom until they feel an urge to void. Then get to the bathroom as soon as possible.
   c. Stay away from the bathroom until urgency or the urge to void occurs. Then they should sit down, practice urge suppression techniques, and once the urge has passed, slowly walk to the bathroom to void.
   d. Wait as long as possible to go to the bathroom to increase bladder capacity.

5. When patients are trying to calm down urgency and prevent leakage, which of the following works BEST?
   a. Crossing the legs
   b. Squeezing the pelvic floor muscles while rushing to the bathroom
   c. Squeezing the pelvic floor muscles while sitting still until the urgency goes away, then walking to the bathroom
   d. Relaxing the pelvic floor muscles to help relax the bladder

6. When using fluid management as a treatment for urgency incontinence, patients are told to:
   a. consume a normal amount of fluid to avoid dehydration as well as sudden urgency.
   b. increase fluid intake to ensure adequate hydration and train the bladder.
   c. decrease fluid intake to minimize bladder filling.
   d. increase fluid intake to prevent the loss of functional bladder capacity.

7. When attempting to identify dietary bladder irritants, the patient should:
   a. avoid spicy foods, tomatoes, and citric fruits
   b. eliminate caffeine
   c. keep a diary to see which foods or beverages increase urgency
   d. all of the above

8. When conducting pelvic floor muscle training, clinicians should:
   a. ensure that patients are contracting the pelvic floor muscles selectively
   b. prescribe a specific set of exercises for the patients to do each day
   c. teach patients to contract pelvic floor muscles whenever they engage in activities that precipitate leakage
   d. all of the above

9. Which of the following is true of caffeine reduction as a lifestyle modification for the treatment of incontinence?
   a. Patients should be told to eliminate caffeine gradually
   b. Patients should be encouraged to try eliminating caffeine for a few days to see how it affects their bladder
   c. Patients should be encouraged to reduce caffeine gradually
   d. Patients should be advised to eliminate coffee only, as it is the main source of caffeine

ANSWERS

1. **c. Bladder training.** Bladder training is an example of "patient-dependent" interventions: it relies on active patient participation. There must be adequate function, learning capability, and motivation of the individual. Bladder training involves patient education regarding lower urinary tract function, setting incremental voiding schedules, and teaching urge control techniques to help patients postpone voiding and adhere to the schedule.

2. **f. b and d.** A bladder diary provides information on the type and amount of fluid intake, type and frequency of symptoms, such as incontinence episodes, frequency of urination, the urgency associated with each, and the circumstances or reasons

for incontinence episodes, which helps the provider plan appropriate components of behavioral intervention. A bladder diary is also the best noninvasive tool available to objectively monitor the patient's voiding habits and the effect of treatment on symptoms guiding the use of various treatment components.

3. **a. Pelvic floor muscle training is effective for treating stress, urge, or mixed incontinence in men and women of any age.** Behavioral interventions are well established for treating stress and urgency UI and OAB. Because behavioral treatments are effective and essentially risk free, they are the mainstay of conservative treatment and are recommended for both men and women of all ages as first-line therapy by several guidelines and consensus panels.

4. **c. Stay away from the bathroom until urgency or the urge to void occurs. Then they should sit down, practice urge suppression techniques, and once the urge has passed, slowly walk to the bathroom to void.** Patients are taught not to feel compelled to rush to the nearest bathroom when they feel the urge to void, believing that they are about to lose control. With behavioral training, they learn how this natural "gotta go" response is actually counter-productive, because it increases physical pressure on the bladder, increases the feeling of fullness, exacerbates urgency, and triggers detrusor contraction. Further, as the patient approaches the toilet, visual cues can trigger urgency and incontinence. To avoid this conditioned response, patients are taught not to rush to the bathroom when they feel the urge to void. Instead, they are advised to stay away from the bathroom, so as to avoid exposure to cues that trigger urgency. They are taught strategies to suppress urgency prior to walking to the toilet.

5. **c. Squeezing the pelvic floor muscles while sitting still until the urgency goes away, then walking to the bathroom.** Patients are taught not to rush to the bathroom when they feel the urge to void. Instead, they are advised to stay away from the bathroom, so as to avoid exposure to cues that trigger urgency. They are encouraged to pause, sit down if possible, relax the entire body, and contract PFM repeatedly, without relaxing in between contractions, to diminish urgency, inhibit detrusor contraction, and prevent urine loss. They focus on inhibiting the urge sensation, giving it time to pass. Once the sensation subsides, they walk at a normal pace to the toilet.

6. **a. Consume a normal amount of fluid to avoid dehydration as well as sudden urgency.** Fluid intake modifications depend on the patients' pattern of intake, which can be assessed by having them complete a 24- to 48-hour diary of intake and output, including voided volumes when possible. Reviewing such a diary can reveal excessive fluid intake, inadequate fluid intake, and diurnal patterns of intake that may be contributing to LUTS. Although it may seem counterintuitive, it is usually good advice to encourage patients to consume at least six 8-ounce glasses of fluid each day to maintain adequate hydration. Fluid intake should be regulated to 6- to 8-ounce glasses or 30 mL/kg body weight per day with a 1500 mL/day minimum at designated times unless contraindicated by a medical condition. The Institute of Medicine issued a report in 2004 with guidelines for total water intake for healthy people.

7. **c. Keep a diary to see which foods or beverages increase urgency.** A diary of food and beverage intake is useful for identifying which substances are in fact irritants for individual patients; and a trial period of eliminating these substances one at a time can be used to confirm the relationship.

8. **d. All of the above.** It is important to verify that patients have identified and can contract the pelvic floor muscles (PFMs) properly before initiating an exercise regimen. Specific exercise regimens vary considerably in frequency and intensity, and the ideal exercise regimen has not yet been determined. However, good results have been achieved in several trials using 45 to 60 paired contractions and relaxations per day. We use an "exercise prescription" to prescribe the daily exercise program. It is important to teach patients how to prevent urine loss in daily life by occluding the urethra using active contraction of PFMs. Although exercise alone can improve urethral pressure and structural support and reduce incontinence, this motor skill enables patients to consciously occlude the urethra at specific times when urine loss is imminent. A careful history or examination of a bladder diary can alert the provider and patient of the circumstances during which each individual patient commonly experiences urine loss. Patients then learn to anticipate these activities and prevent leakage by contracting the PFM to occlude the urethra prior to and during coughing, sneezing, lifting, or any other physical activities that have precipitated urine leakage.

9. **b. Patients should be encouraged to try eliminating caffeine for a few days to see how it affects their bladder.** Many patients are reluctant initially to forgo their caffeinated beverages, but they may be convinced to try it for a short period of time, such as 3 to 5 days, to determine if they are sensitive to its effects. If they experience relief from their symptoms, they are often more willing to reduce or eliminate caffeine from their diet.

CHAPTER REVIEW

1. Conservative behavioral treatments are a group of interventions that improve urinary incontinence and other lower urinary tract symptoms by changing patients' behavior or environment or by teaching new skills.
2. There is strong evidence that conservative interventions are effective first-line treatments for patients with urinary incontinence and other lower urinary tract symptoms.
3. The effectiveness of conservative treatments relies on the active participation of an involved and motivated patient.
4. Intensive behavioral interventions that involve an experienced clinician have been shown to be more effective.

122 Electrical Stimulation and Neuromodulation in Storage and Emptying Failure

John P.F.A. Heesakkers and Bertil Blok

QUESTIONS

1. The current approved indications for sacral neuromodulation include all of the following EXCEPT:
   a. urinary urgency.
   b. urinary frequency.
   c. urgency urinary incontinence.
   d. interstitial cystitis.
   e. idiopathic nonobstructive urinary retention.

2. Which patient is NOT well suited for current neuromodulation therapies?
   a. A 65-year-old insulin-dependent diabetic man with bladder areflexia and nonobstructive urinary retention
   b. A 67-year-old woman who has had a cerebrovascular accident and now has urinary urgency and frequency
   c. A 41-year-old woman with urgency urinary incontinence
   d. A 55-year-old woman who has had vaginal sling surgery and urgency urinary incontinence
   e. A 36-year-old woman with a history of interstitial cystitis with minimal pain who voids between 20 and 25 times per day

3. What reflex or reflexes are responsible for modulation of bladder function?
   a. Guarding reflex
   b. Bladder–Afferent loop reflex
   c. Bladder–Bladder reflex
   d. Bladder–Urethra reflex
   e. a and b

4. Which of the following is (are) considered the major clinical concern(s) associated with performing a sacral rhizotomy?
   a. Pelvic pain
   b. Creation of bladder areflexia
   c. Abnormal sexual function
   d. Pelvic and lower extremity sensory or motor abnormalities
   e. c and d

5. The S3 sensory and motor response pattern to electrical stimulation is best described as having which one of the following?
   a. Plantarflexion of the entire foot with sensation in the leg and buttock
   b. Levator reflex (bellows reflex) and sensations in the leg and buttock
   c. Dorsiflexion of the great toe and bellows reflex and pulling sensation in the rectum, scrotum, or vagina
   d. Plantarflexion of the first three toes of the foot and sensation of pulling in the rectum or vagina
   e. Bellows reflex (levator contraction) and sensation of pulling of the rectum

6. What is the main concern when performing magnetic resonance imaging (MRI) in the setting of neuromodulation and pacemaker-type devices?
   a. Potential of dislodgement of the pacemaker
   b. Heating of the electrical leads
   c. Heating of the pacemaker
   d. Potentially fatal arrhythmias
   e. Significant neuromuscular injury risk

7. Which of the following represents the best clinical scenario for use of neuromodulation therapy in a patient with multiple sclerosis (MS)?
   a. Detrusor sphincter dyssynergy
   b. Bedridden with significant functional incontinence
   c. Mild symptoms with no potential need for future MRI
   d. A poorly compliant bladder
   e. Areflexic bladder

8. What skeletal landmarks are associated with the S3 nerve foramen?
   a. 9 cm from the tip of the coccyx
   b. 11 cm from the tip of the coccyx
   c. 13 cm from the tip of the coccyx
   d. The inferior aspect of the sacral iliac joints
   e. a and d

9. Perhaps the main reason why neuromodulation devices are not currently approved for use in the United States by the Food and Drug Administration in pediatric patients is due to:
   a. lack of efficacy.
   b. potential worsening of neuromuscular function due to bony abnormalities (spina bifida and myelomeningocele).
   c. lack of data on growth of the spinal cord and nerve roots in the setting of neuromodulation devices.
   d. worsening of bowel function (Hinman bladder syndrome).
   e. excellent results with noninvasive therapies (transcutaneous electrical nerve stimulation) and therefore no reason to perform more invasive sacral neuromodulation in the long term.

10. The best option for a patient who has undergone a failed stage I sacral neuromodulation for severe refractory urgency urinary incontinence is:
    a. anticholinergic therapy.
    b. B3 agonist therapy
    c. bilateral stimulation.
    d. botulinum toxin A injections.
    e. bladder augmentation.

11. An implantable pulse generator (IPG) infection would be best treated by:
    a. intravenous antibiotics.
    b. oral antibiotics.
    c. irrigation of the pocket.
    d. removal of the entire device.
    e. a and b.

12. Which of the following statements is FALSE about the Brindley device?
    a. It requires intact neuron pathways between the sacral cord and nuclei, pelvic nerve, and bladder to function.
    b. It works best in a state of long-term areflexic bladder function.
    c. It is used most often in patients with insufficient or nonreflex micturition after spinal cord injury.
    d. It is usually coupled with sacral posterior rhizotomy.
    e. Electrodes are applied to S2, S3, and S4 nerve roots.

13. Direct electrical stimulation of the bladder often results in all of the following EXCEPT:
    a. pelvic musculature contraction.
    b. erection.
    c. defecation.
    d. bladder neck opening.
    e. ejaculation.

14. Which one of the following statements regarding the use of the Brindley device is FALSE?
    a. It requires intact neural pathways between the sacral cord and the bladder.
    b. Sacral posterior rhizotomy is generally performed.
    c. Myogenic decompensation is a contraindication.
    d. Electrodes are applied extradurally to sacral roots S2 to S4.
    e. It utilizes the principle of poststimulation voiding.

15. Which of the following statements regarding neurostimulation or neuromodulation is FALSE?
    a. The desired effect of neurostimulation is through direct stimulation of nerves and muscles.
    b. Neurostimulation is mainly reserved for neurogenic conditions.
    c. Neurostimulation produces a delayed clinical response.
    d. The effect of neuromodulation is achieved through alteration of neurotransmission processes.
    e. Neuromodulation may be useful for neurogenic as well as non-neurogenic conditions.

16. Which of the following studies is (are) the most useful in predicting which patients will or will not respond to sacral neuromodulation?
    a. Uroflow/postvoid residual monitoring
    b. Voiding diary
    c. Urodynamics/electromyography
    d. Percutaneous lead placement and trial stimulation
    e. c and d

17. Which of the following is (are) relative clinical contraindications for excluding potential candidates for neuromodulation and neurostimulation therapies?
    a. Patients with significant anatomic abnormalities in the spine or sacrum that may present challenges to gaining access
    b. Patients who cannot manage their devices or judge the clinical outcomes due to mental incapacitation
    c. Patients with physical limitations that prevent them from achieving normal pelvic organ function such as functional urinary incontinence
    d. Patients who are noncompliant
    e. All of the above

18. Which of the following statements best characterizes bilateral S3 nerve root stimulation for sacral neuromodulation therapy?
    a. It is a rational consideration for salvage therapy or added benefit as the bladder receives bilateral innervation.
    b. It is an approach alternative to failed unilateral stimulation in patients with urinary retention.
    c. Initial basis for this approach produced in spinal cord–injured animal models suggests this may be a potential approach in humans.
    d. All of the above.
    e. a and c only.

19. Potential sites of selective nerve stimulation other than the S3 sacral root for neuromodulation therapies for pelvic health conditions include which of the following?
    a. S4 sacral root
    b. Pudendal nerve
    c. Dorsal genital nerve
    d. Posterior tibial nerve
    e. All of the above

20. When troubleshooting the complication of IPG site discomfort or pain, which of the following statements best describes the necessary action(s) needed?
    a. Rule out IPG site infection by physical examination.
    b. Turn off the device and ask the patient if the discomfort is still present to differentiate IPG pocket site issues from IPG electrical output-related causes.
    c. If the IPG discomfort is output related, check whether bipolar stimulation is better than unipolar stimulation.
    d. If IPG site discomfort is output related, check impedances because a current leak may be present from the neuroelectrode to extension lead connection.
    e. All of the above.

21. When patients report recurrent symptoms after reduction or improvement of symptoms with sacral neuromodulation therapy, which of the following should be undertaken to evaluate the reason for the loss of clinical efficacy?
    a. Check the device settings for inadvertent on/off changes and battery performance.
    b. Evaluate the stimulation perception and anatomic localization for changes.
    c. Check for intermittent stimulation perception via positional changes of the patient because this may suggest lead migration or a loose lead connection.
    d. Obtain a radiograph to detect macro changes in the neuroelectrode position if findings in b and c are evident.
    e. All of the above.

22. What is NOT true for intravesical electrostimulation (IVES)?
    a. It is mainly applied in patients with detrusor underactivity
    b. The mechanism is thought to come from direct efferent nerve stimulation
    c. The effect is higher in patients without underlying neurogenic disease
    d. Patients after hemorrhoidal surgery respond well to IVES.

23. What is true for percutaneous tibial nerve stimulation (PTNS)?
    a. It is one of the few treatments that have a proper sham-controlled study that underlines the efficacy.
    b. Evoked potential studies suggest that PTNS has no adaptive long-term modification in the brain.
    c. There might be some similarities of PTNS with SP5 activation of acupuncture.
    d. PTNS can induce toe flection of the contralateral foot.
    e. All of the above.

24. What is false for PTNS?
    a. There are good urodynamic data that give predictive indications for PTNS efficacy
    b. Efficacy of the known tibial implants is the same as the percutaneous technique.
    c. The PTNS implants have the same result as the SNS implants
    d. Battery life is critical for the PTNS devices
    e. All of the above

ANSWERS

1. **d. Interstitial cystitis.** Although used commonly for interstitial cystitis (IC) symptoms, urgency/frequency IC is not truly an indication for the sacral neuromodulation devices. Several groups have seen benefits of sacral neuromodulation in IC patients, and there may be an expanding indication for this in the future.

2. **a. A 65-year-old insulin-dependent diabetic man with bladder areflexia and nonobstructive urinary retention.** It is implied that the end organ response (bladder in this case) should have good function for sacral neuromodulation and, for that matter, any form of neuromodulation to work. Neurostimulation may be different, but even if neurostimulation were used, simultaneous relaxation of the outlet would be required for a coordinated contraction and emptying phase to ensue.

3. **e. a and b.** Two reflexes may play an important role in modulation of bladder function: the guarding reflex and the bladder afferent loop reflex. Both reflexes promote urine storage under sympathetic tone. The guarding reflex guards or prevents urine loss in times of cough or other physical stress that would normally trigger a micturition episode. Suprapontine input from the brain turns off the guarding reflex during micturition to allow efficient and complete emptying. The bladder afferent reflex works through sacral interneurons that then activate storage through pudendal nerve efferent pathways directed toward the urethral sphincter. Similar to the guarding reflex, the bladder afferent reflex promotes continence during periods of bladder filling and is quiet during micturition.

4. **e. c and d.** Bilateral anterior and posterior sacral rhizotomy or conusectomy converts a hyperreflexic bladder to an areflexic one. This alone may be inappropriate therapy because it also adversely affects the rectum, anal and urethral sphincters, sexual function, and the lower extremities. In an attempt to leave sphincter and sexual function intact, selective motor nerve section was originally introduced as a treatment to increase bladder capacity by abolishing only the motor supply responsible for involuntary contractions.

5. **c. Dorsiflexion of the great toe and bellows reflex and pulling sensation in the rectum, scrotum, or vagina.** The characteristic response of the S3 nerve distribution based on its lower innervation is to the levator musculature (bellows contraction) of the anus and ipsilateral great toe contraction. The other answers suggest either S2 stimulation (leg rotation) or S4 levator contraction.

6. **b. Heating of the electrical leads.** Although many concerns exist for MRI and pacemaker devices, it has been shown that the main concern is heating of the electrical leads. This may, in turn, traumatize blood vessels, nerve roots, or other structures that the leads themselves are next to. Currently, MRI is contraindicated in the presence of a pacemaker.

7. **c. Mild symptoms with no potential need for future MRI.** It is unknown whether subcategories of MS patients (delayed emptying/storage dysfunction, areflexia, poor compliance) would be very good candidates for sacral neuromodulation, although it is doubtful based on disease severity alone. A mildly symptomatic patient without functional issues (e.g., can get to the bathroom in time with no major mobility issues) probably would be the best patient.

8. **e. a and d.** The measurements for the rough vicinity of the S3 nerve foramen have been tested by using the "cross hair" technique (Chai et al., 2000)[a] and simple measurements. The answers b and c are incorrect because they represent measurements from the anal verge (11 cm), and 13 cm is too far in general from the coccyx and would likely place one near S2 or S1.

9. **c. Lack of data on growth of the spinal cord and nerve roots in the setting of neuromodulation devices.** Pediatric patients have undergone sacral neuromodulation in off-label trials, but large-scale use has been limited by lack of data on the growth of the pediatric patient and the relation of the sacral lead with regard to the sacral nerve roots, and so on. Although noninvasive therapies have worked, they are limited by the need for continued repeat therapy to maintain durability of result.

10. **d. Botulinum toxin A injections.** The patient should have tried and failed anticholinergic or β 3 agonist therapy before having the sacral neuromodulation therapy. Scheepens and coworkers have shown that bilateral stimulation, although logical, has not been shown in urgency incontinent patients to lead to much improvement (Scheepens et al., 2002). One could argue that contralateral lead placement should be attempted, but no prospective trials have shown that this makes a difference in outcomes. Because botulinum toxin A therapy has been proven to be as good as sacral neuromodulation, this is the most logical thing to do in this case.

11. **d. Removal of the entire device.** Because an IPG is a foreign body, it could harbor bacteria within a biofilm created by the infection. Accordingly, it is best to have it removed in its entirety. Antibiotics and irrigation for the most part are temporizing measures. Furthermore, there is risk of an infection tracking along the sacral lead, which may create a sacral infection.

12. **b. It works best in a state of long-term areflexic bladder function.** The chief applications of the Brindley device are in patients with inefficient or nonreflex micturition after spinal cord injury. Prerequisites for use are described by Fischer et al. (1993) as the following: (1) intact neural pathways between the sacral cord nuclei of the pelvic nerve and the bladder and (2) a bladder that is capable of contracting.

13. **d. Bladder neck opening.** The spread of current to other pelvic structures the stimulus thresholds of which are lower than that of the bladder has often resulted in (1) abdominal, pelvic, and perineal pain; (2) a desire to defecate or defecation; (3) contraction of the pelvic and leg muscles; and (4) erection and ejaculation in males. It has also been noted that the increase in intravesical pressure was generally not coordinated with bladder neck opening or with pelvic floor relaxation and that other measures to accomplish voiding may be necessary.

14. **d. Electrodes are applied extradurally to sacral roots S2 to S4.** Prerequisites for such use were described in one study as (1) intact neural pathways between the sacral cord nuclei of the pelvic nerve and the bladder and (2) a bladder that is capable of contracting. The chief application is in patients with inefficient or no reflex micturition after spinal cord injury. Simultaneous bladder and striated sphincter stimulation is

---

[a] Sources referenced can be found in *Campbell-Walsh-Wein Urology, 12th Edition,* on the Expert Consult website.

obviated by sacral posterior rhizotomy, usually complete, which also (1) eliminates reflex incontinence and (2) improves low bladder compliance, if present. Electrodes are applied intradurally or extradurally to the S2, S3, and S4 roots, but the pairs can be activated independently. The current Brindley stimulator uses the principle of *poststimulus voiding*, a term first introduced by Jonas and Tanagho (1975). Relaxation time of the striated sphincter after a stimulus train is shorter than the relaxation time of the detrusor smooth muscle. Therefore, when interrupted pulse trains instead of continuous stimulus trains are used, poststimulus voiding is achieved between the pulse trains because of the higher sustained intravesical pressure when compared with the striated sphincter.

15. **c. Neurostimulation produces a delayed clinical response.** In neurostimulation, the use of electrical stimuli on nerves and muscles has mainly been developed for achieving immediate clinical responses in neurogenic conditions of pelvic organ dysfunction, whereas in neuromodulation, the use of electrical stimuli to nerves has been developed for altering neurotransmission processes in cases of non-neurogenic as well as neurogenic conditions.

16. **d. Percutaneous lead placement and trial stimulation.** Despite all the studies done to date, there are no defined preclinical factors such as urodynamic findings that can predict which patients will or will not have a response to sacral neuromodulation. Thus, a trial of stimulation via a temporary or percutaneous lead placement is the best predictor of long-term clinical responsiveness.

17. **e. All of the above.** Whereas most patients who have failed more conservative therapies are considered candidates for neurostimulation and neuromodulation therapies, all of the above clinical considerations for excluding patients from this therapy should be considered. Furthermore, relative contraindications for patients who may be considering or who have an implantable electrical stimulation device are the issues of MRI and pregnancy.

18. **d. All of the above.** Bilateral stimulation has been suggested as an alternative, particularly in failed unilateral lead placements, for potential salvage or added benefit as the bladder receives bilateral innervation. The initial basis to consider bilateral stimulation was based on animal studies demonstrating that bilateral stimulation yielded a more profound effect on bladder inhibition than did unilateral stimulation. Only one clinical study has been performed to demonstrate the potential differences in unilateral versus bilateral stimulation (Scheepens et al., 2002). This study showed no significant difference in outcomes for unilateral versus bilateral stimulation with regard to urgency urinary incontinence, frequency, or severity of leakage in the overactive bladder group, although, overall results were impressive in both categories. The patients in the retention group had better parameters of emptying (volume per void) in bilateral as compared with unilateral stimulation.

19. **e. All of the above.** The introduction of new stimulation methods as well as application of these methods to all the different nerve locations listed will continue to provide improved treatment alternatives, as shown in animal models and human applications. In addition, these innovations will provide the ability to further develop testable hypotheses of more basic questions on electrical neurostimulation, neuromodulation, and neurophysiology of the autonomic, somatic, and central pathways that regulate pelvic organ function.

20. **e. All of the above.** The probable causes of IPG site discomfort or pain are IPG pocket related or IPG output related. Pocket-related causes of discomfort include infection, pocket location (waistline), pocket dimension (too tight, too loose), seroma, and erosion. One should turn off the IPG and determine if the discomfort is still present to differentiate pocket-related from output-related cause. If the discomfort is persistent, the cause is not related to the IPG electrical output. In the absence of clinical signs of infection, IPG pocket-related causes such as pocket size, seroma, and erosion should be considered. If the discomfort disappears, the IPG electrical output is likely causing discomfort or pain. Output-related causes include sensitivity to unipolar stimulation if this mode is used or a current leak as demonstrated by abnormal impedances.

21. **e. All of the above.** When the patient presents with recurrent symptoms, one should evaluate the stimulation perception. The possibilities are that the patient perceives the stimulation in a wrong location as compared with baseline, has no stimulation, or has intermittent stimulation based on lead migration or mechanical issues related to a loose connection or elevated impedances.

22. **b. The mechanism is thought to come from direct efferent nerve stimulation.** The main mechanism underlying IVES is thought to occur from direct field stimulation of Aδ afferents from low-threshold bladder mechanoreceptors, which comprise the sensory system responsible for initiating and maintaining the micturition reflex (Jiang et al., 1998). The other answers are all applicable for IVES.

23. **a. It is one of the few treatments that has a proper sham-controlled study that underlines the efficacy.** This was shown by Peters et al. in 2010. Finazzi Agro showed in 2009 that evoked potential studies suggest that PTNS does have adaptive long-term modification in the brain via SS-LEP changes. There are similarities of PTNS with SP6 (Sanyinjiao) activation of acupuncture, not with SP5. PTNS can only induce toe flection of the ipsilateral foot.

24. **e. All of the above.** Although there are some urodynamic data for prediction of PTNS results (Vandoninck et al.), the overall availability of urodynamic data is scarce and contradictory. So we don't know the real value of this diagnostic tool for prediction of PTNS. There is no direct comparison yet of PTNS with a tibial nerve stimulation implanted device, although the expectation is that the implant is more efficacious. In line with this, there is no direct comparison of tibial nerve devices and sacral nerve devices. One of the assets of tibial nerve implants is that they are small because they lack a battery. Thus battery life is not an issue for the PTNS devices.

CHAPTER REVIEW

1. Electrical stimulation for lower urinary tract dysfunction is in its infancy compared to the standard of care in pain and cardiovascular disorders.
2. Nearly every nerve involved in the innervation of the lower urinary tract could theoretically be used to influence the lower urinary tract.
3. Sacral anterior root stimulation is very effective and improves quality of life dramatically but is also very invasive and irreversible.
4. Future innovation of the Brindley technique should avoid dorsal rhizotomy.
5. Of the peripheral types of neuromodulation, percutaneous tibial nerve stimulation is the best tested and developed one, and it has FDA approval.
6. New initiatives to have more patient- and doctor-friendly techniques are coming up.
7. Sacral neuromodulation is an established third treatment option for idiopathic bladder dysfunction. Sacral neuromodulation does have FDA approval for idiopathic overactive bladder and nonobstructive underactive bladder, but not for bladder or pelvic pain syndrome and neurogenic bladder.

123 Retropubic Suspension Surgery for Incontinence in Women

Siobhan M. Hartigan, Christopher R. Chapple, and Roger R. Dmochowski

QUESTIONS

1. Urodynamic stress urinary incontinence (SUI) refers to:
   a. incontinence that is demonstrated during a cough on clinical examination.
   b. incontinence occurring in the absence of urgency.
   c. incontinence occurring in combination with detrusor overactivity (DO).
   d. incontinence occurring on coughing in association with urgency and demonstrable DO.
   e. incontinence occurring on coughing in the absence of urgency and of urgency incontinence and with no demonstrable DO.

2. Anti-incontinence surgery via the retropubic route:
   a. is an effective approach for primary intrinsic sphincter deficiency (ISD).
   b. works by restoring the same mechanism of continence that was present before the onset of incontinence.
   c. aims to improve the support to the urethrovesical junction and correct deficient urethral closure.
   d. is the most effective form of anti-incontinence surgery.
   e. is carried out laparoscopically as effectively as via an open approach.

3. The most important determinant affecting the outcome of retropubic surgery is:
   a. increasing age.
   b. postoperative activity.
   c. coexisting medical morbidity.
   d. previous surgery.
   e. obesity.

4. ISD is:
   a. present only in 30% of patients presenting with SUI.
   b. most likely present in the majority of women presenting with SUI.
   c. accurately identified on the basis of Valsalva leak point pressure.
   d. an absolute contraindication to a retropubic suspension procedure.
   e. clearly defined in the current literature.

5. Retropubic colposuspension procedures may act via which of the following mechanisms?
   a. Re-creating the normal continence mechanism
   b. Elevating the anterior vaginal wall and paravesical tissues toward the iliopectineal line
   c. Anchoring the obturator internus fascia to the iliopectineal line
   d. Suspending the bladder onto the periosteum of the symphysis pubis
   e. Strengthening the pubourethral ligaments

6. In assessing the outcome of retropubic suspension surgery, which of the following is most important?
   a. Using objective urodynamic-based outcome criteria
   b. Improving symptoms from the patient's perspective
   c. Achieving complete continence
   d. Identifying the degree of improvement in the urethral closure pressure
   e. Having follow-up data of at least 6 months' duration

7. Which of the following is not an indication for retropubic repair of SUI?
   a. A patient who needs a concomitant hysterectomy that cannot be performed vaginally
   b. A patient with urethral descent with straining and SUI
   c. A patient with limited vaginal access
   d. A patient who frequently generates high intra-abdominal pressure due to a chronic cough
   e. A patient with inadequate vaginal length or mobility of the vaginal tissues

8. Which of the following statements is TRUE regarding retropubic procedures for incontinence?
   a. It is important to avoid dissecting the old retropubic adhesions from prior incontinence procedures because these may contribute to continence.
   b. Nonabsorbable sutures are better than absorbable sutures for retropubic suspension procedures.
   c. It may be necessary to open the bladder to facilitate identification of the bladder margins and bladder neck.
   d. A urethral Foley catheter is preferred for bladder drainage because it is more comfortable and associated with fewer urinary tract infections and earlier resumption of voiding.
   e. The retropubic space must be drained after the procedure to prevent bleeding.

9. Which of the following statements is TRUE regarding the Marshall-Marchetti-Krantz (MMK) procedure?
   a. It is important to elevate the midurethra and external sphincter in particular.
   b. It carries little risk of causing urethral obstruction.
   c. It is associated with osteitis pubis.
   d. A better than 90% cure rate can be expected in the long term.
   e. The sutures should incorporate a full thickness of the vaginal wall and lateral urethral wall.

10. Which of the following is TRUE of the Burch colposuspension?
    a. It is appropriate only for patients with adequate vaginal mobility and capacity.
    b. The repair is performed between the vagina and the arcus tendineus fasciae pelvis bilaterally.
    c. It is less effective than a tension-free vaginal tape procedure.
    d. It is less effective than a paravaginal repair.
    e. It is more effectively performed via a vaginal approach.

11. Laparoscopic retropubic colposuspension is advantageous versus open colposuspension because:

    a. it is technically simple to perform.

    b. it provides access for repair of an associated central defect cystocele.

    c. it is more effective than an open colposuspension.

    d. it is associated with shorter hospitalization and recovery times.

    e. it is associated with shorter operating times.

12. Common complications specific to retropubic suspension procedures include:

    a. bladder denervation.

    b. detrusor sphincter dyssynergia.

    c. postoperative voiding difficulty.

    d. detrusor underactivity.

    e. genitourinary tract fistulae.

13. Postoperative voiding difficulty after a retropubic suspension procedure:

    a. is more likely if there is preexisting detrusor dysfunction.

    b. may be due to detrusor sphincter dyssynergia.

    c. is most likely to occur with undercorrection of the urethral axis.

    d. should be managed by ureterolysis within 1 month.

    e. occurs in less than 1% of patients.

14. Which of the following statements is TRUE regarding DO and retropubic suspension procedures?

    a. Preoperative DO is a contraindication to a retropubic suspension because it increases the risk of postoperative DO.

    b. New-onset DO after a suspension procedure performed for SUI invariably resolves within 3 months.

    c. DO occurs de novo, on average in fewer than 2% of the patients reported in the literature.

    d. A history of voiding symptoms and new-onset storage symptoms as well as a retropubically angulated urethra usually suggests obstruction.

    e. DO is not causally related.

15. Prolapse as a reported complication of retropubic repairs:

    a. is rarely associated with a central defect cystocele.

    b. results in genitourinary prolapse as a sequel to Burch colposuspension to occur in less than 10% of women.

    c. may aggravate posterior vaginal wall weakness, predisposing to enterocele.

    d. will be prevented by a synchronous hysterectomy.

    e. occurs only rarely after a paravaginal repair.

16. From comparative studies in the literature, which is correct about open retropubic colposuspension?

    a. It is not as effective as a pubovaginal sling.

    b. It is not effective in patients with a low leak point pressure.

    c. It is no more effective than an anterior colporrhaphy.

    d. It is less effective than a tension-free vaginal tape procedure.

    e. It is no more effective than a paravaginal repair.

ANSWERS

1. **e. Incontinence occurring on coughing in the absence of urgency and of urgency incontinence and with no demonstrable DO.** SUI is the symptom of involuntary loss of urine during situations of increased intra-abdominal pressure such as coughing or sneezing. The International Continence Society defines *urodynamic stress incontinence* as the involuntary loss of urine during increased intra-abdominal pressure during filling cystometry, in the absence of detrusor (bladder wall muscle) contraction (Abrams et al., 2002).[a] Thus urodynamic evaluation is a prerequisite for the diagnosis of urodynamic SUI. It is not clear, however, especially from the clinical management standpoint, whether a urodynamic diagnosis is imperative for successful treatment of SUI.

2. **c. Aims to improve the support to the urethrovesical junction and correct deficient urethral closure.** Surgical procedures to treat SUI generally aim to improve the support to the urethrovesical junction and correct deficient urethral closure. There is disagreement, however, regarding the precise mechanism by which continence is achieved in the "normal asymptomatic female" and therefore, not surprisingly, how restoration of "normality" is reestablished via surgical manipulation. Anti-incontinence surgery is generally used to address the failure of normal anatomic support of the bladder neck and proximal urethra and ISD. Anti-incontinence surgery does not necessarily work by restoring the same mechanism of continence that was present before the onset of incontinence. Rather, it works by a compensatory approach, creating a new mechanism of continence (Jarvis, 1994). The surgeon's preference, coexisting problems, and the anatomic features of the patient and her general health condition often influence the choice of procedure.

   Current evidence would suggest that in adequately experienced hands, there is no difference in overall safety and efficacy between laparoscopic and open colposuspension. Clearly, another concern is how generalizable the data are on laparoscopic colposuspension because the majority of reported studies are from expert laparoscopists or surgeons working in specialized units. The evidence base on both laparoscopic and open colposuspension is limited by relatively short-term follow-up (robust data are needed out to 5 years) and the tendency toward small numbers, and poor methodology limits the interpretation of most studies with the exception of those reported by Carey and coworkers (2006) and Kitchener and colleagues (2006).

3. **d. Previous surgery.** Surgery for recurrent SUI has a lower success rate. One study has reported that Burch colposuspension has an 81% success rate after one previous surgical procedure has failed, but this drops to 25% after two previous repairs and 0% after three previous operations (Petrou and Frank, 2001). Other series report excellent results for colposuspension performed after prior failed surgery. Maher and associates (1999) and Cardozo and colleagues (1999) have both shown good objective (72% and 79%) and subjective (89% and 80%) success rates with repeat colposuspension at a mean follow-up of 9 months. Nitahara and coworkers (1999) reported a 69% subjective success at a mean follow-up of 6.9 years.

   The evidence on the duration of symptoms as a predictor of outcome is conflicting. Age may not be a contraindication to colposuspension (with equivalent success rates in the elderly at long-term follow-up), although others reported less success with increasing age. The influence of levels of postoperative activity has been inadequately studied, so no recommendations can be made. There is limited evidence that medical comorbidity may affect surgical outcomes, depending on the outcomes selected. Obesity as a confounding variable is the subject of conflicting evidence in the literature and has not been studied in a prospective fashion. Approximately one-fourth of women undergoing urodynamic study have mixed urodynamic SUI and DO. It is likely that the presence of concomitant DO lessens the success rate of surgery. There is no

---

[a]Sources referenced can be found in *Campbell-Walsh-Wein Urology, 12th Edition*, on the Expert Consult website.

consensus in the literature as to whether the presence of ISD as assessed by urethral pressure profilometry has any influence in outcome of colposuspension.

4. **b. Most likely present in the majority of women presenting with SUI.** Hypermobility of the bladder neck and proximal urethra results from a weakening or loss of the supporting elements (ligaments, fasciae, and muscles), which in turn may result from aging, hormonal changes, childbirth, and prior surgery. It seems likely that the majority of women with SUI will also have an element of intrinsic sphincteric weakness with a variable degree of loss of the normal anatomic support of the bladder neck and proximal urethra, resulting in hypermobility.

   A standardized test is not, however, available to differentiate the relative contributions of ISD and hypermobility, and therefore few studies have been able to accurately differentiate their individual contributions to the incontinence. Retropubic procedures act to restore the bladder neck and proximal urethra to a fixed, retropubic position and are used when hypermobility is thought to be an important factor in the development of that woman's SUI. This may facilitate the function of a marginally compromised intrinsic urethral sphincter mechanism, but if significant ISD is present, SUI will persist despite efficient surgical repositioning of the bladder neck and proximal urethra.

5. **b. Elevating the anterior vaginal wall and paravesical tissues toward the iliopectineal line.** Retropubic colposuspension urethral repositioning can be achieved by three distinctly different procedure principles. These are all based on a similar underlying principle but in a spectrum in relation to the degree of the support/elevations they achieve, and their outcomes differ somewhat in the longer term. The Burch colposuspension is the elevation of the anterior vaginal wall and paravesical tissues toward the iliopectineal line of the pelvic side wall using two to four sutures on either side (Burch, 1961). The vagino-obturator shelf repair aims to anchor the vagina to the obturator internus fascia and is a modification of a combination of the Burch colposuspension and paravaginal defect repair with placement of the sutures laterally anchored to the obturator internus fascia rather than hitching the vagina up to the iliopectineal line (Turner Warwick, 1986). The paravaginal defect repair aims to close a presumed fascial weakness laterally at the site of attachment of the pelvic fascia to obturator internus fascia (Richardson et al., 1976). The MMK procedure is the suspension of the vesicourethral junction (bladder neck) onto the periosteum of the symphysis pubis (Marshall et al., 1949). It aims to close the fascial defect rather than elevate the tissues in the paravesical area.

6. **b. Improving symptoms from the patient's perspective.** One or more high-quality validated symptom and quality-of-life instruments should be chosen at the outset of a clinical trial representing the patient's viewpoint, accurately defining baseline symptoms, as well as any other areas in which treatment may be beneficial, and assessing the objective severity and subjective impact of bother. Although many, including the author, believe that urodynamic studies are helpful in defining the underlying pathophysiology in cases with incontinence, these tests have not been proven to have adequate sensitivity, specificity, or predictive value (Chapple et al., 2005). The International Consensus Meeting on Incontinence concluded that although urodynamic studies such as frequency-volume charts and pad tests were useful, there was inadequate evidence to justify pressure-flow studies for routine testing as either entry criteria or outcome measures in clinical trials, and they recommended that most large-scale clinical trials should enroll patients by carefully defined symptom-driven criteria when the treatment will be given on an empirical basis (Abrams et al., 2005).

7. **e. A patient with inadequate vaginal length or mobility of the vaginal tissues.** Although it has been suggested that a retropubic colposuspension should be considered in patients who frequently generate high intra-abdominal

pressure (e.g., those with chronic cough from obstructive pulmonary disease and women in strenuous occupations), it has also been argued that these patients may be better served by a pubovaginal sling as well. There may be specific indications for a retropubic approach for the correction of anatomic SUI, namely:
- A patient undergoing a laparotomy for concomitant abdominal surgery that cannot be performed vaginally.
- In cases with limited vaginal access.
Conversely, contraindications include:
- If there is a history of prior failed incontinence procedures, the existence of significant sphincteric deficiency must be suspected, even if hypermobility exists, and consideration given to performing a pubovaginal sling.
- In cases with a pan-pelvic floor weakness, a colposuspension should not be used in isolation but should be used as part of a comprehensive approach to the pelvic floor and be combined as appropriate with other alternative pelvic floor repair procedures. Although lateral defect cystocele and enterocele lend themselves to retropubic repair, central defect cystocele, rectocele, and introital deficiency do not.
- In cases in which there is an inadequate vaginal length or mobility of the vaginal tissues, such as after previous vaginal surgery or irradiation or after a previous vaginal incontinence procedure, a colposuspension should not be used.
- A retropubic colposuspension does not always adequately correct the associated vaginal prolapse that frequently coexists with bladder neck hypermobility.

8. **c. It may be necessary to open the bladder to facilitate identification of the bladder margins and bladder neck.** In open retropubic suspension procedures, good access to the retropubic space is crucial. This is best performed with the patient in the supine position with the legs abducted, in either a low or a modified dorsal lithotomy position using stirrups, allowing access to the vagina during the procedure and a perineoabdominal progression. A urethral Foley catheter is inserted; the catheter balloon is used for subsequent identification of the urethra and bladder neck and is invaluable in allowing palpation of the edges of the bladder by appropriate manipulation. A Pfannenstiel or lower midline abdominal incision is made, separating the rectus muscles in the midline and sweeping the anterior peritoneal reflection off the bladder. It is essential to optimize the access to the retropubic space, and if a Pfannenstiel skin incision is made, it is advisable to utilize the suprapubic V modification described by Turner-Warwick and colleagues (1974). Likewise, whatever incision is made, extra valuable access to the retropubic space is obtained by extending the division of the rectus muscles right down to the pubic bone and elevating the aponeurotic insertion of the rectus muscle right off the upper border of the pubic bone.

   The retropubic space is then developed by teasing away the retropubic fat and underlying retropubic veins from the back of the pubic bone. The bladder neck, anterior vaginal wall, and urethra are then easy to identify—often facilitated by the presence of the Foley catheter balloon. In patients who have had previous retropubic surgery, the dissection is performed sharply, and it is important to take down all old retropubic adhesions, particularly in the presence of a prior failed repair. If difficulty is encountered in the identification of the bladder neck, the bladder may be partially filled or even opened to identify its limits; an examining finger in the vagina is invaluable in aiding the dissection (Symmonds, 1972; Gleason et al., 1976).

   It is important to identify the lateral limits of the bladder as it reflects off the vaginal wall, because only in this manner can one avoid inadvertent suturing of the bladder itself. Dissection over the bladder neck and urethra in the midline is to be avoided so as to not damage the intrinsic musculature. The lateral bladder wall may be "rolled off" medially and cephalad from the vaginal wall using a mounted swab and by using countertraction with a finger in the vagina. In the author's experience, it is necessary to incise the endopelvic fascia. Occasional venous bleeding from the large vaginal veins is controlled by suture ligature, although it often resolves with tying of elevating sutures. To aid in the identification of the lateral margin of the bladder, it is helpful to displace the balloon of the Foley catheter into the lateral recess, where it can be easily palpated through the bladder wall.

Absorbable sutures were used in the original descriptions of the MMK procedure (chromic catgut), Burch colposuspension (chromic catgut), and vagino-obturator shelf procedure (polyglycolic acid or polydioxanone), whereas the original paravaginal repair used nonabsorbable sutures (silicon-coated Dacron). Fibrosis during subsequent healing is likely to be the most important factor in providing continued fixation of the perivaginal fascia to the suspension sites (Tanagho, 1996); nevertheless, some surgeons believe that a nonabsorbable suture material is better because of the risk of suture dissolution before the development of adequate fibrosis (Penson and Raz, 1996). Clearly the choice of suspension suture material is personal, but it must be remembered that nonabsorbent sutures eroding into the lumen of the bladder are a not uncommon complication and a not-uncommon source of medical litigation (Woo et al., 1995).

Some degree of immediate postoperative voiding difficulty can be expected after retropubic suspensions (Lose et al., 1987; Colombo et al., 1996). Immediately postoperatively, bladder drainage may take the form of a urethral or a suprapubic catheter, generally based on surgeon preference. A voiding trial is usually performed around the fifth day postoperatively. However, there is some evidence that a suprapubic catheter may be advantageous with respect to a lower incidence of asymptomatic and febrile urinary tract infection and earlier resumption of normal bladder function (Andersen et al., 1985; Bergman et al., 1987). In addition, the use of a suprapubic tube is generally more comfortable, allows the patient to participate in catheter management, and avoids the need for clean intermittent catheterization. Catheterization can be discontinued when efficient voiding has resumed, which is usually indicated by a postvoid residual volume either less than 100 mL or less than 30% of the functional bladder volume.

A tube drain may be placed in the retropubic space when there is concern about ongoing bleeding from perivaginal veins that may prove difficult to control with suture and electrocautery. Often, tying the suspension sutures is sufficient to stop this bleeding, but when it persists, drainage of the retropubic space is indicated. The drain is generally removed on the first to third day, when minimal output is noted.

9. **c. It is associated with osteitis pubis.** Complications occur in up to 21% of cases (Mainprize, 1988), and the placement of sutures through the pubic symphysis incurs the risk of osteitis pubis, a potentially devastating complication of the MMK procedure that has been reported in 0.9% to 3.2% of patients (Lee et al., 1979; Mainprize, 1988; Zorzos and Paterson, 1996). Patients usually present 1 to 8 weeks postoperatively with acute pubic pain radiating to the inner thighs and aggravated by moving. Physical examination reveals tenderness over the pubic symphysis, and radiography demonstrates haziness to the borders of the pubic symphysis and possibly lytic changes. Treatment is with bed rest, analgesics, and possibly corticosteroids (Lee et al., 1979).

10. **a. It is appropriate only for patients with adequate vaginal mobility and capacity.** The Burch retropubic colposuspension, which has undergone few modifications since its original description, is appropriate only if the patient has adequate vaginal mobility and capacity to allow the lateral vaginal fornices to be elevated toward and approximated to the Cooper ligament on either side.

11. **d. It is associated with shorter hospitalization and recovery times.** Proposed advantages to the laparoscopic approach include improved intraoperative visualization, less postoperative

pain, shorter hospitalization, and quicker recovery times (Liu, 1993). Disadvantages include greater technical difficulty with resultant longer operating times and higher operating costs (Paraiso et al., 1999).

The last major publication in this field was a meta-analysis of all of the comparative studies published between 1995 and 2006 of laparoscopic versus open colposuspension (Tan et al., 2007). End points evaluated were operative outcomes and subjective/objective cure. A random-effect model was used and sensitivity analysis performed to account for bias in patient selection. Sixteen studies matched the selection criteria, reporting on 1807 patients, of whom 861 (47.6%) underwent laparoscopic and 946 (52.4%) underwent open colposuspension. Length of hospital stay and return to normal life were significantly reduced after laparoscopic surgery. These findings remained consistent on sensitivity analysis. Bladder injuries occurred more often in the laparoscopic group, but only with marginal statistical significance. Comparable bladder injury rates were found when studies were matched for quality, year, and randomized trials. Cure rates were similar between the two procedures at 2-year follow-up.

12. **c. Postoperative voiding difficulty.** As with any major abdominal or pelvic surgical procedure, intraoperative and perioperative complications that may occur after a retropubic suspension include bleeding, injury to genitourinary organs (bladder, urethra, ureter), pulmonary atelectasis and infection, wound infection or dehiscence, abscess formation, and venous thrombosis/embolism. Other common complications more specific to retropubic suspension procedures include postoperative voiding difficulty, DO, and vaginal prolapse.

Nevertheless, the reported incidence of these problems is relatively low. In their meta-analysis, Leach and associates (1997) noted a 3% to 8% transfusion rate for retropubic suspensions and no significant difference in the overall medical and surgical complication rates among retropubic suspensions, needle suspensions, anterior colporrhaphy, and pubovaginal slings.

Ureteral obstruction has been reported rarely after Burch colposuspension, and it usually results from ureteral kinking after elevation of the vagina and bladder base, although direct suture ligation of the ureter can occur (Applegate et al., 1987). If identified intraoperatively, it is best remedied by removal of the offending ligature and temporary placement of a ureteral stent. The so-called *post-colposuspension syndrome*, which has been described as pain in one or both groins at the site of suspension, has been noted in as many as 12% of patients after a Burch colposuspension (Galloway et al., 1987). More recently, Demirci and associates (2001) reported the occurrence of groin or suprapubic pain in 15 of 220 women (6.8%) after Burch colposuspension with a follow-up of 4.5 years.

13. **a. Is more likely if there is preexisting detrusor dysfunction.** Postoperative voiding difficulty after any type of retropubic suspension is not uncommon, and undoubtedly its occurrence is more likely if there is preexisting detrusor dysfunction or denervation resulting from extensive perivesical dissection. In most cases, however, it is the result of overcorrection of the urethral axis, owing to sutures being inappropriately placed or excessively tightened. If they are placed too medially, sutures may also transfix the urethra or distort it.

Preoperatively, at-risk patients may be identified by their history of prior voiding dysfunction or episodes of urinary retention. Preoperatively, these women should be counseled carefully about the potential for postoperative voiding difficulty and the possible need for self-catheterization. Their incontinence should be of sufficient magnitude that its correction offsets the risk of the need for self-catheterization.

Women with post-cystourethropexy voiding problems who have obstruction often do not exhibit the classic urodynamic features of obstruction. However, the history of postoperative voiding symptoms and associated new-onset bladder irritative symptoms and a finding of a retropubically angulated and fixed urethra generally indicate that obstruction does exist (Carr and Webster, 1997). In such cases, revision of the retropubic suspension by releasing the urethra into a more anatomic position resolves voiding symptoms in as many as 90% of cases (Webster and Kreder, 1990; Nitti and Raz, 1994; Carr and Webster, 1997).

The meta-analysis by Leach and coworkers (1997) noted that the risk of temporary urinary retention lasting more than 4 weeks postoperatively was 5% for all retropubic suspensions, the risk for permanent retention was estimated to be less than 5%, and these risks were not significantly different from those for needle suspensions or pubovaginal slings.

14. **d. A history of voiding symptoms and new-onset irritative symptoms as well as a retropubically angulated urethra usually suggests obstruction.** Bladder hyperactivity commonly accompanies anatomic SUI, and its incidence preoperatively has been reported to be as high as 30% in patients undergoing either first correction or repeated operations (McGuire, 1981). Provided that it is considered as a diagnosis, urodynamic study is performed to show whether DO is present, an attempt at treatment of the related overactive bladder symptoms has been made (with or without success), and the patient has been advised that the presence of DO will increase the risk of continuing storage symptoms postoperatively, then preoperative bladder overactivity does not contraindicate a retropubic suspension procedure, provided that anatomic SUI has also been demonstrated. In the majority of cases the bladder overactivity symptoms resolve after surgical repair (McGuire, 1988). Leach and coworkers' meta-analysis (1997) found the risk of urgency after a retropubic suspension was 66% if urgency and DO were present preoperatively, 36% if there was urgency but no documented overactivity preoperatively, and only 11% if there was neither urgency nor overactivity preoperatively. There was no significant difference in the incidence of postoperative urgency among retropubic suspensions, needle suspensions, and pubovaginal slings. Postoperative urgency was noted in only 0.9% of MMK procedures in Mainprize and Drutz's meta-analysis of 15 series (1988), although Parnell and associates (1982) reported that 28.5% of their patients developed postoperative storage symptoms. Jarvis's meta-analysis (1994) of Burch colposuspensions found the incidence of de novo bladder overactivity to be 3.4% to 18%. More recently Smith and associates quote a figure for postoperative DO of 6.6% for colposuspension (range 1.0% to 16.6%), whereas the incidence of postoperative urgency or urgency incontinence after the paravaginal/vagino-obturator shelf repair has been reported to be 0% to 6% (Shull and Baden, 1989; German et al., 1994; Colombo et al., 1996).

For those patients in whom postoperative storage symptoms persist, proven to be associated with DO and intractable to management with anticholinergic therapy and behavioral modification, surgical techniques including intravesical botulinum toxin therapy, neuromodulation, augmentation cystoplasty, or detrusor myectomy may be indicated.

Bladder storage symptoms arising de novo after retropubic suspension may be associated with bladder outlet obstruction. This premise is supported by the frequent coexistence of these symptoms with impaired voiding after suspension procedures and confirmed by the finding that ureterolysis, by freeing the urethra from an obstructed position, often resolves both storage and voiding symptoms (Raz, 1981; Webster and Kreder, 1990).

15. **c. May aggravate posterior vaginal wall weakness, predisposing to enterocele.** Retropubic suspensions alter vaginal and bladder base anatomy, and, thus, postoperative vaginal prolapse is a potential complication. Genitourinary prolapse has been reported as a sequel to Burch colposuspension in 22.1% of women (range 9.5% to 38.2%) by Smith and colleagues (2005) in their review of the literature. The Burch colposuspension, because of lateral vaginal elevation, may aggravate posterior vaginal wall weakness, predisposing to enterocele. The incidence varies between 3% and 17% (Burch, 1961, 1968; Galloway et al., 1987; Wiskind et al., 1992), and because of this, prophylactic obliteration of the cul-de-sac of Douglas is

sometimes considered when performing retropubic suspensions (Shull and Baden, 1989; Turner-Warwick and Kirby, 1993). However, simultaneous hysterectomy is not recommended prophylactically because it does not enhance the outcome of a retropubic suspension and should be performed only if there is concomitant uterine pathology (Milani et al., 1985; Langer et al., 1988). Although the Burch colposuspension and paravaginal/vagino-obturator shelf repair both correct lateral defect cystourethroceles, recurrent cystourethroceles were noted in 11% and 39% of Burch colposuspensions and paravaginal repairs, respectively (Colombo et al., 1996). In Mainprize and Drutz's review (1988), postoperative cystocele was noted in only 0.4% of patients after an MMK procedure.

Wiskind and coworkers (1992) noted that 27% of patients who had undergone a Burch colposuspension developed prolapse requiring surgery: rectocele in 22%, enterocele in 11%, uterine prolapse in 13%, and cystocele in 2%. More recently, it has been suggested that most women are asymptomatic and fewer than 5% have been reported to request further surgery (Smith et al., 2005). Ward and associates (2004) reported 4.8% of women needing a posterior repair whereas Kwon and coworkers (2003) reported 4.7% requiring subsequent pelvic reconstruction.

Because retropubic suspensions are unable to correct central defect cystoceles, patients must be carefully examined preoperatively to exclude their presence.

16. **a. It is not as effective as a pubovaginal sling.** A total of 655 women were randomly assigned to study groups: 326 to undergo the sling procedure and 329 to undergo the Burch colposuspension; 520 women (79%) completed the outcome assessment (Aldo et al., 2007). At 24 months, success rates were higher for women who underwent the sling procedure than for those who underwent the Burch colposuspension for both the overall category of success (47% vs. 38%, $P = .01$) and the category specific to SUI (66% vs. 49%, $P < .001$). There was no significant difference between the sling and Burch colposuspension groups in the percentage of patients who had serious adverse events (13% and 10%, respectively; $P = .20$). However, more women who underwent the sling procedure had adverse events than in the Burch colposuspension group, with 415 events among 206 women in the sling group as compared with 305 events among 156 women in the Burch colposuspension group. This difference was due primarily to urinary tract infections: 157 women in the sling group (48%) had 305 events and 105 women in the Burch colposuspension group (32%) had 203 events. When urinary tract infections were excluded, although the rates of adverse events were similar in the two groups, there was more difficulty voiding. The distribution of time to return to normal voiding differed significantly between the two groups: Voiding dysfunction was more common in the sling group than in the Burch colposuspension group (14% vs. 2%, $P < .001$). Consequently, surgical procedures to reduce voiding symptoms or improve urinary retention were performed exclusively in the sling group, in which 19 patients underwent 20 such procedures (63% vs. 47%, $P < .001$). Treatment satisfaction rates for the 480 subjects who answered the satisfaction question at 24 months were significantly higher in the sling group than in the Burch colposuspension group (86% vs. 78%, $P = .02$). A further analysis of this study focused on sexual activity as assessed by the Pelvic Organ Prolapse/Urinary Incontinence Sexual Questionnaire (PISQ-12) among those sexually active at baseline and 2 years after surgery (Brubaker et al., 2009). This report demonstrated that sexual function improves after successful surgery and does not differ between Burch colposuspension and sling procedures.

It can therefore be reliably concluded that in specialist centers working in a standardized fashion, the autologous fascial sling results in a higher rate of successful treatment of SUI but also greater morbidity than the Burch colposuspension.

Comparisons between the MMK and the Burch colposuspension procedures have generally yielded similar results. Three articles that reviewed the literature on incontinence procedures all found retropubic suspensions to be more effective than either needle suspensions or anterior colporrhaphies (Jarvis, 1994; Black and Downs, 1996; Leach et al., 1997). Most studies in the literature have not demonstrated a significant difference in cure rates between retropubic suspensions (generally a Burch colposuspension) and pubovaginal slings (Jarvis, 1994; Black and Downs, 1996; Leach et al.,

1997). The literature on the paravaginal repair is sparse. The only randomized study that compared the Burch colposuspension with a paravaginal repair found significantly greater subjective and objective cure with the Burch colposuspension (Colombo et al., 1996). At this point, the tension-free vaginal tape procedure appears to be at least equivalent to the Burch colposuspension.

CHAPTER REVIEW

1. Anti-incontinence surgery does not work by restoring the normal mechanism of continence but, rather, by a compensatory approach creating a new mechanism of continence.
2. ISD is suggested by a leak point pressure less than 60 cm H_2O or a maximum urethral closure pressure of less than 20 cm H_2O.
3. Approximately 40% of nulliparous 30- to 49-year-old women experience some degree of incontinence with exercise.
4. If nonabsorbable sutures are used in a retropubic suspension, they may migrate into the bladder and serve as a foreign body nidus for stone formation and infection.
5. The postoperative risk of SUI in continent women undergoing an abdominal sacrocolpopexy is substantially reduced by the addition of a Burch colposuspension.
6. A maximum urethral closing pressure of less than 20 cm H_2O is a contraindication to the Burch colposuspension.
7. All patients, before any colposuspension, should be advised about the potential need for intermittent self-catheterization.
8. The Burch colposuspension is regarded as the standard open retropubic procedure for incontinence.
9. If ISD is the primary problem, a fascial sling procedure should be performed rather than a colposuspension.
10. A MMK procedure, a paravaginal defect repair, and needle suspension procedures are not recommended for the treatment of SUI.
11. The majority of women with SUI will also have an element of intrinsic sphincteric weakness with a variable degree of loss of the normal anatomic support of the bladder neck and proximal urethra, resulting in hypermobility.
12. Contraindications for a retropubic colposuspension include significant sphincteric deficiency, pan-pelvic floor weakness, and inadequate vaginal length or mobility. Moreover, it may not correct the associated vaginal prolapse.
13. Bladder hyperactivity commonly accompanies anatomic SUI, and its incidence preoperatively has been reported to be as high as 30%. In the majority of cases, the bladder overactivity symptoms resolve after surgical repair.
14. Simultaneous hysterectomy is not recommended prophylactically because it does not enhance the outcome of a retropubic suspension and should be performed only if there is concomitant uterine pathology.

124 Vaginal and Abdominal Reconstructive Surgery for Pelvic Organ Prolapse

J. Christian Winters, Ryan M. Krlin, and Barry Hallner

QUESTIONS

1. Which of the following statements regarding anterior colporrhaphy is FALSE?
   a. Anterior colporrhaphy is not used to treat stress incontinence.
   b. Recent series report a 40% recurrence rate for standard anterior colporrhaphy.
   c. The most likely contributing factor for failure of anterior compartment repairs is the concomitant presence of other compartmental defects.
   d. Cystoscopy with indigo carmine is not routinely necessary.
   e. Ensuring that the bladder is drained before perforating the endopelvic fascia may decrease bladder injuries.

2. A 50-year-old woman presents with symptoms of voiding difficulty and vaginal bulging. She has had a prior hysterectomy. In the supine position she demonstrates stage 3 prolapse with the Ba point at +4. Her C point is –4 with a TVL of 9 cm, and her Bp is –3. With prolapse reduction there is no stress incontinence. Which of the following repairs would be most appropriate?
   a. Vault suspension alone
   b. Vault suspension with anterior repair
   c. Vault suspension with anterior repair and anti-incontinence procedure
   d. Vault suspension with anterior repair, anti-incontinence procedure, and posterior repair
   e. Anterior repair alone
   f. Anterior and posterior repair

3. Which surgical technique of rectocele repair is most associated with postoperative dyspareunia?
   a. Levator plication
   b. Site-specific repair
   c. Site-specific repair with biologic interposition graft
   d. Transanal repair of rectocele
   e. Perineorrhaphy

4. Which symptom changes the least following site-specific posterior colporrhaphy?
   a. Dyspareunia
   b. Constipation
   c. Vaginal mass
   d. Splinting
   e. Vaginal pressure or pain

5. When planning a multi-compartment repair with an outlet procedure, which of the following is the preferred sequence of compartmental approaches?
   a. Apical, anterior, posterior, sling
   b. Sling, apical, anterior, posterior
   c. Apical, anterior, sling, posterior
   d. Posterior, anterior, apical, sling
   e. Anterior, posterior, sling, apical

6. When performing a posterior repair, the literature currently supports which of the following methods to maximize success rates and decrease complications, namely dyspareunia?
   a. Traditional posterior colporrhaphy
   b. Mesh augmented posterior colporrhaphy
   c. Traditional posterior colporrhaphy with levator plication
   d. Porcine graft augmented posterior colporrhaphy
   e. Cadaveric graft augmented posterior colporrhaphy

7. Which of the following procedures have proven to be ineffective in the treatment of stress urinary incontinence?
   a. Synthetic midurethral sling
   b. Anterior colporrhaphy
   c. Burch colposuspension
   d. Autologous pubovaginal sling
   e. Vaginal paravaginal repair
   f. b and e
   g. All of the above

8. Which of the following statements regarding anterior compartment prolapse and/or repair is false?
   a. An anterior compartment defect may be central, lateral, or combined.
   b. A central defect results from midline separation or attenuation of the pubocervical (perivesical) fascia.
   c. A lateral defect results when the pubocervical fascia detaches from the arcus tendineus fascia pelvis (ATFP).
   d. Most anterior compartment defects have concomitant lateral and/or apical defects.
   e. Isolated anterior colporrhaphy is not recommended when additional defects are present.
   f. Anterior compartment prolapse repair also suspends the vaginal apex.

9. Which of the following defects requires surgical correction?
   a. Ba –1 in an asymptomatic 48-year-old
   b. Bp –3 with complaints of constipation
   c. C –9, TVL 10, Ba –3
   d. Ba 0 with complaint of a vaginal bulge
   e. C –8, TVL 10, Ba –2

10. A 31-year-old woman with a history of four prior vaginal deliveries presents to your office with symptoms of a vaginal bulge. On pelvic exam, you note the cervix is protruding 4 cm beyond the introitus, the anterior vaginal wall bulges just beyond the hymenal ring, and the posterior wall seems to be well supported. Total vaginal length is about 9 cm. The patient

is not interested in using a pessary. She desires future fertility. She wants you to do the operation that will reduce her chance of requiring another surgery for prolapse in the future. The next best step in management is:

a. Vaginal hysterectomy and uterosacral ligament suspension

b. Vaginal hysterectomy and sacrospinous ligament suspension

c. Transvaginal suture hysteropexy

d. Abdominal sacrohysteropexy with mesh

e. Abdominal hysterectomy and sacrocolpopexy

11. A 48-year-old active woman with incomplete uterovaginal prolapse with cervical elongation desires a transvaginal uterine-sparing procedure. POQ point C is +2 and Point D is −7. Select the most appropriate type of uterine-preserving POP reparative surgery for her condition.

a. Le Forte colpocleisis

b. Sacrohysteropexy

c. Manchester procedure

d. Sacrospinous cervicopexy

e. Uterosacral hysteropexy

12. An 89-year-old woman who has failed numerous pessaries has symptomatic complete uterovaginal prolapse. She is frail, lives in a nursing home, and has medical comorbidities making her high risk for general anesthesia. Select the most appropriate surgical procedure.

a. Uterosacral hysteropexy

b. Sacrospinous cervicopexy

c. Sacrohysteropexy

d. Le Forte colpocleisis

e. Manchester-Fothergill operation

13. A 54-year-old woman who has a history of multiple laparotomies for treatment of endometriosis and a history of small bowel obstruction requiring resection and anastomosis presents with symptomatic incomplete uterovaginal prolapse. POPQ C is at 1, Point D is −4. During her small bowel surgery, the surgeon noted significant pelvic adhesions involving the uterus, tubes, and ovaries, which were not addressed during that surgery. Select the most appropriate surgical procedure.

a. Uterosacral hysteropexy

b. Sacrospinous cervicopexy

c. Sacrohysteropexy

d. Le Forte Colpocleisis

e. Manchester-Fothergill operation

14. A 41-year-old woman with symptomatic uterovaginal prolapse with POPQ point C +2, D −6 presents to your office desiring a uterine-sparing procedure. She smokes a half a pack of cigarettes per day and will not quit. She also has a history of two procedures to treat recurrent mid-urethral polypropylene sling exposure. She also has a 5-cm ovarian cyst that appears benign but has been present for 8 months; she desires its removal. She is sexually active and is concerned about pain with intercourse after the procedure. Select the most appropriate surgical procedure.

a. Uterosacral hysteropexy

b. Sacrospinous cervicopexy

c. Sacrohysteropexy

d. Le Forte colpocleisis

e. Manchester-Fothergill operation

15. A 28-year-old woman who has Ehlers-Danlos syndrome presents with symptomatic uterovaginal prolapse. Her relevant POPQ is as

follows: C +1, TVL 8, D −4. She desires future fertility. She has a history of asthma and problems with chronic constipation. Select the most appropriate procedure for this patient.

a. Uterosacral hysteropexy

b. Sacrospinous cervicopexy

c. Sacrohysteropexy

d. Le Forte colpocleisis

e. Manchester-Fothergill operation

16. A 60-year-old patient undergoes a transvaginal hysterectomy (TVH), bilateral salpingo-oophorectomy (BSO), uterosacral ligament suspension, enterocele repair, anterior and posterior repair, and transvaginal tape (TVT) sling procedure for symptomatic uterovaginal prolapse (POPQ point C +3, D-5) and stress urinary incontinence. She presents 6 months postoperative and tells you she is having pain with intercourse. Select the procedure that is the probable cause of her dyspareunia.

a. Vaginal vault suspension

b. Enterocele repair

c. TVT sling

d. Anterior colporrhaphy

e. Posterior colporrhaphy

17. A 46-year-old woman with vaginal vault prolapse undergoes a laparoscopic sacrocolpopexy for symptomatic vaginal vault prolapse. Her BMI is 19 and she has a history of lupus. The patient is positioned by a new nurse circulator. The surgery lasts 5 hours. When seeing her on POD#1, she is unable to flex her knee, has foot drop, and decreased sensation in the calf. Select the likely nerve affected.

a. Femoral

b. Genitofemoral

c. Sciatic

d. Brachial plexus

e. Obturator

f. Common peroneal

g. Ilioinguinal

h. Iliohypogastric

18. A 57-year-old woman with symptomatic uterovaginal prolapse presents desiring surgical correction of her prolapse. She has no significant comorbidities other than well-controlled hypertension. She is sexually active. She has been menopausal for the last 6 years and reports no postmenopausal bleeding. Her last pap smear was negative for malignancy; she has never had an abnormal pap smear. On manual exam her uterus is small and mobile. Her POPQ is as follows: Aa +3, Ba+5, C +7, Gh 5, Pb 1, TVL 10, Ap −1, Bp −1, D+4. Select the best procedure to address her prolapse.

a. Anterior and posterior colporrhaphy

b. Vaginal hysterectomy with an anterior and posterior colporrhaphy

c. Abdominal supracervical hysterectomy with sacrocervicopexy ± anterior and posterior colporrhaphy

d. Abdominal hysterectomy

e. Lefort colpocleisis

19. Which of the procedures listed below to address pelvic organ prolapse has been reported to have the highest risk of ureteral injury?

a. Sacrospinous ligament suspension

b. Uterosacral ligament suspension

c. Anterior colporrhaphy

d. Transvaginal hysterectomy

e. Posterior colporrhaphy

20. A 51-year-old woman presents 2 months after a laparoscopic sacrocolpopexy with persistent low back pain. She states the pain has been present for the last 3 weeks and it does not feel like it is getting better. She describes the pain as constant and achy. Over-the-counter ibuprofen helps, but the pain never goes away. She admits to intermittent fever and chills but denies abdominal pain, nausea, or vomiting. She admits to having regular bowel movements and denies dysuria. Select the most likely diagnosis.

    a. Herniated disc

    b. Bowel obstruction

    c. Osteomyelitis

    d. Spinal stenosis

21. You are instructing your first-year fellow through a sacrospinous ligament suspension and tell your fellow that, to avoid complications related to suture placement, the suture should be placed:

    a. 1 cm lateral and slightly superior to the ischial spine

    b. 3 cm medial to the ischial spine, slightly below the superior edge of the ligament

    c. 3 cm medial to the ischial spine, superiorly and slightly behind the ligament

    d. 1 cm medial to the sacrum, slightly below the superior edge of the ligament

22. An 80-year-old woman has recurrent vaginal vault prolapse. She had a sacrospinous ligament fixation 20 years prior. She has not been sexually active for the last 15 years. She has failed numerous pessary trials. She is interested in a surgical procedure with the lowest likelihood for repeat surgery. Select the best procedure.

    a. Mesh sacrocolpopexy

    b. Vaginal mesh for prolapse

    c. Sacrospinous ligament fixation

    d. Colpocleisis

ANSWERS

1. **d. Cystoscopy with indigo carmine is not routinely necessary.** Cystoscopy after the administration of indigo carmine or methylene blue is recommended as a routine practice after anterior colporrhaphy. If blue-tinged urine is not seen effluxing from each ureteral orifice, catheterization may be considered before taking down the plication sutures. Appropriate steps must be performed to ensure ureteral patency, including takedown of the sutures.

2. **b. Vault suspension and anterior repair.** The patient has stage 3 anterior vaginal wall prolapse at the apical descent. These defects are best addressed by restoring the apical and anterior support. Failure rates for an anterior repair alone are unacceptably high. As no stress urinalysis incontinence was demonstrated, there is no absolute indication for an anti-incontinence procedure. The support of the posterior compartment is intact and posterior repair is not indicated.

3. **a. Levator plication.** Levator plication was associated with high rates of de novo postoperative dyspareunia. As such, it has largely been abandoned.

4. **b. Constipation.** Constipation may be associated with dysmotility disorders of the rectum that do not improve with an anatomic repair. The symptoms most likely to improve are dyspareunia, the need for vaginal splinting, vaginal mass, and pressure.

5. **c. Apical, anterior, sling, posterior.** The apical compartment should always be addressed first. The anterior compartment should preferentially be repaired before the posterior compartment when an anti-incontinence procedure is being performed, should an inadvertent rectal injury occur. Once the

sling incision is closed, a rectal injury can be repaired and the mesh is uninvolved.

6. **a. Traditional posterior colporrhaphy.** Both mesh-augmented repairs and levator plication report a higher incidence of complications, namely dyspareunia. As far as success is concerned, neither porcine nor biologic interposition grafts create a superior outcome when compared to traditional colporrhaphy.

7. **f. b and e.** Neither anterior colporrhaphy nor vaginal paravaginal repair have proven efficacy for the treatment of stress urinary incontinence. The other options are all viable treatment options.

8. **f. Anterior compartment prolapse repair also suspends the vaginal apex.** An anterior colporrhaphy restores the level 2 support, but has no effect on the apex, which is level 1 support. The other statements are true.

9. **d. Ba 0 with complaint of a vaginal bulge.** Only symptomatic prolapse requires repair. Repair of prolapse will have little effect on constipation, as this is usually a motility issue. Choices c and e demonstrate normal vaginal exams.

10. **d. Abdominal sacrohysteropexy with mesh.** Since she desires future fertility, we recommended that a hysterectomy not be performed for the management of her prolapse. This eliminates answers a, b, and e. Of the remaining two choices, the one that has the best potential of long-term success is the sacrohysteropexy. During this operation, a rectangular piece of mesh is sewn to the posterior vaginal wall (all the way down to the perineum), the cervix, and the lower uterine segment. An inverted U-shaped mesh is then sewn to the anterior vaginal wall all the way down to the pubic bone and lower portion of the anterior rectus abdominis fascia. Due to the fact that mesh is fixated to the lower uterine segment, a C-section should be recommended as the mode of delivery.

11. **c. Manchester procedure.** The Manchester-Fothergill operation is the most appropriate transvaginal surgery for treatment of hypertrophic cervical elongation co-existing with a well-supported uterine corpus in a woman desiring uterine preservation.

12. **d. Le Forte colpocleisis.** The Leforte procedure is a partial colpocleisis in which matching rectangular sections of vaginal epithelium are excised from both the anterior and posterior vaginal walls and then fused together by sutures. The procedure can be performed under local anesthesia in patients with significant comorbidities.

13. **b. Sacrospinous cervicopexy.** Sacrospinous hysteropexy is a uterine-sparing procedure for cervical prolapse useful when an abdominal or laparoscopic/robotic procedure may be very difficult, due to presence of intraperitoneal adhesions or previous mesh-augmented ventral hernia repair.

14. **a. Uterosacral hysteropexy.** Uterosacral hysteropexy has been reported using both transvaginal and laparoscopic techniques in which the posterior cul de sac may be closed, the uterosacral ligaments are plicated in the midline, and if severed, then reattached to the cervix. This technique avoids the use of synthetic surgical mesh, for which this patient in the scenario has both known risk factors and complications from previous personal experience. This technique also reduces the risk of dyspareunia that can be associated with deviation of the vaginal axis related to unilateral sacrospinous fixation. The patient also has abdominal pathology and requests it be addressed at this surgery. An abdominal approach to her suspension procedure allows for evaluation and management of abdominal pathology.

15. **c. Sacrohysteropexy.** Sacrohysteropexy using a synthetic mesh bridge to suspend the posterior lower uterine segment/proximal cervix from the anterior sacrum (at S1-2) has been reported to be successful in a small series of women with collagen connective tissue disorders and in young women born with bladder exstrophy.

16. **e. Posterior colporrhaphy.** Posterior colporrhaphy is associated with the highest rate of dyspareunia—on average around 18% (0%–46%). In general, there is a high prevalence of dyspareunia in women with prolapse, but sexual function does improve with prolapse repair. Improvement in sexual function occurs more often in women who did not have a posterior repair. The uterosacral ligament suspension, anterior repair and enterocele

repair are much less likely to cause dyspareunia. However, about 1% to 2% of patients who have undergone high uterosacral ligament suspension can develop sacral nerve entrapment (thigh, buttocks, and low back pain), which can affect sexual function (answer a, b, and d are incorrect). The TVT sling does not affect overall sexual function and satisfaction, but the partners of patients with mesh exposure (<3%) may complain of pain with intercourse (answer C is incorrect). The possible reasons for dyspareunia after posterior repair are the following:

- Inadequate lateral dissection of the rectovaginal septum before plicating
- Aggressive plication of lateral tissue, including levator muscles
- Aggressive trimming of vaginal skin prior to closure
- Poor surgical technique, making introitus too narrow
- Development of vaginal scar tissue, infection, or hematoma
- Vaginal atrophy

17. **c. Sciatic.** Prolonged hyperflexion and external rotation of the hips with knees extended can lead to sciatic nerve injury. This presents with foot drop, inability to flex the knee, and loss in sensation of the calf and lateral foot. One must be careful to properly position the patient; we recommend proper positioning be confirmed by the surgeon. Prolonged hip flexion, abduction, and external rotation may also lead to femoral nerve injury. This presents with weakness of the quadriceps muscle, which makes it difficult to extend the knee (i.e., knee gives out when trying to stand). There is also decrease in sensation of the anterior thigh and medial lower leg. The three big risk factors for neurologic injury because of patient positioning are thinness (BMI <20 kg/m^2), diabetes mellitus, and time (each additional hour in lithotomy position increases risk).

18. **c. Abdominal supracervical hysterectomy with sacrocervicopexy ± anterior and posterior colporrhaphy.** The patient is sexually active, has no history of post-menopausal bleeding, and has a negative pap smear with no history of abnormal pap smears. A supracervical hysterectomy reduces the risk of graft extrusion at the time of the sacrocervicopexy. The procedure can be done open, laparoscopicly, or robotically; a, b, and d are incorrect because none of them address the apex. Answer e is incorrect because it is an obliterative procedure and she is currently sexually active.

19. **b. Uterosacral ligament suspension.** In reported studies uterosacral ligament suspension has a ureteral injury risk of 0% to 11% in prolapse surgery. In a systematic review, the rate of ureteral injury following transvaginal hysterectomy was 0.2 per 1000 surgeries. Ureteral injury can occur with anterior colporrhaphy but is uncommon.

20. **c. Osteomyelitis.** Sacral osteomyelitis is a well-known but fortunately rare complication of sacrocolpopexy, and common presenting symptoms include back pain, fevers, lethargy, and vaginal discharge. Sacral infections after sacrocolpopexies are likely to have a multifactorial origin. One hypothesis is that ischemia from devascularization during surgical dissection provides a microenvironment conducive to infection. It is conceivable that a suture placed too deeply into the vaginal canal or the sacral promontory provides a mechanism by which bacteria can be introduced into the abdominal cavity or into the periosteum of the sacral promontory. Similarly, placement of the sutures into the disc itself can lead to discitis. Sacrocolpopexy presacral sutures are often placed without knowledge of the location of the intervertebral discs. Herniated disc and spinal stenosis are clinical etiologies of back pain, but have not been reported as complications of mesh sacrocolpopexy. Though bowel obstruction can occur after sacrocolpopexy, it would be unusual to present with back pain. This condition more commonly presents with nausea/vomiting.

21. **a. 1 cm lateral and slightly superior to the ischial spine.** In the area, there is decreased chance of injuring the pudendal nerves or vessels. The pudendal nerves and vessels lie directly posterior to the ischial spine. The suture should not be placed as close as these to the ischial spine. Superiorly and just behind the ligament lies the inferior gluteal vessels and hypogastric venous plexus.

22. **d. Colpocleisis.** Obliterative procedures have the lowest rates of prolapse recurrence and low rates of reoperation. When compared to native tissue repairs, the use of mesh in pelvic organ prolapse surgery is associated with increased rates of reoperations.

CHAPTER REVIEW

1. The iliococcygeus and the coccygeus muscles fuse in the midline and attach to the coccyx, forming a complex called the *levator plate* that supports the upper vagina and cervix.
2. The urethra is fused to the anterior vaginal wall for much of its length.
3. Vaginal support is provided by the endopelvic connective tissues.
4. The cardinal and uterosacral ligaments provide level I support of the uterus and upper vagina; the endopelvic and pubocervical fascia provide level II support of the mid-vagina while it attaches to the arcus tendineus fasciae pelvis; the distal vagina attaches to the levator ani muscles and perineal body to provide for level III support.
5. Pelvic organ prolapse is for the most part a quality-of-life issue.
6. Anterior compartment defects can be central, lateral, or both.
7. Anterior colporrhaphy and paravaginal repairs are both ineffective alone in the treatment of stress urinary incontinence. They do not suspend the vaginal apex.
8. Sacrospinous ligament fixation may result in posterior displacement of the vaginal apex and increase the risk of anterior compartment prolapse.
9. If either the bladder or rectum is injured during pelvic organ prolapse repair, mesh should not be used.
10. Reoperation is needed for 29% of women who experience failed incontinence and prolapse surgery.
11. Synthetic mesh grafts erode in 10% of patients in whom they are used for the repair.
12. Sacrospinalis ligament fixation is an effective method of correcting vaginal apical prolapse. It results in posterior displacement of the vaginal apex.
13. Abdominal sacrocolpopexy maximizes functional vaginal length without significant distortion of the anatomic vaginal axis.
14. Colpocleisis obliterates a portion of the vagina and may be used to prevent vaginal vault prolapse. It precludes functional sexual activity.
15. Cystoscopy after the administration of indigo carmine or methylene blue is recommended as a routine practice after anterior colporrhaphy.
16. All women with advanced-stage anterior compartment prolapse should be screened for occult stress urinary incontinence.
17. The pain from sacrospinous ligament suspension is either gluteal or radiates down the leg posteriorly. It is neuropathic, and it occurs in 15% of patients.

125 Slings: Autologous, Biologic, Synthetic, and Midurethral

Alex Gomelsky and Roger R. Dmochowski

QUESTIONS

1. The Integral Theory proposed by Petros and Ulmsten states that:
   a. urethral hypermobility is the primary cause of stress urinary incontinence (SUI).
   b. adequate function of the pubourethral ligaments, the suburethral vaginal hammock, and the pubococcygeus muscle helps to preserve continence.
   c. anchoring a sling to the rectus muscle allows it to respond to changes in intra-abdominal pressure.
   d. dynamic kinking of the urethra during stress preserves incontinence.
   e. synthetic mesh integrates into host tissue.

2. Which of the following statements about the preoperative assessment of a sling patient is TRUE?
   a. It is generally not necessary to perform a focused neurologic examination.
   b. Urgency is not associated with worse outcomes after sling surgeries.
   c. The American Urological Association (AUA) Guidelines state that a postvoid residual (PVR) volume should be checked on all patients.
   d. Cystoscopy should be performed in all patients to rule out bladder pathology.
   e. The abdominal leak-point pressure is traditionally defined by a pressure of less than 80 cm H_2O.

3. As an option for the index patient with SUI, the AUA SUI guidelines strongly recommends that physicians offer:
   a. synthetic MUS.
   b. autologous fascia pubovaginal sling (PVS).
   c. Burch colposuspension.
   d. bulking agents.
   e. all of the above.

4. Which of the following statements regarding PVS materials is TRUE?
   a. Harvesting a thin strip of fascia lata is associated with significant morbidity.
   b. The risk of perforation and exposure associated with synthetic slings is minimal.
   c. The benefit of harvesting fascia lata is that patient position can be maintained for the entire case.
   d. Synthetic sling materials exhibit the least amount of degradation.
   e. Although concerning, disease transmission has never been documented with allograft materials.

5. An autologous PVS is indicated in all of the following conditions EXCEPT:
   a. urethral incompetence in a T12 spinal cord injury.
   b. low urethral resistance with decreased bladder compliance.
   c. urethral incompetence and large urethral diverticulum.
   d. proximal urethral loss secondary to long-standing indwelling Foley catheter.
   e. refractory SUI after failed mid-urethral sling (MUS) and bulking agents.

6. Which of the statements about the normal female urethra and pelvic floor is TRUE?
   a. The female urethra is composed of four separate tissue layers, and the middle seromuscular layer is most important in enhancing the urethral sphincter mechanism during voiding.
   b. The Valsalva pressure of the bladder exceeds the resting closing pressure of the internal sphincter.
   c. The fast-twitch fibers of the external sphincter are responsible for sudden protection against incontinence, and slow-twitch fibers provide passive control through the involuntary guarding reflex.
   d. The levator ani, urethropelvic ligament, and round ligament provide needed support to the bladder neck and undersurface of the bladder.
   e. The PVS is placed at the bladder neck to provide adequate urethral coaptation at rest and to decrease urethral responsiveness to abdominal pressure.

7. Which of the following statements regarding materials for bladder neck PVSs is FALSE?
   a. The ideal material has minimal tissue reaction and complete biocompatibility.
   b. Stiffness and maximal load failure are the same between freeze-dried fascia lata and solvent-dehydrated and dermal grafts.
   c. The estimated risk of human immunodeficiency virus (HIV) transmission by an allograft sling is approximately 1 in 1,660,000.
   d. Porcine small intestinal submucosa has less tensile strength than cadaveric fascia lata.
   e. Synthetic materials are associated with high perforation rates during use for bladder neck PVS.

8. Before final tensioning of the rectus fascial autologous PVS:
   a. the weighted speculum is removed.
   b. the abdominal skin incision should be closed.
   c. vaginal packing should be placed.
   d. the patient should be taken out of lithotomy position.
   e. a drain should be placed in the retropubic space.

9. In outcomes associated with PVS procedures, which of the following is/are TRUE?
   a. Reported cure rates after an autologous PVS procedure are 24% to 97%.
   b. Preoperative Valsalva leak point pressure is a reliable predictor of outcomes after sling surgery.
   c. In the Stress Incontinence Surgical Treatment Efficacy Trial (SISTEr) trial, cure rates and voiding symptoms were greater for the PVS than for the Burch colposuspension.
   d. a and c.
   e. a, b, and c.

10. Which of the following statements about perforation and PVS material is TRUE?

    a. Synthetic slings perforate into the urinary tract 15 times more often than autologous, allograft, or xenograft slings.

    b. Urethral perforations are rarely associated with urinary retention and mixed urinary incontinence.

    c. Synthetic slings are less likely to be associated with vaginal exposure than autologous, allograft, and xenograft slings.

    d. Perforation from synthetic slings requires removal of the entire sling from a vaginal and retropubic approach.

    e. None of the above are true.

11. Which of the following statements is NOT associated with voiding dysfunction after a PVS procedure?

    a. Obstruction, detrusor overactivity, or impaired detrusor contractility are all manifestations of voiding dysfunction for iatrogenic PVS obstruction.

    b. Persistent urgency is more common than urinary retention in bladder outlet obstruction after a PVS procedure.

    c. Fifty percent of affected patients have symptoms of overactive bladder, which can be avoided if sling lysis is performed within 2 weeks of PVS placement.

    d. Urodynamic study is valuable in assessment and planning management.

    e. There is up to a 20% recurrent SUI rate after urethrolysis.

12. Regarding the pathophysiology of incontinence:

    a. hypermobility is the main underlying cause of SUI.

    b. intrinsic sphincter deficiency (ISD) is rarely the primary cause of SUI.

    c. ISD is the primary underlying cause of SUI for women, with hypermobility being a secondary finding.

    d. the levator floor provides active compression to the proximal urethra.

    e. the extrinsic urethral skeletal sphincter is the primary mechanism for urinary continence.

13. Obese patients who undergo MUS surgery:

    a. clearly have a higher rate of sling-related complications.

    b. should have been offered weight loss as an initial management option.

    c. have a significantly higher risk of trocar injury at the time of sling placement.

    d. have been consistently shown to have worse outcomes.

    e. are at a greater risk for voiding dysfunction.

14. All of the following are associated with the MUS procedure EXCEPT:

    a. trocars are inserted and used to transpose the implanted material into position.

    b. the synthetic material used is a mesh with large pores.

    c. loose tension is placed on the sling material.

    d. the sling is sutured to the underlying tissues for fixation purposes.

    e. cystoscopy is a crucial component of the procedure.

15. Common presenting symptoms of voiding dysfunction after PVS surgery are:

    a. urgency and frequency.

    b. painful voiding and suprapubic pain.

    c. incomplete emptying and straining.

    d. recurrent urinary tract infections.

    e. all of the above.

16. The transobturator MUS passes through all of the following structures EXCEPT the:

    a. obturator internus muscle.

    b. obturator membrane.

    c. obturator externus muscle.

    d. rectus fascia.

    e. ischiorectal fascia.

17. In review of the efficacy outcomes obtained with mid-urethral procedures, which of the following is TRUE?

    a. MUSs are less effective than open colposuspension procedures.

    b. MUSs produce inferior results compared with laparoscopic colposuspensions.

    c. Postoperative voiding dysfunction is more common with mid-urethral procedures than with other types of suspension procedures.

    d. Mixed urinary incontinence results are superior to those for pure SUI.

    e. Five-year results demonstrate durability similar to one-year results.

18. Which of the following is theorized to be TRUE regarding patients at risk for voiding dysfunction after PVS surgery?

    a. Failure to relax the external striated sphincter is not associated with postoperative voiding dysfunction.

    b. Patients who habitually void with abdominal straining will not have an increased risk of voiding dysfunction after PVS surgery.

    c. Patients with pure SUI are more likely to have voiding dysfunction after PVS surgery.

    d. Patients with subclinical impaired detrusor contractility are at increased risk for voiding dysfunction after PVS surgery.

    e. Young patients are more at risk for voiding dysfunction after PVS surgery.

19. In placing the single-incision mini sling, the passer punctures the:

    a. obturator internus muscle.

    b. obturator membrane.

    c. obturator externus muscle.

    d. rectus fascia.

    e. ischiorectal fascia.

20. Compared to younger patients, MUSs in elderly patients are associated with:

    a. lower success rates.

    b. lower satisfaction rates.

    c. higher rates of postoperative urgency.

    d. higher rates of mixed incontinence resolution.

    e. higher rates of postoperative urinary retention.

21. In a patient with voiding dysfunction after sling surgery:

    a. it is generally appropriate to wait as long as 3 months after MUS surgery before considering surgical intervention.

    b. it is generally appropriate to wait as long as 3 months after autologous PVS surgery before considering surgical intervention.

    c. loosening a synthetic sling through traction with a cystoscope in the operating room is associated with little risk.

    d. formal urethrolysis has been shown to be superior to sling incision.

    e. intermittent catheterization is not advisable.

22. When MUSs are performed at the time of prolapse surgery:
    a. risks of perforation, exposure, and infection are higher than in cases in which only a sling is performed.
    b. concomitant hysterectomy has an adverse effect on incontinence outcome.
    c. rates of urethrolysis for postoperative retention are higher.
    d. occult incontinence may not be adequately addressed.
    e. rates of retention are slightly higher than in those undergoing a sling procedure only.

23. When MUSs are used as salvage procedures:
    a. complication rates are higher than when MUSs are done primarily.
    b. the technique needs to be altered compared to a primary procedure.
    c. failure rates are unaffected by urethral hypermobility.
    d. bladder perforation is less than in primary cases.
    e. overall efficacy is similar to that of primary implantation.

24. Complications associated with MUSs include:
    a. bladder perforation in up to 5%.
    b. voiding dysfunction in 4% to 20%.
    c. de novo urgency in as many as 12%.
    d. delayed wound healing in approximately 1%.
    e. all of the above.

25. According to International Continence Society (ICS) and International Urogynecological Association (IUGA) terminology pertaining to synthetic (prosthetic) mesh sling complications, which of the following is TRUE?
    a. The term *perforation* should be used when mesh is present within the urinary tract or bowel.
    b. The term *exposure* should be used when mesh is present in the urinary tract or bowel.
    c. The term *erosion* should be used when mesh is found in the urinary tract a year or more after surgery.
    d. a and b.
    e. a and c.

26. Material-related exposures and perforations associated with MUSs are:
    a. decreased by the macroporous nature of the sling material.
    b. unaffected by tension placed on the slings.
    c. associated with vaginal exposures approximately 20% of the time.
    d. associated with bladder perforation rates of 20%.
    e. irrelevant to outcomes or satisfaction.

27. Which of the following statements about the anatomy of MUSs is TRUE?
    a. The obturator nerve and vessels are less than 2 cm away from the transobturator sling at the level of the obturator foramen.
    b. For retropubic slings, the dorsal nerve of the clitoris is typically less than 2 cm away from the sling.
    c. The anatomic position of a single-incision sling is significantly affected by position of the legs.
    d. A branch of the obturator artery that courses along the pubic bone is more likely to be injured with an in-to-out transobturator sling technique.
    e. The periurethral fascia covering the posterior urethra is very thin.

28. Which of the following statements is FALSE regarding the treatment of patients with recurrent SUI with a MUS surgery?
    a. Retropubic slings have been shown to have better outcomes than transobturator slings in patients with recurrent SUI in a few small series.
    b. Repeat MUS surgery is significantly less effective at curing incontinence than primary MUS surgery.
    c. A meta-analysis of MUS surgery for recurrent SUI found that retropubic MUS surgery was significantly better than transobturator MUS surgery.
    d. Recurrent SUI after MUS surgery may be due to ISD.
    e. None of the above statements are false.

29. In regard to perforations associated with MUSs:
    a. bladder perforations cannot be managed endoscopically in well-selected cases.
    b. vaginal exposures cannot be managed conservatively.
    c. exposures and perforations are not related to errant sling placement.
    d. symptoms are not usually associated with exposure.
    e. complete excision of exposed material should be performed.

30. In regard to the mechanics of MUSs, which of the following is TRUE?
    a. MUSs work primarily by compressing the urethra.
    b. There is no evidence to support dynamic kinking of the urethra as a mechanism for continence for MUSs.
    c. Placing a sling tight at the mid-urethra will help eliminate postoperative hypermobility.
    d. It appears that a MUS works by impeding the movement of the posterior urethral wall.
    e. Postoperative urethral hypermobility is associated with failure of the procedure.

31. Which of the following statements is TRUE?
    a. Retropubic MUSs cure SUI better than transobturator MUSs.
    b. The risk of urinary tract trocar injury is higher with retropubic MUSs than transobturator MUSs.
    c. Postoperative voiding dysfunction is higher with transobturator MUSs than retropubic MUSs.
    d. It is not necessary to perform cystoscopy after a transobturator MUS surgery.
    e. It is not necessary to perform cystoscopy after a single-incision MUS surgery.

32. Voiding dysfunction associated with MUSs is:
    a. not associated with changes in urodynamic parameters.
    b. predictable based on unique preoperative voiding parameters such as flow rate.
    c. managed by immediate sling release.
    d. managed initially conservatively, but sling release should be contemplated when persistent voiding trials are not successful.
    e. resolved by complete excision of the sling.

33. In regard to operative management for voiding dysfunction after MUS surgery:
    a. a single incision of the sling results in incontinence in the majority of patients.
    b. it is important to remove the entire sling.
    c. surgery should not be considered until at least 3 months after sling placement as after autologous PVSs,.
    d. voiding dysfunction is usually transient.
    e. loosening the sling in the operating room with a cystoscope is a very safe option.

34. Complications associated with MUSs include:
    a. superficial vaginal material exposure.
    b. vascular perforation.
    c. intestinal perforation.
    d. significant hemorrhage requiring transfusion.
    e. all of the above.

35. Which of the following statements is TRUE regarding sexual dysfunction after MUS surgery?
    a. Postoperative dyspareunia is not associated with MUS surgery.
    b. Sling removal has been shown to improve dyspareunia.
    c. It has been clearly shown that MUS surgery will improve the sexual function of a woman with incontinence.
    d. A decrease in coital incontinence may improve sexual function.
    e. b and d.

36. Which of the following statements is TRUE regarding bleeding and hematomas after MUS surgery?
    a. The rate of undiagnosed hematomas is likely less than 5%.
    b. The majority of postoperative hematomas resolve without intervention.
    c. In the literature, the rate of severe bleeding is consistently less than 1%.
    d. The rate of hematomas and severe bleeding is lower after retropubic MUS surgery than transobturator MUS surgery.
    e. All of the above are true.

37. Regarding the transobturator technique, the:
    a. surgical placement of the tape requires insertion through the adductor longus tendon.
    b. tape never traverses the gracilis or adductor magnus brevis muscles.
    c. anterior branch of the obturator artery is located at the medial aspect of the obturator foramen.
    d. tape remains above the perineal membrane and outside the true pelvis and does not penetrate the levator ani group.
    e. dorsal nerve of the clitoris is in close juxtaposition to the tape.

38. The transobturator technique involves:
    a. either outside-in or inside-out approaches.
    b. no absolute requirement for cystoscopy.
    c. no risk of lower urinary tract injury.
    d. no risk of leg pain or dyspareunia.
    e. similar meshes in all available kits.

39. Reported outcomes with the transobturator MUS:
    a. appear to be relatively similar regardless of whether ISD is present preoperatively.
    b. include bladder, but not urethral, injury being reported.
    c. indicate that vaginal exposure is similar regardless of the type of tape used.
    d. show that voiding dysfunction is significantly less with this technique as compared with the retropubic approach.
    e. are not affected by the presence of urethral hypermobility.

40. Which of the following statements is TRUE regarding pain after MUS surgery?
    a. Groin pain is more commonly associated with the transobturator MUS approach.
    b. When groin pain does occur, it persists longer after retropubic MUS surgery.

    c. Most groin pain resolves after 2 days.
    d. a and c.
    e. a and b.

41. Which of the following statements is TRUE regarding infection after MUS surgery?
    a. Severe infection is a common complication after MUS surgery.
    b. Randomized controlled trials demonstrate a vaginal wound infection rate of approximately 10%.
    c. There are no reports in the literature about delayed presentation of infection after MUS surgery.
    d. Obesity and diabetes are associated with fasciitis after pelvic surgery.
    e. All of the above are true.

42. Which of the following is FALSE regarding the surgical management of mesh perforation and exposure after MUS surgery?
    a. Observational treatment is not recommended for mesh perforation of the bladder.
    b. Endoscopic excision or ablation is an acceptable first step for select patients with small areas of bladder perforation.
    c. A midline vaginal incision is acceptable for patients undergoing removal of mesh that has perforated into the urethra.
    d. Reconstruction should involve nonoverlapping suture lines and may benefit from interposition of tissue such as a labial fat pad, greater omentum, or autologous fascial sling.
    e. In cases of mesh perforation of the urinary tract, the adjacent MUS portions outside the urinary tract should also be removed.

43. Which of the following is FALSE regarding recurrent or persistent SUI after MUS?
    a. Persistent SUI may be due to poor surgical technique, wrong choice of procedure, or suboptimal patient selection.
    b. Cystoscopy and urodynamics are indicated in the workup of recurrent SUI.
    c. Sling tightening is not supported by evidence-based literature.
    d. Periurethral bulking produces inferior outcomes to repeat MUS for recurrent SUI.
    e. The data support the use of autologous PVS over repeat MUS in this population.

44. Which of the following statements is TRUE regarding regulatory and legal issues related to sling mesh complications?
    a. The first MUS had to go through the premarket approval (PMA) process, and then subsequent slings were approved through the 510(k) process.
    b. MUSs can no longer use the 510(k) approval process.
    c. The FDA considers mesh complications to be "rare."
    d. In the legal profession, the § symbol does NOT stand for "section."
    e. Single-incision mini-sling manufacturers are required to perform 522 postmarket surveillance studies.

45. In 2016, the following medical devices have been reclassified as class III:
    a. retropubic midurethral slings.
    b. single-incision mini-slings.
    c. surgical mesh for transvaginal prolapse.
    d. surgical mesh for sacral colpopexy.
    e. b and c.

ANSWERS

1. **b. Adequate function of the pubourethral ligaments, the suburethral vaginal hammock, and the pubococcygeus muscle helps to preserve continence.** They postulated that injury to any of these three components from surgery, parturition, aging, or hormonal deprivation could lead to impaired mid-urethral function and subsequent urinary incontinence.

2. **c. The American Urological Association (AUA) Guidelines state that a postvoid residual (PVR) volume should be checked on all patients.** Based on AUA guidelines, a urinalysis and measurement of PVR volume should be performed on all patients, but more extensive imaging is not part of the routine evaluation of urinary incontinence. However, in some patients abnormal findings in the history, physical examination, or urinalysis may warrant further imaging.

3. **e. All of of above.** All of the following are options for the index patient and are supported by Grade A evidence. The choice of intervention should be individualized based on the patient's symptoms, the degree of bother the symptoms cause the patient, patient goals and expectations, and the risks and benefits for a given patient.

4. **d. Synthetic sling materials exhibit the least amount of degradation.** In 2008, Woodruff et al.[a] examined explanted sling materials and determined that synthetic materials demonstrated the least amount of degradation. They also demonstrated the greatest amount of fibroblast and tissue ingrowth into the specimen.

5. **b. Low urethral resistance with decreased bladder compliance.** Decreased bladder compliance is of concern for upper tract deterioration. The addition of a PVS, by increasing bladder outlet resistance, would cause significant damage to the upper tracts. The compliance should be addressed before or concurrently to anti-incontinence measures. A PVS procedure is indicated for ISD associated with urethral hypermobility, SUI presenting as concomitant cystoceles, SUI associated with urethral diverticulum, urethral damage from previous MUS, SUI associated with urethral defects (e.g., urethrovaginal fistula) in which urethral reconstruction is required, and in women with SUI and associated neurogenic conditions.

6. **c. The fast-twitch fibers of the external sphincter are responsible for sudden protection against incontinence, and slow-twitch fibers provide passive control through the involuntary guarding reflex.** The female urethra is composed of four layers, with the middle muscular layer maintaining the resting urethral closure mechanism and the outer seromuscular layer augmenting this closing pressure. The levator ani, urethropelvic ligament, and pubocervical fascia provide support to the bladder neck and underside of the bladder. The round ligament provides support to the uterus. A PVS is placed at the bladder neck to provide adequate urethral coaptation for increasing urethral responsiveness to abdominal pressure.

7. **b. Stiffness and maximal load failure are the same between freeze-dried fascia lata and solvent-dehydrated and dermal grafts.** Maximum load to failure, maximum load/graft width, and stiffness are significantly lower for the freeze-dried fascia lata group compared with the autologous, solvent-dehydrated, and dermal graft groups. The ideal graft material causes no tissue reaction, is completely biocompatible, leads to significant host fibroblast infiltration and neovascularization, and causes negligible perforation or exposure. The estimated risk of HIV transmission from an allograft is 1 in 1,667,600. The theoretical risk of developing Creutzfeldt-Jakob disease from a non-neural allograft is 1 in 3.5 million. Porcine small intestinal submucosa has less tensile strength than cadaveric fascia lata. Synthetic material is no longer used for bladder neck PVS because of the exceedingly high perforation rates.

8. **a. The weighted speculum should be removed.** Tensioning before the speculum is removed may result in failure of the procedure due to too much or too little tension. The abdominal incision is also closed after the sling is tensioned.

9. **d. a and c.** Cure rates reported in peer-reviewed literature for autologous PVS procedures are 24% to 97%. There are no risk factors that predict outcomes after PVS surgery for primary or recurrent SUI. The SISTEr trial was a multicenter, randomized clinical trial (Albo et al., 2007[a]) that found higher cure rates for the PVS procedure than the Burch colposuspension, but also more associated voiding symptoms (urinary tract infection, difficulty voiding, and postoperative urge incontinence, $P < .001$).

10. **a. Synthetic slings perforate into the urinary tract 15 times more often than autologous, allograft, or xenograft slings.** This includes sutures, bone anchors, and screws. Synthetic slings perforate 15 times more often into the urethra and are exposed 14 times more often into the vagina than autologous, allograft, and xenograft slings. Urethral perforation usually presents at a mean of 9 months as urinary retention, urgency, and mixed urinary incontinence.

11. **c. Fifty percent of affected patients have symptoms of overactive bladder, which can be avoided if sling lysis is performed within 2 weeks of PVS placement.** Transient urinary retention is common, and most patients return to spontaneous voiding within 10 days postoperatively. Obstructive symptoms may improve or resolve with time, which is the reason most physicians prefer waiting 3 months before considering surgical intervention. The incidence of voiding dysfunction after continence surgery varies from 2.5% to 35% and includes obstruction, detrusor overactivity, or impaired detrusor contractility. Persistent postoperative urgency incontinence and urgency present more commonly (8% to 25%) than frank retention. Although urodynamics do not preoperatively predict outcomes after anti-incontinence surgery or urethrolysis, it is useful in diagnosing and treating patients with obstruction after a PVS procedure. There is a 0% to 18% recurrent SUI rate after urethrolysis.

12. **c. ISD is the primary underlying cause of SUI for women, with hypermobility being a secondary finding.** Although urethral hypermobility is present in many women, most do not manifest incontinence, and therefore, ISD is considered to be the most important factor in women who experience urinary loss. The extrinsic urethral sphincter is not considered to be the primary mechanism for urinary continence in women. The ongoing debate regarding hypermobility and ISD is further compounded by the advent of midurethral slings, which clearly address hypermobility during stress events. Given the efficacy of midurethral slings, there has been some confusion regarding the role of hypermobility in promoting continence. However, most believe that the intrinsic urethral mechanism is of primary importance for urinary control.

13. **b. Should have been offered weight loss as an initial management option.** It has been consistently shown in the literature that obese patients with incontinence benefit from weight loss. The literature regarding improvement or cure of incontinence in patients with obesity compared with nonobese patients is mixed. Multiple authors have found a higher rate of bladder trocar injury in nonobese patients during MUS surgery.

14. **d. The sling is sutured to the underlying tissues for fixation purposes.** The tension-free vaginal tape (TVT) procedure incorporates several specific technical components. Insertion trocars are used in either a suprapubic or a vaginal approach to assist in implantation of the material in the retropubic area. It is now well known that type 1 synthetic meshes are best because of their wide porosity. In addition, this mesh should be monofilamentous. Most authorities recommend placement of loose tension only on the TVT, although some authorities now are placing greater tension on the TVT, with success being established in patients with lesser degrees of hypermobility.

---

[a]Sources referenced can be found in *Campbell-Walsh-Wein Urology, 12th Edition,* on the Expert Consult website.

No suture fixation to the underlying periurethral fascia is necessary to anchor the sling. Cystoscopy is a vital component of this procedure to exclude urinary tract injury.

15. **e. All of the above.** The presentation of patients with voiding dysfunction is variable, and the symptoms range from complete urinary retention and urgency incontinence to the less obvious irritative symptoms. Obstruction may also present with recurrent urinary tract infections, prolonged suprapubic pain, and painful voiding, even if emptying is completed.

16. **d. Rectus fascia.** During placement of the transobturator MUS, the trocar must traverse the obturator internus muscle, obturator membrane, and obturator externus muscle as it goes through the obturator foramen. Medially, the transobturator MUS enters the anterior compartment of the ischiorectal fascia, in the area of the levator ani membrane and obturator internus muscle. While the MUS passes through the rectus fascia, the transobturator sling does not.

17. **e. Five-year results demonstrate durability similar to 1-year results.** Five-year (and now 7-year) longitudinal results have shown that midurethral slings have procedural durability in terms of efficacy. This efficacy is not substantially less than results obtained at 1 year. Furthermore, several studies with greater than 10-year outcomes have recently been published and reveal similar durability in the longer term. Randomized trials have demonstrated similar efficacy in patients undergoing either open colposuspensions or laparoscopic colposuspensions. MUSs provide superior results compared with laparoscopic procedures. Although voiding dysfunction may be observed after any type of sling procedure, results suggest that midurethral slings are associated with less voiding dysfunction than either colposuspensions or bladder neck slings. Results with mixed incontinence are acceptable compared with other types of interventions for urinary incontinence but are less than those obtained in pure SUI.

18. **d. Patients with subclinical impaired detrusor contractility are at increased risk for voiding dysfunction after PVS surgery.** It has been shown that preoperative voiding dysfunction affects a patient's ability to empty after antiincontinence surgery. Subclinical preoperative impaired detrusor contractility may manifest symptomatically with voiding dysfunction after PVS surgery. Dysfunctional voiding or failure of relaxation of the external urethral sphincter may also affect emptying after surgery. Also, a patient who habitually voids by abdominal straining may have difficulty emptying after incontinence surgery. Because of the variability of presenting symptoms following a PVS, it is important to ascertain the predominant symptom with a thorough history.

19. **a. Obturator internus muscle.** None of the other structures should be penetrated during the procedure.

20. **c. Higher rates of postoperative urgency.** They are associated with rates of postoperative urgency that are higher than those in young patients. Elderly patients experience higher rates of postoperative urgency associated with any sling material, and this is true for the MUS as well. However, elderly patients have results similar to their younger peers, and therefore satisfaction rates are also similar to those of their younger peers. Mixed urinary incontinence resolution rates are similar to those of the younger population, and actual postoperative retention occurs to a similar degree as in younger patients, but postoperative voiding function may be slightly higher in the older population.

21. **b. It is generally appropriate to wait as long as 3 months after autologous PVS surgery before considering surgical intervention.** Obstruction following an autologous PVS usually improves or resolves with time, therefore, most physicians historically have preferred waiting 3 months before considering surgical intervention after PVS (it may not be suitable to wait this long after midurethral slings). It is appropriate and effective to initially treat persistent voiding dysfunction conservatively. This includes temporary catheter drainage, clean intermittent catheterization, timed voiding, double voiding, biofeedback, pelvic floor muscle training, and anticholinergic therapy.

22. **d. Occult incontinence may not be adequately addressed.** Midurethral slings performed at the time of prolapse surgery have now been shown to be safe and efficacious; however, appropriate MUS tensioning in women with occult SUI (only seen with POP reduction) may be challenging. Risks of perforation, exposure, and infection are no greater than when the midurethral sling is performed as a primary isolated procedure. Concomitant hysterectomy has been shown not to have an adverse effect on continence status associated with these procedures. In addition, rates of postoperative urethrolysis are no greater when the midurethral sling technology is combined with a prolapse correction. Rates of retention are also not appreciably higher in this population, compared with those women undergoing isolated slings only.

23. **e. Overall efficacy is similar to that of primary implantation.** As salvage procedures, midurethral slings have overall efficacy similar to their use in primary implantation procedures. Complications should be no higher than when done as primary procedures. The technique remains the same, and no alteration is required. Success does appear to be reliant on hypermobility, and patients with less hypermobility would appear to have less overall functional success than those patients with greater hypermobility. Rates of bladder perforation may be somewhat higher in this population than in primary cases.

24. **e. All of the above.** Complications with midurethral slings are an important part of informed consent. Bladder perforation rates range as high as 5% and in some studies are somewhat higher. Voiding function rates vary from 4% to 20%, and this variance is largely related to definitional reasons based on literature evidence. De novo urgency occurs with postoperative voiding dysfunction in as many as 12% of patients, and wound healing can be affected in approximately 1% of patients; results represent dramatic improvement compared with historic dense weave meshes.

25. **d. a and b.** In 2010, the IUGA and the ICS released a report clarifying and standardizing the terminology related to complications from insertion of synthetic and biological materials during female pelvic surgery (Haylen et al., 2011[a]). According to that report, synthetic mesh is termed a *prosthesis* and a biologic implant is termed a *graft.* Mesh located in the lower urinary tract is termed a *perforation* and extrusion of mesh through the skin or vagina is termed *exposure.*

26. **a. Decreased by the macroporous nature of the sling material.** Exposure and perforation associated with midurethral slings is clearly decreased by the use of macroporous monofilament sling material (type 1). Tension may have a role in increasing mesh-related complications even in macroporous slings. Vaginal exposure rates and bladder perforation rates are very low and do not exceed 5% to 10% with newer sling materials. When material complications do occur, however, they have an adverse impact on overall patient satisfaction.

27. **b. For retropubic slings, the dorsal nerve of the clitoris is typically less than 2 cm away from the sling.** The left and right dorsal nerves of the clitoris (DNC) run along the inferior surface of the ischiopubic rami and cross under the pubic bone approximately 1.4 cm from the midline. Therefore, when a placing a trocar, it is important to stay at least 2 cm from the midline to avoid injuring the DNC.

28. **c. A meta-analysis of MUS surgery for recurrent SUI found that retropubic MUS surgery was significantly better than transobturator MUS surgery.** In 2013, Agur et al.[a] performed a meta-analysis of the 10 randomized, controlled trials that of MUSs that addressed recurrent SUI. The review included 350 women with a mean follow-up of 18.1 months. The authors found no significant difference in subjective cure rates in patients after retropubic versus transobturator MUS surgery.

29. **e. Complete excision of exposed material should be performed.** Management of exposures and perforations is complex and must be individualized. Primarily, all exposed material, whether it be vaginal or within the urinary tract, must be removed or in some manner covered. There have been

successful reports of bladder management endoscopically, although this is contingent on absolute excision of all exposed material. Some authors have reported successful management of vaginal exposures with conservative use of topical estrogens and delayed primary closure as well as simple secondary intention healing. Exposures and perforations are clearly linked to technique, and errant sling placement has a high significance in creating perforations.

30. **d. It appears that a MUS works by impeding the movement of the posterior urethral wall.** Indeed, it appears that a midurethral sling works by impeding the movement of the posterior urethral wall above the sling, directing its motion in an anteroinferior or anterior direction. In addition, inward movement of the posterior urethral wall after placement of a midurethral sling results in urethral lumen narrowing (compression). This securing of the posterior wall of the urethra (with or without compression during stress maneuvers) is one theory of how midurethral slings achieve continence.

31. **b. The risk of urinary tract trocar injury is higher with retropubic MUSs than transobturator** MUSs. In the majority of published series comparing retropubic and transobturator midurethral slings, the rate of urinary tract trocar injury at the time of sling placement is higher with retropubic slings. However, there are numerous case reports of transobturator sling mesh perforating into the urinary tract. Therefore, cystoscopy should be performed after transobturator sling trocar passage.

32. **d. Managed initially conservatively, but sling release should be contemplated when persistent voiding trials are not successful.** Voiding dysfunction associated with midurethral slings is substantially less than with bladder neck slings but still occurs. Timing of intervention is dependent on surgeon experience but is trending toward earlier intervention. Most experts recommend a period of conservative management of a few days to 1 month. Persistent obstruction will require intervention. Urodynamic parameters are often affected in cases of persistent obstruction. Unfortunately, no preoperative factors are predictive of postoperative voiding dysfunction. Immediate release is not recommended because a short period of observation usually results in resolution of the voiding dysfunction. When sling release occurs, midline incision of the sling is all that is required; the entire sling does not need to be excised.

33. **d. Voiding dysfunction is usually transient.** Urinary obstruction after MUS surgery is usually transient and can be managed with short-term intermittent catheterization, although occasionally symptoms mandate sling release. Long-term retention after retropubic midurethral sling surgery is a rare complication. In these cases, removal or incision of the sling usually improves the patient's symptoms.

34. **e. All of the above.** Complications of technique include injury to surrounding structures and significant hemorrhage due to laceration of perivesical vessels. Intestinal and vascular complications can cause substantial morbidity and mortality.

35. **e. b and d.** The rate of de novo dyspareunia after MUS surgery is between 3% and 14.5%. Some authors attribute improved sexual function after MUS surgery to a significant decrease in coital incontinence. There is contradictory evidence in the literature that MUS surgery improves and worsens sexual function. There is evidence in the literature that sling removal can improve dyspareunia.

36. **b. The majority of postoperative hematomas resolve without intervention.** In 2005, Tseng et al.[a] performed ultrasound on 62 women after MUS surgery and found that 8 (12.9%) patients had significant retropubic hematomas larger than 5 cm on the day after surgery. Repeat ultrasonographic examinations 1 month after surgery revealed all the hematomas except one had resolved. In randomized controlled trials, the majority of bleeding complications occur in patients after retropubic MUS surgery.

37. **d. Tape remains above the perineal membrane and outside the true pelvis and does not penetrate the levator ani group.**

The transobturator technique is unique because (when done correctly) it avoids entry into the true pelvis and the levator group. Errant sling placement through the adductor longus tendon can result in substantial pain. Smaller muscle groups, such as the magnus brevis and gracilis, are often traversed by this technique without substantial complications. The obturator vessels are lateral and superior to the area of insertion of the device. The dorsal nerve of the clitoris is separated from the trajectory of the device by at least 1 to 2 cm.

38. **a. Either outside-in or inside-out approaches.** The transobturator technique can be performed by insertion of the passing needles from either vaginal or obturator approaches. Associated risks of device use include leg pain, dyspareunia, and injury to surrounding structures. Cystoscopy is a useful safety adjunct and should be performed as an integral and necessary part of the transobturator MUS surgery. Different kits use different meshes, and not all meshes are similar. The kit to be used should be evaluated critically for this parameter.

39. **a. Appear to be relatively similar regardless of whether ISD is present preoperatively.** Transobturator MUS surgery outcomes are relatively similar to those seen with the retropubic slings, regardless of urethral function. Any lower urinary tract structure, including the ureter, can be injured by the transobturator trocar, including the urethra and bladder. Vaginal exposure is clearly related to mesh type. Voiding dysfunction is similar to retropubic techniques. Less urethral hypermobility probably militates against success rates with transobturator slings, such as those reported in women with higher degrees of urethral hypermobility.

40. **d. a and c.** Thigh and groin pain appear to be more commonly associated with the transobturator approach. In addition, it appears that groin pain persists longer after the transobturator midurethral slings. Most groin pain resolves after the second postoperative day.

41. **d. Obesity and diabetes are associated with fasciitis after pelvic surgery.** A review of necrotizing fasciitis in gynecologic surgery found that obesity (88%), hypertension (65%), and diabetes (47%) were all factors associated with the development of fasciitis after surgery. In their randomized controlled trial from 2002, Ward and Hilton[a] found a 2% rate of vaginal wound infection after retropubic MUS surgery. In 2010, Richter et al.[a] found a 0.7% rate of vaginal wound infection in both the retropubic and transobturator MUS arms.

42. **c. A midline vaginal incision is acceptable for patients undergoing removal of mesh that has perforated into the urethra.** For slings that perforate into the urethra an inverted-U incision is best because this allows for exposure of the proximal urethra, bladder neck, and endopelvic fascia as well as providing a vaginal epithelial flap that avoids overlapping suture lines.

43. **e. The data support the use of autologous PVS over repeat MUS in this population.** Overall, the data guiding the choice of procedure for recurrent or persistent SUI after MUS is inadequate, with a Cochrane systematic review identifying 12 trials, but none meeting eligibility criteria (Bakali et al, 2013[a]). Both urodynamics and cystoscopy may assist in elucidating the source of failure in this patient with failure of previous anti-incontinence surgery (AUA SUI Guidelines). Sling tightening is not supported by evidence-based literature, and periurethral bulking therapy produces outcomes inferior to repeat MUS for recurrent SUI.

44. **e. Single-incision sling manufacturers are required to perform 522 postmarket surveillance studies.** In January 2012, the Food and Drug Administration (FDA) mandated that all manufacturers of synthetic prosthetic mesh and biologic graft materials marketed for pelvic organ prolapse repair and single-incision sling products perform 522 postmarket surveillance studies. Midurethral sling products (except single-incision slings) were excluded from this mandate because, in September 2011, an FDA advisory panel[a] deemed existing midurethral sling products "safe and effective."

45. **c. Surgical mesh for transvaginal prolapse.** On January 4, 2016, the FDA issued one order to reclassify mesh used for transvaginal prolapse repair from class II device, which generally includes moderate-risk devices, to class III, which includes high-risk devices.[a] A second order requires manufacturers to submit a PMA application to support the safety and effectiveness of surgical mesh for transvaginal POP repair. The PMA pathway will require manufacturers to address safety concerns, including severe pelvic pain and organ perforation, to demonstrate safety and effectiveness. These orders do not apply to surgical mesh used for other indications, such as full-length MUS and mesh for sacral colpopexy, and remain class II devices. Single-incision mini-slings are currently undergoing 522 postmarket surveillance order studies.

CHAPTER REVIEW

1. Urethral slings are the procedure of choice for the surgical correction of female SUI.
2. PVSs should be placed at the bladder neck.
3. Slings are particularly helpful in treating ISD.
4. The majority of patients who require clean intermittent catheterization after PVS placement had a neurogenic bladder preoperatively.
5. Persistent urgency or urgency urinary incontinence are more common than frank urinary retention as presenting symptoms for bladder outlet obstruction after a sling.
6. Maximum urethral closure pressure occurs at the level of the midurethra.
7. Midurethral slings are less successful in patients with a fixed urethra and/or a low abdominal or Valsalva leak-point pressure.
8. Urethral mobility before midurethral sling procedures has been shown to be predictive of success (i.e., the more the proximal urethra moves during a Valsalva maneuver, the better the cure rate for incontinence).
9. For patients with persistently elevated post-void residuals and bothersome symptoms refractory to conservative management after a sling procedure, MUS release procedures consistently provide resolution of symptoms with maintenance of continence in the majority of patients
10. Cystoscopy is an integral part of all urethral sling procedures to visualize and exclude any injury to the urethra or bladder.
11. Periurethral bulking agents have limited success in treating SUI.
12. The use of autologous tissue for a sling has the lowest rate of erosion and infection.
13. The most common reason for patient dissatisfaction following sling surgery is the persistence or development of urgency symptoms and/or urgency urinary incontinence.
14. Synthetic material is no longer used for slings placed at the bladder neck.
15. When synthetic mesh erodes into the urethra or bladder, the mesh must be removed.
16. Obese patients with incontinence benefit from weight loss.
17. When sling release is performed, a midline incision of the sling is all that is required and the entire sling does not need to be excised.

126 Complications Related to the Use of Mesh and Their Repair

Anne P. Cameron

QUESTIONS

1. What is a mesh erosion?
   a. When mesh gradually becomes apparent in the vagina
   b. It is an incorrect term that should not be used
   c. When mesh gradually becomes exposed in the urethra or bladder
   d. Any palpable or visible mesh in any organ
   e. A result of trocar injury to the bladder or urethra

2. Why are large pores essential for mesh to prevent complications?
   a. These make the mesh a lighter weight.
   b. They make the mesh stretch.
   c. They make the mesh cheaper to produce.
   d. They allow macrophages and other cells to penetrate the mesh.
   e. They make the mesh less visible.

3. Mesh is known to increase the long-term risk of
   a. pelvic cancers
   b. systemic (nonpelvic) cancers
   c. autoimmune diseases
   d. chronic fatigue syndrome
   e. none of the above

4. Which of the following is a contraindication for mesh sling placement?
   a. Prior failed mesh sling
   b. Vaginal atrophy
   c. Urethral injury during procedure
   d. History of recurrent urinary tract infections (UTIs)
   e. Fibromyalgia

5. In which of the following procedures can bladder perforations occur?
   a. Retropubic sling
   b. Transobturator sling
   c. Mini/single incision sling
   d. Anterior prolapse mesh
   e. All of the above

6. In a woman with retention immediately after a mesh sling placement, which of the following treatments is contraindicated?
   a. Self-catheterization for 2 weeks
   b. Urethral dilation after 1 week
   c. Indwelling catheter for 3 days
   d. Sling loosening/division in 1 week

7. What is a desirable property for type I mesh?
   a. Low melting point
   b. Knitted
   c. Smaller pore size

   d. Clear colored material
   e. Made of polytetrafluoroethylene

8. Which of the following statements about mesh is true?
   a. New mesh exposures/extrusions cannot occur more than two years after the original surgery
   b. Conservative treatment of mesh exposures with estrogen is never effective
   c. If your technique is meticulous, you can remove the entire mesh
   d. Cystoscopy always needs to be performed after any mesh sling placement
   e. Dyspareunia without mesh exposure should only be treated conservatively

9. What symptom is the most likely to resolve after mesh sling revision?
   a. Urinary retention
   b. Mesh exposure
   c. Stress incontinence
   d. Urgency incontinence
   e. Dyspareunia

10. Abdominal sacrocolpopexy (ASC) mesh presenting with mesh-related abdominal abscess should be treated with:
    a. long-term antibiotics and percutaneous drainage
    b. complete abdominal and vaginal mesh removal
    c. abdominal mesh removal leaving vaginal mesh in place to avoid vaginal tissue loss
    d. vaginal mesh removal and vaginal drainage of the abscess
    e. abdominal exploration and washout

11. Which of the following statements about male mesh slings are true?
    a. The mesh perforation rate of the urethra is underreported.
    b. Retention after catheter removal should quickly be treated by sling incision to prevent bladder remodeling.
    c. If a man requires an artificial sphincter after failed mesh sling, the sling can simply be divided and left in place during artificial urinary sphincter (AUS) placement.
    d. Mesh urethral perforation is often asymptomatic.

ANSWERS

1. **b. It is an incorrect term that should not be used.** *Erosion* is a generic term that implies that tissue has been worn away by friction or pressure. Therefore, the term should not be used.
2. **d. They allow macrophages and other cells to penetrate the mesh.** Pore size is critical to wound healing and mesh integration by the body. Smaller pore size in woven grafts allows bacteria (1 μm) to enter but restricts entry of host macrophages and lymphocytes (50 μm), impeding immune response. When pores are large such as with polypropylene type I mesh (~1500 μm), fibrocollagenous tissue ingrowth can occur, which allows the mesh to integrate into the local tissue providing strength and support.

3. **e. None of the above.** With long-term use of mesh in the vagina, there has been the opportunity to follow women over many years for complications. Mesh has been hypothesized to increase cancer risk due to chronic foreign body response. This theory has been disproved with population-based studies that showed no increase in pelvic or any other cancer diagnoses in women followed for 6 years after implant. Similarly, mesh implantation has not been associated with the development of autoimmune diseases over long-term follow-up.

4. **c. Urethral injury during procedure.** Mesh perforation or later extrusion at the bladder neck or into urethra is a rare complication. It occurs due to an injury to the urethra or bladder neck during either the vaginal dissection or trocar passage. If an intraoperative urethral injury is noted during dissection for placement of the sling, the surgeon must abandon mesh placement. One should repair the urethral injury with absorbable suture and allow healing before undertaking any mesh procedure, given the extraordinary high risk of urethral extrusion of the mesh.

5. **e. All of the above.** Bladder injury is far more common with retropubic than transobturator trocars (4.8% vs. 0.6%) and is typically diagnosed on cystoscopy with a 70-degree lens during the sling placement. The trocar is seen as at the dome/lateral wall of the bladder. Mesh perforation into the bladder (0.7% to 3.5%) in the case of anterior compartment pelvic organ prolapse repair and into the rectum (0.15%) from posterior repair can present with pain, fistula formation, or, in the case of bladder perforation, recurrent hematuria, UTIs, or voiding-related pain.

6. **b. Urethral dilation after 1 week.** Urethral dilation is ineffective in the setting of bladder outlet obstruction (BOO) from an obstructing sling and puts the patient at risk for urethral extrusion of the mesh with the dilation traumatizing the tissue over the inflexible mesh.

7. **b. Knitted.** Type I mesh is macroporous with pore size greater than 75 µm. Examples of type I mesh are polypropylene and Marlex. Marlex is a woven monofilament polypropylene. It is one of the stiffest mesh materials, with a propensity to wrinkle and a high extrusion rate. In contrast, Polypropylene is a monofilament knitted graft that is softer and more compliant than woven configurations and has larger interstices due to the loose knit (1500 vs. 600 µm) increasing elasticity. In addition, its melting point of 160°C allows it to be autoclaved. It is currently the only recommended implantable vaginal mesh for slings and pelvic organ prolapse.

8. **d. Cystoscopy always needs to be performed after any mesh sling placement.** Bladder injury is far more common with retropubic than transobturator trocars (4.8% vs. 0.6%) and is typically diagnosed on cystoscopy with a 70-degree lens during the sling placement. The trocar is seen as at the dome/lateral wall of the bladder. Complete filling of the bladder is required to evaluated for injuries as an underfilled may obscure a small perforation.

9. **b. Mesh exposure.** Mesh re-exposure if these principles are followed is near 0%.

10. **b. Complete abdominal and vaginal mesh removal.** Abdominal mesh removal is sometimes indicated after failed vaginal approach or for patients with intractable mesh-related pain, abscess/infected upper portion of the mesh, or discitis. In the case of infection, the entire mesh should always be removed since residual infected mesh after a failed partial excision causes significant morbidity, including chronic infection, sinus tracts, abscess, and fistula formation. These will require a repeat excision typically via laparotomy, and this is usually a very difficult and morbid procedure.

11. **c. If a man requires an artificial sphincter after failed mesh sling, the sling can simply be divided and left in place during artificial urinary sphincter (AUS) placement.** Sling division without actual removal is sometimes needed when placing an artificial sphincter and can be performed simultaneously without difficulty.

CHAPTER REVIEW

1. One should aim to remove enough mesh to correct the problem and prevent future mesh complications. Removal of all the mesh is rarely required, and removing asymptomatic mesh is never indicated.

2. Mesh slings should be circumscribed and divided lateral to the urethra.

3. The amount of mesh removed depends on the indication: Retention = simple division; exposure/extrusion = divide and remove mesh to at least a centimeter from defect; pain = maximal vaginal removal and rarely removal of retropubic or obturator arms.

4. Bladder and urethral perforations are difficult complications to treat and can be managed endoscopically or open with the open approach being more thorough but potentially more morbid.

5. Transvaginal prolapse mesh has a higher rate of mesh exposure/extrusion than slings given the larger volume of mesh. Small exposures can be treated conservatively. Large exposures and pain are treated with vaginal mesh excision; typically the entire vaginal mesh is excised leaving only the arms in place. Vaginal pain/dyspareunia is the most difficult to treat given the multifactorial etiology of pain.

6. ASC sutures are easily removed vaginally; however, mesh is very difficult to effectively remove transvaginally, often requiring multiple attempts. Open abdominal mesh removal is a potentially very morbid procedure with high risk of bowel injury, vaginal tissue loss, and high blood loss.

7. Male slings often have temporary retention that will typically resolve over time. It is uncommon to require mesh division to resolve it, and urodynamics are helpful in determining obstruction versus bladder dysfunction as the cause.

127 Additional Therapies for Storage and Emptying Failure

Timothy B. Boone, Julie N. Stewart, and Laura M. Martinez

QUESTIONS

1. All of the following patients would be candidates for augmentation cystoplasty EXCEPT:
   a. a patient with a neurogenic bladder and poor bladder compliance who has failed trials of anticholinergic medications and intravesical injections of botulinum toxin.
   b. a patient with a spinal cord injury and detrusor leak point pressures of greater than 40 cm H_2O and subsequent vesicoureteral reflux.
   c. a patient with refractory idiopathic detrusor overactivity.
   d. a patient with significant urinary frequency and a bladder capacity of less than 100 mL.
   e. a patient with rapidly progressing multiple sclerosis and bothersome neurogenic detrusor overactivity causing urinary leakage.

2. What is the minimum threshold for particle size of urethral injectable agents that determines migration risk?
   a. 20 μm
   b. 40 μm
   c. 60 μm
   d. 80 μm
   e. 100 μm

3. Which injectable agent was reported to migrate to pelvic lymph nodes seen in radiograph?
   a. Porcine collagen
   b. Silicone macroparticles
   c. Carbon-coated zirconium beads
   d. Bovine collagen
   e. Autologous fat

4. The Credé maneuver for emptying the bladder is relatively contraindicated in patients:
   a. with decreased outlet resistance.
   b. who are obese.
   c. with vesicoureteral reflux.
   d. with high-pressure detrusor overactivity.
   e. younger than the age of 2 years.

5. All of the following statements are TRUE regarding bladder outlet closure EXCEPT:
   a. Complete closure of the bladder neck is rarely necessary.
   b. The main indication is urethral destruction after prolonged catheter drainage.
   c. An obstructing sling or artificial urinary sphincter (AUS) is rarely feasible, if less than 1 cm of urethra exists.
   d. Reflex sphincteric activity may result in disruption of the bladder neck closure.
   e. The transvaginal approach has decreased the postoperative fistula rate.

6. Of the following statements, which one is FALSE regarding "trigger voiding" in spinal cord–injured patients?
   a. Trigger voiding can be induced by digital rectal stimulation.
   b. Reflex contractions can be generated by using somatic motor axons to innervate parasympathetic bladder ganglia cells.
   c. Rhythmic suprapubic manual pressure is usually the most effective method for trigger voiding.
   d. Trigger voiding induces a reflex decrease in outlet resistance in patients with detrusor-sphincter dyssynergia.
   e. Trigger voiding can be induced by squeezing the clitoris.

7. Common complications associated with a continent catheterizable channel include all of the following EXCEPT:
   a. stomal stenosis.
   b. perforation of the catheterizable channel.
   c. incontinence from the stoma site.
   d. difficulty passing a catheter through the stoma due to stricture.
   e. stomal prolapse.

8. Which of the following statements is FALSE?
   a. Chronic indwelling urethral catheterization protects against poor bladder compliance and upper tract complications.
   b. Chronic indwelling urethral catheterization compared with clean intermittent catheterization (CIC) is associated with a higher incidence of urolithiasis.
   c. Asymptomatic bacteriuria is common in catheterized patients and does not usually require treatment.
   d. Periodic upper and lower tract evaluation is important in all patients managed with chronic indwelling catheters.
   e. There is still a role for anticholinergic medications in patients managing their bladders with a chronic indwelling catheter.

9. Which of the following is FALSE regarding the use of condom catheters?
   a. Similar incidence of bacteriuria and symptomatic UTIs to indwelling urethral catheters
   b. Preferable in patients who cannot perform CIC due to lack of caregiver
   c. Use of a malleable penile prosthesis can facilitate applying and maintaining a condom catheter
   d. Condom catheters should be changed daily to decrease risk for UTI
   e. Skin maceration is more likely to occur in patients with neurogenic LUT dysfunction

10. All of the following statements are TRUE regarding catheterization EXCEPT:
    a. There is no known association with intermittent catheterization and development of squamous cell carcinoma of the bladder.
    b. Gross hematuria in a patient with a chronic indwelling catheter is likely related to infection or inflammation and does not require a thorough hematuria workup.

c. Urinary incontinence may worsen in patients with intrinsic sphincter deficiency who convert from an indwelling urethral to suprapubic catheter.

d. There is a lower incidence of epididymitis in men who have chronic suprapubic catheters compared with urethral catheters.

e. There is a low risk of developing squamous cell carcinoma of the bladder with chronic indwelling catheter use.

11. Incontinence-associated dermatitis (IAD) is associated with the following factors in the incontinent patient EXCEPT:

a. it may be caused by infrequent pad changes.

b. it is manifested by inflammation of the skin with redness and edema.

c. it may lead to malignant lesions of the skin.

d. it predominately occurs in skin folds.

e. it promotes candidiasis and bacterial infections.

ANSWERS

1. **e. A patient with rapidly progressing multiple sclerosis and bothersome neurogenic detrusor overactivity causing urinary leakage.** A patient with a progressive neurologic disease, such as multiple sclerosis, may not have the ability to perform CIC in the future and an alternative treatment plan should be considered. Noncompliance with CIC puts the patient at risk for life-threatening spontaneous bladder perforation.

2. **d. 80 μm.**

3. **c. Carbon-coated zirconium beads.** Pannek and coworkers did report particle migration (2001). This was subsequently attributed to the high pressure necessary to inject the viscous material with large particles, resulting in material displacement into vascular or lymphatic spaces. Durasphere EXP with smaller particles is less likely to lead to this.

4. **c. With vesicoureteral reflux.** The Credé maneuver (manual compression of the bladder) is most effective in patients with decreased bladder tone who can generate an intravesical pressure greater than 50 cm H_2O and have decreased bladder outlet resistance. The Credé maneuver requires good hand control, is easier in a thin individual than an obese one, and is more easily performed in a child than in an adult. Voiding by Credé is unphysiologic, because active opening of the bladder neck does not occur, and increases in outlet resistance by a reflex mechanism may actually occur. If complete emptying does not occur, treatment to decrease outlet resistance can be contemplated, or an alternative method to empty the bladder should be used. Vesicoureteral reflux is a relative contraindication to external compression and straining maneuvers, especially in patients capable of generating a high intravesical pressure.

5. **e. The transvaginal approach has decreased the postoperative fistula rate.** Complete closure of the bladder neck is rarely necessary, because a compressive bladder neck sling is more easily performed, is less morbid, and allows transurethral access if necessary. The main indication for bladder outlet closure is urethral destruction secondary to prolonged catheter drainage in neurogenic bladder patients. A case series using "tight" autologous pubovaginal sling and lower urinary tract reconstruction for urethras destroyed by long-term Foley catheter use reported excellent results with minimal incontinence. The authors concluded that at least 1 cm of normal urethra was required for proper functioning of the sling. The risk of complications, specifically a vesicovaginal fistula, is relatively common and can be difficult to repair. It is important to remember that a bladder neck closure is much more difficult than a simple closure of the bladder wall. The bladder neck is usually hyperactive in patients with neurologic disease, and every voiding reflex includes active opening and closing of the bladder neck, which forcibly attempts to destroy the bladder neck closure. To reduce this risk, postoperative suppression of the voiding reflex using prolonged continuous catheter

drainage (3 weeks) and liberal use of anticholinergics is imperative. In addition, to reduce the risk of fistula, the repair must be watertight from the beginning, and this requires a precise mucosal closure using a running suture and multiple additional layers of muscle to reinforce the strength of the repair.

6. **d. Trigger voiding induces a reflex decrease in outlet resistance in patients with sphincter dyssynergia.** In some types of spinal cord injury or bladder dysfunction characterized by detrusor hyperreflexia, manual pressure may sometimes be used to initiate a reflexive bladder contraction—sometimes called "trigger voiding." The most effective method of initiating a reflex contraction is thought to be rhythmic suprapubic manual pressure, typically seven or eight compressions every 3 seconds. This rhythmic pressure is thought to produce a summation effect on the tension receptors in the bladder wall, resulting in an afferent neural discharge that activates the bladder reflex arc. Trigger voiding can also sometimes be induced by pulling the skin or hair of the pubis, scrotum, or thigh; squeezing the clitoris; or digital rectal stimulation. Surgical procedures to reduce outlet resistance should be considered, if significant obstruction or sphincter dyssynergia are present. In an animal model using neural rerouting, a detrusor contraction without striated sphincter dyssynergia could be initiated by scratching the skin or by percutaneous electrical stimulation in the L7 dermatome. The pathway was found to be mediated by cholinergic transmission at both ganglionic and peripheral levels. The importance of this experimental model is that somatic motor axons were able to innervate parasympathetic bladder ganglion cells and therefore transfer somatic reflex activity to the lower urinary tract.

7. **b. Perforation of the catheterizable channel.** These catheterizable channels are not free of complications, and long-term issues with catheterization, incontinence, and stomal stenosis can occur. A large retrospective study by Leslie et al. (2011) analyzed the long-term outcomes of 169 pediatric patients who had either undergone a Mitrofanoff appendicovesicostomy or a transverse ileal, or Monti, tube. The authors report a 39% revision rate (8% stricture, 4% prolapse, 10% incontinence, and 17% stomal stenosis at skin level). Perforation of the catheterizable channel has not been commonly reported as a complication.

8. **a. Chronic indwelling urethral catheterization protects against poor bladder compliance and upper tract complications.** The exact etiology of upper tract deterioration in patients with long-term indwelling catheters is unclear because the bladder should be well drained by a catheter; however, it is likely related to chronic "occult" or subclinical detrusor overactivity in the face of sphincteric dyssynergy providing a functional obstruction. Regardless of the etiology, it is clinically heralded by the development of poor detrusor compliance demonstrated on urodynamic studies.

9. **a. Similar incidence of bacteriuria and symptomatic UTIs to indwelling urethral catheters.**

10. **b. Gross hematuria in a patient with a chronic indwelling catheter is likely related to infection or inflammation and does not require a thorough hematuria workup.** The long-term risk of carcinoma in the spinal cord injury patient with a chronic catheter has been estimated to be 8% to 10%. This association has not been identified in patients performing intermittent catheterization. The development of gross hematuria in patients with a chronic indwelling catheter should prompt further evaluation, including upper tract imaging, urine cytology, cystoscopy, and consideration of bladder biopsy.

11. **c. It may lead to malignant lesions of the skin.** Prolonged exposure of the skin to a wet environment may lead to supersaturation and disruption of the skin's protective barriers, thus promoting skin maceration, dermatitis, and possibly infection. IAD can be defined as inflammation of the surface of the skin with redness, edema, and, in some cases, bullae containing clear exudate. IAD predominately occurs in skin folds and may promote candidiasis or bacterial skin infections. IAD has not been associated with premalignant or malignant lesions of the skin.

CHAPTER REVIEW

1. The goals of therapy for storage failure are low-pressure storage, improved bladder capacity, decreased incontinence due to detrusor overactivity, and preservation of renal function.
2. Augmentation cystoplasty is an option after failed conservative management such as pharmacologic therapy, intravesical botulinum toxin injection, or CIC.
3. Use of large bowel versus small bowel may lead to more significant metabolic disturbance, increased mucus production, and theoretically heightened risk of malignancy.
4. Goal of urethral injection therapy is to restore urethral mucosal coaptation and its hermetic seal effect, especially during periods of increased abdominal pressure.
5. Injectable agents are an option for patients who are not candidates for more invasive procedures. Efficacy and durability are generally inferior to surgery.
6. Functional urethral closure with pubovaginal sling provides pop-off valve for leakage at higher pressures and allows access for transurethral instrumentation.
7. Bladder neck closure with simultaneous LUT reconstruction may be successful in refractory patients with destroyed bladder outlet.
8. Indications for catheterizable channel include difficulty catheterizing per urethra, urethral scarring, and urethral incompetence requiring outlet closure.
9. Complications of continent catheterizable channels include long-term issues with catheterization, incontinence, and stomal stenosis.
10. Asymptomatic bacteriuria is common in catheterized patients and does not require treatment unless the patient becomes symptomatic.
11. Chronic catheterization (CIC or indwelling) may lead to poor bladder compliance and upper tract deterioration; thus periodic surveillance is recommended.
12. Credé and Valsalva maneuvers may elevate intravesical pressure enough to cause upper tract deterioration, especially in a setting of poor detrusor compliance.
13. Reflex voiding depends on the ability to stimulate detrusor contractions and may be most suitable for patients with spinal cord injury (SCI) or neurogenic detrusor overactivity.
14. Condom catheter use is associated with lower rate of bacteriuria, symptomatic UTIs, and death than indwelling Foley; also more comfortable and less restrictive.
15. Complications of condom catheter include allergic reactions, penile edema; higher risk for pressure sores in patients with impaired sensation or cognition.
16. Consumers spend billions of dollars on absorbent products; selection is often based on trial and error, cost, convenience, and manufacturers' claims.
17. IAD is inflammation of skin with redness, edema, and/or bullae with clear exudate; it is often found in skin folds and may promote candidiasis or bacterial skin infections.

128 Aging and Geriatric Urology

Tomas L. Griebling

QUESTIONS

1. With aging:
   a. renal function increases.
   b. bladder capacity declines.
   c. hepatic function remains relatively stable.
   d. pulmonary function declines.
   e. immunologic function remains stable.

2. Urinary tract infections (UTIs) in elderly women may best be decreased by:
   a. nitrofurantoin prophylaxis.
   b. systemic estrogen administration.
   c. cranberry juice.
   d. vaginal estrogen application.
   e. α-blocker therapy.

3. In demented elderly patients, incontinence:
   a. is inevitable.
   b. is virtually always due to detrusor hyperreflexia.
   c. is unlikely to respond to therapy.
   d. is multifactorial and often reversible.
   e. treatment should focus primarily on preventing skin breakdown.

4. Urinary incontinence (UI) in older people is usually:
   a. brought to a physician's attention by the patient.
   b. detected by the patient's primary physician.
   c. obvious to the urologist.
   d. detected by the physician but ignored.
   e. unknown to the patient's physician.

5. In older patients, involuntary bladder contractions:
   a. are rarely seen in asymptomatic patients.
   b. are primarily due to central nervous system (CNS) pathology.
   c. are almost always the cause of the patient's incontinence.
   d. are inevitable in demented patients.
   e. may not be the cause of the incontinence.

6. After the history and physical examination, evaluation of the incontinent older patient should include:
   a. cystoscopy.
   b. videourodynamics.
   c. postvoid residual assessment.
   d. urinary cytology.
   e. assessment of prostate size in a male.

7. Which of the following occurs as part of normal aging?
   a. Urinary incontinence
   b. A small increase in serum creatinine concentration
   c. Uninhibited detrusor contractions
   d. Increase in bladder capacity
   e. Urinary flow rate is unchanged

8. The cornerstone of treatment for persistent urgency incontinence is:
   a. behavioral therapy.
   b. flavoxate.
   c. oxybutynin.
   d. tolterodine.
   e. solifenacin.

9. Acute urinary retention in an older man:
   a. indicates the need for surgical decompression.
   b. is treated effectively with α-adrenergic blockers.
   c. can be seen with detrusor hyperactivity with impaired contractility (DHIC).
   d. is treated effectively with bethanechol.
   e. requires treatment of the underlying urinary tract abnormality.

10. Incontinence management products (e.g., garments/pads):
    a. are reimbursed by insurance companies.
    b. should include menstrual pads.
    c. generally cost less than a dollar per day.
    d. should be chosen according to the type of incontinence rather than its severity.
    e. should be tailored to the individual.

11. The voiding diary completed by an 83-year-old woman bothered by daytime incontinence discloses 800-mL output between 8:00 am and 11:00 pm, and 1500 mL from 11:00 pm to 8:00 am. The next step should be:
    a. to have her repeat it with a record of fluid intake.
    b. to take furosemide at 7:00 pm each evening to reduce nocturnal excretion.
    c. to use pressure-gradient stockings to minimize peripheral edema.
    d. to advise her to curtail fluid intake after dinner.
    e. none of the above.

12. Anticholinergic bladder relaxants may, ironically, actually exacerbate incontinence through all of the following mechanisms EXCEPT:
    a. causing/exacerbating confusion.
    b. causing/exacerbating impaired mobility.
    c. causing/exacerbating a dry mouth.
    d. causing/exacerbating subacute urinary retention.
    e. precipitating acute urinary retention.

13. A 78-year-old woman with dementia has responded modestly to donepezil (Aricept, a cholinesterase inhibitor) for the past year. The recent onset of urgency incontinence led her primary physician to prescribe tolterodine last month while awaiting your assessment. Her incontinence has responded well. The next appropriate step is to:
    a. discontinue tolterodine due to its interaction with donepezil.
    b. discontinue donepezil because her cognitive function is stable.

c. discontinue both drugs because she is stable and the urgency incontinence may reflect an adverse effect of the donepezil.

d. continue both drugs and monitor her for deterioration in cognitive function.

e. taper the tolterodine.

14. A 68-year-old obese woman with significant daily stress incontinence comes for a follow-up. Her bladder diary shows maximal voided volume of 125 mL during the daytime. Each of these measures is appropriate EXCEPT:

a. adjustment of fluid excretion and voiding intervals.

b. advising weight reduction.

c. teaching her postural maneuvers.

d. consideration of surgical correction.

e. pelvic floor muscle exercises.

15. A 72-year-old man has urinary urgency and postvoid residual (PVR) of 40 mL. He also has hypertension and aortic stenosis that has caused minimal symptoms. His friend suggested that he ask for terazosin because it helped him with similar symptoms. The most appropriate response is:

a. to prescribe terazosin and see him again in 4 weeks.

b. to prescribe alfuzosin instead, because it has a better side-effect profile.

c. to obtain medical consultation before prescribing the drug.

d. to perform urodynamic testing before deciding.

e. to prescribe an anticholinergic agent.

ANSWERS

1. **d. Pulmonary function declines.** Pulmonary surface area for oxygen diffusion decreases, which leads to alterations in the ventilation perfusion ratio. With aging, renal function and renal mass decline, bladder capacity remains relatively stable but elasticity and contractility decline, and hepatic and immunologic function decline.

2. **d. Vaginal estrogen application.** It has been proposed that vaginal estrogens promote the growth of lactobacillus and thereby lower vaginal pH, which helps reduce pathogen colonization. Systemic estrogens are generally not prescribed in the elderly and may in fact cause incontinence in this population. Nitrofurantoin should not be given during the long term in the elderly because it may reduce renal function and lead to pulmonary fibrosis. Cranberry juice has its advocates but has not been shown to be effective in randomized trials, and α-blocker therapy in the female would not be expected to have much of an effect on residual urine as the female has few alpha receptors at the bladder neck.

3. **d. Is multifactorial and often reversible.** Incontinence is never normal, even with dementia. Detrusor overactivity (DO) is the most common type of lower urinary tract dysfunction among demented incontinent nursing home residents, but it is also the most common dysfunction among their dry peers. Moreover, incontinence in 40% of these individuals is not associated with DO but with obstruction (in men), stress incontinence (in women), or a combination of an outlet and a detrusor problem, and the cause does not correlate with either the presence or severity of dementia. Thus it is no longer tenable to attribute incontinence a priori to DO. Because incontinence in the elderly is usually multifactorial, involving urinary tract as well as nonurinary tract contributions, it is often treatable. Even among nursing home patients, studies have documented more than a 50% reduction in incontinent episodes overall and full daytime continence in nearly 40% of residents. Particularly among demented individuals, nonurinary factors are prevalent and commonly include medication

use, depression, fecal impaction, UTI, atrophic vaginitis, and disorders of fluid excretion. It is important to prevent skin breakdown, but this should not be the primary approach to the incontinent nursing home resident.

4. **e. Unknown to the patient's physician.** Despite the fact that incontinence is so common and amenable to therapy, most patients do not mention it to a physician. Reasons include embarrassment, misperception that it is a normal part of aging, belief that it is untreatable, fear of complications associated with its evaluation and treatment, or misconception that only major surgery can cure it. Moreover, when patients do mention it, most physicians either dismiss it as a normal part of aging or merely check a urinalysis. With newer undergarments and pads that better absorb and deodorize, the doctor may be unaware of the problem unless he/she asks about it.

5. **e. May not be the cause of the incontinence.** It is important to realize that involuntary bladder contractions are found commonly in even continent, neurologically intact elderly; the prevalence ranges in various studies between 50% and 55%. This fact underscores the concept that such contractions are a risk factor for UI but not necessarily sufficient. Moreover, even when such contractions are the major contributor to UI, they may be due to a urethral abnormality. More than half of obstructed individuals and approximately 25% of those with stress incontinence have associated DO that usually remits with correction of the urethral abnormality alone. The proportion of elderly individuals in whom DO remits is likely lower, but clearly it is insufficient merely to identify involuntary contractions on cystometry and attribute the incontinence to them. To be considered the cause of the UI, such contractions must reproduce the patient's type of leakage, and urethral abnormalities must be excluded. This is particularly important because a bladder relaxant medication prescribed for DO that is actually due to obstruction may precipitate acute retention.

6. **c. Postvoid residual assessment.** Determining the PVR is essential in all incontinent older individuals, not only because retention can mimic other causes of UI, but also because knowledge of the PVR will affect therapy. For instance, an older woman with DO and PVR of 250 mL would be approached differently from a woman with DO and PVR of 5 mL. The rest of the diagnostic evaluation depends on the need for diagnostic certainty. However, if surgical correction is contemplated, or if the risk of empiric therapy exceeds the benefit, further testing is warranted. Cytology is indicated when bladder carcinoma is suspected and would be treated if found (i.e., not in a bedfast, demented patient). Cystoscopy has many indications, but it is not routinely required for evaluation of incontinence, nor is it alone sufficient to detect or exclude prostatic obstruction. Palpated prostate size correlates poorly with the presence of obstruction.

7. **c. Uninhibited detrusor contractions.** Incontinence is never part of normal aging. Even at age 90 years, at least half of people are continent. Although renal function declines in most older adults, there is no change in serum creatinine because of a concomitant and balanced decrease in muscle mass. Involuntary detrusor contractions are common in continent and even asymptomatic elderly, but are rarely seen during routine cystometry in younger people. Bladder capacity may decrease in the elderly, but there is no evidence for an increase. Flow rate declines, not only because obstruction becomes more likely in aging men, but also because detrusor contractility appears to decrease in both sexes.

8. **a. Behavioral therapy.** Behavioral therapy is the cornerstone of treatment for detrusor overactivity, although the type of therapy must be tailored to the individual. Bladder retraining attempts to restore a normal voiding pattern by progressively lengthening the voiding interval. Scheduled toileting aims to reduce incontinence by frequent voiding, which reduces total bladder volume and the chance of triggering involuntary bladder contractions. Prompted voiding works by regularly and frequently reminding cognitively impaired residents of the

need to void. The role of medications is to supplement behavioral therapy, but only if needed. By reducing bladder irritability, such agents allow the bladder to hold more urine before the spasm occurs. However, even when continence is restored by these drugs, detrusor overactivity is still generally demonstrable. Furthermore, if the drug increases residual urine more than total bladder capacity, it may paradoxically decrease functional capacity, allowing the persistent involuntary contraction to occur at more frequent intervals. Thus before deciding that drug therapy has failed, PVR should be remeasured. Except for flavoxate, each of the agents listed has been proved effective in randomized controlled trials that included a substantial number of elderly patients.

9. **c. Can be seen with detrusor hyperactivity with impaired contractility (DHIC).** The differential diagnosis for urinary retention extends beyond urethral obstruction, particularly in the elderly. Patients with underactive detrusor or DHIC also may develop urinary retention. In addition, fecal impaction, pain (e.g., following hip replacement), and medications with urinary tract side effects (e.g., anticholinergics, sedating antihistamines, decongestants, and opiates) may induce acute urinary retention, particularly in patients with underlying bladder weakness or obstruction. Thus the bladder should be decompressed for at least a week while reversible causes are addressed; the larger the PVR, the longer should be the decompression. Decompression allows some restoration of detrusor strength, which also facilitates urodynamic testing should it be necessary. α-Adrenergic blockers are effective for men with symptoms of prostatism, but clinical trials excluded patients with significant urinary retention. Bethanechol, although originally designed to improve bladder emptying in unobstructed patients, has not proved effective for this purpose (and likely not for nonobstructed patients either). Decompression in some elderly patients can reduce but not eliminate residual urine; provided it does not cause symptoms or renal compromise, subclinical retention need not necessarily be treated in all elderly patients, even if obstruction is present.

10. **e. Should be tailored to the individual.** The cost of pads is rarely covered by insurance and can easily exceed $1/day. Menstrual pads, although often used for incontinence, are usually inappropriate. They are designed to absorb small amounts of slowly leaking viscid fluid rather than rapid gushes of urine. From among the numerous types of pads and garments, selection should be tailored to the individual's needs and comorbidity; the type of incontinence matters less than severity.

11. **e. None of the above.** The patient's altered pattern of fluid excretion may occur for a variety of reasons. The most common is accumulation of peripheral edema due to venous insufficiency, peripheral vascular disease, low albumin states (malnutrition, hepatic disease), congestive heart failure, or medications (e.g., nonsteroidal antiinflammatory drugs [NSAIDs], dihydropyridine calcium channel blockers [e.g., nifedipine], or thiazolidinediones [e.g., rosiglitazone]). Each can be readily addressed. Before doing so, however, it is important to realize that the multiple pathologic conditions so often found in the elderly may be causal, contributory, a consequence, or unrelated to the condition for which the patient seeks help. In this individual, daytime leakage is the problem. Addressing the excess nocturnal excretion will not improve the daytime problem and, if it shifts the excess nocturnal excretion to the daytime (e.g., by use of pressure-gradient stockings), therapy may exacerbate the daytime leakage. If the nocturnal polyuria can be eliminated entirely (e.g., by substituting a drug that does not cause fluid retention), this should be done. If, however, therapy will only shift excretion to the daytime, one may elect not to treat if it is not dangerous (e.g., venous insufficiency). Evening furosemide risks inducing hypovolemia and increasing her risk of falls and fracture. Daytime predominance of incontinence suggests that she has stress incontinence, or DO associated with bladder neck incompetence that is exacerbated when she is upright. Once the cause is sorted out, the appropriate intervention can be prescribed, but in this individual, it should not include alteration of fluid intake: Her daytime output is too small

to contribute to her daytime UI and, unless she is ingesting 2 L after dinner, her intake is also likely unrelated to her nocturnal polyuria. Moreover, the older kidney generally takes twice as long to respond to fluid restriction as the younger one, so restricting fluid after dinner is apt to do little. This case highlights the need to tailor the evaluation and treatment to the patient rather than to a given abnormality.

12. **b. Causing/exacerbating impaired mobility.** All of the currently available bladder relaxant medications have anticholinergic properties and thus can cause anticholinergic side effects. Dry mouth (xerostomia) results from the anticholinergic effect on the salivary and parotid glands. Even the M_3-specific agents have this effect, because M_3 receptors are the predominant receptor in these glands as well as in the bladder. Because bladder relaxants generally do not abolish the involuntary detrusor contractions, the xerostomia-mediated increased fluid intake results in the bladder filling more frequently to the volume at which detrusor contractions may be triggered. Bladder relaxants often impair detrusor contractility and can lead to subacute retention. If the increase in PVR is more than the increase in total bladder capacity, the effective bladder capacity will decrease. In turn, this could allow involuntary contractions to occur at a lower effective volume; an increase in incontinence frequency can ensue.

13. **d. Continue both drugs and monitor her for deterioration in cognitive function.** Because cholinesterase inhibitors block the metabolism of acetylcholine, there is concern that they will provoke urgency incontinence, especially in older adults who already may have underlying age-related involuntary detrusor contractions that have not yet caused incontinence. However, despite prescription of these agents to millions of demented patients, there is little evidence that they cause incontinence. Moreover, because the benefits of these drugs for dementia are modest at best and are not seen in the majority of patients who use them, patients and families may decide that the benefit of the bladder relaxant outweighs the risk. Particularly in this patient, who has already benefited from tolterodine without notable cognitive deterioration, it is worth continuing therapy and monitoring her cognitive status.

14. **a. Adjustment of fluid excretion and voiding intervals.** Recent evidence suggests that weight loss will improve stress incontinence in obese women, and data support the use of postural maneuvers, pelvic floor muscle exercises, and surgical correction as well. Adjusting fluid excretion and voiding intervals can also be useful, especially for women with volume-dependent stress leakage. It can work particularly well for women with a threshold of at least 150 mL and best in those with a threshold greater than 250 mL. However, when the threshold is this low, the extent of fluid restriction required is usually not feasible and might even lead to dangerous dehydration.

15. **c. To obtain medical consultation before prescribing the drug.** Men with these lower urinary tract symptoms and a low PVR generally respond well to an α-adrenergic receptor blocker. However, many of these agents can reduce cardiac preload and thus impede adequate left ventricular filling and cardiac output, especially in individuals whose ventricular filling is already more difficult in the setting of left ventricular hypertrophy. The risk is exacerbated by the normal age-related decline that occurs in baroreflex sensitivity and further compounded in patients who take a β blocker and/or have aortic stenosis. Thus although the overall risks of orthostasis, falls, and fracture appear to be lower with the newer α-adrenergic agents, it would be prudent to obtain medical consultation before prescribing an α-blocker in this clinical setting. Anticholinergic therapy can be used in men with urgency and a low PVR, but because of the risk of inducing a tachycardia in a man with aortic stenosis and thereby also reducing left ventricular filling—combined with the potential risk of inducing urinary retention—prescription of an anticholinergic should not be the next step.

CHAPTER REVIEW

1. Renal blood flow, renal mass, and functional reserve decrease with aging, which results in a 10-mL decrease in glomerular filtration rate (GFR) per decade.
2. Serum creatinine levels do not accurately reflect renal function in the elderly due to decreased muscle mass. The Cockcroft-Gault formula is more accurate than the Modification of Diet in Renal Disease equation for estimating GFR in the elderly population.
3. Antidiuretic hormone secretion decreases in older adults, resulting in increased nocturia.
4. With age, there is a decrease in cardiac output and stroke volume.
5. The majority of deaths in the perioperative period in geriatric patients are due to cardiovascular events; however, pulmonary problems are the major cause of prolonged hospitalization.
6. Hepatic function and immunologic function diminish with age.
7. With aging, there is a loss of muscle mass and an increase in body fat mass.
8. Bladder capacity does not change with age; however, bladder sensation, contractility, and ability to postpone voiding decline in both sexes with age.
9. Increased involuntary detrusor contractions and decreased bladder elasticity and compliance occur with aging. Indeed, detrusor overactivity is the most common type of lower urinary tract dysfunction in incontinent elderly of both sexes.
10. There is a decrease in striated muscle in the rhabdosphincter with age.
11. Urinary incontinence, UTIs, pelvic prolapse, and bladder outlet obstruction all increase with aging.
12. Stress incontinence in elderly women is usually associated with hypermobility and some degree of intrinsic sphincter deficiency.
13. A functional assessment is correlated with health care outcomes and includes: (1) activities of daily living, (2) mobility with a slow gate speed a strong predictor of mortality, and (3) cognition.
14. Cognitive changes are frequently seen following anesthesia in elderly patients.
15. There is no difference in mortality and morbidity between general and regional anesthesia in the elderly.
16. Major geriatric syndromes include frailty, falls, pressure ulcers, multiple medications, delirium, and urinary incontinence.
17. The frailty phenotype may include an unintentional weight loss in excess of 10 lb per year, reduced grip, slowing of the gait, decreased activity, and easy exhaustion with activity.
18. Elderly men on androgen deprivation therapy are at increased risks for fractures.
19. A number of medications should be used with caution or not used at all in the elderly. For example, Demerol and prolonged use of nitrofurantoin should not be given and caution should be exercised when prescribing antimuscarinics. Anticholinergic agents are one of the most common causes of delirium in the elderly, especially in those with preexisting cognitive or functional impairment.
20. Asymptomatic bacteriuria in the elderly does not require treatment; it does not cause incontinence.
21. Peripheral edema may be mobilized when supine and cause nocturia.
22. Conservative measures used to treat excessive fluid output at night include compression stockings, changing the time diuretics are taken or administering a rapid acting diuretic in the late afternoon, and altering the diet.
23. Poststroke fecal and urinary incontinence are not uncommon.
24. Incontinence may be due to impaired mobility and/or cognition.
25. Timed voidings may be helpful in controlling incontinence.
26. An elevated postvoid residual is common in older adults.
27. Decreased fluid consumption may worsen urge incontinence due to the concentrated urine acting as an irritant on the detrusor.
28. Pelvic floor exercises, when done correctly, may be helpful in treating incontinence.
29. If a chronic indwelling catheter is required, a suprapubic tube is preferable to a urethral catheter.
30. α-Blockers are associated with the "floppy iris syndrome," and the ophthalmologist should be informed of their use prior to any ophthalmologic surgery.
31. An underactive bladder characterized by poor bladder emptying is not necessarily due to outlet obstruction and occurs in both men and women. Both structural and functional changes occur in the bladder. Currently there is no effective medication for this condition.
32. Sleep abnormalities may be responsible for nocturia and may worsen the severity of neurologic conditions which affect the bladder.
33. Nocturia once per night in the elderly is considered normal.
34. Nocturia is usually multifactorial in the elderly and thus is often not adequately addressed with a single treatment modality.
35. Hyponatremia is a significant risk factor when desmopressin is given to the elderly.
36. Fecal and urinary problems often coexist, and one may cause the other.
37. UTIs may present atypically in the elderly with symptoms of confusion, agitation, lethargy, and anorexia.
38. Vaginal estrogens are useful for reducing UTIs in elderly women.
39. Elder mistreatment screening is an important part of the urologic evaluation, just as child abuse screening is an important part of the pediatric urologic visit.

129 Urinary Tract Fistulae

Dirk J.M.K. De Ridder and Tamsin Greenwell

QUESTIONS

1. The most common cause of vesicovaginal fistulae in the non-industrialized, developing world is:
   a. cesarean section.
   b. surgical trauma during abdominal hysterectomy.
   c. surgical trauma during vaginal hysterectomy.
   d. obstructed labor.
   e. none of the above.

2. The most common type of acquired urinary fistulae is:
   a. vesicovaginal fistula.
   b. ureterovaginal fistula.
   c. colovesical fistula.
   d. rectourethral fistula.
   e. vesicouterine fistula.

3. Vesicovaginal fistulae (VVF) may occur as a result of:
   a. locally advanced vaginal cancer.
   b. incidentally noted and repaired iatrogenic cystotomy during hysterectomy.
   c. radiotherapy for cervical cancer.
   d. cystocele repair with bladder neck suspension.
   e. all of the above.

4. Intraoperative consultation is requested by a gynecologist for a possible urinary tract injury during a difficult abdominal hysterectomy. There is clear fluid noted in the pelvis. The gynecologist is particularly worried about postoperative VVF formation. All of the following statements are correct regarding counseling this gynecologist EXCEPT:
   a. The incidence of iatrogenic bladder injury during hysterectomy is approximately 0.5% to 1.0%.
   b. Approximately 0.1% to 0.2% of individuals undergoing hysterectomy develop a VVF.
   c. The risk of ureterovaginal fistula is greater than the risk of VVF in this setting.
   d. The absence of blue-stained fluid in the operative field following the administration of intravenous indigo carmine does not eliminate a possibility of a urinary tract injury.
   e. All of the above are true.

5. VVF due to obstructed labor are:
   a. the most common etiology of VVF in sub-Saharan Africa.
   b. usually located at the vaginal apex.
   c. never associated with simultaneous rectovaginal fistula.
   d. typically found in multiparous women.
   e. usually smaller and simpler to repair than those associated with gynecologic surgery.

6. A 47-year-old woman presents with the new onset of constant urinary leakage 5 years after completing radiation therapy for locally advanced cervical carcinoma. All of the following may be considered part of the diagnostic evaluation EXCEPT:
   a. cystoscopy and possible biopsy.
   b. voiding cystourethrography (VCUG).
   c. computed tomographic (CT) scan of the abdomen and pelvis.
   d. urodynamics.
   e. ureteroscopy.

7. A 52-year-old woman with a history of an abdominal hysterectomy 2 months previously presents for the evaluation of a constant clear vaginal discharge since the surgery. Following oral intake of Pyridium, her pads continue to have a clear watery discharge. The most likely diagnosis is:
   a. vesicovaginal fistula.
   b. ureterovaginal fistula.
   c. peritoneovaginal fistula.
   d. vesicouterine fistula.
   e. urethrovaginal fistula.

8. In the industrialized world, postsurgical VVF are associated with ureteral injury in approximately:
   a. 0.01% of cases.
   b. 0.1% of cases.
   c. 10% of cases.
   d. 25% of cases.
   e. 50% of cases.

9. A 68-year-old woman presents with a 1-week history of vaginal leakage 6 months after completion of radiation therapy for locally advanced cervical cancer. VCUG reveals a VVF. On physical examination, the fistula is irregular and indurated, and approximately 3 mm in size. Cystoscopy reveals bullous edema surrounding the fistula, and biopsy of the fistula tract reveals only fibrosis without evidence of malignancy. There is no suggestion of recurrent malignancy on CT scan. She should be counseled that:
   a. the optimal timing for repair of this fistula may be in 5 to 6 months.
   b. the best chance to repair this fistula is with immediate surgical intervention.
   c. a vaginal approach is not indicated.
   d. the use of an adjuvant flap will not be necessary.
   e. the success rate for the repair of this fistula is similar to that of a nonradiated VVF.

10. The abdominal approach to VVF repair:
    a. is the preferred approach in all patients with VVF.
    b. has a higher success rate than the vaginal approach.
    c. is suitable for the use of an omental interpositional flap.
    d. is associated with less morbidity and a shorter hospital stay than the vaginal approach.
    e. is more often associated with postoperative vaginal shortening and dyspareunia than the vaginal approach.

11. The vaginal approach to an uncomplicated VVF repair:
    a. is most often bolstered with use of a gracilis flap.
    b. may be accomplished with a multilayer-layer closure.

c. requires the use of nonabsorbable suture.

d. is not indicated for obstetric-related fistula.

e. is contraindicated if the fistula tract is within 2 cm of the ureter.

12. Principles of urinary fistula repair include all of the following EXCEPT:

a. excision of the fistula tract.

b. tension-free closure.

c. use of well-vascularized tissue flaps.

d. watertight closure.

e. adequate postoperative urinary drainage.

13. Level I evidence (one or more randomized control trials) exists to support which of the following statements?

a. Preoperative administration of topical estrogens improves tissue quality prior to the repair of VVF.

b. Preoperative administration of topical estrogens improves the success rate of transvaginal VVF repair.

c. Preoperative administration of broad-spectrum intravenous antibiotics improves the success rate of all types of VVF repair.

d. Suprapubic bladder drainage is superior to urethral (Foley) catheter drainage in preventing surgical failure following VVF repair.

e. None of the above.

14. Vaginal repair of VVF is contraindicated in:

a. multiparous women.

b. large fistulae.

c. radiation-induced fistulae.

d. fistulae located at the vaginal cuff.

e. none of the above.

15. Potential complications of repair for a VVF following abdominal hysterectomy include all of the following EXCEPT:

a. stress urinary incontinence.

b. dyspareunia.

c. recurrence of the fistula.

d. urinary urgency and frequency.

e. ureteral injury.

16. Advantages of the transabdominal approach to VVF repair as compared with the transvaginal repair include all of the following EXCEPT:

a. ease of mobilization of the omentum as an interpositional flap.

b. decreased rate of intraoperative ureteral injury.

c. preservation of vaginal depth.

d. easier access to the apical VVF in individuals with high narrow vaginal canals.

e. ability to perform an augmentation cystoplasty through the same incision.

17. Seventeen days following a transvaginal VVF repair, a cystogram is performed. The bladder is filled to 100 mL with contrast medium and several images are taken. There is no evidence of a fistula on the filling images; however, the patient was unable to void during the study. A postvoid film was not obtained. This study:

a. demonstrates successful repair of the VVF, and the catheter should be removed.

b. is nondiagnostic, because it was done too soon following repair.

c. is nondiagnostic, because there are no voiding images or postvoid images.

d. is nondiagnostic, because the bladder was not filled to an adequate volume.

e. should be terminated and cystoscopy performed to examine for a persistent fistula.

18. Before surgical mobilization, the blood supply to a potential Martius flap (fibrofatty labial flap) is through the:

a. inferior hemorrhoidal artery.

b. external pudendal artery.

c. uterine artery.

d. inferior epigastric artery.

e. gonadal artery.

19. An interpositional flap of the greater omentum during VVF repair:

a. may be able to reach the deep pelvis without any mobilization in some patients.

b. is most commonly based on the superior mesenteric artery.

c. is contraindicated in the setting of inflammation or infection.

d. should not be divided or incised vertically in the midline because this may compromise the blood supply.

e. is most commonly used during a transvaginal approach.

20. A 39-year-old woman presents with constant vaginal leakage for 1 month following an abdominal hysterectomy. She describes symptoms of stress incontinence before the hysterectomy. She has no urgency and is voiding normally. Physical examination demonstrates no obvious fistula tract at the vaginal cuff. Oral phenazopyridine is given, and the bladder is filled with 100 mL of saline mixed with indigo carmine. A gauze pad is packed from the apex of the vagina proximally to the introitus distally, and the patient is told to ambulate for 90 minutes. Upon the patient's return, the pad is removed and examined. The most proximal portion of the pad is stained yellow-orange, and the most distal portion is blue. This is most consistent with:

a. ureterovaginal fistula.

b. vesicovaginal fistula.

c. urethrovaginal fistula.

d. a and b.

e. a and c.

21. Ureterovaginal fistulae are:

a. not associated with transvaginal hysterectomy.

b. usually associated with normal voiding patterns.

c. best diagnosed on VCUG.

d. found more commonly following hysterectomy for malignancy than for benign indications.

e. usually located in the middle one-third of the ureter.

22. Two weeks following an emergent cesarean section for fetal distress during labor, a 28-year-old woman reports constant leakage per vagina. Analysis of the collected fluid reveals it to have a high creatinine level consistent with urine. Physical examination, including pelvic examination, reveals absolutely no abnormalities or surgical trauma to suggest a urinary fistula. There is no stress incontinence elicited on physical examination. Renal ultrasonography demonstrates no hydronephrosis, and the bladder is empty. The most likely diagnosis is:

a. occult vesicovaginal fistula.

b. occult ureterovaginal fistula.

c. urethrovaginal fistula.

    d. vesicouterine fistula.

    e. peritoneovaginal fistula.

23. Vesicouterine fistulae occur most commonly due to:

    a. low-segment cesarean section.

    b. vaginal delivery.

    c. malignancy.

    d. conization of the cervix.

    e. myomectomy.

24. Potential options for therapy of vesicouterine fistula in a patient desiring long-term preservation of fertility include:

    a. observation.

    b. cystoscopy and fulguration of the fistula tract.

    c. hormonal therapy.

    d. surgical exploration and repair of the fistula with interpositional omental flap.

    e. all of the above.

25. Two months following resection of a large urethral diverticulum extending proximally beyond the bladder neck, a patient complains of urinary leakage. All of the following may be the source of this patient's symptoms EXCEPT:

    a. a urethrovaginal fistula.

    b. a vesicovaginal fistula.

    c. stress urinary incontinence.

    d. a recurrent urethral diverticulum.

    e. a vesicouterine fistula.

26. Urethrovaginal fistulae in the distal one-third of the urethra:

    a. are often asymptomatic.

    b. are associated with significant bladder overactivity.

    c. cannot be repaired using a vaginal flap technique.

    d. can result in severe stress incontinence.

    e. are usually the result of malignant infiltration.

27. The most common cause of a colovesical fistula is:

    a. colon cancer.

    b. bladder cancer.

    c. prostate cancer.

    d. Crohn disease.

    e. diverticulitis.

28. CT scan findings suggestive of a colovesical fistula include:

    a. intravesical mass, air in the bladder, and bladder wall thickening.

    b. air in the bladder, bowel wall thickening adjacent to the bladder, and clear fluid in a bowel segment adjacent to the bladder.

    c. air in the bladder, bladder wall thickening adjacent to a loop of thickened bowel wall, and the presence of colonic diverticula.

    d. air in the colon, colonic mass adjacent to the bladder, and debris within the bladder.

    e. air in the colon, bladder wall thickening, and an intravesical mass.

29. In the evaluation of a possible colovesical fistula, cystoscopy:

    a. has high diagnostic accuracy in revealing the cause of the fistula.

    b. has a high yield in identifying potential fistulae.

    c. should not be performed due to the risk of sepsis.

    d. is usually normal.

    e. most commonly reveals a large connection to the bowel.

30. A 62-year-old man presents with pneumaturia and recurrent urinary tract infections. A cystoscopy is performed, revealing a bullous lesion on the posterior bladder wall. Two hours later, a CT scan is performed, revealing air in the bladder. In this patient, air in the bladder:

    a. suggests colovesical fistula.

    b. may be due to a bacterial infection.

    c. may be due to instrumentation.

    d. is a nonspecific finding.

    e. all of the above.

31. The most common cause of a ureterocolic fistula is:

    a. locally extensive colon cancer.

    b. appendicitis with an associated abscess.

    c. diverticulitis.

    d. Crohn disease.

    e. tuberculosis.

32. The incidence of rectal injury during radical retropubic prostatectomy is:

    a. 0.1%.

    b. 1.0%.

    c. 5.0%.

    d. 10%.

    e. 20-fold higher in patients undergoing laparoscopic radical prostatectomy.

33. Rectourethral fistula (RUF) formation following brachytherapy for prostate cancer:

    a. may require complex reconstructive surgery or urinary diversion for repair.

    b. is located at the level of the prostate.

    c. is associated with fecaluria.

    d. may be associated with recurrent malignancy.

    e. may relate to all of the above.

34. A 61-year-old otherwise healthy man returns to the office with symptoms of mild stress urinary incontinence and fecaluria 3 weeks following radical retropubic prostatectomy. A VCUG is performed and reveals a 1-mm fistula at the vesicourethral junction. The prostate-specific antigen (PSA) is undetectable, and the final pathology reveals organ-confined disease. This patient should be counseled that:

    a. a York-Mason transsphincteric approach to this fistula is associated with a high risk of anal incontinence.

    b. a trial of indwelling catheterization may result in resolution of the fistula.

    c. immediate colostomy is indicated.

    d. the stress incontinence will become more severe following repair of the fistula.

    e. urinary and fecal diversion will be necessary to repair this fistula.

35. Pyelovascular fistulae:

    a. are usually related to percutaneous procedures in the upper urinary tract.

    b. are most often due to renal malignancy.

    c. should be treated by removal of the nephrostomy tube.

    d. usually occur following radiation therapy.

    e. are usually fatal.

36. A 74-year-old woman with a history of colon cancer and external beam radiotherapy develops ureteral obstruction, and a stent is placed. Three months later, she presents with severe anemia and ongoing bright red gross hematuria for several hours. On examination she is pale and tachycardic, with a thready pulse and a systolic blood pressure of 60. As resuscitation is initiated with fluids and blood transfusion, the next step in management is:

   a. a CT scan of the abdomen and pelvis.

   b. cystoscopy, removal of the stent, and retrograde pyelography.

   c. immediate laparotomy and possible nephrectomy.

   d. angiography.

   e. a tagged red blood cell scan to lateralize the bleeding.

IMAGING

1. See Fig. 129.1. A 36-year-old woman presents with increased vaginal discharge 3 weeks after an abdominal hysterectomy. On the axial CT images in the delayed excretory phase, the most likely diagnosis is:

   a. vesicovaginal fistula.

   b. ureterovaginal fistula.

   c. colovesical fistula.

   d. ureteral duplication.

   e. vesicocutaneous fistula.

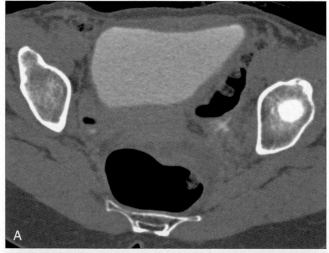

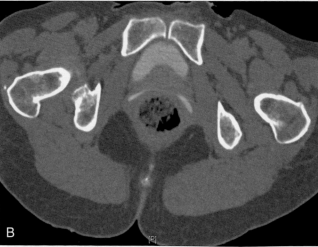

Fig. 129.1

ANSWERS

1. **d. Obstructed labor.** In the industrialized world, the most common cause of VVF is surgical trauma during gynecologic surgery, specifically hysterectomy. In the developing world, untreated obstructed labor results in ischemic necrosis of the anterior vaginal wall and underlying lower urinary tract and is the most common fistula in these geographic areas.

2. **a. Vesicovaginal fistula.** The vast majority of urinary fistulae involve the bladder and vagina in both the industrialized and nonindustrialized world. The other types of fistulae listed are much less common.

3. **e. All of the above.** Causes of VVF in the industrialized world include surgical trauma during hysterectomy, locally advanced gynecologic malignancy, anterior vaginal wall prolapse, anti-incontinence surgery, and pelvic radiotherapy. Intraoperative recognition and repair of bladder injury during hysterectomy should reduce the probability of VVF formation, but it does not eliminate the possibility.

4. **c. The risk of ureterovaginal fistula is greater than the risk of VVF in this setting.** The most common injury to the urinary tract during hysterectomy is a bladder laceration. Although ureteral injuries are not uncommon, they occur far less frequently than bladder injuries. Furthermore, ureterovaginal fistulae are much less common than VVF. The absence of blue-colored fluid in the pelvis does not exclude injury to the urinary tract. For example, a small bladder laceration may not be evident, especially if the bladder is decompressed with a Foley catheter.

5. **a. The most common etiology of VVF in sub-Saharan Africa.** VVF in the developing world occur primarily due to obstructed labor. Typically, these occur in individuals who are young primigravidas with a narrow bony pelvis. These fistulae are usually large; located distally in the vagina, sometimes encompassing large segments of the trigone, posterior bladder wall, and bladder neck; and are often part of a larger complex of presenting signs and symptoms termed the "obstructed labor injury complex," which includes rectovaginal fistulae. Because of their size and extensive ischemia of the surrounding tissues, these fistulae are often difficult to repair.

6. **e. Ureteroscopy.** This individual does not have diagnosis of VVF, and therefore multiple considerations are present. Nevertheless, VVF is a strong possibility given the history of radiation therapy and pelvic malignancy. A VCUG can establish the presence of a fistula. Cystoscopy and biopsy of a fistula, if present, are mandatory to rule out recurrent malignancy. A CT scan of the abdomen and pelvis can evaluate for recurrent malignancy. Urodynamics may be helpful in evaluating for other types of incontinence, as well as assessing for bladder compliance and capacity in this individual, with a risk for impaired compliance due to radiation therapy. There is no indication for ureteroscopy in this individual.

7. **c. Peritoneovaginal fistula.** Clear fluid draining from the vagina following surgery should be properly characterized. A urinary fistula is a possible source; however, urinary incontinence (stress, urge, overflow, etc.) are strong considerations as well. A peritoneovaginal fistula is a rare complication of hysterectomy in which peritoneal fluid leaks through the vaginal cuff. The fluid may be collected and analyzed for creatinine level. A creatinine level similar to that found in serum excludes urinary fistula as the source of the fluid. In addition, if a Pyridium pad test is negative (pads are wet but are not stained orange), then this is highly suggestive of a peritoneal vaginal cuff fistula.

8. **c. 10% of cases.** Approximately 10% to 12% of individuals with VVF are found to have an associated ureteral injury.

9. **a. The optimal timing for repair of this fistula may be in 5 to 6 months.** This patient has a VVF due to radiation therapy. It is recent in onset, suggesting that the fistula is immature and has a possibility of enlarging because the radiation injury has not yet completely demarcated. The optimal timing for repair of this fistula may be in 5 to 6 months. A reevaluation

at that time will be needed to assess whether the VVF is now mature and amenable to repair. Radiation-induced fistulae can be repaired vaginally, and adjuvant flaps are used to bolster the repair. The success rates for radiation-induced VVF are less than those associated with non-radiation-induced VVF, whether they are approached vaginally or abdominally.

10. **c. Is suitable for the use of an omental interpositional flap.** The choice of approach for VVF repair is generally individualized based on the patient's anatomy, clinical circumstances, and the experience of the operating surgeon. In experienced hands, success rates are similar between the two approaches. Advantages of the vaginal approach include a shorter hospital stay and less postoperative morbidity compared with the abdominal approach; however, vaginal shortening may be an issue with some types of vaginal VVF repairs, including the Latzko operation.

11. **b. May be accomplished with a three- or four-layer closure.** The vaginal approach to VVF repair uses a three- or four-layer closure. Absorbable suture is preferred to avoid complications related to foreign bodies in the urinary tract, including stone formation and infection. Gracilis flaps are rarely necessary as peritoneal flaps or Martius labial fat flaps are much more convenient and local. The vaginal approach is not contraindicated in obstetric fistula, or if the ureter is near the fistula tract.

12. **a. Excision of the fistula tract.** Although some authors have suggested that excision of the epithelialized portion of the fistula tract is beneficial, it is not required in all cases.

13. **e. None of the above.** There is no evidence-based medicine to support any of these statements. Although both topical estrogens and intravenous antibiotics are commonly used, this is on the basis of expert opinion. There is no preferred method for postoperative bladder drainage following VVF repair, although unobstructed drainage is critical in preventing disruption of the suture line.

14. **e. None of the above.** The transvaginal approach to VVF repair can be used in most patients with uncomplicated VVF. There are few absolute contraindications to the vaginal approach. Nulliparous individuals with VVF located at the vaginal cuff in a high narrow vagina can be challenging to repair vaginally due to anatomic considerations, but this approach is not contraindicated.

15. **a. Stress urinary incontinence.** Stress urinary incontinence may coexist with VVF; however, it is usually not related to the repair. One exception is the fistula located at the bladder neck or with involvement of the proximal urethra such as obstetric fistulae. These individuals may have new onset stress incontinence following repair due to destruction of the sphincter from the original injury.

16. **b. Decreased rate of intraoperative ureteral injury.** The transabdominal approach to VVF repair has several distinct advantages compared with the transvaginal approach. However, there are no studies to suggest that ureteral injury is less common using a transabdominal approach than a transvaginal approach.

17. **c. Is nondiagnostic, because there are no voiding images or postvoid images.** A postoperative cystogram should include voiding or postvoiding images to ensure that the VVF has been adequately repaired. Voiding may marginally increase the intravesical pressure, thereby providing opacification of some VVF that otherwise would be missed on simple filling cystograms. There is no standard filling volume for cystography. In general, 2 to 3 weeks from surgery is an adequate time period for postoperative imaging. There is no indication for cystoscopy in this patient.

18. **b. External pudendal artery.** The blood supply to the Martius flap is provided from three sources: the internal and external pudendal arteries as well as the obturator artery. In general, the small branches from the obturator artery, supplying the flap from a lateral direction, are sacrificed during mobilization. Furthermore, either the anterior (external pudendal) or posterior (internal pudendal) blood supply is divided in order to tunnel and then position the flap over the fistula.

19. **a. May be able to reach the deep pelvis without any mobilization in some patients.** The greater omentum has several favorable properties that support its use during transabdominal VVF repair. It is based on the right and left gastroepiploic arteries. Because of its rich blood supply and lymphatic properties, it can be a useful adjunctive measure in the setting of infection or inflammation. The blood supply enters the omentum perpendicular to its origin off the greater curvature of the stomach, enabling vertical incisions and mobilization into the deep pelvis. Wide mobilization may be necessary to permit the omentum to reach the deep pelvis in some cases; however, in many individuals the flap will reach into the deep pelvis without mobilization and without tension.

20. **a. Ureterovaginal fistula.** This patient has at least a ureterovaginal fistula, based on the yellow orange staining at the proximal portion of the gauze pad. This would be consistent with the normal voiding pattern. The distal blue staining would be consistent with stress incontinence as noted by the patient preoperatively. Hysterectomy is not associated with formation of urethrovaginal fistula. Vesicovaginal fistula is less likely because the staining would tend to be green (a combination of blue and yellow) and located in the midportion of the pad. A VCUG would be most helpful in definitively ruling out a vesicovaginal fistula.

21. **b. Usually associated with normal voiding patterns.** Ureterovaginal fistulae involve the distal one-third of the ureter. They most commonly occur in the setting of hysterectomy: laparoscopic, abdominal, and vaginal hysterectomy may all result in ureterovaginal fistulae. Most ureterovaginal fistulae occur following hysterectomy for benign indications. Patients often do not complain of voiding dysfunction because the contralateral upper urinary tract provides filling of the bladder. VCUG is used primarily to exclude a concomitant VVF.

22. **d. Vesicouterine fistula.** The most common cause of vesicouterine fistula is low-segment cesarean section. The normal physical examination suggests a lack of surgical trauma to the vagina, which most likely excludes a vaginal fistula. In the postpartum period, urine from a vesicouterine fistula will leak out of the incompetent cervical os, resulting in constant urinary leakage. A VCUG will confirm the diagnosis.

23. **a. Low-segment cesarean section.** The vast majority of vesicouterine fistulae occur following low-segment cesarean section. Rarely, these may occur due to uterine rupture at the time of vaginal delivery.

24. **e. All of the above.** All of the listed options may preserve long-term fertility in patients with vesicouterine fistula. In those not desiring preservation of fertility, hysterectomy is indicated.

25. **e. A vesicouterine fistula.** It is very unlikely that a vesicouterine fistula can result from such a clinical circumstance. Stress incontinence, VVF, urethrovaginal fistula, and a recurrent diverticulum may all result in the described symptoms.

26. **a. Are often asymptomatic.** Distal urethrovaginal fistulae are often asymptomatic, because they originate beyond the sphincter. Vaginal voiding and pseudoincontinence may be present in some patients. A vaginal flap technique is an effective method of repair.

27. **e. Diverticulitis.** Diverticulitis is the most common cause of colovesical fistula in most series. Colon cancer is the second most common cause, followed by Crohn disease.

28. **c. Air in the bladder, bladder wall thickening adjacent to a loop of thickened bowel wall, and the presence of colonic diverticula.** The classic triad found on CT scan, which is suggestive of a colovesical fistula, includes air in the bladder, bladder wall thickening adjacent to a loop of thickened bowel, and the presence of colonic diverticula.

29. **b. Has a high yield in identifying potential fistulae.** The finding of bullous edema during cystoscopy is nonspecific; however, in the appropriate clinical setting, this can be very suggestive of a colovesical fistula. Eighty percent to 100% of cases of colovesical fistulae have an abnormality noted on cystoscopy. Cystoscopy and biopsy are useful to rule out a malignant fistula when this is a consideration.

30. **e. All of the above.** Air can be introduced into the bladder from instrumentation (i.e., cystoscopy or catheterization) or may be present due to infection with a gas-forming organism. Less commonly, air in the bladder results from a colovesical fistula.

31. **d. Crohn disease.** Most ureterocolic fistulae occur on the right side and occur in patients with Crohn disease. Left-sided fistulae in Crohn disease are much less common.

32. **b. 1.0%.** Most large series report a 1.0% to 1.5% incidence of rectal injury during radical retropubic prostatectomy. When recognized and repaired intraoperatively, very few of these injuries result in a rectourethral fistula. The incidence of rectal injury during laparoscopic radical prostatectomy, when performed by experienced surgeons, is similar to that reported in most open series.

33. **e. May relate to all of the above.** RUF commonly present with fecaluria, regardless of the etiology. RUF in the setting of prostatic malignancy should be biopsied to evaluate for the possibility of recurrent disease.

34. **b. A trial of indwelling catheterization may result in resolution of the fistula.** This is a small fistula, and as such, a trial of conservative therapy is warranted. Because this fistula is not associated with signs of local infection or sepsis, immediate colostomy is not indicated. A York-Mason operation is not associated with a high rate of anal incontinence. Furthermore, a single-stage approach may be attempted (without fecal diversion) in this uncomplicated fistula, if conservative measures fail. Finally, urinary incontinence may not worsen following surgical repair of the fistula.

35. **a. Are usually related to percutaneous procedures in the upper urinary tract.** Pyelovascular fistulae are most often related to interventional procedures in the upper urinary tract, especially percutaneous procedures. Renal neoplasms and radiation therapy are not usually causative of these fistulae. Initial treatment consists of tamponade of the bleeding vessel. If this is unsuccessful, angiographic embolization may be necessary.

36. **d. Angiography.** This individual is at high risk for a ureteroarterial fistula at the level of the stent. A CT scan and retrograde pyelography will both most likely be nondiagnostic. Removal of the stent could result in an increase in bleeding and be rapidly fatal. Angiography in the setting of active bleeding will provide both the diagnosis of a ureteroarterial fistula, if present, and a possible therapeutic intervention in the form of embolization or stent graft placement. Nephrectomy will not stop the acute hemorrhage. A red blood cell scan will be too time consuming, and although it may lateralize the side of the bleeding, it will delay a potentially lifesaving intervention.

IMAGING

1. **b. Ureterovaginal fistula.** There is extraluminal contrast around the left distal pelvic ureter with contrast opacification of the vagina on the lower image. The bladder is normal in appearance with no contrast extravasation, making options a, c, and e incorrect. Ureteral duplication does not have this appearance.

CHAPTER REVIEW

1. Vesicovaginal fistulae may occur many years after completion of radiation therapy.
2. Clear vaginal discharge may not invariably represent a urinary fistula but may be a sign of a peritoneal vaginal fistula, lymphatic fistula, vaginitis, or fallopian tube fluid.
3. A fistula that does not heal following primary repair should be suspected of being associated with poor nutrition, a fungal infection, a malignancy, tuberculosis, distal obstruction, or the presence of a foreign body.
4. In the repair of fistulae, multiple layers should be used, and there should be no overlapping suture lines.
5. Long-term complications of vesicovaginal fistula repair include vaginal shortening and stenosis.
6. For an abdominal repair of a vesicovaginal fistula, it is essential to mobilize the bladder caudal to the fistula. Cholinergic agents are used liberally in the postoperative period following repair of a vesicovaginal fistula.
7. A Martius flap may be divided at either its superior or its inferior margin, because the vascular supply is provided at both ends of the graft.
8. A peritoneal flap is mobilized without opening the peritoneum, advancing it and securing it in a tension-free manner between the bladder and the vagina.
9. Following a ureteral injury, decompression of the upper tracks is essential.
10. Vesicouterine fistulae do not always present with urinary incontinence.
11. Soft tissue flaps are an important component of successful urethrovaginal fistula repair.
12. A recurrence of the malignancy should be ruled out in any fistula that develops following treatment of a primary malignancy with radiation therapy.
13. Vesicovaginal fistulae following hysterectomy are usually located on the anterior vaginal wall at the vaginal cuff.
14. Tissue interposition should be considered when repairing a fistula that failed primary closure, very large fistulae, and those occurring following radiation therapy.
15. The gracilis muscle, the rectus abdominis muscle, and a Martius pad are excellent flaps for tissue interposition.
16. An endovascular stent should be considered for ureterovascular (usually iliac) fistula repair.
17. Distal urethrovaginal fistulae are often asymptomatic because they originate beyond the sphincter.
18. Diverticulitis is the most common cause of colovesical fistula in most series. Colon cancer is the second most common cause, followed by Crohn disease.

130 Bladder and Female Urethral Diverticula

Lindsey Cox and Eric S. Rovner

QUESTIONS

1. Congenital bladder diverticula are:
   a. usually multiple.
   b. strongly associated with bladder outlet obstruction.
   c. often found in smooth-walled bladders.
   d. located at the dome.
   e. usually less than 1 cm in size.

2. Acquired bladder diverticula are most commonly located:
   a. near the urethrovesical junction.
   b. adjacent to the ureter.
   c. at the dome.
   d. at the 10 and 2 o'clock positions.
   e. posteriorly.

3. Videourodynamic evaluation in an adult female with a bladder diverticulum will likely reveal:
   a. impaired compliance.
   b. bladder outlet obstruction.
   c. intrinsic sphincter deficiency (ISD).
   d. low-pressure, low-flow voiding.
   e. no abnormality.

4. Pathologic examination of a surgical bladder diverticulectomy specimen will likely reveal:
   a. absence of epithelium.
   b. premalignant or malignant changes.
   c. nephrogenic metaplasia.
   d. a poorly developed muscularis propria layer.
   e. trabeculation of the smooth muscle layer.

5. The most common malignant tumor associated with bladder diverticula is:
   a. urothelial.
   b. squamous cell.
   c. adenocarcinoma.
   d. sarcomatous.
   e. undifferentiated.

6. A 68-year-old man presents with hematuria. Cystoscopy reveals a 15-cm bladder diverticulum with a 3-mm papillary lesion at the base of the diverticulum. The next step is:
   a. biopsy of the papillary lesion.
   b. transurethral resection of the papillary lesion with deep muscle resection.
   c. urodynamics and transurethral prostatectomy (TURP) if bladder outlet obstruction is noted.
   d. bladder diverticulectomy.
   e. radical cystectomy and urinary diversion.

7. Acquired bladder diverticula are commonly found in association with:
   a. prostatic obstruction.
   b. calyceal diverticula.
   c. nephrogenic adenoma.
   d. infection of perivesical glands.
   e. erectile dysfunction (ED).

8. A 65-year-old man with bladder outlet obstruction and a 5-cm bladder diverticulum undergoes uneventful TURP. Postoperatively, the patient's symptoms are resolved, and a voiding cystourethrogram (VCUG) demonstrates satisfactory emptying of the bladder and the bladder diverticulum. The next step is:
   a. annual surveillance with cystoscopy and urine cytology.
   b. discharge from urologic care.
   c. transvesical bladder diverticulectomy.
   d. repeat urodynamics.
   e. computed tomographic (CT) cystogram.

9. Ten years following TURP, a 71-year-old man with congestive heart failure (CHF) and atrial fibrillation who is on warfarin sodium (Coumadin) has recurrent urinary tract infections (UTIs) and an American Urological Association (AUA) symptom score of 25. A videourodynamic study shows a 14-cm poorly emptying bladder diverticulum. The peak subtracted detrusor pressure (Pdet) during micturition is 15 cm H_2O with a Qmax of 3 mL/s. Renal ultrasonography is normal. The next step is:
   a. repeat TURP.
   b. clean intermittent self-catheterization (CIC).
   c. observation.
   d. bethanechol.
   e. CT urography.

10. Endoscopic examination of the lower urinary tract in the setting of bladder diverticula:
    a. is best performed with a rigid cystoscope.
    b. is associated with a high risk of perforation.
    c. should include examination of the entire interior of the diverticulum.
    d. is not indicated if an elective submucosal bladder diverticulectomy is planned.
    e. should always be performed with concomitant bilateral retrograde pyelography (RPG).

11. Bladder diverticula:
    a. often do not produce specific symptoms.
    b. can be associated with UTIs.
    c. are commonly diagnosed incidentally during the evaluation of other symptoms or conditions.
    d. may be associated with persistent pyuria.
    e. all of the above.

12. Bladder diverticula associated with bladder outlet obstruction:
    a. are usually found in the absence of cellules and saccules.
    b. are associated with the universal finding of ipsilateral vesicoureteral reflux.
    c. cannot be imaged by CT.
    d. are associated with medial deviation of the pelvic ureter.
    e. are less likely to be associated with malignancy compared with congenital bladder diverticula.

13. Increased size of urethral diverticula (UDs) at presentation correlates with:
    a. increased symptoms.
    b. risk of UTI.
    c. risk of recurrence postoperatively.
    d. risk of malignancy.
    e. risk of incontinence.

14. Common symptoms associated with UDs include all of the following EXCEPT:
    a. vaginal pruritus.
    b. dysuria.
    c. dyspareunia.
    d. postvoid dribbling.
    e. urinary urgency and frequency.

15. In a 35-year-old woman a 1.5-cm firm anterior vaginal wall mass is noted approximately 2 cm proximal to the urethral meatus at the level of the mid-urethra without distorting the urethral meatus. It is nontender. Urine analysis is unremarkable. This mass may represent any of the following EXCEPT:
    a. vaginal wall cyst.
    b. Skene gland abscess.
    c. UD.
    d. vaginal leiomyoma.
    e. Gartner duct cyst.

16. The ostium of a UD is:
    a. most commonly found in the proximal third of the urethra.
    b. most commonly found at the 10 and 2 o'clock position in the urethral lumen.
    c. usually seen on transvaginal ultrasound imaging.
    d. unable to be visualized with rigid cystoscopy.
    e. usually located in the ventrolateral urethra.

17. Two weeks after removal of a 5-cm proximal UD extending beneath the trigone of the bladder, a 48-year-old woman returns to the office with complaints of urine staining her undergarments. Possible etiologies include:
    a. urethrovaginal fistula.
    b. ureterovaginal fistula.
    c. vesicovaginal fistula.
    d. stress urinary incontinence (SUI).
    e. all of the above.

18. During excision of the epithelial lining (sac) of a UD, a portion of the indwelling urethral catheter is seen at the base of the dissection. The next step is to:
    a. close the urethra and abort the procedure.
    b. perform buccal mucosal urethroplasty and abort the procedure.
    c. complete the urethral diverticulectomy.
    d. construct a vaginal inversion flap and close the urethra.
    e. close the urethra primarily, place a suprapubic tube, and harvest a Martius flap.

19. A VCUG is performed for evaluation of a possible UD. The filling images are nondiagnostic. The radiologist calls you because the patient is unable to void under fluoroscopy in the radiology suite. The patient is taken off the imaging table and is able to void in the adjacent bathroom. The next step is to:
    a. obtain a CT cystogram.
    b. do a transvaginal ultrasound.
    c. obtain postvoid images.
    d. implement endoluminal magnetic resonance imaging (MRI).
    e. positive pressure urethrography (PPU).

20. The most common malignancy found in UDs is:
    a. squamous.
    b. urothelial.
    c. adenocarcinoma.
    d. undifferentiated.
    e. sarcomatous.

21. Principles of surgical urethral diverticulectomy include all of the following EXCEPT:
    a. preservation or creation of urinary continence.
    b. excision of all identifiable periurethral fascia.
    c. identification of the ostium of the UD.
    d. closure of periurethral fascia following removal of the UD.
    e. watertight closure of the urethra.

22. The initial event implicated in the formation of most UDs is:
    a. congenital lack of fusion of the urethral crest.
    b. infection of vaginal cysts.
    c. a traumatic vaginal delivery.
    d. infection of the periurethral glands.
    e. dysfunctional voiding.

23. In a patient with bothersome SUI and UD, anti-incontinence surgery is being considered. Of the choices listed below, the best concomitant surgical procedure to treat the SUI is to provide a:
    a. transobturator midurethral sling.
    b. retropubic midurethral sling.
    c. single-incision synthetic sling.
    d. autologous pubovaginal fascial sling.
    e. polypropylene bladder neck sling.

24. The ostia of UD are most commonly found at:
    a. 12 o'clock.
    b. 6 o'clock.
    c. 4 and 8 o'clock.
    d. 10 and 12 o'clock.
    e. none of the above.

IMAGING

1. A 47-year-old woman presents with dribbling and recurrent UTIs; see Fig. 130.1.
   The most likely diagnosis on this axial and coronal T2-weighted MRI done with an endovaginal coil is:

a. bladder prolapse.

b. urethral diverticulum.

c. bladder diverticulum.

d. ureteral duplication.

e. ectopic ureter.

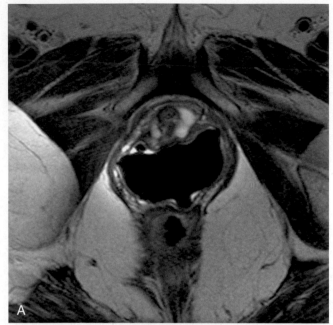

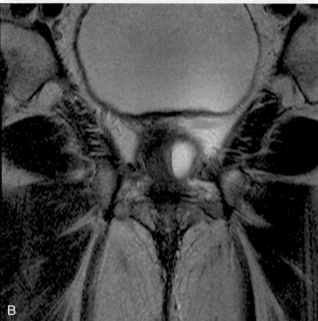

Fig. 130.1 Endovaginal T2 MRI images. (A) Axial. (B) Coronal.

ANSWERS

1. **c. Often found in smooth-walled bladders.** Unlike acquired bladder diverticula, congenital lesions are found in smooth-walled bladders, often adjacent to the ureteric orifice. Congenital bladder diverticula are usually solitary, often large, and not associated with bladder outlet obstruction. Congenital diverticula at the dome may be related to prune-belly syndrome, posterior urethral valves, or urachal anomalies.

2. **b. Adjacent to the ureter.** Similar to congenital bladder diverticula, acquired bladder diverticula are often located near the ureteric orifice. This area of the bladder is thought to be a location of relative anatomic weakness of the bladder wall, predisposing to the formation of bladder diverticula.

3. **b. Bladder outlet obstruction.** Bladder diverticula in adults are most commonly associated with some type of bladder outlet obstruction. In an adult female this may be due to prior anti-incontinence surgery (iatrogenic), dysfunctional voiding, neurogenic causes (e.g., detrusor external sphincter

dyssynergia), or a variety of other conditions such as obstructing vaginal or urethral masses (e.g., malignancy).

4. **d. A poorly developed muscularis propria layer.** Although varying amounts of detrusor muscle fibers may be found on pathologic examination of surgical excised bladder diverticula, the muscularis propria layer is usually incomplete and the fibers are disorganized. Such a lack of a well-developed muscularis propria layer is a hallmark of a bladder diverticulum. Absence of an epithelial layer, nephrogenic metaplasia, and malignant changes are uncommonly reported in the histologic evaluation of bladder diverticula. Typically there is no trabeculation within the wall of a bladder diverticulum.

5. **a. Urothelial.** The most common malignant tumors seen within bladder diverticula are urothelial. The other types of tumors can be seen but are much less common.

6. **a. Biopsy of the papillary lesion.** A papillary lesion in a bladder diverticulum, similar to the rest of the urinary tract, may indicate a malignancy, but it may also represent a benign lesion. Biopsy is warranted. Care should be taken to avoid perforation of the diverticular wall during the biopsy as the wall lacks a muscularis propria layer. A 3-mm lesion can easily be biopsied without the use of a resectoscope. In the event that the biopsy demonstrates malignancy, perforation of the bladder wall risks malignant dissemination.

7. **a. Prostatic obstruction.** Acquired bladder diverticula are most commonly associated with bladder outlet obstruction (approximately 70%). They are also more common in males than in females. The most common cause of bladder outlet obstruction in males is prostatic obstruction. There is no known association of bladder diverticula with calyceal diverticula, ED, nephrogenic adenoma, or perivesical gland infection.

8. **a. Annual surveillance with cystoscopy and urine cytology.** Although the bladder diverticulum drains well and the patient is asymptomatic, long-term follow-up of bladder diverticula is warranted. The natural history of such lesions is unknown, and although the etiology of malignant transformation is thought to involve urinary stasis, this is unproved. Furthermore, it is possible that premalignant changes may have occurred during the time that the diverticulum was not draining well.

9. **b. Clean intermittent self-catheterization (CIC).** This patient is at high risk for major abdominal surgery. Removal of his diverticulum is likely to be a large surgical undertaking with substantial risk and would be ill advised unless other conservative measures failed. Endoscopic treatment with TURP is also a risk because of anticoagulation. His detrusor pressure is low, suggesting that even an adequate outlet procedure (in this patient without definite evidence of obstruction) will not provide satisfactory emptying of the diverticulum. He has normal upper tracts but recurrent UTIs, thus observation would not be optimal. It is likely that his UTIs are due to urinary stasis in the diverticulum. CIC should adequately empty the diverticulum and reduce the risk of ongoing UTIs.

10. **c. Should include examination of the entire interior of the diverticulum.** Periodic endoscopic examination of bladder diverticula is warranted because of the risk of malignant transformation and early transmural involvement. The entire lining of the diverticulum should be examined. Rigid and flexible cystoscopes can be used. The upper urinary tract should be imaged. However, RPGs are not necessary unless otherwise indicated for another reason (e.g., a filling defect on urography).

11. **e. All of the above.** Bladder diverticula are most commonly recognized incidentally on evaluation for other signs and symptoms. There are no symptoms that are specific to bladder diverticula. Bladder diverticula are associated with UTIs and pyuria in some individuals.

12. **d. Are associated with medial deviation of the pelvic ureter.** Bladder diverticula found in association with lower urinary tract obstruction are commonly seen with saccules and cellules. Reflux is not a common finding with acquired bladder diverticula but may be present in some individuals, especially those with "Hutch" diverticula. Congenital bladder

diverticula are not associated with malignancy. Medial deviation of the ureter can be seen on intravenous urography and CT, with some large bladder diverticula due to the location of the diverticula relative to the ureter.

13. **c. Risk of recurrence postoperatively.** Although some UDs can be quite large, symptoms, malignancy risk, incontinence, and risk of UTI are not known to correlate with size. Large diverticula, including those extending in a "saddle bag" configuration, are more likely to recur.

14. **a. Vaginal pruritus.** Vaginal pruritus is not a symptom of UDs. Inflammatory and infectious conditions as well as lichen sclerosis (vulvar dystrophy) may cause vaginal pruritus. The other symptoms listed are often, although not invariably, individually or collectively associated with UDs. The classic triad of symptoms of UDs includes the "3 D's"—dysuria, postvoid dribbling, and dyspareunia—although these are seen only rarely in the same patient.

15. **b. Skene gland abscess.** Skene gland abscess is usually associated with distortion of the urethral meatus due to its distal location. These lesions are also often symptomatic, with associated dyspareunia and tenderness on physical examination. Vaginal wall cysts, vaginal leiomyomas, and Gartner duct cysts are firm anterior vaginal wall masses and are often nontender. UDs in some cases may be asymptomatic and found incidentally in the evaluation of other conditions, but they do not result in distortion of the urethral meatus.

16. **e. Usually located in the ventrolateral urethra.** The ostium (opening) of a UD is most commonly found in the middle or distal third of the urethra, at the 4 and 8 o'clock positions. They are usually too small to be visualized by ultrasound but can often be seen with both rigid and flexible cystoscopy as small openings in the urethral lumen ventrolaterally.

17. **e. All of the above.** Complications of urethral diverticulectomy include urinary fistulas as well as stress incontinence. Large diverticula may extend beneath the trigone of the bladder, and excision of such lesions risks injury to the urethra, bladder, and ureters. De novo SUI may occur following urethral diverticulectomy, which may be due to distortion or injury to the sphincter mechanism.

18. **c. Complete the urethral diverticulectomy.** Successful excision of a UD involves removal of the ostium that connects with the urethral lumen. This often results in direct visualization of the urethral catheter within the urethral lumen during surgery. The urethral defect is closed primarily with absorbable suture in a watertight fashion following completion of the removal of the sac. Additional procedures such as buccal mucosal urethroplasty, Martius flap, or vaginal flaps are not necessary to close the urethra.

19. **c. Obtain postvoid images.** In the absence of voiding images, many UDs will not be visualized during fluoroscopy as there is no contrast in the urethra. This is a nondiagnostic but incomplete study. Postvoid images will often reveal retained contrast in the diverticulum. CT, ultrasound, MRI, and PPU are all potentially useful studies in the evaluation of diverticula, but every effort should be made to maximize the diagnostic potential of each radiographic imaging technique, and a postvoid image in this clinical scenario may provide useful diagnostic information.

20. **c. Adenocarcinoma.** The most common malignant tumor type found in UDs is adenocarcinoma. Although the other malignant tumors listed may be found, adenocarcinoma is the most common.

21. **b. Excision of all identifiable periurethral fascia.** Preservation of periurethral fascia is an important step in urethral diverticulectomy. This tissue is very important in reconstruction of the urethra to prevent fistula formation and close dead space. This tissue should not be excised.

22. **d. Infection of the periurethral glands.** Infection of the periurethral glands is felt to be the initial step in the formation of UDs. Such infection may lead to periurethral abscess formation and development of a cavity or space within the periurethral fascia that then becomes the anatomic location of a UD.

23. **d. Autologous pubovaginal fascial sling.** SUI may accompany UDs. In symptomatic patients, concomitant repair can be considered. UDs connect to the urethral lumen, and therefore the surgical excision of these lesions requires suture repair and closure of the ostium of the UD where it connects to the urethra. In such settings, the use of synthetic material for a sling is not advisable because of the risk of subsequent erosion of the synthetic material into the urethra. Autologous fascia is an excellent choice for a concomitant sling at the time of urethral diverticulectomy.

24. **c. 4 and 8 o'clock.** UDs are thought to originate from infection of the periurethral glands. Such glands are located along the urethra and arborize laterally. They generally drain medially into the urethral lumen ventrolaterally at approximately the 4 and 8 o'clock positions of the middle and distal third of the urethra.

IMAGING

1. **b. Urethral diverticulum.** These images demonstrate a fluid collection surrounding the urethra, compatible with a saddle-bag UD. The coronal image clearly shows that the collection is separate from the bladder. (Options a and c are incorrect. An ectopic ureter would not have a saddlebag configuration.)

CHAPTER REVIEW

1. When the diverticulum encompasses the ureteral orifice in the setting of neurogenic bladder and vesicoureteral reflux, it is termed a *Hutch diverticulum*.
2. Congenital diverticula generally occur lateral and posterior to the ureteral orifice and are often associated with vesicoureteral reflux.
3. Acquired bladder diverticula usually occur in the setting of obstruction or neurogenic vesicular dysfunction.
4. The major complications of diverticula include recurrent UTIs, stones, carcinoma or premalignant change in the diverticulum, and upper tract deterioration as a consequence of obstruction or reflux.
5. Many diverticula are located adjacent to the ureter and may be very adherent to it. This has implications in surgical resection.
6. The urethropelvic ligament in the female is composed of two parts: (1) endopelvic fascia and (2) periurethral fascia. Within these two leaves of fascia lie the urethra, and this is the location of most UDs in women.
7. The etiology of UDs in women has been attributed to recurrent UTI of periurethral glands with obstruction, suburethral abscess formation, and subsequent rupture of the infected gland into the urethra.
8. Skene glands do not communicate with the urethra.
9. Gartner duct cysts are located on the anterolateral vaginal wall from cervix to introitus.
10. Urethral mucosal prolapse occurs in postmenopausal women and prepubertal girls.
11. A distinct layer of periurethral fascia should be preserved in managing excision of UDs for reconstruction.

12. When cancer occurs in a bladder diverticulum, the lack of a defined muscle wall makes biopsy and staging difficult because a deep biopsy may cause perforation; without a deep biopsy, proper staging may not be possible.
13. A UD may extend partially around the urethra, anterior to the urethra, or circumferentially around the urethra.
14. Stress incontinence occurs in approximately 10% of women after a repair of a UD.
15. Congenital bladder diverticula are usually solitary, often large, and not associated with bladder outlet obstruction.
16. The ostium (opening) of a UD is most commonly found in the middle or distal thirds of the urethra, at the 4 and 8 o'clock positions.

131 Surgical Procedures for Sphincteric Incontinence in the Male

Hunter Wessells and Alex J. Vanni

QUESTIONS

1. Male stress urinary incontinence (SUI) may result from all of the following except:
   a. radical prostatectomy
   b. pelvic fracture urethral injury
   c. spinal cord injury
   d. bladder extrophy
   e. multiple system atrophy

2. The Advance male sling is hypothesized to provide continence by:
   a. mucosal coaptation.
   b. elevation of the bulbar urethra.
   c. compression of the membranous urethra.
   d. circumferential occlusion of the bulbar urethra.
   e. repositioning and lengthening of the membranous urethra.

3. Nerve-sparing radical prostatectomy has been associated with which of the following:
   a. Earlier return to urinary continence and improved final urinary continence
   b. Delayed return to urinary continence
   c. Earlier return of urinary continence
   d. Improved final continence
   e. No difference in time to return of continence

4. The initial evaluation of a man with SUI should include all of the following except:
   a. Detailed history and physical exam
   b. Voiding diary and pad test
   c. Post void residual (PVR)
   d. Urinalysis
   e. Pressure flow urodynamics

5. A 65-year-old man status post robotic assisted radical prostatectomy had a direct vision internal urethrotomy for a vesicourethral anastomotic stenosis 6 months ago. He has SUI, wears 6 pads per day, and does not leak at night. Office examination reveals a normal urinalysis, PVR of 175 mL, and positive leak test on Valsalva. What is the next best step?
   a. Cystoscopy
   b. Retrograde urethrogram
   c. Pressure flow urodynamics
   d. Advance sling
   e. Artificial urinary sphincter (AUS)

6. Recurrent moderate SUI 4 years following AUS placement is most likely due to:
   a. detrusor overactivity.
   b. bladder neck stenosis.
   c. subcuff atrophy.
   d. pressure regulating balloon (PRB) herniation.
   e. cuff erosion.

7. A 71-year-old male underwent successful implantation of an Advance sling for stress incontinence. Preoperatively he wore two pads per day, and 1 week postoperatively he is perfectly continent. Two weeks postoperatively he went on a hike with his family and immediately noticed that he was requiring two pads per day again. He is now 3 weeks postop. What is the best option to treat his recurrent incontinence?
   a. Immediate re-exploration, removal of the sling, and replacement with another Advance sling
   b. Placement of a second Advance sling in 3 months
   c. AUS in 3 months
   d. Urethral bulking agent
   e. Removal of the sling in 3 months and placement of a Virtue sling

8. A 57-year-old man presents with SUI 12 months after robot-assisted radical prostatectomy and adjuvant external beam radiation therapy. His PSA is <0.01. His 24 hour pad weight is 600 g, and he has incontinence while sleeping. What is his best option for maximal urinary control?
   a. Advance male sling
   b. Virtue male sling
   c. Urethral bulking agent
   d. AUS
   e. Sacral neuromodulation

9. A 74-year-old man has SUI after radical prostatectomy with a 24-hour pad weight of 600 g. He would like treatment of his SUI and is considered an acceptable surgical candidate. He has poor manual dexterity. Which treatment is his best option for urinary control?
   a. Advance sling
   b. Virtue sling
   c. Urethral bulking agent
   d. AUS
   e. External collecting device

10. A 72-year-old man with incontinence after radical prostatectomy and adjuvant radiation therapy had an AUS implanted 5 years ago and has recurrent incontinence due to subcuff atrophy. He is impotent and not interested in sexual activity. Intraoperatively, the urethra measures <3.5 cm under the previous cuff and the bulbar urethra distal to this appears atrophic as well and likely measures <4.0 cm. What is the next best step?
    a. Place a second cuff in tandem distal to the existing cuff.
    b. Place a transcorporal cuff distal to the existing cuff site.
    c. Place a transcorporal cuff at the existing cuff site.
    d. Place a 3.5-cm cuff distal to the existing cuff site.
    e. Place a 3.5-cm cuff at the existing cuff site.

11. A 63-year-old man underwent uncomplicated 4.0-cm cuff bulbar AUS placement and has failed a series of voiding trials over the first week postoperatively. What is the best option to manage his bladder?
    a. Suprapubic cystostomy drainage
    b. 12 French catheter for an additional week followed by another voiding trial

c. Clean intermittent catheterization (CIC) until able to spontaneously void

d. Re-exploration and upsize of AUS cuff

e. Re-exploration and removal of AUS

12. Artificial urinary sphincter infections are most commonly due to which organisms?

a. *Escherichia coli*

b. Proteus

c. *Streptococcus*

d. *Staphylococcus*

e. Yeast

13. All of the following are established risk factor for AUS erosion except:

a. Prior radiation

b. Urethral catheterization

c. Prior AUS revision

d. Prior urethroplasty

e. Prior Advance sling

14. Management of AUS cuff atrophy can be performed in which way?

a. Cuff downsizing at existing cuff location

b. Repositioning a cuff at a different location

c. Tandem cuff placement

d. Transcorporal cuff placement

e. All of the above

15. A 67-year-old man status who underwent implantation of a 3.5-cm cuff bulbar AUS for post–radical prostatectomy SUI develops a symptomatic vesicourethral anastomotic stenosis. How is this best managed?

a. Urethral dilation with sounds

b. Antegrade incision through a SP cystostomy tract

c. Transurethral incision through a 21 Fr rigid cystoscope

d. Surgically uncouple the cuff followed by endoscopic treatment

e. Robotic or transperineal bladder neck reconstruction

ANSWERS

1. **c. Spinal cord injury.** SUI develops only in men with concomitant internal and external sphincter impairment. Internal sphincter incompetence results from pelvic surgery, such as radical prostatectomy, bladder neck injury, specific sympathetic neuropathic dysfunction, or embryological disruption. Incompetence of the external sphincter occurs most frequently after radical prostatectomy, but also can result from pelvic fracture urethral injuries, traumatic and acquired myelopathy, and congenital disorders such as spinal dysraphism, sacral agenesis, and the exstrophy/epispadias complex. Spinal cord injury leads to external or internal sphincter dyssynergia, which cause failure to empty, not failure to store.

2. **e. Repositioning and lengthening of the membranous urethra.** Transobturator slings are hypothesized to enhance external sphincter function by repositioning and lengthening the membranous urethra without significant compression. Urodynamic studies show an increase in abdominal leak point pressure without other urodynamic evidence of obstruction. Evidence for this comes from fluoroscopic studies and magnetic resonance imaging. The latter studies demonstrate an increase in membranous urethral length and elevation of the bladder neck, posterior bladder wall, and rhabdosphincter.

3. **c. Earlier return of urinary continence.** In systematic review and meta-analysis, nerve-sparing techniques have been associated with more rapid return of continence, although not final continence status, after RP.

4. **e. Pressure flow urodynamics.** The initial evaluation of a man with UI requires a detailed history, physical examination, postvoid residual measurement, and urinalysis. **Pressure flow urodynamics** can be used to evaluate potential bladder neck stenosis, residual sphincteric function, and bladder storage function as indicated, but is not part of the initial evaluation of stress incontinence.

5. **a. Cystoscopy.** Because unrecognized urethral or bladder neck pathology can significantly complicate all surgical approaches, endoscopic evaluation should be considered prior to surgical correction of UI post RP or TURP if there is any suspicion of bladder neck stenosis. Cystoscopy is the best way to evaluate his elevated PVR and determine if he has a recurrent vesicourethral anastomotic stenosis. Urethrography is less useful in delineating posterior urethral strictures. Urodynamics are not indicated unless poor bladder emptying cannot be otherwise explained.

6. **c. Subcuff atrophy.** While detrusor overactivity, PRB herniation and cuff erosion may all result in recurrent UI, subcuff atrophy is the most common cause of recurrent SUI 4 years after AUS placement. Mechanical failure, another cause of recurrent incontinence, is not listed as an option but over time becomes more common.

7. **a. Immediate re-exploration, removal of the sling, and replacement with another Advance sling.** Evaluation of the patient who had prior urethral sling is similar to the evaluation after AUS placement with several caveats. Identifying the type of sling placed (Advance vs. Virtue vs. bone anchored) and the timing of the incontinence are important. In the case of the Advance sling, it is important to determine whether the patient may have loosened the sling in the first 6 weeks postoperatively, whether the incontinence is persistent (ongoing SUI) or the result of detrusor overactivity. If patients give a history of improved UI and a loosening of the sling in the first 6 weeks postoperatively, re-exploration is appropriate. The perineum is opened, the arms of the sling lateral to the bulbar urethra are identified and each arm is cut. The remaining central portion of the sling should be removed from the surface of the corpus spongiosum of the bulbar urethra. Another sling can then be placed in the same manner, as described later.

8. **d. AUS.** Because of limited efficacy, submucosal bulking agents are not part of the treatment algorithm for post-RP UI. Thus the AUS and slings should be considered as first-line surgical therapy for sphincteric incontinence in most men, although a trial of a bulking agent may be appropriate in cases of neurogenic male stress UI. The AUS remains the established device for treatment of moderate to severe UI, supported by numerous publications documenting its benefits. Thus, the transobturator slings should be primarily used in cases with mild to moderate incontinence, which can be defined as a 24-hour pad weight of less than 150 grams for mild UI and less than 400 grams for moderate UI. A sling procedure should be offered with caution to those with prior radiation therapy or urethral erosion, because the degree of urine loss that exists in this group usually exceeds the limits of the procedure. One reason for the lower efficacy in these patients may be the lack of appropriate tissue elasticity for deformation/elongation/compression of the external urinary sphincter apparatus.

9. **a. Advance sling.** Because of limited efficacy, submucosal bulking agents are not part of the treatment algorithm for post-RP UI. Although the patient has severe UI, an AUS is not advised due to his poor manual dexterity, and a perineal sling is the preferred treatment option. The authors recommend the Advance sling based on broader experience with this device in the urological community, more substantial corroborating literature, and personal experience with the device compared to the Virtue sling.

10. **b. Place a transcorporal cuff distal to the existing cuff site.** Indiscriminate use of the tandem cuff approach as first-line surgical treatment should be tempered by higher rates of erosion associated with the distal cuff in several series. Use of the 3.5-cm size has resulted in an increased risk of erosion in patients with a prior history of radiation therapy. Patients with radiation therapy or other adverse risk factors and significant urethral atrophy should be considered for transcorporal placement rather than a 3.5-cm cuff. Placing a transcorporal cuff should be performed at a different location along the bulbar urethra.

11. **a. Suprapubic cystostomy drainage.** If the patient fails a voiding trial at 48 hours, suprapubic cystostomy drainage is recommended to reduce the risk of urethral erosion. Ultrasound or fluoroscopic guidance is recommended to prevent puncture or potential contamination of the PRB. Retention persisting beyond several weeks implies undersizing of the cuff; in such cases reoperation and cuff replacement may be required. Prolonged urethral catheterization or CIC after AUS will result in an increased risk of cuff urethral erosion, even if the device is deactivated.

12. **d. *Staphylococcus*.** Skin pathogens are the most commonly cultured organism, usually *Staphylococcus epidermidis* and *Staphylococcus aureus*.

13. **e. Prior Advance sling.** Prior radiation, urethral catheterization, prior AUS revision, and urethroplasty are all risk factors for AUS urethral erosion. Prior Advance sling has not resulted in an increased risk of AUS erosion.

14. **e. All of the above.** Managing AUS cuff atrophy can be performed in a number of ways and may require any one of the following maneuvers—cuff downsizing at existing cuff location, repositioning a cuff at a different location, tandem cuff placement, or transcorporal cuff placement—depending on intraoperative findings.

15. **d. Surgically uncouple the cuff followed by endoscopic treatment.** First-line management of vesicourethral anastomotic strictures usually involves an endoscopic approach with DVIU or dilation. In the event significant endoscopic manipulation is required proximal to the cuff site, our practice is to surgically uncouple the cuff for the duration of the endoscopic procedure to avoid the risk of urethral erosion or damaging the AUS cuff, which may result from either a balloon dilation or transurethral incision through a 21-Fr rigid cystoscope.

CHAPTER REVIEW

1. A careful history and voiding diary characterize the type and severity of urinary incontinence in most men.
2. Uroflometry and post void residual urine volume measurement should be assessed at minimum.
3. Suspected outlet obstruction, significant bladder overactivity, or impaired bladder contractility should prompt urodynamic studies.
4. Patients with suspected urethral, vesicourethral, or bladder neck pathology should undergo cystoscopy.
5. Urinalysis (and culture, if indicated) is required prior to surgical treatment.
6. Surgical intervention is indicated for SUI due to ISD that fails to improve with conservative management.
7. Implant selection depends on the severity of UI, prior surgical procedures, bladder function, cystoscopic findings, manual dexterity and cognitive function, long-term risk of complications and reoperation, and patient preference.
8. Slings should only be used very selectively in cases of radiation and severe gravitational urinary incontinence.
9. AUS should not be used in cases of poor manual dexterity, cognitive disability, poor urethral tissue integrity, or severely reduced bladder compliance.
10. Standard implantation of the bulbar AUS places the cuff around the corpus spongiosum proximal to the convergence of the corporal bodies.
11. Pressure regulating balloon of 61 to 70 cm H_2O is advised for bulbar urethral cuffs; placement may be via abdominal, scrotal, or perineal approach.
12. Postoperative deactivation of the cuff for 4–6 weeks is essential for proper healing without erosion.
13. Prolonged urinary retention requires suprapubic cystostomy drainage.
14. Revision surgery for nonmechanical causes may require transcorporal cuff placement or other modifications such as using 3.5-cm or tandem cuff.
15. Male bulbar urethral slings are indicated in men with mild to moderate sphincteric UI, intact bladder contractility, and well-vascularized nonradiated urethral anatomy.
16. Transobturator slings reposition and elongate the membranous urethra and depend on the intact external sphincter.
17. Quadratic fixation provides an alternative to the two arm devices with limited data on efficacy and durability.
18. Device infection typically requires total explantation, but salvage procedures in select patients with device removal, antibiotic regimen washout, and reimplantation are feasible.
19. Device erosion requires total explantation and catheter drainage.
20. Troubleshooting of recurrent UI post AUS requires a systematic and exhaustive evaluation.
21. Cuff atrophy requires downsizing, repositioning, tandem cuff, or transcorporal surgery.
22. Artificial urinary sphincter continues to provide a reliable solution to male UI of all degrees of severity across the range of first-time implantation to complex reoperative and high-risk patients.
23. Transobturator slings such as Advance and newer devices provide long-term durable outcomes for mild to moderate male UI after radical prostatectomy.

132 Bladder Surgery for Benign Disease

Paras H. Shah and Lee Richstone

QUESTIONS

1. All of the following are critical to consider in the surgical management of a bladder diverticulum EXCEPT one. Which?

   a. If outlet obstruction is present, it should be managed prior to or at the time of bladder diverticulectomy.

   b. The need for ureteral reimplantation is a contraindication to surgical resection of a bladder diverticulum.

   c. Cystoscopic examination of the diverticulum should be attempted in order to characterize the anatomy of the diverticulum as well as to evaluate for the presence for a bladder tumor within the diverticulum.

   d. A preoperative stent may be placed if there is concern for ureteral injury during bladder diverticulectomy.

2. In patients with ureteral stricture disease, which of the following should ideally be a part of the preoperative evaluation?

   a. Retrograde pyelography

   b. Both retrograde and antegrade evaluation

   c. Computed tomography (CT) urography

   d. None of the above; direct intraoperative visualization of stricture length will suffice.

3. Which of the following maneuvers can be used to reduce tension on the ureterovesical anastomosis?

   a. Ligation of the contralateral bladder pedicles to facilitate cephalad displacement of the bladder

   b. Disengagement of the peritoneal reflection off the bladder dome to enhance bladder mobility

   c. A psoas hitch procedure

   d. Renal mobilization and downward nephropexy

   e. All of the above

4. All of the following are essential surgical aspects of the Boari flap or bladder advancement flap EXCEPT one. Which?

   a. An adequate-sized bladder must be present (200- to 300-mL capacity).

   b. The contralateral vesical pedicle may be transected if necessary.

   c. The bladder flap should be slightly shorter than anticipated because bladder tissue can easily be stretched.

   d. A tension-free anastomosis is important.

   e. Typically, a refluxing ureteral anastomosis is created.

5. What nerves may be injured during a psoas hitch procedure?

   a. Obturator nerve

   b. Genitofemoral nerve

   c. Ilioinguinal nerve

   d. Sciatic nerve

6. Which of the following statements is NOT correct regarding enterocystoplasty?

   a. Subtotal cystectomy is not always mandatory.

   b. The mesenteric pedicle of the selected bowel segment is wide and broad-based.

   c. The mesenteric window is closed.

   d. Reestablishment of bowel continuity is a critical step of the operation and may be performed extracorporeally, if necessary, for added security.

   e. Bowel-to-bladder anastomosis is optimally performed with interrupted serosa-to-serosa sutures.

7. Contraindications for enterocystoplasty include all of the following EXCEPT:

   a. diverticulosis.

   b. inflammatory bowel disease.

   c. renal failure.

   d. noncompliance.

8. Which is the following is a contraindication to partial cystectomy for a bladder leiomyoma?

   a. Need for ureteral reimplantation

   b. Transmural involvement by the neoplastic process

   c. Significant irritative voiding symptoms at baseline

   d. Reduced preoperative bladder capacity

   e. c and d

9. Which of the following with regard to ureteral reimplantation is true?

   a. A nonrefluxing anastomosis is superior to a refluxing anastomosis due to a reduced risk for infection.

   b. The ureter should be skeletonized as much as possible to facilitate maximal ureteral mobility and increase the chance for a tension-free anastomosis.

   c. For a nonrefluxing anastomosis, the length of the submucosal tunnel should be approximately three to five times the diameter of the ureter to be reimplanted.

   d. For ureteral defects greater than 4 cm, a primary ureteroneocystotomy is generally feasible without the need for a psoas hitch or Boari flap.

10. When urachal surgery is performed for a benign indication, which of the following is true?

   a. Wide margins of resection along the peritoneal wing are necessary.

   b. A wide-margin bladder cuff is preferred.

   c. Excision of the umbilicus should be performed.

   d. Narrow peritoneal wings around the urachus and a narrow-margin bladder cuff will suffice.

ANSWERS

1. **b. The need for ureteral reimplantation is a contraindication to surgical resection of a bladder diverticulum.** The need for ureteral reimplantation is not a contraindication to performing bladder diverticulectomy. Rather, careful preoperative planning is necessary to discern the proximity of the ureter to the diverticulum and to gauge whether surgical maneuvers, such as retrograde ureteral stent placement, are necessary to prevent inadvertent ureteral injury. Alternatively, planned ureteral reimplantation may be performed at the time of bladder diverticulectomy. The surgeon should be cognizant of the ureteral anatomy relative to the diverticulum to avoid intraoperative injury. At the conclusion of the case, the ureter should be inspected to ensure its integrity; reimplantation should be performed if there is any concern for ureteral compromise.

2. **b. Both retrograde and antegrade evaluation.** Both antegrade and retrograde evaluation of stricture disease is necessary to accurately assess the length and location of disease as well as whether multiple strictures are present, as these factors heavily influence operative planning. In cases of distal ureteral strictures, retrograde contrast administration alone may fail to opacify more proximal aspects of the ureter, precluding an understanding of the length of stricture disease. Similarly, high-grade proximal strictures may prevent adequate ureteral opacification past the stricture segment with antegrade studies (e.g., contrast administration through a nephrostomy tube or delayed-phase imaging on a CT urogram), hindering adequate characterization of the extent of stricture disease. Obstructive uropathy in the setting of a ureteral stricture may also impair the uptake of intravenous contrast by the kidney during a CT urogram study, rendering this study futile for the anatomic characterization of stricture disease when it is performed in isolation.

3. **e. All of the above.** It is critical to avoid tension at the ureterovesical junction during reimplantation as ischemic injury related to undue traction may result in the formation of scar and subsequent stricture. All the aforementioned techniques can be employed to reduce tension, although they vary in their degree of surgical complexity. In general, a psoas hitch procedure represents the least complex of the options mentioned and is generally all that is needed for ureteral strictures involving the distal third of the ureter. If further length is needed, a Boari flap may be performed prior to more aggressive surgical maneuvers such as ligation of bladder pedicles, disengagement of the peritoneal reflection, and renal mobilization.

4. **c. The bladder flap should be slightly shorter than anticipated because bladder tissue can easily be stretched.** The bladder flap should be slightly shorter than anticipated because bladder tissue can easily be stretched. A tension-free anastomosis of the anterolateral bladder flap based on the ipsilateral vesical pedicle is critical. The bladder flap should be somewhat longer and wider than anticipated because the nondistended bladder shrinks in size, thus placing tension on the anastomosis. Ideally, a flap length-to-breadth ratio of 3:1 ensures good vascularity of its apex.

5. **b. Genitofemoral nerve.** During a psoas hitch procedure, sutures should be placed superficially through the tendon of the psoas minor parallel to the direction of the muscle fibers. This helps to minimize the risk of disrupting the genitofemoral nerve, situated superficially on the psoas muscle, or the femoral nerve, located deeper in the belly of the muscle.

6. **e. Bowel-to-bladder anastomosis is optimally performed with interrupted serosa-to-serosa sutures.** The technical principles of enterocystoplasty are identical between open surgical and laparoscopic techniques. Generous mobilization of the bladder allows creation of an adequate anteroposterior cystotomy. Subtotal cystectomy is necessary only in patients with severely symptomatic interstitial cystitis. An optimal segment of bowel based on a broad, well-vascularized mesenteric pedicle is selected that will reach the pelvis without tension. The bowel segment is isolated and bowel continuity reestablished, either by intracorporeal or extracorporeal techniques, and the mesenteric window is closed. The isolated bowel segment is detubularized and a bowel plate is created appropriately. A tension-free, watertight, full-thickness circumferential running anastomosis of the bowel segment to the bladder is created. Adequate urinary drainage is established.

7. **a. Diverticulosis.** The presence of bowel pathology such as diverticulitis or ulcerative colitis requires the use of alternative, nondiseased bowel segments. Enterocystoplasty should not be performed in the presence of advanced renal or liver failure, inflammatory bowel disease, or short gut syndrome or in a patient who is unable to perform or noncompliant in performing intermittent catheterization reliably. Diverticulosis is not a contraindication for performing enterocystoplasty.

8. **e. c and d.** Bladder leiomyomas are benign tumors of the bladder that most commonly manifest with an endovesical, intramural, or extravesical pattern of growth; therefore they may not be discerned on cystoscopic exam or may appear only as a submucosal growth. Owing to the benign nature of bladder leiomyomas, partial cystectomy represents a reasonable treatment approach, particularly for lesions that are large in size and require wide local excision. Patient selection is critical when partial cystectomy is being considered irrespective of the pathology for which it is being performed. This includes performing the procedure only in patients with adequate preoperative bladder capacity, as further postoperative reduction in capacity can result in significant voiding complaints. Additionally, the presence of baseline irritative voiding complaints is a relative contraindication, as the process of bladder tissue resection and postoperative reduction in bladder capacity may exacerbate these symptoms. Ureteral reimplantation is not an absolute contraindication for partial cystectomy, particularly for benign disease, and can be performed concomitantly if necessary.

9. **c. For a nonrefluxing anastomosis, the length of the submucosal tunnel should be approximately three to five times the diameter of the ureter to be reimplanted.** When a nonrefluxing anastomosis is being performed, a submucosal tunnel is created to support compression of the reimplanted ureter during bladder contraction. The length of this tunnel should be roughly three to five times the diameter of the ureter to be reimplanted. Nonrefluxing anastomoses can be created via an extravesical or transvesical approach. Based on the currently available literature, the use of a refluxing anastomosis does not appear to place individuals at increased risk for accelerated renal functional decline or for stenosis as compared with nonrefluxing anastomoses. Similarly, long-term studies in adults undergoing a refluxing anastomosis do not seem to indicate increased risk for infection. For ureteral defects greater than 4 cm, primary ureteroneocystotomy would likely result in undue traction at the ureterovesical anastomosis and cause stricture secondary to ischemic injury. Therefore additional measures such as psoas hitch and/or Boari flap are often implemented. In addition to creating a tension-free anastomosis during ureteral reimplantation, the ureter should be manipulated delicately so as to minimize devascularization injury. Furthermore, a conscious effort should be made during extravesical mobilization of the ureter to preserve the periureteral fibroadipose tissue and avoid excessive skeletonization, which may also compromise the blood supply.

10. **d. Narrow peritoneal wings around the urachus and a narrow-margin bladder cuff will suffice.** Surgery is indicated for symptomatic or infected urachal anomalies that do not respond to conservative approaches to treatment, such as incision and drainage and/or antibiotic therapy. When surgery is performed, the entire urachus should be excised, including a small area on the dome of the bladder. The practice of incorporating a bladder cuff into the surgical specimen is thought to ensure that no residual tissue will be left in the vicinity of the bladder apex, as this may risk recurrence of symptoms or malignant transformation. In general, a narrow peritoneal wing around the urachus will suffice, as will a narrow bladder cuff because of the noninfiltrative nature of benign urachal lesions. Excision of the umbilicus is not necessary for a benign indication, especially when the lesion is not in the vicinity of the umbilicus.

CHAPTER REVIEW

1. For bladder diverticulectomy, the success of surgery is contingent on a meticulous preoperative workup that characterizes the number, size, and location of diverticula. Specifically, the anatomy relative to the ureter should be defined to ensure preservation of the ureter's integrity during repair.

2. The disease process underlying formation of the bladder diverticulum should be managed prior to or at the time of diverticular repair.

3. The fibrous pseudocapsule surrounding the diverticulum serves as a cleavage plane to free the diverticulum from surrounding extravesical tissue.

4. During minimally invasive bladder diverticulectomy, selective catheterization of the diverticulum with a Council-tip catheter placed over a guidewire allows for selective filling of the diverticulum and aids in intraoperative identification.

5. In ureteral reimplantation, aggressive skeletonizing of the ureter during mobilization should be avoided, as this may lead to ischemia and ureteral stricture formation.

6. A tension-free anastomosis between the bladder and ureter is critical, as the presence of tension risks anastomotic stricture formation.

7. The ureter should be adequately spatulated prior to creation of the anastomosis.

8. When a nonrefluxing ureteral reimplant is being performed, the length of the submucosal tunnel should be three to five times the caliber of the ureteral lumen.

9. Longer ureteral defects may be bridged through maneuvers such as ligation of the contralateral medial umbilical ligament, dissection of the peritoneal reflection off the bladder dome, or ligation of the contralateral bladder pedicle, all of which are conducive to cephalad displacement of the bladder.

10. During creation of a psoas hitch, sutures that fix the extravesical surface of the bladder to the psoas minor tendon should be placed superficially and parallel to the direction of the muscle fibers to avoid entrapment of the femoral and genitofemoral nerves, respectively.

11. Reimplantation of the ureter should be performed prior to tying the anchoring sutures to the psoas muscle tendon during psoas hitch creation.

12. The base of a Boari flap should measure at least 4 cm in width, with longer flaps requiring wider base measurement to maintain adequate blood supply; in this regard, the length-to-base ratio should not exceed 3:1.

13. If a non-refluxing anastomosis is planned into a Boari flap, there should be at least 3 cm of overlap between the flap and the ureteral segment.

14. Due to its relative simplicity and versatility, advancement flaps may be used in lieu of Boari flaps to bridge longer ureteral defects.

15. In enterocystoplasty, the ileum is most frequently utilized for bladder augmentation given its abundance, ease of mobilization, and robust blood supply.

16. The ileum should be isolated approximately 20 cm proximal to the ileocecal valve to spare the terminal ileum and avoid risk for bile salt and vitamin B12 malabsorption.

17. Detubularization of the isolated intestinal segment is necessary to reduce coordinated peristaltic contractions, which may otherwise contribute to high intravesical pressures.

18. A broad mesenteric base to the isolated intestinal segment should be maintained to avoid torsion of the pedicle as well as preserve a rich blood supply.

19. The bladder should be generously bivalved along its dome so as to facilitate a wide-mouth anastomosis with the intestinal patch; a narrow-mouth anastomosis would result in the creation of a pseudo-diverticulum that may poorly empty and cause complications.

20. Patients should be counseled regarding the importance of continuous intermittent catheterization as the failure to do so risks perforation.

21. Preoperative evaluation should confirm the presence of adequate bladder capacity and the absence of significant voiding symptoms prior to proceeding with partial cystectomy.

22. Partial cystectomy for benign disease processes still require adequate margins of resection given the infiltrative nature of many conditions and the propensity for recurrence in cases of inadequate excision.

23. During minimally invasive partial cystectomy, intraoperative flexible cystoscopy by the bedside assistant can aid the surgeon in identification of the site of bladder pathology.

24. Urachal surgery, when being performed for benign indication, does not require a wide margin of resection of the bladder dome around the site of urachal insertion.

25. Approach to bladder stone surgery depends on the size and number of calculi as well as the presence of any associated processes contributing to stone formation that may need to be simultaneously addressed.

26. Percutaneous cystolithotripsy is a minimally invasive alterative to management of large bladder calculi; percutaneous access, however, may be prohibited in patients with prior pelvic or abdominal surgery given concern over intestinal injury.

133 Genital and Lower Urinary Tract Trauma

Allen F. Morey and Jay Simhan

QUESTIONS

1. Which of the following is an absolute indication for open repair of blunt bladder rupture injury?
   a. Significant extraperitoneal bladder rupture with extravasation of contrast agent into the scrotum
   b. Significant extraperitoneal bladder rupture with gross hematuria
   c. Significant extraperitoneal bladder rupture that has not healed after 3 weeks of Foley catheter drainage
   d. Intraperitoneal bladder rupture
   e. Significant extraperitoneal bladder rupture associated with pelvic fracture requiring treatment by external fixation

2. Which of the following statements is TRUE regarding cystography for diagnosis of bladder injury?
   a. If the patient is already undergoing computed tomography (CT) for evaluation of associated injuries, CT cystography should be performed via antegrade filling of the bladder after intravenous administration of radiographic contrast material and clamping the Foley catheter.
   b. If plain film cystograms are obtained, the study is considered negative and complete if there is no extravasation of contrast agent seen on the filling film.
   c. CT cystography is best performed with undiluted contrast medium.
   d. An absolute indication for immediate cystography is the presence of pelvic fracture and microhematuria.
   e. None of the above.

3. Which of the following statements is TRUE about blunt bladder rupture injuries?
   a. They are present in 90% of patients presenting with pelvic fractures.
   b. They coexist with urethral disruption in 50% of cases.
   c. Extraperitoneal ruptures are always amenable to nonoperative treatment.
   d. High mortality rate is primarily related to nonurologic comorbidities.
   e. They are associated with microhematuria or no hematuria in 40% of cases.

4. The risk of complications from nonoperative treatment of extraperitoneal bladder rupture is increased by:
   a. associated orthopedic injury.
   b. associated vaginal injury.
   c. associated urethral injury.
   d. associated rectal injury.
   e. all of the above.

5. Three months after a urethral distraction injury, a patient is found to have a 2-cm obliterative posterior urethral defect. Which of the following is TRUE about the repair?
   a. One-stage, open, perineal anastomotic urethroplasty is preferred.
   b. Orthopedic hardware in the pubic symphysis area is a contraindication to open posterior urethroplasty.
   c. Buccal mucosa graft urethroplasty is recommended.

d. Urethral stent placement is recommended.
   e. The patient is at high risk for incontinence after posterior urethral reconstruction surgery.

6. In a patient with a pelvic fracture from blunt trauma in whom no urine is returned after catheter placement, what is the best initial method to evaluate urethral injury?
   a. Retrograde urethrography
   b. CT of abdomen and pelvis
   c. Filiforms and followers
   d. Bladder ultrasonography
   e. None of the above

7. During exploration after a scrotal gunshot wound, 20% of the left testicular capsule is found to be disrupted. What should be done?
   a. Left orchiectomy
   b. Application of wet dressings and delayed testicular surgery
   c. Left testicular reconstruction with synthetic graft
   d. Closure of the scrotal laceration followed by ultrasonography
   e. Immediate primary repair of the left testis

8. A 23-year-old man is found to have an 80% transection of the proximal bulbar urethra after a gunshot wound with a 22-caliber pistol. A 1-cm urethral defect is visualized during cystoscopy. What is the most appropriate therapy?
   a. Buccal mucosa graft urethroplasty
   b. Spatulated, stented, tension-free, watertight repair of the urethra with absorbable sutures
   c. Suprapubic tube placement
   d. Urethral catheterization alone
   e. Perineal urethrostomy

9. Which of the following statements regarding penile fracture is FALSE?
   a. Most injuries occur ventrolaterally.
   b. Rupture of a superficial vein can sometimes mimic the presentation of a corporal tear.
   c. Retrograde urethrography should be uniformly performed to assess for urethral injury.
   d. Patients with penile fracture who are treated nonoperatively are more likely to have longer hospital stays, a higher risk of infection, and penile curvature than those whose fracture is repaired surgically.
   e. Physical examination is usually sufficient in making the diagnosis or for deciding on surgical exploration.

10. The blood in a hematocele is contained in which of the following?
    a. Tunica albuginea
    b. Tunica vaginalis
    c. Dartos muscle
    d. Camper fascia
    e. Spermatic cord

11. Blunt scrotal trauma that results in testis rupture:
    a. is usually a bilateral process.
    b. is often diagnosed by the presence of intratesticular hypo-echoic areas on ultrasonography.
    c. has a degree of hematoma that correlates with the extent of injury.
    d. requires conservative management that results in acceptable viability and function.
    e. is definitively diagnosed during physical examination alone in most cases.

12. Which of the following statements is TRUE regarding penile amputation injury?
    a. Microscopic reanastomosis of the corporal arteries is recommended.
    b. The severed phallus should be placed directly on ice during transport.
    c. Microscopic dorsal vascular and neural reanastomosis is the best method of repair.
    d. Primary macroscopic reanastomosis invariably results in erectile dysfunction.
    e. Skin loss is rarely a problem after macroscopic repair.

13. What is the best option for coverage of acute penile skin loss?
    a. Foreskin flap for small distal lesions
    b. Meshed skin graft in a young child
    c. Wet-to-dry dressings
    d. Thigh flaps
    e. Burying the penile shaft in a scrotal skin tunnel

14. Which is FALSE about penile fracture?
    a. Penile fracture must be repaired immediately for the best outcomes.
    b. Ultrasonography can identify location of the corporal tear.
    c. Magnetic resonance imaging (MRI) can demonstrate disruption of the tunica albuginea.
    d. Rupture of the dorsal penile artery can have the same presentation as penile fracture.
    e. Bilateral corporal injury is more commonly associated with urethral injury.

15. Advantages of open suprapubic tube placement after posterior urethral disruption injuries include:
    a. inspection of bladder.
    b. an opportunity for controlled antegrade urethral realignment.
    c. allowance for large-bore catheter insertion.
    d. not jeopardizing continence or potency rates.
    e. all of the above.

ANSWERS

1. **d. Intraperitoneal bladder rupture.** When intraperitoneal bladder laceration occurs after blunt trauma, a large laceration of the bladder dome is usually produced that predisposes to urinary ascites and/or peritonitis if it is not repaired promptly.

2. **e. None of the above.** The CT cystogram must be performed via retrograde distention of the bladder with a diluted contrast medium. Most bladder lacerations are associated with gross hematuria, not microhematuria. A drainage film is required to complete a plain film cystogram.

3. **d. High mortality rate is primarily related to nonurologic comorbidities.** Bladder lacerations occur in approximately 10% of pelvic fractures and often occur in the context of multisystemic trauma.

4. **e. All of the above.** All of the listed concomitant injuries increase the risk of complications such as abscess, fistula, or incontinence.

5. **a. One-stage, open, perineal anastomotic urethroplasty is preferred.** Posterior urethral reconstruction including excision of the fibrotic segment with distal urethral mobilization and primary anastomosis is associated with the best long-term outcomes after urethral disruption. Incontinence occurs in less than 5% of patients.

6. **a. Retrograde urethrography.** Retrograde urethrography is the most reliable imaging study for urethral evaluation.

7. **e. Immediate primary repair of the left testis.** Immediate primary repair should be attempted in the setting of subtotal injury to an otherwise viable testis. Even extensive testicular injuries often can be safely salvaged, and tunica vaginalis grafts provide better outcomes than do synthetic grafts for complex repair.

8. **b. Spatulated, stented, tension-free, watertight repair of the urethra with absorbable sutures.** Immediate urethral repair with fine absorbable suture over a Foley catheter is associated with superior outcomes after penetrating injury. A proximal bulbar urethral pathologic process in a young man is uniquely amenable to primary anastomotic repair.

9. **c. Retrograde urethrography should be uniformly performed to assess for urethral injury.** Flexible cystoscopy performed at the time of surgical exploration is the simplest and most sensitive means to assess for urethral injury. Urethrography is of low yield in men with no hematuria, no blood at the meatus, and no voiding symptoms; intraoperative flexible cystoscopy is an appropriate alternative method of urethral evaluation.

10. **b. Tunica vaginalis.** Blood fills the space between the visceral and parietal layers of the tunica vaginalis.

11. **b. Is often diagnosed by the presence of intratesticular hypoechoic areas on ultrasonography.** Testicular rupture is often difficult to detect clinically. Ultrasound evaluation usually shows intratesticular heterogeneity as a sentinel finding; detection of a defect of the tunica albuginea is less common.

12. **c. Microscopic dorsal vascular and neural reanastomosis is the best method of repair.** Microvascular reanastomosis of the dorsal neurovascular structures is suggested as the preferred treatment modality whenever possible. Reanastomosis of the corporal arteries is not recommended.

13. **a. Foreskin flap for small distal lesions.** Redundant foreskin provides excellent closure when ample viable tissue exists.

14. **a. Penile fracture must be repaired immediately or there is a decrement in erectile function.** Recent data have shown that a delay in surgery of as long as 7 days has no effect on the outcomes of penile fracture.

15. **e. All of the above.** Antegrade urethral realignment may simplify treatment of the defect, and a large-bore suprapubic catheter placed near the midline will promote subsequent identification of the prostatic apex during delayed reconstruction while preventing tube encrustation or obstruction.

CHAPTER REVIEW

1. Penile fracture generally occurs at the base of the penis in a ventrolateral location where the tunica albuginea is thinnest.
2. If the location of the penile fracture is evident, a vertical ventral penile incision over the injury may be used thus avoiding a degloving incision. If the location of the injury is uncertain or there is an associated urethral injury, a distal circumcising incision should be made; if this incision is used in an uncircumcised patient, a limited circumcision should be performed before closure to prevent persistent edema of the foreskin.
3. Dog bites of the penis are treated with copious irrigation, debridement, and primary closure. Human bites should be irrigated, debrided, treated with antibiotics, and left open.
4. A fractured testis should be explored and repaired because the salvage rate is higher than when conservative nonoperative therapy is used.
5. Ninety percent of bladder ruptures are associated with pelvic fractures; 10% of pelvic fractures are associated with a bladder rupture.
6. Noncomplicated extraperitoneal bladder ruptures may be treated with urethral catheter drainage alone.
7. The bulbomembranous junction is more vulnerable to injury during pelvic fracture than is the prostatomembranous junction; thus the external sphincter is often intact. In children, urethral disruptions generally occur at the bladder neck. In females, the urethral avulsion usually occurs proximally.
8. In females, urethral disruptions should be primarily repaired and vaginal lacerations should be closed.
9. Initial suprapubic cystostomy is the standard of care for major straddle injuries involving the urethra.
10. When intraperitoneal bladder laceration occurs after blunt trauma, a large laceration of the bladder dome is usually produced that predisposes to urinary ascites and/or peritonitis if it is not repaired promptly.
11. CT cystogram must be performed via retrograde distention of the bladder with a dilute contrast medium. A drainage film is required to complete a plain film cystogram.
12. Flexible cystoscopy performed at the time of surgical exploration is the simplest and most sensitive means to assess for urethral injury.
13. In posterior urethral disruptions, patients may undergo urethral realignment or immediate suprapubic tube placement with planned delayed urethroplasty. Patients undergoing urethral realignment are at high risk for developing stricture recurrence.

134 Special Urologic Considerations in Transgender Individuals

Nicolas Lumen, Anne-Françoise Spinoit, and Piet Hoebeke

QUESTIONS

1. What is the most common urologic complication after phallic reconstruction?
   a. Urethral fistula
   b. Urethral stricture
   c. Stress incontinence
   d. Urge incontinence
   e. Urinary tract infection

2. What is the most frequent site of urethral stricture in transmen?
   a. The anastomotic region between the fixed and phallic parts of the urethra
   b. The fixed part of urethra
   c. The phallic part of urethra
   d. The bladder neck
   e. The neomeatus

3. Rectal injury as a consequence of vaginectomy occurs in approximately what percent of procedures?
   a. 0.09%
   b. 0.9%
   c. 9%
   d. 19%
   e. 25%

4. The scrotum in transmen is made of the:
   a. labia majora
   b. labia minora
   c. anterior vaginal wall
   d. perineal skin
   e. labia majora and minora

5. Urologic preoperative assessment in transmen should absolutely include:
   a. uroflowmetry.
   b. ultrasound of the urinary tract.
   c. the patient's urologic history.
   d. all of the above.
   e. only c.

6. Transmen are usually difficult to catheterize transurethrally after surgery because of:
   a. the sharp curve between the female native urethra and the pars fixa of the neourethra.
   b. the presence of a vaginal recessus close to the native female urethra.
   c. hairy skin in the phallic urethra.
   d. the presence of the clitoris dorsally in the perineal urethra.
   e. the difference in elasticity between the phallic and the perineal urethra.

7. Overall, the complication rate in gender-confirming surgery for transmen is:
   a. 0.4%.
   b. 4%.
   c. 40%.
   d. 80%.
   e. 25%.

8. An erectile and testicular prosthesis is implanted:
   a. at the time of phalloplasty.
   b. 1 year after phalloplasty.
   c. 3 months after phalloplasty.
   d. 2 years after phalloplasty.
   e. first a testicular and 3 months later an erectile prosthesis.

9. When gender identity and sex do not match in a person, it is called:
   a. transsexualism.
   b. sex reversal.
   c. gender dysphoria.
   d. gender nonconformity.
   e. homosexuality.

10. In transwomen, ultrasound examination of the prostate is best done:
    a. transrectally.
    b. transabominally.
    c. transvaginally.
    d. perineally.
    e. by CT scan only.

11. Which statement is correct about gender identity disorder?
    a. It can be diagnosed at pediatric age.
    b. Is more frequent in biological females than males.
    c. Is based on hormonal imbalance.
    d. Always calls for psychotherapy before any hormonal or surgical treatment.
    e. Is not mentioned in the fifth edition of the *Diagnostic and Statistical Manual of Mental Disorders* (DSM-5).

ANSWERS

1. **a. Urethral fistula.** Urethral fistula is the most common urologic complication after phallic reconstruction.
2. **a. The anastomotic region between the fixed and phallic parts of the urethra.** Multiple retrospective studies in large cohorts of patients show that the anastomotic region between the fixed and phallic parts of the urethra is the most frequent site of urethral stricture in transmen.
3. **b. 0.9%.** Multiple retrospective studies in large cohorts of patients show that rectal injury as a consequence of vaginectomy occurs in approximately 0.9% of patients.
4. **a. Labia majora.** The labia majora are the embryologic counterpart of the scrotum, so using them for scrotal reconstruction is logical and gives the best aesthetic outcomes.

5. **d. All of the above.** In order to exclude any major urologic problem that could interfere with the reconstructive surgery, all three assessments are necessary.
6. **a. Tthe sharp curve between the female native urethra and the pars fixa of the neourethra.** Transmen are usually difficult to catheterize transurethrally after surgery because of the sharp curve between the female native urethra and the pars fixa of the neourethra.
7. **c. 40%.** Based on studies published in the field, the main complication rate including all parts of the surgery is 40%.
8. **b. 1 year after phalloplasty.** The implantation is done when sensitivity is observed in the phallus. As the sensitivity is based on a nerve anastomosis, it takes about a year before this anastomosis becomes functional.
9. **c. Gender dysphoria.** This term is based on the International Classification of Disease and DSM classifications and definitions.
10. **c. Transvaginally.** The neovagina is reconstructed between the rectum and the prostate; thus this new structure allows easy access of the ultrasound probe to examine the prostate.
11. **a. It can be diagnosed at pediatric age.** Gender identity disorder (GID), which is mentioned in DSM-5, can be diagnosed in childhood. GID is more frequent in males and is not based on hormonal imbalance. Psychotherapy as treatment has bad results and is no longer recommended in the standards of care.

CHAPTER REVIEW

1. The urologist has an important role in the treatment and follow-up of transgender individuals.
2. Urinary incontinence is the most frequent complication in transwomen.
3. Be aware of prostate pathology in transwomen.
4. Discuss whether or not to perform vaginectomy in transmen.
5. Urethral fistulas and strictures are frequent complications in transmen and most often occur at the anastomosis between the fixed and phallic part of the urethra.
6. Metoidioplasty is an alternative to phalloplasty in transmen who refuse to accept the complications of phalloplasty.
7. Implantation of an erectile prosthesis in transmen is associated with a higher risk of complications compared to native males.

135 Tumors of the Bladder

Max Kates and Trinity J. Bivalacqua

QUESTIONS

1. The average age of patients with bladder cancer in the United States is:
   a. 65.
   b. 69.
   c. 73.
   d. 76.
   e. 78.

2. Inverted papillomas are:
   a. a benign tumor of the bladder.
   b. a precursor to low-grade papillary cancer.
   c. chemotherapy resistant.
   d. an invasive tumor.
   e. best treated with antibiotics.

3. The incidence rate of urothelial cancer:
   a. has been decreasing recently because of less smoking.
   b. is higher in women than in men.
   c. is highest in developed countries.
   d. peaks in the fifth decade of life.
   e. is higher in Asia than Europe.

4. The mortality rate of urothelial cancer:
   a. is primarily related to lack of health care access.
   b. has been decreasing since 1990.
   c. is highest in underdeveloped countries.
   d. is proportionally higher in women than in men.
   e. is proportionally higher in white men than in African American men.

5. What is the risk of a white male developing urothelial cancer in his lifetime?
   a. Less than 5%
   b. 20%
   c. 40%
   d. 60%
   e. 80%

6. The most common histologic bladder cancer cell type is:
   a. squamous.
   b. adeno.
   c. urothelial.
   d. small cell.
   e. leiomyosarcoma.

7. The mortality rate from bladder cancer is highest in:
   a. the United States.
   b. England.
   c. South America.
   d. China.
   e. Egypt.

8. Recent evidence suggests that physician practice may be related to bladder cancer deaths in the elderly. What percentage of deaths could be avoided?
   a. Less than 5%
   b. 30%
   c. 50%
   d. 70%
   e. 90%

9. Which gene is most commonly mutated in high-grade muscle invasive urothelial cancer?
   a. *Cyclin A*
   b. *TP53*
   c. *FGFR-3*
   d. *HRAS*
   e. *PTEN*

10. Which gene is most commonly mutated in carcinoma in situ (CIS)?
    a. *PI3K*
    b. *RB*
    c. *FGFR-3*
    d. *HRAS*
    e. *CD-44*

11. Which gene is most commonly mutated low-grade papillary urothelial carcinoma (LgTa)?
    a. *PTEN*
    b. *RB*
    c. *FGFR-3*
    d. *HRAS*
    e. *CD-44*

12. The chemotherapy proven to cause urothelial cancer is:
    a. doxorubicin.
    b. bleomycin.
    c. ifosfamide.
    d. etoposide.
    e. cyclophosphamide.

13. The increased risk of developing bladder cancer for a man who has a sister with bladder cancer is:
    a. twofold.
    b. 10-fold.
    c. 20-fold.
    d. 40-fold.
    e. 60-fold.

14. The risk of a family member developing bladder cancer if a first-degree relative has the disease is:
    a. related to secondhand smoke.
    b. higher in men.
    c. higher in smokers.

d. related to inheritance of low-penetrance genes.

e. most common in high-grade cancer.

15. The percent of patients presenting with non–muscle-invasive disease is:

    a. less than 5%.

    b. 20%.

    c. 40%.

    d. 60%.

    e. 80%.

16. A 30-year-old man has gross hematuria, and cystoscopy reveals a papillary tumor. Transurethral resection of the tumor reveals a noninvasive 2-cm papillary low-malignant-potential urothelial tumor. Muscle is present in the resected specimen. All of the tumor is resected. The best treatment is:

    a. intravesical bacille Calmette-Guérin (BCG).

    b. repeat cystoscopy with random bladder biopsies.

    c. radical cystectomy because of the patient's young age.

    d. immediate mitomycin C intravesical therapy.

    e. observation.

17. The external agent most implicated in causing urothelial cancer is:

    a. β-naphthylamine.

    b. 4-aminobiphenyl.

    c. perchloroethylene.

    d. trichloroethylene.

    e. 4,4′-methylene bis(2-methylaniline).

18. If a woman stops smoking for 10 years after 30 pack-years of smoking, her risk of developing bladder cancer:

    a. is the same as if she still smoked.

    b. is the same as if she never smoked.

    c. is unrelated to the intensity of smoking.

    d. is very low because of her gender.

    e. gradually decreases with time.

19. A man exposed to high doses of radiation (more than 500 mSv):

    a. has the same risk of urothelial cancer formation as a nuclear plant worker.

    b. will likely develop urothelial cancer within 5 years.

    c. is more likely to develop urothelial cancer if he is younger than 20 years.

    d. is two times more likely to develop urothelial cancer.

    e. should be quarantined for 3 months.

20. One of the main changes between the AJCC 7th edition and AJCC 8th edition for bladder cancer is:

    a. there should be two grades of non-muscle-invasive bladder cancer.

    b. multiple positive pelvic lymph nodes is considered stage 3 disease.

    c. perivesical fat involvement by tumors is stage T3.

    d. CIS can be low or high grade.

    e. Ta grade 1 tumors should be considered cancerous.

21. Genetic abnormalities associated with low-malignant potential Ta tumors include:

    a. fibroblast growth factor receptor-3 (*FGFR-3*).

    b. TP53.

    c. retinoblastoma (RB) gene.

    d. PTEN.

    e. loss of chromosome 17.

22. A 40-year-old man has a T1 high-grade urothelial cancer on initial presentation. Muscle was present in the biopsy specimen. The next treatment is:

    a. BCG.

    b. repeat transurethral resection of a bladder tumor (TURBT).

    c. radical cystectomy.

    d. immediate mitomycin C instillation.

    e. neoadjuvant chemotherapy followed by radical cystectomy.

23. A 73-year-old man with a history of Ta bladder cancer is found to have a 0.5-cm papillary lesion in the prostatic urethra and undergoes extensive transurethral resection of the prostate, revealing high-grade noninvasive disease of the prostatic urethra without ductal or stromal involvement. The next best step is:

    a. perioperative mitomycin C.

    b. surveillance cystoscopy every 3 months.

    c. mitomycin C therapy.

    d. induction of and maintenance with BCG therapy.

    e. radical cystectomy.

24. A 62-year-old man undergoes a transurethral biopsy of a bladder tumor at the dome. Final pathology reveals muscle-invasive urothelial and small cell carcinoma. Metastatic workup is negative. The next step is:

    a. intravesical gemcitabine therapy.

    b. partial cystectomy.

    c. radical cystoprostatectomy.

    d. external beam radiotherapy.

    e. chemoradiation therapy.

25. When cisplatin-based chemotherapy is used, which of the following genetic mutations is associated with the worst prognosis?

    a. *FGFR-3* mutations

    b. *PTEN*

    c. *TP53*

    d. *RB*

    e. *PTEN*, *TP53*, and *RB*

26. When cisplatin-based neoadjuvant chemotherapy is used, which of the following genetic mutations is associated with an improved response?

    a. *FGFR-3* mutations

    b. *ERCC2*

    c. *TP53*

    d. *RB*

    e. *ERCC2*, *FANCC*, and *ATM*

27. Tumor suppressor genes are activated by:

    a. gene amplification.

    b. translocation.

    c. point mutations.

    d. DNA methylation.

    e. microsatellite instability.

28. The risk of urologic malignancy in a man with recurrent gross hematuria, but who had a previous negative evaluation, is:

    a. less than 5%.

    b. 20%.

    c. 40%.

    d. 60%.

    e. 80%.

29. Which of the following is not a high-risk factor in urothelial cancer formation in patients with microscopic hematuria?
    a. Age younger than 40 years
    b. Smoking
    c. History of pelvic radiation
    d. Urinary tract infections
    e. Previous urologic surgery

30. Commercially available fluorescence in situ hybridization kits test for abnormalities in which of the following chromosomes?
    a. 3, 7, 9, 17
    b. 2, 5, 8
    c. 4, 6, 9
    d. 1, 10, 12
    e. 13, 14, 16

31. Microsatellite analysis:
    a. detects telomeric repeats.
    b. amplifies DNA repeats in the genome.
    c. evaluates abnormalities on chromosome 9.
    d. detects DNA methylation.
    e. identifies hereditary urothelial cancer.

32. Smoking is responsible for what percent of bladder cancer in males?
    a. 5%
    b. 20%
    c. 40%
    d. 60%
    e. 80%

33. Which of the following is not sensitive to cisplatin chemotherapy?
    a. High-grade urothelial cancer
    b. Micropapillary cancer
    c. Squamous cell cancer
    d. Adenocarcinoma
    e. Small cell cancer

34. Nested variant of urothelial cancer can be confused with:
    a. cystitis cystica.
    b. micropapillary cancer.
    c. squamous cell cancer.
    d. small cell cancer.
    e. high-grade urothelial cancer.

35. The most common sarcoma involving the bladder is:
    a. angiosarcoma.
    b. chondrosarcoma.
    c. leiomyosarcoma.
    d. rhabdomyosarcoma.
    e. osteosarcoma.

36. Signet ring cell cancers:
    a. have a good prognosis.
    b. are sensitive to doxorubicin chemotherapy.
    c. usually present in advanced stage.
    d. are responsive to radiation therapy.
    e. are low-grade at initial presentation.

37. The risk of bladder cancer formation in a spinal cord–injured patient is:
    a. less than 5%.
    b. 20%.
    c. 40%.
    d. 60%.
    e. 80%.

38. For patients undergoing radical cystectomy for urothelial cancer, the risk of identifying prostatic urethral disease is:
    a. less than 5%.
    b. 20%.
    c. 40%.
    d. 60%.
    e. 80%.

39. Which of the following is NOT a risk factor for prostatic urethral cancer?
    a. Previous intravesical therapy
    b. CIS of the trigone
    c. CIS of the distal ureters
    d. Low-grade urothelial cancer
    e. Recurrent bladder tumors

PATHOLOGY

1. A 70-year-old man has microscopic hematuria. Cytology and computed tomography (CT) scan are negative. Cystoscopy reveals a raised 3-mm lesion on the trigone. The lesion is biopsied and is depicted in Fig. 135.1A and B, and is reported as adenocarcinoma. The next step in management is:
    a. review the pathology slides with the pathologist.
    b. cystectomy.
    c. intravesical chemotherapy.
    d. bone scan.
    e. ask for special stains from pathology.

2. A 65-year-old man has gross hematuria. He has a history of tuberculosis. Cytology is suspicious, CT scan is normal, and cystoscopy reveals a papillary lesion cephalad to the trigone. The lesion is visually completely resected (Fig. 135.2) and is reported as high-grade invasive urothelial carcinoma. The next step in management is:
    a. intravesical BCG.
    b. immediate intravesical mitomycin C.
    c. repeat transurethral resection of bladder at the previous biopsied site.
    d. a cystectomy.
    e. ask the pathologist if there is muscularis propria in the specimen.

IMAGING

1. See Fig. 135.3. The depicted findings have an association with:
    a. bladder carcinoma.
    b. previous trauma.
    c. recurrent urinary tract infections.
    d. urolithiasis.
    e. ureteral spasm.

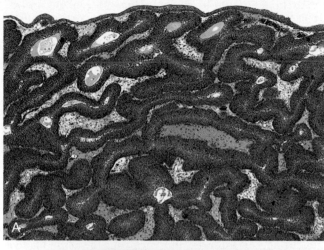

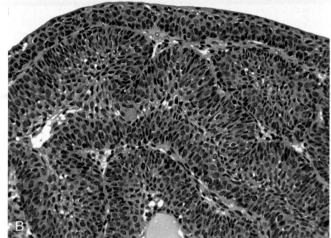

Fig. 135.1 (From Bostwick DG, Cheng L: *Urologic surgical pathology*, ed 2, Mosby, 2008, Edinburgh.)

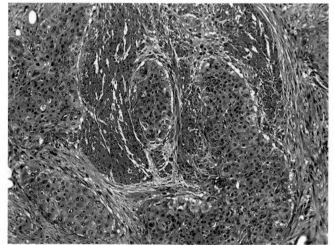

Fig. 135.2 (From Bostwick DG, Cheng L: *Urologic surgical pathology*, ed 2, Mosby, 2008, Edinburgh.)

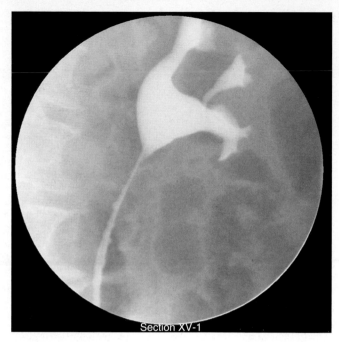

Section XV-1

Fig. 135.3

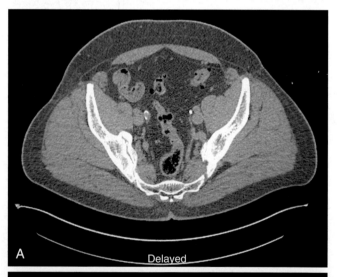

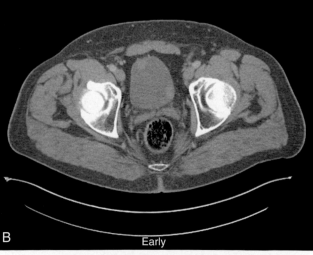

Fig. 135.4

2. Fig. 135.4A is a delayed contrast-enhanced image through the pelvic ureters, and Fig. 135.4B is an early contrast-enhanced image through the bladder. The next step in management is:

   a. shockwave lithotripsy.

   b. percutaneous nephrostolithotomy.

   c. cystoscopy.

   d. cystoscopy with ureteroscopy.

   e. follow-up with imaging in 6 months.

ANSWERS

1. **c. 73.** In the United States, the mean age of diagnosis is 73.[a]

2. **a. A benign tumor of the bladder.** When diagnosed according to strictly defined criteria (e.g., lack of cytologic atypia), inverted papillomas behave in a benign fashion with only a 1% incidence of tumor recurrence (Sung et al., 2006; Kilciler et al., 2008). Occasionally, inverted papillomas are present with coexistent urothelial cancer elsewhere in the urinary system, occurring more commonly in the upper tract than the bladder (Asano et al., 2003). The use of fluorescence in situ hybridization to evaluate chromosomal changes can distinguish between an inverted papilloma and a urothelial cancer with an inverted growth pattern (Jones et al., 2007).

3. **c. Is highest in developed countries.** Sixty-three percent of all bladder cancer cases occur in developed countries, with 55% occurring in North America and Europe. There is a geographic difference in bladder cancer incidence rates across the world, with the highest rates in Southern and Eastern Europe, parts of Africa, Middle East, and North America, and the lowest in Asia and underdeveloped areas in Africa (Ferlay et al., 2007). The incidence of urothelial cancer peaks in the seventh decade of life.

4. **b. Has been decreasing since 1990.** The mortality rate of urothelial cancer has decreased by 5% since 1990, primarily because of smoking cessation, changes in environmental carcinogens, and healthier lifestyles (Jemal et al., 2008).

5. **a. Less than 5%.** A white male has a 3.7% chance of developing urothelial cancer in his lifetime, which is roughly 3 times the probability in white females or African American males and more than 4.5 times the probability of an African American female (Hayat et al., 2007; Jemal et al, 2008).

6. **c. Urothelial.** Histologically, 90% of bladder cancers are of urothelial origin, 5% squamous cell, and less than 2% adenocarcinoma or other variants (Lopez-Beltran, 2008). Urothelial carcinoma is the most common malignancy of the urinary tract and is the second most common cause of death among genitourinary tumors.

7. **e. Egypt.** The mortality rate from bladder cancer in Egypt is three times higher than in Europe and eight times higher than in North America because squamous cell carcinoma is highly prevalent in Egypt (Parekh et al., 2002).

8. **b. 30%.** Mortality from bladder cancer is highest in elderly persons, particularly those past the age of 80, accounting for the third most common cause of cancer deaths in men over the age of 80 (Jemal et al., 2008). Whether this increase in mortality rate is related to tumor biology or changes in physician practice with the elderly is unclear. Recent evidence suggests that physician practice may be related to bladder cancer deaths in the elderly (Morris et al., 2009). These authors estimated that 31% of all bladder cancer deaths were avoidable, more commonly in noninvasive than invasive disease.

9. **b. TP53.** High-malignant potential, non–muscle-invasive bladder cancer is more likely associated with deletions of tumor suppressor genes such as TP53 and RB (Chatterjee et al., 2004a; George et al, 2007; Sanchez-Carbayo et al, 2007).

10. **b. RB.** All CIS is high grade by definition. The genetic abnormalities associated with CIS include alterations to the RB, TP53, and PTEN genes (Cordon-Cardo et al., 2000; Lopez-Beltran et al, 2002; Cordon-Cardo, 2008).

11. **c. FGFR-3.** Low-grade urothelial carcinoma is typically papillary in nature with a fibrovascular stalk and frequent papillary branching with increased cellular size, some nuclear atypia, and occasional mitotic figures. These tumors almost universally display alterations of genes in chromosome 9 and frequent mutations in FGFR3, PI3K or, alternatively, Ras genes.

12. **e. Cyclophosphamide.** The only chemotherapeutic agent that has been proven to cause bladder cancer is cyclophosphamide (Travis et al., 1995; Nilsson and Ullen, 2008). The risk of bladder cancer formation is linearly related to the duration and intensity of cyclophosphamide treatment, supporting a causative role. Phosphoramide mustard is the primary mutagenic metabolite that causes bladder cancer in patients exposed to cyclophosphamide.

13. **a. Twofold.** First-degree relatives of patients with bladder cancer have a twofold increased risk of developing urothelial cancer themselves, but high-risk urothelial cancer families are relatively rare (Aben et al., 2002; Murta-Nascimento et al., 2007; Kiemeney, 2008).

14. **d. Related to inheritance of low-penetrance genes.** The hereditary risk seems to be higher for women and nonsmokers, but it is not related to secondhand exposure to smoking in families. Most likely, there are a variety of low-penetrance genes that can be inherited to make a person more susceptible to carcinogenic exposure, thus increasing the risk of bladder cancer formation.

15. **e. 80%.** At initial presentation, 80% of urothelial tumors are non–muscle-invasive. There are multiple growth patterns of urothelial cancer, including flat carcinoma in situ (CIS), papillary tumors that can be low or high grade, and sessile tumors with a solid growth pattern. Non–muscle-invasive cancers can be very large because of lack of the genetic alterations required for invasion.

16. **d. Immediate mitomycin C intravesical therapy.** PUNLMP is a papillary growth with minimal cytological atypia that is more than seven cells thick and is generally solitary and located on the trigone (Holmang et al., 2001; Sauter et al., 2004). PUNLMP is composed of thin papillary stalks where the polarity of the cells is maintained and the nuclei are minimally enlarged. PUNLMP has a low proliferation rate and is not associated with invasion or metastases. Tumor recurrence is common, and thus perioperative treatment with mitomycin C is warranted.

17. **a. β-naphthylamine.** One of the first and most common chemical agents implicated in the formation of bladder cancer in dye and rubber workers is β-naphthylamine (Case and Hosker, 1954). Activation of aromatic amines allows DNA binding by enzymes that are selectively expressed in the population, making some subjects more susceptible to cancer formation, as described earlier related to the NAT-2 and the GSTM1 polymorphisms.

18. **e. Gradually decreases with time.** Smoking cessation does make a difference in urothelial cancer formation. Smokers who have stopped for 1 to 3 years have a 2.6 relative risk, and those who have stopped for more than 15 years have a 1.1 relative risk of bladder cancer formation (Wynder and Goldsmith, 1977; Smoke IAfRoCT, 2004).

19. **d. Is two times more likely to develop urothelial cancer.** There is a significant increased risk of dying from any cancer if a person is exposed to greater than 50 mSv. The relative risk of urothelial cancer formation is 1.63 in men and 1.74 in women. Interestingly, urothelial cancer formation after radiation is not age related, but the latency period is 15 to 30 years. However, there is no association with low-dose or industrial exposure of radiation therapy and bladder cancer formation. Importantly, urologic technicians and nuclear radiation workers do not have an increased risk of urothelial cancer formation.

20. **b. Multiple positive pelvic lymph nodes is considered stage 3 disease.** Broadly speaking, non–muscle-invasive bladder cancer is composed of stage 0 (noninvasive) and stage 1 (invasion into subepithelial connective tissue), muscle-invasive organ-confined bladder cancer is of stage 2, muscle-invasive locally advanced bladder cancer is stage 3, and metastatic disease is stage 4. Whereas prior AJCC editions viewed positive lymph nodes as stage 4 regardless of the quantity or location, the 2017 AJCC staging update now views nodal disease in the absence of systemic metastases as stage 3.

[a]Sources referenced can be found in *Campbell-Walsh-Wein Urology, 12th Edition*, on the Expert Consult website.

21. **a. Fibroblast growth factor receptor-3 (*FGFR-3*).** Genetic abnormalities associated with low-grade cancer include deletion of 9q and alterations of *FGFR-3*, *HRAS*, and *PI3K* (Holmang et al, 2001; Cordon-Cardo, 2008). Low-grade carcinomas are immunoreactive for cytokeratin-20 and CD-44. The *TP53*, retinoblastoma *(RB)*, and *PTEN* genes and loss of chromosome 17 are all associated with high-grade cancer.

22. **b. Repeat transurethral resection of a bladder tumor (TURBT).** Because of this understaging, the American Urological Association (AUA) guidelines call for a repeat transurethral resection in patients with T1 tumors to assess for muscle-invasive disease even if muscle was present in the specimen (Hall et al, 2007).

23. **d. Induction of and maintenance with BCG therapy.** For patients with noninvasive prostatic urethral cancer, transurethral resection of the prostate with BCG therapy is appropriate (Palou et al, 2007). For patients with prostatic ductal disease, a complete TURP is warranted, plus BCG therapy. Although a radical cystectomy could be performed, a more conservative organ-sparing treatment is recommended.

24. **e. Chemoradiation therapy.** Small cell carcinoma of the bladder should be considered and treated as metastatic disease, even if there is no radiologic evidence of disease outside the bladder. Small cell carcinoma of the bladder accounts for much less than 1% of all primary bladder tumors. In general, small cell carcinoma of the bladder is very chemosensitive, and the primary mode of therapy is chemoradiation therapy or chemotherapy followed by cystectomy.

25. **e. *PTEN*, *TP53*, and *RB*.** Overall genetic instability is the hallmark of invasive urothelial cancer, but, specifically, alterations of *TP53*, *RB*, and *PTEN* carry a very poor prognosis (Chatterjee et al, 2004a). *FGFR-3* mutations are associated with noninvasive bladder cancer.

26. **e. *ERCC2*, *FANCC*, and *ATM*.** The recent application of genomics to large cohorts of MIBCs has produced major breakthroughs in disease heterogeneity with obvious implications for clinical management. Whole transcriptome studies identified basal and luminal molecular subtypes (Choi et al., 2014; TCGAR, 2014; Damrauer et al., 2014), and patients with basal tumors appeared to derive the most benefit from neoadjuvant chemotherapy (NAC) (Seiler et al 2017; McConkey et al., 2018). In parallel, two other groups demonstrated that inactivating mutations in DNA damage repair genes (including ERCC2, FANCC, ATM) were associated with response to NAC (Van Allen et al., 2014; Serebriiskii et al., 2015). These findings are now being prospectively examined within the context of the Southwest Oncology Group's (SWOG's) completed S1314 trial. In addition, two groups have designed prospective clinical trials to test whether DDR mutations can be used to guide bladder preservation in patients treated with NAC, and several groups are considering clinical trials to select MIBC patients for NAC based on basal molecular subtype membership.

27. **c. Point mutations.** Tumor suppressor genes are mainly activated by allelic deletion of one allele followed by point mutations of the remaining allele. Tumor suppressor genes are recessive or have a negative effect, resulting in unregulated cellular growth. Proto-oncogenes are generally activated by point mutations in the genetic code, gene amplification, and gene translocation. The activated proto-oncogenes become oncogenes that can cause cancer, and this is considered a positive or dominant growth effect (Lengauer et al, 1998; Wolff et al, 2005; Cordon-Cardo, 2008).

28. **a. Less than 5%.** Gross, painless hematuria is the primary symptom in 85% of patients with a newly diagnosed bladder tumor (Khadra et al, 2000; Alishahi et al, 2002; Edwards et al, 2006). The gross hematuria is usually intermittent and can be related to Valsalva maneuvers; therefore any episode of gross hematuria should be evaluated even if subsequent urinalysis is negative. Fifty percent of patients with gross hematuria will have a demonstrable cause, 20% will have a urological malig-

nancy, and 12% will have a bladder tumor (Khadra et al, 2000). The risk of malignancy in patients with recurrent gross or microscopic hematuria that had a full, negative evaluation is near zero within the first 6 years (Khadra et al, 2000).

29. **a. Age younger than 40 years.** The guidelines recommend consideration for reevaluation of low-risk individuals with microscopic hematuria, but repeat evaluation every 6 months with a urinalysis, cytology, and blood pressure (to detect renal disease) is recommended for high-risk patients. Age younger than 40 years is the only factor that is not associated with an increased risk of malignancy.

30. **a. 3, 7, 9, 17.** Fluorescence in situ hybridization (FISH) identifies fluorescently labeled DNA probes that bind to intranuclear chromosomes. The current commercially available probes evaluate aneuploidy for chromosomes 3, 7, 17, and homozygous loss of 9p 21 (Zwarthoff, 2008). The median sensitivity and specificity of FISH analysis is 79% and 70%, respectively (van Rhijn et al, 2005).

31. **b. Amplifies DNA repeats in the genome.** There are multiple markers available to identify short DNA repeats present throughout the chromosomes that are lost in some tumor cells. Microsatellite analysis amplifies these repeats in the genome that are highly polymorphic, and PCR amplification can detect tumor-associated loss of heterozygosity by comparing the peak ratio of the two alleles in tumor DNA in a urine sample with that ratio in a blood sample from the same individual (Steiner et al, 1997; Wang et al, 1997). The sensitivity and specificity of microsatellite analysis for the detection of urothelial carcinoma range from 72% to 97% and 80% to 100%, respectively (Steiner et al, 1997; Wang et al, 1997). Microsatellite analysis evaluates abnormalities on all chromosomes.

32. **c. 40%.** Smoking is responsible for 30% to 50% of all bladder cancers in males, and smokers have a twofold to sixfold greater risk for bladder cancer (Brennan et al, 2000; Boffetta, 2008). Smoking cessation will decrease the risk of eventual urothelial cancer formation in a linear fashion. After 15 years of not smoking, the risk of cancer formation is the same as for a person who never smoked (Smoke IAfRoCT, 2004). The strong influence of smoking in bladder cancer formation prevents accurate determination of other, less significant dietary, micronutrient, or lifestyle changes that may alter bladder cancer formation.

33. **b. Micropapillary cancer.** The most effective treatment for all stages of micropapillary urothelial carcinoma is surgical resection. Treatment with transurethral resection and BCG therapy is ineffective unless the tumor is completely resected (Kamat et al, 2007). Neoadjuvant chemotherapy does not appear effective in micropapillary urothelial carcinoma, similar to ovarian cancer (Bristow et al, 2002; Kamat et al, 2007). Neoadjuvant chemotherapy may actually worsen survival by delaying therapy when compared with immediate cystectomy. Cisplatin is effective against urothelial cancer and the associated variants of squamous cell, adenocarcinoma, and small cell cancer.

34. **a. Cystitis cystica.** The nested variant of urothelial cancer is a rare but aggressive cancer that has a male-to-female ratio of 6:1 and can be confused with benign lesions, such as Von Brunn nests that are in the lamina propria, cystitis cystica, and inverted papillomas (Holmang and Johansson, 2001). There is little nuclear atypia in nested variant urothelial carcinoma, but the tumor cells will often contain areas with large nuclei and mitotic figures. The mortality rate from nested variant urothelial carcinoma, despite aggressive therapy, is significant, with 70% dying of their disease within 3 years (Paik and Park, 1996).

35. **c. Leiomyosarcoma.** Leiomyosarcoma is the most common histologic subtype, followed by rhabdomyosarcoma and then, rarely, angiosarcomas, osteosarcomas, and carcinosarcomas. The male-to-female ratio is 2:1, and the average age at presentation is in the sixth decade of life. There are no clear agents that cause bladder sarcomas, although there is an association with pelvic radiation and systemic chemotherapy for

other malignancies (Spiess et al, 2007). Importantly, bladder sarcomas are not smoking related.

36. **c. Usually present in advanced stage.** Primary signet ring cell carcinoma of the bladder is extremely rare, making up less than 1% of all epithelial bladder neoplasms (Morelli et al, 2006). Signet ring cell carcinoma can be of urachal origin and directly extend into the bladder. These tumors generally present as high-grade, high-stage tumors and have a uniformly poor prognosis. The primary treatment is radical cystectomy; however, in the majority of cases there are regional or distant metastases at the time of presentation, and the mean survival time is less than 20 months (Torenbeek et al, 1996). There are reports of elevated carcinoembryonic antigen (CEA) in patients with signet ring cell carcinoma. The prognostic significance of this elevated serum marker is unclear (Morelli et al, 2006). Understaging is very common in signet ring cell carcinoma, with peritoneal studding common at the time of surgical exploration.

37. **a. Less than 5%.** Spinal cord–injured patients are at risk for developing squamous cell carcinoma, most likely due to chronic catheter irritation and infection. Older studies have suggested a 2.5% to 10% incidence of squamous cell carcinoma in the spinal cord–injured population, with a mean delay of 17 years after the spinal cord injury (Kaufman et al., 1977). More recent analysis of the association of spinal cord injury and bladder cancer formation has shown a remarkably lower risk of bladder cancer formation of 0.38%, most likely because of better catheter care (Bickel et al., 1991). This supports the concept that chronic infection and foreign bodies can lead to bladder cancer formation.

38. **c. 40%.** Prostatic urethral cancer is associated with urothelial cancer of the bladder in 90% of cases, primarily CIS, and most will have multifocal bladder tumors. However, the incidence of prostatic urethral disease in patients with primary urothelial cancer is only 3% (Rikken et al., 1987; Millan-Rodriguez et al., 2000). Secondary prostatic urethral involvement in patients with a history of urothelial cancer is approximately 15% at 5 years and 30% at 15 years, almost uniformly associated with extensive intravesical therapy (Herr and Donat, 1999). For patients undergoing radical cystectomy for urothelial cancer, the risk of identifying prostatic urethral disease is 40%.

39. **d. Low-grade urothelial cancer.** Risk factors for prostatic urethral involvement are CIS of the trigone, bladder neck, distal ureters, recurrent bladder tumors, and a history of intravesical chemotherapy (Wood et al., 1989b). Low-grade tumors rarely involve the prostatic urethra.

PATHOLOGY

1. **a. Review the pathology slides with the pathologist.** This is a classic inverted papilloma, and the inexperienced pathologist might mistake it for an adenocarcinoma. The location of the lesion would be unusual for adenocarcinoma, particularly in a patient with no risk factors, and should alert the clinician to review the slides with the pathologist.

2. **e. Ask the pathologist if there is muscularis propria in the specimen.** There are clear bundles of muscularis propria in the micrograph making the tumor at least a T2.

IMAGING

1. **a. Bladder carcinoma.** Pseudodiverticulosis of the ureter is associated with bladder carcinoma in 30% of cases. This association has led many to recommend that patients with this diagnosis undergo surveillance of their bladder for the development of urothelial neoplasms. The etiology is unknown.

2. **d. Cystoscopy with ureteroscopy.** There are multiple enhancing masses in the fluid-filled urinary bladder on the early image. On the delayed image, the ureters are opacified with contrast, and there is a filling defect seen in the mildly dilated right ureter, suspicious for a synchronous ureteral lesion.

CHAPTER REVIEW

1. Inverted papillomas are associated with chronic inflammation.
2. Cystitis glandularis may be associated with pelvic lipomatosis.
3. Bladder cancers in adolescents and young adults generally are well differentiated and noninvasive.
4. The intensity and duration of smoking is linearly related to the risk of developing bladder cancer with no plateau; cessation of smoking reduces the risk.
5. There is a clear association between a healthy diet and a decreased risk of urothelial cancer.
6. There is no convincing evidence that alteration in fluid intake, alcohol consumption, ingestion of artificial sweeteners, or analgesic abuse increase the risk of bladder cancer; however, chronic irritation, bacterial infection, and radiation have all been associated with the development of bladder cancer.
7. Eighty percent of the time, low-grade, low-stage urothelial neoplasia (papillary urothelial neoplasia of low malignant potential) is associated with loss of chromosome 9.
8. Low-grade (stage 1), low-stage urothelial neoplasia is called papillary urothelial neoplasia of low malignant potential (PUNLMP); the terms low grade and high grade replace the old system of grades 2 and 3.
9. Prostatic urethral involvement by transitional cell carcinoma without invasion carries a relatively good prognosis; when it invades the prostatic stroma, the prognosis is less good, and when it directly invades the substance of the prostate from the bladder, the prognosis is poor.
10. Low-grade papillary lesions have a 60% recurrence rate but less than a 10% rate of progression to muscularis propria invasion, whereas high-grade lesions, particularly T1, may have a stage progression in as many as 50% of cases. Moreover, high-grade non-muscularis propria invasive tumors have an 80% incidence of recurrence.
11. Angiolymphatic invasion is a poor prognostic sign.
12. In muscularis propria invasive urothelial cancer, alterations in *TP53*, *RB*, and *PTEN* are poor prognostic indicators.
13. Genetic alterations in low-grade non-muscularis propria invasive disease include alterations in *FGFR-3* and deletions in chromosome 9.
14. Porphyrin-induced fluorescent cystoscopy and narrow-band imaging cystoscopy have been used to increase the sensitivity of cystoscopy.
15. To date, none of the urinary markers are sensitive or specific enough to replace cystoscopy for monitoring bladder cancer.
16. Sarcomas of the bladder, in decreasing order of frequency, include leiomyosarcoma, rhabdomyosarcoma, angiosarcoma, osteosarcoma, and carcinosarcoma.
17. *Schistosoma haematobium* is the causative agent of squamous cell carcinoma in endemic regions.
18. Altered growth patterns, such as micropapillary and nested patterns, carry a poor prognosis.
19. Normal bladder urothelium is less than seven cell layers thick: papillary lesions are greater than seven cell layers thick.
20. The incidence of urothelial cancer peaks in the seventh decade of life.

21. There is some evidence to indicate that BCG plus oral administration of vitamins A, B_6, C, E, and zinc result in a reduced risk of recurrent transitional cell carcinoma.

22. Histologically, 90% of bladder cancers are of urothelial origin, 5% squamous cell, and less than 2% adenocarcinoma or other variants.

23. All CIS is high grade by definition. The genetic abnormalities associated with CIS include alterations to the *RB*, *TP53*, and *PTEN* genes.

24. The only chemotherapeutic agent that has been proven to cause bladder cancer is cyclophosphamide.

25. First-degree relatives of patients with bladder cancer have a two-fold increased risk of developing urothelial cancer themselves.

26. Urothelial cancer formation after radiation is not age related; the latency period is 15 to 30 years.

27. A repeat transurethral resection in patients with T1 tumors to assess for muscle-invasive disease should be performed, even if muscle was present in the original specimen.

28. Small cell carcinoma of the bladder is very chemosensitive.

29. The risk of malignancy in patients with recurrent gross or microscopic hematuria who had a full, negative evaluation is near zero within the first 6 years.

30. Neoadjuvant chemotherapy does not appear effective in micropapillary urothelial carcinoma.

136 Management Strategies for Non–Muscle-Invasive Bladder Cancer (Ta, T1, and CIS)

Joseph Zabell and Badrinath Konety

QUESTIONS

1. Postoperative intravesical chemotherapy (administered in the recovery room) is most appropriate for which of the following patients?
   a. Initial presentation of a solitary 3.0-cm, low-grade–appearing tumor on the posterior bladder wall
   b. Multifocal high-grade Ta lesions with associated urothelial carcinoma in situ (CIS)
   c. 6.5-cm high-grade, broad-based tumor on lateral wall with deep resection
   d. a and b
   e. a, b, and c

2. Which of the following agents is contraindicated for immediate postoperative intravesical chemotherapy (administered at time of transurethral resection of bladder tumor [TURBT])?
   a. Thiotepa
   b. Bacille Calmette-Guérin (BCG)
   c. Mitomycin C (MMC)
   d. Epirubicin
   e. b and c

3. Potential advantage(s) of tumor markers such as, BTA, stat NMP-22, and UroVysion (FISH) when compared with urinary cytology for monitoring patients with bladder cancer is (are) improved:
   a. sensitivity.
   b. specificity.
   c. positive predictive value.
   d. a and c.
   e. a, b, and c.

4. Progression rates for low-grade Ta tumors range from:
   a. 3% to 10%.
   b. 12% to 17%.
   c. 17% to 25%.
   d. 25% to 35%.
   e. Over 35% and higher

5. General anesthesia can be advantageous compared with spinal anesthesia when a bladder tumor is being resected in which setting?
   a. Large mobile papillary tumor
   b. Tumor in a posterior wall diverticulum
   c. Lateral location at approximately 4 or 8 o'clock
   d. Extensive CIS
   e. Tumor at dome and along anterior bladder wall

6. A healthy 55-year-old man undergoes resection of a 2.0-cm bladder tumor in a posterior wall bladder diverticulum. Pathology demonstrates a pT1G3 bladder tumor with associated areas of CIS. Muscularis mucosa is involved, but there is no definite muscularis propria in the specimen. Optimal management includes

   a. repeat resection to stage the cancer.
   b. intravesical BCG therapy.
   c. partial cystectomy with excision of the diverticulum.
   d. radical cystectomy and urinary diversion.
   e. chemotherapy and radiation therapy.

7. The most important principle to follow when tumor is resected near or overlying a ureteral orifice is which?
   a. A ureteral stent must be placed at time of resection.
   b. In most cases resection is to be avoided.
   c. Coagulating current should not be used in this area.
   d. Resection and fulguration may be done at will—a stent or nephrostomy tube can be placed later.
   e. If hydronephrosis is found, an ultrasound should be obtained preoperatively and a nephrostomy tube placed.

8. A restaging TURBT is indicated in which of the following situations?
   a. pT1 high-grade tumor with no muscularis propria identified
   b. pTa low-grade tumor that is multifocal ($n = 5$), for which resection appeared to be complete but postoperative intravesical therapy was *not* administered
   c. pT1 high-grade tumor with muscularis propria identified and negative
   d. a and c
   e. a, b, and c

9. Intravesical mitomycin C chemotherapy for high-risk superficial bladder cancer:
   a. reduces the risk of progression.
   b. reduces the risk of recurrence.
   c. is preferred over BCG, particularly for CIS.
   d. is virtually free of side effects.
   e. is less expensive than BCG.

10. Relative contraindications to intravesical BCG therapy include which of the following?
    a. cirrhosis
    b. history of tuberculosis (TB)
    c. total incontinence
    d. immunosuppression
    e. all of the above

11. The combination of reduced-dose BCG and interferon alpha for intravesical therapy is:
    a. more effective than BCG alone.
    b. more toxic than BCG alone.
    c. preferred first-line therapy for patients with multifocal CIS.
    d. less effective than BCG alone.
    e. a reasonable option for BCG failures after one course of therapy.

12. Common side effects of thiotepa include:
    a. irritative voiding symptoms and fever.
    b. hematuria and irritative voiding symptoms.
    c. bladder contraction and myelosuppression.
    d. irritative voiding symptoms and myelosuppression.
    e. flu-like symptoms and fever.

13. Long-term (15 years) outcomes after intravesical BCG therapy for patients with high-risk non–muscle-invasive bladder cancer include which of the following?
    a. approximately 50% progression rate
    b. approximately 25% alive and with bladder intact
    c. a high incidence of recurrence in extravesical sites (prostatic urothelium and upper tracts)
    d. approximately 33% cancer-related mortality rates
    e. all of the above

14. Understaging for patients with pT1 high-grade bladder cancer is approximately:
    a. 5% to 10%.
    b. 10% to 20%.
    c. 20% to 30%.
    d. 30% to 50%.
    e. 50% to 70%.

15. A patient is diagnosed with a 1.0-cm pTa low-grade bladder cancer. What about imaging of the upper tracts?
    a. Not indicated
    b. Indicated only at diagnosis
    c. At diagnosis and 5 years later
    d. At diagnosis and every other year thereafter
    e. At diagnosis and every year thereafter:

16. For patients with a stage pTa low-grade bladder tumor and a negative cytology, random bladder biopsies:
    a. are more likely to be positive in the prostatic fossa than the bladder.
    b. must be done in a systematic manner.
    c. should include sampling of the muscularis mucosa and preferably also the muscularis propria.
    d. are indicated at initial diagnosis and need not be repeated if negative.
    e. are not indicated in most cases.

17. The risk of progression to muscle-invasive disease for patients with untreated CIS of the bladder is approximately:
    a. 5% to 15%.
    b. 15% to 25%.
    c. 25% to 35%.
    d. 35% to 45%.
    e. higher than 45%.

18. The most important factor determining the long-term impact of BCG on progression is:
    a. using a full dose with each instillation.
    b. adding interferon.
    c. maintenance therapy.
    d. rolling the patient side to side to ensure that BCG covers the entire urothelium.
    e. washing the toilet with bleach after voiding each dose.

19. According to the American Urological Association (AUA) risk stratification tables from the 2016 AUA/Society of Urologic Oncology (SUO) guideline of non–muscle-invasive bladder cancer (NMIBC), which of the following tumor characteristics would classify as an intermediate risk tumor?
    a. HG T1
    b. Any CIS
    c. Solitary LG Ta >3 cm
    d. PUNLMP
    e. Any variant histology

20. Which of the following represents an appropriate surveillance algorithm for high-risk NMIBC according to the 2016 AUA/SUO guideline?
    a. Cystoscopy every 3 to 4 months for 2 years, every 6 months for the subsequent 2 years, and annually for life
    b. Cystoscopy every 3 to 6 months for 2 years, then stop
    c. Imaging unnecessary unless hematuria is present
    d. Upper tract imaging annually for at least 2 years
    e. Cystoscopy at 3 months and then again 9 months later

21. A 76-year-old male with a history of urothelial CIS begins induction BCG. Following his second instillation, he notes severe urinary urgency and dysuria as well as a fever to 102°F that is present 2 days after instillation. Appropriate management of this BCG toxicity includes which of the following?
    a. Continue BCG instillations unchanged at next instillation
    b. Start isoniazid and rifampin
    c. Start ciprofloxacin
    d. Consider infectious disease consult
    e. b and d

22. Which of the following genetic mutations is commonly linked to low-grade NMIBC?
    a. Rb
    b. Fibroblast growth factor receptor 3 (FGFR3)
    c. p53
    d. RAS
    e. PTEN

23. In the setting of initial BCG failure, a second course of BCG provides a response rate of approximately:
    a. 5% to 10%
    b. 10% to 20%
    c. 30% to 50%
    d. 60% to 80%
    e. >90%

ANSWERS

1. **a. Initial presentation of a solitary 3.0 cm, low-grade–appearing tumor on the posterior bladder wall.** Postoperative intravesical chemotherapy should be considered for most cases of new, apparently low-grade non–muscle-invasive bladder cancer because it has been shown to reduce recurrence rates and to improve outcomes for this disease. One major exception is the patient in whom an extensive resection has been performed or whenever there is a possible perforation. In these patients intravesical chemotherapy should be withheld owing to concern about local extravasation and absorption. The benefit of postoperative intravesical chemotherapy is reduced in patients with recurrent or multiple tumors, and there is no clear benefit in patients with high-grade disease.

2. **b. Bacillus Calmette-Guérin (BCG). BCG should never be given in association with known trauma to the urinary tract, such as after transurethral resection of a bladder tumor (TURBT), owing to concern over systemic absorption and sepsis.** All of the other agents have shown efficacy in this setting with a favorable morbidity profile.

3. **a. Sensitivity.** Tumor markers such as BTA stat, NMP-22, and UroVysion (FISH) provide increased sensitivity, particularly for low-grade tumors. High specificity is the strength of urinary cytology. This approaches 90% to 100% in many series and has not been improved on with these other markers. Positive predictive value is highest for urinary cytology because the number of false positives is low.

4. **a. 3% to 10%.** Recurrence is common (50%–70%) for patients with low-grade pTa tumors, but progression to higher tumor stage is uncommon, occurring in about 5% to 10% of patients.

5. **c. Lateral location, at approximately 4 or 8 o'clock. Resection along the lateral bladder wall posterolaterally places one in proximity to the obturator nerve, which can lead to an obturator reflex and increased risk of bladder wall perforation.** In this situation, general anesthesia with complete paralysis is sometimes beneficial to allow the procedure to be performed in a safe and simple manner.

6. **d. Radical cystectomy and neobladder urinary diversion.** This patient should be strongly considered for radical cystectomy. Partial cystectomy is not a good option because of the presence of CIS, which indicates a high risk of field-effect disease and subsequent recurrence. Deeper biopsies will risk perforation and would be unlikely to influence management. Understaging is common with tumors in diverticula, and high-grade invasive tumors like this are best managed with radical cystectomy to ensure local disease control and optimize outcomes on a long-term basis.

7. **c. Coagulating current should not be used in this area.** A stent should be avoided if possible to prevent theoretical risk of reflux of tumor cells into the upper tracts. In most cases this area can be resected, and most ureters will remain unobstructed as long as the orifice is identified and coagulating current is not used in this area. Preoperative placement of a nephrostomy tube is often unnecessary as long as renal function is stable. Many patients with hydronephrosis will have invasive disease and will be undergoing urinary diversion in the near future, and this will relieve the obstruction. Hence, temporary nephrostomy tube placement is usually not required.

8. **d. a and c.** Patients with pT1 tumor for whom the muscularis propria was not identified are understaged about 50% of the time and a repeat resection is clearly indicated. Repeat resection of patients with pT1G3 tumor with muscularis propria present and negative are found to have residual or invasive disease 30% of the time. A repeat TURBT is thus indicated in both of these patient populations to accurately stage the tumor and to optimize patient management.

9. **b. Reduces the risk of recurrence.** Mitomycin C (MMC) can reduce the risk of recurrence, but there is no convincing evidence that it can reduce progression rates, which is true for all forms of intravesical chemotherapy. Most comparative studies and meta-analyses suggest an advantage to BCG, particularly for CIS. MMC can lead to local bladder irritation and a number of other side effects and is thus far from risk free.

10. **e. All of the above.** BGC is contraindicated in patients with liver disease (isoniazid cannot be given if they develop BCG sepsis), have a personal history of TB, have total incontinence (they cannot retain the BCG, so efficacy would be poor). Immunosuppression represents a relative contraindication as the mechanism of action is to stimulate an immune response. Although small series have demonstrated this to be safe, it may be less effective than in immunocompetent patients. Other contraindications include disrupted urothelium, gross hematuria, or active or persistent symptomatic urinary tract infection (UTI).

11. **d. Less effective than BCG alone.** BCG plus interferon alpha has shown activity in BCG failures; this is a viable option for this challenging patient population. However, it is more expensive, and a randomized trial demonstrated that it is less effective than BCG alone in BCG-naive patients. BCG remains the treatment of choice for CIS. BCG plus interferon alpha is well tolerated with a side-effect profile that is better on average than BCG alone, because most of the side effects are related to the BCG and its dose is reduced in this regimen.

12. **d. Irritative voiding symptoms and myelosuppression.** Irritative voiding symptoms are reported by 12% to 69% of patients receiving intravesical thiotepa. The low molecular weight of this agent (189 kD) predisposes to systemic absorption and myelosuppression. These are the two most common side effects of this agent.

13. **e. All of the above.** Data about long-term outcomes for patients with high-risk superficial bladder cancer treated with intravesical BCG therapy are derived primarily from the experience at Memorial Sloan Kettering (Cookson et al., 1997).[a] In this series, 50% of patient progressed and one-third died of cancer progression. Approximately one-third developed disease in the prostatic fossa or upper tracts and only 27% survived with an intact bladder. Such data should be considered when patients are being counseled about treatment options for high-risk disease.

14. **d. 30% to 50%.** The risk of understaging a pT1 high-grade bladder tumor is approximately 30%, but it is even higher if there is no muscularis propria in the specimen. Overall, the risk is about 30% to 50% in this high-risk patient population.

15. **a. Not indicated.** The incidence of upper tract tumor associated with pTaG1 bladder cancer is extremely low (0.3%–2.3%), and current consensus is that upper tract imaging is not indicated in this patient population (Oosterlinck et al., 2005). If hematuria is present, however, upper tract imaging is indicated for its evaluation regardless of the finding of bladder tumor.

16. **e. Are not indicated in most cases.** The yield of random bladder biopsy in patients with low-grade low-stage bladder tumors and a negative cytology is very low and is not indicated unless high-risk features are present.

17. **e. Higher than 45%.** Untreated CIS is very high risk (>50%) for progressing to muscle-invasive disease. Even patients with a complete response to intravesical BCG will experience progression in 30% to 40% of cases on longitudinal follow-up (Sylvester et al., 2005).

18. **c. Maintenance therapy.** Maintenance therapy is the only proven scenario demonstrating reduction of tumor progression. Dose reduction studies appear to support similar benefit for lower doses, which are usually better tolerated if side effects are identified with full dosing. Interferon is incrementally beneficial in certain circumstances. Options d and e are both without scientific basis but are commonly recommended.

19. **c. Solitary LG Ta >3 cm.** According the 2016 AUA/SUO guidelines, cases of NMIBC. can be classified as low-, intermediate-, or high-risk tumors (Table 136.2). LG Ta with recurrence within 1 year, solitary LG Ta tumors larger than 3 cm, multifocal LG Ta tumors, HG Ta tumors smaller than 3 cm, and LG T1 tumors are all considered to be of intermediate risk.

20. **e. a and d.** Appropriate surveillance for high-risk tumors includes cystoscopy every 3 to 4 months for 2 years, semiannually for 2 years, and annually for life with cytology on the same schedule. The clock should be restarted with each recurrence. Upper tract imaging should be done annually for 2 years and considered on a less frequent basis after that.

---

[a]Sources referenced can be found in *Campbell-Walsh-Wein Urology, 12th Edition*, on the Expert Consult website.

21. **e. b and d.** The clinical scenario described represents a grade 3 complication given the persistent high-grade fever. This patient should be started on treatment with isoniazid and rifampin for 3 to 6 months (choice b) along with vitamin B6 or pyridoxine. Furthermore, consultation with an infectious disease specialist (choice d) should be considered in this setting, particularly if symptoms are severe. This patient should also be provided with symptomatic management with anticholinergics and/or nonsteroidal anti-inflammatory drugs (NSAIDs), etc. The dose of BCG should be reduced to a half or one-third dose or stopped completely if there is any evidence of solid organ involvement.

22. **b. Fibroblast growth factor receptor 3 (FGFR3).** Fibroblast growth factor receptor 3 is a commonly mutated cellular proliferation gene that is mutated in low-grade NMIBC. RB and p53, along with a number of mutations on chromosome 9, are commonly associated with high-grade tumors.

23. **c. 30% to 50%.** For patients who fail initial BCG, a second course provides a 30% to 50% chance of response.

CHAPTER REVIEW

1. Malignant tumors are classified as low grade or high grade, regardless of invasion.
2. High- and low-grade cancers are often considered essentially separate diseases based on disparate genetic development, biologic behavior, and management strategies.
3. The most important risk factor for progression is grade.
4. CIS is a precursor as well as a risk factor for progression, invasion, and metastasis.
5. Papillary tumors with orderly cellular arrangement, minimal architectural abnormalities, and minimal nuclear atypia are designated papillary urothelial neoplasm of low malignant potential (PUNLMP).
6. TURBT is performed both to remove all visible tumors and provide specimens for pathologic examination to determine stage and grade.
7. Repeat resection within 2 to 6 weeks is usually indicated in patients with high-grade disease, especially if no muscle was present in the initial TURBT.
8. All suspicious lesions should be sampled, but random biopsies are not required in low-risk patients.
9. Office-based fulguration and observation may be applied to certain low-risk patients.
10. Fluorescence cystoscopy with 5-aminolevulinic acid (5-ALA) derivatives and narrow-band imaging improves the ability to visualize inconspicuous tumors and could reduce short- and long-term recurrence rates after TUR.
11. Single-dose intravesical chemotherapy administered within 6 hours of resection reduces recurrence of low-risk tumors, with significant impact in the setting of initial presentation of solitary low-grade papillary tumors.
12. The incremental benefit in patients with recurrent or multiple tumors is limited.
13. No benefit has been found in patients with high-grade disease.
14. Intravesical BCG has higher efficacy and side effects compared to intravesical chemotherapy.
15. BCG should be used cautiously for patients with low-risk disease because of concern about side effects.
16. BCG is the only agent shown to delay or reduce high-grade tumor progression.
17. The optimal dose and the treatment schedule for BCG are undetermined, but results are better with maintenance therapy, if tolerated.
18. BCG is contraindicated in the setting of a disrupted urothelium because of the risk of intravasation and BCG sepsis.
19. Intravesical chemotherapy has a clear impact on tumor recurrence when immediately instilled after TURBT and in the adjuvant setting. There is no clear evidence of an impact on progression.
20. Combinations of various chemotherapeutic agents and chemotherapy combined with BCG have not demonstrated major benefit combined with single-agent treatment with the exception of interferon.
21. In general, side effects of chemotherapy tend to be less common and less severe than those for BCG, but BCG is more efficacious.
22. Combination intravesical chemotherapy may have a role in treating BCG-refractory cancers.
23. Patients who experience failure of an initial course of intravesical therapy after TURBT are at high risk for recurrence or progression.
24. Failure of initial chemotherapy or BCG is most appropriately treated with a subsequent course of BCG because its efficacy in this setting is significantly greater than that of chemotherapy.
25. Following failure of a second course of intravesical therapy, patients can be enrolled in clinical trials of new agents, consider combination intravesical therapy, or proceed to cystectomy.
26. Patients at high risk for progression should be considered for cystectomy.
27. Failure to respond to an initial course of intravesical therapy is occasion to reconsider cystectomy.
28. Failure to respond to a second course is an indication for immediate cystectomy unless contraindicated or the patient chooses to pursue clinical trials or newer proven intravesical options if evidence builds for their use.
29. Cystoscopy is the hallmark of surveillance. The surveillance schedule should be individualized on the basis of risk stratification of the most recently resected tumor.
30. A number of tumor markers have shown the ability to improve the sensitivity of cytology, but specificity is lower for most.
31. Increased fluids, smoking cessation, and a low-fat diet are recommended.

137 Management of Muscle-Invasive and Metastatic Bladder Cancer

Thomas J. Guzzo, John Christodouleas, and David J. Vaughn

QUESTIONS

1. Important components in the clinical staging of patients with muscle-invasive bladder cancer include which of the following?
   a. Transurethral resection with adequate detrusor muscle in the specimen
   b. Bimanual examination under anesthesia
   c. Cross-sectional imaging of the abdomen and pelvis
   d. Laboratory studies including liver function tests
   e. All of the above

2. The most important pathologic predictor of outcome following radical cystectomy for muscle-invasive bladder cancer is
   a. pT2a versus pT2b substaging.
   b. soft tissue margin status.
   c. nodal metastasis.
   d. ureteral margin status.
   e. prostatic urethral involvement.

3. All of the following have been reported to provide prognostic information with regard to pelvic lymphadenectomy EXCEPT
   a. absolute number of lymph nodes removed.
   b. laterality of a single positive lymph node.
   c. lymph node density.
   d. extranodal extension.
   e. anatomic extent of the lymph node dissection.

4. A 52-year-old male with cT2N0Mx urothelial carcinoma is undergoing a radical cystoprostatectomy and planned orthotopic urinary diversion. What intraoperative finding would be an absolute contraindication to orthotopic diversion?
   a. Positive ureteral frozen section for carcinoma in situ (CIS)
   b. Positive apical urethral frozen section for urothelial carcinoma
   c. Suspicious lymphadenopathy
   d. Greater than 1.5-L blood loss during the cystectomy
   e. None of the above

5. All of the following are true statements regarding neoadjuvant chemotherapy for muscle-invasive bladder cancer EXCEPT which?
   a. Meta-analysis of available randomized trial data has reported an absolute 5% survival advantage for patients who receive neoadjuvant chemotherapy.
   b. Neoadjuvant chemotherapy is likely underutilized in the US-based studies that use administrative data sets.
   c. Patients who are pT0 on final pathology following neoadjuvant chemotherapy have excellent oncologic outcomes.
   d. In patients in whom a cisplatin-based regimen is contraindicated, carboplatin-based chemotherapy provides similar oncologic efficacy.
   e. All of the above.

6. A 65-year-old woman with normal renal function undergoes up-front radical cystectomy, extended pelvic lymphadenectomy, and ileal conduit urinary diversion for bacille Calmette-Guérin–refractory bladder carcinoma in situ (CIS). Final pathology is notable for T2N1M0 disease. The next step in management should be
   a. enrollment in a clinical vaccine trial.
   b. adjuvant cisplatin-based chemotherapy.
   c. adjuvant pelvic external beam radiation therapy.
   d. combination chemotherapy/external beam radiation therapy.
   e. adjuvant carboplatin-based chemotherapy.

7. All of the following are contraindications to trimodal bladder preservation EXCEPT
   a. a solitary, completely resected tumor.
   b. hydronephrosis.
   c. diffuse bladder CIS.
   d. T3 disease on cross-sectional imaging.
   e. multifocal tumors.

8. Predictors of a poor response to chemotherapy in patients with locally advanced or metastatic bladder cancer include
   a. Karnofsky performance status below 80%.
   b. visceral metastasis.
   c. both a and b.
   d. neither a nor b.

9. Gemcitabine/cisplatin systemic therapy is often used in preference to MVAC (methotrexate, vinblastine, doxorubicin, and cisplatin) for patients with locally advanced and metastatic bladder cancer because of
   a. studies demonstrating improved progression-free survival.
   b. studies demonstrating improved overall survival.
   c. a better toxicity profile.
   d. oral administration compared with intravenous administration.
   e. cost.

10. An orthotopic neobladder in a woman undergoing anterior pelvic exenteration for muscle-invasive bladder cancer is contraindicated in the setting of
    a. age older than 75 years.
    b. nodal metastasis.
    c. recurrent urinary tract infection.
    d. a serum creatinine of 1.5.
    e. tumor invading the anterior vaginal wall.

ANSWERS

1. **e. All of the above.** Important components of staging patients with muscle-invasive bladder cancer include adequate transurethral resection, bimanual examination under anesthesia

to assess local extent of disease, cross-sectional imaging, and serum laboratory values.

2. **c. Nodal metastasis.** Approximately 25% of patients with clinical T2 disease will have lymph node metastasis at the time of radical cystectomy. Lymph node status following surgery is a powerful predictor of long-term recurrence-free and overall survival. Of patients with lymph node involvement, 70% to 80% will ultimately experience a recurrence following radical cystectomy.

3. **b. Laterality of a single positive lymph node.** Although some surgical series have demonstrated improved survival in patients with one positive lymph node compared with those with multiple positive nodes, the laterality of a single positive lymph node has no prognostic significance.

4. **b. Positive apical urethral frozen section for urothelial carcinoma.** The only contraindication to performing an orthotopic neobladder is a positive apical urethral margin and inability to achieve a negative margin of the retained urethra.

5. **d. In patients in whom a cisplatin-based regimen is contraindicated, carboplatin-based chemotherapy provides similar oncologic efficacy.** Although carboplatin is a reasonable choice for patients in whom cisplatin is contraindicated, it should not be considered a first-line therapy. Patients who cannot undergo neoadjuvant cisplatin-based chemotherapy should be considered for immediate cystectomy.

6. **b. Adjuvant cisplatin-based chemotherapy.** Adjuvant cisplatin-based combination chemotherapy should be considered. Randomized trials have thus far not been definitive in overall survival results on this subject. A meta-analysis suggests a 9% absolute benefit in overall survival, but the trials often closed early or because of poor accrual, a small number of patients, and inability to represent all of the patients in adjuvant chemotherapy trials.

7. **a. A solitary completely resected tumor.** Patients with solitary completely resected tumors are ideal candidates for bladder preservation.

8. **c. Both a and b.** The Memorial Sloan Kettering Cancer Center group published their data on 203 patients with unresectable or metastatic bladder cancer treated with MVAC (Bajorin et al., 1999). They found a Karnofsky performance status below 80% and visceral (lung, liver, bone) metastasis to be independent predictors of poor outcome. Median survival times for patients who had zero, one, or two risk factors were 33, 13.4, and 9.3 months, respectively.

9. **c. A better toxicity profile.** The toxicity of MVAC led to trials of alternative, less toxic chemotherapy regimens. Most notably, a phase III randomized trial comparing gemcitabine/cisplatin with MVAC was conducted in 405 patients (von der Maase et al., 2000, 2005).[a] There was no difference in response rates (49% vs 46%), time to progression (7.4 vs 7.4 months), and overall survival rates (13.8 vs 14.8 months) between the two study arms. The updated study analysis confirmed equivalence of the two regimens (hazard ratio, 1.09, 95% confidence interval, 0.88 to 1.34, $P = .66$). The gemcitabine/cisplatin regimen was better tolerated, with only 37% of patients in that arm requiring dose modifications compared with 63% in the MVAC arm. Patients in the gemcitabine/cisplatin arm also experienced less grade 3/4 neutropenia, neutropenic fever, neutropenic sepsis, and mucositis. The toxicity-related death rate was also lower in the gemcitabine/cisplatin group (1% vs 3%). Because of its equivalent efficacy and better tolerability, gemcitabine/cisplatin is the most widely used chemotherapeutic regimen for muscle-invasive and metastatic bladder cancer.

10. **e. Tumor invading the anterior vaginal wall.** The distal two-thirds of the female urethra may serve as an adequate sphincter mechanism provided that the risk of cancer in the retained urethra is low. Anterior vaginal wall involvement—by a posterior-based bladder tumor or bladder neck or urethral involvement—is a contraindication to urethral sparing and orthotopic bladder replacement because one cannot get an adequate distal vaginal margin and urethral margin (Stein et al., 1998). Age is not a contraindication as long as there is good pelvic support minimizing the risk of stress incontinence and the patient is capable of intermittent catheterization should the need arise. Nodal metastasis is associated with a 15% local recurrence rate with only a modest risk of invasion of the neobladder, and a thorough node dissection minimizes this risk (Lerner, 2009). Bilateral hydronephrosis, although indicating a deeply invasive cancer, is not a de facto contraindication (Stimson et al., 2010).

---

[a]Sources referenced can be found in *Campbell-Walsh-Wein Urology, 12th Edition*, on the Expert Consult website.

CHAPTER REVIEW

1. Among those with muscularis propria–invasive bladder cancer, 80% are seen with the disease at initial presentation.
2. Deaths due to bladder cancer invariably occur as a result of distant metastases present at the time of local regional therapy and usually occur within the first 2 years following treatment. Therefore muscularis propria–invasive bladder cancer should be considered a systemic disease.
3. The micropapillary variant is an aggressive disease and does not respond particularly well to chemotherapy.
4. T1 grade 3 bladder tumors should routinely be re-resected because understaging is not an uncommon event.
5. Fat can be observed in the bladder wall and should not be confused with perivesical fat.
6. Lymphatic and vascular invasion are risk factors for metastases.
7. Following chemotherapy, metastases may occur in unusual locations, such as the central nervous system.
8. The incidence of pelvic node metastases is directly related to the depth of invasion and the presence of lymphovascular invasion.
9. As many as 50% of patients with muscularis propria–invasive bladder cancer succumb to their disease.
10. Of the randomized trials evaluating neoadjuvant therapy, most have not shown a definite survival advantage; however, a meta-analysis has shown a small survival advantage for those receiving neoadjuvant chemotherapy. The evidence for adjuvant chemotherapy conferring a survival advantage is less convincing.
11. Appropriate candidates for bladder preservation (transurethral tumor resection, chemotherapy, and radiation therapy thereby preserving the bladder) are those who have a solitary T2 lesion of small diameter with no associated hydronephrosis and a visibly complete resection. Such patients should have normal renal function.
12. As many as 15% of patients with tumors invading the muscularis propria have no residual disease following transurethral tumor resection.
13. Factors that affect outcome include stage, performance, status, lymphovascular invasion, age, gender, and histology.
14. Predictors of a poor prognosis include poor performance status and the presence of visceral metastases.
15. Treatment of neuroendocrine bladder tumors includes neoadjuvant chemotherapy and surgical resection; neuroendocrine tumors may be associated with a paraneoplastic syndrome (hypercortisolism and hypercalcemia).

16. There is a significant survival benefit to those who are rendered P0 at the time of radical cystectomy.

17. The highest concentration of prostatic ducts are located from the mid-prostate to the veru at the 5 and 7 o'clock positions and are the locations where CIS of the prostatic urethra is most likely to be found (biopsy should be performed in this location).

18. In women, bladder neck biopsies are a good surrogate for urethral biopsies when an orthotopic bladder is being considered.

19. Skip metastases in nodal disease for bladder cancer are rarely seen; this is not true of prostate cancer.

20. Ureteral margin status is a predictor of upper tract recurrence.

21. Prostatic stromal invasion carries a high risk of recurrent disease.

22. Patients who are not good candidates for cisplatin chemotherapy are those with a poor performance status, a creatinine clearance less than 60 mL/min, hearing loss, peripheral neuropathy, and heart failure.

23. Although carboplatin is a reasonable choice for patients in whom cisplatin is contraindicated, it should not be considered a first-line therapy.

138 Surgical Management of Bladder Cancer: Transurethral, Open, and Robotic

Neema Navai and Colin P.N. Dinney

QUESTIONS

1. The administration of neoadjuvant chemotherapy has improved survival in muscle-invasive bladder cancer from:
   a. 16 to 42 months.
   b. 23 to 54 months.
   c. 37 to 51 months.
   d. 46 to 77 months.
   e. 75 to 85 months.

2. Upper-tract imaging for urothelial carcinoma may include all of the following EXCEPT:
   a. renal ultrasound.
   b. computed tomography (CT) abdomen and pelvis.
   c. whole-body positron emission tomography (PET)/CT.
   d. magnetic resonance imaging (MRI) abdomen and pelvis.
   e. retrograde pyelogram.

3. MRI-based contrast agents are absolutely contraindicated at which glomerular filtration rate (GFR) level?
   a. <15 mL/min
   b. <20 mL/min
   c. <30 mL/min
   d. <35 mL/min
   e. <60 mL/min

4. The improvement in 5-year survival and median survival when more than 10 lymph nodes are removed is approximately:
   a. 15%, 24 months.
   b. 10%, 36 months.
   c. 20%, 24 months.
   d. 5%, 15 months.
   e. 15%, 15 months.

5. Which of the following statements is TRUE?
   a. Urethral recurrence following radical cystectomy is approximately 8% at 5 years.
   b. Even patients with a negative intraoperative urethral frozen section are at high risk for recurrence.
   c. The negative predictive value of urethral frozen section is poor.
   d. Orthotopic neobladder is protective against urethral recurrence and therefore a positive urethral margin is not a contraindication.
   e. Orthotopic neobladder can only be performed after nerve-sparing radical cystectomy.

6. Which of the following statements is FALSE regarding nerve-sparing radical cystectomy?
   a. A technique analogous to radical prostatectomy is used.
   b. Sexual function is similar for capsular-sparing and conventional nerve-sparing techniques.
   c. Age is a strong predictor of the return of erectile function.
   d. Nerve sparing does not increase local recurrence rates.
   e. Ejaculatory function can be maintained with subtotal prostate resection.

7. Anterior pelvic exenteration includes removal of the following EXCEPT:
   a. uterus.
   b. cervix.
   c. ovaries.
   d. urethra.
   e. vaginal introitus.

8. Partial cystectomy is appropriate in which of the following settings?
   a. 4-cm T2 lesion in the trigone
   b. 1-cm T2 lesion in the dome
   c. 3-cm T2 lesion in the dome with carcinoma in situ (CIS) in one location
   d. 1-cm T2 lesion with pelvic lymphadenopathy on imaging
   e. CIS in two locations

9. Enhanced recovery includes all of the following EXCEPT:
   a. alvimopan.
   b. neostigmine.
   c. pharmacologic thromboembolism prophylaxis.
   d. nasogastric suction.
   e. early enteral feeding.

10. Thromboembolism prophylaxis is needed:
    a. immediately before incision.
    b. postprocedure for 1 day.
    c. postprocedure for 1 week.
    d. postprocedure for 1 month.
    e. both a and d.

11. The RAZOR trial demonstrated which of the following:
    a. Inferior 2-year progression-free survival for open radical cystectomy
    b. Inferior 2-year progression-free survival for robotic radical cystectomy
    c. Superior oncologic outcomes for robotic radical cystectomy
    d. Noninferior 5-year progression-free survival for robotic radical cystectomy
    e. None of the above

12. Which of the following statements is supported by level 1 evidence?
    a. Robotic radical cystectomy with minimally invasive urinary diversion has a similar complication rate to an open approach.

b. Robotic radical cystectomy results in decreased blood loss when compared to open radical cystectomy.

c. Robotic radical cystectomy and open urinary diversion is oncologically inferior to an open approach.

d. Robotic radical cystectomy and minimally invasive urinary diversion is more costly than an open approach.

e. None of the above.

ANSWERS

1. **d. 46 to 77 months.** In a seminal randomized trial, Grossman and colleagues compared the treatment of muscle-invasive bladder cancer with radical cystectomy alone or surgery followed by three cycles of MVAC chemotherapy (methotrexate, vinblastine, doxorubicin, and cisplatin). They demonstrated a significant improvement in survival (46 vs. 77 months) in the neoadjuvant chemotherapy arm. This study serves as the basis for current treatment paradigms in muscle-invasive bladder cancer (Grossman et al., 2003).[a]

2. **c. Whole-body positron emission tomography (PET)/CT.** Conventional staging evaluation for upper-tract urothelial carcinoma should include evaluation of both the kidney parenchyma and the urothelial lumen. Although PET/CT can be useful for a staging evaluation, the resolution of imaging within the urinary tract is limited by the excretion of contrast material and lack of granular resolution.

3. **c. <30 mL/min.** Although gadolinium contrast should be administered with caution in patients whose GFR is between 30 and 60 mL/min, it is absolutely contraindicated in those with GFR <30 mL/min. This is due to the risk of nephrogenic systemic sclerosis.

4. **e. 15%, 15 months.** In a study of surgical factors that influence outcomes in bladder cancer treatment, Herr and colleagues found that a lymph node dissection inclusive of more than 10 nodes was associated with improvement in survival of 15 months (Herr et al., 2004).

5. **a. Urethral recurrence following radical cystectomy is approximately 8% at 5 years.** Factors that influence the risk of recurrence after radical cystectomy include orthotopic substitution with a positive urethral margin on frozen section analysis. This should be considered a contraindication for such a diversion. In addition, the negative predictive value is useful in the evaluation of urethral margins, and the risk of recurrence is only 8% at 5 years (Freeman et al., 1996).

6. **b. Sexual function is similar for capsular-sparing and conventional nerve-sparing techniques.** The rate of natural potency after radical cystectomy with conventional nerve sparing is lower than that of analogous prostatectomy series. Studies examining sexual function after subtotal resection (e.g., prostate sparing) have demonstrated improved results (Spitz et al., 1999); however, caution is advised because of the high risk of concurrent occult prostate cancer and potential for increased local recurrence.

7. **e. Vaginal introitus.** The vaginal introitus should be maintained for routine anterior exenteration. Satisfactory vaginal capacity can be maintained with both non–vaginal-sparing and vaginal-sparing approaches. In neither instance should a colpocleisis be performed as a matter of routine.

8. **b. 1-cm T2 lesion in the dome.** In the setting of muscle-invasive bladder cancer, partial cystectomy can be considered in very select patients. In those with small lesions and a lack of concurrent CIS, the results of partial cystectomy approach those of radical cystectomy (Kassouf et al., 2006; Capitanio et al., 2009).

9. **d. Nasogastric suction.** Postoperative nasogastric suction should be considered in patients with compromised airway protection; however, this has not been demonstrated to enhance recovery and need not be incorporated to facilitate return of bowel function postoperatively. Early enteral feeding, neostigmine, and alvimopan have all demonstrated efficacy in improving return of bowel function following abdominal surgery.

10. **e. Both a and d.** In addition to the administration of prophylaxis prior to incision, a reduction in postoperative thromboembolic events from 4.6% to 0.8% was observed in patients treated for 4 weeks following abdominal or pelvic surgery (Kakkar et al., 2010).

11. **e. None of the above.** The RAZOR trial was designed as a prospective multiinstitutional noninferiority trial and demonstrated non-inferior progression-free survival at 2 years for robotic radical cystectomy when compared to open radical cystectomy (Parekh et al., 2018).

12. **b. Robotic radical cystectomy results in decreased blood loss when compared to open radical cystectomy.** The results of the RAZOR trial (Parekh et al., 2018) and the randomized study performed at Memorial Sloan Kettering Cancer Center (Bochner et al., 2014) demonstrated improvements in blood loss for robotic radical cystectomy. Notably both studies utilized an open technique for the urinary diversion.

---

[a] Sources referenced can be found in *Campbell-Walsh-Wein Urology, 12th Edition*, on the Expert Consult website.

CHAPTER REVIEW

1. Before endoscopic treatment of bladder cancer, the patient should have upper-tract imaging.
2. Initial transurethral resection of a bladder tumor should routinely be performed to include muscle. There should be a 2-cm visibly negative margin on the surface.
3. Immediately following transurethral resection of bladder tumors, intravesical installation of epirubicin or mitomycin C modestly reduces recurrences but has little effect on progression.
4. Bacille Calmette-Guérin should never be instilled immediately following bladder tumor resection.
5. Before a cystectomy, the site of the abdominal stoma should be marked by an enterostomal therapist with the patient awake so that the proper location may be ascertained.
6. If prostate- or prostate capsule–sparing techniques are to be used in orthotopic bladder construction, preoperative evaluation to rule out occult cancer—either transitional cell or prostate adenocarcinoma—should be performed.
7. A radical cystectomy in the female includes complete removal of the urethra including the meatus.
8. Patients amenable to partial cystectomy should have a solitary lesion without associated CIS in which a 2-cm margin may be obtained, which is far enough away from the ureteral orifices and bladder neck that closure can be accomplished without compromising these structures.
9. Sixty-four percent of patients undergoing radical cystectomy have at least one perioperative complication in the first 3 months postoperative; 13% experience high-grade complications. The majority of complications are gastrointestinal.
10. The boundaries of a standard lymph node dissection are the genitofemoral nerve laterally, internal iliac artery medially, Cooper ligament caudally, and crossing of the ureter at the common iliac artery cranially.
11. The 90-day mortality rate for radical cystectomy is approximately 3%.

12. Routine administration of antibiotic prophylaxis in patients undergoing a transurethral resection of a bladder tumor is recommended and should be given 30–60 minutes before the procedure.
13. Transurethral resection of tumors on the lateral wall may initiate the obturator reflex and result in bladder perforation. This may be minimized by minimally distending the bladder, using bipolar cautery, and using general anesthesia with muscle paralysis.
14. Routine stenting of a resected ureteral orifice with cutting current is not necessary.
15. In preparation for a cystectomy and urinary diversion, mechanical and antibiotic bowel prep is controversial. The data to justify omitting this preparation come, for the most part, from the general surgical literature in which the bowel is not opened in the peritoneal cavity as it is in urology, particularly in continent diversions. Administration of intravenous antibiotic prophylaxis 30–60 minutes before the incision is recommended.
16. In women, the vagina should be prepped into the surgical field.
17. Care should be taken when using sealing instruments near the rectum because that organ may be injured by radiating heat.
18. Early enteral feeding, neostigmine, and alvimopan have all demonstrated efficacy in improving return of bowel function following abdominal surgery.

139 Use of Intestinal Segments in Urinary Diversion

Anton Wintner and Douglas M. Dahl

QUESTIONS

1. When a portion of stomach is to be used for augmentation, it should:
   a. always be based on the right gastroepiploic artery.
   b. include only the antrum.
   c. never extend to the pylorus.
   d. include a significant portion of the lesser curve.
   e. be mobilized with the omentum.

2. The ileum differs from the jejunum in that:
   a. it has a larger diameter.
   b. the mesentery is thinner.
   c. it has multiple arcades.
   d. the vessels in the mesentery are larger.
   e. the mesentery is longer.

3. When stomach is used for urinary diversion, the electrolyte abnormality that may occur is most commonly what type of metabolic alkalosis?
   a. Hyperchloremic
   b. Hypochloremic
   c. Hyperkalemic
   d. Hypernatremic
   e. Hypocalcemic

4. Postoperative bowel obstruction is most common when which of the following segments is used for diversion?
   a. Right colon
   b. Stomach
   c. Sigmoid
   d. Ileum
   e. Transverse colon

5. Mechanical bowel preparation results in a reduction in:
   a. bacterial counts per gram of enteric contents.
   b. bacterial count in the jejunum.
   c. total number of bacteria in the bowel.
   d. bacterial counts in the stomach.
   e. bacterial counts in the ileum.

6. Systemic antibiotics in elective surgery should be given:
   a. before the patient is anesthetized.
   b. before the skin incision is made.
   c. intraoperatively before closure commences.
   d. at any time in the perioperative period.
   e. postoperatively for 3 to 5 days.

7. The most common cause of a lethal bowel complication is:
   a. use of previously irradiated bowel.
   b. lack of mechanical bowel prep.
   c. lack of antibiotic bowel prep.
   d. placement of a drain adjacent to the anastomosis.
   e. failure to give preoperative antibiotics.

8. When stapled anastomoses are compared with sutured anastomoses, there is/are:
   a. fewer leaks.
   b. less compatibility with urine.
   c. reduced overall operative time.
   d. lesser incidence of bowel obstruction.
   e. earlier return of bowel function.

9. The use of a nasogastric tube in the postoperative period:
   a. hastens the return of intestinal motility.
   b. reduces the incidence of bowel leak.
   c. reduces postoperative vomiting.
   d. increases the risk of aspiration.
   e. reduces the incidence of anastomotic leak.

10. The abdominal stoma for a conduit should be:
    a. flush with the skin.
    b. placed through the belly of the rectus muscle.
    c. made as a loop to reduce parastomal hernia.
    d. made with the colon for the lowest complication rate.
    e. placed in the right lower quadrant.

11. The loop end ileostomy is best used in:
    a. the obese patient.
    b. the thin patient.
    c. when a stoma is revised.
    d. in female patients.
    e. in spinal cord injury patients.

12. Ureteral strictures occurring after an ileal conduit not associated with the ureteral intestinal anastomosis most frequently occur:
    a. at the ureteropelvic junction.
    b. in the right ureter several centimeters proximal to the ureteral intestinal anastomosis.
    c. on the left side where the ureter crosses the aorta.
    d. in the mid-ureter.
    e. in either ureter within several centimeters proximal to the anastomosis.

13. Renal deterioration after a conduit diversion with normal kidneys occurs in what percent of renal units?
    a. 20%
    b. 40%
    c. 50%
    d. 70%
    e. 80%

14. The most common cause of death in patients with ureterosigmoidostomies during the long term is:
    a. cancer.
    b. renal failure.
    c. acid–base abnormalities.
    d. the primary disease.
    e. ammonium intoxication.

15. The minimal glomerular filtration rate (GFR) in mL/min necessary for a continent diversion is:
    a. 70.
    b. 60.
    c. 35.
    d. 25.
    e. 20.

16. The urinary diversion with the fewest intraoperative and immediate postoperative complications is:
    a. ileal conduit.
    b. colon conduit.
    c. Koch pouch.
    d. Indiana pouch.
    e. neobladder.

17. The jejunal conduit syndrome is manifested by:
    a. hyperchloremic metabolic acidosis.
    b. hypochloremic metabolic alkalosis.
    c. hyperkalemic, hyponatremic metabolic acidosis.
    d. hypokalemic, hyponatremic metabolic alkalosis.
    e. hyperkalemic metabolic alkalosis.

18. The primary advantage of a transverse colon conduit is:
    a. its ease of construction.
    b. the ability to perform a non-refluxing anastomosis.
    c. less likely to be injured by radiation.
    d. reduced electrolyte problems.
    e. equidistant from each kidney, allowing for short ureteral length on both sides.

19. Total body potassium depletion is most common in:
    a. ureterosigmoidostomy.
    b. ileal conduit.
    c. colon conduit.
    d. sigmoid conduit.
    e. gastrocystoplasty.

20. In urinary intestinal diversion, serum creatinine may not be an accurate reflection of renal function because of:
    a. interfering substances.
    b. tubule secretion.
    c. tubule reabsorption.
    d. bowel reabsorption.
    e. decreased renal elimination.

21. Patients with urinary diversions who have a hyperchloremic metabolic acidosis with time:
    a. retain the ability to maintain the acidosis.
    b. lose the ability for electrolyte transport in the intestinal segments.
    c. compensate for the metabolic acidosis, thus eliminating risk.
    d. intermittently absorb ammonia when infection is present.
    e. tend to retain potassium.

22. Bone density abnormalities:
    a. are unlikely to occur with ileum.
    b. are most likely to occur with colon.
    c. are more common in patients with persistent hyperchloremic metabolic acidosis.
    d. are common in patients with total body potassium depletion.
    e. are unlikely to occur in patients with conduits.

23. Urinary intestinal diversion in children:
    a. increases the need for vitamin D.
    b. increases the need for calcium.
    c. limits linear growth.
    d. decreases epiphyseal growth.
    e. results in premature epiphyseal closure.

24. Cancer occurring in urinary intestinal diversion is most likely to occur in:
    a. augmentations.
    b. colon conduits.
    c. ileal conduits.
    d. ureterosigmoidostomies.
    e. sigmoid conduits.

25. Reconfiguring the bowel during the long term results in:
    a. decreased motor activity.
    b. increased volume.
    c. decreased metabolic complications.
    d. decreased absorption of solutes.
    e. increased absorption of solutes.

26. The syndrome of severe metabolic alkalosis in patients who have had a gastrocystoplasty is most likely to occur in patients who have:
    a. decreased aldosterone levels.
    b. jejunum interposed in the urinary tract.
    c. total body potassium depletion.
    d. elevated gastrin levels.
    e. decreased renin levels.

27. There is direct evidence from cystectomy patients that the following can be safely omitted from an enhanced recovery after surgery (ERAS) protocol:
    a. preoperative fasting
    b. thrombosis prophylaxis
    c. mechanical bowel prep
    d. pelvic drain
    e. preoperative intravenous antibiotics

28. Arginine hydrochloride infusion can be used to treat life-threatening complications caused by the following type of conduit:
    a. stomach
    b. jejunum
    c. ileum
    d. colon
    e. all of the above

ANSWERS

1. **c. Never extend to the pylorus.** When a wedge of fundus is used, it should not include a significant portion of the antrum and should never extend to the pylorus or all the way to the lesser curve of the stomach.
2. **c. It has multiple arcades.** The ileum, more distal in location, has a smaller diameter. It has multiple arterial arcades, and the vessels in the arcades are smaller than those in the jejunum.

3. **b. Hypochloremic.** Complications specific to the use of stomach include the hematuria-dysuria syndrome and uncontrollable metabolic alkalosis in some patients. When stomach is used, a hypochloremic, hypokalemic metabolic alkalosis may ensue.

4. **d. Ileum.** The incidence of postoperative bowel obstruction is 4% to 10%. Colon, stomach, and sigmoid obstruction result in a 4% incidence, less than that occurring with ileum.

5. **c. Total number of bacteria in the bowel.** The mechanical preparation reduces the amount of feces, whereas the antibiotic preparation reduces the bacterial count. A mechanical bowel preparation reduces the total number of bacteria but not their concentration.

6. **a. Before the patient is anesthetized.** Systemic antibiotics must be given before the operative event if they are to be effective.

7. **a. Use of previously irradiated bowel.** In one study of urinary intestinal diversion, 75% of the lethal complications that occurred in the postoperative period were related to the bowel. Eighty percent of these patients had received radiation before the intestinal surgery.

8. **b. Less compatibility with urine.** In general, anastomoses using reabsorbable sutures or reabsorbable staples are preferable for intestinal segments that are exposed to urine.

9. **c. Reduces postoperative vomiting.** In several studies there was no significant difference in major intestinal complications between those who had postoperative nasogastric tubes and those who did not; however, those who did not have gastric decompression showed a much greater incidence of abdominal distention, nausea, and vomiting.

10. **b. Placed through the belly of the rectus muscle.** All stomas should be placed through the belly of the rectus muscle and be located at the peak of the infraumbilical fat roll.

11. **a. The obese patient.** The loop end ileostomy is usually easier to perform than the ileal end stoma in the patient who is obese.

12. **c. On the left side where the ureter crosses the aorta.** Of importance is that ureteral strictures also occur away from the ureterointestinal anastomosis. This stricture is most common in the left ureter and is usually found as the ureter crosses over the aorta beneath the inferior mesenteric artery.

13. **a. 20%.** Patients who are studied during the long term show a significant degree of renal deterioration. Indeed, 20% of renal units have shown significant anatomic deterioration.

14. **b. Renal failure.** The most common cause of death in patients who have had a ureterosigmoidostomy for more than 15 years is acquired renal disease (i.e., sepsis or renal failure).

15. **b. 60.** If the patient is able to achieve a urine pH of 5.8 or less, can establish a urine osmolality of 600 mOsm/kg or greater in response to water deprivation, has a GFR that exceeds 60 mL/min, and has minimal protein in the urine, he or she may be considered for a retentive diversion.

16. **a. Ileal conduit.** It is the simplest type of conduit diversion to perform and is associated with the fewest intraoperative and immediate postoperative complications.

17. **c. Hyperkalemic, hyponatremic metabolic acidosis.** The early and long-term complications are similar to those listed for ileal conduit except that the electrolyte abnormality that occurs is hyperkalemic, hyponatremic metabolic acidosis instead of the hyperchloremic metabolic acidosis of ileal diversion.

18. **c. Less likely to be injured by radiation.** The transverse colon is used when one wants to be sure that the segment of conduit used has not been irradiated in individuals who have received extensive pelvic irradiation.

19. **a. Ureterosigmoidostomy.** Hypokalemia and total body depletion of potassium may occur in patients with urinary intestinal diversion. This is more common in patients with ureterosigmoidostomies than it is in patients who have other types of urinary intestinal diversion.

20. **d. Bowel reabsorption.** Because urea and creatinine are reabsorbed by both the ileum and the colon, serum concentrations of urea and creatinine do not necessarily accurately reflect renal function.

21. **a. Retain the ability to maintain the acidosis.** The ability to establish a hyperchloremic metabolic acidosis appears to be retained by most segments of ileum and colon over time.

22. **c. Are more common in patients with persistent hyperchloremic metabolic acidosis.** Osteomalacia in urinary intestinal diversion may be due to persistent acidosis, vitamin D resistance, and excessive calcium loss by the kidney. It appears that the degree to which each of these contributes to the syndrome may vary from patient to patient.

23. **c. Limits linear growth.** There is considerable evidence to suggest that urinary intestinal diversion has a detrimental effect on growth and development.

24. **d. Ureterosigmoidostomies.** The highest incidence of cancer occurs when the transitional epithelium is juxtaposed to the colonic epithelium and both are bathed by feces.

25. **b. Increased volume.** Reconfiguring bowel usually increases the volume, but its effect on motor activity and wall tension over the long term is unclear at this time.

26. **d. Elevated gastrin levels.** The syndrome of severe metabolic alkalosis is most likely to occur in patients with high resting gastrin levels who are dehydrated and fail to empty their pouch in a timely manner.

27. **c. Mechanical bowel prep.** There is direct evidence for omission of a mechanical bowel can be safely omitted from cystectomy and urinary diversion patients on an ERAS pathway. Thrombosis prophylaxis (b.) and perioperative antibiotics (e.) should never be omitted. There is is evidence that preoperative fasting (a.) and a pelvic drain (d.) may be safely omitted in colorectal surgery patients, but this has not be studied in depth in cystectomy population.

28. **a. Stomach.** Only urinary diversion consisting of stomach result in metabolic alkalosis. Arginine hydrochloride infusion plays no role in the management of acidosis caused by other bowel segments.

CHAPTER REVIEW

1. Perioperative care. The use of a preoperative mechanical bowel prep, oral antibiotic bowel prep, and postoperative nasogastric tube decompression in patients undergoing bowel surgery is controversial, and can be safely omitted in appropriately selected patients. Administering intravenous antibiotics 1 h before the surgical incision is not controversial and is supported by many studies. Patients undergoing elective intestinal surgery in the studies that show no advantage to a mechanical and/or antibiotic bowel prep received preoperative intravenous antibiotics. It should be appreciated that the majority of these studies involve isolated anastomoses—not large segments of bowel that are opened, as is the case in urologic procedures.

2. Ureteral intestinal anastomotic strictures. Antirefluxing anastomoses have a 10%–20% stricture rate; refluxing anastomoses have a 3%–10% stricture rate. The Wallace ureteral intestinal anastomosis has the lowest stricture rate.

3. Renal function and urinary diversion. Serum creatinine and blood urea nitrogen do not accurately reflect renal function in patients with intestine in the urinary tract because these substances, when excreted by the kidney, are reabsorbed by the bowel. This is more likely to be a problem in continent

Continued

CHAPTER REVIEW—cont'd

diversions. A glomerular filtration rate (GFR) of at least 60 mL/min and an ability to acidify the urine are necessary prerequisites for a continent diversion.

4. The electrolyte abnormality that occurs when ileum or colon are used for the diversion is a hyperchloremic metabolic acidosis (Table 139.1). These patients may have a potassium deficiency as well.

5. Significant perioperative infectious complications occur in up to 10% of patients undergoing cystectomy and urinary diversion.

6. The most common cause of mortality in urologic procedures when the gut is used relates to complications involving the bowel.

7. Complications specific to the use of stomach include the hematuria-dysuria syndrome and uncontrollable metabolic alkalosis in some patients.

8. The incidence of postoperative bowel obstruction is 4%–10%. Colon, stomach, and sigmoid obstruction result in a 4% incidence, less than that occurring with ileum.

9. The mechanical preparation reduces the amount of feces and therefore total bacteria, whereas the antibiotic preparation reduces the bacterial count and therefore the concentration of bacteria.

10. If the patient is able to achieve a urine pH of 5.8 or less, can establish a urine osmolality of 600 mOsm/kg or greater in response to water deprivation, has a GFR that exceeds 60 mL/min, and has minimal protein in the urine, he or she may be considered for a retentive diversion.

11. Osteomalacia in urinary intestinal diversion may be due to persistent acidosis, vitamin D resistance, and excessive calcium loss by the kidney.

12. In patients with gastric tissue in the urinary tract (usually gastrocystoplasty), the syndrome of severe metabolic alkalosis is most likely to occur in those with high resting gastrin levels who are dehydrated and fail to empty their pouch in a timely manner.

TABLE 139.1 Syndromes of Electrolyte Disturbances in Patients in Whom the Bowel Is Interposed in the Urinary Tract

SEGMENT	SYNDROME	NA+	K+	CL-	PH	ASSOCIATED ABNORMALITIES	SYMPTOMS	TREATMENT
Stomach	Severe metabolic alkalosis	--	↓	↓	↑	Elevated aldosterone	Lethargy, muscle weakness, respiratory insufficiency, seizures, ventricular arrhythmia	H₂ blocker, proton pump inhibitor; if life-threatening, arginine hydrochloride infusion and/or removal of segment
Jejunum	Hyperkalemic, hypochloremic metabolic acidosis	↓	↑	↓	↓	Elevated renin and angiotensin	Lethargy, nausea, vomiting, dehydration, muscle weakness	IV hydration, sodium bicarbonate, thiazide; if life threatening, removal of segment
Ileum/Colon	Hyperchloremic metabolic acidosis	--	↓	↑	↓	Total-body potassium depletion, hypocalcemia	Fatigue, anorexia, lethargy, weakness	Potassium citrate, sodium citrate, citric acid, sodium bicarbonate, chlorpromazine, nicotinic acid

140 Cutaneous Continent Urinary Diversion

Guarionex Joel DeCastro, James M. McKiernan, and Mitchell C. Benson

QUESTIONS

1. A 45-year-old man had an ileal conduit diversion as a child for bladder exstrophy. He requests a continent diversion. Serum creatinine is 2 mg/dL. Loopogram shows bilaterally thin ureters with small kidneys. Which is the best procedure?
   a. Ureterosigmoidostomy
   b. T pouch using the ileal conduit
   c. Abandon continent diversion
   d. Penn pouch using the ileal conduit
   e. Indiana pouch

2. A 45-year-old man underwent ileal conduit urinary diversion as a child for bladder exstrophy. He presents requesting continent diversion. Serum creatinine is 2 mg/dL. Loopogram shows bilateral hydronephrosis and a pipestem conduit. What is the best course of action?
   a. Mainz II to avoid problems with dilated ureters
   b. T pouch abandoning the disease conduit
   c. No continent diversion
   d. Drain the upper tracts and reassess renal function
   e. Proceed to neobladder construction

3. A patient undergoing a cystectomy and planned continent cutaneous diversion has positive ureteral margin biopsies up to 2 cm above each iliac artery, at which point negative biopsies are obtained. What is the best course of action?
   a. Use the terminal ileum for ureteral implantation and a Mitrofanoff continence mechanism
   b. No continent diversion
   c. Mobilize the kidneys and stretch the ureters to the reservoir
   d. Use a T pouch with a long chimney
   e. Cutaneous ureterostomies

4. Preservation of the ileocecal valve can be maintained with which catheterizable pouch?
   a. T pouch or Kock pouch
   b. Le Bag
   c. Indiana pouch
   d. Mainz I or II
   e. Penn pouch

5. In which procedure to repair a nipple valve would resection of additional bowel be routinely required?
   a. Stones on exposed staples
   b. Nipple valve slippage
   c. Nipple valve atrophy
   d. Pinhole leak
   e. Anastomotic leak

6. A 10-year-old child has an ileal conduit for myelomeningocele. The conduit was replaced on two occasions for pipestem conduit development. The conduit is again affected by the same process. The patient's family wants a continent diversion. Which is the best procedure?
   a. Ureterosigmoidostomy
   b. Revise the conduit
   c. T pouch using the ileal conduit
   d. Penn pouch using the ileal conduit
   e. Indiana pouch using the ileal conduit

7. A patient with chronic active hepatitis and invasive bladder cancer associated with intravesical carcinoma in situ is scheduled for a cystoprostatectomy. The serum creatinine concentration is 1 mg/dL. Prostatic urethral biopsy shows mild atypia. What is the best diversion?
   a. T pouch
   b. Ileal conduit
   c. Right colon reservoir
   d. Mainz II
   e. Cutaneous ureterostomies

8. The highest reoperation rate in catheterizable pouches occurs with what type of sphincter?
   a. In situ appendix
   b. Imbricated terminal ileum
   c. Plicated terminal ileum
   d. Nipple valves
   e. Transposed appendix

9. Which of the Mitrofanoff sphincter deficiencies can be corrected surgically?
   a. Length of the appendix
   b. Absence of the appendix
   c. Stenosis of the appendix
   d. All of the above

10. Hematuria and skin breakdown may occur with what type of pouch?
    a. T
    b. Gastric
    c. Mainz
    d. Right colon
    e. All of the above

11. Preoperative colonoscopy is indicated in candidates for which reservoir procedures?
    a. Ileal
    b. Jejunal
    c. Rectal
    d. Gastric
    e. All of the above

12. What condition is more common in absorbable stapled ileal pouches?
    a. Urine leaks
    b. Valve failure
    c. Hydronephrosis
    d. Ischemic pouch contraction
    e. Ureteral stricture

13. Anastomotic transitional cell carcinoma develops in a patient who has undergone cystectomy and continent cutaneous urinary diversion. What is the best treatment?
    a. Distal ureterectomy and reimplantation
    b. Conversion to ileal conduit
    c. Ileal ureter interposition
    d. Nephroureterectomy
    e. Cutaneous ureterostomies

14. Drainage of mucus is most difficult with which sphincteric mechanism?
    a. Kock valve
    b. In situ appendix
    c. Imbricated ileum
    d. Plicated ileum
    e. Transposed appendix

15. Which continent cutaneous diversion allows for a refluxing ureteroenteric anastomosis?
    a. Mitrofanoff with implantation of the ureters into terminal ileum
    b. Mitrofanoff with implantation of the ureters into the colon
    c. T pouch
    d. Kock pouch
    e. Indiana pouch

16. Three years after radical cystectomy and construction of a Kock pouch, a patient presents with right lower quadrant discomfort and associated spurts of urinary leakage. The test most likely to diagnose the condition is:
    a. computed tomography (CT).
    b. intravenous pyelogram (IVP).
    c. urine culture and sensitivity.
    d. cystogram of pouch.
    e. urodynamics.

17. Three years after cystectomy and Kock pouch for bladder cancer, a patient presents with recurrent episodes of bilateral pyelonephritis. The test most likely to provide the correct diagnosis is:
    a. CT.
    b. IVP.
    c. urine culture and sensitivity.
    d. cystogram of the pouch.
    e. magnetic resonance imaging (MRI).

18. What is the most important feature in preventing nipple valve slippage?
    a. Absorbable staples
    b. Length of the intussusception
    c. Resecting adequate mesentery
    d. Attaching the nipple valve to the side wall of the reservoir
    e. Length of staple line

19. In a patient with pipestem conduit and bilateral hydronephrosis requesting conversion to continent urinary diversion, nephrostomy drainage results in clearance values of 40 mL/min on the right and 10 mL/min on the left. Serum creatinine is 1.8 mg/dL. The next step in management is:
    a. Mainz II to avoid problems with the dilated ureters.
    b. T pouch abandoning the disease conduit.
    c. no continent diversion.
    d. ureterosigmoidostomy.
    e. neobladder.

20. A patient with squamous cell cancer of the bladder desires cystectomy and continent diversion. He has lost 20 pounds in the month before surgery. The next step in management is:
    a. increased oral intake.
    b. conduct preoperative hyperalimentation.
    c. conduct postoperative hyperalimentation.
    d. proceed directly with surgery.
    e. count calories.

21. Preoperative evaluation with an oatmeal enema is required in which procedure?
    a. Right colon reservoir
    b. Mainz I pouch
    c. Mainz II procedure
    d. Le Bag pouch
    e. Indiana pouch

22. Follow-up urinary cytology and colonoscopy should be used in which type of continent diversion?
    a. Ureterosigmoidostomy
    b. Mainz II procedure
    c. Right colon reservoir
    d. All of the above

23. Nocturnal emptying of the patient's reservoir is required in which type of diversion?
    a. Ureterosigmoidostomy
    b. T pouch
    c. Right colon reservoir
    d. Penn pouch
    e. Ileal conduit

24. The appendix is sacrificed in patients undergoing which pouch construction?
    a. Indiana
    b. Le Bag
    c. Mainz I
    d. All of the above

25. Pouch stone development occurs most commonly with which pouch?
    a. T pouch
    b. Kock pouch
    c. Penn pouch
    d. Gastric-ileal composite pouch
    e. Le Bag

26. What is the typical catheter used for appendiceal sphincters?
    a. 22-French (Fr) straight-tipped
    b. 22-Fr coudé-tipped
    c. 14-Fr straight-tipped
    d. 14-Fr coudé-tipped
    e. 20-Fr coudé-tipped

27. Urinary retention resulting from continent diversion occurs most commonly with what type of sphincter?
    a. Appendiceal stoma
    b. Benchekroun hydraulic valve
    c. Nipple valve sphincter
    d. Imbricated Indiana mechanism

28. Immediate postoperative initial pouch capacity is least in which pouch?
    a. T or Kock ileal
    b. Right colon
    c. Gastric
    d. Mainz I
    e. Transverse colon

29. Elevated pouch pressures would potentially facilitate the continence mechanism seen with which valve or sphincter?
    a. Benchekroun ileal valve
    b. Kock valve
    c. Appendiceal tunnel
    d. Imbricated Indiana mechanism
    e. All of the above

30. The long-term failure rate of continence mechanisms is greatest with which mechanism?
    a. T pouch valve
    b. Appendiceal tunnel
    c. Benchekroun hydraulic valve
    d. Imbricated terminal ileum

31. Absorbable staples in continent urinary diversion are best suited to what type of reservoir pouch?
    a. Ileal
    b. Right colon reservoir
    c. Gastric-ileal composite
    d. Gastric
    e. None of the above

32. When creating a large intestinal reservoir from absorbable staples, why is bowel eversion necessary?
    a. Because staples should not be used in reservoir construction
    b. To inspect the inside of the reservoir
    c. To avoid injury to the mesenteric blood supply
    d. To allow application of the second row of staples
    e. None of the above

33. Which of the following conditions make patients unsuitable candidates for continent urinary diversion?
    a. Multiple sclerosis
    b. Quadriplegia
    c. Mental impairment
    d. Severe physical impairment
    e. All of the above

34. Which of the following sutures should NOT be used in the construction of a reservoir?
    a. Chromic catgut
    b. Plain catgut
    c. Silk
    d. Polyglycolic acid (Dexon)
    e. Polyglactin (Vicryl)

35. Which of the following diversions place the patient at risk for the development of a late malignancy?
    a. Ureterosigmoidostomy
    b. T pouch
    c. Mainz II
    d. Indiana pouch
    e. All of the above

36. Which of the following diversions places the patient at greatest risk for the development of a late malignancy?
    a. Ureterosigmoidostomy
    b. T pouch
    c. Mainz II
    d. Indiana reservoir
    e. Le Bag

37. Continent urinary diversion has which of the following effects?
    a. Results in a psychotic depression
    b. Results in an improved psychosocial adjustment
    c. Results in violent behavior
    d. Bipolar behavior
    e. None of the above

38. According to most randomized studies, which type of urinary diversion is associated with the highest reported quality of life?
    a. Ureterosigmoidostomy
    b. Continent ileal reservoir (Kock pouch)
    c. Ileal conduit
    d. Orthotopic neobladder
    e. None—no conclusive studies have established higher satisfaction or quality of life with any one specific continent diversion

39. Which of the following is NOT true of continent urinary diversion?
    a. It is the gold standard of urinary diversion.
    b. It is a safe and reliable urinary diversion.
    c. It is associated with an increased complication rate.
    d. It is appropriate for selected individuals.
    e. It requires stricter selection criteria than incontinent diversion.

40. Which of the following circumstances would contraindicate a rectal bladder?
    a. Prior pelvic irradiation
    b. Unilateral ureteral dilation
    c. Bilateral ureteral dilation
    d. Lax anal sphincter tone
    e. All of the above

41. During the construction of a continent cutaneous urinary diversion, the surgeon should:
    a. not be concerned about the continence mechanism because the mechanism will mold to the catheter.
    b. not test the continence mechanism for ease of catheterization.
    c. not be concerned about pouch integrity because the pouch will seal itself.
    d. do none of the above.
    e. do all of the above.

42. If the urine in a continent cutaneous reservoir is found to be infected, what should be done?
    a. Nothing needs to be done in the absence of symptoms.
    b. The urine should always be sterilized with appropriate antibiotics.
    c. The infection should be eradicated, and prophylactic antibiotics prescribed.
    d. Administer an intravenous pyelogram to check for upper tract damage.
    e. Perform a pouch-o-gram.

43. The most appropriate and conservative care for pouch rupture is:
   a. broad-spectrum antibiotic therapy.
   b. careful radiologic imaging and antibiotic therapy.
   c. surgical exploration for repair of the rupture and broad-spectrum antibiotic therapy.
   d. pouch drainage and broad-spectrum antibiotic therapy.
   e. bilateral percutaneous nephrostomies.

44. The first pouch to use the Mitrofanoff principle was the:
   a. Mainz I.
   b. Penn.
   c. Kock.
   d. Indiana.
   e. Le Bag.

45. Which of the following represents the advantage of the gastric pouch?
   a. Electrolyte reabsorption is reduced.
   b. Absorptive malabsorption is avoided.
   c. Acid urine may reduce the risk of infection.
   d. All of the above
   e. None of the above

46. When converting from an ileal conduit to a continent diversion, the conduit should be:
   a. discarded because it is older and subject to higher complications.
   b. preserved for the ureteroileal anastomosis.
   c. incorporated into the continent diversion when possible.
   d. discarded because it is a potential nidus of infection.
   e. None of the above

47. Which of the following is TRUE of absorbable staples?
   a. Their use has been shown to shorten operative time.
   b. They are safe and reliable.
   c. Unlike nonabsorbable staples, they must not be overlapped.
   d. All of the above.
   e. None of the above.

ANSWERS

1. **c. Abandon continent diversion.** A creatinine level greater than 1.8 mg/dL indicates a level of renal function insufficient for continent diversion.

2. **d. Drain the upper tracts and reassess renal function.** The best course of action is to place ureteral cutaneous stents bilaterally (bypassing the pipestem segment) and reassess urinary function. In evaluating the hydronephrotic patient with impaired renal function for continent diversion, upper tract drainage is advised. If necessary, bilateral nephrostomy tubes can be used.

3. **a. Use the terminal ileum for ureteral implantation and a Mitrofanoff continence mechanism.** The best course of action is to perform a right colon reservoir with anastomosis of the ureters to the terminal ileum. The appendix or other pseudo-appendiceal (Mitrofanoff) mechanisms can be used for continence. The terminal ileum can accommodate short ureters.

4. **a. T pouch or Kock pouch.** Preservation of the ileocecal valve can be maintained with the T or Kock pouch. All other pouches use the right colon, so that the ileocecal valve is sacrificed.

5. **c. Nipple valve atrophy.** Nipple valve atrophy requires that a new nipple valve be made of additional bowel.

6. **b. Revise the conduit.** With significant small bowel compromise, as well as loss of the ileocecal valve in a neurogenic bladder patient, severe diarrhea may ensue.

7. **b. Ileal conduit.** The best approach is cystoprostatectomy and a conduit. Normal hepatic function is mandated in any patient undergoing continent diversion.

8. **d. Nipple valves.** The highest reoperation rate is associated with nipple valve sphincter failure.

9. **d. All of the above.** The caliber of Mitrofanoff mechanisms, the length of the appendix, stenosis, and even absence of the appendix can be resolved by surgical variations.

10. **b. Gastric.** Hematuria and cutaneous skin erosion may occur with a gastric pouch. With gastric reservoirs or composite reservoirs, the low pH of the urine may lead to hematuria and cutaneous breakdown.

11. **c. Rectal.** Preoperative colonoscopy is relatively indicated in candidates for any pouch. Any pouch using colon mandates preoperative colonic evaluation.

12. **d. Ischemic pouch contraction.** Because of the overlap of staple lines in absorbable stapled ileal pouches, ischemic pouch contraction may occur.

13. **a. Distal ureterectomy and reimplantation.** An additional segment of ileum can serve as a proximal limb to the reservoir. If nephrectomy is necessary, careful attention must be paid to the residual renal function.

14. **b. In situ appendix.** The small-diameter catheter used in draining appendiceal sphincter pouches allows for less effective mucus drainage.

15. **a. Mitrofanoff with implantation of the ureters into terminal ileum.** The implantation of the ureters into the terminal ileum may allow for reflux. The ileocecal valve and the isoperistaltic ileal segment may either prevent or diminish reflux.

16. **c. Urine culture and sensitivity.** The most important diagnostic test is urine culture. The symptoms described are those of pouchitis. This is treated by appropriate antibiotic therapy.

17. **d. Cystogram of the pouch.** The proximal nipple valve may have failed, leading to reflux and pyelonephritis. This is tested by the pouch-o-gram.

18. **d. Attaching the nipple valve to the side wall of the reservoir.** This results in a relative lengthening of the valve rather than a foreshortening of the valve with pouch filling.

19. **c. No continent diversion.** In this case, although the serum creatinine level returns to 1.8 mg/dL, the clearance value measured is less than the 60 mL/min required for continent diversion. Continent diversion should be abandoned, and simple replacement of the conduit considered.

20. **b. Conduct preoperative hyperalimentation.** The 20-pound weight loss indicates a potential for nutritional depletion or metastatic disease. A careful search for metastatic disease should be undertaken. For the patient with nutritional depletion, preoperative hyperalimentation is suggested to be of value.

21. **c. Mainz II procedure.** Any procedure that relies on the intact anal sphincter for continence (i.e., the Mainz II pouch) requires an assessment of the sphincter before carrying out the operation. This can be assessed by an oatmeal enema, which mimics the constitution of a combination of the urinary and fecal streams.

22. **d. All of the above.** Follow-up urinary cytology and colonoscopy is mandatory with any procedure that combines urinary and fecal streams. Because of an increased risk of malignancy even in the absence of admixture of urine and stool, all large intestinal pouches should be subjected to annual investigation by pouchoscopy and cytology.

23. **a. Ureterosigmoidostomy.** Nocturnal reservoir emptying may be required with any of the continent cutaneous reservoirs to prevent overdistention and possible rupture but is mandatory with ureterosigmoidostomy owing to the additional risk of fecal incontinence and metabolic acidosis.

24. **d. All of the above.** The appendix is sacrificed in patients undergoing Indiana, Le Bag, and Mainz I pouch reconstruction because it can serve as a nidus for infection and abscess formation.

25. **b. Kock pouch.** Pouch stone development occurs most commonly with the Kock pouch. Despite the exclusion of distal staples, the stapling techniques used to secure nipple valves will lead to a higher potential for stone development than in pouches not requiring nipple valves.
26. **d. 14-Fr coudé-tipped.** Larger catheters will not fit into the appendix. A straight catheter is more difficult to pass.
27. **c. Nipple valve sphincter.** Urinary retention occurs most commonly with nipple valve sphincters. If the chimney of the nipple valve is not near the surface of the abdomen, the catheter can be misdirected into folds of bowel rather than through the nipple valve.
28. **a. T or Kock ileal.** Immediate postoperative initial pouch capacity is least in ileal reservoirs (i.e., the T or Kock pouch). Small bowel pouches have initial capacities that are much lower than right colon pouches.
29. **a. Benchekroun ileal valve.** Because the Benchekroun ileal valve is hydraulic, higher pouch pressures would facilitate continence, whereas lower pouch pressures might lead to incontinence.
30. **c. Benchekroun hydraulic valve.** The long-term outcome of Benchekroun hydraulic ileal valve mechanisms is possibly the worst of all reported sphincteric mechanisms.
31. **b. Right colon reservoir.** The use of absorbable staples is best suited to large bowel pouches. With large bowel pouches there is no problem with staple lines causing subsequent bowel ischemia.
32. **d. To allow application of the second row of staples.** In an absorbable-stapled right colon pouch, bowel eversion is required to allow for the application of the second row of staples. Staple lines must not cross because this will prevent the bulky, absorbable staples from seating properly. The bowel is everted, a cut is made beyond the end of the staple line, and the next line of staples is applied.
33. **e. All of the above.** Patients with multiple sclerosis, quadriplegia, frailty, or mental impairment will at some point in their lives require the care of family members or visiting nurses, so they are poor candidates for any form of continent diversion.
34. **c. Silk.** All sutures used in the urinary tract should be absorbable.
35. **e. All of the above.** Late malignancy has been reported in all bowel segments exposed to the urinary stream, whether or not there is a commingling with feces.
36. **a. Ureterosigmoidostomy.** Although late malignancy has been reported in all bowel segments exposed to the urinary stream, whether or not there is a commingling with feces, the mixture of urothelium, urine, and feces poses the greatest risk.
37. **b. Results in an improved psychosocial adjustment.** Many studies from throughout the world have suggested an improved psychosocial adjustment of the patient undergoing continent urinary and fecal diversion compared with those patients with diversions requiring collecting appliances.
38. **e. None—no conclusive studies have established higher satisfaction or quality of life with any one specific continent diversion.** There are insufficient quality-of-life data from randomized studies comparing continent and incontinent urinary diversions to establish the superiority of any one technique.
39. **a. It is the gold standard of urinary diversion.** Ileal conduit should be considered the "gold standard" of urinary diversion.
40. **e. All of the above.** Dilated ureters, pelvic irradiation, and lax anal sphincteric tone are all contraindications to the procedure.
41. **d. Do none of the above.** The continence mechanism must be catheterized intraoperatively to ensure ease of catheter passage. This is an extremely important and crucial maneuver because the inability to catheterize is a serious complication that will often result in the need for reoperation.
42. **a. Nothing needs to be done in the absence of symptoms.** Most authors would suggest that bacteriuria in the absence of symptomatology does not warrant antibiotic treatment.
43. **c. Surgical exploration for repair of the rupture and broad-spectrum antibiotic therapy.** In general, these patients require immediate pouch decompression, radiologic pouch studies, and surgical exploration with pouch repair. If the amount of urinary extravasation is small and the patient does not have a surgical abdomen, catheter drainage and antibiotic administration may suffice in treating intraperitoneal rupture of a pouch. Patients managed with this conservative approach require careful monitoring.
44. **b. Penn.** The Penn pouch was the first continent diversion to use the Mitrofanoff principle, wherein the appendix served as the continence mechanism.
45. **d. All of the above.** Electrolyte reabsorption is greatly diminished, shortening of the absorptive bowel does not occur, and the acid urine may decrease the likelihood of reservoir colonization.
46. **c. Incorporated into the continent diversion when possible.** The authors prefer to use the conduit in some form whenever possible. The use of an existing bowel segment has the potential to diminish metabolic sequelae and may result in a lower complication rate.
47. **d. All of the above.** The use of absorbable staples has substantially reduced the time required to fashion bowel reservoirs and has demonstrated short-term and long-term reliability with respect to reservoir integrity and volume. They must not be overlapped because overlapping will prevent the proper close of the staple.

CHAPTER REVIEW

1. The ability to self-catheterize is essential in patients who are to be considered for a continent cutaneous diversion.
2. All patients should be prepared for the possibility of a traditional ileal conduit if intraoperative circumstances warrant it.
3. A patient should have a minimum creatinine clearance of 60 mL/min to undergo a continent urinary diversion.
4. Single J ureteral stents are used in all continent diversions. The stents are brought out through a separate abdominal stab wound, and a Malecot catheter should be placed into the reservoir and brought out through a separate stab wound as well.
5. In continent diversions, it is not clear at this time whether antirefluxing ureteral intestinal anastomoses are necessary to preserve the upper tracts; however, antirefluxing procedures are associated with a higher incidence of stricture over the long term.
6. Most patients are satisfied with the type of urinary diversion, irrespective of whether it is continent or not.
7. It is often useful to secure the reservoir to the anterior abdominal wall to prevent the reservoir from migrating. This is conveniently done where the Malecot exits the reservoir onto the anterior abdominal wall.
8. Renal and hepatic function must be carefully evaluated before a continent diversion is performed. Significant abnormalities in either are a contraindication to continent diversion. The glomerular filtration rate should be 60 mL/min or greater.
9. Patients with rectal bladders are very prone to the complication of hyperchloremic acidosis and total body potassium depletion. These patients also have an increased incidence of rectal cancer.

Continued

CHAPTER REVIEW—cont'd

10. The loss of the ileocecal valve in patients with neurologic or intestinal disorders subjects the patient to a significant risk of debilitating diarrhea.
11. Any procedure that relies on the intact anal sphincter for continence (i.e., the Mainz II pouch) requires an assessment of the sphincter before carrying out the operation. This can be assessed by an oatmeal enema.
12. Because of an increased risk of malignancy even in the absence of admixture of urine and stool, all large intestinal pouches should be subjected to annual investigation by pouchoscopy and cytology.
13. Nocturnal reservoir emptying may be required with any of the continent cutaneous reservoirs to prevent overdistention

and possible rupture, but it is mandatory with ureterosigmoidostomy because of the additional risk of fecal incontinence and metabolic acidosis.
14. Small bowel pouches have initial capacities that are much lower than those of right colon pouches.
15. The use of absorbable staples is best suited to large bowel pouches. With large bowel pouches there is no problem with staple lines causing subsequent bowel ischemia.
16. Although late malignancy has been reported in all bowel segments exposed to the urinary stream, whether or not there is a commingling with feces, the juxtaposition of urothelium, urine, and feces poses the greatest risk.

141 Orthotopic Urinary Diversion

Eila C. Skinner and Siamak Daneshmand

QUESTIONS

1. Which of the following was the key finding that allowed application of orthotopic urinary diversion to women undergoing cystectomy?
   a. Confirmation that an intact bladder neck is required for continence
   b. Demonstration in cystectomy specimens that urethral involvement was rare in the absence of tumor at the bladder neck
   c. Understanding of the relationship between estrogen levels and continence in elderly women
   d. Studies showing that direct invasion into the uterus is relatively rare in women with invasive bladder cancer
   e. Quality of life studies showing that men with continent diversion had better quality of life than those with ileal conduit

2. The risk factor most predictive for urethra recurrence following cystectomy for urothelial carcinoma is:
   a. prostatic stromal invasion.
   b. node-positive disease.
   c. carcinoma-in-situ in females.
   d. pathologic stage pT3b tumor at the trigone.
   e. history of multiple prior tumors.

3. A 80-year-old man with clinical cT2 bladder cancer lives alone but is active. His serum creatinine is 1.0 following neoadjuvant gemcitabine and cisplatin chemotherapy. He is interested in an orthotopic diversion. Which of the following would you tell him about that option?
   a. Neoadjuvant chemotherapy increases the early complications of orthotopic diversion.
   b. Older patients take longer to regain continence than younger patients.
   c. Ileal conduit will be easier for him to take care of than a continent diversion.
   d. Continent diversion is contraindicated in men over 75 years old.
   e. His risk of renal deterioration with continent diversion is higher than with ileal conduit.

4. Which of the following patients should NOT be offered an orthotopic neobladder?
   a. An 82-year-old healthy woman with recurrent cT1 and CIS following intravesical BCG and a prior vaginal hysterectomy
   b. A 53-year-old woman with an eGFR of 55 following neoadjuvant chemotherapy
   c. A 50-year-old man 2 years following low anterior colon resection with adjuvant chemotherapy and external beam radiation to the pelvis
   d. A 60-year-old woman with diabetes and hypertension
   e. A 58-year-old woman with palpable induration of the anterior vaginal apex

5. Which of these is a key requirement for construction of an orthotopic diversion?
   a. It should prevent vesicoureteral reflux to preserve renal function.
   b. It should be made of ileum or a combination of colon and ileum.
   c. The bowel used should be detubularized and fashioned into a spherical shape.
   d. It should be made with the smallest amount of bowel possible.
   e. The ureters should be plugged into an isoperistaltic segment of bowel.

6. Which of the following have been suggested to decrease the risk of urinary retention following ileal neobladder in women?
   a. Regular urethral dilation
   b. Tack the pouch to the anterior abdominal wall
   c. Biofeedback training in the early postop period
   d. Preservation of the uterus
   e. Construct a W pouch rather than a Studer type pouch

7. In performing a cystectomy and orthotopic ileal neobladder in a male, the most important step in preserving continence is to:
   a. construct a large capacity reservoir.
   b. avoid excess dissection anterior to the urethra.
   c. perform a nerve-sparing procedure in all cases.
   d. avoid removal of the presacral lymph nodes.
   e. place a suprapubic catheter during the early postoperative period.

8. A 64-year-old man with recurrent CIS who strongly prefers an orthotopic or continent cutaneous diversion is found to have grossly node-positive disease at surgery. The next step is:
   a. close and refer for chemotherapy and radiation.
   b. complete the cystectomy but do an ileal conduit.
   c. complete the cystectomy but do a continent cutaneous diversion.
   d. complete the cystectomy and neobladder and refer for adjuvant chemotherapy.
   e. complete the cystectomy and neobladder and refer for adjuvant radiation therapy.

9. Prior to considering a continent orthotopic diversion, what evaluation is mandatory?
   a. Prostatic urethral biopsy
   b. Evaluation of renal function
   c. Colonoscopy to rule out colon polyps
   d. Biopsy of the bladder neck in a female
   e. Video urodynamics to test the integrity of the external sphincter

10. The primary innervation of the rhabdosphincter responsible for continence in men and women following an orthotopic diversion is:

    a. parasympathetics from S2 to S4.

    b. anterior branches of the sciatic nerve.

    c. sympathetic nerves from the hypogastric plexus.

    d. pudendal nerve.

    e. femoral nerve.

11. Use of metallic surgical staples should be avoided in construction of a continent diversion because:

    a. it is less secure than a hand-sewn closure.

    b. they tend to be buried in the bowel mucosa.

    c. the staples increases the risk of subsequent infection.

    d. the staples can become a nidus for stone formation.

    e. they increase the risk of cancer developing in the segment.

12. A 71-year-old male is found on routine follow-up to have a pelvic recurrence 13 months after cystectomy and ileal neobladder. The mass is 2.5 cm in the obturator fossa, abutting the pouch. There is no hydronephrosis. He has good daytime continence but occasionally leaks at night. The next step is:

    a. resection of the mass with removal of the pouch and conversion to an ileal conduit.

    b. cystoscopy to look for invasion of the reservoir.

    c. placement of a permanent suprapubic tube.

    d. resection of the mass with preservation of the neobladder.

    e. systemic chemotherapy with or without external beam radiation.

13. Asymptomatic bacteruria in patients with orthotopic diversion:

    a. carries a high risk of subsequent pyelonephritis.

    b. leads to an increase in urethral recurrence.

    c. does not generally require treatment.

    d. is very rare in most reported series.

    e. suggests probable outlet obstruction.

14. A 59-year-old man is 6 years out from a radical cystectomy and neobladder. He had excellent day and nighttime continence and no problems with infections, but recently has started to leak at night. The next step is:

    a. fluorourodynamics.

    b. CT scan looking for local recurrence.

    c. check postvoid residual.

    d. trial of long-term antibiotics.

    e. MRI of the spine.

15. A 66-year-old male 2 years after a cystectomy and Hautmann ileal neobladder for pathologic stage T2N0M0 bladder cancer is found on routine CT scan to have a very distended neobladder and mild bilateral hydronephrosis. He has a postvoid residual of over 800cc. Cystoscopy and digital rectal exam are normal. The next step is:

    a. teach the patient intermittent catheterization.

    b. dilate the urethra with van Buren sounds.

    c. instruct the patient to Crede while Valsalva voiding.

    d. convert the diversion to an ileal conduit

    e. decompress the neobladder with a catheter for 2 weeks and then resume regular voiding.

16. Quality-of-life studies of patients with orthotopic diversion

    a. are best done by the physician asking the patient about the function of his/her neobladder.

    b. have consistently shown that patients with continent diversions have a better quality of life than those with ileal conduits.

    c. can be easily done with currently available questionnaires used for other populations.

    d. have often been underpowered or affected by selection bias.

    e. have shown that most patients with any urinary diversion have very poor quality of life.

17. A 70-year-old man who is 10 days s/p cystectomy and neobladder is readmitted with fever, and CT scan shows a large fluid collection near the reservoir that fills with contrast on delayed images. The catheter and ureteral stents are still in place. The next step is:

    a. IV antibiotics and observation with frequent catheter irrigation.

    b. exploration and repair of the pouch.

    c. bilateral percutaneous nephrostomy tube placement.

    d. percutaneous drainage of the fluid collection.

    e. percutaneous placement of a suprapubic catheter.

18. A 53-year-old woman had an anterior exenteration and neobladder with omental flap interposition 3 months previously. She still has total incontinence day and night. The next step is:

    a. reassurance and reinforce Kegel exercises.

    b. refer for physical therapy for pelvic floor strengthening.

    c. evaluate for possible vesicovaginal fistula.

    d. prescribe extended-release oxybutynin.

    e. fluorourodynamics.

19. A 70-year-old woman had a cystectomy and ileal neobladder diversion 5 years ago for pT2N0 urothelial cancer. CT scan is normal, and she has excellent continence and empties well with negative urine culture. The next step is:

    a. refer her to her primary care physician for routine health maintenance.

    b. continue annual CT abdomen and pelvis out to 10 years.

    c. annual endoscopy of the pouch to screen for secondary malignancy.

    d. annual cystogram and serum creatinine to evaluate for reflux nephropathy.

    e. renal ultrasound, chemistry panel, and vitamin B12 level every 1 to 2 years.

20. Which of the following is NOT usually part of an Early Recovery After Surgery (ERAS) protocol applied to patients undergoing radical cystectomy?

    a. Alvimopan BID beginning AM of surgery

    b. Early feeding

    c. No mechanical or antibiotic bowel prep

    d. Continuous IV narcotics to optimize pain management

    e. Early removal of nasogastric tubes

21. An otherwise healthy 90-year-old man had a cystectomy and ileal neobladder 15 years previously with a hemi-Kock pouch to the urethra. He presented with a creatinine of 4.0 and bilateral hydronephrosis on renal ultrasound that did not resolve with catheter drainage. The most likely cause of his problem is:

    a. bilateral ureteral stones.

    b. stenosis of the afferent nipple valve.

    c. reflux nephropathy.

    d. urinary retention.

    e. cancer recurrence in the reservoir.

22. Which of the following is true about robotic cystectomy with extracorporeal neobladder construction compared with standard open cystectomy?

    a. Patients undergoing robotic-assisted laparoscopic radical cystectomy (RARC) have significantly fewer early and late complications.

    b. Continence has been shown to be improved.

    c. Long-term cancer control has been proven to be equivalent.

    d. The surgery can be performed through a smaller incision with lower blood loss.

    e. Hospital stay is consistently shorter.

23. A 66-year-old man had a cystectomy and sigmoid neobladder 4 years previously and has good continence. He was noted on recent CT scan to have two 0.7 cm calcifications in the pouch. The next step is:

    a. reassurance that the stones will probably pass.

    b. shock wave lithotripsy.

    c. metabolic stone evaluation.

    d. begin intermittent catheterization

    e. cystoscopy and laser lithotripsy of the stone.

24. A 49-year-old man had a cystectomy and neobladder 4 months previously. He has excellent continence in the daytime but still has accidents at night even though he gets up twice to empty. The next step is:

    a. reassurance that the nighttime continence will likely improve with more time.

    b. trial of extended release oxybutynin.

    c. strict fluid restriction to no more than 1500cc per day.

    d. intermittent catheterization.

    e. refer for physical therapy for pelvic floor strengthening.

ANSWERS

1. **b. Demonstration in cystectomy specimens that urethral involvement was rare in the absence of tumor at the bladder neck.** The two findings that paved the way for orthotopic diversion in women were retrospective pathologic studies showing that urethral involvement was rare in the absence of bladder neck involvement (in other words, "skip lesions" were rarely seen, suggesting oncologic safety), and studies showing that women could be continent without an intact bladder neck (previously thought to be required).

2. **a. Prostatic stromal invasion.** Two large studies have demonstrated conclusively that urethral recurrence in men is associated with prostatic stromal invasion in the cystectomy specimen.

3. **b. Older patients take longer to regain continence than younger patients.** Older men regain continence more slowly than younger men, but the majority of fit older men will ultimately have good control, especially in the daytime. Older men often have difficulty becoming independent in managing an ileal conduit, and in a man living alone a neobladder may actually be simpler.

4. **A 58-year-old woman with palpable induration of the anterior vaginal apex.** Women with palpable invasion of the anterior vaginal wall have a high risk of urethral tumor and should not undergo orthotopic diversion.

5. **c. The bowel used should be detubularized and fashioned into a spherical shape.** Orthotopic diversions can be made from small or large bowel. The key to obtaining a low-pressure reservoir with good volume is to detubularize the segment and reconfigure it into a spherical shape.

6. **d. Preservation of the uterus.** Late urinary retention ("hyper-continence") in women appears to be primarily due to posterior displacement of the pouch into the vagina resulting in a kinking at the urethral anastomosis. A number of maneuvers have been suggested such as sacrocolpopexy, but preservation of the uterus appears to be the most promising.

7. **b. Avoid excess dissection anterior to the urethra.** In preserving the urethra for an orthotopic bladder in males, one should be careful of the dorsal venous complex and avoid deep bites into the pelvic floor, especially anterior to the urethra where the rhabdosphincter is the most developed.

8. **d. Complete the cystectomy and neobladder and refer for adjuvant chemotherapy.** Patients with node-positive disease have a poor prognosis, but up to 30% may be long-term survivors, especially with adjuvant chemotherapy. Orthotopic diversion should not impact survival, and if a patient is highly motivated to avoid a stoma this option can still be pursued.

9. **b. Evaluation of renal function.** In order to consider a patient a candidate for a continent diversion, he/she must have a GFR in excess of 35 mL/min and his/her kidneys must be capable of concentrating and acidifying the urine.

10. **d. Pudendal nerve.** The rhabdosphincter is innervated by the pudendal somatic nerve. The contribution to continence from the pelvic autonomic plexus is uncertain, though some nonrandomized studies suggest that preserving the neuro-vascular bundle posterolateral to the prostate may improve continence.

11. **d. The staples can become a nidus for stone formation.** Metallic staples have a high association with subsequent stone formation, as was seen in the long-term experience with the hemi-Kock pouch. Recent efforts to perform intracorporeal neobladder using minimally invasive techniques have advocated using metal staplers to construct the pouch, but early results have suggested a high risk of stones.

12. **e. Systemic chemotherapy with or without external beam radiation.** Local recurrence of urothelial cancer will not usually impact the neobladder function. Rarely, direct invasion of the reservoir will cause bleeding or outlet obstruction. Prognosis is poor, and local resection is rarely successful in eradicating the tumor, so primary treatment should be systemic chemotherapy and possibly radiation (which can be safely applied around a neobladder).

13. **c. Does not generally require treatment.** In patients with orthotopic bladders, approximately one quarter have asymptomatic bacteriuria. After the initial 6 months, it is rare for patients to have symptomatic infections or pyelonephritis, and bacteriuria does not require treatment.

14. **c. Check postvoid residual.** Patients who have a change in their continence after initial good function should be evaluated for possible urinary retention. This is often the first sign of incomplete emptying. Urodynamics are not necessary unless the pouch is made from colon, since ileal neobladders are very reliably low-pressure with good compliance.

15. **a. Teach the patient intermittent catheterization.** All patients who are considered for a continent diversion should be willing and capable of doing self-catheterization. The likelihood of needing self-catheterization is lower in men than in women, with reported rates of 10% to 40% in most series.

16. **d. Have often been underpowered or affected by selection bias.** Quality-of-life surveys have not shown one type of urinary diversion to be superior over another, though the vast majority of studies have serious methodological flaws. Obviously randomized studies in this area have been impossible. Most patients are reasonably well adapted socially, physically, and psychologically to their diversion. The key to this adaptation is appropriate and realistic preoperative education.

17. **d. Percutaneous drainage of the fluid collection.** If a patient has an undrained urine leak postoperatively, percutaneous drainage is the first step. Nephrostomy tubes can be placed if a large urine leak does not respond to percutaneous drainage with optimal catheter drainage. Open surgical repair should be avoided if possible because the complication rate is high and success in closing the leak in the face of acute postsurgical inflammation is low.

18. **c. Evaluate for possible vesicovaginal fistula.** A woman with persistent incontinence should be evaluated for a pouch vaginal fistula. This is most common when the anterior vaginal wall is removed with the specimen. It is best prevented by interposition of an omental pedicle but still can occur. Evaluation is easily performed with a speculum exam with methylene blue in the bladder.

19. **e. Renal ultrasound, chemistry panel and vitamin B12 level every 1 to 2 years.** Long-term risks in diversion patients include late ureteral stricture, stones, and vitamin B12 deficiency. All of these can be silent, so long-term routine follow-up is required. Most primary care physicians are not familiar with this.

20. **d. Continuous IV narcotics to optimize pain management.** New ERAS protocols have resulted in shorter hospital stay. Avoidance of bowel prep and the use of the μ opioid inhibitor alvimopan have been proven effective in randomized trials.

21. **b. Stenosis of the afferent nipple valve.** Afferent nipple stenosis is a well-documented late complication of the classic hemi-Kock pouch with an intussuscepted nipple valve antireflux mechanism. Treatment includes nephrostomy tube placement and endoscopic incision of the valve mechanism.

22. **d. The surgery can be performed through a smaller incision with lower blood loss.** A large series of patients undergoing robotic-assisted cystectomy with extracorporeal diversion showed no decrease in hospital stay or early or late complications compared to open series, and this was confirmed in one recent randomized trial from Memorial Sloan Kettering. Oncologic efficacy appears to be similar but long-term results are not yet available.

23. **e. Cystoscopy and laser lithotripsy of the stone.** Stones can occur in all types of continent diversions. These stones should be removed endoscopically while they are still small because they will inevitably grow and be more difficult to manage when larger.

24. **a. Reassurance that the nighttime continence will likely improve with more time.** Patients typically attain nighttime continence more slowly than daytime, with patients reporting improvement out to 1 to 2 years. Early on there is an obligate nocturnal diuresis from the pouch that aggravates this. If the patient has good daytime control, further efforts to strengthen the sphincter are unlikely to help the nighttime continence. There is no role for anticholinergics or urodynamics in this setting.

CHAPTER REVIEW

1. Urinary diversion has developed along three paths: conduit, continent cutaneous diversion, and most recently orthotopic diversion.

2. Long-term complications of the ileal and colon conduits include stomal stenosis, peristomal hernia, pyelonephritis, calculus formation, ureteral obstruction, and renal deterioration.

3. The major long-term problems with continent cutaneous diversion relate to function of the efferent continence mechanism, and surgical revision is often required.

4. The orthotopic neobladder allows for volitional voiding, avoids the need for an appliance and only require self-catheterization in a minority of patients.

5. 80%–90% of males and 75% of females undergoing cystectomy are potential candidates for orthotopic reconstruction.

6. Patient must have a healthy urethra and adequate external sphincter function to maintain continence.

7. The bowel segment used for the reservoir should be completely detubularized and reconstructed into a spherical shape.

8. Ultimate storage volume of the mature pouch should be at least 300–500 mL at low pressure.

9. The presence of CIS, multifocal tumor, or extravesical disease should not preclude orthotopic diversion if frozen section of the urethral margin is negative at surgery.

10. The most significant risk factor for a urethral tumor recurrence in men after orthotopic diversion is the presence of prostatic stromal invasion on final pathology.

11. The most important risk factor in women for urethral tumor involvement is bladder neck or anterior vaginal wall involvement with cancer, best evaluated on bimanual examination under anesthesia.

12. Intraoperative frozen-section analysis of the urethral margin accurately identifies urethral involvement in both men and women. Preoperative biopsy of the prostatic urethra or bladder neck is not mandatory.

13. Local pelvic recurrence should occur in less than 10% of patients undergoing cystectomy and rarely interferes with the function of the neobladder.

14. Adequate renal function (eGFR exceeding 35 or 40 mL/min) is recommended for patients considering continent diversion.

15. Older age and obesity are not contraindications to orthotopic diversion.

16. Orthotopic diversion can be performed after prior pelvic irradiation or radical prostatectomy in carefully selected male and female patients.

17. In patients with prior bowel resection the prior anastomosis should be taken down and that segment used for the orthotopic diversion rather than choosing a new site, to avoid devascularization of the bowel.

18. The striated rhabdosphincter muscle fibers and associated innervation from the pudendal nerve are concentrated in the area anterior and lateral to the proximal urethra in both males and females.

19. In male patients, one should obtain careful control of the dorsal venous complex, and avoidance of deep suture bites into the pelvic floor muscles is critical.

20. In female patients, the endopelvic fascia and levator muscles should not be disturbed.

21. Reservoirs made from ileum or combined ileum and colon appear to have the best physiologic properties for orthotopic diversion.

22. Isolation of the segment of bowel to be used for the diversion must be performed carefully to preserve blood supply to the pouch and bowel anastomosis.

23. The addition of an antireflux mechanism does not appear to be necessary for preservation of the upper tracts and prevention of infections, at least in the intermediate term.

24. Daytime continence develops gradually over 3–6 months in most patients and is ultimately achieved in 80%–90% of both male and female patients.

25. Persistent nocturnal incontinence is common, observed in 20%–50% of patients. Nocturnal continence may continue to improve beyond 12 months from surgery and may improve with timed voiding.

26. Factors influencing continence rates include age, intestinal segment used, and application of a prostate-sparing technique.

27. Failure to empty or urinary retention has been reported in 4%–10% of men and 20%–60% of women.

28. Early morbidity and mortality of cystectomy and orthotopic diversion are not increased compared with ileal conduit.

29. Undrained urine leak is best managed using percutaneous drains and bilateral nephrostomy tubes when necessary. Early open surgical revision should be avoided.
30. The majority of late urologic complications related to the neobladder can be managed using endoscopic techniques.
31. Patients require regular follow-up imaging to identify upper tract obstruction and stones, which may be clinically silent.
32. Follow-up should include physical and pelvic examination and urethral cytology to identify urethral recurrence, which occurs in approximately 10% of males and rarely in females.
33. Most quality-of-life studies that have evaluated and compared patients undergoing various forms of urinary diversion have been criticized for methodologic problems that limit their conclusions.
34. The current body of published literature is insufficient to conclude that any form of urinary diversion is superior to another on the basis of health-related quality-of-life outcomes, though most studies report better body image with neobladders.

142 Minimally Invasive Urinary Diversion

Khurshid A. Guru

QUESTIONS

1. Regarding perioperative thrombo-prophylaxis treatment after robot-assisted radical cystectomy (RARC), which of the following is true?
   a. Pneumatic compressions and leg stockings only are adequate.
   b. Low molecular weight heparin can be used as a single dose before the operation
   c. Low molecular weight heparin should be continued up to 4 weeks after surgery.
   d. Both mechanical and pharmacological prophylaxes are adequate for 48 hours perioperative.
   e. No prophylaxis.

2. Criteria for patient selection for intracorporeal urinary diversion during RARC include all of the following except:
   a. high body mass index.
   b. locally advanced disease.
   c. older age.
   d. prior abdominal surgery.
   e. none of the above.

3. Enhanced recovery after surgery (ERAS) includes which of the following?
   a. Allow clear liquids up to 2 hours prior to the surgery.
   b. Allow solid food up to 6 hours prior to the surgery.
   c. Maintain positive balance during the procedure.
   d. Mechanical bowel preparations and oral antibiotics should be omitted.
   e. All of the above.

4. During RARC and intracorporeal urinary diversion,
   a. usage of 30° up lens is advantageous for deep female pelvis.
   b. a 0-degree lens can be used for the entire procedure.
   c. the camera port is inserted below the umbilicus.
   d. the camera can be easily switched to another robotic port.
   e. a five-port configuration is used.

5. During intracorporeal urinary diversion, the benefit of marionette stitch is to:
   a. identify the distal and proximal ends of the conduit.
   b. help in retaining orientation of the bowel.
   c. allow free movement of the bowel segment for creation of the conduit.
   d. prevent leakage of bowel contents during the creation of the conduit.
   e. allow free movement of the bowel segment and prevent inadvertent movements of the robotic instruments.

6. To avoid the risk of uretero-ileal strictures, which of the following is correct?
   a. Button-hole enterotomy is done using cold scissors.
   b. Spatulation is omitted.

   c. Slit-like enterotomy.
   d. Using electrocautery in creating the enterotomy.
   e. None of the above.

7. During creation of the neobladder, mobilization of the bowel to reach the urethra can be achieved by all of the following except:
   a. reducing Trendelenburg position.
   b. using Penrose drain for gentle traction and stretching.
   c. mobilization of the urethra cephalad.
   d. incising the peritoneum over the mesentery.
   e. dissection of the ileum around the ileocecal junction.

8. All of these factors that may affect operative time during RARC except:
   a. female gender.
   b. higher body mass index.
   c. prior abdominal surgery.
   d. approach to urinary diversion (intracorporeal versus extracorporeal).
   e. urinary diversion type (ileal conduit vs neobladder).

9. Regarding the approach for nerve sparing cystectomy in men, which of the following is incorrect?
   a. Preservation of the proximal neurovascular complex.
   b. Athermal approach of the seminal vesicles.
   c. Control of the proximal prostatic pedicles near the prostate.
   d. Lateral nerve preservation is done after dissection of the prostatic apex.
   e. Computer-assisted reconstruction does not help.

10. It is critical to avoid injury to the neural pathway for continence and sexual function in the following area:
    a. common iliac bifurcation.
    b. tip of seminal vesicles.
    c. lateral prostatic fascia.
    d. dorsal venous complex and ureters.
    e. all of the above.

11. The ileal surgical maneuvers for continence after creation of neobladder are:
    a. adequate de-tubularization and double-folding.
    b. capacity (length of bowel used).
    c. preservation of urethral length.
    d. sphincter complex.
    e. all of the above.

12. The most common cause of complications after RARC and intra-corporeal urinary diversion is:
    a. bleeding.
    b. sepsis.
    c. necrosis of the bowel segment.
    d. enteroenteric anastomotic leak.
    e. port site and parastomal hernia.

ANSWERS

1. **c. Low-molecular-weight heparin should be continued until 4 weeks after surgery.** Based on 939 patients who underwent robot-assisted radical cystectomy, the incidence of hematologic and vascular complications was 10%. A survey of urologists who were aware of the American Urological Association (AUA) Best Practice Statement guidelines revealed that 51% were likely to use thromboprophylaxis (odds ratio, 1.4, confidence interval, 1.2 to 1.6). Eighteen percent of urologic oncologists and/or laparoscopic/robotic specialists and 34% of non-urologic oncologists and/or laparoscopic/robotic specialists avoided routine thromboprophylaxis in patients undergoing radical cystectomy. The former were more likely to use thromboprophylaxis ($P < .0001$) than other respondents. Urologists graduating after the year 2000 used thromboprophylaxis in high-risk patients undergoing radical cystectomy more often than did earlier graduates (79.2% vs. 63.4%, $P < .0001$). Based on the American College of Surgeons NSQIP (National Surgical Quality Improvement Program) database from 1307 patients who underwent radical cystectomy, the mean time to venous thromboembolism diagnosis was 15.2 days postoperatively; 55% of all venous thromboembolism events were diagnosed after patient discharge home. It is recommended to consider extended duration pharmacologic prophylaxis (4 weeks) in this high-risk surgical population.

2. **e. None of the above.** The selection criteria (including high body mass index, locally advanced disease, older age, prior abdominal surgery) have significantly broadened as learning curve has flattened. Reduction in cardiac and pulmonary compliance due to the inability to tolerate steep Trendelenburg position especially with prolonged operative duration during intracorporeal urinary diversion (ICUD) has also been addressed. Newer technology available is the Xi model of the da-Vinci Surgical System and use of the AirSeal has allowed surgeons to operate in less steep Trendelenburg position. Absolute and relative contraindications for neobladder are similar to open surgery.

3. **e. All of the above.** ERAS has evolved with more than 20 key components and has been tailored by several cystectomy experts. Recent modifications include early use of alvimopan, intraoperative goal-oriented fluid optimization, immediate initiation of oral diet, and reduced narcotic use. Xu and colleagues (2015) compared traditional pathway to an enhanced recovery protocol and reported decreased opioid usage per day, incidence of ileus, and hospital stay. Opioid use for breakthrough pain underwent a radical change from opioid patient controlled analgesia (PCA) and epidurals to high-dose acetaminophen and/or ketorolac. Patients who underwent RARC with ICUD and participated in the ERAS pathway had shorter length of stay and were more likely to receive a neobladder. The ERAS group was associated with significantly lower overall, gastrointestinal-related complications and readmission rates at 90 days. Participating in the ERAS pathway and younger age were independently associated with a hospital stay of less than 10 day. Pooled meta-analysis of 13 studies with 1493 patients showed that implementation of ERAS protocols after surgery reduced complications, length of stay without impacting overall readmission rates.

4. **b. A 0-degree lens can be used for the entire procedure.** The majority of robot-assisted radical prostatectomy procedures use different lenses for the procedure. During robot-assisted radical cystectomy, surgeons prefer a 0-degree lens. Special situations of a narrow, deep pelvis in association with obesity can require a 30-degree down lens for better visualization, especially for the proximal portion of the extended lymph node dissection.

5. **c. Allow free movement of the bowel segment for creation of the conduit.** Because of the multiple detailed steps required during intracorporeal urinary diversion in a narrow operative space, the marionette stitch helps in controlling the area of focus by acting as a retraction and exposing the correct surgical space to perform the right and left uretero-ileal anastomosis.

6. **a. Button-hole enterotomy is done using cold scissors.** To avoid risk of strictures, it is advisable to avoid the use of electrocautery; instead, it is better to use a cold scissors to create a wide button-hole enterotomy by removing the serosa in the proximal end of the ileum. We also have started to preserve a flap of peritoneum while dissecting the right ureter (periureteral space) at the time of RARC and extended lymph node dissection. This peritoneal flap helps in covering the proximal uretero-ileal anastomosis and retroperitonealize it, to avoid an inflammatory response at the site of the anastomosis.

7. **c. Mobilization of the urethra cephalad.** Traditionally, a steep Trendelenburg position has been used to avoid bowel in the operative field and also to gain direct access to the deeper pelvis. Unfortunately this works against intracorporeal neobladder because urethral-neobladder anastomosis is difficult if the bowel tries to retract back into the abdominal cavity and is in tension. Several options used to reduce tension and ease anastomosis include reducing Trendelenburg, performing the urethra-neobladder anastomosis at the beginning of the procedure, incising the peritoneum over the mesentery, dissection of the ileum around the ileocecal junction, and, finally, using temporary traction for stretching and holding the bowel in place for anastomosis.

8. **d. Approach to urinary diversion (intracorporeal versus extracorporeal).** No significant difference between intracorporeal and extracorporeal approaches to urinary diversion was found based on the recent International Robotic Cystectomy Consortium (IRCC) study of 2134 patients. One possible explanation is that the additional time for undocking, patient positioning and then redocking for extracorporeal diversion may have reduced the difference between both approaches. High-volume institutions had shorter operative times for radical cystectomy. This may be attributed to the experience of the surgeon and the teams at those institutions.

9. **e. Computer-assisted reconstruction does not help.** Computer-assisted dissection that involved 3D reconstruction of the inferior hypogastric plexus has demonstrated the precise location and distribution of pelvic nerves helping in both continence and erectile function. Approximately one-third of cross-sectional external urethral sphincter area has shown to be laterally overlapped by the dorsal venous complex at the prostatic apex. Doppler studies have shown dorso-cavernous anastomoses play an important role in the cavernous arterial hemodynamics. Vascular anastomoses have also been found between different arterial supplies (dorsal, the cavernous and the bulbourethral) of the penis. These arteries, except for bulbo-urethral arteries, have been shown to have function of contractibility based on their muscular walls and accompanying nerves. At the site of the external urethral sphincter, cavernosa nerves converge close to the urethra before they penetrate the muscular pelvic floor.

10. **e. All of the above.** Nerve-sparing approach should only be utilized in patients who have anatomically safe location of tumor, lower tumor burden, and adequate baseline sexual function making such patients more amenable to nerve-sparing not only for sexual preservation but also for continence after creation of a neobladder. The nerves are at risk at their origin in the medial aspect of the common iliac vessels and the presacral area. It is critical to keep in mind the course of the pelvic plexus while performing an extended lymph node dissection as it can risk both sexual function and continence. The approach to nerve-sparing has to also start early on from the high ligation of the bladder vascular pedicle (ensuring preservation of the proximal neurovascular complex) to the incision of the peritoneum in the pouch of Douglas overlying the recto-vesical space. Once the ampullae of the vasa are identified and safely dissected an athermal approach of the seminal vesicles, while sparing the Denonvilliers fascia (where the pelvic plexus is mostly concentrated), should be attempted. It is safe to avoid manipulation and sometimes spare the middle to lower part of the seminal vesicles. The complete

lateral nerve preservation (i.e., veil of Aphrodite) and its distal extent are difficult to complete without dissecting the apex of the prostate after dropping of the bladder.

11. **e. All of the above.** Several other key steps include mobilizing the sigmoid colon out of the true pelvis, and occasionally a stay suture is used to keep it temporarily fixed laterally until the neobladder is created. It is also critical to reduce the steep Trendelenburg position after undocking the robot. The new advances with the da-Vinci Xi Surgical System with an integrated operating room table will make this easier without undocking the surgical robot. Application of perineal pressure at the time of anastomosis with insertion of Foley catheter to guide the needle towards the urethral opening has already been used consistently during robot-assisted radical prostatectomy. The utilization of barbed suture, especially the V-Loc, has helped reduce time and complexity of neobladder creation as well as the urethral anastomosis. Detubularization of the ileal segment, opening and stretching of the bowel helps in adding length to the ileum. The peritoneal covering of the ileum can be also incised and the mesenteric fat is released to help add length. This should be performed with care as it exposes the mesenteric vessels and can lead to annoying bleeding which can jeopardize the vascular supply to the neobladder. The Karolinska group has used Penrose drains in their early experience for gentle stretching and traction of bowel for ease of anastomosis.

12. **b. Sepsis.** A study evaluated 935 patients in the IRCC database who had robot-assisted radical cystectomy and pelvic lymph node dissection with both intracorporeal (ileal conduit: 106; neobladder: 61), and extracorporeal urinary diversion (ileal conduit: 570; neobladder: 198). The 90-day complication rate was not significantly different between the two groups, but there was a trend favoring the intracorporeal group (41% vs. 49%, $P = .05$). Gastrointestinal complications and sepsis constituted the majority of the complications in all robot-assisted radical cystectomy series comparing intracorporeal and extracorporeal urinary diversion. Although both complications were significantly lower in the intracorporeal group, sepsis was the most common complication in that group.

CHAPTER REVIEW

1. Advantages of robot-assisted approaches for bladder cancer include less pain, minimal blood loss, and earlier return of bowel function.
2. Incorporation of intracorporeal urinary diversion has recently increased (annual increase of 11%).
3. Ileal conduit is the most commonly performed diversion with robot-assisted approach.
4. Mechanical bowel preparation and oral antibiotics should be avoided.
5. Anticoagulant treatment can help avoid significant thrombo-embolic complications.
6. Preoperative broad-spectrum intravenous antibiotics are preferably given up to 1 h within the procedure.
7. Enrollment in the ERAS pathway helps with reduction in length of stay, complications, and readmissions.
8. A six- to seven-port transperitoneal approach in a more cephalad position helps in maneuvering the small bowel.
9. The robotic arm could be used alternatively with an assistant instrument by inserting an additional robotic arm inside 15-mm laparoscopic port.
10. A zero-degree lens is used during the entire procedure.
11. Robotic arms can be undocked and steep Trendelenburg position is reduced for ease of urethra-neobladder anastomosis.
12. The marionette stitch is not tied but held together using a surgical instrument to allow free movement of the bowel segment.
13. Adequate length on the ileocecal end should be preserved to avoid metabolic disturbances and kinking once the conduit is exteriorized.
14. The guidewire is removed only after the anchoring suture is placed as it is difficult to identify the stent due to lack of tactile feedback.
15. We recommend avoid using thermal approach in creating an enterotomy in ileum at site of ureteral anastomosis and retroperitonealize the anastomosis.
16. Optimizing fluid balance and avoiding over hydration should help manage fluid shift in this patient population with advanced age.
17. Adequate pelvic drainage and stenting of ureters especially at the anastomosis has shown to help in bowel recovery and avoid metabolic abnormalities.
18. Irrigation of the neobladder is recommended every 8 h to avoid mucus plugging and catheter blockage.

143 Development, Molecular Biology, and Physiology of the Prostate

Brian W. Simons and Ashley E. Ross

QUESTIONS

1. Which of the following is NOT considered a sex accessory tissue?
   a. Prostate gland
   b. Seminal vesicles
   c. Tunica albuginea
   d. Ampullae
   e. Bulbourethral gland

2. Which fetal hormone stimulates the development of the wolffian ducts?
   a. Estradiol
   b. Dihydrotestosterone (DHT)
   c. Estrone
   d. Testosterone
   e. Inhibin

3. Which one of the following statements about fetal development of the lower urogenital tract is FALSE?
   a. The urogenital sinus derives from the cloaca.
   b. The cloaca gets its name (L. "sewer") because it receives input from the gastrointestinal and urinary tracts.
   c. The seminal vesicles derive from the posterior portion of the wolffian ducts, whereas the prostate derives from the anterior portion.
   d. Sox9 is an early molecular marker of prostate development.
   e. The urogenital sinus is a primordial structure that contributes to bladder *and* prostate development.

4. Which fetal hormone is most important in stimulating the growth of the prostate during development?
   a. Estradiol
   b. DHT
   c. Estrone
   d. Testosterone
   e. Inhibin

5. Which one of the following statements is TRUE regarding the role of androgens in prostate development?
   a. Males will develop prostates in the presence of sufficiently high levels of androgens, but females will not.
   b. Females will develop prostates in the presence of sufficiently high levels of androgens, but males will not.
   c. Both males and females will develop prostates in the presence of sufficiently high levels of androgens.
   d. Prostate tissue rudiments with a normal androgen receptor in the epithelium but mutant androgen receptor in the

   mesenchyme will develop into normal prostates in the presence of sufficiently high levels of androgen.
   e. Prostate tissue rudiments with androgen receptor overexpression in the epithelium but mutant androgen receptor in the mesenchyme will develop into normal prostates in the absence of androgen.

6. Which α_1-adrenergic receptor subtype is linked to smooth muscle contraction in the prostate?
   a. α_D
   b. α_{1A}
   c. α_{1B}
   d. α_2
   e. α_{2B}

7. Which of the following is TRUE regarding testosterone?
   a. Testosterone is synthesized by the Sertoli cells of the testes.
   b. Testosterone is synthesized by the Leydig cells of the testes.
   c. Testosterone is a direct precursor of pregnenolone.
   d. 5α-Reductase is an enzyme that converts DHT into testosterone.
   e. Aromatase converts estrogens into testosterone.

8. Dehydroepiandrosterone (DHEA) has been suggested as a major source of testosterone within the plasma. What percentage of total testosterone has been determined to be derived from DHEA?
   a. 1%
   b. 2%
   c. 5%
   d. 15%
   e. 20%

9. To what is the majority of testosterone in the plasma bound?
   a. Insulin
   b. Cholesterol
   c. Prostaglandins
   d. TP53
   e. Sex hormone-binding globulin (SHBG)

10. Which 5α-reductase isoform predominates in the prostate gland?
    a. Type 1
    b. Type 2
    c. Type 3
    d. Type 4
    e. Type 5

11. What is the source of fructose in seminal plasma?
    a. Prostate gland
    b. Bulbourethral gland
    c. Vas deferens
    d. Seminal vesicles
    e. Basal cells

12. Compartmentalization of the androgen receptor from the cytosol to the nucleus is dependent on:
    a. dimerization.
    b. adenosine triphosphate (ATP).
    c. RAN-mediated transport.
    d. nuclear localization and nuclear export signals.
    e. all of the above.

13. Which feature of the androgen receptor polymorphisms is thought to impact on the overall activity of androgen target gene induction?
    a. Zinc finger motifs
    b. Poly CAG repeats
    c. Nuclear export signals
    d. Ligand binding domain

14. Which of the following is TRUE with regard to the effects of estrogens in prostate development?
    a. Estrogens are not required for the development of a prostate because ER-α and ER-β knockout mice have phenotypically normal prostates.
    b. ER-α regulates ductal formation.
    c. ER-β is required for prostates to allow sperm to mature to an active form.
    d. b and c

15. When the androgen receptor binds to an androgen response element, which of the following is (are) true?
    a. The dimerization of the receptor is always head to head, regardless of whether the sequence is a direct repeat or an inverted repeat.
    b. The dimerization occurs head to head for an inverted repeat and head to tail for a direct repeat.
    c. The dimerization of the androgen receptor occurs on the DNA template in a process that requires ATP and heat shock proteins.
    d. The androgen receptor can bind to a target androgen response element in either a head-to-head or a head-to-tail orientation, depending on the orientation of the structural gene.

ANSWERS

1. **c. Tunica albuginea.** Sex accessory tissues include the prostate gland, seminal vesicles, ampullae, and bulbourethral glands. They are believed to play a major, but unknown, role in the reproductive process.
2. **d. Testosterone.** The wolffian ducts develop into the seminal vesicles, epididymis, vas deferens, ampulla, and ejaculatory duct; the developmental growth of this group of glands is stimulated by fetal testosterone and not DHT.
3. **c. The seminal vesicles derive from the posterior portion of the wolffian ducts, whereas the prostate derives from the anterior portion.** The prostate develops from the urogenital sinus, not the wolffian duct.
4. **b. DHT.** The prostate first appears and starts its development from the urogenital sinus during the third month of fetal growth, and development is directed primarily by DHT, not testosterone.
5. **c. Both males and females will develop prostates in the presence of sufficiently high levels of androgens.** If androgen (testosterone or DHT) levels are sufficiently high at the right time in fetal development, prostate development will proceed in the urogenital sinus regardless of whether the embryo is male or female. For prostate development to proceed, androgen receptor is required to be functional in the mesenchyme.
6. **b. α_{1A}.** Research work has demonstrated three subtypes of the α_1-adrenergic receptor (α_{1A}, α_{1B}, and α_{1D}), of which the α_{1A} receptor appears to be linked to contraction.
7. **b. Testosterone is synthesized by the Leydig cells of the testes.** Foremost among the hormones and growth factors that stimulate the prostate is the prohormone testosterone, which must be converted within the prostate into the active androgen DHT. Testosterone is synthesized in the Leydig cells of the testes from pregnenolone by a series of reversible reactions; however, once testosterone is reduced by 5α-reductase into DHT or to estrogens by aromatase, the process is irreversible. In other words, whereas testosterone can be converted into DHT and into estrogens, estrogens and DHT cannot be converted into testosterone.
8. **a. 1%.** Less than 1% of the total testosterone in the plasma is derived from DHEA.
9. **e. Sex hormone-binding globulin (SHBG).** The majority of testosterone bound to plasma protein is associated with SHBG.
10. **b. Type 2.** The type 2 isoform is mutated in 5α-reductase deficiency and is the dominant isoform present in the prostate gland.
11. **d. Seminal vesicles.** The source of fructose in human seminal plasma is the seminal vesicles. Patients with congenital absence of the seminal vesicles also have an associated absence of fructose in their ejaculates.
12. **e. All of the above.** After binding ligand, the androgen receptor dissociates from chaperonins, dimerizes, and then is transported to the nucleus via a nuclear localization motif, which activates Ran-dependent active transport, a process that is ATP dependent.
13. **b. Poly CAG repeats.** The shorter the length, the more actively the androgen receptor is thought to function.
14. **a. Estrogens are not required for the development of a prostate because ER-α and ER-β knockout mice have phenotypically normal prostates.**
15. **a. The dimerization of the receptor is always head to head, regardless of whether the sequence is a direct repeat or an inverted repeat.** Although most models predicted that inverted repeat and direct repeat androgen response elements would have dimers that bind with opposite polarity, this prediction was not observed in x-ray crystallography studies.

CHAPTER REVIEW

1. The seminal vesicles are extremely resistant to disease.
2. There are two major cellular components in the prostate: epithelial and stromal.
3. The stromal component consists of connective tissue, smooth muscle cells, and fibroblasts.
4. The epithelial component consists of basal cells, intermediate cells, and neuroendocrine cells.
5. The prostate contains a rich plexus of autonomic nerves.
6. Because of the diurnal variation of serum testosterone, to avoid inconsistency it should be measured in the morning.
7. The role of circulating adrenal androgens on prostate growth is minor.
8. Because the plasma half-life of testosterone is 10 to 20 minutes, patients who undergo bilateral orchiectomy are functionally castrate within 1 to 2 hours after surgery.
9. The androgen receptor is transported to the nucleus and then back to the cytoplasm; nuclear matrix is the major target for androgen and estrogen receptor binding in the nucleus.
10. The longer the CAG repeat in the androgen receptor, the lower its activity in activating target genes.
11. The source of prostaglandins, fructose, and semenogelin is the seminal vesicle.
12. The seminal vesicle contributes the most volume to the seminal fluid.
13. The source of citrate, zinc, spermine, and choline is the prostate.
14. Prostate-specific antigen is a serine protease and degrades semenogelin. Semenogelin gives rise to the coagulation of semen.
15. Complexed PSA is irreversibly bound to α1-antichymotrypsin and α2-macroglobulin.
16. Increases in human kallikrein 2, pro-PSA, and bound PSA are associated with prostate cancer.
17. Few drugs reach concentrations in the prostatic secretions that approach or surpass their concentrations in the serum. The exceptions include erythromycin, oleandomycin, sulfonamides, tetracycline, clindamycin, trimethoprim, and the fluoroquinolones.
18. Prostatic fluid is more acidic than is serum.
19. Acid phosphatase produced in the prostate may be elevated in prostate cancer; it is also produced in the bone and may be elevated in diseases that affect the bone such as Paget disease, osteoporosis, and bone metastases.
20. The wolffian ducts develop into the seminal vesicles, epididymis, vas deferens, ampulla, and ejaculatory duct; the developmental growth of this group of glands is stimulated by fetal testosterone and not DHT.
21. Testosterone is reduced by 5α-reductase into DHT or to estrogens by aromatase; the process is irreversible.

144 Benign Prostatic Hyperplasia: Etiology, Pathophysiology, Epidemiology, and Natural History

Claus G. Roehrborn and Douglas W. Strand

QUESTIONS

1. Which statement is correct regarding the role of androgenic hormones in the etiology of benign prostatic hyperplasia (BPH)?

   a. Testosterone and dihydrotestosterone (DHT) are the sole causes of the hyperplasia taking place in the prostate after the age of 40 years.

   b. The total amount of androgen receptors in the prostate decreases with aging, leading to a lesser response to androgenic stimuli.

   c. DHT is considered the more potent of the androgenic steroid hormones by a factor of approximately 10:1.

   d. Of the two 5α-reductase isoforms, type 1 is most commonly found in the prostate.

   e. Only testosterone produced in the testis and not in the adrenal gland enters into the prostate gland.

2. Regarding genetic and familial factors in the etiology of BPH, which statement is TRUE?

   a. There is no evidence that BPH is a familial disease.

   b. Any man who has undergone transurethral resection of the prostate (TURP) should alert his sons that their chances of requiring TURP is three times greater than age-matched controls.

   c. Cases of familial BPH tend to occur in men with smaller prostates than the sporadic cases of BPH.

   d. Approximately 50% of cases of BPH in men who undergo surgery when younger than the age of 60 years are estimated to be inheritable.

   e. The most likely inheritance pattern is autosomal recessive.

3. The prevalence of a disease is defined as the number of:

   a. diseased people per 100,000 population per year.

   b. existing cases per 100,000 population at a distinct target date.

   c. deaths per 100,000 population per year.

   d. deaths per number of diseased.

   e. cumulative cases of a disease over a specified time period.

4. Concerning the autopsy prevalence of BPH or stromoglandular hyperplasia of the prostate, which statement is correct?

   a. No adequate studies have been done to date.

   b. It is commonly found in men of all ages.

   c. It is very uncommon in men younger than 30 years.

   d. It is found in 100% of men beginning at the age of 40 years.

   e. International comparisons are impossible because of a lack of its definition.

5. Which of the following statements regarding the International Prostate Symptom Score (IPSS) is TRUE?

   a. Moderate symptom severity is defined as a score from 12 to 22 points.

   b. The IPSS score addresses voiding and storage symptoms as well as questions regarding incontinence.

   c. Quantitative symptom scores in BPH are not as important as are objective measures such as a flow rate recording.

   d. The IPSS score has been translated and validated in many languages.

   e. Physicians and nurses may fill out the IPSS score for their patients after consultation.

6. Which statement is TRUE regarding prostate volume?

   a. International studies show significant similarity in prostate volume in white, age-stratified men.

   b. Prostate volume assessment by digital rectal examination (DRE) is reproducible across examiners.

   c. Although there is a steady increase in total prostate volume with age, the transition zone volume increases only marginally.

   d. Magnetic resonance imaging (MRI) measurements are, in general, smaller compared with transrectal ultrasound measurements.

   e. DRE estimation of prostate volume is fairly accurate when done by an experienced urologist.

7. Concerning liver disease and BPH, which of the following statements is TRUE?

   a. Ethanol consumption increases circulating levels of estrogens.

   b. The risk of having surgery for BPH is increased in heavy drinkers.

   c. The intake of ethanol can decrease serum testosterone levels by a variety of mechanisms.

   d. Most autopsy studies find a higher prevalence of BPH in men with liver cirrhosis.

   e. In men with liver disease, histologic specimens of the prostate show a similar influence of estrogen such as seen in hormonally treated prostate cancer.

8. How do medications influence symptoms and flow rate?

   a. There is no documented influence of any medication on symptoms or flow rate.

   b. Antihistamines and bronchodilators significantly decrease urinary flow rates.

   c. Calcium channel blockers and β-adrenergic blockers reduce urinary flow rates significantly.

   d. Antidepressants, antihistamines, and bronchodilators increase the symptom score by several points.

   e. Anticholinergic agents decrease the peak urinary flow rate markedly.

9. Concerning correlations between baseline parameters, which statement is TRUE?

   a. A clinically useful correlation exists between prostate volume and serum prostate-specific antigen (PSA) level.

   b. Many studies have shown a significant correlation between the transition zone volume and symptom severity.

   c. Correlation of symptoms, bother, interference, and quality of life are poor.

d. Urinary flow rate and prostate volume correlate highly with serum PSA level.

e. Serum PSA level shows a strong correlation with symptom frequency and bother.

10. Which statement is correct regarding the study of the natural history of BPH?

a. Placebo groups from treatment trials are useful because they do not have treatment biases.

b. A longitudinal population-based study has the fewest biases and is the most useful type of study.

c. Control groups from intervention or medical therapy trials reflect the natural history of the disease in unselected community-dwelling men.

d. Placebo groups have fewer selection biases compared with population-based studies.

e. No such studies have been conducted.

11. Regarding the magnitude of the placebo response and its perception, which of the following statements is TRUE?

a. Placebo response is not dependent on the baseline severity score.

b. Most patients report subjective improvement when the drop from baseline is 30%.

c. The higher the baseline score, the more of a drop is required for patients to subjectively feel improved.

d. Perception of improvement is independent of baseline score.

e. There are convincing data to demonstrate that the final score after treatment is more important than the baseline score or the drop from baseline.

12. Descriptive studies of the incidence rates of acute urinary retention (AUR) have demonstrated that:

a. depending on the population studied, incidence rates less than 5 to more than 130 cases/1000 man-years have been reported.

b. the incidence rates reported do not differ significantly between various studies and populations.

c. AUR has been poorly defined, and therefore no incidence rate can be calculated.

d. incidence rates of approximately 10/1000 man-years have been reported in all watchful waiting studies.

e. incidence rates of AUR have not been reported in the urologic literature, only prevalence rates.

13. What is the most significant finding regarding analytical epidemiology of AUR?

a. Serum PSA level is a more powerful predictor of AUR than is age.

b. Serum PSA level and prostate volume have limited ability to predict episodes of AUR.

c. Urinary flow rates in placebo control groups are strong predictors of AUR episodes.

d. Age has been found to be the most significant risk factor for AUR in population-based studies.

e. There is virtually no relationship between symptom frequency and bother and AUR episodes.

14. Which statement regarding surgery for BPH is TRUE?

a. The incidence rates of surgery are similar across wide geographic regions and ethnic backgrounds.

b. AUR is a harder and more objective end point compared to surgery.

c. Surgery is a less common end point compared with AUR.

d. Most patients with BPH eventually require surgery for their condition.

e. Surgery rates for BPH have remained stable since approximately 1990.

ANSWERS

1. **c. DHT is considered the more potent of the androgenic steroid hormones by a factor of approximately 10:1.** The androgenic steroid hormones testosterone and DHT have a permissive role in the development of BPH but are not the sole cause. The androgen receptor remains at high levels in the prostate in aging men and specifically in BPH tissues, maintaining responsiveness to androgenic stimuli. The most common of the two 5α-reductase isoforms in the benignly enlarged prostate gland is type 2.

2. **d. Approximately 50% of cases of BPH in men who undergo surgery when younger than the age of 60 years are estimated to be inheritable.** There is significant evidence to suggest that some cases of BPH are familial, with autosomal dominant being the most likely inheritance pattern. An increased risk for BPH surgery exists mostly for men who come to BPH surgery when younger than the age of 60 years, and men with familial cases of BPH have larger glands than men with sporadic cases.

3. **b. Existing cases per 100,000 population at a distinct target date.** When studying diseases by descriptive or analytical epidemiologic methods, it is important to have a good understanding of the definitions that apply. Most epidemiologic terms are expressed as rates, which are the number of cases for persons expressed over the population. The definitions that are of relevance are incidence rates, which are equal to the number of people/100,000 population/year getting a certain disease; prevalence, which is the number of existing cases of the disease of interest/100,000 at a distinct target date; mortality rate, which is the number of deaths/100,000 population/year; and fatality, which equals the number of deaths due to the disease/ number of diseased people.

4. **c. It is very uncommon in men younger than 30 years.** The autopsy prevalence of BPH has been studied as early as 1984 by Berry and colleagues.[a] Since then, many studies have been done on virtually all continents in many ethnic groups. It is astonishing that these studies find a very significant agreement in terms of the actual prevalence of histologic BPH or stromoglandular hyperplasia around the world. Stromoglandular hyperplasia or BPH is very uncommon in men younger than the age of 30 years, but then increases steadily in an almost linear manner. In fact, approximately 90% of men in their 80s have evidence of stromoglandular hyperplasia.

5. **d. The IPSS score has been translated and validated in many languages.** The IPSS symptom score is a seven-question, self-administered questionnaire that yields a total score ranging from 0 to 35 points. Men who score 0 to 7 points are classified as mildly symptomatic, those scoring from 8 to 19 points as moderately symptomatic, and those scoring from 20 to 35 points as severely symptomatic. The IPSS score addresses both voiding and storage, but not incontinence symptomatology. It is widely accepted that quantitative symptom scores are more important than, for example, urinary flow rate recordings. The IPSS score, the most widely utilized instrument, has been translated and culturally validated in many languages. Providers should abstain from filling in the questionnaire for their patients as it is validated as a self-reported symptom severity instrument.

6. **a. International studies show significant similarity in prostate volume in white, age-stratified men.** Prostate volume can relatively easily be assessed by transrectal ultrasonography

---

[a]Sources referenced can be found in *Campbell-Walsh-Wein Urology, 12th Edition*, on the Expert Consult website.

(TRUS). TRUS has been found to be a reliable measure that is reproducible across examiners, in contrast to DRE, which is only poorly reproducible. MRI is very expensive and it yields in general a larger volume compared with TRUS measurements. Of note is the fact that international studies show significant similarity in regard to total and transitional zone prostate volume in white, age-stratified men.

7. **c. The intake of ethanol can decrease serum testosterone levels by a variety of mechanisms.** It is known that alcohol intake may decrease plasma testosterone levels by reducing production of and increasing clearance of testosterone. However, despite this hypothetical reason for a lower incidence, an inverse relationship has been described. The age-adjusted multivariate relative risks for undergoing surgery for BPH in men drinking more than three or four glasses of alcohol per day is lower than in age-matched controls. Of course, this could be due to a bias against surgery in patients who are heavy drinkers and therefore in poor health. It is interesting to note, however, that in the majority of studies, namely, four of five, a lower prevalence of BPH is found in men with cirrhosis compared with those without cirrhosis.

8. **d. Antidepressants, antihistamines, and bronchodilators increase the symptom score by several points.** There is only one study that systematically assessed the effect of medications on urinary symptoms and flow rate. Cold medications containing α-sympathomimetics tend to exacerbate lower urinary tract symptoms by the expected effect on the smooth muscle of the bladder outlet. Data from the Olmsted County Study of Urinary Symptoms and Health Status Among Men show that daily use of antidepressants, antihistamines, or bronchodilators is associated with a 2- to 3-point increase in the symptom score. However, only the daily use of antidepressants is associated with a decrease in the age-adjusted urinary flow rate.

9. **a. A clinically useful correlation exists between prostate volume and serum prostate-specific antigen (PSA) level.** In general there is an absence of useful baseline correlations between subjective and objective parameters such as symptoms, frequency, quality of life, and urinary flow rate measures of obstruction and prostate volume. However, symptom, bother, and interference with quality of life show excellent correlation with each other, and a clinically useful correlation exists between total and transition zone prostate volume and serum PSA in men with BPH.

10. **b. A longitudinal population-based study has the fewest biases and is the most useful type of study.** There are several ways to study the natural history of BPH. One can look at watchful waiting cohorts or placebo-controlled groups of medication trials, or study population-based groups of men longitudinally over time. The latter is clearly the best way of studying the natural history of the disease because it incurs the fewest biases. However, it is also the most tedious and most expensive method. Placebo groups in medication trials clearly suffer from enrollment biases but do provide useful information.

11. **c. The higher the baseline score, the more of a drop is required for patients to subjectively feel improved.** The placebo response is partially a regression to the mean and partially an effect induced by the interaction between patient and doctor. The response is clearly dependent on the baseline severity score, with patients' higher scores having a larger decrease from baseline. The perception of subjective improvement has been shown to be dependent on the drop from baseline as well as on the baseline itself. For example, the higher the baseline score, the more of a drop from baseline is required for patients to have a subjective perception of improvement. Overall, a 3-point decrease is associated with a subjective perception of improvement.

12. **a. Depending on the population studied, incidence rates less than 5 to more than 130 cases/1000 man-years have been reported.** AUR has been studied during the past few years in population-based studies as well as in placebo-control groups from long-term treatment trials. The incidence rates differ significantly between different studies because of the inclusion and exclusion criteria and selection biases. Fortunately, AUR is a very clearly defined outcome and, thus, incidence rates can easily be calculated and compared.

13. **d. Age has been found to be the most significant risk factor for AUR in population-based studies.** In population-based studies such as the Olmsted County Study of Urinary Symptoms and Health Status Among Men, age is the most significant predictor of AUR. Data from placebo groups of long-term medical treatment trials demonstrate that serum PSA is the most powerful predictor of AUR together with prostate volume. Although this appears on the surface to be a contradiction, it can be relatively easily explained by the fact that in BPH treatment trials, elderly men with already an existing diagnosis of BPH are enrolled. Thus, age plays a lesser factor in terms of predicting AUR. In population-based studies in which men stratified by age are followed during long periods of time, age plays a more significant factor compared with PSA.

14. **b. AUR is a harder and more objective end point compared with surgery.** Incidence rates of surgery vary significantly across geographic regions and patients with different ethnic backgrounds. Depending on the interaction between patient and physician, the physician can convince the patient to undergo surgery or, based on the patient's comorbidities, talk him out of surgery. The same cannot be said for urinary retention. It is clear that a vast majority of patients do not require surgery in the course of their disease but, rather, can be treated effectively with reassurance alone or medication.

CHAPTER REVIEW

1. BPH is characterized by an increased number of epithelial and stromal cells, not an increase in their size.
2. Androgens are required for normal cell proliferation and differentiation and actively inhibit cell death.
3. Serum estrogen levels increase in men with age.
4. Early periurethral nodules are stromal; transition zone proliferation is glandular.
5. Prostatic stroma represents 40% of the gland. Smooth muscle is a prominent component of the stroma.
6. Autonomic system overactivity may contribute to lower urinary tract symptoms in men with BPH; the alpha 1a receptor is the most abundant form in the prostate.
7. Symptoms that use the AUA Symptom Index are classified as mild if the score is 0 to 7, moderate if it is 8 to 19, and severe if it is 20 to 35. A change of 3 points or more from time to time is subjectively discernible.
8. Men and women experience a decrease in maximum urinary flow rate as they age.
9. Bladder fibrosis is seen in both sexes with advancing age.
10. After spontaneous acute urinary retention (AUR), 15% of patients will have another episode and three fourths will undergo surgery; after precipitated AUR, 9% will have another episode and 26% will undergo surgery.
11. A significant portion of male lower urinary tract symptoms is related to age-related detrusor dysfunction and other conditions unrelated to the prostate.
12. DHT, the most potent androgen in the prostate, and androgen receptors remain high with age.
13. Androgen withdrawal results in apoptosis of prostate cells.
14. Estrogen receptors are found in the prostate and may play a role in BPH.

Continued

15. The size of the prostate does not correlate with the degree of obstruction.
16. Trabeculation is due to an increase in detrusor collagen.
17. A maximum flow rate less than 10 mL/sec in the male indicates a high probability of obstruction.
18. There is no relationship between vasectomy and BPH; however, there is a positive relationship between lack of physical activity, obesity, BMI, and LUTS/BPH.
19. Hydronephrosis is found in 7.6% of patients having surgery for BPH, one third of whom have renal insufficiency.
20. Some cases of BPH are familial, with autosomal dominant being the most likely inheritance pattern. Patients with familial BPH tend to have larger glands than those with sporadic BPH.
21. Cold medications containing α-sympathomimetics tend to exacerbate lower urinary tract symptoms by the expected effect on the smooth muscle of the bladder outlet.
22. A clinically useful correlation exists between total and transition zone prostate volume and serum PSA in men with BPH.

145 Evaluation and Nonsurgical Management of Benign Prostatic Hyperplasia

Paolo Capogrosso, Andrea Salonia, and Francesco Montorsi

QUESTIONS

1. Lower urinary tract symptoms (LUTSs) may arise as a consequence of:
   a. benign prostatic enlargement.
   b. bladder outlet obstruction.
   c. neurologic disease.
   d. detrusor underactivity.
   e. all of the above.

2. Medications that may exacerbate LUTSs include:
   a. loop diuretics.
   b. α adrenergic antagonists.
   c. β-3 adrenergic agonists.
   d. muscarinic receptors agonists.
   e. phytotherapy.

3. Digital rectal examination at the time of the assessment of patients with LUTSs:
   a. should always be performed with the only aim to rule out prostate cancer.
   b. allows estimation of prostate volume, which is useful for planning further management.
   c. does not provide reliable information, and therefore should not be performed.
   d. may be used to obtain prostatic secretion.
   e. has the main goal of estimating the rectal tone.

4. Frequency-volume charts:
   a. should always be used when patients with LUTSs are being assessed.
   b. should cover at least a 72-hour period.
   c. are particularly useful to assess obstructive symptoms.
   d. allows estimation of the average postvoid residual volume.
   e. should be requested only when a diagnosis of detrusor overactivity has been established.

5. It is advisable in a man with LUTSs/benign prostatic hyperplasia and a slightly elevated creatinine level to perform:
   a. transurethral resection of the prostate.
   b. an intravenous pyelogram.
   c. renal ultrasound imaging.
   d. a urodynamic study.
   e. flexible cystoscopy.

6. Which test should always be considered in a man with prevalent storage symptoms and a history of smoking?
   a. Urinalysis.
   b. Serum prostate-specific antigen (PSA) test.
   c. Urine cytology.
   d. Frequency-volume charts.
   e. Noninvasive urodynamic tests.

7. Serum PSA testing should be requested in which of the following clinical scenarios?
   a. A patient older than 75 years with a family history of prostate cancer.
   b. A 55-year-old patient with negative digital rectal examination findings and no previous PSA measurements.
   c. Serum PSA should be performed every case to rule out prostate cancer.
   d. A patient with severe symptoms regardless of age.
   e. A patient with a recent episode of macrohematuria.

8. What is the gold standard for the assessment of bladder outlet obstruction?
   a. Invasive urodynamic tests.
   b. Uroflowmetry.
   c. Transrectal prostate ultrasound imaging.
   d. Flexible urethrocystoscopy.
   e. Cystourethrogram.

9. What is the suggested first treatment approach for a 50-year-old patient with an International Prostate Symptom Score (IPSS) score of 7 without risk factors for disease progression?
   a. Phytotherapy.
   b. α Adrenergic blockers.
   c. Watchful waiting.
   d. No treatment.
   e. β3 Adrenergic agonists.

10. Which of the following strategies should be part of watchful waiting management?
    a. Regular patient monitoring.
    b. Education and reassurance.
    c. Fluid management.
    d. Concurrent medication adjustment.
    e. All of the above.

11. Which of the following is an indication for surgical treatment in patients with LUTSs?
    a. Severe symptoms.
    b. Postvoid residual volume urine of 300 mL or more.
    c. Recurrent episodes of acute urinary retention.
    d. Elevated PSA level.
    e. Lack of response to an α-blocker.

12. Detrusor overactivity:
    a. is always an indicator of overactive bladder syndrome.
    b. is rarely observed in patients with benign prostatic enlargement.
    c. may be observed in up to 83% of men with severe bladder outlet obstruction.
    d. should always be reduced by LUTS treatment.
    e. None of the above sentences are true.

13. Which of the following receptors is not relevant for LUTS treatment?

    a. $\alpha\text{-}1_a$.

    b. $\alpha\text{-}1_b$.

    c. $\alpha\text{-}1_d$.

    d. $\beta\text{-}3$.

    e. $\beta\text{-}1$.

14. Which of the following is considered a uroselective α adrenergic blocker?

    a. Terazosin.

    b. Sildenafil.

    c. Tamsulosin.

    d. Doxazosin.

    e. None of them.

15. In the first placebo-controlled phase III trial, terazosin showed a symptom-reduction rate of approximately:

    a. 22%.

    b. 13%.

    c. 85%.

    d. 40%.

    e. 8%.

16. One of the most commonly reported side effects with terazosin therapy is:

    a. retrograde ejaculation.

    b. anejaculation.

    c. headache.

    d. dyspepsia.

    e. dizziness.

17. Pooled data analysis of randomized trials showed that the relative risk of postural hypotension with doxazosin treatment as compared with placebo is:

    a. approximately 2.7.

    b. approximately 5.6.

    c. approximately 7.8.

    d. approximately 1.1.

    e. not different.

18. The Medical Therapy of Prostatic Symptoms (MTOPS) trial showed that treatment with doxazosin was associated with:

    a. reduced risk of clinical progression as compared with placebo.

    b. increased risk of acute urinary retention as compared with placebo.

    c. no change in the risk of clinical progression as compared with placebo.

    d. reduced risk of surgical treatment as compared with finasteride.

    e. none of the above.

19. Which of the following drugs needs dose titration at first prescription:

    a. Finasteride.

    b. Alfuzosin.

    c. Terazosin.

    d. Doxazosin gastrointestinal therapeutic system.

    e. Tamsulosin.

20. An effect of tamsulosin on patient symptoms should be expected after approximately:

    a. 1 month of treatment.

    b. 6 months of treatment.

    c. 1 week of treatment.

    d. 3 months of treatment.

    e. 1 day of treatment.

21. What is the magnitude of the change of the bladder outlet obstruction index (BOOI) after treatment with silodosin?

    a. −30.4.

    b. −5.4.

    c. −11.1.

    d. −2.1.

    e. Treatment with α adrenergic blockers is never associated with an improvement of urodynamic parameters.

22. Naftopidil has demonstrated high affinity for which of the following receptors?

    a. $\alpha\text{-}1_b$.

    b. $\alpha\text{-}1_a$.

    c. $\alpha\text{-}1_a$ and $\alpha\text{-}1_b$.

    d. $\beta3$.

    e. $\alpha\text{-}1_d$.

23. Randomized active-controlled trials comparing the effect of different α adrenergic blockers demonstrated that:

    a. tamsulosin at a dose of 0.4 mg is as effective as silodosin at a dose of 8 mg in terms of symptom relief.

    b. alfuzosin at a daily dose of 10 mg has lower overall efficacy as compared with tamsulosin at a dose of 0.4 mg.

    c. tamsulosin at a dose of 0.4 mg showed the greatest BOOI reduction among all available α adrenergic blockers.

    d. uroselective α adrenergic blockers are generally more effective than doxazosin and terazosin.

    e. there is no clinically relevant difference in the efficacy and tolerability profile among α adrenergic blockers.

24. Physicians should warn patients regarding the risk of first-dose hypotension when prescribing:

    a. silodosin.

    b. tamsulosin.

    c. terazosin.

    d. alfuzosin.

    e. all of the above.

25. What is the likely mechanism for dizziness after $\alpha\text{-}1$ adrenergic blocker therapy?

    a. Reduced cardiac output.

    b. Central nervous system.

    c. Carotid baroreceptor.

    d. Both a and c.

    e. None of the above.

26. Before they undergo cataract surgery, patients should be advised to:

    a. discontinue treatment with α-blockers to reduce the risk of intraoperative floppy iris syndrome (IFIS).

    b. report the use of α-blockers to the ophthalmologist.

    c. discontinue treatment with tamsulosin and switch to a nonuroselective α-blocker.

    d. reduce the dosage of the α-blocker at least 1 month before surgery.

    e. do none of the above.

27. Which of the following effects should be expected after 1 month of treatment with finasteride?
    a. Significant decrease in serum dihydrotestosterone (DHT) level.
    b. Significant decrease in prostate volume.
    c. Significant increase in the peak urinary flow.
    d. 70% decrease in serum PSA level.
    e. None of the above.

28. What is the expected decrease in prostate volume with 5-α reductase inhibitors (5-ARIs)?
    a. 15% to 30%.
    b. More than 50%.
    c. 10%.
    d. 80%.
    e. 5%.

29. Regarding the safety profile of 5-ARIs:
    a. 5-ARIs may increase the risk of diabetes mellitus.
    b. patients treated with 5-ARIs showed higher risk of cardio-vascular events.
    c. 5-ARIs may increase the overall risk of prostate cancer.
    d. patients should be warned regarding a higher risk of de-pressive symptoms associated with 5-ARI treatment.
    e. none of the above are true.

30. Tolterodine should not be prescribed to a patient with:
    a. a total IPSS score suggestive of severe symptoms.
    b. postvoid residual volume greater than 200 mL.
    c. evidence of detrusor overactivity.
    d. low cystometric capacity.
    e. prostate volume greater than 50 mL.

31. Who is the best candidate for treatment with mirabegron?
    a. A 75-year-old patient with prevalent storage symptoms.
    b. A 65-year-old patient with moderate LUTSs and a postvoid residual volume of 250 mL.
    c. A 70-year-old patient with moderate LUTSs and a previous episode of acute urinary retention.
    d. A 45-year-old patient with mild LUTSs and erectile dysfunc-tion.
    e. None of the above.

32. Which of the following is considered a possible biologic effect of phosphodiesterase type 5 inhibitors (PDE5is) on the lower urinary tract?
    a. Relaxation of smooth muscle at the level of the prostate and bladder neck.
    b. Decreased blood flow at the level of the bladder and pros-tate resulting in decreased local inflammation.
    c. Increased activity of afferent nerves in the bladder wall.
    d. Inhibition of the 5α-reductase type 2 isoenzyme at the level of the prostate.
    e. All of the above.

33. What is the effect of PDE5i monotherapy in patients with LUTSs?
    a. There is no evidence of a significant reduction in the IPSS score with PDE5i monotherapy alone.
    b. PDE5i monotherapy resulted in a significant increase in the peak urinary flow after 1 month of treatment.
    c. PDE5i monotherapy has been shown to significantly de-crease the IPSS score as compared with placebo.

    d. Tadalafil is the only PDE5i that has resulted in relief of symptoms in randomized trials.
    e. PDE5i monotherapy can decrease the risk of acute urinary retention in the long term.

34. Pooled data analysis has shown that the mean difference in the posttreatment IPSS between PDE5is and placebo is:
    a. approximately 2 to 4 points.
    b. approximately 6 to 8 points.
    c. approximately 1 to 2 points.
    d. not significant.
    e. none of the above.

35. The MTOPS trial showed that:
    a. the combination of doxazosin and finasteride is superior to placebo in reducing the risk of clinical progression.
    b. doxazosin is not superior to placebo in reducing the risk of clinical progression.
    c. finasteride alone does not reduce the risk of subsequent invasive therapy as compared with placebo.
    d. combination therapy is not superior to doxazosin mono-therapy in terms of symptom relief.
    e. doxazosin is superior to placebo in reducing the risk of subsequent invasive therapy.

36. The Combination of Avodart and Tamsulosin (CombAT) study showed that:
    a. tamsulosin monotherapy significantly reduces the risk of acute urinary retention.
    b. dutasteride alone reduces the risk of surgical treatment as compared with tamsulosin.
    c. combination therapy is not superior than dutasteride monotherapy in reducing the risk of disease progression.
    d. tamsulosin is superior to dutasteride in reducing the IPSS score at long-term assessment.
    e. None of the above.

37. According to international clinical guidelines, a patient with a large prostate volume and predominantly bothersome voiding symptoms should be counseled for:
    a. surgical treatment.
    b. α-blocker plus 5-ARI therapy.
    c. α-blocker monotherapy.
    d. 5-ARI monotherapy.
    e. α-blocker plus antimuscarinic drug therapy.

38. The definitive mechanism of action for *Serenoa repens* is:
    a. inhibition of 5α-reductase.
    b. inhibition of cyclooxygenase.
    c. inhibition of lipoxygenase.
    d. prostate smooth muscle relaxation.
    e. inconclusive.

39. The results of placebo-controlled trials assessing treatment with *S. repens* showed:
    a. a significant reduction of symptom scores.
    b. a reduction of the IPSS score only at triple the usual dose.
    c. no difference in the urinary flow parameters but significant relief symptoms.
    d. no difference in both symptoms and urinary flow param-eters as compared with placebo.
    e. None of the above.

40. In a patient with a first episode of acute urinary retention, what is the probability of a successful trial without catheter?

    a. Approximately 60%.

    b. Less than 50%.

    c. Approximately 10%.

    d. Very low without concomitant α-blocker therapy.

    e. More than 80%.

ANSWERS

1. **e. All of the above.** LUTSs are considered a clinical manifestation with a multifactorial pathophysiology arising from different conditions, including benign prostatic enlargement, bladder outlet obstruction, neurologic disease, and bladder dysfunction.

2. **a. Loop diuretics.** Loop diuretics may increase urinary output, exacerbating symptoms in patients with bladder outlet obstruction.

3. **b. Allows estimation of prostate volume, which is useful for planning further management.** Digital rectal examination should always be performed at the first assessment of patients with LUTS. It can provide an estimate of prostate volume and at the same time rule out locally advanced prostate cancer.

4. **b. Should cover at least a 72-hour period.** A 3-day period is considered a reasonable compromise to increase the accuracy of frequency-volume charts without decreasing patient adherence.

5. **c. Renal ultrasound imaging.** International clinical guidelines suggest upper urinary tract imaging in the case of elevated serum creatinine level.

6. **c. Urine cytology.** This test should be considered in patients presenting with storage symptoms and a history of smoking to rule out urothelial neoplasms.

7. **b. A 55-year-old patient with negative digital rectal examination findings and no previous PSA measurements.** Among patients with LUTSs, PSA testing should be suggested if a diagnosis of prostate cancer would change the clinical management.

8. **a. Invasive urodynamic tests.** The diagnosis of bladder outlet obstruction relies on urodynamic tests.

9. **c. Watchful waiting.** Patients with mild symptoms without factors suggesting a high risk of disease progression (e.g., large postvoid volume, large prostate volume) should be counseled for conservative management.

10. **e. All of the above.** Watchful waiting is mainly based on lifestyle modifications, education, and reassurance and monitoring.

11. **c. Recurrent episodes of acute urinary retention.** Surgical treatment of LUTSs is indicated for patients with recurrent acute urinary retention because they may not benefit from medical treatment.

12. **c. May be observed in up to 83% of men with severe bladder outlet obstruction.** Detrusor overactivity is extremely common in the case of bladder outlet obstruction; however, LUTS treatment may not reduce detrusor overactivity.

13. **e. β-1.** Among adrenergic receptors, the β-1 subfamily is poorly represented in the lower urinary tract and is not targeted by any of the currently available treatments for LUTSs.

14. **c. Tamsulosin.** Uroselective agents have high affinity for the $\alpha\text{-}1_a$ and $\alpha\text{-}1_d$ receptors; as such, they have greater selectivity for prostatic and urethral tissue.

15. **a. 22%.** The first phase II multicenter, placebo-controlled trial showed a 22.4% reduction in symptom score from the baseline for patients treated with terazosin.

16. **e. Dizziness.** As a consequence of the vascular side effects associated with the inhibition of $\alpha\text{-}1_b$ receptors, dizziness is frequently reported after treatment with terazosin and doxazosin.

17. **a. Approximately 2.7.** A meta-analysis of 10 placebo-controlled trials showed that the relative risk of postural hypotension associated with doxazosin treatment was 2.72 (95% confidence interval 1.21–6.15).

18. **a. Reduced risk of clinical progression as compared with placebo.** In the MTOPS trial, doxazosin therapy resulted in a significant decrease in the risk of clinical progression as compared with placebo, although it was inferior to both finasteride monotherapy and combination therapy.

19. **c. Terazosin.** Given the high risk of first-dose hypotension, nonuroselective α-blockers need dose titration over the first few weeks of treatment.

20. **c. 1 week of treatment.** Randomized trials have shown that tamsulosin leads to symptom relief after 1 week of treatment and to changes in urinary flow parameters after only a few hours.

21. **a. –30.4.** In a recent study pooling data from trials assessing urodynamic changes associated with α-blocker treatment, silodosin showed the greatest BOOI reduction as compared with the other compounds.

22. **e. $\alpha\text{-}1_d$.** Naftopidil is the only developed compound with a distinct selectivity for the $\alpha\text{-}1_d$ receptor subtype.

23. **a. Tamsulosin at a dose of 0.4 mg is as effective as silodosin at a dose of 8 mg in terms of symptom relief.** Data from two meta-analyses of randomized controlled trials comparing silodosin with tamsulosin showed no difference in terms of efficacy.

24. **e. All of the above.** Despite the lower risk of vascular side effects associated with uroselective α-blockers, patients should be always warned regarding the risk of first-dose hypotension.

25. **b. Central nervous system.** The α-1–mediated dizziness and asthenia are likely due to effects at the level of the central nervous system.

26. **b. Report the use of α-blockers to the ophthalmologist.** IFIS cannot be prevented, but the ophthalmologist should be notified regarding the use of α-blockers so as to properly manage complications.

27. **e. None of the above.** As a type 1 5-ARI, finasteride does not lower the serum level of DHT. Moreover, 1 month of treatment is not enough to observe a significant change in prostate volume and urinary flow parameters. Conversely, PSA level may change after 1 month of treatment.

28. **a. 15% to 30%.** Randomized trials assessing treatment with dutasteride and finasteride have shown a prostate volume reduction ranging from 15% to 30% after 6 to 24 months of treatment.

29. **d. Patients should be warned regarding a higher risk of depressive symptoms associated with 5-ARI treatment.** Large prospective trials have shown a higher prevalence of depressive symptoms among patients treated with 5-ARIs.

30. **b. Postvoid residual volume greater than 200 mL.** All trials investigating antimuscarinic drugs included only patients with a postvoid residual volume lower than 200 mL.

31. **a. A 75-year-old patient with prevalent storage symptoms.** Given its more favorable tolerability profile as compared with antimuscarinic drugs, mirabegron therapy could be preferred in old men with prevalent storage symptoms.

32. **a. Relaxation of smooth muscle at the level of the prostate and bladder neck.** This effect is associated with the increase in nitric oxide signaling from nerve fibers close to the muscle fibers.

33. **c. PDE5i monotherapy has been shown to significantly decrease the IPSS score as compared with placebo.** Several randomized trials demonstrated significant relief of symptoms associated with PDE5i monotherapy. Conversely, there is no evidence of improved urinary flow parameters with PDE5is alone.

34. **a. Approximately 2 to 4 points.** Meta-analyses of placebo-controlled trials have shown a mean difference in the posttreatment IPSS score, between PDE5is and placebo, ranging from 2 to 4 points.

35. **a. The combination of doxazosin and finasteride is superior to placebo in reducing the risk of clinical progression.** The MTOPS trial demonstrated that combination therapy of an α-blocker and a 5-ARI can significantly reduce the risk of disease progression at long-term follow-up. This effect was greater than with both placebo and monotherapy.
36. **b. Dutasteride alone reduces the risk of surgical treatment as compared with tamsulosin.** The CombAT study showed a greater reduction in the risk of surgical treatment for patients treated with dutasteride as compared with tamsulosin.
37. **b. α-Blocker plus 5-ARI therapy.** Treatment algorithms suggest a combination of an α-blocker and a 5-ARI to treat patients with large gland volumes and bothersome voiding symptoms.
38. **e. Inconclusive.** Although experimental data have suggested numerous possible mechanisms of actions for the phytotherapeutic agents, it is uncertain which, if any, of these proposed mechanisms is responsible for the clinical responses.
39. **d. No difference in both symptoms and urinary flow parameters as compared with placebo.** Although meta-analysis of randomized trials of *S. repens* did not show significant relief of LUTSs, it has been recognized that those results could be affected by the heterogeneity of the extracts used in the different trials and may not be applicable to all marketed products.
40. **a. Approximately 60%.** Prospective studies have shown that a successful trial without catheter after a first episode of acute urinary retention could be achieved in 60% of cases.

CHAPTER REVIEW

1. Assessing symptom severity is the first step in the workup of patients with LUTSs.
2. The PSA test should be considered for patients with a life expectancy longer than 10 years.
3. Ultrasound imaging and uroflowmetry should be performed for patients with moderate to severe symptoms.
4. Invasive urodynamic tests should be considered if bladder motility alterations (e.g., detrusor overactivity, detrusor underactivity) are suspected.
5. Conservative management is the preferred approach for patients with mild symptoms and without complicating factors.
6. Watchful waiting is based on patient education, lifestyle interventions, and disease monitoring.
7. Lifestyle modifications include proper daily fluid intake, tea, caffeine, and alcohol avoidance/restriction, and concurrent medication adjustment.
8. Patients should be followed up yearly to detect worsening of symptoms or the occurrence of complications.
9. α1-Blockers are the first line treatment for patients with moderate to severe LUTSs.
10. The uroselective α1-blockers tamsulosin, silodosin, and alfuzosin showed the best tolerability profile.
11. 5-ARIs are effective in reducing the risk of disease progression and the need for invasive treatment.
12. Patients with predominant storage symptoms may benefit from a combination therapy with antimuscarinic drugs.
13. PDE5is are effective in relieving LUTSs, either alone or in combination with α1-blockers.
14. There is no consensus on the efficacy of phytotherapy for LUTS treatment, although encouraging results have been published for the hexane extract of *S. repens* and for the combination of *S. repens* with lycopene and selenium.
15. Acute urinary retention (AUR) is a common complication of benign prostatic hyperplasia progression.
16. A trial without catheter (TWOC) is the preferred management after initial decompression by bladder catheterization.
17. The use of α1-blockers is recommended to increase the odds of a successful TWOC.
18. Dutasteride and finasteride have been shown to significantly decrease the risk of AUR in patients with moderate to severe LUTSs.

146 Minimally Invasive and Endoscopic Management of Benign Prostatic Hyperplasia

Sevann Helo, R. Charles Welliver, Jr., and Kevin T. McVary

QUESTIONS

1. In the conduct of performing a transurethral resection of the prostate (TURP) on a 65-g prostate using a continuous flow instrument, the urologist notes a disturbing amount of dark blood from the rectoscope efflux. In carefully and repeatedly observing the prostate fossa he notes no obvious bleeding sites. The likely etiology of such blood is:
   a. venous bleeding from prostatic fossa.
   b. unstable blood pressure resulting in intermittent arterial bleeding.
   c. inadvertent use of chromogen dyes (methylene blue or indocarmine) by anesthesia.
   d. perforation of the bladder.
   e. previous unrecognized coagulopathy.

2. A patient is 6 weeks post-TURP for long-standing obstruction and detrusor overactivity; voices marked concern over his persistent symptoms, wondering if there was an incomplete resection. A urine culture is negative. The next best sequence of care is:
   a. measure post void residual, provide reassurance, and monitor symptom improvement.
   b. measure post void residual volume and schedule formal urodynamics.
   c. restart a course of 5-alpha reductase inhibitors (5ARIs) and antibiotics.
   d. perform immediate cystoscopy looking for residual tissue.
   e. prescribe 90-day supply of phenazopyridine HCl

3. In the course of performing a monopolar TURP under spinal block, the nurse anesthetist reports the patient is suddenly markedly confused, brachycardic, and hypertensive. An emergent serum sodium level is 110 mEq/L. The following are the next best steps:
   a. Switch to bipolar TURP equipment and finish the case.
   b. Drop the height of the irrigating fluid to <60 cm above the patient, control bleeding, terminate the case, administer furosemide, and begin a calculated dose of hypertonic saline.
   c. Convert to an open simple prostatectomy
   d. Measure serum levels of illicit drugs and ammonia.
   e. Swap irrigating fluid form glycine to sorbitol.

4. Risk factors for development of the TUR syndrome include:
   a. prostate volume less than 45 g.
   b. failure to use isotonic, iso-osmolar irrigating solution and the bipolar electroresection system.
   c. underlying hepatic dysfunction.
   d. irrigating fluid above the patient should be ideal be >60 cm.
   e. preoperative use of opioids.

5. Transurethral resection (TUR) syndrome is caused by:
   a. absorption of fluid during procedures such as holmium laser enucleation of the prostate (HoLEP) and bipolar TURP.
   b. absorption of non–sodium-containing irrigating fluid, leading to an acute dilutional hyponatremia.
   c. irrigating fluid placed at a less than ideal height above the patient.
   d. a serum sodium of greater than 130 mEq/L.
   e. intraoperative ureteral injury.

6. TURP should begin with resection of the:
   a. apical portion of the prostate.
   b. prostate floor.
   c. bladder neck.
   d. median lobe, if present.
   e. anterior portion of the prostate.

7. Which of the following is TRUE of bipolar compared with monopolar TURP?
   a. In a meta-analysis of patients undergoing bipolar TURP, authors concluded that by treating 50 patients with bipolar TURP, one case of TUR syndrome could be prevented.
   b. A relative risk of 0.53 for blood transfusion with bipolar resection was found in meta-analysis.
   c. Improved visualization during bipolar TURP may also lead to a decrease in capsular perforations and operating time.
   d. Late complications such as bladder neck contracture and need for retreatment of benign prostatic hyperplasia (BPH) do not appear to be much different from those found with conventional TURP.
   e. All of the above.

8. Sham studies on urologic procedures for lower urinary tract symptoms (LUTS) due to BPH:
   a. frequently show statistically significant decreases in AUASS (American Urological Association Symptom Score).
   b. are poorly tolerated by the patient.
   c. have significant side effects and should not be performed as part of research.
   d. have never shown a statistically significant improvement in objective measures such as peak urinary flow.
   e. have never been performed.

9. Which of the following is TRUE regarding transurethral incision of the prostate (TUIP)?
   a. It commonly results in TUR syndrome.
   b. It is generally only used in prostates larger than 60 mL.
   c. It causes retrograde ejaculation in 80% of cases.
   d. It results in removal of a large volume of prostate adenoma.
   e. It may have a lower rate of ejaculatory dysfunction in patients when done unilaterally.

10. With regard to laser safety, which of the following statements is correct?

    a. Eye protection is required for the surgeon only.

    b. All windows or wall openings from the operating room (OR) must be covered.

    c. Signs denoting that a laser is in use need only be displayed on the most commonly used door for that OR.

    d. Eye protection is required only when a video camera is not used during the case.

    e. All laser energy is readily absorbed by air/irrigating fluid, making it safe to use in the OR.

11. Patients on anticoagulation who undergo photoselective vaporization of the prostate (PVP) have an increased risk of:

    a. erectile dysfunction.

    b. blood transfusion.

    c. TUR syndrome.

    d. ejaculatory dysfunction.

    e. time in the hospital after procedure.

12. When using the prostate lift for treatment of LUTS due to BPH, implants are placed where in the prostate anatomically?

    a. Anterolaterally

    b. Posterolaterally

    c. Anteriorly

    d. Posteriorly

    e. In the peripheral zone

ANSWERS

1. **a. Venous bleeding from prostatic fossa.** Venous bleeding can be more vexing and generally appears darker in color than arterial bleeding. Venous bleeding will often disappear with a full bladder as it applies pressure to the prostatic fossa. Identifying venous sinuses may be difficult due to the lack of persistent bleeding with rapid irrigation influx and controlling of the bleeding with fulguration may be even more challenging. Once again, the cutting loop may be used to temporarily tamponade any bleeding with precise fulguration. If the venous bleeding is unable to be completely controlled (as is frequently the case) a catheter may be inserted, the balloon overinflated and pulled to traction for tamponade of venous bleeding.

2. **a. Measure post void residual, provide reassurance, and monitor symptom improvement.** Patients with long-standing obstruction (particularly those with urgency and frequency preoperatively) will often experience a continuation or exacerbation of these symptoms in the postoperative period. If proper bladder emptying can be verified, an anticholinergic or beta-3 agonist medication during this time may help the patient feel more comfortable. It is our practice to warn those men with preoperatively documented detrusor overactivity that patience will be required in the months following surgery to see if this will resolve. Such caution goes a long way in assuring patients to adopt a strong coping mechanism rather than a polypharmacy approach.

3. **b. Drop the height of the irrigating fluid to <60 cm above the patient, control bleeding, terminate the case, administer furosemide, and begin a calculated dose of hypertonic saline.** Patient is likely experiencing TUR syndrome; thus rapid termination is needed. The height of the irrigating fluid above the patient should be carefully chosen. Investigators have demonstrated that the ideal height of the fluid was 60 cm above the patient. This appears to be the minimal height to maintain good vision but also not lead to excessive systemic fluid absorption. Increasing the height 10 cm above this leads to increased pressure in the prostatic fossa and a greater than twofold increase in systemic fluid absorption. Diagnosis of this condition is made by assessment of neurologic status and comparison to laboratory values. Serum sodium should be obtained in long, large resections postoperatively (or intraoperatively if concern exists). A serum sodium of less than 120 mEq/L indicates a significant dilution and may lead to coma or seizures. Transient visual disturbances or blindness indicate central nervous system (CNS) toxicity and are obviously very distressing to all the parties involved. If profound central nervous symptoms are noted, judicious administration of hypertonic saline should be instituted and formulas exist to help guide this resuscitation as overly rapid correction of hyponatremia may lead to a demyelinating lesion of the brain (central pontine myelinolysis).

4. **b. Failure to use isotonic, iso-osmolar irrigating solution and the bipolar electroresection system.** The absorption of the hypo-osmolar irrigating fluid leads to an acute dilutional hyponatremia with resulting neurologic changes (confusion, nausea, vomiting, visual changes, hypertension, tachypnea, and bradycardia). Now with the use of isotonic, iso-osmolar irrigating solution and the bipolar electroresection system this risk has theoretically been eliminated. While most authors agree that TUR syndrome is caused by dilutional hyponatremia, there have been alternate etiologies proposed. Excessive glycine absorption can lead to liberation of ammonia from metabolic pathways leading to immediate or delayed encephalopathic symptoms. Several steps can be taken to prevent this complication. Use of a bipolar resection method should certainly be considered. The height of the irrigating fluid above the patient should be carefully chosen. Use the minimal height to maintain good vision but also not lead to excessive systemic fluid absorption.

5. **b. Absorption of non–sodium-containing irrigating fluid, leading to an acute dilutional hyponatremia.** Absorption of non–sodium-containing irrigating fluid into the prostatic venous system that is exposed during resection is the etiology of the disease. This risk appears to be unique to monopolar TURP; other BPH techniques (such as bipolar TURP, HoLEP, and laser vaporization) use isotonic/iso-osmolar irrigating fluid such as normal saline. The ideal height of irrigating fluid was determined to be 60 cm above the patient, as this balanced the benefits of visualization with systemic absorption. Heights above this level will lead to an increased systemic absorption. In general, symptoms of TUR syndrome begin with a serum sodium of less than 120 mEq/L. Ureteral injury is not associated with TUR syndrome.

6. **d. Median lobe, if present.** Although many different plans for resection exist, resection of the median lobe (when present) is generally accepted as the first step.

7. **e. All of the above.** All of the findings in a through d have been demonstrated in studies. The use of a sodium-containing iso-osmolar irrigating fluid has essentially eliminated the risk of TUR syndrome in bipolar TURP. The "cut and seal" action of the technology improves intraoperative hemostasis with better visualization, leading to less blood transfusion and quicker operating times. Differences in many late complications such as bladder neck contracture and need for retreatment have not been demonstrated in comparison to monopolar technology.

8. **a. Frequently show statistically significant decreases in AUASS (American Urological Association Symptom Score).** Multiple sham studies have been performed as part of clinical trials on transurethral microwave thermotherapy and prostate lift. Significant improvements in both AUASS and peak flow have been shown. Side effects of treatment are infrequent, and the sham procedures are well tolerated.

9. **e. It may have a lower rate of ejaculatory dysfunction in patients when done unilaterally.** The procedure is relatively short and does not cause TUR syndrome. The procedure is only appropriate for small prostate glands (generally less than 30 mL), and no prostate adenoma is removed. Retro-

grade ejaculation occurs in up to 37% of patients. Although this is controversial, most authors believe that the risk of retrograde ejaculation is lower if done unilaterally as opposed to bilaterally.

10. **b. All windows or wall openings from the operating room (OR) must be covered.** Eye protection is required for all classes of lasers used in urology currently. Eye protection should be utilized by the patient and all personnel in the room even if a video camera is used during the case. Signs should be placed on all entries to the OR. Any and all openings to the OR from which laser energy could escape should be covered to preclude injury to persons outside of the OR. Although holmium laser energy is absorbed in irrigating fluid, potassium-titanyl-phosphate/lithium-triborate (KTP/LBO) laser energy is not readily absorbed in either fluid. Both of these

lasers can damage the eye when outside the body as neither are readily absorbed/dispersed in air.

11. **e. Time in the hospital after procedure.** Patients who undergo PVP while on anticoagulation appear to be more likely to require longer times in the hospital. They also appear to require more continuous bladder irrigation and a longer time with a urethral catheter. Blood transfusions do not appear to be more frequent. TUR syndrome does not occur with PVP, as normal saline is used. Erectile dysfunction and ejaculatory dysfunction in patients on anticoagulation during PVP are not well studied.

12. **a. Anterolaterally.** The implants in the prostate lift system are placed anterolaterally to avoid the neurovascular bundles (posterolateral) and the prostate veins (anterior). The implants work by primarily compressing the transition zone of the prostate and leading to an increased opening of the urethral lumen.

CHAPTER REVIEW

1. The incorporation of medical management and new technologies has changed which treatment options are selected for the treatment of LUTS/BPH.
2. LASER based treatments are increasingly used although multiple factors have affected acceptance. Multiple factors have changed the usual patient that advances to surgical management of BPH in the preceding decades. Increasingly these are more challenging clinical scenarios.
3. Patients should generally be trialed on medical management before proceeding to surgical intervention. Patients failing medical management may be considered for surgical therapy.
4. Perioperative antibiotic coverage should not be neglected as serious adverse outcomes still occur.
5. Both patient and physician factors should be considered when selecting the appropriate surgical treatment for patients.
6. PUL is an option for patients with LUTS/BPH provided prostate volume <80 g when the clinician has verified the absence of a middle lobe.
7. Patients electing PUL or water vapor thermal ablation therapy should be warned that long-term durability is uncertain, though long-term uncontrolled data is available.
8. In the appropriate patients, PUL and water vapor thermal ablation therapy are less likely to impact erection and ejaculation than conventional therapies.
9. LASER treatments are the fastest growing option in treatment of LUTS/BPH but should be used as part of a "culture of safety" in the operating room.
10. HoLEP is a very effective treatment option with excellent results that are often comparable to those historically seen with open prostatectomy. There is a significant learning curve associated with the procedure and catastrophic complications (mostly due to the morcellator) have been observed.
11. Photoselective vaporization of the prostate is a growing and very safe treatment option for BPH/LUTS. Results in patients on anti-coagulation have been encouraging.
12. Thulium is the newest addition to the LASER family and has some theoretical advantages although scientific data is lacking.

147 Simple Prostatectomy: Open and Robot-Assisted Laparoscopic Approaches

Misop Han and Alan W. Partin

QUESTIONS

1. The major advantage of simple prostatectomy over transurethral resection of the prostate (TURP) in the management of prostatic adenoma includes:
   a. removal of the prostatic adenoma under direct vision.
   b. decreased risk of hypernatremia.
   c. shortened convalescence period.
   d. decreased perioperative hemorrhage.
   e. enhanced preservation of erectile function.

2. The suprapubic simple prostatectomy, in comparison to the retropubic simple prostatectomy, allows:
   a. direct visualization of the prostatic adenoma during enucleation.
   b. better visualization of the prostatic fossa after enucleation to obtain hemostasis.
   c. easier management of a large median lobe and/or bladder calculi.
   d. an extraperitoneal approach.
   e. possible management of concomitant ureteral calculi.

3. The suprapubic approach to the prostatectomy is ideal for the patient with a large prostatic adenoma and:
   a. multiple small bladder calculi.
   b. total prostate-stimulating antigen (PSA) greater than 10.0 ng/mL.
   c. erectile dysfunction.
   d. symptomatic bladder diverticulum.
   e. presence of dilated renal pelvis.

4. The most appropriate definitive treatment options for the patient with a 120-g prostatic adenoma and a symptomatic bladder diverticulum are:
   a. radical retropubic prostatectomy with the fulguration of bladder diverticulum.
   b. long-acting α-adrenergic antagonist and prophylactic antibiotics.
   c. TURP followed by bladder diverticulectomy in 3 months.
   d. TURP and partial cystectomy.
   e. simple prostatectomy with bladder diverticulectomy.

5. The contraindications to simple prostatectomy include:
   a. multiple cores of Gleason 8 prostate cancer.
   b. bladder diverticulum.
   c. large bladder calculi secondary to obstruction.
   d. recurrent urinary tract infection.
   e. acute urinary retention.

6. Both retropubic and suprapubic simple prostatectomies:
   a. are performed in the space of Retzius.
   b. are ideal for patients with a large, obstructive prostatic adenoma and a concomitant, small bladder tumor.
   c. require no blood transfusion.
   d. cause no trauma to the urinary bladder.
   e. require control of the dorsal vein complex before the enucleation of an obstructive prostatic adenoma.

7. Compared with open simple prostatectomy, robot-assisted laparoscopic simple prostatectomy has:
   a. quicker operative time.
   b. longer hospital stay.
   c. decreased need for blood transfusion.
   d. shorter learning curve.
   e. decreased need for anesthesia.

ANSWERS

1. **a. Removal of the prostatic adenoma under direct vision.** When compared with TURP, simple prostatectomy offers the advantages of lower retreatment rate and more complete removal of the prostatic adenoma under direct vision and avoids the risk of dilutional hyponatremia (the TUR syndrome).

2. **c. Easier management of a large median lobe and/or bladder calculi.** The major advantage of suprapubic simple prostatectomy over the retropubic approach is that it allows direct visualization of the bladder neck and bladder mucosa. As a result, this operation is ideally suited for patients with a large median lobe protruding into the bladder or a clinically significant bladder diverticulum.

3. **d. Symptomatic bladder diverticulum.** Suprapubic simple prostatectomy is ideally suited for patients with a large median lobe protruding into the bladder, a clinically significant bladder diverticulum that requires repair, or large bladder calculi. It also may be preferable for obese men, in whom it is difficult to gain direct access to the prostatic pseudocapsule and dorsal vein complex.

4. **e. Simple prostatectomy with bladder diverticulectomy.** Combined suprapubic simple prostatectomy and bladder diverticulum is the best option for the patient with a massive benign prostatic hyperplasia (BPH) and a symptomatic bladder diverticulum because of easy access to both prostatic adenoma and bladder diverticulum. If the prostatectomy is performed without the diverticulectomy, incomplete emptying of the bladder diverticulum and subsequent, persistent infection may occur.

5. **a. Multiple cores of Gleason 8 prostate cancer.** Contraindications to simple prostatectomy include a small fibrous gland, the presence of significant prostate cancer, and previous prostatectomy or pelvic surgery that may obliterate access to the prostate gland.

6. **a. Are performed in the space of Retzius.** Both retropubic and suprapubic simple prostatectomies are performed in the space of Retzius. The dorsal vein complex does not have to be controlled before the enucleation of an obstructive prostatic adenoma during suprapubic simple prostatectomy.

7. **c. Decreased need for blood transfusion.** Compared with open simple prostatectomy, robot-assisted laparoscopic simple prostatectomy can be performed with smaller incisions with shorter hospital stay and decreased risk for perioperative hemorrhage and blood transfusion.

CHAPTER REVIEW

1. Of the indications for simple prostatectomy—(a) acute urinary retention, (b) recurrent or persistent urinary tract infections, (c) significant symptoms of bladder outlet obstruction not responsive to medical therapy, (d) persistent gross hematuria from the prostate, (e) pathologic changes of the kidneys secondary to prostatic obstruction, and (f) bladder calculi—the only absolute indication for prostatectomy is pathologic changes of the kidneys secondary to prostatic obstruction. All the others are relative indications because they may on occasion be corrected without the need for simple prostatectomy.

2. One should not consider doing a simple prostatectomy for glands of less than 75 g. A simple prostatectomy on small glands carries a high complication rate.

3. Simple prostatectomy should be considered in patients who cannot be placed in the lithotomy position and who have a sufficiently large gland that can be enucleated. Small fibrous glands, the presence of significant prostate cancer, previous prostatectomy, and pelvic surgery are contraindications to open simple prostatectomy.

4. Although a cystoscopic examination is not indicated for routine evaluation of obstructive voiding symptoms, one must estimate the size of the prostate adenoma preoperatively to schedule the patient appropriately. Cystoscopy may be a crucial component of that estimation. Moreover, in patients who have hematuria or a urethral stricture, or in whom one needs to evaluate a known bladder calculus or diverticulum, cystoscopy is indicated.

5. The risks of simple prostatectomy include urinary incontinence, erectile dysfunction, retrograde ejaculation, urinary tract infections, bladder neck contracture, urethral stricture, and the need for a blood transfusion.

6. Suprapubic simple prostatectomy is ideally suited for patients with a large median lobe protruding into the bladder, a clinically significant bladder diverticulum that requires repair, or large bladder calculi. It also may be preferable for obese men, in whom it is difficult to gain direct access to the prostatic pseudocapsule and dorsal vein complex.

7. Continuous bladder irrigation and blood transfusion are less frequently used following robot-assisted laparoscopic simple prostatectomy.

148 Epidemiology, Etiology, and Prevention of Prostate Cancer

Andrew J. Stephenson, Robert Abouassaly, and Eric A. Klein

QUESTIONS

1. Since 2008, the incidence of prostate cancer in the United States:
   a. is decreasing.
   b. is stable.
   c. is increasing.
   d. increased initially, then decreased.
   e. is fluctuating.

2. In the United States, the highest prostate cancer incidence rates are seen in:
   a. Caucasians.
   b. African Americans.
   c. Hispanic/Latinos.
   d. Asian Americans
   e. American Indians.

3. Worldwide, prostate cancer:
   a. is the leading cancer diagnosis in men.
   b. is the leading cause of cancer-related mortality.
   c. incidence is highest in countries with the highest rates of screening
   d. is entirely genetic in origin.
   e. has the lowest age-adjusted mortality rates per 100,000 men in North America.

4. With respect to two large randomized trials assessing the effect of prostate specific antigen (PSA) screening on prostate cancer mortality:
   a. overall incidence rates were higher in European Randomized Study of Screening for Prostate Cancer (ERSPC,) but overall mortality rates were higher in Prostate, Lung, Colorectal and Ovarian PLCO
   b. the ERSPC showed no significant difference in survival between screened and unscreened men.
   c. the PLCO cancer screening trial demonstrated a 20% risk reduction in prostate cancer mortality in screened men compared to unscreened men.
   d. contamination of the control arm with PSA screening is a limitation of the PLCO cancer screening trial.
   e. both studies clearly show no benefit to PSA screening for prostate cancer.

5. Compared with a man with no family history of prostate cancer, the risk of developing prostate cancer in a man with one affected first-degree relative is:
   a. unchanged.
   b. 1.5 times higher.
   c. 2 to 3 times higher.
   d. 5 times higher.
   e. 100%

6. High body mass index is associated with:
   a. protection against oxidative stress.
   b. higher circulating androgens.
   c. lower serum PSA levels.
   d. better cancer-specific survival after radical prostatectomy.
   e. lower free IGF-1.

7. Which of the following statements regarding gene fusions in prostate cancer are correct?
   a. The most frequent fusions are between the TMPRSS2 serine protease to members of the E26 transformation-specific (ETS) family of oncogenic transcription factors.
   b. The TMPRSS2-ERG fusion gene is present in prostate stem cells.
   c. TMPRSS2 expression is induced by androgens.
   d. TRMPSS2-related gene fusions are highly specific to prostate cancer.
   e. All of the above

8. Which of the following statements about androgens and the prostate are correct?
   a. Testosterone is the primary androgen affecting prostate cell growth.
   b. Higher circulating serum levels of androgens increase the risk of developing prostate cancer.
   c. Men with hypogonadism never develop prostate cancer.
   d. Exposure to androgens before or at puberty are necessary for the development of prostate cancer.
   e. Type I 5 alpha reductase is the enzyme primarily responsible for converting T to DHT in the prostate.

9. Prostate tumors defined by mutations in the *SPOP* gene and overexpression of *SPINK1*:
   a. May also contain ETS family gene fusions
   b. Are frequently hypermethylated
   c. Are more common in African American men
   d. Are associated with lower Gleason scores
   e. Account for 25% of all prostate cancer.

10. Epigenetic mechanisms active in prostate cancer include:
    a. chromatin remodeling
    b. promoter hypo- and hypermethylation
    c. microRNAs that lead to gene silencing
    d. long noncoding RNAs
    e. all of the above.

11. Findings of the Selenium and Vitamin E Cancer Prevention Trial (SELECT) include:
    a. A significant reduction in the incidence of prostate cancer in the combination arm.
    b. A significant effect of selenium and vitamin E on reducing the risk of cardiovascular disease and non-prostate malignancies.
    c. A significant increased incidence of diabetes mellitus in the selenium arm.
    d. A reduction in prostate cancer–specific mortality
    e. An increased risk of prostate cancer in those taking vitamin E alone

12. In two large randomized controlled intervention trials (Prostate Cancer Prevention Trial [PCPT] and Reduction by Dutasteride of Prostate Cancer Events [REDUCE]), the use of 5ARIs in healthy men resulted in:
    a. significant toxicity leading to high dropout rates
    b. no improvement in symptoms related to benign prostatic hypertrophy (BPH)
    c. an excess of high-grade cancers, leading to higher rates of prostate cancer–specific and all-cause mortality
    d. higher rates of biopsy than those taking placebo
    e. a 25% reduction in the risk of being diagnosed with prostate cancer.

ANSWERS

1. **a. Is decreasing.** According to Surveillance, Epidemiology, and End Results (SEER) estimates, the incidence of prostate cancer peaked in 1992, approximately 5 years after introduction of PSA as a screening test, fell precipitously until 1995, increased slowly at a slope similar to that observed prior to the PSA era until 2001, has fluctuated year-to-year since 2001, and has been consistently decreasing since 2008.

2. **b. African Americans.** African American men have one of the highest reported incidences of prostate cancer in the world, with an incidence of 186.8 per 100,000 person-years and a relative incidence of 1.75 compared to white men in the United States (American Cancer Society). Although African Americans have experienced a greater decline in mortality than white men since the early 1990s, their death rates remain 2.2 times higher than whites. Many biological, environmental, and social hypotheses have been advanced to explain these differences, ranging from postulated differences in genetic predisposition; differences in mechanisms of tumor initiation, promotion and/or progression; higher fat diets, higher serum testosterone levels, or higher body mass index; structural, financial, educational, and cultural barriers to screening, early detection and aggressive therapy; and physician bias. There are currently no data that clearly indicate any of these hypotheses are the determinants of the observed differences in incidence or mortality, and it seems likely that the source of the disparity is multifactorial, although emerging data indicate a clear biologic underpinning.

3. **c. Incidence is highest in countries with the highest rates of screening.** The age-standardized incidence rates per 100 000 men are highest in the highest income regions of the world where PSA screening is more commonly practiced.

4. **d. Contamination of the control arm with PSA screening is a criticism of the PLCO cancer screening trial.** The trial has been criticized for high rates of pre-screening (44% reported undergoing PSA testing prior to enrollment), poor compliance with prostate biopsy, and 52% contamination by ad hoc screening in the control arm. A follow-up study in which PLCO participants were questioned about PSA testing reported a 15% non-PSA testing rate in the control arm of PLCO, which is identical to the non-compliance with screening in the screening arm. Another study showed that when analyzed by actual screening status, rather than an intent to screen analysis, results of the PLCO were similar to that of the ERSPC with respect to the benefit of PSA screening in reducing prostate cancer mortality.

5. **c. 2 to 3 times higher.** In someone with a positive family history of prostate cancer, the relative risk increases according to the number of affected family members, their degree of relatedness, and the age at which they were affected. There have been more than 100 single nucleotide polymorphisms (SNPs)

identified in germline genome-wide association study (GWAS) studies that influence the risk of prostate cancer, and multi-SNP panels can identify individuals at very low and very high risk, although none have shown to be correlated with disease aggressiveness.

6. **c. Lower serum PSA levels.** Higher body mass index has been associated with increased biologic measures of oxidative stress, lower circulating androgen levels, lower serum PSA (perhaps as a consequence of lower circulating androgens), higher serum-free IGF-1 levels, and worse cancer specific survival after radical prostatectomy. Obese men have lower PSA levels and larger prostates, which together may lead to fewer biopsies and more sampling error, potentially contributing to an increased risk of high-grade disease.

7. **e. All the above.** Gene fusions, once thought to be the exclusive domain of hematologic malignancies, are common in prostate cancer and are fundamental drivers of prostate cancer growth and progression. The most commonly observed fusion results from the fusion of the 5' untranslated end of TMPRSS2 serine protease to members of the ETS family of oncogenic transcription factors, bringing the latter growth-promoting genes under androgen control. The most common fusion identified in localized prostate cancer involves TMPRSS2 fused to ERG (ETS-related gene, 21q22.3) in approximately 50% of patients. The TMPRSS2 gene is prostate specific, and is expressed in both benign and malignant prostatic epithelium. TRMPSS-related gene fusions are highly specific for the presence of prostate cancer.

8. **d. Exposure to androgens before or at puberty are necessary for the development of prostate cancer.** All of the other statements are false. DHT, derived from T by Type II 5 alpha reductase (not type I which is predominantly located in skin and liver), is the primary androgen that spurs prostate growth. Intraprostatic levels of androgens are tightly regulated by local mechanisms and are not affected by the level of circulating androgens. Hypogonadal men can develop prostate cancer, likely by pathways independent of androgens.

9. **c. Are more common in African American men.** Tumors with SPOP mutations account for about 10% of primary prostate cancers and have average levels of methylation. A subclass of SPOP-mutated tumors that overexpress the *SPINK1* gene occur more commonly in African Americans and are associated with higher Gleason scores, and may in part underlie the increased incidence and mortality of prostate cancer in this group.

10. **e. All of the above.** Epigenetic events affect gene expression without altering the actual sequence of DNA, and in prostate cancer all of the listed mechanisms are important.

11. **e. An increased risk of prostate cancer in those taking vitamin E alone.** SELECT demonstrated no beneficial effect of vitamin E or selenium on the risk of prostate cancer (alone or in combination). Hazard ratios for prostate cancer were 1.13 (99% CI: 0.95 to 1.13) for vitamin E, 1.04 (99% CI: 0.87 to 1.24) for selenium, and 1.05 (99% CI: 0.88 to 1.25) for selenium and vitamin E. A follow-up study that included an additional 54,464 person-years showed that dietary supplementation with vitamin E significantly increased the risk of prostate cancer among healthy men (HR 1.17; 95% CI: 1.004 to 1.36; $P = 0.008$).

12. **e. A 25% reduction in the risk of being diagnosed with prostate cancer.** Both these trials showed a significant reduction in the risk of being diagnosed with prostate cancer with drugs (finasteride and dutasteride) that were well tolerated and reduced both short- and long-term symptoms of BPH. Although there seemed to be an excess of high-grade cancers diagnosed in men who took these drugs, this had no effect on the risk of dying or dying specifically from prostate cancer.

CHAPTER REVIEW

1. In the United States, prostate cancer is the most common visceral malignancy in men and the third leading cause of cancer-related deaths.
2. Prostate cancer mortality has declined since 1991 and for Caucasians is now lower than before PSA testing was introduced.
3. Worldwide, prostate cancer incidence and mortality rates vary significantly between countries and regions but are highest in African American and Jamaican men.
4. PSA has induced a significant downward migration in age and both clinical and pathological stage at diagnosis.
5. PSA screening reduces prostate cancer mortality; however, the absolute effect is small relative to the number needed to screen and treat to cure a single individual.
6. Both genetics and environment are important in the origin and evolution of prostate cancer.
7. Genome-Wide Association Studies have identified multiple chromosomal loci and variant alleles in germline DNA that confer risk of getting prostate cancer.
8. Because the predictive value of single loci is small, models with multiple risk loci or less common alleles with greater risk are needed for individual risk prediction.
9. HOXB13 and BRCA are two genes that substantially increase individual risk. BRCA-related tumors present with more aggressive clinical features.
10. Chronic inflammation leading to cellular hyperproliferation to replace damaged tissue appears to contribute to the development of prostate cancer.
11. Both genetic and histologic observations suggest that compromised cellular defenses against inflammatory oxidants are important in prostate cancer initiation and promotion.
12. Inflammation may be triggered by diet, infection, estrogens, or other environmental agents.
13. Histologic evidence of inflammation, as manifested by proliferative inflammatory atrophy (PIA), is common in prostate cancer and may represent a key pathobiologic process in its development.
14. Androgen exposure of the prostate plays an important but incompletely defined role in prostate carcinogenesis.
15. Long-term absence of androgen exposure protects against cancer, but a dose-response relationship between androgen levels and prostate cancer risk has not been established.
16. Polymorphisms in genes encoding for the androgen receptor and various enzymes related to androgen metabolism may be important determinants of prostate cancer risk.
17. Vitamin D and its interaction with its receptor modulate risk and disease aggressiveness.
18. Smoking increases the risk of disease recurrence and death due to prostate cancer.
19. Obesity is associated with lower PSA, increases risk for getting high-grade disease, and is associated with higher treatment failure rates and mortality.
20. The primary androgen of the prostate is dihydrotestosterone (DHT). Exposure to DHT is a prerequisite for developing prostate cancer.
21. Stem cells are precursors with multilineage differentiation potential that populate epithelium of prostatic acini and are the origin of clonal epithelial expansion.
22. Primary prostate cancer has a distinct molecular taxonomy characterized by seven distinct subtypes, including four defined by gene fusions and three by mutations.
23. Variations in gene methylation profiles further distinguish the molecular subtypes of prostate cancer.
24. The androgen receptor plays a central role in prostate cancer development and progression.
25. There are distinct biological differences in the genomics of prostate cancers of African American and European American men.
26. The goal of primary chemoprevention is to decrease the incidence of a given cancer, simultaneously reducing both treatment-related side effects and mortality.
27. Effective chemoprevention requires the use of nontoxic agents that inhibit specific molecular steps in the carcinogenic pathway.
28. Prostate cancer is an attractive target for primary prevention because of its incidence, prevalence, treatment-related morbidity, and mortality.
29. The Prostate Cancer Prevention Trial demonstrated that finasteride reduces the period prevalence of prostate cancer by 25% with no effect on overall mortality.
30. SELECT demonstrated that neither vitamin E nor selenium prevents prostate cancer, and that use of vitamin E was associated with an increased risk of prostate cancer.

149 Prostate Cancer Biomarkers

Todd M. Morgan, Ganesh S. Palapattu, and Simpa S. Salami

QUESTIONS

1. Serum prostate-specific antigen (PSA) levels are specific for the presence of prostate:
   a. disease.
   b. cancer.
   c. enlargement.
   d. inflammation.
   e. none of the above.

2. Most detectable PSA in sera is bound to:
   a. albumin.
   b. α_1-antichymotrypsin (ACT).
   c. α_2-macroglobulin.
   d. human kallikrein.
   e. none of the above.

3. TRUE or FALSE: As many as 75% of men presenting with elevated PSA levels are found not to have prostate cancer after transrectal ultrasonography (TRUS) biopsy.
   a. True
   b. False

4. Compared with prostatic tissue PSA levels, prostatic tissue levels of hK2 are:
   a. elevated in well-differentiated prostate cancer tissue.
   b. elevated in poorly differentiated prostate cancer tissue.
   c. depressed in well-differentiated prostate cancer tissue.
   d. depressed in poorly differentiated prostate cancer tissue.
   e. not measurable in prostatic cancer tissue.

5. The serum urine prostate cancer biomarker PCA-3 represents a:
   a. gene on chromosome 20q13.4.
   b. noncoding gene in the *TP53* cluster.
   c. noncoding mRNA with no known protein product.
   d. glycosylated protein of molecular weight 60 kD.
   e. high-molecular-weight nuclear matrix protein.

6. TRUE or FALSE: Evaluation of tissue from prostate cancer specimens has demonstrated higher mRNA expression levels compared with normal prostate tissue, suggesting that prostate cancer cells make more PSA than normal prostatic tissue.
   a. True
   b. False

7. A man with a PSA of 4 ng/mL while taking finasteride for 2 years stops this medication and begins taking saw palmetto. What should his PSA be on his next annual check-up?
   a. 2 ng/mL
   b. 4 ng/mL
   c. 6 ng/mL
   d. 8 ng/mL
   e. 10 ng/mL

8. Which of the following biomarkers has the greatest specificity for the presence of prostate cancer in patients with an elevated PSA?
   a. PCA3
   b. TMPRSS2:ERG
   c. fPSA
   d. phi
   e. 4Kscore

9. proPSA represents:
   a. the early form of the PSA protein in urine.
   b. PSA that has been autocleaved by another molecule several times.
   c. an early form of bound PSA found within the nucleus.
   d. an uncleaved free PSA molecule with a leader sequence.
   e. PSA that gets paid a high salary for hitting home runs.

10. Compared with men without prostate cancer, the fraction of free or unbound PSA in serum from men with prostate cancer:
    a. is equal.
    b. is lower.
    c. is greater.
    d. is undetectable by current assays.
    e. varies depending on which assay is used.

11. The value percentage of free PSA has been approved by the U.S. Food and Drug Administration (FDA) for use in improving:
    a. cancer detection in men with PSA levels less than 4 ng/mL.
    b. cancer detection in men with benign digital rectal examinations and PSA levels of 4 to 10 ng/mL.
    c. the determination of prognosis.
    d. cancer detection in men found to have atypical small acinar proliferation (ASAP).
    e. cancer detection in men with a family history of prostate cancer.

12. After starting finasteride, serum PSA should _____ and the percentage of free PSA should _____.
    a. increase, not change
    b. increase, increase
    c. decrease, not change
    d. decrease, decrease
    e. not change, not change

13. The products of hypermethylated genes evaluated in prostate cancer development are:
    a. UROC28 and hepsin.
    b. GSTP1, APC, RARβ2, and RASSF1A.
    c. PCA3, PAC, ERG, and NMP 48.
    d. all of the above.

14. Commercially available tissue-based prognostic tests performed on prostate cancer tissue to predict disease aggressiveness assess genes involved in which of the following?

   a. Androgen pathway, stromal response, immune response.

   b. Cell cycle progression (CCP).

   c. Cellular organization, adhesion, motility, and structure.

   d. Cell proliferation, differentiation.

   e. All of the above.

ANSWERS

1. **e. None of the above.** Although PSA is widely accepted as a prostate cancer tumor marker, it is organ specific and not disease specific. Unfortunately, there is an overlap in the serum PSA levels among men with cancer and benign disease. Thus elevated serum PSA levels may reflect alterations within the prostate secondary to tissue architectural changes, such as cancer, inflammation, or benign prostatic hyperplasia (BPH).

2. **b. α_1-antichymotrypsin (ACT).** The current clinically relevant immunodetectable complexed forms of PSA are bound to ACT and, to less extent, to α_1-protease inhibitor (API). The sum of these and other presently unknown PSA complexes is represented by the term complexed PSA (cPSA). The major form of cPSA in serum, PSA bound to ACT, is found in greater serum concentrations in men with cancer than in men with benign disease.

3. **a. True.** Although up to 30% of men presenting with an elevated PSA level may be diagnosed after this invasive procedure, as many as 75% to 80% will not be found to have cancer.

4. **b. Elevated in poorly differentiated prostate cancer tissue.** Immunohistochemical studies reveal different tissue expression patterns for hK2 and PSA. In benign epithelium, PSA is intensely expressed compared with the minimal immunoreactivity of hK2. This is in contrast to cancerous tissue, in which more intense expression of hK2 is seen.

5. **c. Noncoding mRNA with no known protein product.** Using differential display and Northern blot analysis to compare normal and prostate cancer tissue, investigators identified the *PCA3* prostate-specific gene on chromosome 9q21-22. Study of this gene has determined that it may function as noncoding mRNA, because it has been found to be alternatively spliced, contains a high density of stop codons, and lacks an open reading frame.

6. **b. False.** Although prostate cancer cells do not necessarily make more PSA than do normal prostate cells, elevated serum levels are likely a result of cancer progression and destabilization of the prostate histologic architecture (Stamey et al., 1987). Studies have demonstrated that prostate cancer cells do not make more PSA but rather less PSA than normal prostatic tissue (Meng et al., 2002). Evaluation of tissue from prostate cancer specimens have demonstrated up to 1.5-fold lower mRNA expression levels compared with normal prostate tissue (Meng et al., 2002).

7. **d. 8 ng/mL.** Finasteride (5 mg) and other 5α-reductase inhibitors for treatment of BPH have been shown to lower PSA levels by an average of 50% after 6 months of treatment (Guess et al., 1993). Thus one can multiply the PSA level by 2 to obtain the "expected" PSA level of a patient who has been on finasteride for 6 months or more. Although saw palmetto has not been shown to affect PSA levels, possible contamination of these unregulated supplements may include compounds that can alter PSA levels (i.e., PC-SPES, currently off the market).

8. **b. TMPRSS2:ERG.** This gene fusion is one of the earliest events that occurs in prostate carcinogenesis and is therefore close to 100% specific for prostate cancer, when present. However, it is only present in approximately 50% of PSA-screened prostate cancers, and therefore its sensitivity is substantially lower.

9. **d. An uncleaved free PSA molecule with a leader sequence.** PSA originates with a 17–amino acid chain that is cleaved to yield a precursor inactive form of PSA termed proPSA (pPSA). The precursor form of PSA contains a 7–amino acid proleader peptide, in addition to the 237 constituent amino acids of mature PSA, and it is termed [−7]pPSA. Once released, the proleader amino acid chain is cleaved at the amino terminus by hK2, converting pPSA to its active 33-kD PSA form. In addition to hK2, pPSA may be activated to PSA by other prostate kallikreins, including hK4. Incomplete removal of the 7–amino acid leader chain has led to the identification of various other truncated or clipped forms of pPSA. These include pPSAs with 2-, 4-, and 5-leader amino acids ([−2]pPSA, [−4]pPSA, and [−5]pPSA). With cellular disruption, these inactive forms circulate as free PSA and may constitute the majority of the circulating free PSA in patients with prostate cancer.

10. **b. Is lower.** Although prostate cancer cells do not produce more PSA than benign prostate epithelium, the PSA produced from malignant cells appears to escape proteolytic processing. Thus men with prostate cancer have a greater fraction of serum PSA complexed to ACT and a lower percentage of total PSA that is free compared with men without prostate cancer (Christensson et al., 1993; Leinonen et al., 1993; Lilja et al., 1993; Stenman et al., 1994).

11. **b. Cancer detection in men with benign digital rectal examinations and PSA levels of 4 to 10 ng/mL.** Currently the percentage of free PSA is FDA approved for use to aid PSA testing in men with benign digital rectal examinations and minimal PSA elevations, within the diagnostic gray zone of 4 to 10 ng/mL.

12. **c. Decrease, not change.** Free PSA and total PSA both decrease in men on finasteride. Because both decline, the percentage of free PSA is not altered significantly by this medication (Keetch et al., 1997; Panneck et al., 1998).

13. **b. GSTP1, APC, RARβ2, and RASSF1A.** The products of hypermethylated genes that have been evaluated in prostate cancer development are glutathione S-transferase P1 (GSTP1), APC, RARβ2, and RAS-association domain family protein isoform A (RASSF1A).

14. **e. All of the above.** The Prolaris test assesses 31 CCP genes and 15 housekeeping genes to predict the risk of progression and death from prostate cancer. The Oncotype Dx Prostate classifier uses 12 cancer-related genes in four biologic pathways (androgen pathway, cellular organization, proliferation, and stromal response) and five housekeeping genes to predict the likelihood of aggressive pathologic features at the time of prostatectomy. The Decipher assay is a 22-marker genomic classifier assessing cell structure and various cellular processes such as cell proliferation, differentiation, adhesion, motility, mitosis, CCP, and immune response.[a]

---

[a]Sources referenced can be found in *Campbell-Walsh-Wein Urology, 12th Edition*, on the Expert Consult website.

1. Prostate–specific membrane antigen (PSMA) has been identified in the central nervous system, intestine, and prostate and currently serves as an important target for advanced molecular imaging.
2. PSA is a member of the human kallikrein gene family. PSA and human kallikrein-2 have been used in prostate cancer detection.
3. Ectopic expression of PSA occurs in breast tissue, adrenal, and renal carcinomas.
4. PSA is organ specific not disease specific; its half-life is 2 to 3 days.
5. 5α-Reductase inhibitors reduce serum PSA by 50%.
6. Prostate cancer cells make less PSA than normal prostate tissue, gram for gram. PSA expression is strongly influenced by androgens. Ejaculation can lead to a false increase in PSA.
7. Seventy percent of serum PSA is bound to three proteins: α_2-macroglobulin, API, and ACT. Patients with prostate cancer have a higher fraction of circulating PSA bound to these proteins (i.e., they have a lower free PSA).
8. When PSA is released from the cell, a portion of an attached amino acid chain is cleaved, leaving a smaller amino acid chain attached, which inactivates its biologic activity. This molecule is termed proPSA. When this amino acid chain is cleaved from proPSA, PSA becomes active as a serum protease. ProPSA may be used to diagnose prostate cancer.
9. PCA-3 is a urine-based marker used in the diagnosis of prostate cancer. It can be combined with detection of the TMPRSS2:ERG gene fusion to improve diagnostic accuracy.
10. Circulating tumor cells and circulating tumor DNA are promising sources of biomarkers, particularly in advanced prostate cancer.
11. Tissue-based gene expression signatures are commercially available and can be performed on small amounts of formalin-fixed paraffin-embedded tissue and may provide additional prognostic information beyond Gleason score and other clinical parameters.
12. Prostate cancer susceptibility genes that have been located on a number of chromosomes increase the risk of developing prostate cancer.
13. Key inherited genes with moderate penetrance that increase the risk of aggressive prostate cancer are BRCA1, BRCA2, and ATM. These are all DNA damage repair genes.

150 Prostate Biopsy: Techniques and Imaging

Edouard J. Trabulsi, Ethan J. Halpern, and Leonard G. Gomella

QUESTIONS

1. Prostatic corpora amylacea are calcifications:
   a. always associated with prostate infection.
   b. pathognomonic for acute prostatitis.
   c. most commonly seen between the transition and peripheral zone of the prostate.
   d. associated with hypoechoic lesions and prostate cancer.
   e. in the peripheral zone exclusively and are located in blood vessels.

2. Calcifications diffusely seen in the prostate on transrectal ultrasound are:
   a. called corpora amylacea.
   b. always considered abnormal and mandate biopsy.
   c. considered diagnostic for prostate cancer.
   d. incidental findings usually due to advanced age.
   e. the walls of blood vessels.

3. Which of the following statements is TRUE about transrectal ultrasonography (TRUS) of the seminal vesicles?
   a. Masses in the seminal vesicles are the most common lesion seen on TRUS of the prostate.
   b. The seminal vesicles are usually asymmetrical and normally measure less than 2 cm in length in the adult.
   c. Most cystic masses in the seminal vesicle are malignant and related to prostate cancer.
   d. A solid mass in the seminal vesicle is always associated with malignancy.
   e. Solid masses in the seminal vesicle can be caused by schistosomiasis in endemic regions.

4. Which of the following statements about the seminal vesicle (SV) when imaged by ultrasound is TRUE?
   a. The average seminal vesicle is approximately 4.5 to 5.5 cm in length.
   b. A unilaterally absent seminal vesicle suggests an undescended testicle on the ipsilateral side.
   c. Seminal vesicles are usually asymmetric.
   d. The ejaculatory ducts run alongside the seminal vesicles and cannot be visualized on transrectal ultrasound.
   e. The seminal vesicles are difficult to image using standard TRUS probes.

5. Which of the following statements concerning ultrasonographic estimates of prostate size/volume is TRUE?
   a. Only one formula (prolate ellipse) is acceptable to determine prostate volume.
   b. There is a poor correlation between radical prostatectomy specimen weights and volume as measured by TRUS.
   c. The mature average prostate is between 20 and 25 g and remains relatively constant until approximately age 50, when the gland enlarges in many men.
   d. Prostate cancer is always associated with an increase in overall volume of the prostate.
   e. Planimetry with a stepping device should be used for routine prostate volume determinations.

6. A hypoechoic lesion of the prostate can be caused by all of the following EXCEPT:
   a. granulomatous prostatitis.
   b. transition zone, benign prostatic hyperplasia nodules.
   c. prostate cancer.
   d. hematologic malignancies.
   e. normal urethra.

7. Which of the following statements is TRUE about anesthesia for TRUS prostate biopsy?
   a. Intrarectal lidocaine gel is as effective as the injection of lidocaine.
   b. It is not necessary even with extended-core biopsies, owing to the small size of the needle.
   c. It is best performed using direct injection of lidocaine into the prostate gland.
   d. It is typically performed using lidocaine, a long 22-gauge spinal needle, and the biopsy channel of the ultrasound probe.
   e. It is typically performed using digital guidance to ensure that the base of the prostate near the seminal vesicles is infiltrated.

8. When performing TRUS prostate biopsy:
   a. the left lateral decubitus position is most commonly used.
   b. the right lateral decubitus position is most commonly used.
   c. enemas should not be used before the procedure and may increase the risk of bleeding.
   d. intravenous antibiotic prophylaxis is necessary in all patients to prevent urosepsis.
   e. the dorsal lithotomy position with the use of stirrups increases the diagnostic accuracy of the prostate biopsies.

9. When performing TRUS prostate biopsy:
   a. only hypoechoic lesions should be sampled.
   b. sextant biopsy represents the current standard of care for the diagnosis of prostate cancer.
   c. the transition zone should be included in all initial biopsies because of the high incidence of cancer in this area.
   d. a minimum of 12 systematic biopsies is currently recommended.
   e. isoechoic lesions are rarely cancerous and should not be sampled unless they are calcified.

10. Which of the following statements is TRUE concerning TRUS appearance after treatment?
    a. With an ideal permanent implant, seeds should be distributed evenly throughout the gland with periurethral sparing.
    b. TRUS findings are accurate in determining residual cancer following external beam radiation.
    c. Androgen ablation will always reduce the size of the prostate by more than 50% regardless of baseline size.

d. With prostate-specific antigen (PSA) recurrence following radical prostatectomy, the anastomosis should be biopsied.

e. Prostate volume decreases by more than 50% at 6 months using agents such as finasteride.

11. Which of the following statements about antibiotic prophylaxis for TRUS biopsy is TRUE?

a. It eliminates the risk of any infection.

b. It reduces the risk of febrile urinary tract infection requiring hospitalization but does not prevent them.

c. It is not necessary if the probe is sterilized and an enema is given.

d. Epididymitis is the most common infection after TRUS biopsy even if antibiotics are used.

e. Bacteriuria is the only indication for antibiotics after TRUS prostate biopsy.

12. Hematospermia after TRUS biopsy:

a. usually requires hospitalization.

b. is eliminated with the routine use of antibiotics.

c. usually clears immediately after TRUS biopsy.

d. can persist for up to 4 to 6 weeks after TRUS biopsy.

e. is eliminated if the probe is held firmly against the prostate after the needle is passed.

13. Which of the following statements is TRUE in men with a negative prostate biopsy?

a. They can be assured that no cancer is present.

b. They will require repeated biopsy if one of the cores contains seminal vesicle.

c. Transurethral biopsy is the next step after an initial negative biopsy.

d. Additional biopsies demonstrate decreasing yield of detecting cancer, and the cancer tends to be of lower grade and stage.

e. They should undergo transperineal biopsy for all future biopsies because these have been shown to be the most accurate approach in large randomized European trials.

14. Risk factors for prostate biopsy related infection include all of the following EXCEPT:

a. recent antibiotic use.

b. diabetes mellitus.

c. prostate enlargement.

d. foreign travel.

e. White race.

15. Which of the following statements is TRUE concerning TRUS/magnetic resonance imaging (MRI) fusion biopsy?

a. It must be performed in an "in-bore MRI."

b. The MRI must be obtained within 24 hours of the prostate biopsy.

c. TRUS/MRI fusion biopsy relies on coregistration of the MRI and TRUS images at the time of biopsy.

d. It relies on a method known as "cognitive fusion."

e. Any MRI of the prostate can be used for the fusion biopsy.

16. Concerning prostate cancer on transrectal ultrasound, which statement is FALSE?

a. Thirty-nine percent of cancers are isoechoic.

b. One percent may be hyperechoic.

c. A hypoechoic lesion is malignant up to 57% of the time.

d. An irradiated prostate is diffusely hypoechoic.

e. Hypoechoic lesions are all high Gleason score and suggest extraprostatic disease.

IMAGING

1. See Fig. 150.1.

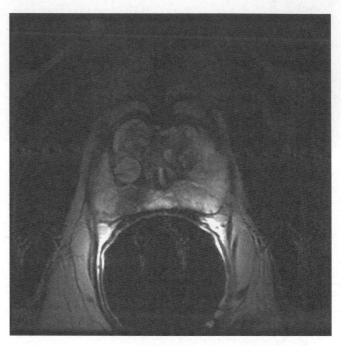

Fig. 150.1

A 62-year-old man with a PSA of 4.5 ng/dL has this axial T2-weighted endorectal coil MRI. The most likely diagnosis is:

a. extracapsular spread of prostate cancer.

b. cancer confined to the gland.

c. enlarged central gland due to benign prostatic hypertrophy.

d. neurovascular bundle involvement.

e. seminal vesicle involvement.

PATHOLOGY

1. A 52-year-old black male whose father died of prostate cancer has a PSA of 3 ng/mL for which he has a 12-core biopsy. The pathology on 8 of the cores is benign; however, 4 of the cores were read as normal seminal vesicle without prostate tissue, the pathology of which is depicted in Fig. 150.2. The next step in management is:

a. inquire as to the presence of lipofuscin because it is not shown on this slide to confirm that it is seminal vesicle.

b. reassure the patient that the biopsy is benign.

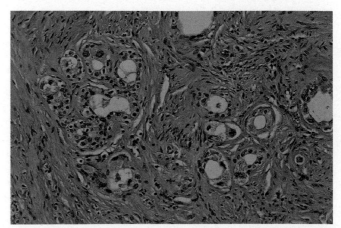

Fig. 150.2 (From Bostwick DG, Cheng L: *Urologic surgical pathology*, ed 2, Edinburgh, 2008, Mosby.)

c. ask the pathologist to stain for PSA to be sure this is not a poorly differentiated adenocarcinoma.

d. repeat the biopsy.

e. obtain a computed tomography (CT) scan to evaluate the seminal vesicles.

ANSWERS

1. **c. Most commonly seen between the transition and peripheral zone of the prostate.** Corpora amylacea develop in the surgical capsule between the transition and peripheral zones of the prostate.

2. **d. Incidental findings usually due to advanced age.** Small, multiple diffuse calcifications are a normal result of age rather than a pathologic entity. Larger prostatic calculi associated with symptoms may be related to underlying infection or inflammation and require further evaluation.

3. **e. Solid masses in the seminal vesicle can be caused by schistosomiasis in endemic regions.** Although cystic lesions of the seminal vesicle can be presumed to be benign, solid masses represent a small chance of malignancy. Schistosomiasis should be considered in the differential diagnosis of a solid seminal vesicle mass, especially in endemic regions (i.e., Nile river valley, South East Asia).

4. **a. The average seminal vesicle is approximately 4.5 to 5.5 cm in length.** The normal SV measures 4.5 to 5.5 cm in length and 2 cm in width, has a smooth, saccular appearance, and should be symmetric.

5. **c. The mature average prostate is between 20 and 25 g and remains relatively constant until approximately age 50, when the gland enlarges in many men.** The prostate size increases at puberty. Many men develop symptomatic enlargement of the prostate that typically begins after age 50.

6. **d. Hematologic malignancies.** Many lesions can be hypoechoic, and many will prove to be malignant, reinforcing the need for biopsy of these lesions if seen. Many cancers, including hematologic malignancies of the prostate, are isoechoic.

7. **d. It is typically performed using lidocaine, a long 22-gauge spinal needle, and the biopsy channel of the ultrasound probe.** All recent studies indicate that infiltration of lidocaine around the neurovascular bundles increases tolerability of TRUS prostate biopsy.

8. **a. The left lateral decubitus position is most commonly used.** TRUS biopsy has become the "gold standard" to diagnose prostate cancer. It is most commonly performed with the patient in the left lateral decubitus position. Dorsal lithotomy may also be used in certain circumstances.

9. **d. A minimum of 12 systematic biopsies is currently recommended.** Sextant biopsy revolutionized the utility of TRUS biopsy to diagnose prostate cancer. However, significant numbers of cancers were missed based on the analysis of radical prostatectomy specimens. Increasing to a minimum of 12 systematic biopsies has increased the diagnostic yield and is endorsed based on a recent white paper from the American Urological Association.

10. **a. With an ideal permanent implant, seeds should be distributed evenly throughout the gland with periurethral sparing.**

Even distribution of seeds and urethral sparing is the hallmark of proper seed placement for interstitial brachytherapy.

11. **b. It reduces the risk of febrile urinary tract infection requiring hospitalization but does not prevent them.** Short-term use of prophylactic antibiotics can reduce the incidence of serious infections. Unfortunately, it does not completely eliminate the risk of infection.

12. **d. Can persist for up to 4 to 6 weeks after TRUS biopsy.** This can be a concerning side effect of prostate biopsy and is of no clinical consequence. Patients should be counseled about the likelihood of hematospermia after TRUS biopsy.

13. **d. Additional biopsies demonstrate decreasing yield of detecting cancer, and the cancer tends to be of lower grade and stage.** Data from the large European screening study suggested that as the number of biopsy sessions increased to ultimately diagnose prostate cancer, the cancers diagnosed after several biopsy sessions were generally of lower grade and stage.

14. **e. White race.** Risk factors for prostate biopsy–related infection include non-white race, increased number of comorbidities, diabetes mellitus, prostate enlargement, foreign travel, and recent antibiotic use.

15. **c. TRUS/MRI fusion biopsy relies on coregistration of the MRI and TRUS images at the time of biopsy.** TRUS/MRI fusion requires a specific software platform. It combines the familiarity of real-time TRUS guidance with detailed information from a diagnostic multiparametric MRI and superimposes both images via software image reconstruction. The reconstruction involves "image registration" or "image matching." A prebiopsy MRI must identify target lesions suspicious for cancer based on imaging characteristics.

16. **e. Hypoechoic lesions are all high Gleason score and suggest extraprostatic disease.** There is a need to biopsy hypoechoic lesions, but these lesions are not pathognomonic for cancer as once thought and do not correlate with the aggressiveness of the disease as measured by Gleason score.

IMAGING

1. **b. Cancer confined to the gland.** The small focus of prostate cancer is seen as a well-demarcated low-signal-intensity area in the right peripheral zone. The seminal vesicles are not included on this image and therefore cannot be accessed. The low-signal-intensity capsule is well seen, bordering the tumor focus (options [a] and [d] are incorrect). Although there are a few enlarged nodules in the central gland, the gland itself is small in size (option [c] is incorrect).

PATHOLOGY

1. **d. Repeat the biopsy.** Although obtaining normal seminal vesicle on a prostate biopsy is not unusual, four cores is unusual and probably means that the systematic biopsy was not well directed. This patient is at high risk for prostate cancer in view of his race, family history, and elevated PSA for age. The biopsy needs to be repeated and done systematically by an experienced clinician.

CHAPTER REVIEW

1. There are five divisions of the prostate: (1) anterior fibromuscular stroma, (2) transition zone, (3) central zone, (4) periurethral zone, and (5) peripheral zone.
2. Calcifications may be seen along the surgical capsule, which is the junction between the transition zone and peripheral zone. Multiple diffuse calcifications are often found incidentally and are not diagnostic of a specific entity.
3. A mass in the seminal vesicle that is cystic is usually benign, whereas a solid lesion has a small probability of being malignant. Schistosomiasis may cause solid lesions in the seminal vesicles.
4. Increasing the frequency of the ultrasound probe increases the resolution; decreasing the frequency increases the depth of penetration. It is important to eliminate an air interface between the ultrasound probe and the tissue being visualized.
5. A volume calculation of the prostate should always be performed and requires measurement of three dimensions: anteroposterior (AP) and sagittal. The former is performed at the mid-gland transversely and the latter just off the midline sagittally. Formulas used to calculate volume include those for an ellipse, a sphere, or a prolate (egg) shape. When a more accurate determination is required, multiple sections of the prostate must be measured using the technique of planimetry.
6. Thirty-nine percent of cancers are isoechoic; 1% are hyperechoic. A hypoechoic lesion contains cancer approximately 20% of the time.
7. All hypoechoic lesions should be biopsied; however, they may be caused by granulomatous prostatitis, infarct, or lymphoma in addition to cancer.
8. There is no PSA threshold at any age that can absolutely rule out cancer.
9. The preferred antibiotic prophylaxis for prostate biopsy is a fluoroquinolone given 2 hours prior to the procedure and for 48 hours following the procedure. For those at risk for endocarditis or those who have a prosthesis requiring additional coverage, intravenous ampicillin or vancomycin, if penicillin allergic, and gentamicin followed by fluoroquinolones is the appropriate prophylaxis.
10. Proper analgesia is performed by injection of 5 mL lidocaine bilaterally at the level of the seminal vesicles near the bladder base.
11. The best visualization of the biopsy path is in the sagittal plane.
12. Risk factors for prostate biopsy–related infection include non-white race, increased number of comorbidities, diabetes mellitus, prostate enlargement, foreign travel, and recent antibiotic use.
13. For individuals lacking a rectum, an ultrasound directed transperineal or CT-guided biopsy may be performed.
14. The benefit of a transperineal versus a transrectal biopsy approach is improved sampling of the prostatic apex and potential for less infectious complications.
15. A 12-core biopsy is standard on initial biopsy; increasing the number of cores to 18 to 20 at initial biopsy has minimal benefit.
16. Most suggest a self-administered enema be given before the biopsy.
17. The initial cancer detection rate for patients with a PSA between 4 and 10 µg/mL is 22%; subsequent biopsies for an elevated PSA result in a cancer detection rate of 10% on the second biopsy, 5% on the third, and 4% on the fourth.
18. Isolated transition zone tumors without peripheral zone involvement occur less than 5% of the time.
19. For patients who have had multiple biopsies and no imaging abnormalities and who are suspect of harboring cancer, the two areas found most likely to be involved if cancer is present are the anterior zone and the apex. These areas may reliably be approached with a template biopsy or fusion biopsy.
20. Complications of prostate biopsy include febrile urinary tract infection, bacteremia, acute prostatitis, bleeding, hematospermia, acute urinary retention, and sepsis.
21. Newer imaging modalities allowing for the potential of targeted biopsy include Doppler to determine vessel density, determination of the elasticity of an area, endorectal MRI with dynamic contrast enhancement and diffusion weighting, and MRI spectroscopy.
22. Newer imaging modalities such as fusion biopsy, which couples the MRI image with the real-time ultrasound image, have the potential for allowing the clinician to target specific suspicious areas.

151 Pathology of Prostatic Neoplasia

Jonathan I. Epstein

QUESTIONS

1. All of the following statements are true about high-grade prostatic intraepithelial neoplasia (PIN), EXCEPT:
   a. glands are architecturally benign.
   b. if unifocal, PIN is not associated with an increased risk of cancer on rebiopsy.
   c. PIN shares some of the molecular findings with prostatic adenocarcinoma.
   d. PIN is the same as intraductal carcinoma.
   e. PIN does not by itself give rise to elevated serum prostate-specific antigen (PSA) levels.

2. Which of the following is TRUE about the pathologic staging of prostate adenocarcinoma?
   a. pT1c can be assigned to radical prostatectomy specimens.
   b. The difference between T1a and T1b is based on perineural and/or vascular invasion.
   c. pT2c by definition represents more advanced cancer than pt2a.
   d. pt2x refers to prostatectomy specimens with intraprostatic incision.
   e. Microscopic bladder neck muscle invasion is pT3b.

3. Which of the following is TRUE about prostate cancer tumor volume/location?
   a. Posterior/posterolateral in 85% of T1c cases
   b. Multifocal in 30% of cases
   c. Transition zone carcinomas extend out of the prostate at smaller volumes than peripheral zone cancers.
   d. Tumor volume is an independent predictor of prognosis, factoring in other pathological variables at radical prostatectomy.
   e. The number of involved chips distinguishes stages T1a and T1b.

4. All of the following are true about the Gleason grading system, EXCEPT:
   a. on needle biopsy, it sums the most common and highest patterns.
   b. on radical prostatectomy, it sums the most common and second most common patterns.
   c. it factors in cytology as well as glandular architecture.
   d. Gleason score 6 is for the most part the lowest score assigned on biopsy.
   e. Gleason score 6 cancers do not have the ability to metastasize.

5. Which of the following Gleason grade groupings is the most prognostically accurate?
   a. 2-4; 5; 6; 3 + 4; 4 + 3; 8-10
   b. 2-4; 5-6; 3 + 4; 4 + 3; 8, 9-10
   c. ≤6; 7; 8, 9-10
   d. ≤6, 3 + 4; 4 + 3; 8-10
   e. ≤6; 3 + 4; 4 + 3; 8; 9-10

6. All of the following findings at radical prostatectomy adversely affect prognosis, EXCEPT:
   a. tertiary grades.
   b. subdividing extraprostatic extension into focal and non-focal.
   c. the extent of positive margins.
   d. perineural invasion.
   e. vascular invasion.

PATHOLOGY

1. a. See Fig. 151.1.
   A 68-year-old man with an abnormal digital rectal exam (DRE) has a PSA of 4.2 ng/mL and has a needle biopsy of the prostate depicted in the figure. The tissue is stained with high-molecular-weight cytokeratin, and the pathologist reports the biopsy is consistent with benign prostatic hyperplasia (BPH). The next step is to:
   a. repeat the biopsy.
   b. ask the pathologist for additional molecular marker stains.
   c. follow up the patient with a PSA and DRE in 3 to 6 months.
   d. obtain endorectal magnetic resonance imaging (MRI).
   e. obtain a PCA3.

2. See Fig. 151.2.
   A 55-year-old man has a prostate biopsy depicted in the figure for a PSA of 4.5 and is reported as adenocarcinoma. The next step in management is:
   a. ask the pathologist for a Gleason score and volume of cancer.
   b. radical prostatectomy.
   c. metastatic workup with abdominal computed tomography (CT) and bone scan.

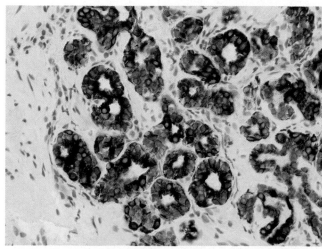

Fig. 151.1 (From Bostwick DG, Cheng L: *Urologic surgical pathology*, ed 2, Edinburgh, 2008, Mosby.)

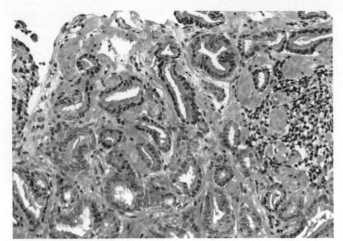

Fig. 151.2 (From Bostwick DG, Cheng L: *Urologic surgical pathology*, ed 2, Edinburgh, 2008, Mosby.)

d. endorectal MRI.

e. active observation.

ANSWERS

1. **d. PIN is the same as intraductal carcinoma.** Intraductal carcinoma is morphologically worse than high-grade PIN and is typically associated with high-grade carcinoma. Whereas high-grade PIN is either just followed clinically or leads to a repeat biopsy, intraductal carcinoma is treated the same as high-grade invasive prostate adenocarcinoma.

2. **d. Pt2x refers to prostatectomy specimens with intraprostatic incision.** Pt2x means that the tumor is organ confined everywhere in the prostate except in the area of the positive margin where extraprostatic extension cannot be assessed because there is an intraprostatic incision and the edge of the prostate is not visualized in this area.

3. **a. Posterior/posterolateral in 85% of T1c cases.** Even though T1c tumors are nonpalpable, the majority are still in the posterior or posterolateral region.

4. **c. It factors in cytology as well as glandular architecture.** Gleason grading assesses only the architectural pattern.

5. **e. ≤ 6; 3 + 4; 4 + 3; 8; 9-10.** There is a progressive increase in adverse outcome in this sequence of Gleason scoring.

6. **d. Perineural invasion.** Perineural invasion in the radical prostatectomy specimen has no prognostic significance; however, there are conflicting data on whether it has any predictive value in biopsy specimens.

PATHOLOGY

1. **c. Follow up the patient with a PSA and DRE in 3 to 6 months.** The patient has BPH as demonstrated by the presence of a basal layer with the positive cytokeratin stain. Because of the abnormal DRE, close follow-up is indicated.

2. **a. Ask the pathologist for a Gleason score and volume of cancer.** The figure demonstrates a straightforward Gleason 6 adenocarcinoma. The pathologist needs to report the Gleason score and the volume of cancer in the biopsy specimen for the physician to make an informed decision about management.

CHAPTER REVIEW

1. PIN is classified into low and high grade.
2. Low-grade PIN does not increase the risk of prostate cancer.
3. Rebiopsying patients with PIN is unnecessary unless there are multiple cores involved with high-grade PIN or there are other clinical indications.
4. Eighty-five percent of prostate adenocarcinomas are in the peripheral zone, and 85% are multifocal.
5. Peripherally located cancers tend to extend outside the prostate through the perineural space. The presence of perineural invasion within the prostatectomy specimens does not worsen the prognosis. By contrast, vascular invasion increases the risk of metastatic disease.
6. Prostate cancer metastasizes, in descending order, to lymph nodes, bone, lung, bladder, liver, and adrenal glands.
7. Subdividing pathologic T2 disease has no prognostic significance.
8. Transition zone tumors require larger volumes than peripheral zone tumors for comparable rates of extraprostatic extension and/or distant metastases.
9. For needle biopsy specimens, the primary pattern (dominant pattern) and the highest grade (irrespective of volume) should be reported as the Gleason sum.
10. Adverse findings on needle biopsy generally accurately predict adverse findings in radical prostatectomy specimens. However, favorable findings on needle biopsy do not necessarily predict favorable findings in the radical prostatectomy specimen.
11. Benign glands are differentiated from malignant glands in that the former contain basal cells. These can be labeled, if necessary, with high-molecular-weight cytokeratin and p63. Patients with atypical glands reported on biopsy specimens have a high likelihood of cancer on rebiopsy. Follow-up is warranted with serum or urine tests, imaging, and, in some cases, repeat biopsy with relative increased sampling of the atypical site.
12. Adenosis (atypical adenomatous hyperplasia) is characteristically found in the transition zone, and although it may mimic carcinoma histologically, there is no increased risk for adenocarcinoma in patients with this diagnosis.
13. Only 25% of men with seminal vesicle invasion and few with lymph node metastases are biochemically free of disease following radical prostatectomy 10 years postoperatively.
14. Tumor volume correlates well with pathologic stage and Gleason grade in clinical T2 cancers; however, it is not an independent predictor of cancer progression once grade, stage, and margins are accounted for.
15. The prostate lacks a discrete histologic capsule.
16. Involvement of the seminal vesicles is almost always due to direct extension (T3b); it carries a poor prognosis.
17. Only 50% of men with positive margins progress following radical prostatectomy.
18. Endocrine therapy results in atrophic changes with squamous metaplasia in the prostate. Carcinomas in patients who have had endocrine therapy may appear artifactually higher in grade.
19. Primary urothelial carcinomas of the prostate show a propensity to infiltrate the bladder neck and surrounding tissue such that more than 50% of the patients are stage T3 or T4, and 20% have distant metastases at the time of presentation.
20. Intraductal carcinoma is morphologically worse than high-grade PIN and is typically associated with high-grade carcinoma.

152 Diagnosis and Staging of Prostate Cancer

Stacy Loeb and James A. Eastham

QUESTIONS

1. Most immunodetectable prostate-specific antigen (PSA) in serum is bound to which of the following?
   a. Albumin.
   b. α_1-Antichymotrypsin (ACT).
   c. α_2-Macroglobulin (MG).
   d. Human kallikrein.
   e. Globulin.

2. Serum PSA levels vary with which factor?
   a. Age.
   b. Race.
   c. Prostate volume.
   d. ACT concentration.
   e. Age, race, and prostate volume.

3. Serum PSA elevations may occur with prostate:
   a. manipulation.
   b. cancer.
   c. enlargement.
   d. inflammation.
   e. all of the above.

4. Which of the following should be recommended for an elevated PSA?
   a. Repeat the measurement after cystoscopy.
   b. Give a 2-week course of fluoroquinolones, then repeat PSA.
   c. Give a 4-week course of doxycycline, then repeat PSA.
   d. Repeat the PSA measurement after a period of observation.
   e. All of the above.

5. Which of the following represent ways to adjust the PSA measurement?
   a. PSA density.
   b. PSA velocity.
   c. PSA transition zone density.
   d. Percent free PSA.
   e. All the above.

6. A 60-year-old man taking finasteride (Proscar) for 2 years with a PSA value of 4 ng/mL would most likely, if he were not taking finasteride, have which PSA value?
   a. 2 ng/mL
   b. 6 ng/mL
   c. 8 ng/mL
   d. 12 ng/mL
   e. 4 ng/mL

7. Which of the following tests has the highest positive predictive value for prostate cancer?
   a. PSA.
   b. Digital rectal exam (DRE).
   c. Transrectal ultrasonography (TRUS).
   d. Combination of DRE and TRUS.
   e. Human glandular kallikrein (hK2).

8. Which of the following statements about prostate cancer staging is FALSE?
   a. A goal of staging is to predict prognosis.
   b. Staging facilitates the selection of rational therapy based on predicted extent of disease.
   c. Imaging can accurately identify all cases of pelvic lymph node metastases.
   d. PSA and DRE are components of the staging evaluation.
   e. Pelvic lymphadenectomy is the gold standard for the detection of pelvic lymph node metastases.

9. The currently available modalities for assessing disease extent in men with prostate cancer include:
   a. DRE.
   b. serum PSA.
   c. histologic grade.
   d. bone scan.
   e. all of the above.

10. Pathologic staging is superior to clinical staging because all the following factors are confirmed in the final pathologic examination EXCEPT:
    a. PSA.
    b. surgical margin status.
    c. seminal vesicle involvement.
    d. tumor volume.
    e. capsular penetration.

11. What pathologic finding or findings at radical prostatectomy are highly predictive of the presence of occult metastatic disease?
    a. Positive surgical margins.
    b. Seminal vesicle involvement.
    c. Lymph node involvement.
    d. Both b and c.
    e. Both a and b.

12. In 2017, which group recommends shared decision making about PSA screening?
    a. United States Preventive Services Task Force.
    b. American Urological Association.
    c. American Cancer Society.
    d. European Association of Urology.
    e. All of the above.

13. As general guidelines regarding PSA levels and pathologic stage, which of the following statements is TRUE?
    a. Twenty-five percent of men with a PSA value less than 4 ng/mL have organ-confined disease.
    b. One hundred percent of men with a PSA value greater than 50 ng/mL have pelvic lymph node involvement.

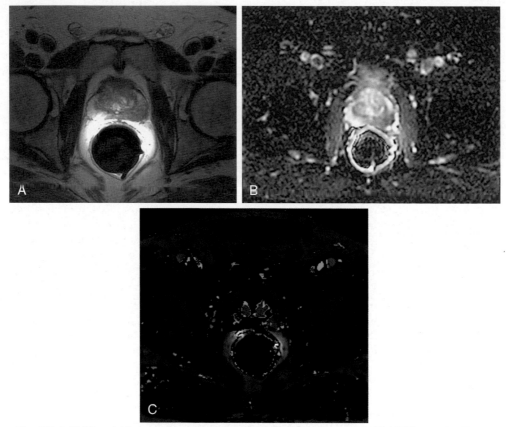

Fig. 152.1 (A) T2-weighted axial image of prostate MRI with endorectal coil. (B) MRI image A, diffusion weighted. (C) MRI image A with dynamic contrast enhancement.

c. Ten percent of men with a PSA value greater than 10 ng/mL have extraprostatic extension.

d. Serum PSA has no predictive value for staging.

e. Seventy percent or more of men with a PSA value between 4 and 10 ng/mL have organ-confined disease.

14. With respect to the grade groups, all of the following statements are TRUE EXCEPT:

a. Grade groups range from 1 to 5.

b. Gleason 3 + 3 disease is considered grade group 1.

c. Gleason 4 + 5 = 9 disease is considered grade group 5.

d. Gleason 4 + 4 disease is considered grade group 3.

e. Gleason 4 + 3 disease is considered grade group 3.

15. Which of the following variables are used to predict pathologic stage in the Partin tables?

a. PSA.

b. Number of positive biopsy cores.

c. Gleason score.

d. Clinical stage.

e. a, c, and d are all correct.

IMAGING

1. A 55-year-old man with a family history of prostate cancer had a 12-core prostate biopsy 1 year ago for a PSA of 2.6 ng/mL. Currently his PSA is 2.7 ng/mL and his DRE reveals a smooth soft minimally enlarged prostate with no nodules or firm areas. Prostate magnetic resonance imaging (MRI) is obtained and is depicted in Fig. 152.1A: T2-weighted axial image of the prostate; Fig. 152.1B: diffusion-weighted image of panel A; and

Fig. 152.1C: dynamic contrast enhancement image of 1A. The patient should be:

a. reassured and scheduled for yearly PSA and rectal examination.

b. sent back to his primary care physician for follow-up.

c. scheduled for a directed prostate biopsy.

d. scheduled for a saturation biopsy.

e. followed with a PSA every 4 months and an MRI in a year.

ANSWERS

1. **b. α₁-Antichymotrypsin (ACT).** Most detectable PSA in sera (65% to 90%) is bound to ACT.

2. **e. Age, race, and prostate volume.** In the absence of prostate cancer, serum PSA levels vary with age, race, and prostate volume.

3. **e. All of the above.** Serum PSA elevations may occur as a result of disruption of the normal prostatic architecture that allows PSA to diffuse into the prostatic tissue and gain access to the circulation. This can occur in the setting of prostate disease (benign prostatic hyperplasia [BPH], prostatitis, and prostate cancer) and with prostate manipulation (prostate massage, prostate biopsy). The presence of prostate disease (prostate cancer, BPH, and prostatitis) is the most important factor affecting serum levels of PSA. PSA elevations may indicate the presence of prostate disease, but not all men with prostate disease have elevated PSA levels. Furthermore, PSA elevations are not specific for cancer.

4. **d. Repeat the PSA measurement after a period of observation.** The American Urological Association does not recommend giving empiric antibiotics for an elevated PSA. Manipulation of the urinary tract such as cystoscopy can lead to PSA elevations. Repeating an abnormal test after a period of observation is a good practice.

5. **e. All of the above.** Many different variations on the PSA test have been proposed to improve specificity. These include dividing by total prostate volume (PSA density) or volume of the transition zone (PSA transition zone density), examining changes over time (PSA velocity), and determining the proportion circulating in the free form (percent free PSA).

6. **c. 8 ng/mL.** Finasteride (a 5α-reductase inhibitor for treatment of BPH) at 5 mg has been shown to lower PSA levels by approximately 50% after 12 months of treatment. Thus, one can multiply the PSA level by 2 to obtain the "true" PSA level of a patient who has been taking finasteride for 12 months or more. After 2 and 7 years of finasteride therapy, the PSA level should be multiplied by a factor of 2.3 and 2.5, respectively. Men who are to be treated with finasteride should have a baseline PSA measurement before initiation of treatment and should be followed with serial PSA measurements. If there is a rise in the PSA value when the patient is taking finasteride, these men should be suspected of having an occult prostate cancer.

7. **a. PSA.** PSA is the single test with the highest positive predictive value for cancer.

8. **c. Imaging can accurately identify all cases of pelvic lymph node metastases.** The goals in staging of prostate cancer are twofold: (1) to predict prognosis and (2) to rationally select therapy based on predicted extent of disease.

9. **e. All of the above.** The currently available modalities for assessing disease extent in men with prostate cancer include DRE, serum tumor markers, histologic grade, radiographic imaging, and pelvic lymphadenectomy.

10. **a. PSA.** Pathologic staging is more useful than clinical staging in the prediction of prognosis because tumor volume, surgical margin status, extent of extracapsular spread, and involvement of seminal vesicles and pelvic lymph nodes can be determined.

11. **d. Both b and c.** The finding of seminal vesicle invasion or lymph node metastases on pathologic evaluation after radical prostatectomy is associated with a high risk of distant disease.

12. **e. All of the above.** All of these groups recommend shared decision making or a discussion of risks and benefits between the patient and provider about PSA screening.

13. **e. Seventy percent or more of men with a PSA value between 4 and 10 ng/mL have organ-confined disease.** As a general guideline, the majority of men (80%) who have prostate cancer with PSA values less than 4 ng/mL have pathologically organ-confined disease, two-thirds of men with PSA levels between 4 and 10 ng/mL have organ-confined cancer, and more than 50% of men with PSA levels more than 10 ng/mL have disease beyond the prostate. Pelvic lymph node involvement is found in nearly 20% of men with PSA levels greater than 20 ng/mL and in most men (75%) with serum PSA levels greater than 50 ng/mL.

14. **d. Gleason 4 + 4 disease is considered grade group 3.** The new grade groups of 1 to 5 represent Gleason scores of ≤6, 3 + 4, 4 + 3, 8 and 9 to 10). Thus, Gleason 4 + 3 is considered grade group 3 and Gleason 4 + 4 is considered grade group 4.

15. **e. a, c, and d are all correct.** The "Partin tables" are probability tables for the determination of pathologic stage that are based on three parameters: preoperative clinical stage, serum PSA level, and Gleason sum. In the Partin tables, numbers within the nomogram represent the percent probability of having a given final pathologic stage based on logistic regression analyses for all three variables combined; dashes represent data categories in which insufficient data existed to calculate a probability. This information is useful in counseling men with newly diagnosed prostate cancer with respect to treatment alternatives and probability of complete eradication of tumor.

IMAGING

1. **c. Scheduled for a directed prostate biopsy.** The T2-weighted image (Fig. 152.1A) shows a well-demarcated low-signal-intensity area in the left peripheral zone with likely extracapsular extension. The diffusion-weighted image (B) shows restricted diffusion (dark area) in the same location as the abnormality seen in A and the dynamic contrast enhanced image (C) shows rapid uptake and loss of contrast (red area) in the same location of the abnormal left peripheral zone seen in A. These findings are highly suggestive of prostate cancer. The patient should have a directed biopsy to this area.

CHAPTER REVIEW

1. PSA levels are lower in hypogonadal men; statins may reduce PSA, whereas BPH, prostatitis, prostate manipulation, and prostate cancer increase serum levels of PSA.

2. PSA may be elevated within 24 hours following ejaculation; DRE does not result in a significant fluctuation of PSA.

3. Surgical therapy for BPH may reduce PSA.

4. A PSA velocity of more than 0.75 ng/mL/year in patients with levels between 4 and 10 prompts a concern for prostate cancer; a PSA density (PSAD) may also be used in this group for risk assessment.

5. A low noncomplexed PSA (free PSA) has a higher association with prostate cancer than does a high level of free PSA (>25%) in patients with PSAs between 4 and 10 ng/mL.

6. Prostate cancer screening was found in one study to reduce the rate of advanced disease at the time of diagnosis and reduce prostate-specific mortality; however, in another prospective study there was no reduction in prostate-specific mortality with screening. Moreover, it may increase morbidity due to increased unnecessary biopsies or treatment in some men.

7. There is some evidence that a PSA less than 1 ng/mL in patients aged 40 to 45 years may be used to inform the frequency of screening.

8. African Americans have higher PSA values than whites.

9. A tertiary pattern of Gleason grade is reported if there is a small focus of a higher grade than the primary and secondary grades. The Gleason sum is a combination of the primary grade and the highest grade.

10. Bone scans are not appropriate for staging unless the PSA is greater than 20 ng/mL, the clinical stage is T3 or T4, or the patient has specific complaints referable to the bones.

11. MRI with diffusion-weighting and dynamic contrast enhancement has improved the specificity of MRI to predict cancer.

12. Specific criteria for who should have a pelvic lymphadenectomy as a preliminary staging procedure or combined with a radical prostatectomy have not been firmly established. At the very least, it probably should be done in patients with a Gleason score greater than 8, enlarged nodes on imaging, T3 disease on rectal exam, and/or a PSA greater than 20 ng/mL.

13. The majority of men (80%) who have prostate cancer with PSA values less than 4 ng/mL have pathologically organ-confined disease, two-thirds of men with PSA levels between 4 and 10 ng/mL have organ-confined cancer, and more than 50% of men with PSA levels more than 10 ng/mL have disease beyond the prostate. Pelvic lymph node involvement is found in nearly 20% of men with PSA levels greater than 20 ng/mL and in most men (75%) with serum PSA levels greater than 50 ng/mL.

14. The "Partin tables" are probability tables for the determination of pathologic stage that are based on three parameters: preoperative clinical stage, serum PSA level, and Gleason sum.

153 Active Management Strategies for Localized Prostate Cancer

Samir S. Taneja and Marc A. Bjurlin

QUESTIONS

1. Decisions regarding the benefit of prostate cancer treatment should be primarily rooted in:
   a. life expectancy calculation of greater than 10 years.
   b. the expertise of the managing physician.
   c. assessment of the risk of prostate cancer mortality relative to other competing risks for death over time.
   d. the prostate-specific antigen (PSA) level at time of diagnosis.
   e. selection of candidates with low risk for metastatic progression.

2. Appropriate candidate selection for prostate cancer treatment may be improved through:
   a. use of validated comorbidity indices and life tables.
   b. exclusion of men who are obese.
   c. exclusion of men over the age of 70.
   d. inclusion of men with high-risk disease features.
   e. psychosocial assessments with validated instruments.

3. The instrument that considers comorbidities with prostate cancer patients in making predictions of 10-year longevity is the:
   a. Kattan nomogram.
   b. PCPT calculator.
   c. WHO Life Tables.
   d. CAPRA score.
   e. prostate cancer-specific Charlson Comorbidity Index (CCI).

4. Men with a high risk of metastatic progression or mortality within 10 years of diagnosis:
   a. are not likely to be helped by active treatment.
   b. are unlikely to develop symptoms of prostate cancer progression.
   c. may benefit from curative-intent treatment, regardless of age.
   d. are most often more likely to die of competing risks.
   e. should empirically be offered androgen deprivation.

5. Which of the following increases the risk of early urinary toxicity after external beam radiation therapy to the prostate?
   a. Previous urinary tract infection
   b. Nocturia
   c. History of hematospermia
   d. Previous transurethral resection of prostate (TURP)
   e. Prior urethroplasty

6. Decision regret in prostate cancer therapy selection is reduced by:
   a. robotic surgery.
   b. less aggressive therapy.
   c. second-opinion consultation.
   d. shared decision-making.
   e. physician bias.

7. The 2005 ISUP modifications in prostate cancer grading resulted in:
   a. characterization of cribriform pattern as Gleason grade 4.
   b. downward migration in Gleason score.
   c. characterization of intraductal variant as Gleason grade 3.
   d. limits on number of cancers deemed Gleason grade 5.
   e. creation of Gleason grade groups.

8. In its initial description, the UCSF-CAPRA score was able to widely discriminate:
   a. risk of extraprostatic extension.
   b. likelihood of Gleason upgrade.
   c. risk of mortality from competing causes.
   d. recurrence-free survival.
   e. response to adjuvant therapy.

9. The Scandinavian Prostate Cancer Group Study Number 4, comparing radical prostatectomy and watchful waiting, demonstrated improved survival among men undergoing radical prostatectomy. The study was limited by:
   a. predominant inclusion of indolent, low-risk disease.
   b. high rates of death from competing causes.
   c. increased age at time of accrual.
   d. excessive complications from surgery.
   e. primary enrollment in the pre-PSA era.

10. The PIVOT trial, comparing radical prostatectomy and watchful waiting, demonstrated no difference in survival among men undergoing radical prostatectomy or watchful waiting. The study was limited by:
    a. predominant inclusion of indolent, low-risk disease.
    b. high rates of death from competing causes.
    c. increased age at time of accrual.
    d. excessive complications from surgery.
    e. primary enrollment in the pre-PSA era.

11. The Prostate Testing for Cancer and Treatment (ProtecT) trial, a randomized trial of prostatectomy, external-beam radiation with androgen deprivation, or prostate-specific antigen–based active monitoring, demonstrated no difference in mortality between the three study groups at 10 years of follow-up. The study was limited by:
    a. predominant inclusion of indolent, low-risk disease.
    b. high rates of death from competing causes.
    c. increased age at time of accrual.
    d. excessive complications from surgery.
    e. primary enrollment in the pre-PSA era.

12. Whole-gland prostate ablation with high-intensity focused ultrasound is characterized by:
    a. demonstration of durable disease control at 15 to 20 years of follow-up.
    b. rates of erectile dysfunction comparable to radical prostatectomy.

c. substantial requirement for re-treatment within 5 years.

d. higher rates of erectile dysfunction than cryoablation.

e. urinary toxicity comparable to radiation therapy.

13. In risk assessment, the prostate MRI parameter most predictive of disease outcomes is:

a. T2-weighted signal attenuation.

b. diffusion weighted image.

c. contrast wash-in.

d. apparent diffusion coefficient (ADC).

e. hemorrhage on T1-weighted image.

14. Initial risk stratification and staging workup for a man with newly diagnosed clinically localized intermediate risk prostate cancer (T2b, GG 2, PSA 8) includes:

a. imaging is not indicated in this patient.

b. cross-sectional abdominopelvic imaging.

c. bone scan and cross-sectional abdominopelvic imaging.

d. bone scan and cross-sectional abdominopelvic imaging only if a nomogram predicts greater than 10% probability of pelvic lymph node involvement.

e. bone scan, cross-sectional abdominopelvic imaging, and fluciclovine PET.

15. Prediction of seminal vesical invasion by prostate MRI is characterized by a high:

a. false-positive rate.

b. positive predictive value.

c. sensitivity.

d. negative predictive value.

e. diagnostic accuracy.

ANSWERS

1. **c. Assessment of the risk of prostate cancer mortality relative to other competing risks for death over time.** Evaluation of the relative benefit of prostate cancer treatment in the individual patient should be based upon a determination of the relative probability of prostate cancer metastatic progression and cancer-specific mortality, as compared to the risk of death from other causes, within the expected natural longevity of the patient. A number of tools are available for assessing the risk of prostate cancer progression including nomograms, predictive models, and long-term observational cohorts. Most of these are based upon biopsy characteristics (including Gleason score and disease volume), serum PSA, imaging characteristics, genomic markers, and metastatic staging, in combination, rather than individually. The optimal candidate likely to benefit from treatment is the individual who has a reasonable likelihood of metastatic progression within his lifetime, if not treated. A number of tools exist for predicting life expectancy on the basis of age, adjusted for baseline comorbidities. While a life expectancy of 10 years is often used as a benchmark for benefit from therapy, life expectancy should be considered within the context of disease aggressiveness and the likelihood of disease progression within 5, 10, 15 years and beyond.

2. **a. Use of validated comorbidity indices and life tables.** The perception of longevity in clinical practice is often based solely upon age rather than comorbidity. Daskivich et al. have previously demonstrated that among men with low-risk prostate cancer diagnosed in the VAMC, treatment rates were higher for men with CCI ≥ 3 than those with age greater than 75 (54% vs. 16%), despite a much higher likelihood of other cause mortality within 10 years (70% vs. 24%). Additionally, among men in the SEER-Medicare database, aggressive treatment for men with less than 10 years life expectancy, based upon CCI, was dependent upon age, with 68% to 69% of men aged less than 75 receiving aggressive therapy compared to only 57% and 24% of those aged 75 to 79, or greater than or equal to 80. Similarly, Bratt et al. demonstrated that among men with high-risk prostate cancer in the National Prostate Cancer Register of Sweden, 50% of men aged less than 70 received radical treatment, as compared to only 10% of men aged 70 to 80, despite a 52% likelihood of 10-year longevity. Improvements in appropriate candidate selection for treatment, and secondarily survival benefit, can be achieved through age-adjusted assessment of longevity on the basis of validated comorbidity indices and life tables.

3. **e. Prostate cancer-specific Charlson Comorbidity Index (CCI).** The most widely utilized scale of comorbidity is the CCI. The CCI was designed to weigh comorbidities in prediction of one-year mortality among inpatients, but ultimately has been shown to be a significant prognostic indicator in the treatment of many types of cancer. In 2011, Daskivich et al. created a prostate cancer-specific CCI (PCCI) weighting comorbidities to predict 10-year risk of mortality among prostate cancer patients. When adjusting for age, and applying the PCCI to men with prostate cancer in the Veteran's Administration health care system (VAMC), segregated PCCI score at 0, 1–2, 3–4, 5–6, 7–9, and 10, the 10-year cumulative incidence of other cause mortality was 10%, 19%, 35%, 60%, 79%, and 99%, respectively.

4. **c. May benefit from curative-intent treatment, regardless of age.** Longevity assessment must be contemplated within the context of cancer aggressiveness. Men with aggressive malignancies may benefit from diagnosis and treatment regardless of a shortened longevity, particularly if presenting at an advanced stage. In men with high-risk, poorly differentiated prostate cancer, within the SEER-Medicare dataset, when comparing cancer-specific survival, aggressive treatment resulted in mortality improvements of 11.3%, 7.9%, 8.6%, and 2.8% at 10-year follow-up for men with Charlson scores of 0, 1, 2, and 3+, respectively, and numbers needed to treat to prevent 1 cancer death at 10 years were 9, 13, 12, and 36 men. Lead time from diagnosis to symptoms and eventual cancer-related mortality is heavily influenced by Gleason score and tumor stage, and this suggests that the relevance of expected longevity in treatment decision-making must be framed within a temporal estimate of cancer progression and mortality risk. Men with a high risk of metastatic progression or mortality within 10 years of diagnosis should be considered for aggressive therapy despite the presence of one or more competing risks for mortality within the same time period.

5. **d. Previous transurethral resection of prostate (TURP).** For men who have had a previous aggressive TURP for outlet obstruction, the risk of *urinary toxicity* may be higher in those that undergo radiotherapy, but the rates of long-term severe urinary symptoms may be lower. Delay of radiation for 6 to 8 weeks after TURP may reduce the risk of incontinence and bladder neck contracture.

6. **d. Shared decision-making.** Shared decision-making involves a collaborative process in which patients and clinicians make decisions together. Given the controversy surrounding the relative benefit of prostate cancer screening and treatment, shared decision-making, both with regard to PSA testing and prostate cancer treatment, has been strongly advocated by a number of governing bodies. This shared decision-making model has been adopted into guidelines on localized prostate cancer management supported by the AUA, ASTRO, and the SUO. More recently, consensus has been achieved regarding strategies for implementation of shared decision-making in clinical practice. In a recent multicenter, prospective, observational study of 454 men undergoing prostate cancer counseling and treatment, regardless of whether men expressed an initial desire to be actively or passively involved in decision-making or not, after treatment, men who perceived their involvement in decision-making as active were more well-informed with regard to the disease and expressed less decisional regret in follow-up after treatment. The available evidence suggests that

interventions aimed at informing patients regarding the comparative effectiveness of prostate cancer management alternatives should include the influence of physician recommendations and family members' desires on patient decision-making. The urologist's recommendation for treatment, however, continues to have the most influence on the decision-making.

7. **a. Characterization of cribriform pattern as Gleason grade 4.** In 2005, the International Society of Urologic Pathology (ISUP) recommended against the use of patterns 1 and 2, leaving a shortened scoring scale of 6 to 10. Additionally, the consensus recommended that a number of variant patterns previously graded as 3, and all cribriform patterns, should be considered pattern 4. In doing so, there has been an observation of Gleason scoring migration, with a greater number of cancers designated as Gleason score 3+4 or 4+3, as compared to historical cohorts. This migration has led to a reassessment of the accuracy of Gleason scoring in contemporary practice, with most such evaluations demonstrating improved prognostic accuracy. While the grading system appears to be more prognostically accurate, it has created difficulty in comparing historical outcomes of treatment to contemporary cohorts, given the difference in what is meant by Gleason 3+3 and 3+4/4+3.

8. **d. Recurrence-free survival.** The UCSF-Cancer of the Prostate Risk Assessment (CAPRA) score was developed for predicting clinical outcomes using age, PSA level, clinical stage, biopsy Gleason score, and percentage of positive biopsy cores. In its initial description, the UCSF-CAPRA score was able to widely segregate risk from a 5-year recurrence free survival of 85% among low-risk to 8% among high-risk patients. This stratification scheme has subsequently been shown to additionally predict prostate-cancer-specific mortality independently of the treatment given.

9. **e. Primary enrollment in the pre-PSA era.** SPCG-4 was the first to publish a randomized intention-to-treat analysis comparing watchful waiting and radical prostatectomy using informative clinical endpoints such as overall and cancer-specific survival. Furthermore, the SPCG-4 offered the long-term follow-up necessary to characterize between-group differences in survival and employed rigorous study design methods such as blinded histopathologic review. However, because this trial enrolled men predominantly during the pre-PSA era, nearly 90% of the 695 participants harbored palpable disease. Although a number of important observations regarding the comparative effectiveness of radical prostatectomy in the treatment of localized prostate can be made from the SPCG-4 data, this trial does not reflect current prostate cancer screening, detection, and treatment paradigms.

10. **b. High rates of death from competing causes.** The follow-up of the original PIVOT analysis was published in 2017, after 19.5 years of follow-up, demonstrating an absolute risk reduction (ARR) of 5.5% (95% confidence interval [CI]; −1.5% to 12.4%, $P = .06$) for all-cause mortality (61.3% vs. 66.8%) through prostatectomy. An ARR of 4.0% (95% CI; −0.2 to 8.3%, $P = .06$) was found for prostate cancer-specific mortality (7.4% vs. 11.4%). On subgroup analysis, surgery reduced all-cause mortality among men with intermediate-risk disease (ARR = 14.5%, 95% CI 2.8% to 25.6%). By contrast, no benefit was seen in the low- or high-risk groups. While surgery reduced the need for treatment of progressive disease, there were increased incidences of therapy-related long-term complications such as urinary incontinence and erectile and sexual dysfunction. One of the major concerns regarding the PIVOT study design was that the inclusion criterion for the study was life expectancy of greater than 10 year. However, according to the analysis of all-cause mortality after 10-year follow-up, nearly 40% of the study population had died, with only approximately 5% from prostate cancer. After 15 years, up to 60% had died, with ~10% from prostate cancer. These considerations suggest poor risk assessment at baseline inclusion and lessen the impact of the study. Since the design of the study, it is now well understood that patients with low-risk prostate cancer and comorbidities do not benefit within 10 years from radical interventions.

11. **a. Predominant inclusion of indolent, low-risk disease.** In the ProtecT trial, a total of 82,429 men 50 to 69 years of age received a PSA test; 2664 received a diagnosis of localized prostate cancer, and 1643 agreed to undergo randomization to active monitoring (545 men), surgery (553 men), or radiotherapy (plus 3 to 6 months androgen deprivation therapy, 545 men). The primary outcome was prostate-cancer mortality at a median of 10 years of follow-up. In total, 62% of eligible men accepted randomization, comprising a cohort with mostly low- to intermediate-risk tumors. The primary outcome of prostate cancer mortality was not different between the three arms at a median follow-up of 10 years. However, the incidence of metastases was higher in the active monitoring group. The majority of included patients had a low PSA and Gleason 6 tumors (grade group 1). As the chance of low-risk patients dying from prostate cancer within 10 years is very low, longer follow-up may be needed to draw firm conclusions. The mortality in the study was approximately 1% which is low in comparison to the predicted mortality of 15% at the time the study was designed, thereby reducing the power of the study to assess its intended purpose.

12. **c. Substantial requirement for re-treatment within 5 years.** The primary attraction of whole-gland ablation is the potential to preserve sexual and urinary function more frequently than radical prostatectomy or radiation therapy. While whole-gland cryoablation almost always results in erectile dysfunction, preservation of function with whole-gland high-intensity focused ultrasound (HIFU) is more common, but may vary with the aggressiveness and oncologic efficacy of the procedure. Additionally, the need for re-treatment is 29% to 38% with an increased rate of erectile dysfunction and stricture following a second treatment. As such, men considering whole-gland ablation by HIFU should be counseled with regard to the paucity of long-term outcomes and the potential need for re-treatment.

13. **d. Apparent diffusion coefficient (ADC).** The apparent diffusion coefficient, measured on diffusion-weighted imaging, has been shown to correlate with clinical outcomes and thus can be used as a risk stratification tool. Recent data have explored the value of MRI in monitoring tumors in patients on an active surveillance protocol. In patients with low-risk, localized disease, tumor ADC on diffusion-weighted imaging (DWI) may be a useful marker of prostate cancer progression and may help to identify patients who stand to benefit from radical treatment. As a preoperative imaging tool, tumor ADC and PI-RADS may also be useful to predict biochemical recurrence after radical prostatectomy and radiation therapy. MRI data improves the prediction of biochemical failure within nomograms after external-beam radiation therapy. Pretreatment MRI findings have also been found to predict for biochemical recurrence in intermediate- and high-risk prostate cancer patients treated with combination brachytherapy and external-beam radiotherapy.

14. **d. Bone scan and cross-sectional abdominopelvic imaging only if a nomogram predicts greater than 10% probability of pelvic lymph node involvement.** Guidelines for initial diagnostic imaging in the newly diagnosed prostate cancer patient vary considerably. While most definitions support radionuclide bone scan for the initial staging of high-risk prostate cancer, not all specifically address imaging for soft tissue metastases. Those that do commonly endorse pelvic CT or MRI. Current NCCN guidelines recommend the use of technetium 99m bone scan and cross-sectional imaging (CT or MRI) among high-risk and unfavorable intermediate-risk men deemed to be at high risk for occult metastasis on the basis of clinical parameters or nomograms. In cases of equivocal bone scans, PET/CT or MRI have been endorsed by several professional organizations.

15. **b. Positive predictive value.** For identifying extraprostatic extension (EPE) or seminal vesical invasion (SVI), MRI is the only examination with sufficient accuracy to be used in clinical practice given its combination of both high spatial and contrast resolution. Historically, assessment for EPE on MRI was based on T2-weighted imaging (T2WI) which provides the best spatial resolution of the MR sequences typically employed. The identification of EPE on T2WI alone is dependent on the amount of EPE present. Gross extension or disruption of the capsule is highly predictive of EPE, but more subtle findings such as irregularity or bulging of the "capsule" have a lower predictive value. As such, when deemed positive for seminal vesical invasion, MRI is generally correct resulting in low rates of false-positive and high positive predictive value. In general, MRI is poor for the detection of focal ECE, as demonstrated by the majority of patients with ECE, resulting in poor sensitivity and low negative predictive value. More subtle findings, such as linear length of capsular contact at the region of suspicion, may improve the pre-treatment prediction of the likelihood of ECE. Accuracy for more subtle EPE is improved when T2WI is combined with diffusion-weighted imaging (DWI) or dynamic contrast enhanced (DCE) imaging primarily because these additional sequences improve dominant tumor localization, which in turn helps predict presence of EPE, however, uncertainty remains because these ancillary sequences have lower spatial resolution than T2WI.

CHAPTER REVIEW

1. Prostate cancer treatment outcomes may be influenced by the malignant potential of the tumors as well as by the treatment used. Furthermore, outcome measurements are not necessarily comparable among different forms of therapy, confounding comparisons.

2. Traditionally, deferred treatment has been reserved for men with a life expectancy of less than 10 years and a low-grade prostate cancer. Additional research is needed to define the parameters for safe use of active surveillance in younger men, including the appropriate selection criteria, follow-up procedures, and trigger points for intervention.

3. A prospective, randomized clinical trial reported that patients with clinically localized prostate cancer managed with watchful waiting have significantly higher rates of local cancer progression, metastases, and death from prostate cancer than do those treated initially with radical prostatectomy. In addition, as discussed earlier, a prospective, randomized screening trial reported that prostate cancer screening with PSA and DRE reduces prostate cancer–specific mortality by 20% to 27% with early follow-up and up to 44% with longer follow-up. Because many of these patients were treated with radical prostatectomy, it may also be inferred to be evidence of the efficacy of radical prostatectomy for localized prostate cancer.

4. Radical prostatectomy was the first treatment used for prostate cancer, and it still remains the gold standard. An ideal candidate for radical prostatectomy is a healthy man with a life expectancy of at least 10 years. Preoperative clinical and pathologic parameters are often used to predict the pathologic stage and thus to identify patients most likely to benefit from the operation.

5. A rising serum PSA level is usually the earliest evidence of tumor recurrence after radical prostatectomy and is frequently an intermediate end point for treatment outcomes. However, not all patients with biochemical recurrence ultimately develop metastases or die of prostate cancer.

6. The most common late complications of radical prostatectomy are erectile dysfunction, urinary incontinence, hernia, and urethral stricture. The return of erectile function after surgery correlates with age of the patient, preoperative potency status, extent of nerve-sparing surgery, and era of surgery; the return of urinary continence is associated with the patient's age.

7. The long-term outcome of cancer control is better documented for open prostatectomy.

8. External beam radiotherapy uses gamma radiation beams directed at the prostate and surrounding tissues through multiple fields. To minimize radiation injury to the bladder and the rectum, 3D-CRT, IMRT, image-guided radiotherapy, SBRT, and proton beam radiotherapy have been developed. Patients with a high PSA level, high Gleason score, or large-volume tumor benefit from ADT in conjunction with radiotherapy. Currently, the most frequently used definition to determine treatment success after radiation therapy is the Phoenix definition, which requires PSA increases of 2 ng/mL above the nadir PSA level.

9. With brachytherapy, radioactive seeds or needles are implanted directly into the prostate gland to deliver a high dose of radiation to the tumor while attempting to spare the bladder and the rectum. Brachytherapy is used primarily for the treatment of patients with clinically localized prostate cancer, but it is seldom used for the treatment of high-volume, high-risk prostate cancers. Urinary symptoms are more common after brachytherapy than after external beam radiotherapy, especially in patients with prostatic hyperplasia.

10. Adjuvant radiotherapy shortly after surgery is most likely to benefit patients with extensive positive surgical margins or extracapsular tumor extension without seminal vesicle invasion or lymph node involvement. Patients most likely to have favorable responses to salvage radiotherapy are those with PSA recurrence long after surgery, slowly rising PSA level, low-grade tumor, and no seminal vesicle invasion or lymph node metastases. However, mortality benefits have also been demonstrated in patients with rapid PSA doubling times and high-risk tumors. Adjuvant radiotherapy reduces relapse rates in patients with high-risk tumor features but does not increase overall survival. Early salvage radiotherapy produces durable responses in most patients with intermediate-risk tumor features. It is unknown whether early adjuvant radiation is better than delayed salvage therapy in patients with adverse pathology findings after radical prostatectomy.

154 Active Surveillance of Prostate Cancer

Laurence Klotz

QUESTIONS

1. Which of the following is true about low-risk prostate cancer?
   a. The major concern is biological grade progression over time (from GG 1 to GG 2-5).
   b. About 25% of patients harbor occult higher-grade cancer at diagnosis.
   c. 30% of middle-aged Caucasian men harbor some prostate cancer.
   d. Most low-risk prostate cancers harbor significant genetic mutations.
   e. GG 1 cancer metastasizes in 3% to 5% of cases.

2. In men with low-risk prostate cancer on active surveillance:
   a. With long-term follow-up, local progression of disease resulting in outflow obstruction, retention, and hydronephrosis is common.
   b. Delayed treatment is less likely to be effective.
   c. Approximately 40% will have a signal for treatment by 10 years.
   d. The likelihood of metastasis of low-grade prostate cancer is 0.5% to 5% at 15 years.
   e. A PSA above 10 is a significant risk factor for metastatic disease.

3. Clinical parameters which predict for the likelihood of upgrading include:
   a. Extent of core involvement.
   b. Bilaterality.
   c. PSA density.
   d. Proportion of cores involved.
   e. All of the above.

4. Which of the following parameters should preclude active surveillance?
   a. Extensive GG1 disease.
   b. High PSA density.
   c. Baseline PSA >10.
   d. Presence of any Gleason pattern 4.
   e. None of the above.

5. The switch from active surveillance to watchful waiting should be based on:
   a. More than 10 years stable on surveillance.
   b. More than 2 successive negative biopsies and negative MRI.
   c. An estimated life expectancy of <5 to 7 years.
   d. Presence of cardiovascular co-morbidity.
   e. Patient refuses further biopsies.

6. For patients on surveillance, the trigger for intervention should be:
   a. Short PSA doubling time (<3 years) or PSA velocity >2.0/year.
   b. Progression in lesion size or conspicuity on MRI.
   c. Grade group progression.
   d. Volume progression of GG 1.
   e. Tissue-based biomarker showing >15% risk of high-grade cancer.

7. Most national guidelines (Cancer Care Ontario, AUA, ASCO) state which of the following regarding active surveillance?
   a. For low-risk disease, it is one of several recommended options.
   b. Patients should be followed with serial PSA, DRE, and biopsy.
   c. MRI is a useful diagnostic test in these patients and should be incorporated into routine clinical practice.
   d. Tissue-based biomarkers have a clear role in the low-risk patient in identifying those at risk.
   e. Patients with intermediate risk disease should not be offered surveillance.

ANSWERS

1. **b. About 25% of patients harbor occult higher-grade cancer at diagnosis.** Grade progression over time occurs in 1% to 2% per year; this is much less of a concern than coexistent high-grade cancer. Fifty to sixty percent of middle-aged men have microfocal prostate cancer. Most low-risk cancers have a very low mutational burden. GG1 cancer is a non-metastasizing lesion; low-grade cancers in men with metastasis invariably have an underlying higher-grade cancer.

2. **c. Approximately 40% will have a signal for treatment by 10 years.** Local progression of cancer is rare. Delayed treatment in this cohort does not reduce effectiveness of therapy. In published series, 20% to 30% are treated by 5 years and 30% to 40% by 10 years. Metastasis occurs from higher-grade cancer (which may be occult). PSA is not a strong predictor for metastasis.

3. **e. All of the above.** These are all clinical parameters that predict for the likelihood of upgrading.

4. **e. None of the above.** None of these parameters should exclude a patient from surveillance. Small amounts of pattern 4 may represent artefactual upgrading and is not an exclusion.

5. **c. An estimated life expectancy of <5 to 7 years.** A patient refusing biopsy may still be followed actively with, for example, MRI.

6. **c. Grade group progression.** None of the other criteria have been demonstrated to predict for an adverse outcome with reliable accuracy.

7. **b. Patients should be followed with serial PSA, DRE, and biopsy.** It is THE recommended option for low-risk disease; MRI and biomarkers are not recommended routinely; and AS can be offered to selected intermediate-risk patients.

CHAPTER REVIEW

1. Microfocal Gleason pattern 3 occurs in most men with age, in all races and regions of the world.
2. The mutational burden of Gleason 3 is very favorable, and dramatically different from higher-grade cancer. Most oncogenic pathways characterized by specific genetic alterations are normal in Gleason pattern 3 and aberrant (deleted/amplified/mutated/overexpressed, etc.) in Gleason 4 and 5.
3. Gleason 6 (Grade Group 1) has no metastatic potential.
4. Cancer deaths reported in men with low-risk cancer managed conservatively are thought to be due to the co-existence of higher-grade cancer missed on the diagnostic biopsy.
5. Misattribution of grade (25% to 30% of cases) is much more common than true biological progression from Gleason 3 to 4 or 5 (1% to 2.3% per year).
6. Factors that increase the risk of coexistent higher-grade cancer include PSA density (>0.15), race (African American), and volume of cancer on biopsy (number of positive cores, extent of core involvement).
7. Newly diagnosed men on active surveillance should have a confirmatory biopsy within 1 year, targeting the undersampled areas of the prostate.
8. Following this, they should have PSA q 6 months, and periodic repeat biopsy (every 3 to 5 years).
9. MRI and targeted biopsy may replace serial systematic biopsies in very low-risk men. Since the NPV of MRI is a function of underlying risk, those at higher risk still warrant systematic biopsies.
10. Clinicians managing patients on AS should use the opportunity of regular follow-up visits to counsel patients about the benefits of dietary and lifestyle modifications.

155 Open Radical Prostatectomy

Edward M. Schaeffer, Alan W. Partin, and Herbert Lepor

QUESTIONS

1. What is the arterial blood supply to the prostate?
   a. The pudendal artery.
   b. The superior vesical artery.
   c. The inferior vesical artery.
   d. The external iliac artery.
   e. The obturator artery.

2. What vessels are located in the neurovascular bundle?
   a. Capsular arteries and veins.
   b. Pudendal artery and vein.
   c. Hemorrhoidal artery and vein.
   d. Santorini plexus.
   e. Accessory pudendal artery.

3. A radical prostatectomy may compromise the arterial blood supply to the penis by injuring the aberrant blood supply from which artery?
   a. The obturator artery.
   b. The inferior vesical artery.
   c. The superior vesical artery.
   d. The penile artery.
   e. All of the above.

4. The main parasympathetic efferent innervation to the pelvic plexus arises from:
   a. S1.
   b. S2 to S4.
   c. T11 to L2.
   d. L3 to S1.
   e. T5 to T8.

5. What is the relationship of the neurovascular bundle to the prostatic fascia?
   a. Inside Denonvilliers fascia.
   b. Outside the lateral pelvic fascia.
   c. Inside the prostatic fascia.
   d. Between the layers of the prostatic fascia and the levator fascia.
   e. Both inside and outside the prostatic fascia.

6. Which anatomic structure is responsible for the maintenance of passive urinary control after radical prostatectomy?
   a. Bladder neck.
   b. Levator ani musculature.
   c. Preprostatic sphincter.
   d. Striated urethral sphincter.
   e. Bulbar urethra.

7. What is the major nerve supply to the striated sphincter and levator ani?
   a. The neurovascular bundle.
   b. The sympathetic fibers from T11 to L2.

   c. The pudendal nerve.
   d. The obturator nerve.
   e. The accessory pudendal nerve.

8. What is the posterior extent of the pelvic lymph node dissection?
   a. The hypogastric vein.
   b. The obturator nerve.
   c. The obturator vessels.
   d. The sacral foramen.
   e. The pelvic sidewall musculature.

9. In opening the endopelvic fascia, there are often small branches traveling from the prostate to the pelvic sidewall. These branches are tributaries from the:
   a. Obturator artery.
   b. External iliac artery.
   c. Inferior vesical artery.
   d. Pudendal artery and veins.
   e. Neurovascular bundle.

10. How extensively should the puboprostatic ligaments be divided?
    a. Superficially, with just enough incised to expose the junction between the anterior apex of the prostate and the dorsal vein complex.
    b. Extensively, down to the pelvic floor, including the pubourethral component.
    c. Not at all; the puboprostatic ligaments should be left intact.
    d. Widely enough to permit a right angle to be placed around the dorsal vein complex.
    e. Not at all; the puboprostatic ligaments do not need to be divided to perform a radical prostatectomy.

11. When the dorsal vein complex is divided anteriorly, what is the most common major structure that can be damaged, and what is the most common adverse outcome?
    a. Aberrant pudendal arteries; impotence.
    b. Neurovascular bundle; impotence.
    c. Striated urethral sphincter; incontinence.
    d. Levator ani musculature; incontinence.
    e. Both a and b.

12. What is the most common site for a positive surgical margin and when does this occur?
    a. Posterolateral; during release of the neurovascular bundle.
    b. Posterior; when the prostate is dissected from the rectum.
    c. Apex; during division of the striated urethral sphincter-dorsal vein complex.
    d. Bladder neck; during separation of the prostate from the bladder.
    e. Seminal vesicles.

13. How should the back-bleeders from the dorsal vein complex on the anterior surface of the prostate be oversewn and why?
    a. The edges should be pulled together in the midline to avoid bleeding.
    b. Bunching sutures should be used to avoid excising too much striated sphincter.
    c. The edges should be oversewn in the shape of a V to avoid advancing the neurovascular bundles too far anteriorly on the prostate.
    d. They should be oversewn horizontally to avoid a positive surgical margin.
    e. Oversewing the proximal dorsal vein complex is not required.

14. After the dorsal vein complex has been ligated and the urethra has been divided, what posterior structure, other than the neurovascular bundles, attaches the prostate to the pelvic floor?
    a. Rectourethralis.
    b. Denonvilliers fascia.
    c. Rectal fascia.
    d. Posterior portion of the striated sphincter complex.
    e. Neurovascular bundles.

15. What are the advantages of releasing the levator fascia higher at the apex (more than one answer may be correct)?
    a. More soft tissue on the prostate.
    b. Less traction on the neurovascular bundles as they are released.
    c. Preservation of anterior nerve fibers.
    d. Less blood loss.
    e. Better visualization of the location of the cancer.

16. Once the apex of the prostate has been released, what is the best way to retract the prostate for exposure of the neurovascular bundle?
    a. Traction on the catheter, producing upward rotation of the apex of the prostate.
    b. Use of a sponge stick to roll the prostate on its side.
    c. Downward displacement of the prostate with a sponge stick.
    d. Use of finger dissection to release the prostate posteriorly.
    e. Dissection with the sucker.

17. To avoid a positive surgical margin, what is the best way to release the neurovascular bundle?
    a. Right-angle dissection beginning on the posterior surface of the prostate and dissecting anterolaterally.
    b. With sharp dissection, laterally dissecting toward the rectum.
    c. With finger dissection to fracture the neurovascular bundle from the prostate.
    d. With electrocautery to separate the neurovascular bundle from the prostate.
    e. Elevation of the prostate with traction on the Foley catheter.

18. What is the latest point at which a decision can be made regarding preservation or excision of the neurovascular bundle?
    a. When perineural invasion is identified on the needle biopsy specimen.
    b. When the neurovascular bundle is being released from the prostate and fixation is identified.
    c. When the prostate has been removed and tissue covering the posterolateral surface of the prostate is thought to be inadequate.

    d. When the patient is found to have a positive biopsy result at the apex.
    e. When the Partin tables indicate a greater than 50% chance of extraprostatic extension.

19. Before the lateral pedicles are divided, what is the last major branch of the neurovascular bundle that must be identified and released?
    a. Apical branch.
    b. Posterior branch.
    c. Capsular branch.
    d. Bladder neck branch.
    e. Seminal branch.

20. When the vesicourethral anastomosis sutures are being tied, if tension is found, what is the best way to release it?
    a. Creating an anterior bladder neck flap.
    b. Placing the Foley catheter on traction postoperatively.
    c. Releasing attachments of the bladder to the peritoneum.
    d. Using vest sutures.
    e. Releasing the urethra from the pelvic floor.

21. If there is excessive bleeding from the dorsal vein complex while it is being divided, what should be done?
    a. Abandon the operation and close the incision.
    b. Ligate the hypogastric arteries.
    c. Inflate a Foley balloon and place traction on it.
    d. Divide the dorsal vein complex completely over the urethra and oversew the end.
    e. Deflate the Foley catheter.

22. If a rectal injury occurs during the operation, the most appropriate next step is:
    a. To create a loop colostomy.
    b. To create an end colostomy.
    c. To create a Hartman pouch.
    d. To ensure interposition of the omentum following repair of the injury.
    e. To repair the rectal injury in two layers.

23. In postoperative patients who require transfusions of blood for hypotension, the best approach is to:
    a. Avoid re-exploration because it might damage the anastomosis.
    b. Perform re-exploration.
    c. Place the Foley catheter on traction.
    d. Administer fresh frozen plasma.
    e. Serially monitor the patient in an intensive care unit setting.

24. What is the best way to ensure good coaptation of the anastomotic mucosal surfaces to avoid a bladder neck contracture?
    a. Hold the catheter on traction while tying the sutures.
    b. Use a sponge stick in the perineum.
    c. Use a Babcock clamp to hold the bladder down.
    d. Use vest sutures.
    e. Evert the bladder mucosa.

25. What is the most common cause of incontinence after radical prostatectomy?
    a. Intrinsic sphincter deficiency.
    b. Detrusor instability.
    c. Failure to reconstruct the bladder neck.
    d. Injury to the neurovascular bundles.
    e. Bladder neck contracture.

26. Preservation of the seminal vesicles during radical prostatectomy has demonstrated:
    a. Improved erectile function in most men.
    b. No increase in biochemical recurrence.
    c. Improved early and late urinary control.
    d. Increased rate of pelvic abscess.
    e. None of the above.

27. Preservation of the bladder neck during radical prostatectomy has demonstrated:
    a. Improved erectile function.
    b. Improved long term urinary control.
    c. Decreased surgical margins.
    d. Improved anastomotic stricture rate.
    e. None of the above.

28. What percentage of men who had bilateral sural nerve grafting demonstrated full erections capable of penetration?
    a. 9%
    b. 13%
    c. 26%
    d. 38%
    e. 57%

29. Sural nerve grafts are placed:
    a. End to end on the ipsilateral side from the tumor.
    b. Above the bladder neck and below the pubic arch.
    c. In reverse to the natural position (proximal to distal and distal to proximal).
    d. In a circle to enhance nerve growth factor release.
    e. Next to the prostatectomy specimen in the pelvis until it is time for anastomosis.

30. Which complication has changed dramatically with experience with salvage prostatectomy?
    a. Overall urinary incontinence.
    b. Potency.
    c. Blood loss.
    d. Rectal injury.
    e. Stricture rate.

31. Concerning postoperative neurapraxia, which of the following statements is TRUE?
    a. The literature supports that it is almost always transient.
    b. It usually results in a motor deficit that is transient.
    c. Most studies show that a self-limited neurapraxia occurs in approximately 25% of patients.
    d. The same rates of neurapraxia tend to occur in retropubic prostatectomy as well.
    e. This is a major source of morbidity and the reason many surgeons do not use this approach.

32. Which of the following statements concerning rectal injury associated with perineal prostatectomy is FALSE?
    a. If unrecognized, it may result in the occurrence of a rectocutaneous or urethrocutaneous fistula.
    b. Despite the close proximity of the rectum in the initial dissection, the incidence is fairly low.
    c. It can be avoided when an assistant places gentle downward pressure on the Lowsley tractor while the rectourethralis muscle is divided.
    d. If repaired with a two-layer closure, most clinical sequelae are avoided.

e. After repair with a two-layer closure, the operation can continue without a problem.

33. Which of the following statements concerning postoperative care is TRUE?
    a. The diet is rapidly advanced to a regular diet.
    b. Most patients are discharged from the hospital by postoperative day 2.
    c. A rectal suppository is administered on a scheduled basis while in the hospital to minimize Foley catheter discomfort except in cases of intraoperative rectal injury.
    d. a and b only.
    e. All of the above.

34. Which of the following statements concerning the technique of urethral anastomosis is TRUE?
    a. The presence of the Lowsley retractor assists in identifying the membranous urethral stump for the initial placement of interrupted sutures.
    b. A running suture technique is advocated for a watertight anastomosis.
    c. The visualization of the anastomosis is difficult, one of the few disadvantages of the radical perineal prostatectomy.
    d. The sutures are interrupted in a tennis-racquet fashion.
    e. The indwelling Foley catheter is not passed until after the anterior vesicourethral anastomotic sutures are placed and tied down.

ANSWERS

1. **c. The inferior vesical artery** The prostate receives arterial blood supply from the inferior vesical artery.
2. **a. Capsular arteries and veins.** The capsular branches run along the pelvic sidewall in the lateral pelvic fascia posterolateral to the prostate, providing branches that course ventrally and dorsally to supply the outer portion of the prostate. Histologically, the capsular arteries and veins are surrounded by an extensive network of nerves. These capsular vessels provide the macroscopic landmark that aids in the identification of the microscopic branches of the pelvic plexus that innervate the corpora cavernosa.
3. **e. All of the above.** The major arterial supply to the corpora cavernosa is derived from the internal pudendal artery. However, pudendal arteries can arise from the obturator, inferior vesical, and superior vesical arteries. Because these aberrant branches travel along the lower part of the bladder and anterolateral surface of the prostate, they are divided during radical prostatectomy. This may compromise arterial supply to the penis, especially in older patients with borderline penile blood flow.
4. **b. S2 to S4.** The autonomic innervation of the pelvic organs and external genitalia arises from the pelvic plexus, which is formed by parasympathetic visceral efferent preganglionic fibers that arise from the sacral center (S2 to S4).
5. **d. Between the layers of the prostatic fascia and the levator fascia.** The neurovascular bundles are located in the lateral pelvic fascia between the prostatic and levator fasciae.
6. **d. Striated urethral sphincter.** The striated sphincter contains fatigue-resistant, slow-twitch fibers that are responsible for passive urinary control.
7. **c. The pudendal nerve.** The pudendal nerve provides the major nerve supply to the striated sphincter and levator ani.
8. **a. The hypogastric vein.** The obturator artery and vein are skeletonized but are usually left undisturbed and are not ligated unless excessive bleeding occurs. The dissection then continues down to the pelvic floor, exposing the hypogastric veins.

9. **d. Pudendal artery and veins.** The incision in the endopelvic fascia is carefully extended in an anteromedial direction toward the puboprostatic ligaments. At this point, one often encounters small arterial and venous branches from the pudendal vessels, which perforate the pelvic musculature to supply the prostate. These vessels should be ligated with clips to avoid coagulation injury to the pudendal artery and nerve, which are located just deep to this muscle as they travel along the pubic ramus.

10. **a. Superficially, with just enough incised to expose the junction between the anterior apex of the prostate and the dorsal vein complex.** The dissection should continue down far enough to expose the juncture between the apex of the prostate and the anterior surface of the dorsal vein complex at the point where it will be divided. The pubourethral component of the complex must remain intact to preserve the anterior fixation of the striated urethral sphincter to the pubis.

11. **c. Striated urethral sphincter; incontinence.** The goal is to divide the complex with minimal blood loss while avoiding damage to the striated sphincter.

12. **c. Apex; during division of the striated urethral sphincter-dorsal vein complex.** The exact plane on the anterior surface of the prostate can be visualized, avoiding inadvertent entry into the anterior prostate and ensuring minimal excision of the striated sphincter musculature. This is the most common site for positive surgical margins because it can be difficult to identify the anterior apical surface of the prostate.

13. **c. The edges should be oversewn in the shape of a V to avoid advancing the neurovascular bundles too far anteriorly on the prostate.** To avoid back-bleeding from the anterior surface of the prostate, the edges of the proximal dorsal vein complex on the anterior surface of the prostate are sewn in the shape of a V with a running 2-0 absorbable suture. If one tries to pull these edges together in the midline, the neurovascular bundles can be advanced too far anteriorly on the prostate.

14. **d. Posterior portion of the striated sphincter complex.** The posterior band of urethra is now divided to expose the posterior portion of the striated urethral sphincter complex. The posterior sphincter complex is composed of skeletal muscle and fibrous tissue.

15. **b. Less traction on the neurovascular bundles as they are released, and c. Preservation of anterior nerve fibers.** The purpose of this technique is to speed up recovery of sexual function by reducing traction on the branches of the nerves to the cavernous bodies and striated sphincter and/or avoiding inadvertent transection of the small branches that travel anteriorly. However, because there is less soft tissue at the apex, the risk of positive margins may be increased.

16. **b. Use of a sponge stick to roll the prostate on its side.** When the surgeon releases the neurovascular bundle, there should be no upward traction on the prostate. Rather, the prostate should be rolled from side to side.

17. **a. Right-angle dissection beginning on the posterior surface of the prostate and dissecting anterolaterally.** After the plane between the rectum and prostate in the midline has been developed, it is possible to release the neurovascular bundle from the prostate, beginning at the apex and moving toward the base, by using the sponge stick to roll the prostate over on its side. Beginning on the rectal surface, the bundle is released from the prostate by spreading a right angle gently. With use of this plane, Denonvilliers fascia and the prostatic fascia remain on the prostate; only the residual fragments of the levator fascia are released from the prostate laterally.

18. **c. When the prostate has been removed and tissue covering the posterolateral surface of the prostate is thought to be inadequate.** Clues that indicate that wide excision of the neurovascular bundle is necessary include inadequate tissue covering the posterolateral surface of the prostate once the prostate has been removed, leading to secondary wide excision of the neurovascular bundle. This last point is important to understand. The surgeon does not have to make the decision about whether to excise or preserve the neurovascular bundle until the prostate is removed, and, if there is not enough soft tissue covering the prostate, one can excise the neurovascular bundle then.

19. **b. Posterior branch.** The surgeon should look for a prominent arterial branch traveling from the neurovascular bundle over the seminal vesicles to supply the base of the prostate. This posterior vessel should be ligated on each side and divided. By this method, the neurovascular bundles are no longer tethered to the prostate and fall posteriorly.

20. **c. Releasing attachments of the bladder to the peritoneum.** The anterior suture is tied initially. There should be no tension. If there is, the bladder should be released from the peritoneum.

21. **d. Divide the dorsal vein complex completely over the urethra and oversew the end.** If there is troublesome bleeding from the dorsal vein complex at any point, the surgeon should completely divide the dorsal vein complex over the urethra and oversew the end. This is the single best means to control bleeding from the dorsal vein complex. Any maneuver short of this will only worsen the bleeding. To gain exposure for the prostatectomy, one must put traction on the prostate. If the dorsal vein is not completely divided, traction opens the partially transected veins and usually worsens the bleeding.

22. **d. To ensure interposition of the omentum following repair of the injury.** It is wise to interpose omentum between the rectal closure and the vesicourethral anastomosis to reduce the possibility of a rectourethral fistula.

23. **b. Perform re-exploration.** Our findings suggest that patients requiring acute transfusions for hypotension after radical prostatectomy should undergo exploration to evacuate the pelvic hematoma in an effort to decrease the likelihood of bladder neck contracture and incontinence.

24. **c. Use a Babcock clamp to hold the bladder down.** We have found that the use of a Babcock clamp to approximate the bladder neck and urethra while the anastomotic sutures are tied has virtually eliminated bladder neck contractures in our practice.

25. **a. Intrinsic sphincter deficiency.** After radical prostatectomy, incontinence is usually secondary to intrinsic sphincter deficiency.

26. **e. None of the above.** Sparing of the seminal vesicles has not improved incontinence, potency, or margin status, and there have been no reported cases of pelvic abscess.

27. **e. None of the above.** Sparing of the bladder neck has not improved incontinence, potency, margin status, or stricture rates.

28. **c. 26%.** The percentage of men who had bilateral sural nerve grafting and demonstrated full erections (capable of penetration) was 26%.

29. **c. In reverse to the natural position (proximal to distal and distal to proximal).** Sural nerve grafts are placed in reverse to the natural position (proximal to distal and distal to proximal).

30. **d. Rectal injury.** Only rectal injury rates have dramatically changed.

31. **a. The literature supports that it is almost always transient.** Sensory neurapraxia of the lower extremity is reported to occur in approximately 2% of radical perineal prostatectomy cases. However, one study did report an incidence of 25%. This is reported significantly more often than with retropubic prostatectomy. True motor deficits are rare. Because of the transient nature, this is not a major source of morbidity.

32. **c. It can be avoided when an assistant places gentle downward pressure on the Lowsley tractor while the rectourethralis muscle is divided.** Traction on the Lowsley tractor during division of the rectourethralis muscle tents the rectum upward and increases the likelihood of injury. Traction should not be placed until after the rectourethralis muscle is divided. When unrecognized, a fistula may ensue. Although one report showed an incidence of rectal injury in 11% of cases, most series recognize an incidence of 1% to 5%. When the injury is

recognized and repaired at the time of occurrence, the operation can continue without a problem.

33. **d. a and b only.** Postoperatively, the diet is advanced rapidly as tolerated, patients ambulate early, and the overwhelming majority of patients are discharged by the second postoperative day. However, rectal stimulation or manipulation is prohibited in the postoperative period.

34. **e. The indwelling Foley catheter is not passed until after the anterior vesicourethral anastomotic sutures are placed and tied down.** During placement of the anterior vesicourethral anastomotic sutures, a red rubber catheter is placed transurethrally and used to identify the membranous urethral stump and provide traction on the urethra to assist in placement of the sutures. The red rubber catheter is then removed, and the indwelling Foley catheter is then placed retrograde into the bladder. Simple interrupted sutures are placed for the anastomosis. A tennis-racquet technique is used for bladder neck reconstruction if necessary.

CHAPTER REVIEW

1. The dorsal vein has three major branches: a superficial branch in the midline and two lateral branches that span over the lateral aspects of the prostate.
2. The prostate is covered with three distinct fascial layers: Denonvilliers fascia, prostatic fascia, and levator fascia.
3. Denonvilliers fascia is most prominent and dense near the base of the prostate and overlying the seminal vesicles and thins dramatically more caudad at its termination at the striated sphincter.
4. Laterally, the prostatic fascia fuses with the levator fascia.
5. Following radical prostatectomy, 15% to 20% of men develop an inguinal hernia. It is usually an indirect inguinal hernia.
6. The final decision whether to preserve the neurovascular bundles is made at surgery.
7. Findings that would indicate a neurovascular bundle should be resected include palpable induration in the lateral pelvic fascia, a neurovascular bundle that appears fixed to the prostate, and insufficient tissue on the posterolateral aspect of the specimen.
8. Thermal energy should never be used on or near the neurovascular bundles.
9. Bladder neck contractures occur in less than 10% of patients.
10. Factors important for recovery of erectile function include patient age, preoperative potency status, and preservation of the neurovascular bundles.
11. Potency improves with time such that in one study, 42% of patients were potent at 3 months and 73% at a year.
12. In a randomized study using sural nerve grafting to preserve potency in patients in whom a neurovascular bundle needed to be sacrificed, there was no difference in those grafted versus those who were not.
13. Salvage radical prostatectomy should only be considered in men who have unequivocally clinically localized prostate cancer.
14. Complications following salvage radical prostatectomy include 50% incontinence, 24% anastomotic stricture, and nearly universal erectile dysfunction, with approximately a 45% recurrence rate at 5 years.
15. Complete excision of the seminal vesicle during radical prostatectomy is recommended for cancer control.
16. Surgery should be deferred for 6 to 8 weeks after biopsy and 3 months after a transurethral resection of the prostate.
17. During pelvic lymphadenectomy, one should preserve the lymphatic tissue covering the external iliac artery, which drains the lower extremity.
18. Accessory pudendal arteries should be preserved.
19. The most common site of a positive margin occurs at the apex, followed by the posterior and the posterolateral prostate.
20. The bladder mucosa should be advanced so that the urethral vesicle anastomosis opposes mucosa to mucosa, is watertight, and is tension free.
21. If postoperative phosphodiesterase type 5 inhibitors are to be used, on demand is preferred to daily dosing.
22. Aberrant pudendal arteries may arise from the obturator, inferior vesical, and superior vesical arteries and should be preserved so as not to compromise the blood supply to the penis.
23. Wide excision of the neurovascular bundle should be considered when there is inadequate tissue covering the posterolateral surface of the prostate once the prostate has been removed. The surgeon does not have to make the decision about whether to excise or preserve the neurovascular bundle until the prostate is removed, and, if there is not enough soft tissue covering the prostate, one can excise the neurovascular bundle then.
24. If there is troublesome bleeding from the dorsal vein complex at any point, the surgeon should completely divide the dorsal vein complex over the urethra and oversew the end.
25. Patients requiring acute transfusions for hypotension after radical prostatectomy should undergo exploration to evacuate the pelvic hematoma in an effort to decrease the likelihood of bladder neck contracture and incontinence.
26. Rectal stimulation or manipulation is prohibited in the postoperative period.

156 Laparoscopic and Robotic-Assisted Radical Prostatectomy and Pelvic Lymphadenectomy

Li-Ming Su, Brandon J. Otto, and Anthony Costello

QUESTIONS

1. With laparoscopic/robotic prostatectomy, a continuous suture for the vesicourethral anastomosis:
   a. avoids incontinence.
   b. has a high rate of bladder neck contracture.
   c. can be performed with the need for only a single knot.
   d. requires an indwelling catheter for at least 2 weeks.
   e. eliminates the need for a pelvic drain.

2. With laparoscopic/robotic radical prostatectomy, positive margin rates are not influenced by:
   a. surgical technique.
   b. patient selection.
   c. the method of pathologic analysis.
   d. transperitoneal versus extraperitoneal exposure.
   e. tumor grade and stage.

3. Compared with open surgical approaches, laparoscopic/robotic prostatectomy has been consistently shown to decrease:
   a. postoperative pain.
   b. urinary incontinence.
   c. bleeding.
   d. erectile dysfunction.
   e. positive margins.

4. Positive surgical margins with laparoscopic/robotic prostatectomy:
   a. decrease as technical experience is gained.
   b. are rare at the prostatic apex.
   c. occur only when extracapsular disease is present.
   d. are seen most commonly at the prostate base.
   e. can be avoided by using a robotic-assisted approach.

5. An advantage of extraperitoneal versus transperitoneal approach to laparoscopic/robotic prostatectomy is:
   a. faster operating room time.
   b. shorter hospitalization.
   c. increased working space.
   d. avoidance of bowel manipulation.
   e. fewer positive margins.

6. Minimally invasive pelvic lymph node dissection:
   a. is difficult to perform along with robotic radical prostatectomy.
   b. should always be performed transperitoneally.
   c. has an increased risk of thromboembolic complication compared with open approaches.
   d. should only be performed for tumors lower than or equal to Gleason grade 7.
   e. can allow lymph node removal comparable with open surgery.

7. Rectal injury with laparoscopic/robotic radical prostatectomy:
   a. is best avoided by antegrade release of the rectum from the posterior prostate.
   b. is usually from trocar placement.
   c. can be avoided by bluntly dividing Denonvilliers fascia.
   d. should be treated with an immediate diverting colostomy.
   e. is often unrecognized and heals spontaneously.

8. Bleeding during laparoscopic/robotic radical prostatectomy is usually minimal because:
   a. the plane of periprostatic tissue dissection is different than with open surgery.
   b. the dorsal vein complex does not have to be divided.
   c. the pneumoperitoneum tamponades venous bleeding.
   d. suturing is easier than with open surgery.
   e. the Trendelenburg position decreases venous pressure.

9. Robotic assistance with laparoscopy is most useful in:
   a. trocar insertion and removal.
   b. maintaining a steady insufflation pressure.
   c. decreasing operating room costs.
   d. facilitating suturing.
   e. eliminating the need for a tableside assistant.

10. The neurovascular bundle lies within which two periprostatic fascial planes?
    a. Prostate capsule and prostatic fascia.
    b. Prostate capsule and levator fascia.
    c. Prostatic fascia and levator fascia.
    d. Denonvilliers fascia and prostate capsule.
    e. Denonvilliers fascia and endopelvic fascia.

11. Antegrade laparoscopic dissection of the prostate results in less blood loss as compared with the retrograde approach due in part to:
    a. early division of the dorsal venous complex and prostatic pedicles.
    b. early division of the prostatic pedicles and late division of the dorsal venous complex.
    c. less tissue manipulation.
    d. better visualization.
    e. late division of the dorsal venous complex and prostatic pedicles.

12. The higher cost of laparoscopic/robotic-assisted as compared with open radical prostatectomy is mostly a consequence of:
    a. higher blood loss and transfusion rates.
    b. a higher complication rate.
    c. a longer operative time and disposable equipment.
    d. longer hospital stays.
    e. higher surgical and anesthesia charges.

13. As a consequence of the CO_2 pneumoperitoneum used during minimally invasive prostatectomy, the anesthesia team must be most aware of the potential for:

    a. bleeding and hypotension.

    b. hypoxia and acidosis.

    c. tachycardia and hypertension.

    d. bradycardia and hypotension.

    e. hypercarbia and oliguria.

14. Positive margins at the prostatic apex:

    a. are more common with the robotic-assisted technique as compared with open surgery.

    b. can occur due to protrusion of the posterior prostatic apex beneath the urethra.

    c. can occur more commonly with retrograde versus antegrade dissection of the prostate.

    d. are less common in laparoscopic versus open surgery.

    e. are less common than at the prostatic base.

15. Men who are not candidates for laparoscopic/robotic-assisted laparoscopic radical prostatectomy include those with:

    a. palpable tumors.

    b. history of prior pelvic surgery.

    c. morbid obesity.

    d. uncorrectable bleeding diatheses.

    e. prior neoadjuvant hormonal therapy.

16. The following are true about robotic salvage prostatectomy except:

    a. Higher risk of rectal injury than standard robotic-assisted laparoscopic prostatectomy (RALP).

    b. Higher risk of urinary incontinence than standard RALP.

    c. Need to rule out metastatic disease prior to performing.

    d. Should be attempted early in one's experience.

    e. The Foley catheter should be left in place longer than with a standard RALP.

ANSWERS

1. **c. Can be performed with the need for only a single knot.** The vesicourethral anastomosis may be accomplished using either an interrupted closure or a running continuous suture with a single knot.

2. **d. Transperitoneal versus extraperitoneal exposure.** Comparison of margin status between high-volume centers with the operations performed by experienced surgeons has shown no definitive advantage for one surgical approach over the other in achieving negative surgical margins.

3. **c. Bleeding.** Because most of the blood loss that occurs during radical prostatectomy is from venous sinuses, the tamponade effect from the pneumoperitoneum helps diminish ongoing blood loss during laparoscopic robotic prostatectomy (LRP)/RALP. Blood loss of less than a few hundred milliliters is routinely reported.

4. **a. Decrease as technical experience is gained.** In most series of LRP and RALP, positive margin percentages decrease as greater familiarity with the procedure is obtained.

5. **d. Avoidance of bowel manipulation.** As the extraperitoneal technique avoids violation of the peritoneal envelope, bowel manipulation is avoided. It is for this reason that patients with extensive prior abdominal surgery can undergo successful laparoscopic and robotic prostatectomy by the extraperitoneal route.

6. **e. Can allow lymph node removal comparable with open surgery.** Pelvic lymphadenectomy can be performed by open or laparoscopic techniques with no significant difference in nodal yield.

7. **a. Is best avoided by antegrade release of the rectum from the posterior prostate.** Thorough dissection of the rectum off of the posterior prostate is critical to minimize the risk of rectal injury during subsequent steps such as division of the urethra and dissection of the prostatic apex. With LRP and RALP, sharp and complete incision of the posterior layer of Denonvilliers fascia is necessary after seminal vesicle dissection to allow adequate mobilization of the rectum.

8. **c. The pneumoperitoneum tamponades venous bleeding.** Because most of the blood loss that occurs during radical prostatectomy is from venous sinuses, the tamponade effect from the pneumoperitoneum helps diminish ongoing blood loss during LRP/RALP. Blood loss of less than a few hundred milliliters is routinely reported.

9. **d. Facilitating suturing.** Most surgeons, however, believe that the robotic technology significantly facilitates suturing (especially for the vesicourethral anastomosis) and other aspects of the surgical dissection.

10. **c. Prostatic fascia and levator fascia.** The neurovascular bundle travels between two distinct fascial planes that surround the prostate, namely, the prostatic fascia and levator fascia.

11. **b. Early division of the prostatic pedicles and late division of the dorsal venous complex.** Because the dorsal venous complex is divided early in the operation and the prostatic pedicles late, there is potentially a greater risk of ongoing bleeding with the retrograde technique. In contrast, during the antegrade neurovascular bundle dissection, the arterial blood supply to the prostate (via the prostatic pedicles) is divided early and the dorsal venous complex is divided near the end of the operation, thus reducing blood loss during the operation.

12. **c. A longer operative time and disposable equipment.** In the study by Link and colleagues (2004), the factors that most influenced overall cost in order of importance included operative time, length of hospital stay, and consumable items (e.g., disposable laparoscopic equipment and trocars).

13. **e. Hypercarbia and oliguria.** The anesthesiologist must be aware of the potential consequences of CO_2 insufflation and pneumoperitoneum including oliguria and hypercarbia.

14. **b. Can occur due to protrusion of the posterior prostatic apex beneath the urethra.** Before division of the posterior urethra, great care must be taken to inspect the contour of the posterior prostatic apex. In some patients, the posterior prostatic apex can protrude beneath the urethra, resulting in an iatrogenic positive margin if not identified.

15. **d. Uncorrectable bleeding diatheses.** Contraindications to minimally invasive laparoscopic prostatectomy include uncorrectable bleeding diatheses or the inability to undergo general anesthesia due to severe cardiopulmonary compromise.

16. **d. Should be attempted early in one's experience.** These cases are perhaps best performed in high-volume centers by experienced robotic surgeons, as they can be very challenging with a higher risk of intraoperative and postoperative complications.

CHAPTER REVIEW

1. Regarding patient selection, it is strongly advised that patients with more complex anatomic challenges (e.g., large prostate size, large median lobe, morbid obesity, prior pelvic surgery, after radiation, after transurethral resection of prostate [TURP]) be avoided in a surgeon's early experience with LRP and RALP; however, these patient features are not by themselves absolute contraindications for a minimally invasive approach to prostatectomy.

2. Having a skilled bedside assistant who is well versed in basic laparoscopy, but also specifically in the mechanics, setup, and troubleshooting of the robotic system, can greatly facilitate RALP procedures.

3. Both surgeon and anesthesiologist must be aware of the unique physiologic effects of prolonged pneumoperitoneum with patients in the steep Trendelenburg position, including hypercarbia and acidosis, corneal edema, increased intraocular pressure, and neurapraxia and take proper steps to prevent such complications.

4. Use of a transperitoneal or extraperitoneal approach is based primarily on surgeon preference because there does not appear to be a significant advantage of one approach over the other.

5. The robotic technology facilitates suturing and dissection for surgeons who may not have advanced laparoscopic skills.

6. Identification of the precise margin between the bladder neck and prostate can be accomplished by using a set of physical maneuvers and visual cues.

7. After division of the anterior bladder neck, the presence or absence of a median lobe should be defined before division of the posterior bladder neck.

8. Complete mobilization of the plane between the posterior prostate and rectum is an important step in avoiding rectal injury and defining the medial aspect of the prostatic pedicles and neurovascular bundles (NVBs).

9. Use of thermal energy should be minimized during control of the prostatic pedicles and dissection near the NVBs, as thermal energy has been shown to be deleterious to cavernous nerve function in both animal and human studies.

10. An interfascial dissection of the NVB is preferred in patients with presumed organ-confined cancer who desire NVB preservation for potency.

11. An anterior or posterior protruding lip of prostate should be anticipated when dividing the prostatic apex from the urethra to avoid an iatrogenic positive apical margin.

12. Bladder neck reconstruction may be required if there is a size discrepancy between the bladder neck and urethra, especially in patients with prior TURP, median lobe, or large prostate gland.

13. The vesicourethral anastomosis is most efficiently accomplished with a running continuous suture.

14. Complications and Outcomes of RALP: (1) **Patient positioning**: Care must be taken when positioning in the Trendelenburg position that any potential, area of neural compression is padded. (2) **Blood loss**: Blood loss of robotic prostatectomy is usually minimal, and transfusion requirements should be less than 2%. (3) **Bowel injury**: Injury to the rectum is well reported but rare, and should be repaired when recognized. The rectal injury rate is higher in salvage surgery. (4) **Urine leak**: This occasionally occurs through a non-watertight anastomosis and requires a longer urinary catheter period. (5) **Bladder neck stricture**: The occurrence of bladder neck stricture is much reduced since the introduction of robotic anastomotic technique. The rate should be less than 5%. (6) **Machine failure**: Machine failure is rare and impacts less than 0.5% of cases. (7) **Oncologic outcomes**: There is equivalence in oncologic outcomes between robotic and open radical prostatectomy. The robotic oncologic outcomes (margin negative) are better when surgery is performed in a high-volume centers. (8) **Potency outcomes**: This is a statistically better outcome for potency recovery following robotic prostatectomy versus the open method. (9) **Continence outcomes**: Even in the best hands, at least 20% of men following robotic prostatectomy will not be pad free, and 5% will have severe incontinence irrespective of technical excellence. (10) **Minimally invasive surgery outcomes.** Following robotic prostatectomy, patients can be discharged in 24 hours and return to normal activity within 3 weeks. This is a significant advantage of the minimally invasive surgical approach.

15. Pelvic lymph node dissection (PLND) is generally recommended in patients with intermediate- or high-risk prostate cancer or by having a >5% risk of nodal metastasis using a clinical nomogram.

16. Although an extended PLND may yield a higher lymph node count, debate continues as to the extent of PLND and the clinical benefit of removing cancerous nodes, given the increased time and complications rates.

17. Use of clips on identifiable lymphatic channels can minimize the occurrence of postoperative lymphoceles.

18. A transperitoneal approach is not protective against the formation of a lymphocele because loculation of lymphatic fluid can still occur within the peritoneal cavity.

19. Symptomatic lymphoceles, which cause local problems such as venous or bladder compression, may require percutaneous or laparoscopic drainage.

157 Radiation Therapy for Prostate Cancer

Ryan Phillips, Sarah Hazell, and Daniel Y. Song

QUESTIONS

1. When managed with radiation alone, patients with high-risk prostate cancer have a 5-year prostate-specific antigen (PSA) failure-free survival rate of approximately:
   a. 75%.
   b. 60%.
   c. 33%.
   d. 10%.

2. Which of the following represents unfavorable intermediate-risk disease?
   a. Gleason 3 + 4, PSA 9.5, cT2a
   b. Gleason 4 + 3, PSA 9.5, cT3a
   c. Gleason 4 + 4, PSA 9.5, cT1c
   d. Gleason 4 + 3, PSA 12.8, cT2a

3. A 58-year-old man presents with a T2b, Gleason 7 (4 + 3: 80% pattern 4, 2/6 sextants positive, 4/10 cores), PSA 7.8 ng/mL. He is treated with 6 months combined androgen deprivation therapy (ADT) + 78 Gy intensity-modulated radiation therapy (IMRT). Testosterone recovers 6 months following completion of IMRT. At 12 months, PSA is 0.8 ng/mL; at 18 months, 2.6 ng/mL; at 24 months, 3.2 ng/mL; and now at 30 months, following IMRT, PSA is 5.4 ng/mL. The best next step in management is:
   a. because the most likely explanation for the rising PSA is testosterone recovery, reassure the patient and continue to follow up.
   b. arrange biopsy for presumed local failure.
   c. because patient clearly has failed radiotherapy, advise radical local salvage.
   d. because patient's PSA doubling time and time to biochemical failure make him an unlikely candidate for local salvage because they are indicative of systemic failure, arrange systemic staging with or without multiparametric magnetic resonance imaging (MRI) of the prostate.
   e. The PSA kinetics are compatible with a benign increase or "bounce." Reassure the patient and continue to monitor.

4. A 53-year-old man presents with T2a, Gleason 7 (3 + 4: 20% pattern 4, 1/6 sextants positive, 2/10 cores), PSA 5.9 ng/mL. He is treated with iodine-125 (^{125}I) permanent seed prostate brachytherapy. At 12 months, PSA has fallen to 1.2 ng/mL. At 15 months, PSA is 1.8 ng/mL; at 18 months, it is 3.2 ng/mL. He is sexually active and asymptomatic. Which is the best next step?
   a. Brachytherapy has failed. Start ADT.
   b. Brachytherapy has failed. Arrange radical local salvage.
   c. Brachytherapy has failed. Arrange biopsy before radical local salvage.
   d. Recognizing that this is classic timing for a benign PSA bounce, contact his radiation oncologist, review the dosimetry of the implant, and continue to monitor the PSA every 3 months, planning for eventual biopsy if the PSA has not started to decline again by 30 months.

   e. Given his time to nadir of 12 months and PSA doubling time of 4 months, explain to the patient that this is almost certainly distant failure and discuss timing of ADT.

5. In two large trials that randomized patients with high-risk and locally advanced prostate cancer to ADT with versus without radiation therapy, the addition of radiation improved what outcome by an absolute of 8% to 10%?
   a. Biochemical recurrence-free survival
   b. Clinical recurrence-free survival
   c. Metastasis-free survival
   d. Disease-specific survival
   e. Overall survival

6. Modern radiation therapy for prostate cancer differs from the technology used in the 1980s to 1990s in what ways? Modern radiation uses:
   a. computed tomography (CT)-based treatment planning.
   b. intensity-modulated radiation delivery.
   c. image guidance.
   d. dose-escalated radiation.
   e. all of the above.

7. A randomized trial comparing 76 Gy in 38 fractions to 70.2 Gy in 26 fractions found:
   a. the shorter regimen improved 5-year biochemical failure and had comparable rectal and urinary toxicity.
   b. the shorter regimen improved 5-year biochemical failure and had higher late urinary toxicity.
   c. the shorter regimen improved 5-year biochemical failure and had higher late rectal toxicity.
   d. the shorter regimen did not improve 5-year biochemical failure and had higher late urinary toxicity in men with poor baseline urinary function.
   e. the shorter regimen did not improve 5-year biochemical failure and had higher late rectal toxicity.

8. In 2013, radium-223 was approved by the U.S. Food and Drug Administration (FDA) for use in the treatment of men with _____ because of a prolongation in _____.
   a. castrate-resistant metastatic prostate cancer, overall survival
   b. castrate-resistant metastatic prostate cancer, disease-free survival
   c. castrate-resistant nonmetastatic prostate cancer, overall survival
   d. castrate-resistant metastatic prostate cancer, PSA failure–free survival
   e. castrate-resistant nonmetastatic prostate cancer, PSA failure–free survival

Imaging

1. A voiding cystourethrogram on a 72-year-old man who presents with urinary tract infections 2 years after combination external beam radiation therapy and brachytherapy for

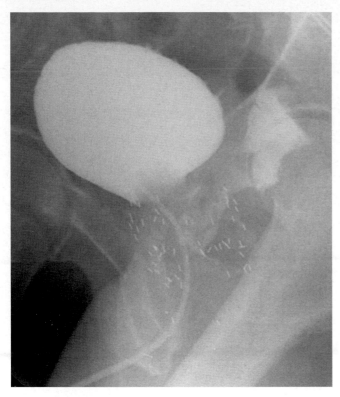

Fig. 157.1

prostate cancer is depicted in Fig. 157.1. The most likely diagnosis is:

a. brachytherapy seed migration.

b. urethra rectal fistula.

c. vesico sigmoid fistula.

d. urethra cutaneous fistula.

e. vesico rectal fistula.

ANSWERS

1. **c. 33%.** (see D'Amico AV, Whittington R, Malkowicz S, et al: Biochemical outcome after radical prostatectomy, external beam radiation therapy, or interstitial radiation therapy for clinically localized prostate cancer. *JAMA* 280:969–974, 1998.)
2. **d. Gleason 4 + 3, PSA 12.8, cT2a.** (see Zumsteg ZS, Spratt DE, Pei I, et al: A new risk classification system for therapeutic decision making with intermediate-risk prostate cancer patients undergoing dose-escalated external-beam radiation therapy. *Eur Urol* S0302-2838[13]00257-1, 2013.)
3. **d. Because patient's PSA doubling time and time to biochemical failure make him an unlikely candidate for local salvage because they are indicative of systemic failure, arrange**

systemic staging with or without multiparametric magnetic resonance imaging (MRI) of the prostate. This PSA increase is much too high to be due to testosterone recovery. Because this patient was treated with IMRT and not brachytherapy, this is not a benign increase. A 58-year-old man should not be denied potentially curative salvage, but his PSA kinetics are strongly suggestive of distant failure. Although ADT may well be the correct maneuver, systemic staging should be undertaken first. A posttreatment biopsy of the prostate should be interpretable 30 months after completion of treatment, but even if residual disease is demonstrated, this patient is at very high risk of also harboring systemic disease because of his PSA kinetics and should fully understand this before consenting to further local treatment.

4. **d. Recognizing that this is classic timing for a benign PSA bounce, contact his radiation oncologist, review the dosimetry of the implant, and continue to monitor the PSA every 3 months, planning for eventual biopsy if the PSA has not started to decline again by 30 months.** This is classic timing for a benign PSA bounce after brachytherapy monotherapy. Bounces are seen in 65% of men younger than 55 years, especially those who are sexually active, and can be quite dramatic, with kinetics characteristic of distant failure because of the early onset and rapid doubling. Reassurance, close monitoring, biopsy if the bounce has not resolved by 30 months, and systemic staging if the PSA approaches 10 ng/mL are appropriate.
5. **e. Overall survival.** In the NCIC/MRC trial of 1205 patients, the addition of radiation therapy significantly improved overall survival: 7-year survival 66% for ADT versus 74% ADT/RT (P = .033). In a Scandinavian trial (SPCG-7/SFUO-3) of 875 patients, radiation therapy decreased overall mortality: 10-year mortality was 39.4% for ADT versus 29.6% for ADT/RT ($P < .05$).
6. **e. All of the above.** CT-based treatment planning was developed in the 1990s, IMRT in the early 2000s, and image guidance more recently. Four randomized trials consistently demonstrated improved cancer control with "dose-escalated" radiation, which has changed the standard of care in prostate cancer radiation.
7. **d. The shorter regimen did not improve 5-year biochemical failure and had higher late urinary toxicity in men with poor baseline urinary function.** (See Pollack A, Walker G, Buyyounouski MK, et al: Five year results of a randomized external beam radiotherapy hypofractionation trial for prostate cancer. *Int J Radiat Oncol Biol Phys* 81[2]:S1, 2011.)
8. **a. Castrate-resistant metastatic prostate cancer, overall survival.** (See Parker C, Nilsson S, Heinrich D, et al: ALSYMPCA Investigators. Alpha emitter radium-223 and survival in metastatic prostate cancer. *N Engl J Med.* 369[3]:213–223, 2013.)

Imaging

1. **b. Urethra rectal fistula.** There is partial opacification of the irregular prostatic urethra with immediate filling of the rectum. The bladder is normal in appearance, making option e incorrect. The contrast is in the rectum, making a urethra cutaneous fistula and vesico sigmoid fistula incorrect. The seeds are located in the area one would expect following brachytherapy.

CHAPTER REVIEW

1. The advantage of brachytherapy is that there is a rapid falloff of dose within a few millimeters of the seed implant.
2. A pretreatment PSA velocity of greater than 2 ng/mL/yr is associated with an increased risk of biochemical failure following radiation therapy.
3. The American Society for Radiation Oncology (ASTRO) definition of failure following radiation therapy is three consecutive rises in PSA following the nadir. It is recommended that these determinations be obtained 3 to 4 months apart. The Phoenix definition of failure is a 2 ng/mL or more increase in PSA above the nadir.
4. A PSA nadir of less than 0.5 ng/mL is correlated with successful treatment.
5. PSA nadir is the strongest predictor of outcome.
6. Approximately 50% of potent men are impotent at 5 years following conformal external beam radiation therapy; 10% will have some rectal bleeding. Less common complications include urinary and fecal incontinence, hemorrhagic cystitis, and urethral stricture.
7. Conformal radiation therapy (CRT) uses a computerized algorithm to conform the dose of radiation to the contours of the prostate.

8. IMRT uses a set of radiation beams with changing intensities distributed across the field.

9. When IMRT is compared with CRT, lower doses are delivered to critical tissues such as rectum, bladder, and small bowel.

10. Heavy particle beams such as neutrons and protons exhibit a Bragg effect. This is manifested by a sharp falloff beyond the particle's tissue range, thus delivering little radiation beyond that point.

11. ^{125}I has a half-life of approximately 60 days; palladium-103 has a half-life of 17 days.

12. Treatment of impending spinal cord compression due to prostate cancer consists of immediate ablation of androgens (most effectively accomplished by bilateral orchiectomy), steroids, and radiation therapy. Occasionally a decompression laminectomy is required emergently.

13. The dose delivered to the prostate with IMRT is 75 to 79 Gy; for brachytherapy with ^{125}I is 140 to 160 Gy; and for ^{103}Pd is 110 to 125 Gy.

14. Pretreatment risk stratification may be divided as follows: low risk—T1c-T2a, PSA less than 11 ng/mL and no Gleason score higher than 6; intermediate risk—T2b, PSA 11 to 20 ng/mL or Gleason score of 7; and high risk—T2c, PSA greater than 20 ng/mL or Gleason score greater than 7.

15. The percentage of positive biopsies and the PSA velocity have also been used for risk stratification.

16. Radiation causes significant changes in cell architecture that can make interpretation of biopsy specimens after radiation therapy difficult.

17. At present there does not appear to be any advantage of proton therapy over conventional photon IMRT.

18. Radium-223 used to treat metastatic prostate cancer to bone is an alpha particle emitter and as such there is less damage to hematopoietic marrow elements when compared with strontium-89.

19. A postradiation treatment biopsy of the prostate should be interpretable 30 months after completion of treatment.

158 Focal Therapy for Prostate Cancer

Kae Jack Tay and Thomas J. Polascik

QUESTIONS

1. Advantages of using mpMRI to identify suitable candidates for prostate focal therapy include all the following EXCEPT:
   a. It improves the detection of anterior zone cancers
   b. It preferentially detects high-grade lesions
   c. It accurately estimates lesion size for determination of ablation margin
   d. It improves the detection of extra-prostatic extension
   e. It helps accurately identify the index lesion

2. Selection of an ablative energy source for prostate focal therapy is predicated on:
   a. availability of ablative technology.
   b. lesion location.
   c. presence of extensive intra-prostatic calcifications.
   d. both (a) and (b).
   e. all of the above.

3. Technical innovations improving focal cryotherapy for prostate cancer include all EXCEPT the use of:
   a. transrectal ultrasound.
   b. urethral warming catheters.
   c. warming of neurovascular bundles.
   d. thermocouples placed in critical areas of the prostate.
   e. smaller-diameter cryoprobes allowing percutaneous insertion.

4. What is the most clinically important parameter of tissue ablation other than lowest temperature achieved by cryotherapy?
   a. The diameter of the cryoprobe
   b. The number of freeze/thaw cycles
   c. The velocity of tissue thawing
   d. The velocity of tissue freezing
   e. The duration of freezing

5. What is the characteristic appearance of ice ball created during prostate focal cryotherapy on ultrasound?
   a. Mixed echogenicity
   b. Hyperechogenicity
   c. Anechogenicity with a hypochogenic rim
   d. Hypoechogenicity with a hyperechogenic rim
   e. None of the above

6. Prostate cell death is likely to occur completely in a single freeze cycle when tissue temperature reaches:
   a. $20°C$.
   b. $0°C$.
   c. $-20°C$.
   d. $-40°C$.
   e. none of the above.

7. High-intensity focused ultrasound (HIFU) exerts what effect on prostate tissue?
   a. Tissue fragmentation with disruption of vascular architecture
   b. Coagulative necrosis
   c. Nuclear injury
   d. Cavitation
   e. Disruption of protein synthesis

8. There exists level 1 evidence that prostate focal therapy:
   a. is equivalent to radical therapy in terms of cancer control.
   b. is superior to active surveillance for progression free survival.
   c. is superior to active surveillance for overall survival.
   d. is equivalent to active surveillance for overall survival.
   e. is superior to radical therapy in terms of sexual function outcomes.

9. The following modalities all employ a thermal form of ablation EXCEPT:
   a. MRI-guided transurethral ultrasound ablation.
   b. focal laser ablation.
   c. focal cryotherapy.
   d. vascular-targeted photodynamic therapy.
   e. none of the above.

10. Reliable markers of post-focal therapy treatment success include:
    a. post-treatment PSA levels.
    b. digital rectal examination.
    c. post-treatment mpMRI alone.
    d. targeted biopsy of the treated area only.
    e. targeted biopsy of the treated area plus a systematic biopsy.

ANSWERS

1. **c. It accurately estimates lesion size for determination of ablation margin.** mpMRI has been consistently shown to underestimate the actual tumor volume by 5% to 30% in historadiological correlation studies.

2. **e. All of the above.** The oncological premise of focal therapy is to completely destroy the index lesion while preserving as much function as possible. As such, selection of the ablative technology will depend on availability, operator experience, desired approach, and the suitability of the technology to deliver a lethal dose of energy to the desired location in order to successfully ablate the lesion.

3. **c. Warming of neurovascular bundles.** Use of transrectal ultrasonography (TRUS) for real-time monitoring of the freezing process, use of a urethral warming catheter, use of thermocouples placed in critical areas of the prostate, and improved cryoprobes allowing percutaneous insertion are technical innovations that have all contributed to improving cryotherapy for prostate cancer.

4. **b. The number of freeze/thaw cycles.** In a clinical setting, the number of freezing cycles, the lowest temperature achieved, and the existence of any regional "heat sinks" may be more important factors relating to cancer destruction. Repeating a freeze/thaw cycle results in more extensive tissue damage compared with a single cycle.

5. **d. Hypoechogenicity with a hyperechogenic rim.** Frozen tissue is significantly different from unfrozen tissue in sound impedance, resulting in strong echo reflection at the interface of frozen and normal tissue. The frozen area can be seen as a well-marginated hyperechoic rim with acoustic shadowing by ultrasonography. Sonography provides no information about the temperature distribution within the ice, nor does it show the extent of freezing at the lateral or anterior aspects of the prostate.

6. **d. −40°C.** Complete cell death is unlikely to occur at temperatures higher than −20°C, and temperatures lower than −40°C are required to completely destroy cells.

7. **b. Coagulative necrosis.** Highly focused sound energy results in mechanical and thermal effects on tissue. In the case of HIFU, the primary mechanism of tissue ablation is by raising the temperature in the tissue above the level needed to create coagulative necrosis.

8. **b. Is superior to active surveillance for progression free survival.** Azzouzi et al. randomized 415 men with low-risk prostate cancer to focal VTP or active surveillance demonstrating that FT significantly improved negative biopsy at 2 years and decreased disease progression and those requiring definitive disease intervention. Of the 216 men assigned to VTP, 196 received the treatment and 195 completed 24 months of follow-up. In the AS arm, 174 men completed 24 months of follow-up. Overall, cancer progression rate (volume, grade, or PSA progression) in the AS arm was 58% compared to 28% in the VTP arm. This is the first randomized trial with level 1 evidence comparing focal therapy to an accepted management strategy demonstrating a meaningful clinical benefit.

9. **d. Vascular-targeted photodynamic therapy.** In VTP, low-power near-infrared laser light of specific wavelength destroys targeted tissues that have been photosensitized with an intravascular agent preferentially taken up by tumor cells. This occurs via the production of reactive oxygen species in the target zone causing irreversible damage to cell membranes and small arterioles leading to tumor necrosis.

10. **e. Targeted biopsy of the treated area plus systematic biopsy.** A 2015 ICUD consensus on follow-up after focal therapy recommended an mpMRI with mandatory targeted biopsy of 4 to 6 cores in the treated area at 3 to 6 months, then mpMRI at 1 to 2 and 5 years with targeted biopsy as needed, especially if a new lesion should become manifest. A systematic biopsy was also recommended at 1 to 2 and 5 years to provide further histological evaluation of the untreated zone for potential outfield recurrence.

CHAPTER REVIEW

1. Gleason patterns 4 and 5 demonstrate many of the hallmarks of malignancy compared to Gleason pattern 3 and represent priority targets for elimination. The feasibility of focal therapy for a multifocal disease such as prostate cancer is based on the presumption that an index lesion is primarily responsible for disease progression and metastases.

2. The index lesion as the focus of disease progression and/or metastases is supported by: (1) most of the time, the grade/stage of the cancer is determined by the index lesion, (2) most of the tumor volume is often contributed by the index lesion, (3) majority of satellite tumors are small (<0.5 mL) and low grade, and (4) genetic studies suggest a monoclonal origin of metastatic or lethal prostate cancer.

3. A successful focal therapy strategy depends on a multidisciplinary team to accurately determine the disease extent/location through advanced imaging and biopsy, ascertain that the patient will be compliant to follow-up, completely ablate the index lesion(s), and monitor the patient post-treatment with a view to future targeted treatment of either persistent or de novo disease, or conversion to whole-gland treatment as necessary.

4. The use of TRUS-guided biopsy to guide focal therapy is fraught with the following difficulties: it overdiagnoses clinically insignificant cancer; it misses clinically significant cancers in 30% of cases—usually in the anterior or apical regions; it may underrepresent true cancer burden; and repeat biopsies do not give consistent results.

5. mpMRI has become a key enabler for prostate focal therapy due to its ability to preferentially detect high-grade lesions, improve the detection of anterior zone cancers, improve the detection of extra-prostatic extension, and accurately identify the index lesions for targeted biopsy. However, systematic biopsy remains necessary to evaluate the prostate gland prior to focal therapy due to the 10% to 15% miss rate with mpMRI. Other imaging modalities such as multiparametric ultrasound or PSMA-PET CT/MRI have potential use in this area but remain to be further evaluated.

6. Focal therapy can be applied in various patterns (hemi-ablation, quadrant-ablation, lesion-ablation) using different technologies (cryotherapy, HIFU, IRE, laser, etc.). The chosen approach depends on the location of the tumor, the desired ablative technology that is available, and other anatomical considerations that may be peculiar to the patient.

7. Cryotherapy is a thermal ablative modality achieving cell kill through extraction of heat producing lethal cold temperatures. Cryosurgery kills target tissues via physical and physiological changes including mechanical forces resulting in membrane disruption created by intra- and extracellular ice formation, recrystallization, vascular stasis/ischemia, apoptosis, and immune effects.

8. Recent developments have made cryotherapy increasingly suited for focal therapy. First, new third-generation cryoprobes are as fine as 17-gauge, allowing them to be maneuvered to the appropriate position within the prostate. Second, variable ice length adjustment allows the ice ball to be contoured exactly to the lesion that is to be ablated. Third, the ice edge can be clearly seen using transrectal ultrasound allowing for the extent of ablation and the ablation margin to be monitored and adjusted in real time. Fourth, the use of a urethral warmer has greatly reduced the risk of urethral complications arising from cold injury to the urethral mucosa.

9. Cell destruction is determined by the cooling rate, warming rate, and the nadir temperature attained. Slow thawing is generally more effective in tissue destruction compared to rapid thawing. A nadir temperature of −40°C and a double freeze/thaw cycle are recommended for adequate cell death in the target zone.

10. High-intensity focused ultrasound (HIFU) is a process where multiple ultrasound beams are focused onto a preset point generating a temperature of at least 55°C to produce coagulative necrosis within the desired target. The transducer is typically built into the transrectal ultrasound probe which is also used for treatment planning and monitoring making it well suited for treatment of posterior zone lesions. However, the anterior gland may be more difficult to treat due to energy dissipation over the intervening prostate tissue and displacement of anterior zone targets with gradual edema of the prostate tissue as treatment progresses.

CHAPTER REVIEW—cont'd

11. In-bore MRI guided HIFU (MRgFUS) and MRI-guided transurethral ultrasound ablation of the prostate (TULSA) are new developments being actively studied.

12. Focal laser ablation (FLA) refers to the creation of coagulative necrosis using an interstitially placed laser fiber. The ablation zone is guided by the laser fiber, and tissue destruction occurs only within a fixed distance from the fiber tip, offering the possibility of true focal ablation where accurate and predictable tissue destruction zones can theoretically be safe within close proximity to vital structures. The disadvantages are that longer procedure times or extra laser fibers may be necessary for ablation of larger lesions, and early studies show that additional care may be needed to treat the lesion with an adequate margin.

13. Irreversible electroporation (IRE) is a non-thermal ablative technique that uses short pulses of direct current electricity to produce irreversible pores in the cell membrane, leading to cell death, and preferentially damages cells while preserving connective tissue architecture that could theoretically serve as a scaffolding for new cells to grow.

14. Vascular-targeted photodynamic therapy (VTP) employs the use of a low-power near-infrared laser light of specific wavelength producing reactive oxygen species in tissues that have been photosensitized with an intravascular agent preferentially taken up by tumor cells causing irreversible damage to cell membranes and small arterioles leading to tumor necrosis.

15. A randomized trial (Azzouzi et al.) of 415 men with low-risk prostate cancer compared focal VTP or active surveillance demonstrating that FT significantly improved negative biopsy at 2 years and decreased disease progression and those requiring definitive disease intervention. Of the 216 men assigned to VTP, 196 received the treatment and 195 completed 24 months of follow-up. In the AS arm, 174 men completed 24 months of follow-up. Overall, cancer progression rate (volume, grade, or PSA progression) in the AS arm was 58% compared to 28% in the VTP arm. This is the first randomized trial with level 1 evidence comparing focal therapy to an accepted management strategy demonstrating a meaningful clinical benefit.

16. Brachytherapy, stereotactic body radiotherapy (SBRT), toxins, and various nanoparticles are currently being investigated for use in prostate focal therapy.

17. After prostate focal therapy, PSA, which is a traditional marker of therapeutic success, is less relevant due to its levels being affected by the amount of residual prostate epithelia that may continue to grow. MRI and prostate biopsies are recommended in order to assess the treated (infield) area as well as the untreated (outfield) area.

18. Future research endeavors should focus on better patient selection using clinical, imaging, and/or genetic biomarkers, cost-effectiveness studies, and the investigation of adjuvant agents to improve the efficacy of focal therapy in prostate cancer.

159 Treatment of Locally Advanced Prostate Cancer

Maxwell V. Meng and Peter R. Carroll

QUESTIONS

1. Identification of patients with high-risk prostate cancer is best achieved by:
   a. transrectal ultrasonography.
   b. serum prostate-specific antigen (PSA).
   c. digital rectal examination.
   d. serum PSA, biopsy grade, clinical stage.
   e. PSA kinetics.

2. By using the Kattan postoperative nomogram, which of the following contributes most to the risk of biochemical recurrence after radical prostatectomy?
   a. Positive surgical margin
   b. Pretreatment serum PSA of 17 ng/mL
   c. Gleason 4 + 3 disease
   d. Established capsular penetration
   e. Seminal vesicle invasion

3. Neoadjuvant androgen deprivation (AD) before radical prostatectomy leads to:
   a. improved biochemical-free survival.
   b. improved overall survival.
   c. reduced positive surgical margins.
   d. reduced local recurrence.
   e. increased operative morbidity.

4. In men with locally advanced prostate cancer undergoing prostatectomy, clinical overstaging (i.e., pathologically organ confined disease) occurs in:
   a. less than 10%.
   b. 15% to 30%.
   c. 40% to 60%.
   d. 70% to 80%.
   e. more than 90%.

5. The use of high-dose antiandrogen monotherapy after prostatectomy in men with locally advanced disease:
   a. reduces disease progression.
   b. increases cardiac morbidity.
   c. does not have an impact on sexual function.
   d. improves overall survival.
   e. improves local disease control.

6. In men with locally advanced/high-risk prostate cancer, the most effective treatment among the following options is:
   a. brachytherapy + external-beam radiation therapy.
   b. neoadjuvant AD + external-beam radiation therapy.
   c. neoadjuvant AD + external-beam radiation therapy + adjuvant AD.
   d. concurrent AD plus external-beam radiation therapy.
   e. long-term AD alone.

7. Risk assessment schemes for prostate cancer are most accurate for patients with:
   a. low-risk disease.
   b. high-risk disease.
   c. the disease.
   d. metastatic disease.
   e. locally advanced cancers.

8. The current appropriate dose for adjuvant radiation therapy after radical prostatectomy is:
   a. less than 45 Gy.
   b. 45 to 50 Gy.
   c. 51 to 55 Gy.
   d. 56 to 60 Gy.
   e. greater than 60 Gy.

9. The use of AD in combination with radiation therapy for those with high-risk cancers is associated with all of the following EXCEPT:
   a. improved local control.
   b. improved biochemical-free survival.
   c. less gastrointestinal toxicity.
   d. worsened sexual function.
   e. more urinary frequency.

10. The benefits of early radiation therapy after radical prostatectomy in men with locally advanced disease are observed:
    a. for improved local control.
    b. for improved overall survival.
    c. in men with positive surgical margins.
    d. none of the above.
    e. all of the above.

11. After radical prostatectomy in those with loco-regional disease, overall survival may be optimized by adjuvant treatment with:
    a. androgen deprivation.
    b. radiation therapy.
    c. sipuleucel-T.
    d. docetaxel.
    e. radiation therapy + androgen deprivation.

12. Over the past decade, the trend in the treatment of men with higher-risk disease (CAPRA 6-10) has shown:
    a. increase in primary androgen deprivation.
    b. decrease in primary androgen deprivation.
    c. increase in radiation therapy.
    d. decrease in radical prostatectomy.
    e. decrease in active surveillance/watchful waiting.

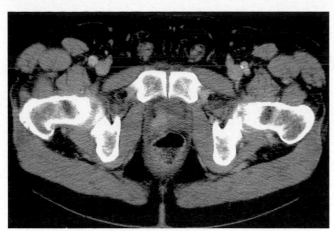

Fig. 159.1 **Computed Tomography Scan of Pelvis.**

IMAGING

1. A 65-year-old man underwent a radical retropubic prostatectomy 4 years ago for a pT3a N0 Gleason 8 adenocarcinoma of the prostate. Two years postoperatively, his PSA first became detectable and has slowly risen since then to its current value of 1.2 ng/mL. A computed tomography (CT) scan of the pelvis is obtained and is depicted in Fig. 159.1. The most likely diagnosis is:

   a. retained seminal vesicle.

   b. enlarged lymph node.

   c. recurrence in the prostatectomy bed.

   d. rectal mass.

   e. rectal diverticulum.

ANSWERS

1. **d. Serum PSA, biopsy grade, clinical stage.** Although clinical stage, serum PSA, and Gleason score all individually predict pathologic stage and prognosis, the combination of these three variables increases the accuracy of this assessment.

2. **b. Pretreatment serum PSA of 17 ng/mL.** Despite the trend toward lower serum PSA at the time of diagnosis, PSA remains an important predictor of treatment failure, and greater elevations (>8 ng/mL) of PSA contribute significantly to calculated biochemical recurrence.

3. **c. Reduced positive surgical margins.** The randomized and nonrandomized studies of neoadjuvant androgen deprivation in men with lower clinical stage (cT1-T2) clearly demonstrate a reduction in the rate of positive surgical margins; however, this advantage has not been observed in men with cT3c and has not translated into improved long-term PSA-free survival.

4. **b. 15% to 30%.** Recent data suggest that clinical overstaging occurs in approximately 27% of men with clinical stage T3 disease undergoing prostatectomy, consistent with the range in the literature of 7% to 26%.

5. **a. Reduces disease progression.** Bicalutamide at greater dose (150 mg) appears to have a positive effect in those men with locally advanced disease, with 43% reduction in disease progression and potential benefit of improved survival; however, it should be remembered that high-dose bicalutamide given to men with localized prostate cancer is associated with increased risk of death (hazard ratio: 1.23).

6. **c. Neoadjuvant AD + external-beam radiation therapy + adjuvant AD.** The accumulated data from multiple Radiation Therapy Oncology Group (RTOG) and European Organisation for Research and Treatment of Cancer (EORTC) trials suggest that improved outcomes are achieved with greater duration of administration of androgen deprivation in combination with external-beam radiation therapy, with apparent benefit of both neoadjuvant and adjuvant therapy.

7. **a. Low-risk disease.** Validation has confirmed the general accuracy of the available risk assessment tools, but there is a tendency to overestimate the risk of cancer recurrence in men with high-risk disease features.

8. **e. Greater than 60 Gy.** There is a trend to improve response to adjuvant radiation therapy, and most contemporary series report doses greater than 60 Gy, with potential threshold of either 61.2 or 64 Gy. Similarly, for primary radiation therapy, improved outcomes have been shown for higher doses (78 Gy or greater).

9. **c. Less gastrointestinal toxicity.** The longer application (longer than 6 to 9 months) of AD in conjunction with radiation therapy may be associated with increased rectal morbidity as well as sexual dysfunction.

10. **e. All of the above.** Data from EORTC 22911 and Southwest Oncology Group (SWOG) 8794 clearly demonstrate a benefit of adjuvant radiation therapy in men with pT3 disease, after radical prostatectomy, with respect to biochemical relapse-free, metastasis-free, and overall survival, as well as improved local control. The EORTC study suggests that patients who benefit the most are those with positive surgical margins.

11. **e. Radiation therapy + androgen deprivation.** The traditional approach to those patients with N+ disease after radical prostatectomy has been androgen deprivation therapy, based on results from ECOG 3886 showing improved overall survival for immediate versus delayed treatment. More recent studies suggest that the combination of androgen deprivation and radiotherapy may yield the best outcomes with respect to overall survival, even when compared with androgen deprivation alone. There is no evidence that adjuvant immunotherapy or chemotherapy improves outcomes in these patients after surgery.

12. **b. Decrease in primary androgen deprivation.** There has been significant evolution in the management of high-risk prostate cancer. A contemporary analysis of the CaPSURE database has shown a significant increase in the number of men undergoing radical prostatectomy with concomitant decrease in primary androgen deprivation as well as radiation therapy. Rates of surveillance/watchful waiting appear stable.

IMAGING

1. **c. Recurrence in the prostatectomy bed.** The pelvic CT scan demonstrates a mass in the prostatectomy bed on the right at the level of the urethra-vesicle anastomosis. Because the mass is anterior to the rectum, it is not likely to be a lymph node or seminal vesicle. In view of the radical prostatectomy specimen and the rising PSA, the mass is likely a prostate cancer recurrence in the prostatectomy bed.

CHAPTER REVIEW

1. At least 10% of men with newly diagnosed prostate cancer have locally advanced disease.
2. Risk assessment for locally advanced disease is best determined by a combination of PSA, T stage, cancer grade, and extent of cancer in the biopsy.
3. PSA recurrence following radical prostatectomy is influenced by Gleason score, extracapsular extension, seminal vesicle invasion, positive lymph nodes, and positive surgical margins.
4. Neoadjuvant androgen deprivation therapy before radical prostatectomy has no role.
5. Early androgen deprivation therapy appears to have a potential survival advantage in subsets of men with more aggressive disease. Unfortunately, side effects of the therapy may be a sequela.
6. The role of adjuvant radiation therapy following radical prostatectomy is controversial. A subset of patients apparently benefits from adjuvant radiation therapy. Unfortunately, all studies to date are flawed such that specific subsets of patients who will benefit have not been adequately defined.
7. Patients with seminal vesicle involvement or regional lymph node metastases are highly likely to develop progressive disease despite adjuvant local therapy.
8. EORTC trials suggest that improved outcomes are achieved with greater duration of administration of androgen deprivation in combination with external-beam radiation therapy for selected patients with high-grade disease.

160 Management Strategies for Biochemical Recurrence of Prostate Cancer

Eugene K. Lee and J. Brantley Thrasher

QUESTIONS

1. What have the American Urological Association (AUA) and European Association of Urology (EUA) determined as the definition of prostate-specific antigen (PSA) failure following radical prostatectomy?
   a. Any level of detectable PSA following radical prostatectomy.
   b. Two values of 0.1 ng/mL or higher.
   c. 0.2 ng/mL.
   d. 0.2 ng/mL with a confirmatory value.
   e. 0.4 ng/mL with a confirmatory value.

2. Which imaging modality in PSA recurrence following radical prostatectomy has the highest sensitivity at the lowest PSA values?
   a. Radionucleotide bone scan.
   b. Computed tomography (CT) of abdomen/pelvis.
   c. Fluorodeoxyglucose-positron emission tomography (FDG-PET) scan.
   d. Prostascint scan.
   e. Multiparametric magnetic resonance imaging (MRI).

3. What is the minimum recommended dosage for salvage radiotherapy?
   a. 43 Gy
   b. 54 Gy
   c. 64 Gy
   d. 72 Gy
   e. 78 Gy

4. Candidates for salvage prostatectomy following failed radiation therapy of the prostate should have all but which factor before treatment?
   a. Negative metastatic workup.
   b. At least 10 years of life expectancy.
   c. Biopsy-proven local recurrence.
   d. Negative pelvic lymph node sampling.
   e. PSA value less than 10 ng/mL.

5. Which has the highest sensitivity in detecting recurrent local disease following radiation therapy for prostate cancer?
   a. Rectal exam.
   b. Transrectal ultrasound.
   c. MRI.
   d. Prostascint scan.
   e. PET scan.

6. Which of these is NOT a commonly known side effect of androgen deprivation therapy (ADT)?
   a. Decreased bone mineral density.
   b. Mania.
   c. Hot flashes.
   d. Fatigue.
   e. Sexual side effects.

7. The most important therapeutic consideration in selecting either local salvage therapy or systemic therapy for a patient with a rising PSA value after definitive local therapy is:
   a. patients with a rising PSA level after definitive local therapy should be started on hormonal therapy because they are destined to experience systemic relapse.
   b. patients with a rising PSA level should undergo salvage local procedures, such as radiation or cryotherapy or prostatectomy, before undergoing any systemic treatment.
   c. patients with a rising PSA level and no metastatic disease should be started on chemotherapy.
   d. patients with a rising PSA level should undergo neither systemic nor local treatments, because the only appropriate context in which to begin any intervention is when radiographic metastases have developed.
   e. patients with a rising PSA level should be risk stratified and treated with a modality of therapy that matches their risk of relapse, risk of developing local versus systemic disease, and risk of dying of other causes.

ANSWERS

1. **d. 0.2 ng/mL with a confirmatory value.** Throughout the radical prostatectomy literature, there have been more than 50 individual definitions for PSA failure. In 2007, the AUA Guidelines panel for localized prostate cancer released its recommendations for PSA failure following radical prostatectomy as 0.2 ng/mL with a confirmatory value greater than 0.2 ng/mL (Cookson et al., 2007).[a] Although higher values would result in greater specificity for disease recurrence and progression, the value of 0.2 ng/mL resulted in higher sensitivity and generalizability. The panel reported that in no way should this individual definition be used for determining the usage of adjuvant/salvage therapies and reiterated that this definition is not predictive of death outcomes.

2. **e. Multiparametric magnetic resonance imaging (MRI).** Traditional imaging techniques such as CT scan and bone scan demonstrate limited value at PSA values less than 10 ng/mL (Dotan et al., 2005; Okotie et al., 2004). Multiparametric MRI has shown reliability in identifying local recurrence even at low levels of PSA. In fact, MRI sensitivity may be as high as 86% at PSA values between 0.4 and 1.4 ng/mL and has also demonstrated an ability to perform better than PET-CT (Panebianco et al., 2012; Sciarra et al., 2008).

3. **c. 64 Gy.** In 1999, the American Society for Therapeutic Radiation Oncology (ASTRO) guidelines panel concluded that a minimum of 64 Gy should be used for salvage radiation following radical prostatectomy (Cox JD et al., 1999). This dosage was confirmed by the AUA guidelines in 2013 (Thompson IM

---

[a]Sources referenced can be found in *Campbell-Walsh-Wein Urology, 12th Edition,* on the Expert Consult website.

et al., 2013). Modern reports suggest that salvage radiation dosages as high as 76 Gy may demonstrate effective biochemical recurrence-free survival with reasonable toxicities (De Meerleer et al., 2008; Ost, Lumen et al., 2011). It is hoped that studies such as SAKK 09/10 will clarify the role of dose escalation and identify an optimal therapeutic window for salvage radiation (http://clinicaltrials.gov/show/NCT01272050).

4. **d. Negative pelvic lymph node sampling.** Although modern series of salvage prostatectomy demonstrate improved morbidity, patient selection is of the utmost importance (Heidenreich et al., 2010; Stephenson, Scardino et al., 2004). Patients who are candidates for salvage surgery must have at least 10 years of life expectancy, a negative metastatic workup, biopsy-proven local recurrence, and ideally a PSA value less than 10 ng/mL. A separate negative pelvic lymph node sampling is not imperative before undergoing salvage surgery, although sending lymph nodes for frozen section before prostatectomy would not be unreasonable.

5. **c. MRI.** Traditional imaging modalities have not demonstrated consistent ability to detect radiorecurrent prostate cancer. Transrectal ultrasonography (TRUS) demonstrates sensitivities no better than digital rectal exam, and CT scans are not relevant at PSA values less than 20 ng/mL (Crook J et al., 1993).

Alternatively, MRI with contrast enhancement, spectroscopy, and diffusion-weighted imaging has demonstrated improved sensitivity (Haider et al., 2008; Hara et al., 2012; Westphalen et al., 2010). In fact, diffusion-weighted imaging has demonstrated a sensitivity and specificity of 100% using a 22-core biopsy as a reference (Hara et al., 2012).

6. **b. Mania.** All other answers are commonly reported side effects of patients undergoing ADT.

7. **e. Patients with a rising PSA level should be risk stratified and treated with a modality of therapy that matches their risk of relapse, risk of developing local versus systemic disease, and risk of dying of other causes.** In the setting of biochemical recurrence following radical prostatectomy, patients' risks of metastasis and death are variable (Pound et al., 1999). Both metastasis-free and prostate-cancer survival depend on several factors such as Gleason score, PSA doubling time, and time from surgery to biochemical recurrence (Antonarakis et al., 2012; Freedland et al., 2005, 2006). All of these factors must be considered in salvage therapies. Clearly, patients with significant comorbidities and limited life expectancy are not good candidates for salvage local therapies, and this should be taken into consideration. The use of nomograms to help in decision-making processes is paramount.

CHAPTER REVIEW

1. The AUA and the EAU have defined biochemical recurrence following radical prostatectomy as a value of ≥0.2 ng/mL with a second confirmatory value.
2. Salvage radiation therapy should be discussed with patients with non-metastatic prostate cancer and a rising PSA following radical prostatectomy.
3. Androgen deprivation therapy should be considered in patients receiving salvage radiation therapy, especially in those with high-risk features.
4. Multiparametric MRI can be a useful tool for detection of local recurrence following radical prostatectomy.
5. Patients who undergo a transient rise in their PSA should be closely monitored, because not all men are destined for biochemical failure, let alone clinical failure.
6. The ideal candidates for salvage radical prostatectomy have at least 10 years of life expectancy, lack of metastasis on imaging, and a PSA less than 10 ng/mL.

161 Hormonal Therapy for Prostate Cancer

Scott Eggener

QUESTIONS

1. The effectiveness of estrogen as a hormone therapy for prostate cancer is primarily based on:
   a. direct cytotoxic effects of estrogen on prostate cancer cells.
   b. competitive binding of estrogen to the androgen receptor.
   c. inhibition of the conversion of cholesterol to pregnenolone.
   d. desensitizing luteinizing hormone–releasing hormone (LHRH) receptors in the anterior pituitary.
   e. negative feedback on luteinizing hormone (LH) secretion by the pituitary.

2. The expected response of a man to the administration of the nonsteroidal antiandrogens is:
   a. LH increases, testosterone decreases, estrogen decreases.
   b. LH increases, testosterone increases, estrogen decreases.
   c. LH increases, testosterone increases, estrogen increases.
   d. LH decreases, testosterone decreases, estrogen increases.
   e. LH decreases, testosterone increases, estrogen increases.

3. All of the following therapeutic approaches for androgen axis blockade are in current clinical use, EXCEPT:
   a. inhibition of androgen synthesis.
   b. blocking androgen action by binding to the androgen receptor in a competitive fashion.
   c. ablating the source of androgens.
   d. direct inhibition of androgen receptor–mediated pathways.
   e. inhibition of LHRH and LH release.

4. Nonsteroidal antiandrogens:
   a. do not act as agonists for prostate cancer cells when used in combination with LHRH agonists.
   b. allow long-term maintenance of erectile function and sexual activity at rates similar to men undergoing surgical castration.
   c. commonly induce gastrointestinal toxicity, manifest as constipation leading, on occasion, to fecal impaction.
   d. have pancreatic toxicity, ranging from reversible mild to fulminant, life-threatening suppurative pancreatitis, and require periodic monitoring of serum amylase and lipase.
   e. cause fluid retention and thromboembolism in the majority of patients.

5. Which of the following nonsteroidal antiandrogens is associated with interstitial pneumonitis and a delayed adaptation to darkness after exposure to bright illumination?
   a. Bicalutamide
   b. Flutamide
   c. Hydroxyflutamide
   d. Nilutamide
   e. Cyproterone acetate

6. Which of the following statements is TRUE concerning LHRH agonists?
   a. Based on a review of 24 trials, involving more than 6600 patients, survival after therapy with an LHRH agonist was significantly better than after surgical castration.
   b. Although depot preparations and osmotic pump devices allow dosing to extend from 28 days to 1 year, the most effective dosing regimen is daily.
   c. Current LHRH agonists are based on analogues of the native LHRH decapeptide by amino acid substitutions, particularly position 6 of the peptide.
   d. Widespread use of orally effective LHRH agonists has been limited by severe allergic reactions in some patients, even after previously uneventful treatment.
   e. The use of LHRH agonists is limited to combined androgen blockade.

7. Each of the following has been associated with a favorable initial response to androgen deprivation therapy (ADT), EXCEPT:
   a. the magnitude of the PSA decline.
   b. the rapidity of the PSA decline.
   c. the PSA doubling time before initiating ADT.
   d. the Gleason score of the primary tumor.
   e. the maintenance of a detectable PSA.

8. Which of the following statements about the complications of ADT is TRUE?
   a. Most men undergoing ADT have normal bone mineral density before initiating therapy, and it usually takes at least a decade of treatment before the average man will develop osteopenia.
   b. Hot flashes occur in about one quarter of men on ADT but should always be treated because of the associated rare but life-threatening cardiovascular side effects.
   c. Erectile dysfunction after surgical castration or use of an LHRH is common but not inevitable: Although 1 in 5 men maintains some sexual activity, only 1 in 20 maintains high levels of sexual interest (libido).
   d. Because most men on ADT maintain lean muscle mass, the increase in weight is due to increases in adipose tissue.
   e. Gynecomastia and mastodynia are common with estrogenic compounds and antiandrogens but are effectively treated by external beam radiation after they occur.

9. Which of the following statements about the combination of 3 months of neoadjuvant ADT before radical prostatectomy is TRUE?
   a. Positive surgical margin rates are significantly reduced with ADT-treated patients.
   b. There is a significant reduction in biochemical (PSA) progression with ADT-treated patients.
   c. The benefit of neoadjuvant ADT appears to be in men with locally advanced disease and/or those with high-grade disease.

d. Antiandrogen monotherapy has not shown a significant reduction of biochemical failure, but LHRH agonists have demonstrated this reduction.

e. Although the results of prospective randomized studies of this combination are mixed, the overall body of evidence supports the use of ADT in this setting.

10. Combined androgen blockade:

a. is designed to address the low levels of testicular androgens remaining after the use of LHRH agonists or antagonists.

b. typically uses an antiandrogen at the time of PSA rise after treatment with an LHRH agonist.

c. has not shown a survival advantage compared with an LHRH agonist alone.

d. significantly benefits men with minimally metastatic disease when used in combination with surgical castration.

e. using cyproterone acetate has a slightly worse outcome.

11. Compared with deferred ADT, early ADT instituted before the development of objective metastatic disease:

a. provides an overall survival advantage in all clinical disease states.

b. has an equivalent quality of life.

c. does not increase overall death rates.

d. does not prevent the emergence of castration-resistant prostate cancer.

e. should be offered to men with PSA recurrence after radical prostatectomy because of the rapid disease progression in this clinical setting.

12. In men with lymph-node metastatic prostate cancer discovered at the time of radical prostatectomy:

a. significant overall survival benefits of immediate ADT are limited to those with extrapelvic positive nodes.

b. a significant overall survival benefit of immediate ADT has been demonstrated in men who have also undergone subsequent radical prostatectomy.

c. a significant overall survival benefit of immediate ADT has been demonstrated in men who have not undergone subsequent radical prostatectomy.

d. b and c are correct.

e. a, b, and c are correct.

13. From a strictly financial point of view, which of the following forms of ADT is the least expensive?

a. Scrotal orchiectomy

b. LHRH agonist

c. Diethylstilbestrol (DES)

d. Antiandrogen monotherapy

e. LHRH antagonist

14. In a trial studying continuous ADT to intermittent ADT for men with rising PSA after radiation therapy:

a. prostate cancer–specific death was more common in the continuous ADT arm.

b. death unrelated to prostate cancer was more common in the intermittent ADT arm.

c. attrition from the intermittent arm was rare throughout the cycles.

d. duration of intermittent ADT progressively shortened over time.

e. quality of life was not improved in the intermittent arm.

15. There is general consensus that ADT should always be initiated in a hormonally intact patient in which of the following clinical settings?

a. Before radical prostatectomy with a clinical T2 tumor.

b. In all clinical stages of men undergoing external beam radiation therapy.

c. In those with clinically localized prostate cancer who do not want local treatment.

d. In those with symptomatic metastatic disease.

e. In those with high-grade prostatic intraepithelial neoplasia (PIN) on needle biopsy who refuse a subsequent biopsy.

ANSWERS

1. **e. Negative feedback on luteinizing hormone (LH) secretion by the pituitary.** After the success of surgical castration in treating prostate cancer, the first central inhibition of the hypothalamic-pituitary-gonadal axis exploited the potent negative feedback of estrogen on LH secretion. Estradiol is a 1000-fold more potent at suppressing LH and follicle-stimulating hormone (FSH) secretion by the pituitary compared with testosterone. Although estrogen has some direct cytotoxic effects on prostate cancer cells, this is not its primary mode of action. All antiandrogens competitively bind to the androgen receptor. Aminoglutethimide inhibits the conversion of cholesterol to pregnenolone, an early step in steroidogenesis. The LHRH agonists desensitize LHRH receptors in the anterior pituitary.

2. **c. LH increases, testosterone increases, estrogen increases.** Unlike the steroidal antiandrogens, such as cyproterone acetate, which have central progestational inhibitory effects, the nonsteroidal antiandrogens simply block androgen receptors, including those in the hypothalamic-pituitary axis. Because those central androgen receptors no longer sense the normal negative feedback exerted by testosterone, both LH levels and—as the normal testicular response to increased LH—testosterone levels increase. Peripheral conversion of this excessive testosterone also increases estrogen levels, leading to the gynecomastia and mastodynia associated with the nonsteroidal antiandrogens.

3. **d. Direct inhibition of androgen receptor–mediated pathways.** There are four therapeutic approaches for androgen axis blockade in current clinical use. All current forms of ADT function by reducing the ability of androgen to activate the androgen receptor, whether through lowering levels of androgen or by blocking androgen–androgen receptor binding. Therefore, the androgen receptor is not directly affected by ADT, leading many to hypothesize that hormone-refractory prostate cancer is a reactivation of androgen receptor–mediated pathways.

4. **b. Allow long-term maintenance of erectile function and sexual activity at rates similar to men undergoing surgical castration.** By blocking testosterone feedback centrally, the nonsteroidal antiandrogens cause LH and testosterone levels to increase, allowing antiandrogen activity without inducing hypogonadism and potency can be preserved. In clinical trials specifically examining erectile function and sexual activity in men on antiandrogen monotherapy, however, long-term preservation of those domains was 20% and not significantly different from that in men undergoing surgical castration. All antiandrogens can act agonistically on prostate cancer cells and, when used in combination with LHRH agonists, withdrawal of the antiandrogen can lead to declines in PSA and even objective responses. The common gastrointestinal toxicity is diarrhea, most often seen with flutamide. Liver toxicity, ranging from reversible hepatitis to fulminant hepatic failure, is associated with all nonsteroidal antiandrogens and requires periodic monitoring of liver function tests. The steroidal antiandrogen cyproterone acetate is associated with fluid retention and thromboembolism.

5. **d. Nilutamide.** About one quarter of men on nilutamide therapy will note a delayed adaptation to darkness after exposure to bright illumination, and in approximately 1% of patients, nilutamide is also associated with interstitial pneumonitis, which can progress to pulmonary fibrosis. Hydroxyflutamide is the active metabolite of flutamide. Cyproterone acetate is a steroidal antiandrogen.

6. **d. Widespread use of orally effective LHRH agonists has been limited by severe allergic reactions in some patients, even after previously uneventful treatment.** The LHRH agonists exploit the desensitization of LHRH receptors in the anterior pituitary following chronic exposure to LHRH, thereby shutting down the production of LH and, ultimately, testosterone. Analogues of native LHRH increase their potency and half-lives. The initial flare in LH and testosterone may last 10 to 20 days, and co-administration of an antiandrogen is required for only 21 to 28 days. Survival after therapy with an LHRH agonist was equivalent to that for orchiectomy. The clinical utility of the first LHRH agonists was hampered by their short half-lives, requiring daily dosing. The LHRH antagonist abarelix has been associated with severe allergic reactions: All LHRH agonists are administered either IM or subcutaneously. LHRH can be used without combination with an antiandrogen.

7. **e. The maintenance of a detectable PSA.** The odds ratio of progressing to androgen-refractory progression at 24 months after starting ADT was 15-fold higher in those who did not achieve an undetectable PSA. The magnitude and rapidity of PSA decline, the pre-ADT PSA doubling time, and pretreatment testosterone levels are all associated with the ability to predict the response to ADT. For each unit increase in Gleason score, the cumulative hazard of castration-resistant progression was nearly 70%.

8. **c. Erectile dysfunction after surgical castration or use of an LHRH is common but not inevitable: Although 1 in 5 men maintains some sexual activity, only 1 in 20 maintains high levels of sexual interest (libido).** The loss of sexual functioning is not inevitable with surgical or chemical castration, with up to 20% of men able to maintain some sexual activity. Libido is more severely compromised, with approximately 5% maintaining a high level of sexual interest. More than half of men undergoing ADT meet the bone mineral density criteria for osteopenia or osteoporosis; it is estimated osteopenia will develop in the average man within 4 years of initiating ADT. Hot flashes are among the most common side effects of ADT, affecting between 50% and 80% of patients. Hot flashes should be treated only in those who find them bothersome. Loss of muscle mass and increase in percent fat body mass are common in men undergoing ADT. Prophylactic radiation therapy (10 Gy) has been used to prevent or reduce gynecomastia and mastodynia, but it has no benefit once these side effects have already occurred.

9. **a. Positive surgical margin rates are significantly reduced with ADT-treated patients.** In both nonrandomized and randomized clinical trials, the pathologic positive surgical margin rate is significantly reduced. In one study, the positive surgical margin rate fell from nearly 50% in hormonally intact patients to 15% in ADT-treated patients. Despite this improvement, there has not been a corresponding significant reduction in biochemical (PSA) progression in ADT-treatment patients, a finding in four separate prospective randomized studies. The benefit of ADT in men with locally advanced disease and/or high-grade disease has been in combination with external beam radiation therapy. There is no evidence that any form of 3-month neoadjuvant ADT before radical prostatectomy reduces biochemical failure rates.

10. **e. Using cyproterone acetate has a slightly worse outcome.** In studies of combined androgen blockade using the steroidal antiandrogen cyproterone acetate compared to LHRH agonists alone, the outcomes were slightly worse with the combination,

suggesting increased non–prostate cancer deaths with this agent. Combined androgen blockade is designed to block the possible contribution of adrenal androgens to prostate cancer progression. Combined androgen blockade uses an antiandrogen along with an LHRH agonist: Addition of an antiandrogen at the time of PSA rise (evidence of hormone-refractory disease) is considered secondary hormonal manipulation. Several clinical trials have shown a slight but significant survival advantage for combined androgen blockade. A landmark randomized clinical trial comparing surgical castration alone with surgical castration combined with flutamide did not show a significant benefit in men with minimal metastatic disease.

11. **d. Does not prevent the emergence of castration-resistant prostate cancer.** The timing of the initiation of ADT has not prevented the development of castration-resistant prostate cancer. Although early ADT may provide an overall survival advantage in certain clinical disease states, in most studies there is no significant overall survival advantage. Indeed, in localized, low-risk prostate cancer, early ADT is associated with an increase in overall death rates. The natural history of disease progression after biochemical failure following radical prostatectomy is protracted: Median time to bone metastases is 10 years.

12. **b. A significant overall survival benefit of immediate ADT has been demonstrated in men who have also undergone subsequent radical prostatectomy.** A randomized prospective study of men with positive regional pelvic lymph nodes discovered at the time of radical prostatectomy showed an overall survival advantage to immediate ADT. In that study, all men also underwent the radical prostatectomy. A similar study, performed by the European Organisation for Research and Treatment of Cancer (EORTC) in men who did not undergo radical prostatectomy if positive nodes were discovered did not show a significant survival advantage to immediate ADT.

13. **c. Diethylstilbestrol (DES).** At a dose of 1 to 3 mg/day with no prophylactic breast irradiation, DES is the cheapest form of ADT. LHRH agonists would be cheaper than scrotal orchiectomy only if the patient lived a few months after the administration of ADT. Combined androgen blockade is the most expensive form of ADT.

14. **d. Duration of intermittent ADT progressively shortened over time.** The duration of intermittent ADT progressively shortened over time: the median interval of the "off cycle" was 20.1 months for the first interval, 13.2 months for the second cycle, 9.1 months for the third, and 4 to 5 months thereafter. Disease-specific death (prostate cancer and related treatments) was more common in the intermittent-therapy arm compared to the continuous-therapy, 120 versus 94, respectively; conversely, deaths unrelated to prostate cancer were more common in the continuous-therapy arm compared with the intermittent-therapy arm, 162 versus 148, respectively. Attrition from intermittent androgen deprivation progressively increased over time as patients either developed castration-resistant prostate cancer or died of another cause. Attrition occurred in only 5% of men in the first interval, whereas 68% had stopped intermittent therapy by the third interval. A secondary end point, improved quality of life in the intermittent-therapy arm, was associated with significantly better scores for hot flashes, desire for sexual activity, and urinary symptoms.

15. **d. In those with symptomatic metastatic disease.** In hormonally intact men with symptomatic metastatic prostate cancer, ADT is always indicated. There is no significant biochemical (PSA) disease-free advantage in men treated with neoadjuvant ADT. The benefits of ADT in combination with external beam radiation therapy are in men with locally advanced and/or high-grade disease. The use of ADT in men with low-risk, localized prostate cancer is associated with a significantly lower overall survival. There is no indication for ADT in the management of PIN.

CHAPTER REVIEW

1. Antiandrogens bind to the androgen receptor in a competitive fashion. They are either steroidal or nonsteroidal.
2. Steroidal antiandrogens suppress LH release. Thus the steroidal antiandrogens block the effects of testosterone on the receptor as well as lower testosterone through their progestational central inhibition effect. The nonsteroidal antiandrogens simply block androgen receptors.
3. When performing an orchiectomy, double-ligating the transected segments of the cord with one being a transfixion suture is advised.
4. Initial exposure to LHRH agonists results in a flare of testosterone that may last for up to 20 days, the clinical effects of the flare may be blocked by the simultaneous administration of an antiandrogen. The two drugs should be administered together, and the antiandrogen therapy should be continued for 3 weeks.
5. After 4 years of androgen deprivation, the average man is osteopenic.
6. Bothersome hot flashes can be treated with megestrol, cyproterone, DES, estradiol, medroxyprogesterone, or gabapentin.
7. ADT may result in bone loss, sexual dysfunction, hot flashes, decreased cognitive function, loss of muscle mass, increase in body fat, anemia, gynecomastia, diabetes, and increased cardiovascular mortality.
8. Twenty percent of individuals with metastatic prostate cancer die of nonprostate cancer causes.
9. Bilateral orchiectomy reduces testosterone by 90% within 24 hours.
10. The androgen receptor remains responsive to androgen even in the castration-resistant state; therefore, ADT should be continued in the patient who has castration-resistant prostate cancer.
11. The steroid synthesis inhibitors aminoglutethimide, ketoconazole, and abiraterone require simultaneous glucocorticoid replacement. Aminoglutethimide requires mineral corticoid replacement as well, whereas abiraterone results in increased mineral corticoid production that may result in hypokalemia and hypertension.
12. Intermittent ADT compared with continuous therapy is not superior and may be worse.
13. Many men with prostate cancer will never require ADT because of the protracted course of the disease.
14. Estradiol is a 1000-fold more potent at suppressing LH and FSH secretion by the pituitary compared to testosterone.
15. Therapies that block the androgen receptor but do not lower testosterone, such as nonsteroidal antiandrogens, may produce excessive amounts of testosterone, which is peripherally converted to estrogens, leading to the gynecomastia and mastodynia.
16. All antiandrogens can act agonistically on prostate cancer cells and, when used in combination with LHRH agonists, withdrawal of the antiandrogen can lead to declines in PSA and even objective responses.
17. The LHRH agonists exploit the desensitization of LHRH receptors in the anterior pituitary following chronic exposure to LHRH, thereby shutting down the production of LH and, ultimately, testosterone.
18. Prophylactic radiation therapy (10 Gy) has been used to prevent or reduce gynecomastia and mastodynia, but it has no benefit once these side effects have already occurred. Once they are present, a simple mastectomy may be required in some men for cosmetic and symptomatic relief.
19. A clinical trial comparing surgical castration alone with surgical castration combined with flutamide did not show a significant benefit in men with minimal metastatic disease.
20. Although early ADT may provide an overall survival advantage in certain clinical disease states, in most studies there is no significant overall survival advantage. Indeed, in localized, low-risk prostate cancer, early ADT is associated with an increase in overall death rates.
21. The benefits of ADT in combination with external beam radiation therapy are limited to men with locally advanced and/or high-grade disease.

162 Treatment of Castration-Resistant Prostate Cancer

Emmanuel S. Antonarakis and Michael A. Carducci

QUESTIONS

1. The term "castration-resistant disease" has replaced the older classification of "hormone-resistant disease" used to define all patients who demonstrate evidence of disease progression after initial androgen deprivation treatment because:

   a. androgen deprivation treatment focusing on medical/surgical castration is the initial systemic approach for patients with metastatic prostate cancer.

   b. in patients with castration-resistant disease, responses to subsequent androgen receptor (AR)-targeted treatments continue to show a benefit.

   c. current data indicate that the AR continues to play a major role in the control of prostate cancer growth even when serum levels of testosterone are in the castrate range (<50 ng/dL).

   d. castration resistance does not equal hormone resistance.

   e. all of the above adequately describe the castration-resistant state.

2. Patients eventually stop benefiting from primary and secondary hormonal treatments and become refractory. Which of the following statement(s) INCORRECTLY defines the "castration-resistant" paradigm?

   a. Careful clinical monitoring of patients in clinical practice, including regular physical exams and sequential assessments of radiologic parameters and serum prostate-specific antigen (PSA) levels, facilitates early identification of patients who are becoming resistant to secondary hormonal manipulations.

   b. The definition of castration resistance is based on well-defined clinical and pathologic criteria such as Gleason score and extent of disease.

   c. Determination of castration resistance requires clinical evidence of PSA or disease progression to primary and secondary hormonal manipulations.

   d. The vast majority of patients treated with endocrine manipulations will develop evidence of disease progression and eventually require chemotherapy.

3. Docetaxel remains the standard first-line chemotherapy treatment for patients with metastatic castration-resistant prostate cancer considered candidates for this modality. Which of the following statement(s) is NOT true?

   a. Docetaxel infusion every 3 weeks (for as many as 10 cycles) given in conjunction with daily oral prednisone is the standard schedule that has been shown to prolong survival and improve quality of life compared with mitoxantrone.

   b. Significant clinical benefits are seen in patients regardless of their age, functional status, and presence or absence of pain.

   c. Patients with metastatic castration-resistant disease who have favorable functional status (fully ambulatory, asymptomatic), no visceral involvement, and normal hemoglobin and serum lactate dehydrogenase (LDH) have survival outcomes using docetaxel that frequently exceed 2 years.

   d. Frequent toxicities associated with docetaxel treatment include fatigue, myelosuppression, neuropathy, lacrimation, and nail changes, among others. Routine clinical and laboratory evaluation before each cycle is indicated.

   e. Patients demonstrating rising serum PSAs during the first three to four cycles of treatment should probably be taken off treatment because it is not effective.

4. Cabazitaxel is another taxane approved for metastatic castration-resistant prostate cancer. In preclinical studies that used cancer cell lines and mouse xenograft models, cabazitaxel was shown to be active in docetaxel-sensitive tumors, as well as those with primary or acquired docetaxel resistance. Which of the following statements adequately describes the clinical experience with this compound?

   a. Cabazitaxel was shown to prolong survival compared with mitoxantrone in patients previously treated with docetaxel.

   b. The toxicity pattern of cabazitaxel suggests a lower incidence of neuropathy, fatigue, lacrimation, and nail changes but has a higher incidence of neutropenic fever and diarrhea compared with docetaxel.

   c. Data on the TROPIC trial suggest that patients who fail to respond or develop early evidence of disease progression after docetaxel may benefit from cabazitaxel.

   d. Patients demonstrating disease progression after docetaxel can still survive longer than 12 months with cabazitaxel treatment.

   e. All of the above are correct.

5. After initial gonadal suppression, AR signaling is upregulated in castration-resistant disease and continues to play a major role in tumor growth. Which of the following statement(s) adequately describes AR-targeted treatments?

   a. CYP17 inhibitors target androgen synthesis both of adrenal and intracrine source and yield significant benefit in patients treated with first-line gonadal suppression who subsequently develop evidence of disease progression. This effect has been shown in patients with or without previous treatment with docetaxel.

   b. The side effects with abiraterone acetate include a mineralocorticoid excess state (efficiently prevented by a concomitant administration of prednisone), fatigue, abnormal liver function tests, possible cardiac toxicity, and potential drug interactions.

   c. Enzalutamide is a nonsteroidal antiandrogen that differs from the first-generation compounds (flutamide, bicalutamide, and nilutamide) based on a greater AR affinity, AR nuclear translocation, and DNA binding. Most patients with castration-resistant disease benefit from treatment, which was shown to be significantly superior to placebo in prospective randomized trials.

   d. The benefits from CYP17 inhibitors (abiraterone) and AR antagonists (enzalutamide) are most likely more pronounced in patients who have not received prior docetaxel treatment.

   e. All of the above are correct.

6. Which of the following statements is correct regarding patients with widely metastatic prostate cancer who present with back pain?

   a. Administration of narcotic analgesics is the appropriate management, and if pain management becomes more challenging, patients should be referred to hospice.

   b. All patients with known bone metastasis should be carefully assessed clinically for the possibility of epidural cord or nerve root compression. Administration of high-dose dexamethasone and early magnetic resonance imaging (MRI) should be used, and more definitive treatment with radiation or neurosurgical decompression should be considered.

   c. Patients with back pain and stable skeletal radiographs should be treated with narcotic analgesics and corticosteroids. If improvement occurs, no further evaluation is necessary.

   d. If the PSA is not rising and the workup with a bone scan and computed tomography (CT) scans reveal stable disease, it can be assumed that cord compression or other complex neurologic involvement is unlikely.

   e. Most current systemic treatments are effective for managing extensive bone metastasis even if there is evidence of nerve root or cord compression.

7. A small proportion of patients with advanced-stage disease develop a syndrome of rapid and dramatic development of severe symptoms (pain, obstruction, weight loss) and clinical evidence of rapidly growing disease with soft tissue and organ involvement. In these patients, typically serum PSA levels are either below detectable levels or grossly disproportionate to the other extent of disease parameters. Which statement is correct regarding this rare event in castration-resistant prostate cancer?

   a. These patients usually benefit from hormonal therapy including all AR-targeted compounds.

   b. Serum PSA is low or undetectable, and the PSA stains in tumor biopsies are usually negative. These tumors do not express AR.

   c. A small proportion of patients demonstrate evidence of a rapidly progressing disease predominantly involving visceral sites, with low or no PSA expression. Biopsy is indicated because it will affect treatment decisions.

   d. Patients with this clinical syndrome often demonstrate anaplastic tumors at biopsy, some with small-cell features, and most stain positive for neuroendocrine markers. Platinum-based chemotherapy has been shown to offer some benefits for patients with the small-cell variety, whereas those with anaplastic tumors that are not of the small-cell subtype should be treated with taxane-based chemotherapy.

   e. All statements are correct except a.

8. The radiopharmaceutical radium-223 was approved for the treatment of patients with metastatic castration-resistant disease. Which statement regarding 223Ra is FALSE?

   a. Radium-223 is an α-emitting radiopharmaceutical that has recently shown to be associated with a survival advantage compared to symptomatic/palliative care.

   b. α particles are approximately 7000 times heavier than β particles, and as few as one or two hits can be sufficient to cause cell death, in comparison with hundreds or thousands of hits required from β particles. In addition, α particles have a very short path length (<100 μm), which may spare surrounding healthy bone marrow, thereby limiting hematologic toxicities.

   c. Radium-223 infusion has shown a very favorable toxicity spectrum with low hematologic toxicity rates.

   d. It is indicated for patients with bone metastasis, hemoglobin greater than 10 g/L, and lymph-node metastasis smaller than 3 cm.

   e. It was approved only for patients who have received prior docetaxel treatment.

9. Sipuleucel-T is a personalized vaccine derived from autologous CD54 + dendritic cells, the major class of antigen-presenting cells, which are apheresed from individuals and processed with a recombinant fusion protein made up of prostatic acid phosphatase (PAP) and granulocyte-macrophage–colony-stimulating factor (GM-CSF). Which statement is TRUE regarding this treatment?

   a. Sipuleucel-T is approved for all patients with castration-resistant disease as long as they are symptomatic.

   b. Sipuleucel-T treatment results in PSA declines and prolongation of progression-free survival but no survival improvements.

   c. Sipuleucel-T should be offered to patients with no evidence of metastasis as long as their disease is castration resistant.

   d. Sipuleucel-T is a treatment option for patients with minimally or asymptomatic metastatic prostate cancer. Treatment is generally very safe. There is no evidence that sipuleucel-T treatment causes symptomatic relief, any clinically meaningful PSA declines, or delay in disease progression. The drug was approved based on a survival benefit compared with placebo.

10. The nonmetastatic castrate-resistant prostate cancer state, also known as M0 CRPC, is an evolving disease entity with its own therapeutic considerations. Which of these statements about the nonmetastatic CRPC state is FALSE?

   a. This clinical state is defined by a rising PSA level, castrate testosterone levels (<50 ng/dL), and a lack of radiographic metastases on conventional CT/MRI and nuclear medicine bone scans.

   b. Apalutamide was the first drug to be U.S. Food and Drug Administration (FDA) approved specifically for men with nonmetastatic (M0) CRPC.

   c. Enzalutamide is FDA approved for all patients with CRPC, including both those with metastatic (M1) CRPC and nonmetastatic (M0) CRPC.

   d. Abiraterone acetate has also recently received FDA approval for use in men with M0 CRPC, as well as its prior approval for M1 mCRPC.

   e. All of these statements are true, and none are false.

ANSWERS

1. **e. All of the above adequately describe the castration-resistant state.**
2. **b. The definition of castration resistance is based on well-defined clinical and pathologic criteria such as Gleason score and extent of disease.**
3. **e. Patients demonstrating rising serum PSAs during the first three cycles of treatment should be taken off treatment because it is not effective.**
4. **e. All of the above are correct.**
5. **e. All of the above are correct.**
6. **b. All patients with known bone metastasis should be carefully assessed clinically for the possibility of epidural cord or nerve root compression. Administration of high-dose dexamethasone and early magnetic resonance imaging (MRI) should be used, and more definitive treatment with radiation or neurosurgical decompression should be considered.**
7. **e. All statements are correct except a.**
8. **e. It was approved only for patients who have received prior docetaxel treatment.**

9. d. Sipuleucel-T is a treatment option for patients with minimally or asymptomatic metastatic prostate cancer. Treatment is generally very safe. There is no evidence that sipuleucel-T treatment causes symptomatic relief, any clinically meaningful PSA declines, or delay in disease progression. The drug was approved based on a survival benefit compared with placebo.

10. d. Abiraterone acetate has also recently received FDA approval for use in men with M0 CRPC, as well as its prior approval for M1 mCRPC. The only agents with regulatory approval for M0 CRPC are apalutamide and enzalutamide.

CHAPTER REVIEW

1. Androgen ablation induces apoptosis.
2. The AR may be stimulated by hormones other than androgens, including estrogens and progestins, as well as growth factors and cytokines.
3. Patients with castration-resistant disease are not androgen independent and should be maintained on ablative hormonal therapy.
4. PSA doubling time (PSADT) may be used to predict bone scan progression and survival; a PSADT of less than 3 months is associated with a rapid clinical course.
5. When evaluating therapeutic agents, progression-free survival is a better end point than response rate.
6. PSA may or may not be affected by drugs that are efficacious, and therefore it is not a good marker to evaluate new drugs—perhaps circulating tumor cells will become a better marker.
7. Docetaxel is the first-line chemotherapeutic agent for metastatic castration-resistant prostate cancer.
8. Abiraterone inhibits enzymes involved in androgen synthesis. It does result in secondary mineralocorticoid excess with resultant hypertension and hypokalemia, and as such it is commonly given with prednisone. Occasionally, when secondary mineralocorticoid excess causes significant abnormalities, a mineralocorticoid antagonist may be necessary.
9. Bone metastases in prostate cancer are usually blastic; hypercalcemia is rare.
10. Suspected spinal cord compression from prostate metastases may be diagnosed with a spinal MRI. Those with compression or impending compression, if they are not androgen suppressed, should have an immediate orchiectomy, or be given aminoglutethimide or ketoconazole and high-dose corticosteroids. A decompression laminectomy and radiation therapy should be considered.
11. Bisphosphonates or denosumab is used to limit skeletal events. Oral calcium supplements and vitamin D may be necessary.
12. Radiopharmaceuticals used to treat bone pain due to prostate metastases include the β-emitters strontium-89 and samarium-153. These agents may cause severe myelotoxicity. The α-emitter radium-223 shows promise in palliating bone pain and improving survival without the myelosuppressive effects of the β-emitters.
13. Rarely, patients with advanced prostate cancer may have a transformation of their tumor to a neuroendocrine/anaplastic variant. These tumors are endocrine resistant, frequently involve the viscera and brain, have little impact on PSA, and are treated with platinum-based chemotherapy.
14. After initial gonadal suppression, AR signaling is upregulated in castration-resistant disease and continues to play a major role in tumor growth.
15. Sipuleucel-T is a treatment option for patients with minimally or asymptomatic metastatic prostate cancer. Treatment is generally very safe. There is no evidence that sipuleucel-T treatment causes symptomatic relief, any clinically meaningful PSA declines, or delay in disease progression. The drug was approved based on a survival benefit compared with placebo.
16. Apalutamide and enzalutamide, but not abiraterone, are specifically approved by the FDA for use in men with M0 CRPC. Enzalutamide, but not apalutamide, is also FDA approved for M1 CRPC. Abiraterone is only approved for M1 CRPC.